ACSM's Primary Care Sports Medicine

SECOND EDITION

EDITORS

DOUGLAS B. MCKEAG, MD, MS, FACSM

OneAmerica Professor and Chair, Department of Family Medicine
Director, IU Center for Sports Medicine
Indiana University School of Medicine
Indianapolis, Indiana

JAMES L. MOELLER, MD, FACSM

Sports Medicine Associates, PLC
Auburn Hills, Michigan
Chief, Ambulatory Division of Sports Medicine
William Beaumont Hospitals
Troy, Michigan

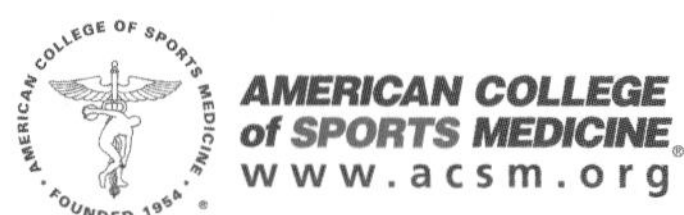

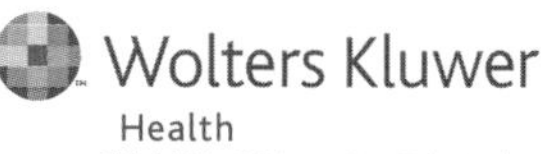

Philadelphia • Baltimore • New York • London
Buenos Aires • Hong Kong • Sydney • Tokyo

Lippincott Williams & Wilkins

Acquisitions Editor: Robert Hurley
Managing Editor: Dave Murphy
Project Manager: Nicole Walz
Senior Manufacturing Manager: Benjamin Rivera
Marketing Director: Sharon Zinner
Creative Director: Doug Smock
Cover Designer: Karen Klinedinst
Production Services: Laserwords Private Limited, Chennai, India
Printer: Gopsons Papers Ltd.
ACSM Medical Education Committee
ACSM's Publications Committee Chair: Jeffrey L. Roitman, EdD, FACSM
ACSM Group Publisher: D. Mark Robertson
ACSM Editorial Assistant: Angela Chastain

530 Walnut Street
Philadelphia, PA 19106 USA
LWW.com

Library of Congress Cataloging-in-Publication Data

ACSM's primary care sports medicine / editors, Douglas B. McKeag, James Moeller.—2nd ed.
p. ; cm.
Rev. ed. of: Primary care sports medicine / Douglas B. McKeag, David O. Hough with Eric D. Zemper. c1993.
Includes bibliographical references and index.
ISBN 978-0-7817-7028-6
1. Sports medicine. 2. Sports injuries. I. McKeag, Douglas, 1945- II. Moeller, James L. III. American College of Sports Medicine. IV. Primary care sports medicine. V. Title: Primary care sports medicine.
[DNLM: 1. Athletic Injuries—therapy. 2. Primary Health Care. 3. Sports Medicine. QT 261 A187 2007]
RC1210.P73 2007
617.1'027—dc22

2007006369

To purchase additional copies of this book, call our customer service department at (800) 638-3030 or fax orders to (301) 223-2320. International customers should call (301) 223-2300.

Visit Lippincott Williams & Wilkins on the Internet: at LWW.com. Lippincott Williams & Wilkins customer service representatives are available from 8:30 am to 6 pm, EST.

10 9 8 7 6 5 4 3 2 1

This volume has two dedications as the reader will notice below.

It is dedicated to the most important people in our lives. For all the lost weekends, late nights, and frustrations endured during the preparation of this book, and for the constant support and love given us, we dedicate this book to our families:

DI, JILL, AND MARLO

HANNAH, HEATHER, IAN, JEFFREY, KELLY, KELSEY, KRISTEN, AND LINDSAY

In addition:

This book is dedicated by the editors and all of the contributing authors to the memory of David O. Hough, MD, a colleague, teacher and mentor at Michigan State University for more than 18 years. Dave passed away in 1996 ending a career that was simply too short. He was a key leader in the field of Primary Care Sports Medicine from the onset of the movement. At his funeral this tribute was read:

DAVID O. HOUGH, MD

1946–1996

I lost a friend yesterday. Actually more than a friend, Dave Hough was my professional colleague, my personal confidante, my sometimes rival but really more of a "comrade in arms." I was close enough to him to be the best man at his wedding. He was close enough to me to be the godfather of my firstborn child. We shared it all together. The ups and downs of starting, or helping to start the movement of Primary Care Sports Medicine and starting the program at Michigan State University. We shared our pride in watching our efforts and dreams come to fruition and to see the area of Primary Care Sports Medicine come into its own as a legitimate endeavor. We shared our families and more personal experiences than anyone will ever know. He was the soft side of our team, a competent physician, an outstanding lecturer, an adroit politician, a caring and loving father and a wonderful friend. He was a class act from the day that we both started at Michigan State until yesterday when he died. I've never worked with anybody that I complemented so well. There is no way that the success at Michigan State or that the area of Primary Care Sports Medicine could possibly have succeeded as much as it did, if it wasn't for the efforts of this man. He was a giant in his field and somebody that I will miss very, very much. Dave, sit the rest of this game out—I'll cover for you.

DBMc—SEPTEMBER, 1996

Contents

List of Contributors

Eric J. Anish, MD, FACP, FACSM
Assistant Professor
Department of Medicine
University of Pittsburgh School of Medicine;
Attending Physician
Department of Medicine
University of Pittsburgh Medical Center—Presbyterian Shadyside
Pittsburgh, Pennsylvania

Benjamin B. Betteridge, MD, ABFM, Sports Medicine CAQ
Staff Physician
Department of Orthopedics and Sports Medicine
Intermountain Healthcare
Bountiful, Utah

Delmas J. Bolin, MD, PhD
Associate Professor
Family and Sports Medicine
Virginia College of Osteopathic Medicine;
Team Physician
Virginia Tech
Blacksburg, Virginia

Leslie Bonci, MPH, RD, LDN
Director of Sports Nutrition
Department of Orthopedic Surgery
University of Pittsburgh Medical Center for Sports Medicine
Pittsburgh, Pennsylvania

Kenneth A. Buckwalter, MD
Professor of Radiology
Indiana University Hospital
Indianapolis, Indiana

Christopher M. Carr, PhD, HSPP
Sport and Performance Psychologist
St. Vincent Hospital
Indianapolis, Indiana

C. Edward Clark, III, MD
Team Physician, Arizona Diamondbacks
University Sports Medicine
Phoenix, Arizona

Katherine L. Dec, MD
Medical Director
Women' s Sports Medicine
Chippenham and Johnston Willis Sports Medicine, LLC
Richmond, Virginia

Randall W. Dick, MS, FACSM
Associate Director of Research—Injury Surveillance System
Department of Research
National Collegiate Athletic Association
Indianapolis, Indiana

Scott W. Eathorne, MD
Program Director
Providence Athletic Medicine
Providence Hospital and Medical Centers
Novi, Michigan

Matthew J. Faber, MS
Graduate Student
Department of Exercise and Sport Science
University of Wisconsin-La Crosse
La Crosse, Wisconsin

Richard T. Ferro, MD
Director, Duke Primary Care Sports Medicine Fellowship Program;
Head, Medical Team Physician, Duke University;
Assistant Professor, Department of Community and Family Medicine;
Assistant Professor, Division of Orthopedic Surgery
Durham, North Carolina

Carl Foster, PhD, FACSM
Professor, Department of Exercise and Sport Science;
Director, Human Performance Laboratory
University of Wisconsin-La Crosse
La Crosse, Wisconsin

Kevin B. Gebke, MD
Assistant Professor of Clinical Family Medicine
Primary Care Sports Medicine
Fellowship Director
Department of Family Medicine
IU Center for Sports Medicine
Indiana University
Indianapolis, Indiana

Scott H. Grindel, MD
Physician
Department of Orthopedics
Spectrum Health-Reed City Campus;
Head Team Physician
Department of Sports Medicine
Ferris State University
Big Rapids, Michigan

Diana L. Heiman, MD
Associate Sports Medicine Fellowship Director;
Assistant Professor, Department of Family Medicine;
Team Physician Connecticut Sun, Hartford FoxForce
University of Connecticut
Saint Francis Hospital and Medical Center
Hartford, Connecticut

Michael D. Jackson, MD
Divisional Medical Director
Delphi Corporation
Troy, Michigan

Neeru Jayanthi, MD
Assistant Professor
Department of Family Medicine
Orthopaedic Surgery & Rehabilitation
Loyola University Medical Center
Maywood, Illinois

Umar Khan, MBBS
Department of Internal Medicine
University of Utah
Salt Lake City, Utah

Chris A. Klenck, MD, PharmD
Head Team Physician
Men's Athletic Department
University of Tennessee;
Staff Physician
Primary Care Sports Medicine
Knoxville Orthopedic Clinic
Knoxville, Tennessee

Aravind Rao Kokkirala, MD
Clinical Assistant
Cardiology Hospitalist
Department of Cardiology
Hartford Hospital
Hartford, Connecticut

Jeffrey R. Kovan, DO
Assistant Professor
Department of Radiology
Division of Sports Medicine
Michigan State University Sports Medicine
East Lansing, Michigan

Wade A. Lillegard, MD
Section Chief, Medical Orthopedics
Department of Orthopedics
Duluth Clinic;
Assistant Clinical Professor
Department of Family Medicine
University of Minnesota
Duluth, Minnesota

Vivien Lim, MD
Fellow in Cardiology
Hartford Hospital
Hartford, Connecticut

Christopher Madden, MD
Clinical Faculty
Department of Family Medicine
University of Colorado Health Sciences
Longs Peak Sports and Family Medicine
Longmont, Colorado

Roger L. McCoy, II, MD
Private Practice
Head Primary Care Sports Medicine
Team Physician
Arizona Diamondbacks
University Sports Medicine;
Team Physician
Assistant Clinical Instructor Primary Care
Sports Medicine Fellowship
Campus Health Service
Arizona State University
Tempe, Arizona

Christopher A. McGrew, MD, FACSM
Professor
Department of Orthopedics and Rehabilitation
Department of Family and Community Medicine
University of New Mexico Health Sciences Center
Albuquerque, New Mexico

Douglas B. McKeag, MD, MS, FACSM
OneAmerica Professor and Chair
Department of Family Medicine;
Director, IU Center for Sports Medicine
Indiana University School of Medicine
Indianapolis, Indiana

James L. Moeller, MD, FACSM
Sports Medicine Associates, PLC
Chief, Ambulatory Division of Sports Medicine
William Beaumont Hospitals
Troy, Michigan

Jeffrey S. Monroe, MS, ATC
Specialist in Athletic Training
Department of Kinesiology
Head Athletic Trainer
Assistant Director of Athletics
Michigan State University
East Lansing, Michigan

Michael P. Montico, MD
Faculty, Department of Family Practice
Associate Program Director
Sports Medicine Fellowship
Providence Hospital
Milford, Michigan

Joanne Nguyen, DO
Providence Athletic Medicine
Primary Care Sports Medicine
Fellowship
Providence Hospital

Sally E. Nogle, PhD, ATC
Associate Athletic Trainer/Adjunct Faculty
Athletic Department/Kinesiology Department
Michigan State University
East Lansing, Michigan

Scott A. Paluska, MD
Clinical Assistant Professor
Department of Family Medicine
University of Illinois
Urbana, Illinois

David M. Peck, MD, FACSM
Team Physician
Athletic Department
Madonna University;
Educational/Research Director
Providence Primary Care Sports Medicine
Providence Sports Medicine Fellowship Program
Providence Hospital
Novi, Michigan

David J. Petron, MD
Assistant Professor
Department of Orthopedics
Director, Primary Care Sports Medicine;
University of Utah
Salt Lake City, Utah

John P. Porcari, PhD, FACSM
Director, Clinical Exercise Physiology Graduate Program;
Professor, Department of Exercise and Sport Science
University of Wisconsin-La Crosse
La Crosse, Wisconsin

Margot Putukian, MD, FACSM
Director of Athletic Medicine, Head Team Physician
University Health Services
Princeton University;
Associate Clinical Professor
Family Practice, Internal Medicine
Robert Wood Johnson UMDNJ
New Brunswick, New Jersey

Brent S.E. Rich, MD, ATC
Director of Sports Medicine Fellowship;
Director, Sports Medicine,
Urban South Region;
Faculty, Utah Valley Family Practice Residency;
Intermountain Health Care
Utah Valley Regional Medical Center;
Team Physician
Department of Intercollegiate Athletics
Brigham Young University
Provo, Utah

Spencer E. Richards, MD, ABFM
Staff Physician
Department of Orthopedics and Sports Medicine
Intermountain Healthcare
Bountiful, Utah

Sami F. Rifat, MD, FACSM
Clinical Associate Professor
School of Health Sciences
Oakland University;
Director, Sports Medicine Fellowship Program
Department of Sports Medicine
William Beaumont Hospitals
Troy, Michigan

Jonathan A. Staser, MD
Department of Radiology
Indiana University
Indianapolis, Indiana

Martha A. Steele, MD
Fellow
Department of Sports Medicine
Providence Hospital
Southfield, Michigan

E. James Swenson, Jr., MD, FACSM
University of Rochester Sports Medicine
Rochester, New York

Thomas R. Terrell, MD, MPhil
Assistant Clinical Professor of Family Medicine;
Assistant Fellowship Director, ECU Primary care sports medicine fellowship;
Assistant Team Physician, Kinston Indians Minor league baseball team
Department of Family Medicine
Brody School of Medicine at East Carolina University.
Admitting Physician
Department of Family Medicine
Pitt County Memorial Hospital
Greenville, North Carolina

Paul D. Thompson, MD, FACSM
Director of Cardiology
Department of Medicine
Hartford Hospital
Hartford, Connecticut

Thomas H. Trojian, MD, FACSM
Sports Medicine Fellowship Director
Department of Family Medicine
University of Connecticut1 School of Medicine
Hartford, Connecticut

Philip D. Zaneteas, PhD, MD
Medical Director
Rehabilitation Hospital of Indiana
Indianapolis, Indiana

Eric D. Zemper, PhD
Research Assistant Professor
Physical Medicine and Rehabilitation
University of Michigan;
Medical Education Consultant
College of Osteopathic Medicine
Michigan State University
East Lansing, Michigan

ACSM Medical Education Committee

CHAIR

Sandra J. Hoffmann, MD, FACSM
Idaho State University
Pocatello, Idaho

REVIEW PANEL

Elizabeth Arendt, MD, FACSM
University of Minnesota
Department of Orthopedic Surgery
Minneapolis, Minnesota

Robert J. Baker, MD, FACSM
MSU/KCMS
Kalamazoo, Michigan

Thomas M. Best, MD, PhD, FACSM
The Ohio State Sports Medicine Center
Columbus, Ohio

Mark P. Bouchard, MD, FACSM
Maine Medical Center
Portland, Maine

William W. Dexter, MD, FACSM
Maine Medical Center
Sports Medicine Program
Portland, Maine

Greg D. Ewert, MD
Northwestern University
Chicago, Illinois

Peter G. Gerbino, MD, FACSM
Monterey Joint Replacement
and Sports Medicine
Monterey, California

Mark R. Hutchinson, MD, FACSM
University of Illinois at Chicago
Chicago, Illinois

Jeff Konin, PhD
University of South Florida
Department of Orthopedics
Tampa, Florida

James MacIntyre, MD, FACSM
Center of Orthopedic
and Rehabilitation Excellence
West Jordan, Utah

Christopher C. Madden, MD
Longmont, Colorado

Susan M. Ott, DO, FACSM
Plant City, Florida

Scott A. Paluska, MD
OAK Orthopedics
Urbana, Illinois

Dilipkumar R. Patel, MD, FACSM
MSU/KCMS
Kalamazoo, Michigan

Stephen M. Simons, MD, FACSM
Saint Joseph Regional Medical Center
Mishawaka, Indiana

Preface

The generation of the Second Edition of *Primary Care Sports Medicine* mercifully did not take the same amount of time as the generation of the First Edition. As editors, it was our intent to update and replicate all of the strong points of the First Edition.

This book remains organized in a similar fashion to the First Edition. However, where the First Edition had two authors, the Second Edition has two editors and many authors. By necessity, a number of different writing styles are present when compared to the First Edition, as this is a compilation work. However, there is a common thread—most of the authors of this text book are graduates or faculty of the Primary Care Sports Medicine Fellowship Program at Michigan State University, University of Pittsburgh, or Indiana University.

Our goals for this book have not changed from its predecessor. We continue to hope that it will serve as a compendium of **how to do things right** in sports medicine. We have continued to emphasize the concepts of **prevention** and **rehabilitation**.

The book continues to take a philosophical approach to Sports Medicine and should not be thought of purely as a reference work. In order for a physician to work within his or her profession, he/she needs a philosophical approach. This remains extremely important in the area of Primary Care Sports Medicine. We feel this book emphasizes such important points.

We want to take this opportunity to thank our colleagues for all the support they have provided us through the years in the field of Sports Medicine. This is especially true for our "learners"—students, residents, and fellows—that have honored us with their interest and enthusiasm for Primary Care Sports Medicine. Finally, and perhaps most importantly, we'd like to thank the athletes who have served not only as our patients, but as our teachers.

Special acknowledgment needs to be given to many people including those mentioned in the Preface to Edition 1. Others include: Jim Moriarity, MD; Steve Simons, MD; Al Tomchaney, MD; Mark Walsh, MD; John Downs, DO; Matthew Roush, MD; Harry Galanty, MD; William "Sandy" Quillen, PT; John L. Turner, MD; Jim Herndon, MD; Donald B. Middleton, MD.

We are grateful to several people who helped make this book possible. At Lippincott Williams & Wilkins, a phenomenal job of organizational prodding and editing was done by Jenny Koleth. She definitely set a high standard and this text is a tribute to her effort. At the American College of Sports Medicine, D. Mark Robertson, Assistant Executive Vice-President, was instrumental in giving this project direction and encouragement. Finally, thanks to the ACSM Medical Education Committee Review Panel, chaired by Sandra Hoffman, MD, for providing timely overview and suggestions concerning text accuracy.

Medicine is facing enormous challenges today. Sports Medicine is not immune from these challenges. Integrated holistic care of the athlete is no longer a model, but an expectation. Exercise, the most powerful provocateur of health known to mankind has been recognized as such. The job of teaching our colleagues is not done.

It is our hope that this book provides a complete look at the field of Sports Medicine, both philosophically and contextually.

PS: The sophistication of Sports Medicine has grown since the First Edition of this book was published. The Sports Medicine Certificate of Added Qualification [CAQ] is now basically recognized as a subspecialty of the American Boards of Family Practice, Pediatrics, Internal Medicine, Emergency Medicine, and, most recently, physical medicine and rehabilitation. The establishment of the Sports Medicine CAQ offers consumers of sports medicine care a quality assurance heretofore not seen. This book continues to use an updated and amended version of the curriculum upon which the CAQ is based.

Douglas. B. McKeag
Indianapolis, Indiana
James L. Moeller
Auburn Hills, Michigan

Preface to the First Edition

Alas, we finally come to the end of the academic road after pursuing this project for 12 years. In 1981, you could count on one hand the number of primary care sports medicine training programs in the country; and the other hand would represent the number of reasonable and useful reference texts in sports medicine. Things seemed to be a little bit simpler then, including our approach to the care of the competitive athlete. A dozen years have produced dozens of surprises and changes. This 12-year period of time has seen the proliferation of training and fellowship programs, the formalization of education in the area of primary care, and a true, measurable improvement in the quality of health care given to the recreational and competitive athlete. Primary care has taken a dominant role in this movement, a situation not ignored by the "medical establishment." The newly formed American Medical Society for Sports Medicine (AMSSM) joined other organizations such as American Orthopedic Society for Sports Medicine (AOSSM) and the American College of Sports Medicine (ACSM) in addressing controversial, clinical concerns and providing practicing physicians with answers to difficult, thought provoking problems. The disciplines of Family Practice, Pediatrics, Internal Medicine, Emergency Medicine, and Physical Medicine and Rehabilitation have all begun to include, as part of training in their respective discipline, experiences in sports medicine.

How does one define "Sports Medicine"? We feel that this special interest area of medicine is nothing more than "medicine in motion." The physiologic intricacies of the human body become even more complex when this body is placed in motion. Yet, we are not stagnant animals. We move, we turn, we bend, we stoop, we run, and we swim. With movement, we do what the human body was built to do. With movement, we enhance our lives. We feel good. We help our psyche, our lungs; but we also strain tendons, dislocate joints, stress hearts, and concuss brains. We have discovered that exercise is a double-edged sword.

We hope that this book will serve as a compendium of **how to do things right** in sports medicine. As primacy care physicians, we have always felt that we brought a somewhat unique perspective to an area of medicine dominated by musculoskeletal injury. From our family practice training we have borrowed the concepts of **prevention** and **rehabilitation** and brought them to the forefront of treatment of sports-induced injury and illness. Hopefully, this book reflects that type of thinking. This book is not merely another reference text in sports medicine, but is an outline of a philosophy and a perspective. It was never meant to be a complete text, but one that would evolve constantly over time as principles of diagnosis and management change. It is our gift to those who come after us; those whose interest in sports and sports medicine can be met with a recommended, organized approach to learning the subject, something the authors and our colleagues never had.

After teaching over 500 residents and medical students the principles of sports medicine, and having the honor of training 14 incredibly competent primary care sports medicine fellows, we have begun to realize just how important this area truly is. We have always felt that you really did not have to know the difference between a basketball and a baseball; your patients surely will. More and more of our general population continue to interests in sports beyond youth in many forms of recreational activity. We must all become "team physicians" of a sort to those recreational exercisers we call our patients.

It is important to acknowledge those who have helped and stimulated us to produce this text. First and foremost, Frederick Bakker-Arkema, Ph.D., Professor of Agricultural Engineering at Michigan State University, has remained an academic role model and source of encouragement for us. He was most responsible for planting the "seed" that became this text. Acknowledgement is necessary to our colleagues with whom we shared ideas and a strong sense of teaching each other: William Anderson, Ph.D., Ronnie Barnes, AT, C., Henry Barry, M.D., John Bergfeld, M.D., Howard Brody, M.D., Vicky Curley, R.N., Brian Halpern, M.D., John Henderson, D.O., Warren Howe, M.D., Al Jacobs, D.O., Rob Johnson, M.D., Ed Kowaleski, M.D., James Kyle, M.D., John Lombardo, M.D., William Moats, M.D., Jeff Monroe, A.T., C., Sally Nogle, AT, C., James O'Brien, M.D., Randy Pearson, M.D., James Potchen, M.D., James Puffer, M.D., Lee Rice, D.O., Lon Rosen, M.D., Herb Ross, D.O., Vern Seefeldt, Ph.D., and Carol Smookler, Ph.D.

We also want to take this opportunity to thank all of the residents, medical students, private physicians, and, most importantly, former sports medicine fellows who provided the stimulus to push on with this project: Tom Morgan, M.D., Marie Schafle, M.D., Jim Swenson, M.D., Chris McGrew, M.D., Wade Lillegard, M.D., Dave Petron, M.D., Jeff Kovan, D.O., Neil Spiegel, D.O., Dave Peck, M.D., Brent Rich, M.D., Phil Zaneteas, M.D., Scott Eathorne, M.D.,

Scott Naftulin, D.O., Margo Putukian, M.D. Some of their work is reflected in this text.

We would like to gratefully acknowledge the assistance and help of Bud Schultz, Anne Schultz, the Michigan State University Training Staff and Athletes for their assistance in the development of this book, its figures, and illustrations.

Appreciation also needs to go to Butch Cooper, executive editor, Jan Edmondson, project coordinator, and Virginia Cowart, copy editor, for lending assistance and "direction" on this long and winding road.

Lastly, we want to acknowledge the effort of Susan Curtis, MA., who coordinated this project acting as typist, graphic artist, and manuscript editor for the entire text. Without question, this book is a testament to her hard work and dedication.

Douglas B. McKeag
David O. Hough

1
Basic Science and Sports Medicine

Primary Care Perspective

1

Douglas B. McKeag James L. Moeller

SECTION A

PHILOSOPHY OF PRIMARY CARE SPORTS MEDICINE

JUSTIFICATION

Despite the recent proliferation of sports medicine textbooks and information regarding this specialty area, we believe there is a need for a single source of appropriate and practical sports medicine information for the primary care physician, resident, medical student, and allied health practitioner.

Primary care physicians can find many justifications for studying and practicing sports medicine:

- Health care delivery in the United States, if it is to be effective, must continue toward community-oriented medicine. This trend places much of the burden of health care delivery, including sports medicine health care delivery, on the shoulders of primary care practitioners.
- Many sources of information about sports medicine for the primary care physician remain poorly organized—the direct result being too much specialization and not enough "big picture" thinking. Although good, practical concepts for treating patients with athletic injuries occasionally appear in primary care medical journals, there are a few practical reference works for the primary care physician that approach sports medicine in a complete, easily referenced manner.
- Sports medicine is a rapidly changing field. Technological advances have an impact on both treatment and rehabilitation. Changes in equipment, techniques, rules, and training that allow athletes to perform better have made it difficult for practitioners, even those well versed in sports medicine, to remain current.
- Most physicians continue to receive little, if any, formal sports medicine education either in medical school or at the postgraduate level. This is in spite of the growing level of musculoskeletal problems currently confronting the primary care physician. The natural result of this situation is inconsistency in patient care. There are encouraging changes. Several organizations—American College of Sports Medicine (ASCM), American Medical Society for Sports Medicine (AMSSM), American Academy of Family Physicians (AAFP), and the American Orthopedic Society for Sports Medicine (AOSSM)—are presenting quality postgraduate courses in sports medicine. The formation of the AMSSM and the advent of the Sports Medicine's Certificate of Added Qualification (CAQ) have added professional definition to this important new specialty. The foundation for these changes was built by sports medicine teaching programs that established the curricula to teach. The legacy of these programs will be the definition of sports medicine as a discipline. Recent changes in Family Medicine Residency educational requirements in the area of sports medicine underlie the importance of this specialty area.
- Injured athletes are not always treated in the same manner as injured nonathletes. Time constraints, patient motivation, and accessibility to highly technical therapy modalities are factors that contribute to this dichotomy of injury care. What we have learned in treating athletes has been successfully translated to treatment of the nonathlete population.
- The number of sports-related injuries has increased. Improved equipment and better supervision have reduced injury rates in certain organized sports settings, but the

total number of sports injuries has been on the rise. Many factors contribute to this increase in injuries, including the following:

(a) An increase in participation. With more people involved in sports, more will be injured.
(b) The disappearance of "natural selection". Most adults involved in recreational sports 25 years ago were individuals who had learned proper training techniques as youngsters. They had developed their exercise regimens over time. Currently, many middle-aged individuals are beginning to participate in exercise after 15 to 25 years of sedentary life. Their lack of knowledge or experience of appropriate training methods generates more injuries.
(c) Increased variety of sports is available. The rising popularity of such sports as lacrosse, soccer, gymnastics, and aerobics has generated a whole new subpopulation of recreational athletes.
(d) Individuals have increased opportunities for participation. The "positive economy" of sports has provided more avenues for participation. The increase in recreational sports has created a demand for biking trails, jogging clubs, skateboard parks, tennis facilities, and fitness centers. This, in turn, makes participation in sports more accessible.
(e) An increased sophistication has gradually developed along with increasing knowledge of the biomechanical aspects of sport. Researchers help players become more successful through better technical skills development. Greater sophistication can, however, lead to cheating, abuse, and the production of additional injuries.
(f) An increase in intensity usually accompanies increases in level of play. It takes more effort to succeed; more commitment and practice time are required to train. Increased exercise exposures at high intensity increase the risk of injury.
(g) Many athletes specialize at a young age, playing a sport yearlong. Early specialization can result in overuse injuries, as constant repetition breaks down muscle–tendon units.
(h) Professionalism in coaching has not kept pace with the increased popularity of sports. Despite scientific revelations in training, poor coaching and training methods remain major factors in the generation of sports injuries.

- The educational level of patients with sports injuries has risen. The lay public obtains information about sports medicine from many sources, reliable and unreliable. Much information is contradictory and some are potentially harmful. Often, it is based on studies of elite athletes, not the type of athletes seen by most primary care physicians.
- Even those individuals with ill health or chronic disease can benefit from exercise as a component of a medical therapeutic plan. Treatments of psychological disorders, chronic pulmonary disease, hypertension, obesity, coronary artery disease, and even some cancers may include exercise as a powerful adjunct to conventional therapy.
- Exercise has a positive effect on every major organ system of the body. Studies have shown that it is not just the cardiovascular and musculoskeletal systems that receive a protective benefit. Exercise holds the promise of decreased morbidity and mortality. Its health promotion potential is staggering. The impact of physical activity in the primary and secondary prevention of chronic disease states is magnified by the ability of primary care physicians to prescribe it to patients.
- Sports medicine principles can be used to benefit patients, active or otherwise, as they could encounter maladies and injuries in any of their activities of daily living. Active interest or knowledge of sports is not a requirement of an effective sports medicine practitioner; an understanding and appreciation of the effects of exercise on the human condition is.
- There continues to be a lack of quality assurance in sports medicine. Sports medicine is still a young specialty area. To obtain a CAQ in Sports Medicine, practitioners must first be board certified in a primary specialty (Family Practice, Internal Medicine, Pediatrics, Emergency Medicine), successfully complete an accredited fellowship in Sports Medicine, and then pass the CAQ examination. This should be enough to assure quality. Unfortunately, there are many practitioners in various specialties who continue to advertise as "Sports Medicine" practitioners without completing more than their primary training.
- Sports medicine care can be an excellent marketing tool. Accepting patients with sports injuries is an effective method for a practitioner to capture new patients.

Primary care residents may find that a general knowledge of sports medicine has additional advantages beyond those already cited:

1. Sports medicine training allows the resident to integrate a number of medical disciplines previously studied (e.g., cardiology, physiology, nutrition, orthopedics).
2. The experience of a formal sports medicine rotation gives residents an opportunity to place appropriate primary care emphasis on areas traditionally thought of as secondary or tertiary care. Many concepts of office musculoskeletal medicine are either absent or not emphasized during general orthopedic rotations.
3. A formal background in sports medicine training can be a definite asset in gaining rapid entrance into a community.
4. New physicians with a sports medicine interest and background are perceived as more current, knowledgeable, and interested in community affairs. They may be asked to make presentations on exercise and sports to lay groups. They may be asked to serve on committees to establish guidelines for the conduct of community sports programs. The list of potential opportunities is unending.

Medical students now realize the value of exercise in their own lives. Many have a profound interest in the area of sports medicine as early as the first quarter of the first year of medical school. Many medical students come from areas of interest that embrace sports medicine (e.g., kinesiology, nutrition, psychology). It is unfortunate that medical school curricula do not change as readily as society. As has been the case with nutrition, the importance of sports medicine has been overlooked in most medical school curricula. Our experience tells us that because of its interdisciplinary nature, sports medicine offers a natural integrative bridge between disciplines. Where else can the integration of the basic sciences (e.g., physiology, pharmacology) be so naturally incorporated into such clinically related fields as cardiology and orthopedics? Furthermore, psychosocial sciences such as biomedical ethics and psychology also assimilate well. Because of its popularity and preventive medicine aspects, sports medicine becomes a natural common pathway for medical school curricular integration.

INTERDISCIPLINARY APPROACH TO SPORTS MEDICINE

As we have said, sports medicine draws upon and integrates a variety of disciplines. But what of the approach to sports medicine? It is important to state that this book deals specifically with a primary care perspective of sports medicine. In our view, the first-contact, comprehensive, continuing care given by most primary care physicians to athletes is sports medicine. The primary physician as leader in an ever-evolving well-defined athlete health care system is the philosophy underlying the organization of this book.

Is there an overemphasis on the musculoskeletal injury in the athlete? When some think of sports medicine, do they really mean sports orthopedics? When the public thinks of a sports medicine "specialist" are they really referring to an orthopedic surgeon? Orthopedic surgeons have done much to advance and upgrade the care of musculoskeletal injuries in the athlete. Their contributions include (a) arthroscopic surgery (e.g., knee, ankle, shoulder, elbow), (b) adaptation of conservative approaches to previously operable injuries (e.g., severe ankle sprains, third-degree ligament tears), (c) further definition of many subtle yet common syndromes (e.g., patellofemoral dysfunction, shoulder impingement, cervical stenosis), and (d) delineation of more appropriate diagnostic testing to better examine the musculoskeletal system (e.g., Lachman's test, shoulder augmentation/relocation tests). Musculoskeletal injuries require a great deal of emphasis in the study of sports medicine. They account for more than 50% of all sports-related injuries.

However, other disciplines have contributed as well. Physical medicine and rehabilitation (PM&R) and athletic training are areas where new modalities have been discovered and new treatment regimens generated. More defined rehabilitation programs for specific injuries have evolved. The principles of biomechanics have been applied to injury etiology and subsequently to the rehabilitative process. Emphasis now is on rehabilitation of isolated muscles or muscle groups. This has produced specific techniques that allow athletes to return to play more quickly than ever before.

Cardiology has made its contributions to sports medicine. Cardiologists first recognized the importance of physical activity as therapy to improve cardiac function. What began as scientifically documented improvement after myocardial insult has evolved into sophisticated rehabilitative programs following cardiac events. The need for a defined cardiac rehabilitation program first spurred the study of exercise physiology. The guidelines of such programs have been applied with modification to the healthy population.

Physiology has long studied the effects of exercise on various body systems, describing what exercise can and cannot do. This basic science has defined the various types of exercise that we do, what is appropriate, in what circumstances, and what specific biologic changes take place that are exercise dependent. The definition of minimal exercise requirements has been of major importance because it gives the lay public an opportunity to use guidelines that are applicable and practical on an everyday basis.

Nutrition, as an applied science, has contributed much to the understanding of sports and performance. These contributions include (a) the realization that diet does affect performance; (b) the further realization that manipulation of diet can improve performance; (c) the delineation of the nutritional costs of exercise; (d) the role of various nutrients, minerals, and fluids in exercise performance; and (e) the sometimes adverse effects of eating disorders on vulnerable exercising individuals.

Psychology as an applied behavioral science has begun to examine how the mind can interact with the exercising body. The realization that exercising individuals have an enhanced sense of well-being has led to the use of exercise as therapy for many psychiatric disturbances. The fascinating research on the effect of competition on an individual's mental outlook remains an area of great interest. Future work may show that psychological well-being is a major predictor of athletic performance.

Many other disciplines are involved, including pharmacology (the appropriate and inappropriate use of drugs by athletes), optometry (the prevention of eye injuries), and podiatry (studies of the interface between foot and running surface).

Musculoskeletal injury remains the single most important type of injury of concern to the sports medicine physician although it is far from the only system. It is safe to say that every body system can and has been affected by exercise or exercise-induced injury or illness. Each has been shown to benefit from exercise, just as each can be adversely affected by it.

An important concept needs to be emphasized—the athlete is not merely a movable bony skeleton upon which musculotendinous units are draped. Each sports injury is not just an orthopedic injury. The athlete is a human being with multiple systems, each capable of reacting to movement. Precisely for this reason, the athlete or exerciser should receive the type of comprehensive care that only the primary care physician can give. The entire person, not just the body part or system, should be considered.

This book advocates an interdisciplinary approach to sports medicine. The authors believe strongly that a comprehensive continuing care approach to the athlete can only be directed by the primary care specialist, usually a family physician, internist, or pediatrician. The primary care practitioner should then gather a cadre of additional specialists (e.g., athletic trainer, physical therapist, nutritionist, or podiatrist) to complete the creation of the sports medicine network.

FUTURE DIRECTIONS

Sports medicine as a special interest area and, eventually, as the specialty it is currently was born from primary care roots. We firmly believe that these roots should not be forgotten. From the earlier information, however, it is obvious that sports medicine has grown into an exciting and rapidly changing, important area of medicine. As previously discussed, due to the rapid changes in the field, it is difficult for practitioners, even those well versed in sports medicine, to remain current.

The time is quickly approaching where we will need to consider the creation of a full sports medicine specialty that incorporates the necessary multidisciplinary training for sports medicine practitioners and gives practitioners in this field the opportunity to obtain their primary Board Certification in the field of Sports Medicine.

The creation of such a specialty would not eliminate the importance of Sports Medicine training in the classic primary care fields of Family Medicine, Internal Medicine, Pediatrics and Emergency Medicine, but would serve to enhance the educational opportunities in these fields. Practitioners in the classic primary care specialties will always have a need for skills in sports medicine and will always see patients with sports medicine issues. However, if we continue to expect advancement in the field of sports medicine, excellence in education and delivery of sports medicine care, and continue to hold sports medicine practitioners to a higher standard of care, we will need to recognize the difficulties of this in the current system.

SECTION B

SPORTS MEDICINE AND THE LAW

As our society becomes more litigious, the medical/legal aspects of sports medicine take on increasing importance. A fair question to ask might be: Is there truly any difference in risk between serving the athletic population and the nonathletic population? The answer is arguably "yes." At this time, the risk is not significant in the context of all sports-related lawsuits. Most often, local boards of education, coaches, and equipment manufacturers are the target of sports injury lawsuits. Physicians have been remarkably free of involvement in such actions but this should not lull the practitioner into a false sense of security. There is a trend in the opposite direction. As sports medicine becomes a more recognized specialty area, it is only natural that all its practitioners will be held to higher medical standards commensurate with the increased duties and responsibilities they have assumed. A summary of important areas of medical–legal interaction in sports medicine includes the following.

NEGLIGENCE

Team physicians must treat athletes the same as other patients. It is immaterial whether care is provided for a fee or not. Furthermore, the statute of limitations is no safeguard, as a suit can be withheld until a young athlete reaches maturity. Tort liability is the prevalent concept. This is a liability for personal injury that is alleged to be the result of the defendant's negligence. Because negligence is the principal charge, its definition is of interest: "failure to act as a prudent physician would under similar circumstances." Generally speaking, four elements must be present to prove negligence:

1. The physician had a duty to act to avoid unreasonable risk to others.
2. The defendant failed to observe that duty.
3. Failure to observe that duty was the proximate cause of damage.
4. Actual damage or injury did occur.

The "standard of care" concept is applied to most of these situations. For a primary care practitioner, the standard of care incorporates what would normally be done by a primary care specialist in this locale, in this situation. Legal defenses in this case usually encompass one or two strategies: assumption of risk—in other words, the athlete assumed a certain degree of risk with his or her participation in the activity; contributory negligence—the athlete in question was participating in a reckless or negligent manner.

AVOIDING LAWSUITS

The risk of litigation over medical treatment of athletes can be reduced if sports physicians are guided by the following:

1. Follow established guidelines (that you may have helped formulate).
2. Generate a written contract with the school or group with which you are working.

3. If at all possible, work with athletic trainers.
4. Generate a thorough preparticipation sports physical examination.
5. Always use sound judgment concerning return to competition.
6. Institute early, proper care.
7. Seek informed consent for treatment.
8. Be careful with release of information.

Make sure to follow standard procedures and established methods in the treatment of injuries. The playing field and/or locker room are no place for experimentation. Reserve the right to await developments before making a final judgment about any injury.

The contract with the sponsoring organization should be an agreement spelling out the responsibilities and limits of the team physician. The agreement should acknowledge that the team physician has the final word in all medical decisions, including return to participation after injury or illness. Encourage communication by meeting with parents, athletes, and coaches before the start of each season to discuss how injuries will be handled and what the line of authority will be. At such meetings, indicate your plans for reducing the incidence of injuries.

Obtaining the services of an athletic trainer is an important step in establishing a comprehensive sports medicine network. The athletic trainer is a very important member of the community sports medicine "team" and should act as the on-site coordinator for all sports medicine activities, and as a liaison between team physician, athlete, and/or school officials. Athletic trainers should be responsible for the initial treatment and early triage of the injury. They should also be responsible for the implementation of injury prevention programs.

The importance of the preparticipation examination is underlined by its function not only as a screening examination but also as a base of referral. It is important to avoid statements, either written or verbal, that say: "It is safe for _____ to participate in _____." More appropriate terminology might be: "I can find no medical reason why _____ should not participate in _____." In the event of a disqualification, it is important to remember that even if parents wish to give permission for the disqualified athlete to participate, the law gives parents no authority to release future claims on behalf of the child.

It should be standard policy that all injuries are reported to the team physician and that no return to play should occur until assessment is complete. A sound judgment will incorporate both the physician's clinical impression of the seriousness of the injury and the trainer's impression of how it occurred and how well the athlete has progressed in rehabilitation.

It is important to institute early proper care. Because it is impractical for most physicians to be in attendance at practices, early institution of proper care should, by necessity, fall into the hands of the athletic trainer or other capable personnel. It is important to arrange for availability of medical coverage during practices and competition and to make sure transportation from sites of participation is practical in the event of serious injury. The physician should instruct athletic trainers and other personnel in the proper use of the stretcher or other means of emergency transport.

The principle of informed consent is especially important in the treatment of athletic injuries. Injuries should be explained and proposed treatment options discussed with the athlete and parents (if appropriate). Good records should be maintained as to what was said and decided. Treatment should not end prematurely because of a desire to return an athlete to play.

The doctor–patient relationship has been and continues to be a foundation for all of medicine. This is no different in treating athletes. Such a relationship must be confidential. Barring specific permission from the athlete, no part of the written medical record or verbal impressions of an injury should be disclosed to other interested parties. Of particular concern to the team physician is the relationship between himself and the athlete's primary care physician, if one has been identified. From a professional standpoint, communication and consultation should also involve this physician colleague.

Team physicians should provide athletic trainers with ongoing medical updates and evaluation to ensure against negligence on the part of the trainer. They also should familiarize themselves with the safety limits of equipment to be used by athletes in the sports to be covered.

SECTION C

HEALTH INSURANCE PORTABILITY AND ACCOUNTABILITY ACT

On April 14, 2003, Health Insurance Portability and Accountability Act (HIPAA) of 1996 went into effect for most health care groups. HIPAA is designed to ease the electronic flow of medical information while protecting patient privacy. Although the bulk of the law applies to electronic transmissions, there are privacy laws contained in the act which also apply to oral and written communications. This, of course, creates significant concerns, especially in the area of sports medicine, as these new layers of bureaucracy and potential obstacles to treatment are imposed.

Sports medicine involves frequent interactions and consultations with orthopedic surgeons, athletic trainers, coaches, athletic directors, physical therapists, and many others in sports medicine systems. Player injury reports, although they remain part of the culture in both professional and college teams, are just one example in which the sports culture *may* violate the new act.

Major points of concern have been outlined and discussed by various groups and include (but are not limited to) the following:

1. Are reports about injured players on teams released?
2. Are medical communications between team physicians, consultants, and others and the school and team illegal?

3. What will be the appropriate interaction between team physicians and consultants regarding player injuries?

The U.S. Department of Health and Human Services (DHHS) has begun to clarify some of these issues. It has been determined that physicians, as *covered* entities, are free to share patient's private health information for treatment purposes. This applies to *uncovered* entities as well.

Communication among medical team members and coaches appears to be on safe legal ground as well. Many team physicians are said to work at "hybrid entity institutions," places where sports medicine crosses academic, athletic, clinical, and hospital lines. Team physicians working in such institutions need to probably attend to the following:

1. Computer systems need to ensure secure transmissions within the sports medicine system.
2. Such institutions need to incorporate privacy policies and disclosures into the preparticipation examination before students receive such examinations.

HIPAA remains a broad-based policy in which questions remain unanswered at a local level. It appears that this act has resulted in more codification of privacy issues and assurances of only appropriate release of medical information across most institutions. Common sense has always played a role in the release of medical information for sports medicine physicians. The formalization of this common sense seems to be the most significant effect of HIPAA at the present time.

SECTION D
ETHICS AND MEDICAL DECISION MAKING

Sports medicine, like any other specialty area, is subject to patient care problems that require ethical analysis for rational solution. These can be called *conflict of interest* or *divided loyalty dilemmas*. Such dilemmas result from being situated between two or more parties, each evoking a strong sense of commitment and duty from the care provider. Such conflicts may differ depending upon the level of sport covered (professional, college, high school, or youth programs), but remain a continuing problem and major factor in medical decision making.

Just what are these conflicts?

1. *Role of team physician versus role of a fan.* The fact remains that most sports physicians are involved because they are fans (interested parties). At times this can create a conflict of interest in the treatment of injury and judgment concerning return to play. Obviously, the role of the fan/booster must be subservient to the role of team physician.
2. *Welfare of the athlete versus welfare of the team.* This is probably the most common dilemma occurring at all levels. It becomes more of a conflict as the pressure to win takes priority over medical values in a program. Established return to play criteria can help tremendously.
3. *Welfare of the athlete versus wishes of the athlete.* The principle that should prevail in confronting this problem is—"Physician, do no harm." The team physician must think about long-term harm versus short-term benefit. Is the athlete making this decision in the presence of coercion, either overt or covert? Is the athlete old enough to fully consider the ramifications of his/her actions?
4. *Welfare of the athlete versus welfare of the family.* Occasionally, the wishes of an athlete's family unit conflict with the long-term welfare of the athlete.

How does one minimize such divided loyalty dilemmas? It is important to avoid ambiguity and that can be achieved as follows:

1. Clarify the nature of the relationship between you and other parties at the outset (e.g., coaches, parents, athletes, school administrators, team owners).
2. Insist upon professional autonomy over all medical decisions.
3. Anticipate, identify, and then insulate yourself formally from all possible coercive pressures to ensure such autonomy.
4. Communicate those principles and guidelines under which you intend to deliver care and make decisions before becoming the care provider.
5. Eliminate, or at least recognize and minimize any personal biases you may have that might adversely affect your function as team physician.

Lastly, it is important to realize that adroit initial handling of a potential problem can eliminate more complicated conflicts of interest later. With the onset of any injury:

1. Remove the athlete from the field/court of play to a quieter environment.
2. Carry out an unhurried, thorough examination.
3. Decide whether return to play is possible, considering potential further risk of injury. If the decision concerning return to play is "no," inform the coach of your decision. If the decision is "yes," follow steps a to e.
   (a) Discuss return to play with the athlete only, exclusive of others.
   (b) In the case of a young athlete, insist on discussion to clarify the athlete's wishes and then confer where appropriate with other family members.
   (c) Any doubts expressed by the athlete about return to play should strongly bias the physician toward elimination of the athlete from further play in that contest.
   (d) Act as the athlete advocate when dealing with the coach concerning a decision not to play.
   (e) Be very clear on the limits of your responsibility as team physician. If a physician concludes that an athlete can return to play, but at a diminished level of performance, it becomes the coach's decision as to whether the athlete is more valuable than a healthy backup.

HELPFUL HINTS

Finally, consider the following list before becoming or agreeing to become team physician. Although these are only recommendations, they may help put your participation as team physician in perspective.

- Do you have current training in cardiopulmonary resuscitation (CPR) or basic cardiac life support (BCLS)?
- Do you know how to manage an acutely traumatized athlete with an injury to the head, neck, or back?
- Will your malpractice insurance extend to sports medicine?
- Does the team or program sponsoring the activity you are covering have liability insurance to cover a team physician?
- Are the athletes to be covered provided with a consent form for treatment of nonemergency injuries?
- Are you comfortable with your knowledge base concerning re-entry into a sporting event following injury?
- Can you recognize your own limitations and call in other specialists when necessary?

REFERENCES

Philosophy of Primary Care Sports Medicine

1. Accreditation Council for Graduate Medical Education. *Program Requirements for Graduate Medical Education in Family Medicine (approved 9/05, effective 7/06)*. http://www.acgme.org/acWebsite/downloads/RRC_progReq/120pr706.pdf, 07/06.
2. American Academy of Pediatrics Committee on Sports Medicine and Fitness Policy Statement. Intensive training and sports specialization in young athletes. *Pediatrics* 2000;106(1):154–157.
3. Centers for Disease Control and Prevention (CDC). Nonfatal sports and recreation-related injuries treated in emergency departments—United States, July 2000–June 2001. *MMWR Morb Mortal Wkly Rep* 2002;51(33):736–740.

Sports Medicine and the Law

4. Hurt WT. Elements of tort liability as applied to athletic injuries. *J Sch Health* 1976;XLVI(4):200.
5. Lowell CH. Legal responsibilities and sports medicine. *Phys Sportsmed* 1977;5(7):60.
6. Weistant JC, Lowell CH. *Law of sports*. Charlottesville, Virginia: Merril, 1979.
7. Willis GC. The legal responsibilities of the team physician. *J Sportsmed* 1972;1:28.

Health Insurance Portability and Accountability Act

8. United States Department of Health and Human Services. *Summary of the HIPAA Privacy Rule, last revised 5/03*. http://www.hhs.gov/ocr/privacysummary.pdf, 07/06.

Ethics and Medical Decision Making

9. Johnson R. The unique ethics of sports medicine. *Clin Sportsmed* 2004;23(2):175–182.
10. McKeag DB, Brody H, Hough DO. Medical ethics in sport. *Phys Sportsmed* 1984;12(8):145.
11. Murray TH. Divided loyalties in sports medicine. *Phys Sportsmed* 1984;12(8):134.
12. McKeag DB. *Proceedings of "Ethics in Sports Medicine" Symposium*. Hartford: University of Connecticut, May 1986.
13. Stovitz SD, Satin DJ. Professionalism and the ethics of the sideline physician. *Curr Sports Med Rep* 2006;5(3):120–124.

Epidemiology of Athletic Injuries

2

Eric D. Zemper *Randall W. Dick*

This chapter will introduce some fundamental concepts of epidemiology, the basic science of preventive medicine, and its application to sports medicine, specifically the epidemiology of athletic injuries. The word "epidemiology" is comprised of three Greek root terms: epi (meaning "upon"), demos ("people"), and logos ("study"). Therefore, epidemiology is the study of what is upon, or befalls, a people or population. A more formal definition is that provided by Duncan (1):

> Epidemiology is the study of the distribution and determinants of the varying rates of diseases, injuries, or other health states in human populations.

The basic method of studying and determining these distributions and determinants is comparing groups within a population (the sick and the well; the injured and the noninjured). Doing an epidemiological study is a lot like being a detective, using logic to discover cause and effect relationships for illnesses or other medical conditions in a population. In many ways it is similar to diagnosing an illness, but it is done with a large population rather than with an individual patient.

Duncan (1) lists seven major uses for epidemiological data:

- Identifying the causes of disease
- Completing the clinical picture of a disease
- Allowing identification of syndromes
- Determining the effectiveness of therapeutic and preventive measures
- Providing the means to monitor the health of a community or region, that is, input for rational health planning
- Quantifying risks (health hazard appraisals)
- Providing an overview of long-term disease trends

The initial development of the theory and methods of epidemiology focused on applications to communicable diseases, and guidelines for public health surveillance systems for communicable diseases have been published by the Centers for Disease Control and Prevention (CDC) (2). However, in recent years epidemiological theory and methodologies have been applied to a broader range of subject areas, including athletic injuries. One of the primary tools in applying epidemiological theory and methods to the study of athletic injuries is the use of the techniques of injury surveillance.

Sports injury surveillance applies the well-established principles of public health surveillance to the problem of athletic injury. Injury surveillance is not the same as injury research, although the two are similar. Injury research involves the slow and thorough accumulation of very precise data and can take years to come to fruition. By contrast, injury surveillance uses methods for the rapid collection and dissemination of data and evolves and develops to meet the ever-changing needs of the sports medicine community in general, and users of the data in particular (3). A thorough review of injury surveillance definitions and guidelines has been developed by the World Health Organization in conjunction with the CDC (4).

Meeuwisse and Love (5) suggest that researchers should take the following general recommendations into consideration when collecting and publishing injury data:

- Maximize comparability of data between systems through clear indication of reporting system design and the methods used to collect data.
- Clearly define what constitutes a reportable event.
- Collect outcome information on each reportable event.
- Acknowledge any potential source of error.

The same authors (5) suggest that an "ideal" system for assessing athletic risk would include the following:

- Simplicity and ease of use
- Flexibility to address changing patterns of injury
- Collection of athletic exposure data
- Standardized documentation of injury diagnosis, severity, treatment, and associated risk factors
- Data collection by team athletic trainers who work with the team on a daily basis

A recent publication by Fuller et al. (6) contains recommendations for appropriate injury definitions and data collection procedures for injury surveillance, specifically for the sport of soccer, which involve many of the above concepts.

EPIDEMIOLOGICAL RATES

The basic tool of epidemiology is the calculation of rates of occurrence of medical cases of interest in a given population. The two most commonly used rates are prevalence and incidence. The prevalence rate includes all cases of the medical condition of interest that exist at the beginning of the study period and all new cases that develop during the study period. Incidence rates include only the newly developed cases. In sports medicine, the incidence rate is predominantly used to study athletic injuries, because it is assumed that all athletes are uninjured at the beginning of the season and it is the incidence of new injuries during the season that is of interest. Therefore, we will deal only with incidence rates here. The incidence rate is a measure of the rate at which new events (illnesses, injuries, etc.) occur during a specified time in a defined population:

$$\text{Incidence Rate} = (\text{number of new events during specified period} \times k) \div \text{number in the population at risk}$$

The numerator is simply a count of the number of new cases that occur during the study period. The denominator is the total number of people in the population under study who are "at risk" or exposed to the possibility of infection, injury, and so on. To provide reasonable numbers that are neither extremely large nor extremely small, and to make comparisons easier, this ratio is transformed to a common metric by multiplying by a convenient multiple of 10 (represented by the constant **k** in the preceding equation). If $k = 1{,}000$ the result would be a rate per 1,000 in the population; if $k = 100{,}000$ the result would be a rate per 100,000. For example, suppose 24 cases of measles were reported on a college campus of 34,000 students. A moment's thought will show that stating a rate of 24/34,000 is not the most informative way of presenting this information. The probability of an individual having the disease is not readily apparent, and it is not easy to compare the rate with the five cases that occurred in the population of 630 student-athletes on that campus. The base ratio of 24/34,000 is 0.000706, which is the probability that any one individual has measles. But obviously this is not an easy number to work with. Using $k = 100{,}000$ we transform this rate to 70.6 cases per 100,000, which is a little more manageable. If we make the same calculation for student-athletes, we get a case rate of 793.7 cases per 100,000. Now it is easier to see that student-athletes had a much higher rate of measles, so immediate preventive measures might be in order for this special population.

Determining the numerator of the case rate equation is usually relatively easy. The most critical part of the calculation is determining the denominator, or the "population at risk." This should include everyone in the population who could be affected by the disease or condition of interest, and should exclude those who could not be affected or are not really a member of the population of interest. For instance, in calculating a case rate for pregnancy, males, females past menopause, and females who have not reached menarche should not be used in the denominator. In calculating a case rate for football injuries during games, only those who actually played and were exposed to the possibility of injury, not the whole team, should be included in the denominator.

In sports medicine, case rates are generally used to present epidemiological information about athletic injuries. In the past, these rates have been presented most often as injuries per 100 athletes, which is analogous to the rate per 100,000 population used for reporting disease rates. However, there is a difference between the continuous exposure of a population to a disease and the discrete exposure of an athlete to injury, which occurs only during practices or games. The number of practices and games varies considerably from one sport to another, and often varies from one team to another, or even from one year to another in a given sport. In addition, not every player participates in every practice and every game, and the number of participants on a team may change considerably as the season progresses. Therefore, the common practice of reporting athletic injuries as a rate per 100 participants can lead to questionable conclusions, particularly when results from different sports, or even from different studies of the same sport, are compared. A more precise method is to report case rates per 1,000 athlete-exposures (A-Es). An A-E is defined as one athlete participating in one practice or game where there is the possibility of sustaining an athletic injury. If a football team of 100 players has five practices during the week, there are 500 A-Es to the possibility of being injured in practice during that week. If 40 players get into the game on Saturday, the team has 40 A-Es in the game, and the weekly total is 540 A-Es to the possibility of being injured.

Using A-Es as the denominator allows more accurate and precise comparisons of injury rates between sports and in different years (7). Case rates per 1,000 A-Es are currently used by the National Collegiate Athletic

Association (NCAA) Injury Surveillance System (ISS) (8) and the Athletic Injury Monitoring System (AIMS) (9). An even more precise approach would base the exposure rate on the amount of time actually spent in practices or games. Case rates per 1,000 hours of participation exposure might be possible in small local studies, and should be done at this level if possible. But, in most cases, the amount of record keeping required for a national-scale surveillance system would be prohibitive and impractical for those doing the on-site data recording. Case rates per 1,000 A-Es are therefore believed to be a reasonable compromise that gives a more accurate picture of the epidemiology of athletic injuries than the use of simple rates per 100 athletes.

CONCERNS REGARDING PUBLISHED LITERATURE ON SPORTS INJURY RATES

A major weakness commonly seen in the published literature on athletic injury rates is that the denominator data for the incidence rate equation is poorly defined or has not been determined. This reduces these articles to simple case series reports that have little or no epidemiological value (10). Unless the calculation of rates is based on the population at risk, it is impossible to generalize the results beyond the specific population used in the study. This highlights a major problem in much of the earlier research literature on athletic injury rates, and even some of the current literature: most authors have little or no training in epidemiology, so these articles often are not of any great use on a broader scale in that the information cannot be generalized to other places and situations. For example, several years ago Powell et al. (11) did a thorough review of the literature on running injuries and found only two published articles and one meeting presentation that met minimal criteria for factors such as definition of injury, selection of subjects, and use of proper denominator data ("population at risk") in calculating injury rates.

Two to three decades ago the research literature on the epidemiology of athletic injuries was very sparse, but since the mid 1960s there has been a slow growth in sports injury rate research as the need for this type of data has become more apparent. Even so, many studies cover only one year (or season), occasionally two. Nearly all studies have limitations imposed by sample size, covering one school, one city, or one geographical area. Some studies are limited to injuries of one anatomical site, such as the knee, or one type of injury, such as fatalities or ankle sprains. Getting a clear national perspective by combining results from different studies are greatly hindered by differences in methodologies, such as dissimilar definitions of a reportable injury or different means of collecting and reporting data. Combining study results would be ill advised in any case, because it would be highly unlikely that the various data sources that are combined are truly representative of athletes and teams across the whole country.

Still another problem with many studies is the source used to obtain injury data. Some rely on insurance claim forms, which has the disadvantage of not representing the true injury rate as not all athletic injuries result in insurance claims. Also, these records seldom contain much detail on the circumstances and mechanisms of injury or even the diagnosis itself. Some studies rely on a coach's assessment or recognition of an injury although it has been shown that, unless coaches have received specific training, they do a poor job of recognizing most treatable injuries (12). Studies that depend on recall of injuries at the end of a season have the obvious problems of inaccuracy and incompleteness of recall. One recent study (13) compared weekly recording of soccer injuries with a retrospective questionnaire completed by the athletes at the end of the season, and showed that although more than 80% of the players were injured during the season, less than half the players reported being injured. Only 73% of serious injuries, approximately one third of the moderate injuries, and less than 10% of the mild injuries recorded by medical staff during the season were reported by the athletes in the retrospective questionnaire at the end of the season.

Another example where the source of information has limitations is the National Electronic Injury Surveillance System (NEISS) which compiles injury information related to consumer products. The Consumer Product Safety Commission (CPSC) initiated the system in 1971 utilizing a national stratified probability sample of 100 U.S. hospital emergency departments. In 2000, the CPSC in collaboration with the CDC's National Center for Injury Prevention and Control expanded NEISS to include all injuries, regardless of being consumer product related. The expanded system called the *National Electronic Injury Surveillance System All Injury Program (NEISS-AIP)*, utilizes a national stratified probability sample of 66 of the original 100 NEISS emergency departments to track injuries, including athletic injuries (14).

The hospitals selected for NEISS-AIP were chosen as a nationally representative sample of emergency departments, and therefore the system should be sensitive to those injuries that are seen by an emergency department (15). However, many, if not most, athletic injuries never make it to the emergency department and so are not captured by the system. A second limitation is that no true exposure values of individuals at risk for athletic injuries are associated with the system. Although this system can outline the relative proportion of more serious injuries in certain activities, it still falls short of a sport-specific surveillance system with associated appropriate exposure information.

It has become evident over the past 25 years that there is a need for accurate, reliable data on injury rates for various sports and exercise activities. With the increase in participation in organized sports and in fitness activities, participation that is encouraged by the medical community as a public health intervention, it is often not realized that even today there still is little or no dependable risk data available for these activities. A great deal of effort is focused on defining the benefits of participation of sports and fitness activities, but little is done to assess risk (16). This information is needed to make informed decisions about the value of taking part in a particular activity, and to provide information on how injury rates can be reduced. Therefore, it is desirable to collect data for all types of exercise and fitness activities as well as all levels of sports participation. Unfortunately, although there has been improvement in recent years in the data available for some sports activities, little or no data are available at this time for anything other than college and high school sports. A comprehensive compilation and review of the literature on sports injury epidemiology can be found in the book by Caine et al. (17).

MODEL SPORTS INJURY DATA COLLECTION SYSTEMS

Several sports injury data collection systems have been developed using the concept of rates discussed earlier. The following examples meet most of the criteria noted earlier for an "ideal" system, and the published reports from these systems avoid the problems noted in the previous section.

National Center for Catastrophic Sports Injury Research

In 1931, the American Football Coaches Association initiated the First Annual Survey of Football Fatalities and this research has been conducted at the University of North Carolina, Chapel Hill, since 1965. In 1977, the NCAA initiated a National Survey of Catastrophic Football Injuries, which is also conducted at the University of North Carolina. As a result of these research projects important contributions to the safety of the sport of football have been made. Most notable have been the 1976 rule changes, prohibiting spearing and initial contact with the head and face when tackling and blocking, the implementation of the football helmet standard, improved medical care for the participants, and better coaching techniques.

Because of the success of these two football projects, the research was expanded to all sports for both men and women, and a National Center for Catastrophic Sports Injury ResearchNCCSIR) was established in 1982. In 1987, a joint endeavor was initiated with the section on sports medicine of the American Association of Neurological Surgeons by involving a physician to assist in the collection of medical data. Since 1982, the Center has attempted to collect information on all catastrophic high school and collegiate sports-related injuries (18). Although a primary goal of this system is to understand the cause of these events, participation data can also be used as a denominator to arrive at rates for risk comparison across activities.

The decision to expand the research was based on the following factors:

1. Research based on reliable data is essential if progress is to be made in sports safety
2. The paucity of information on injuries in all sports
3. The rapid expansion and lack of injury information in women's sports

Definitions

The Center uses consistent, clear injury definitions to create a catastrophic injury database with significant application. Injury definitions include:

Catastrophic injury. Any severe injury incurred during participation in a school/college sponsored sport involving a fatality, permanent severe functional disability, or severe head or neck trauma.

Direct injury. Those injuries resulting directly from participation in the skills of the sport, such as paralysis resulting from a football tackle.

Indirect injury. Those injuries caused by systemic failure as a result of exertion while participating in a sport activity or by a complication that was secondary to a nonfatal injury. Catastrophic heat illness or cardiac problems would fit into this category.

Data Collection

As the absolute number of catastrophic injuries is small, the goal is to collect information on every event. Data are compiled with the assistance of coaches, athletic trainers, athletic directors, executive officers of state and national athletic organizations, a national newspaper clipping service, and professional associates of the researchers. On receiving information concerning a possible catastrophic sports injury, contact by telephone, personal letter, and questionnaire is made with the injured player's coach or athletic director. Data collected include background information on the athlete (age, height, weight, experience, previous injury, etc.), accident information, immediate and postaccident medical care, type of injury, and equipment involved. Autopsy reports are used when available.

Applications

Specific data may be obtained by accessing the Center's most recent annual report at www.unc.edu/depts/nccsi. It provides data on a variety of sports and is one of the few resources on catastrophic injuries in the activity of cheerleading. Examples of sport-specific applications of this data collection as noted in the annual report are presented later in this chapter.

The NCAA Injury Surveillance System

Established in 1982, the NCAA ISS (8) is the largest continuous collegiate injury surveillance system in North America and possibly the world. Its mission is to provide current and reliable data on injury trends in intercollegiate athletics in order to optimize student-athlete health and safety. From 1988 to 2003, injury data for 15 intercollegiate sports were collected annually from a representative sample of NCAA member institutions through the volunteer efforts of certified athletic trainers. Since 2003, the ISS has been updated from a paper-based to a web-based format that has the capability of collecting data on all NCAA championship sports as well as club sport activities. This web-based system allows the athletic trainer at an individual school to have a real-time electronic record of athletic training room activities while also contributing to an aggregate national database. The NCAA ISS includes many of the qualities noted previously by Meeuwisse and Love (5).

Sports monitored. All NCAA championship sports and a variety of club activities.

Seasons. The traditional sports seasons are used for data collection and are divided into the following three subcategories:

(a) Preseason—full team practices/competitions before first regular season contest.
(b) In-season—all practice and games from the first regular season contest through last regular season contest.
(c) Postseason—all practice and games following the last regular season contest through the last postseason contest.

Definitions

Injury. A reportable injury according to the NCAA ISS is defined as one that:

(a) Occurs as a result of participation in an organized intercollegiate practice or game
(b) Requires medical attention by a team athletic trainer or physician
(c) Results in any restriction of the student-athlete's participation or performance for one or more days beyond the day of injury

Exposures. An A-E, the unit of risk in the ISS, is defined as one athlete participating in one practice or game where he or she is exposed to the possibility of athletic injury.

Injury rate. An injury rate is a ratio of the number of injuries in a particular category to the number of A-Es in that category. In the ISS, this value is expressed as injuries per 1,000 A-Es. For example, six reportable injuries during 563 practice exposures result in an injury rate of $(6/563) \times 1{,}000$ or 10.7 injuries/1,000 A-Es. In this example, one would anticipate 10.7 injuries if one athlete participated in 1,000 practices, if 50 athletes participated in 20 practices, or if 100 athletes participated in 10 practices.

Sampling

Participation in the NCAA ISS is voluntary and limited to the 1,026 NCAA member institutions (as of September 2005). Before the web-based system was established in 2003, ISS participants were selected from the population of institutions sponsoring a given sport. A convenience sample of those schools indicating a willingness to participate was generated with a goal of establishing an appropriate weighted sample of each NCAA division (I, II, and III) and at least 10% of all schools sponsoring the particular sport. With the introduction of the web-based system, all schools have the ability to participate and contribute data to as many sports as they wish. Schools submitting an appropriate amount of exposure weeks and completed injury forms are included in the national sample with appropriate divisional weighting. It is important to emphasize that this system does not identify *every* injury that occurs at NCAA institutions in a particular sport. Rather, it collects a sampling that is representative of a national cross-section of NCAA institutions.

Data Reporting

Injury and exposure data are recorded in the web-based system on an ongoing basis by certified athletic trainers and student athletic trainers from participating institutions. Information is collected from the first official day of preseason practice to the final tournament contest.

Applications

One of the unique features of the ISS is the annual mechanism for data review and policy development that benefits not only collegiate athletics but also the general sports medicine community. The primary audience for this system was originally envisioned to be the NCAA Committee on Competitive Safeguards and Medical Aspects of Sports, and relevant NCAA sport rules committees, who used the information as a resource upon which to base recommendations, rules, and policies impacting student-athlete health and welfare. However, over the last decade the audiences interested in this information have expanded to include individual colleges and universities, sports medicine researchers, other administrative and sports medicine organizations, media, and the general public. The system's data have been applied to development or modification of sports rules, policies, and issues by organizations such as the American Medical Society for Sports Medicine (AMSSM), American College of Sports Medicine (ACSM), American Orthopaedic Society for Sports Medicine (AOSSM), CDC, and the National Athletic Trainers' Association (NATA). Such efforts have benefited not only collegiate athletics but also the entire sports medicine community. Some specific examples are noted later. Data collection through the ISS followed by annual review through the NCAA sport rules and sports medicine committee structure is a unique mechanism that has led to significant advances in health and safety policy within and beyond college athletics. Basic comparative injury information across sports and general information about the ISS is available on the NCAA Web site (www.ncaa.org/ISS).

Athletic Injury Monitoring System

The AIMS was established in 1986 as a national sports injury data collection system capable of doing injury surveillance on a variety of sports. The structure and methodology of AIMS is very similar to the NCAA ISS. It was designed to complement the NCAA ISS in that it would cover noncollegiate sports as well as collegiate sports, and cover other levels of competition, from youth and high school to elite and older recreational athletes. AIMS meets the major criteria for reliable studies of sports injury rates outlined in 1987 by the AOSSM (19). Data collected by AIMS has been used for published reports on a number of issues in sports medicine, including general injury rates (9,20–25), concussion rates (26–30), prophylactic knee braces (31–33), and football helmets (34,35).

National Athletic Injury/Illness Reporting System

A predecessor to both ISS and AIMS was the National Athletic Injury/Illness Reporting System (NAIRS), developed by Kenneth S. Clarke at Pennsylvania State University in the mid-1970s. This first major attempt at a national sports injury data collection system incorporated many important new design features such as longitudinal data collection from a much larger sample than previously had been attempted, standardized definitions and procedures, and the use of case rates per 1,000 A-Es. However, there were concerns about the number and complexity of the data collection forms and the lack of a truly representative national sample. NAIRS stopped collecting high school and college data in 1983, but it produced by far the best and most comprehensive sports injury data available up to that time. As NAIRS was completing its data collection efforts, the NCAA instituted its own ISS. The NCAA ISS was designed and implemented in 1982 by Eric D. Zemper, as a member of the NCAA staff. Since 1985, ISS has been under the direction of Randall W. Dick. ISS essentially is a direct descendent of NAIRS, being similar in many ways to NAIRS, but utilizing two simplified basic data collection forms, and using a representative national sample of NCAA member schools (8–36). The AIMS was also designed and implemented by Zemper, while at the University of Oregon. AIMS was developed in 1986, utilizing the same basic format as NAIRS and ISS, with the intent of covering a wider variety of sports at all levels of participation (20–28,28–35,37,39).

SUMMARY OF DATA FROM NATIONAL DATA COLLECTION SYSTEMS

As NAIRS, ISS, and AIMS are basically similar in format and use the same definition of a reportable injury (one occurring in a practice or contest that prevents an athlete from participating for 1 day or more), with data provided by on-site athletic trainers, and injury rates reported as cases per 1,000 A-Es, it is possible to summarize and compare data from these three collection systems. The one sport for which data is available from all three systems is college football. Table 2.1 summarizes the overall (practice and games combined) football injury rates over a total of 30 seasons. The cumulative injury rates for ISS and AIMS are quite similar, whereas the earlier NAIRS rate is higher. There are several possible explanations for this difference. As noted earlier, the NAIRS sample was not as representative as the ISS and AIMS samples. It also appears that there has been a general downward trend in college football injury rates over the years (40), although the most recent ISS data for the 2005 season shows a reversal of that trend. This long-term downward trend may be due to the major rule changes in the mid- to late 1970s that were aimed at reducing the risk of major head and neck injuries (a direct result of data from the ongoing annual football fatality studies that showed an increase in major injuries during the 1960s). Along with the rule changes came shifts in coaching philosophy and technique, which have had a positive impact on injury risk, as have continuing improvements in protective equipment. Any or all of these factors may have contributed to this difference between the NAIRS data from the 1970s and the ISS/AIMS data from more recent years.

TABLE 2.1
INJURY RATES IN COLLEGE FOOTBALL FROM THREE NATIONAL DATA COLLECTION SYSTEMS

System	Injury Rate/1,000 Athlete-Exposures	Seasons
NAIRS	10.1	1977–1981
ISS	6.6	1982–1989
	6.6	2001
	8.7	2005
AIMS	6.6	1986–1989
	5.9	1997–1998

NAIRS = National Athletic Injury/Illness Reporting System; ISS = Injury Surveillance System; AIMS = Athletic Injury Monitoring System.
Source: Buckley (41); NCAA (8); Zemper (9,23,27); Zemper (unpublished data).

On the basis of these data showing 6.6 injuries/1,000 A-Es for college football, the average college team of 100 players can expect approximately two time-loss injuries every three times they take to the field for a practice or game. (As we will show later, there can be major differences in injury rates between practices and games, particularly for football.) As would be expected, the body parts injured most often in college football are the knees, ankles, and shoulder, in that order. The most common types of injuries are ligament sprains, muscle strains, and contusions.

NAIRS and ISS have data from other college sports, and AIMS has data from other levels of participation in addition to college. Table 2.2 summarizes the male and female injury

TABLE 2.2
INJURY RATES FOR VARIOUS SPORTS FROM THREE NATIONAL DATA COLLECTION SYSTEMS

	Injury Rate/1,000 Athlete-Exposures				
Sport	NAIRS (1976–1982)	ISS (1985–1989)	ISS (2001–2002)	ISS (2005–2006)	AIMS
College					
Baseball—Men's	1.9	3.3	3.0	3.8	—
Basketball—Men's	7.0	5.1	4.9	6.6	—
Basketball—Women's	7.3	5.0	4.7	6.3	—
Cross-country—Men's	1.6	—	—	4.9	—
Cross-country—Women's	6.7	—	—	5.0	—
Field hockey—Women's	5.4	4.9	4.0	6.7	—
Football—Men's	10.1	6.6	6.6	8.7	6.6 (1986—1990) 5.9 (1997—1998)
Gymnastics—Men's	4.3	5.1	2.1	—	—
Gymnastics—Women's	7.0	8.0	6.9	8.5	—
Ice hockey—Men's	9.1	5.7	6.2	5.6	—
Ice hockey—Women's	—	—	7.6	4.5	—
Lacrosse—Men's	5.7	6.2	4.4	5.8	—
Lacrosse—Women's	4.2	4.1	4.4	4.1	—
Soccer—Men's	9.8	7.7	7.3	10.2	—
Soccer—Women's		8.0	7.5	8.9	—
Softball—Women's	1.7	4.0	2.7	4.6	—
Swimming—Diving—Men's	0.9	—	—	—	—
Swimming—Diving—Women's	0.6	—	—	—	—
Tennis—Men's	1.3	—	—	3.3	—
Tennis—Women's	3.3	—	—	3.7	—
Outdoor track and field—Men's	3.4	—	—	6.3	—
Outdoor track and field—Women's	4.1	—	—	4.6	—
Ultimate frisbee—Men's	—	—	—	—	5.0
Ultimate frisbee—Women's	—	—	—	—	3.7
Volleyball—Men's	2.4	—	—	—	—
Volleyball—Women's	4.8	—	3.6	5.1	—
Wrestling—Men's	7.7	9.6	7.8	9.3	—
Elite					
Gymnastics—Women's	—	—	—	—	3.7
Taekwondo—Men's (competition only)	—	—	—	—	27.2
Taekwondo—Women's (competition only)	—	—	—	—	22.2
Youth (6–17 years old)					
Football—High school	—	—	—	—	4.9
Soccer—Boy's	—	—	—	—	2.7
Soccer—Girl's	—	—	—	—	2.1
Taekwondo—Boy's (competition only)	—	—	—	—	25.5
Taekwondo—Girl's (competition only)	—	—	—	—	28.6
Recreational (45–70 years old)					
Running—Men's	—	—	—	—	11.1
Running—Women's	—	—	—	—	12.3
Walking—Men's	—	—	—	—	12.7
Weightlifting—Men's	—	—	—	—	7.0

Buckley (67); Caine et al. (20); NAIRS (unpublished data); NCAA (8);Watkins (68); Zemper (24,27); Zemper (unpublished data).

rates for sports covered by these systems. The data in this table cover from 1 to 15 seasons, at least 2 or 3 seasons in most cases. As these are reported in the common metric of rate per 1,000 A-Es, direct comparisons are possible between sports, males and females, and different levels of a sport, as well as the different periods represented in the table. The exceptions in this table are injury rates for taekwondo (a Korean full-contact martial art form), which are competition data only, unlike the other sports that show injury rates for practice and competition combined.

From Table 2.2, we can see that participants in men's wrestling, soccer, and football, and women's soccer and gymnastics currently have the highest overall injury rates. The injury rates for corresponding men's and women's sports are generally similar, the exception being the higher rate in gymnastics for women. Younger women gymnasts in a full-time elite training program are less likely to be injured than older collegiate gymnasts. The injury rates for youth soccer players were considerably lower than those at the collegiate level. Injury rates for middle-aged and older recreational athletes were noticeably higher, although the older recreational athlete presumably does not have as much pressure to participate, and therefore may be more willing to take a few days off when injured at a level of severity that a high school or collegiate athlete would tend to ignore.

Comparing the rates reported by the NCAA ISS for the late 1980s and for the more recent 2005 to 2006 academic year indicates that injury rates for most sports have remained relatively stable, although a few appear to have increased (e.g., men's and women's basketball, football, and men's soccer). The large drop in the men's gymnastics rate seen in 2001 to 2002 may be more the result of only three teams reporting to the NCAA during 2001. When looking at these data, one should keep in mind that the data from the 1980s covers 4 years, and is probably relatively more stable than the data from the single years represented by the 2000 to 2001 and 2005 to 2006 columns. Data for the noncollegiate levels must be considered preliminary because these databases are relatively small in comparison with the amount of collegiate data available, but they do indicate the possibility of some interesting trends.

Data across all the sports show that the most frequently injured body part is the ankle, followed by the knee and then the shoulder (17). All are major joints that undergo considerable stress in most sports. Sprains, strains, and contusions are the most frequent types of injuries. Overall, ankle sprains are the most frequently occurring injuries in most sports.

An interesting point that can be highlighted when data are reported in rates per 1,000 A-Es, which is not evident when rates are reported per 100 participants, is the difference in injury risk between practices and competitions. Table 2.3 breaks down the injury rates for 17 collegiate sports into practice and competition rates, along with their relative rankings within each column. The competition injury rate for senior (18–30 years old) taekwondo athletes is included for comparison. Also included in the right-most column of the table is an indication of the relative risk of injury in practice and in competition; in each case injury risk is higher in competition.

It is often reported that most injuries occur in practices, giving the impression that practices are at least as risky as competitions. Most injuries in a given sport usually do occur during practices, but the actual risk of an individual athlete being injured is much higher in competition. As an example, in college football approximately 60% of the recorded injuries occur in practice (8,9). However, although the total *number* of injuries in college football over a season may be higher in practices, the *rate* of injuries is considerably higher in games, in this case 8.8 times higher (see Table 2.3). In other words, a college football player is approximately nine times as likely to be injured in a game as he is in a practice session. Bear in mind that there are at least five to six times as many practices as games in a football season, and there are usually more players participating in practices than play in games, which accounts for the fact that the raw numbers of injuries may be higher in practices. The most obvious explanation for the difference in risk between practices and games is the continuously higher intensity of play during games.

Football represents the upper extreme in the difference between practice and competition injury rates. At the other end of the spectrum is women's volleyball, where the risk of injury in games is only slightly higher than in practices (see Table 2.3). This seems reasonable considering that, at the collegiate level, volleyball practices are often as intense as the games. The data presented in Table 2.3 show that most sports at the collegiate level have a competition injury rate approximately two to four times higher than for practice.

USES OF SPORTS INJURY RATE DATA

Sports injury databases are important information resources that can be applied to the development of sport rules and sport safety equipment, and to sports medicine administration and policy. The major uses of epidemiological data listed at the beginning of this chapter can be adapted for our purposes in athletic medicine. Specifically, sports injury epidemiological data can be used to:

- Identify causes of injuries.
- Provide a more accurate picture of clinical reality. Clusters of injuries (and the resulting media attention they often generate) give a distorted view of reality; on the other hand, data may reveal a previously unsuspected injury problem.
- Determine the effectiveness of preventive measures (on a local or national scale), whether they are rule changes, new or modified equipment, or modifications of training techniques.

TABLE 2.3
INJURY RATES IN PRACTICES VERSUS COMPETITION IN 17 COLLEGE SPORTS

Sport	Injury Rate/1,000 Athlete-Exposures (Column Rank)		
	Practice	Competition	Relative Risk[a]
Baseball (M)	2.1 (16)	6.1 (14)	2.9
Basketball (M)	4.4 (7)	10.0 (9)	2.3
Basketball (W)	4.6 (5)	9.2 (10)	2.0
Field Hockey	4.1 (9)	8.5 (11)	2.1
Football (M)	4.1 (9)	36.0 (1)	8.8
Gymnastics (M)	4.4 (7)	16.5 (7)	3.8
Gymnastics (W)	7.5 (1)	18.5 (4)	2.5
Ice Hockey (M)	2.2 (15)	17.6 (5)	8.0
Lacrosse (M)	3.6 (11)	14.6 (8)	4.1
Lacrosse (W)	3.6 (11)	7.5 (12)	2.1
Soccer (M)	4.7 (4)	20.2 (3)	4.3
Soccer (W)	5.7 (3)	17.6 (5)	3.1
Softball (W)	3.1 (14)	4.9 (16)	1.5
Ultimate Frisbee (M)	3.5 (13)	7.0 (13)	2.0
Ultimate Frisbee (W)	2.0 (17)	5.6 (15)	2.8
Volleyball (W)	4.5 (6)	4.8 (17)	1.1
Wrestling (M)	6.9 (2)	29.7 (2)	4.3
Taekwondo (M)	—	27.2	—
Taekwondo (W)	—	22.2	—

[a]Relative risk = higher rate divided by lower rate.

Example: Men's lacrosse—14.6 injuries/1,000 athlete-exposures in games divided by 3.6 injuries/1,000 athlete-exposures in practices equals a relative risk of 4.1; that is, a men's lacrosse player participating in a game is 4.1 times as likely to be injured as he would be if he were participating in a practice session.

Sources: NCAA (8); NCAA (unpublished data); Watkins (42); Zemper (unpublished data).

- Monitor the health of athletes, which will assist in rational medical planning.
- Quantify the risks of various types, frequencies, and intensities of exercise activities.
- Provide an overview of long-term injury trends in specific sports.

Examples of each of these applications are discussed in the following sections, primarily referencing the model databases noted earlier.

Identify Causes of Injuries

Pole vaulting—NCCSIR. The pole vault was associated with most fatal track and field injuries, and on an injury rate basis it is the most dangerous activity monitored by the NCCSIR. There have been 18 high school pole vaulting fatalities from 1983 to 2004 (18,43). This does not include the coach who while demonstrating (in 1998) bounced out of the pit, struck his head on concrete, and died. In addition to the fatalities there were also seven permanent disability injuries and six serious injuries. All 31 of these accidents involved the vaulter bouncing out of or landing out of the pit area. Requiring a common cover or pad to extend over all sections of the pit and expanding the size of the pit have been policy modifications resulting from this data collection.

Swimming pool starts—NCCSIR. Catastrophic injuries in swimming were all directly related to the racing dive in the shallow end of pools (18). There has been a major effort by both schools and colleges to make the racing dive safer and the catastrophic injury data support that effort. These efforts have involved increasing the minimum depth of water in the starting end and reducing the height of the starting blocks.

Men's basketball—ISS. At an August 2002 sports medicine conference held in conjunction with the Men's World Basketball Championships, NCAA ISS data on the epidemiology of collegiate basketball injuries were presented (44). Five-year within-sport analysis revealed that most of the men's collegiate basketball game injuries occurred from player contact when within the lane. Ankles (29%) and knees (11%) were also reported to be the two most frequently injured body parts in games. However, more detailed analysis revealed that most ankle injuries resulted from rebounding and player contact, and most knee injuries occurred from rebounding and noncontact defending. With the additional specific causes of injury information, preventive measures ranging from rule modifications (possible wider lanes) and officials' points of emphasis (enforcing player contact) to shoe design (addressing noncontact issues) and focused practice techniques are possible.

Field hockey injuries—ISS. The sport of women's field hockey is played with a hard ball that can travel up to 40 mph propelled by a hard stick. Field players wear minimal protective equipment (shin guards, mouth guards) and the sport has a moderate injury rate compared to other collegiate activities (see Table 2.2). However, ISS data show that when injuries do occur, impact from a ball (mostly elevated) accounts for 25% of all reported game injuries and contact with the stick accounts for another 18%. This information can be evaluated by sport rules committees when considering possible rule modifications or protective equipment in the sport.

Provide A More Accurate Picture of Clinical Reality

Human immunodeficiency virus (HIV), bleeding, and sports (ISS). As concern about HIV in intercollegiate and professional athletics grew in the early 1990s following the revelations of Magic Johnson, athletic organization responses ranged from indifference to overreaction. Science scrambled to provide a fact-based recommendation in response to the range of reactionary proposals. Using data from a modified ISS form (frequency of bleeding injuries) and information from the CDC (risk of HIV transmission in a hospital setting) a study was performed to determine the risk of HIV transmission in college athletics (45). Results indicated that the risk of HIV transmission during participation in NCAA sport was less than one chance in 1 million exposures. Similar results were found in an analysis of professional football players (46). Subsequently, policies were developed for all NCAA and other sports organization activities to address bleeding on the field of play in a reasonable and medically sound manner.

Anterior cruciate ligament (ACL) injuries (ISS). ACL injuries pose a significant threat to a student-athlete, not only in the time away from the sport but also in the economic cost to repair and rehabilitate the injury. Early studies had suggested that the risk of such an injury in females might be greater than their male counterparts. In 1995, Sports Illustrated (47) noted that "Knee injuries of the most serious kind—tears of the anterior cruciate ligament, one of the two central ligaments that support the knee—are virtually epidemic in women's college basketball." Such statements led some to question whether participation in sports was worth the risk, especially for female athletes. Yet most medical research has focused on the repair of this injury rather than preventive efforts.

A 5-year study of NCAA ISS data (48) showed a two- to threefold increased risk of ACL injury to female collegiate soccer and basketball student-athletes relative to their male counterparts. With its large national sample over a 5-year period, this study validated the anecdotal evidence that women were at higher risk of such an injury, at least in certain sports. However, by quantifying the risk, the authors were also able to show that although the risk was higher in females, it was still relatively infrequent (estimated one ACL injury for every 247 female basketball practices or games with 15 participants/event). Subsequent studies (49,50) reported similar results. Further presentation and discussion of these findings noted the many benefits of participating in physical activities (51) that far outweighed the risk of ACL injury portrayed in the media. Once the increased risk was identified, researchers began discussion of identifying the causative factors involved in ACL injuries (52).

Head injuries in taekwondo—AIMS. The previous example illustrated a case where data showed how a perceived problem was not as severe as thought. In the case of head injuries in the sport of taekwondo, there was a belief that the sport had no injury problems, until there was an effort to collect injury data. AIMS collected injury data at national taekwondo competitions for the U.S. Olympic Committee and the U.S. Taekwondo Union, the national governing body for this sport (21,22,25,26,28,29,37,39). The major result was to draw immediate attention and concern to the high rate of cerebral concussions recorded during taekwondo competitions (26,28,29,37). The cerebral concussion rate over a 2-year period for taekwondo compared with AIMS data for college football showed that the rate for taekwondo competition (5.45 cerebral concussions/1,000 A-Es) is 3.2 times as high as the rate seen in college football games (1.69 cerebral concussions/1,000 A-Es). On the basis of time of exposure, taekwondo (1.2/1,000 minutes of exposure) has a cerebral concussion rate 9.2 times that of college football games (0.13/1,000 minutes of exposure). These rates are essentially the same for Junior (6–17 years old) and Senior (18 years and older) taekwondo competitors. The data uncovered a previously unsuspected problem with head injuries in this sport. The primary suggestions for addressing the problem include working with the manufacturers of the helmet used in taekwondo to develop a more protective product; changing the rules to require mouthguards, rather than just recommending their use; establishing and enforcing standards for competition mats; and adopting rules similar to those of amateur boxing, which require a minimum period before an athlete is allowed to return to participation after a loss of consciousness from a blow during a bout.

Determine the Effectiveness of Preventive Measures

Adding protective equipment. Epidemiological studies can be used to evaluate the effectiveness of a rule or equipment change. Having baseline data before a change allows for the possibility of evaluating the impact of the intervention, if other possible confounding variables can be controlled. Specific applications of this analysis could assist in the evaluation of protective equipment effectiveness on the nature of competition in sport. A model example of such a study was the work by Benson et al., in evaluating head and neck injuries among ice hockey players wearing full and half shields (53). This prospective cohort study evaluated injuries among college hockey players playing in the same hockey league over one season. Eleven teams wore full face shields while another 11 wore half shields. Results showed that the use of full face shields was associated with a significantly reduced risk of sustaining facial and dental injuries without an increase in the risk of neck injuries, concussions, or other injuries. This study should be considered a template to follow when evaluating the possible effect of protective equipment on injuries. Laprade et al. recorded similar findings in an ice hockey face mask evaluation (54), whereas Marshall et al. (55) studied protective equipment and injury in North American college football and club level New Zealand Rugby Union.

Protective eyewear, women's lacrosse—ISS. The sport of women's lacrosse has a relatively low overall game injury rate compared with other sports monitored by the NCAA ISS (see Table 2.3). Until the 2003–2004 academic year, minimal protective equipment (a mouthguard) was mandated, as the playing rules prohibit intentional contact with another player. However, the sport is played with a small, hard ball that can travel up to 60 mph, often at head level, which has the potential to cause a significant injury to the face, particularly the eye. Hard sticks are also used that sometimes inadvertently make contact with the head as defenders confront a dodging attacker or opponents battle for a loose ball. ISS data indicated that almost 25% of all game injuries occurred above the neck and there was a small but definable risk of eye injury that had the potential to be severe under the right circumstances. In 2003–2004, the NCAA mandated that protective eyewear be worn by all collegiate players. The national governing body for the sport adopted the rule for most levels the following year. Table 2.4 shows the frequency and rate of eye injuries and all above-the-neck injuries for the 3 years before the addition of protective eyewear and for the first year following implementation. No eye injuries were reported in the sample following the mandate and the rate of all above-the-neck injuries were reduced by more than half. The concern that players might become more aggressive, based on the addition of the eye protection, also appeared unfounded. The overall game injury rate

TABLE 2.4

HEAD INJURIES IN WOMEN'S LACROSSE BEFORE (2001–2003) AND AFTER (2004) MANDATORY EYE PROTECTION

	Games Injuries/1,000 Athlete-Exposures				
		2001–2003			2004
Average Number of Schools/Year		73			67
	Total No. of Injuries—3 Years	**Average Injuries/Year**	**Rate over 3 Years**	**No. of Injuries**	**Rate**
Eye(s)	12	4	0.23	0	0.00
Ear(s)	2	1	0.04	0	0.00
Nose	26	9	0.50	1	0.06
Mouth, teeth, tongue	5	2	0.95	1	0.06
Face, chin, jaw	10	3	0.09	4	0.24
Head	54	18	1.03	13	0.78
Total Above Neck	109	36	2.84	19	1.14
Overall injury rate			**8.40**		**6.10**

NCAA ISS.

did not increase with the addition of the protective equipment. In summary, ISS data validated that the addition of protective eyewear achieved its primary goal of reducing the risk of eye injuries. In addition, a possible unforeseen consequence of more aggressive play was not borne out after the first year, at least based on above-the-neck or overall game injury rates.

Spring football—ISS. In 1997, spring football practice injuries at NCAA Division I and II football programs were more than double the regular season practice rates (8,56). The football and sports medicine communities collaborated to develop a policy that would allow coaches to teach the skills of the game while reducing the threat of serious injury. This policy included allowing for initial acclimatization and providing opportunities for contact practice while reducing full tackle activities. Since the resulting NCAA legislation was enacted in 1998, the injury rate in Division I spring football has decreased by 27%, from 11.2 to 8.1 injuries/1,000 A-Es (see Figure 2.1).

ACL injuries (ISS). The 1999 Hunt Valley Consensus Conference on Prevention of Noncontact ACL Injuries, funded by the Orthopedic Research and Education Foundation, AOSSM, National Athletic Trainers' Association Research and Education Foundation, and the NCAA, was a landmark meeting that began the integration of ACL incidence and causative information into prevention efforts. Before that time, Garrick and Requa (57) noted that only 133 of 3,572 MedLine citations under the ACL topic heading were placed under subheading "prevention" and less than 10 of the citations actually dealt with injury prevention rather than prevention of some surgical complication. The meeting resulted in a consensus publication that identified risk factors and offered prevention strategies (52). A special issue of the *Journal of Athletic Training* devoted to ACL injury in the female athlete provides further epidemiology and causative research on this subject (58). Current ongoing prevention studies will use several

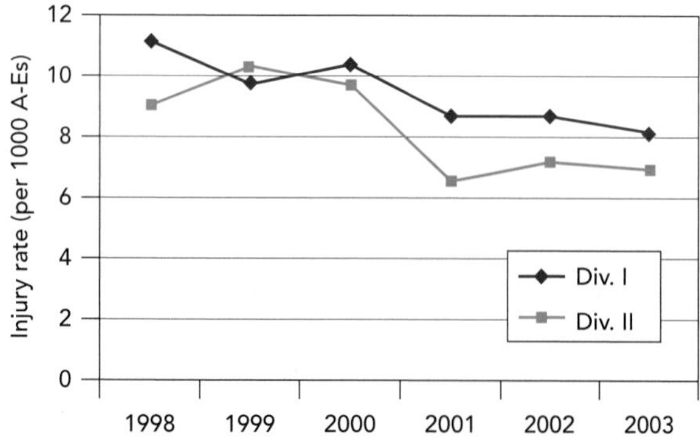

Figure 2.1 Football spring practice injury rates by division—1998 to 2003. (Source: National Collegiate Athletic Association. NCAA injury surveillance system reports. Indianapolis: NCAA, (www.ncaa.org/iss.html), 2002.)

epidemiology and surveillance techniques to assess the effectiveness of these programs.

Assessing protective equipment—football helmets—AIMS. Epidemiological studies of sports injuries may be used to evaluate new protective equipment or monitor the performance of existing equipment, if the study is properly designed to collect the necessary data. An example of this use for existing equipment is the AIMS monitoring of concussion rates in users of various brands and models of football helmets (34,35). By collecting enough detail about helmets in use and concussions during general data collection on football injuries, AIMS is able to assess whether specific brands and models of football helmets are performing within expectations with regard to the occurrence of concussions. When this data was first analyzed, there was one older model of helmet that had a higher than expected rate of concussions, but it was no longer manufactured by the time the report was released. Since then, all helmet models have been performing within expectations, through the 1998 season (Zemper, unpublished data).

Assessing protective equipment—preventive knee braces—AIMS. Another example, evaluating new protective equipment, is a study of preventive knee braces in college football conducted by AIMS (31–33) as a part of general data collection on football injuries. Braces designed to prevent medial collateral ligament (MCL) injuries from lateral blows to the knee came into widespread use in the 1980s, before any studies were performed to see if they actually worked. The only "data" available were a lot of anecdotes and a few one- or two-season, one-team studies. There are many variables that could have an impact on the results of any study like this, such as brand or type of brace, position played, proper placement of brace, whether it was actually worn at the time of injury, previous history of knee injury, intensity of practices, condition of playing surface, or weather, to name a few.

From an epidemiological perspective, the only way to "control" these numerous variables is to do a large-scale, long-term study with as many teams as possible so that the impact of the uncontrollable and essentially unrecordable variables (proper brace placement, practice intensity, condition of playing surface, weather) will "wash out" in the data collection process. At the same time, the more easily recordable variables (position played, whether the brace was worn at the time of injury, brand or type of brace, previous history) will be recorded in sufficient numbers to provide more reliable results than could ever be possible with a study of a single team or a small number of teams. The results of earlier, small-scale studies were mixed, with some showing that braces reduced the number of MCL injuries and others showing they did not. However, the later large-scale studies, such as those of Teitz (59) and the AIMS study (31–33), show that wearing preventive knee braces appears to have no effect on reducing the number or severity of MCL injuries, or on the time lost due to injury.

A well-controlled smaller-scale study done at the U.S. Military Academy (60) does show some positive effect in reducing MCL injuries by wearing preventive knee braces, but only with defensive players. This indicates that position played may be an important factor. There was no effect on the severity of knee injuries. However, the subjects were cadets playing intramural football rather than larger and heavier intercollegiate players, so the study may indicate a possible size/weight and, therefore, a force threshold involvement. Obviously, much more data must be collected from large-scale epidemiological studies, as well as biomechanical studies, before complex issues such as this can be resolved.

Catastrophic football injuries—NCCSIR. Football is associated with the greatest number of catastrophic injuries of all sports, but the total incidence of injury per 100,000 participants is higher in both gymnastics and ice hockey. In 1968 there were 36 fatalities associated with football. There have been dramatic reductions in the number of football fatalities and nonfatal catastrophic injuries since 1976 and the 1990 data illustrated a historical decrease in football fatalities to zero (18). This dramatic reduction, particularly in head and neck neurological problems, can be directly related to data collection and subsequent recommendations based on that data, including the 1976 rule changes that prohibited initial contact with the head and face when blocking and tackling, the National Operating Committee on Standards in Athletic Equipment (NOCSAE) helmet standard that went into effect in colleges in 1978 and high schools in 1980, better coaching in the techniques of blocking and tackling, and improved medical care.

Monitor the Health of Athletes, Which Will Assist In Rational Medical Planning

Nontraumatic cardiac deaths—NCCSIR. Data from the NCCSIR report have been further analyzed to assist the sports medicine community in addressing preventive issues more effectively. An example of this is the 1995 work by Van Camp et al. (61) on nontraumatic deaths in high school and college athletes. The authors noted that the study provides information that may assist in three important sports medicine issues: (a) appropriate athletic preparticipation examinations, (b) eligibility recommendations for athletic participation, and (c) evaluation and medical treatment of athletes. Maron et al. (62) also have published on this subject, with the principal cause of sudden death in young competitive athletes being cardiovascular disease, most commonly hypertrophic cardiomyopathy.

Marathon running. A 12-year profile of medical injury and illness for the Twin Cities Marathon was conducted, with the objective to summarize the medical encounters (injury/illness) for runners and monitor weather conditions (63). Finish line medical encounter rates were 18.3/1,000 entrants and 25.3/1,000 finishers. The study concluded that marathon racing in cool conditions is a safe activity and most medical encounters are of minor severity. More than 99.9% of runners who finish the race leave the finish area without hospital or emergency room care. The injury/illness profile can be used to tailor appropriate medical care at the finish area of a marathon.

Special populations—ISS. Since the incorporation of women's athletics into the NCAA in 1982, participation has increased from approximately 80,000 to more than 165,000 in 2004, a 106% increase (64). Women's soccer participation alone has increased from less than 2,000 to more than 21,000 in this time frame, with softball, volleyball, lacrosse and basketball also showing large gains. Although these participants should reap health benefits that extend beyond collegiate athletics, increased participation brings with it issues such as sports injuries, which have not been well documented. As part of the 1999 Women's Health in Sport and Exercise Workshop, cosponsored by the American Academy of Orthopaedic Surgeons and the National Institutes of Health, 10 years of ISS data were analyzed to assess injury risks and issues of women participating in college athletics. The subsequent publication (65), which was part of a thorough review of women's health issues in sports and exercise, included the following recommendations:

- Medical issues unique to women will continue to develop with increased participation. Research efforts that are able to identify, isolate, and affect such issues are needed now and in the future.
- Expand injury surveillance to more sports, develop acute and overuse collection instruments where applicable, and create a system for review and application of findings for the benefit of participants in these activities.
- Develop and apply injury surveillance to individual and individual/team sports, such as swimming, cross-country, and track and field, with a particular emphasis on overuse issues. Develop strategies to affect change through educational efforts rather than rule changes or equipment modification.
- Include women in the current and future research associated with head trauma in sport. Consider mechanisms to address player contact issues if they become a concern. Consider the potential costs and benefits of protective head equipment for selected activities that currently do not use such equipment.

- Identify causative factors for injuries that may have gender as a risk variable. Develop controlled studies to verify the effect of any proposed modifications. Reflect the significant benefits of athletic participation in any reports or educational efforts associated with specific injury issues.

Quantify the Risks of Various Types, Frequencies, and Intensities of Exercise Activities

Sports sponsorship/athletics health care and coverage—ISS. Because the ISS uses identical exposure and injury definitions for each sport, it is easy to compare injury rates across different activities (8). Such information can be applied by administrators in the following:

- Evaluating the potential comparative medical costs associated with adding new sports or athletics-related activities
- Considering delegation of athletics' health care and coverage resources. Medical or athletic administrators can use injury rates to make an information-based decision on where to assign limited resources when numerous simultaneous athletic activities are occurring. The National Athletic Trainers' Association has used ISS data to develop guidelines for appropriate medical coverage for intercollegiate athletics (55).

Specific injury risk and return to play—ISS. Evaluation and return to play decision sometimes involve a medical risk assessment of repeat or further damage to a particular area. In situations where the absence or nonfunction of a set of paired organs is a concern, the probability of injury to the remaining organ should be considered. The ISS can provide definitive injury risk data on organs such as eyes and kidneys to assist the student-athlete and the team physician in assessing the overall risks and benefits of athletic participation.

Relative risk of a second concussion—AIMS. Return to play decisions following a concussion are another area where protocols are still evolving. One element in formulating these recommendations is information about the risk of a second concussion following an initial concussion. For many years it was believed that there is an increased risk following an initial injury, but solid evidence for this increased risk and its magnitude was not available. As part of its process of monitoring the effectiveness of football helmets, AIMS has been able to provide data demonstrating that there indeed is an increased risk of a second concussion following an initial one, and the increased risk is approximately six times greater. Factors not related to previous history of concussion, such as player position, do not appear to impact this added risk. This level of increased risk was first noted in an AIMS published report on college injury data from the 1988 to 1990 seasons (35), and recently was replicated with high school and college football injury data from the 1997 to 1998 seasons (27).

Heat illness and injury in preseason football practice—ISS. In 2001, the NCAA began developing a preseason practice model for college football that had several health and safety components. The model, which was implemented at the start of the 2003 football season, included a 5-day single-practice acclimatization period at the start of fall practice. This time-period would focus on acclimating the student-athletes to environmental conditions, exercise intensity, and equipment. During the first 2 days, helmets would be the only allowable piece of protective equipment. The second 2 days would allow helmets and shoulder pads, whereas the fifth day would be a single practice in full equipment. Subsequent practices could have multiple practices on 1 day, but these "double sessions" could not occur on consecutive days. ISS data (see Table 2.5) was used to justify this model (8).

TABLE 2.5
NATIONAL COLLEGIATE ATHLETIC ASSOCIATION (NCAA) FOOTBALL—HEAT ILLNESS DURING EARLY FALL PRACTICE (2001)

Division	Number of Schools	Number of Heat Illnesses	Rate/1,000 A-Es	First 3 Days
I	53	88	0.22	Helmets, shoulder pads
II	29	58	0.33	Helmets, shoulder pads
III	46	19	0.08	Helmets only

A-Es = athlete-exposures.
Sources: National Collegiate Athletic Association. NCAA injury surveillance system reports. *Indianapolis: NCAA, (www.ncaa.org/iss.html), 2002.*

As Table 2.5 indicates, ISS data showed that Division I and II institutions averaged 1.5 to 2 heat illnesses/school. These events restricted participation for at least 1 day. By legislation, these institutions were allowed to initiate their fall preseason practice in helmets and shoulder pads. Division III institutions reported time-loss heat illnesses at a rate one third to one fourth that of Division I and II schools. By legislation, the Division III schools were required to practice with helmets as the only piece of protective equipment for the first 3 days. These data, as well as the findings of Kulka and Kenney (66), show the importance of acclimating to protective equipment as well as the environment.

In addition, ISS data showed that in 2002, a student-athlete was almost four times as likely to receive a time-loss injury in preseason as opposed to the regular season. Eighty-seven percent of all reported time-loss heat illnesses and 49% of ANY time-loss practice injury for the entire season occurred on the 10 to 12 preseason days in which a school conducted a multiple session practice. These findings provided the rationale for alternating double- and single-practice days after the 5-day acclimatization period to emphasize recovery and rehydration.

Provide an Overview of Long-Term Injury Trends

Trend analysis for administrative decisions—ISS. Historically, the role of the physician has been to address an injury after it occurs. The ISS data allows the entire medical community to critically evaluate the injury trends in college athletics and to respond proactively. ISS final reports allow physicians and athletic trainers at participating schools to annually evaluate individual school injury patterns and discuss results with the coaching staff. The ability to compare an individual school injury rate to conference, division, or national values can be a convincing tool in modifying practice techniques.

Concussions in men's collegiate ice hockey—ISS. The game concussion injury rate in men's collegiate ice hockey has doubled since 1990 (see Figure 2.2). On the basis of these data, the NCAA Ice Hockey Rules Committee has created stricter penalties associated with noncompliance with the mouthpiece rule, hitting from behind, and checking into the boards. In addition, a mechanism for recertification of the hockey helmet and the addition of a four-point chinstrap were considered. Officials were educated that the helmet is not designed to prevent concussion and that any contact to the head should be penalized. The ISS will be used as an evaluation tool to assess the effectiveness of these rules and equipment modifications on injury rates. Concussions in many sports have become a research focus in sports medicine. The July–September

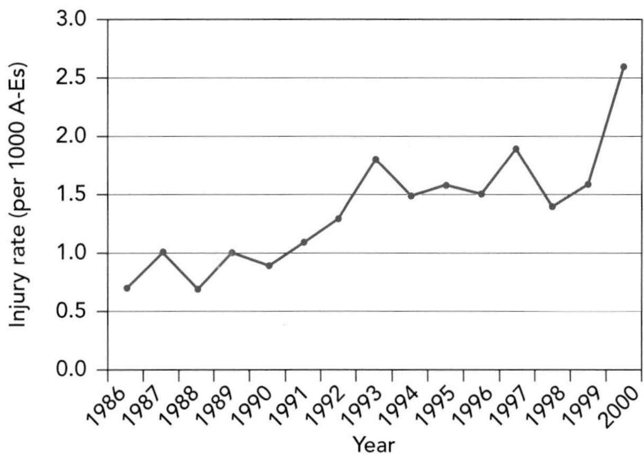

Figure 2.2 Ice hockey game concussion injury rates—1986 to 99. (Source: National Collegiate Athletic Association. NCAA injury surveillance system reports. Indianapolis: NCAA, (www.ncaa.org/iss.html), 2002.)

2001 issue of the *Journal of Athletic Training* (67) is devoted to concussions in athletes, and includes concussion injury trends in several other athletic activities.

LOCAL SPORTS INJURY DATA COLLECTION

Although the importance of longitudinal, national-scale epidemiological data collection to adequately address major sports injury issues has been emphasized here, the small-scale local data collection effort also has an important place in sports medicine. A primary care physician who is responsible for the medical care of a high school or other local sports program, or who is part of a local sports medicine network (see Chapter 38), is in a good position to track local injury patterns, across sport seasons as well as at mass participation episodic events (e.g., marathons and other road races). At a minimum, this will require some form of centralized records of all sports injuries treated. Forms such as those suggested in Chapter 38 for the records of a local sports medicine network would serve this purpose very well.

An alternative to normal patient files, which would make data compilation much easier, is a brief check-off form describing the athlete, injury, and circumstances. This would be similar to those used by larger data collection systems. These forms could be filled out by the physician, nurse, or athletic trainer at the high school for every sports injury treated, and kept in a single file. As mentioned earlier, this data is only a case series and cannot be used to make comparisons across sports or with data from other sources. However, they might alert the physician if an unexpected number of injuries of a certain type or injuries that happen under specific circumstances are noted.

If comparisons are desired, some form of exposure or "denominator" data is required to calculate injury rates, as discussed earlier. The simplest denominator data to obtain are the number of athletes on the team, so that injury rates per 100 athletes can be calculated. The fact that many teams have more athletes at the beginning of the season than at the end presents a problem. The most reasonable solution is to use an average number of athletes if the rate of attrition is fairly stable over the season, or use the number of athletes on the team during most of the season if the dropouts tend to occur at the beginning of the season and the numbers stabilize as the season progresses.

For reasons presented previously, rates per 100 athletes are not the most accurate way to calculate sports injury rates. With some extra effort and on-site assistance from a student athletic trainer or coach, it is feasible to get data at the local level on the number of athletes participating in practices and competitions, or possibly even the amount of time of participation, so that rates per 1,000 A-Es or rates per 100 hours or 1,000 minutes can be calculated.

In some team sports, the time of exposure in games is relatively easy to estimate, because the games last a specified length of time and involve a specified number of players at any one time. A high school football game will involve four quarters of 12 minutes each, and 11 players from a team are on the field at any given time. Therefore, the amount of exposure time for a single team in a single game will be 528 player-minutes/game (4 quarters/game × 12 minutes/quarter × 11 players). It is more difficult to get data on time of exposure in practices, but it basically means keeping track of the number of players participating in each practice and the length of the practices. When collecting A-E data, the time element is ignored, and data are recorded only on the number of players at each practice and the number who actually get into the games and are exposed, however briefly, to the possibility of injury (not the number who dress for the game).

Once appropriate denominator data on the population at risk are available, the rate equation presented earlier can be used to calculate injury rates that can be used in comparisons across local sports teams or with data from other sources that are calculated in a similar manner. When comparing local data with injury data from other sources (or when comparing injury data from any sources), always note any differences in methodologies used (data sources and collection procedures, definition of an injury, type of rate calculated, etc.). If there are any major differences, conclusions drawn from the comparisons may not be valid. Of particular importance are the type of rate calculated and the definition of an injury. Obviously, trying to compare injury rates per 100 athletes with rates per 1,000 A-Es would be meaningless. Less obvious is the need to ensure that the same definition of a reportable injury is being used. If one set of data includes everything seen by the medical staff and another includes only injuries that cause 3 or more days of time lost from participation, comparisons would be meaningless. The most commonly used definition of a reportable injury is based on time loss:

> A reportable injury is any injury (a) occurring in a scheduled practice or competition, (b) requiring medical attention, and (c) resulting in the athlete being restricted from further normal participation for the remainder of that practice or competition or for the following day or more.

This is essentially the basic definition of a reportable time-loss injury used by ISS and AIMS, and we recommend its use in local data collection systems. By basing the definition on time loss of 1 day or more before a return to unrestricted participation, all minor scrapes, bumps, and bruises that do not cause time loss are eliminated, so they do not overburden the data collection system. (The only exception to this in AIMS is that any mild concussion is reported, although it may not cause time loss.)

Rates for specific types of injuries or body parts can also be calculated for local injury data. For example, the total number of knee injuries could be the numerator rather than the total number of all injuries. If game and practice exposure data are available, separate game and practice injury rates can be calculated. Make sure the appropriate denominator is matched with the numerator. If a game injury rate is being calculated, be sure to divide the number of game injuries by the number of game exposures. As with large-scale sports injury data collection systems, the more local data collected over time, the more useful and valuable the information becomes.

CONCLUSION

Applying the principles of epidemiology to sports injuries is a relatively recent development, and national-scale data collection systems such as NCCSIR, ISS, and AIMS are making important contributions to current sports medicine issues. As Mueller (68) notes, "injury data collection plays an important role in the prevention of (catastrophic football) injuries... There is no question that the beneficial changes are the result of reliable data collection and the publication of the results in the athletic and medical literature. Persistent surveillance of sports injury data is mandatory if progress is to continue in the prevention of fatalities. Continuous data are needed to observe the development of specific trends, to implement in-depth investigation into areas of concern, and to carry out preventive measures. If continued progress in sports injury prevention is to be made, reliable data is a must."

There will be ample opportunity for contributions from others as well, such as the primary care physician working with a local sports program. Understanding the basic principles of epidemiology presented in this chapter will allow the primary care physician to be more discriminating in reading the literature, and will also be useful in setting up a system for keeping track of local injury patterns. These efforts on the part of the primary care physician can play an important role in reducing the number and severity of injuries in the local community.

REFERENCES

1. Duncan DF. *Epidemiology: basis for disease prevention and health promotion*. New York: Macmillan, 1988.
2. German RR, Armstrong G, Birkhead GS, et al. Updated guidelines for evaluating public health surveillance systems: recommendations from the Guidelines Working Group. *MMWR* 2001;50(RR13):1–35.
3. Teutsch SM, Churchill RE, eds. *Principle and practice of public health surveillance*. New York: Oxford University Press, 1994.
4. Holder Y, Peden M, Krug E, et al., eds. *Injury surveillance guidelines*. Geneva, Switzerland: World Health Organization, www.who.int/violence_injury_prevention/index.html, 2001.
5. Meeuwisse WH, Love EJ. Athletic injury reporting: development of universal systems. *Sports Med* 1997;24(3):184–204.
6. Fuller CW, Ekstrand J, Junge A, et al. Consensus statement on injury definitions and data collection procedures in studies of football (soccer) injuries. *Br J Sports Med* 2006;40:193–201.
7. De Loes M. Exposure data: why are they needed. *Sports Med* 1997;24(3):172–175.
8. National Collegiate Athletic Association. *NCAA injury surveillance system reports*. Indianapolis, IN: NCAA, (www.ncaa.org/iss.html), 2006.
9. Zemper ED. Injury rates in a national sample of college football teams: a two-year prospective study. *Phys Sportsmed* 1989;17(11):100–113.
10. Walter SD, Sutton JR, McIntosh JM, et al. The aetiology of sports injuries: a review of methodologies. *Sports Med* 1985;2:47–58.
11. Powell KE, Kohl I-IW, Casperson CJ, et al. An epidemiological perspective on the causes of running injuries. *Phys Sportsmed* 1986;14(6):100–114.
12. Rice SG, Schlotfeldt JD, Foley WE. The athletic health care and training program. *West J Med* 1985;142:352.
13. Junge A, Dvorak J. Influence of definition and data collection on the incidence of injuries in football (soccer). *Am J Sports Med* 2000;28(5 Suppl):S40–S46.
14. Gotsch K, Annest JL, Holmgreen P, et al. Nonfatal sports- and recreation-related injuries treated in emergency departments - United States, July 2000-June 2001. *MMWR* 2002;51(33):736–740.
15. Quinlan KP, Thompson MP, Annest JL, et al. Expanding the National Electronic Injury Surveillance System to monitor all nonfatal injuries treated in US hospital emergency departments. *Ann Emerg Med* 1999;34:637–645.
16. Koplan JP, Siscovick DS, Goldbaum GM. The risks of exercise: a public health view of injuries and hazards. *Public Health Rep* 1985;100:189–195.
17. Caine D, Caine C, Lindner K, eds. *Epidemiology of sports injuries*. Champaign, IL: Human Kinetics, 1996.
18. National Center for Catastrophic Sports Injury Research (NCCSIR). *22nd Annual Report: Fall 1982—Spring 2004*. Chapel Hill, North Carolina: University of North Carolina, www.unc.edu/depts/nccsi, 08/06.
19. Thompson N, Halpern B, Curl WW, et al. High school football injuries: evaluation. *Am J Sports Med* 1987;15:117–124.
20. Caine D, Cochrane B, Caine C, et al. An epidemiologic investigation of injuries affecting young competitive female gymnasts. *Am J Sports Med* 1989;17(6):811–820.
21. Pieter W, Zemper ED. Injury rates in children participating in taekwondo competition. *J Trauma* 1997;43(1):89–95.
22. Pieter W, Zemper ED, Heijmans J. Taekwondo blessures (taekwondo injuries). *Geneeskd Sport* 1990;23(6):222–228.
23. Zemper ED. A prospective study of injury rates in a national sample of American College Football Teams. *Proceedings of the First International Olympic Committee World Congress on Sport Sciences*. Colorado Springs: U.S. Olympic Committee, 1989:194–195.
24. Zemper ED. Exercise and injury patterns in a sample of active middle-aged adults. *International Congress and Exposition on Sport Medicine and Human Performance*. Vancouver, BC: April 1991. Programme/Abstracts, 1991:98.
25. Zemper ED, Pieter W. Injury rates at the 1988 U.S. Olympic Team Trials for taekwondo. *Br J Sports Med* 1989;23(3):161–164.
26. Pieter W, Zemper ED. Incidence of reported cerebral concussion in adult taekwondo athletes. *J R Soc Health* 1998;118(5):272–279.
27. Zemper ED. A two-year prospective study of relative risk of a second cerebral concussion. *Am J Phys Med Rehabil* 2003;82(9):653–659.
28. Zemper ED, Pieter W. Cerebral concussion rates in taekwondo competition. *Med Sci Sports Exerc* 1990;22(2-Suppl):S130.
29. Zemper ED, Pieter W. Cerebral concussion in taekwondo athletes. In: Hoerner EF, ed. *Head and neck injuries in sports ASTM STP 1229*. Philadelphia: American Society for Testing and Materials, 1994:116–123.
30. Zemper ED. A two-year prospective study of cerebral concussion in American football. *Res Sports Med: An Int J* 2003;11(3):157–172.
31. Zemper ED. A prospective study of prophylactic knee braces in a national sample of American college football players. *Proceedings of the First International Olympic Committee World Congress on Sport Sciences*. Colorado Springs: U.S. Olympic Committee, 1989:202–203.
32. Zemper ED. A two-year study of prophylactic knee braces in a national sample of college football players. *Sports Train Med Rehabil* 1990;1:287–296.
33. Zemper ED. A four-year prospective study of preventive knee braces and MCL injuries in a national sample of college football players. In: Hoerner EF, ed. *Safety in American football ASTM STP 1305*. Philadelphia: American Society for Testing and Materials, 1996.
34. Zemper ED. Cerebral concussion rates in various brands of football helmets. *Athl Train* 1989;24(2):133–137.
35. Zemper ED. Analysis of cerebral concussion frequency with the most commonly used models of football helmets. *J Athl Train* 1994;29:44–50.
36. Zemper ED. NCAA injury surveillance system: initial results. *Paper Presented at the 1984 Olympic Scientific Congress, July 1984*. Eugene, OR: University of Oregon, 1984.
37. Pieter W, Zemper ED. Head and neck injuries in young taekwondo athletes. *J Sports Med Phys Fitness* 1999;39(2):147–153.
38. Zemper ED. Four-year study of weight room injuries in a national sample of college football teams. *Natl Strength Cond Assoc J* 1990;12(3):32–34.
39. Zemper ED, Pieter W. Two-year prospective study of injury rates in national taekwondo competition. *International Congress and Exposition on Sport Medicine and Human Performance*. Vancouver, BC: April 1991. Programme/Abstracts, 1991:99.
40. Mueller FO, Zemper ED, Peters A. American football. In: Caine D, Caine C, Lindner K, eds. *Epidemiology of sports injuries*. Champaign, IL: Human Kinetics, 1996:41–62.
41. Buckley WE. Five year overview of sport injuries: the NAIRS model. *JOPERD* 1982;53:36–40.
42. Watkins RJ. *An epidemiological study: injury rates among collegiate ultimate frisbee players in the western United States*. PhD Thesis, University of Oregon, 1990.
43. Boden BP, Pasquina P, Johnson J, et al. Catastrophic injuries in pole-vaulters. *Am J Sports Med* 2001;29(1):50–54.
44. Dick RW. Epidemiology of basketball injuries. *World Basketball Sports Medicine Conference sponsored by American College of Sports Medicine and Indiana University Center for Sports Medicine*. Indianapolis, IN: August 28, 2002.
45. Dick RW. Frequency of bleeding and risk of HIV transmission in intercollegiate athletics. *American College of Sports Medicine 40th Annual Convention*. Indianapolis, IN: June 1–4, 1994.
46. Brown LS, Drotman DP, Chu A, et al. Bleeding injuries in professional football: estimating the risk for HIV transmission. *Ann Intern Med* 1995;122(4):271–274.
47. McCallum J, Gelin D. Out of joint. *Sports Illus* 1995;82(6):44–49.
48. Arendt EA, Dick RW. Knee injury patterns among men and women in collegiate basketball and soccer: NCAA data and review of literature. *Am J Sports Med* 1995;23:694–701.
49. Arendt EA, Agel J, Dick RW. Anterior cruciate ligament injury patterns among collegiate men and women. *J Athl Train* 1999;34(2):86–92.
50. Harmon KG, Dick RW. The relationship of skill level to anterior cruciate ligament injury. *Clin J Sports Med* 1998;8(4):260–265.
51. U.S. Department of Health and Human Services. *Physical activity and health: a report of the surgeon general*. Atlanta, GA: U.S. Department of Health and Human Services, Centers for Disease Control and Prevention, National Center for Chronic Disease Prevention and Health Promotion, 1996.
52. Griffin LY, ed. *Prevention of noncontact ACL injuries*. Chicago: American Academy of Orthopedic Surgeons, 2001.
53. Benson BM, Mohtadi NGH, Rose MS, et al. Head and neck injury risk among hockey players wearing full versus half face shields. *JAMA* 1999;282(24):2328–2332.
54. LaPrade RF, Burnett QM, Zarzour R, et al. The effect of the mandatory use of face masks on facial lacerations and head and neck injuries in ice hockey. *Am J Sports Med* 1995;23(6):773–775.
55. Marshall SW, Waller AE, Dick RW, et al. An ecologic study of protective equipment and injury in two contact sports. *Int J Epidemiol* 2002;31:587–592.
56. Dick RW. A comparison of injuries that occur during collegiate fall and spring football using the NCAA Injury Surveillance System. In: Hoerner EF, ed. *Safety in American football ASTM STP 1305*. Philadelphia: American Society for Testing and Materials, 1996:9–18.
57. Garrick JG, Requa RK. Anterior cruciate ligament injuries in men and women: how common are they? In: Griffin LY, ed. *Prevention of noncontact ACL injuries*. Chicago: American Academy of Orthopedic Surgeons, 2001:1–9.
58. Special issue: anterior cruciate ligament injury in the female athlete. *J Athl Train* 1999;34(2):86–201.
59. Teitz CC, Hermanson BK, Krommal HA, et al. Evaluation of the use of braces to prevent injury to the knee in collegiate football players. *J Bone Joint Surg* 1987;69A(1):3–9.
60. Stitler M, Ryan J, Hopkinson W, et al. The efficacy of a prophylactic knee brace to reduce knee injuries in football. *Am J Sports Med* 1990;18(3):310–315.
61. Van Camp SP, Bloor CM, Mueller FO, et al. Nontraumatic sports death in high school and college athletes. *Med Sci Sports Exerc* 1995;27:641–647.
62. Maron BJ, Shirni J, Poliac LC, et al. Sudden death in young competitive athletes: clinical, demographic and pathological profiles. *JAMA* 1996;276:199–204.
63. Roberts WO. A 12-year profile of medical injuries and illnesses for the Twin Cities Marathon. *Med Sci Sports Exerc* 2000;32(9):1549–1555.

64. National Collegiate Athletic Association. *1981–82 - 2004–05 NCAA sports sponsorship and participation rates report.* Indianapolis, IN: NCAA, 2006.
65. Dick RW. Epidemiology of women's collegiate sports injuries. In: Garrett WE Jr, Lester GE, McGowan J, et al. eds. *Women's health in sports and exercise.* Chicago: American Academy of Orthopedic Surgeons, 2001:23–36.
66. Kulka TJ, Kenney WL. Heat balance limits in football uniforms. *Phys Sportsmed* 2002;30(7):29–39.
67. Special issue: concussion in athletes. *J Athl Train* 2001;36(3):228–341.
68. Mueller FO. Fatalities from head and cervical spine injuries occurring in tackle football: 50 years' experience. *Clin Sports Med* 1998;17(1):169–181.

Exercise Physiology and Exercise Testing

3

Carl Foster *Matthew J. Faber* *John P. Porcari*

BASICS OF EXERCISE PHYSIOLOGY

Exercise is about skeletal muscle contraction. Exercise physiology is about how skeletal muscles contract, how the rest of the body arranges to deal with the disturbance in homeostasis provoked by skeletal muscle contraction, how these physiological mechanisms adapt to repetitive skeletal muscle contraction (exercise training), and (for the clinician) how these physiological mechanisms are deranged in pathological states. However, without the obligatory requirement for skeletal muscle, there is no exercise.

At the simplest level skeletal muscle contraction involves a linkage of the actin and myosin filaments that are part of the architecture of the basic unit of every muscle, the sarcomere. This is mediated by calcium released from the sarcoplasmic reticulum in response to the depolarization induced when acetylcholine is released at the motor end plate. This process leads to a cascade of reactions that results in the formation of an actin-adenosine triphosphate (ATP)-myosin complex, leading to a conformational change in the myosin unit, which in turn causes traction to be exerted on the actin filament. Because the architecture of the muscle is symmetrical, the process leads to the actin filament pulling on the rudiments of the connective tissue architecture of the sarcomere, resulting in shortening the muscle. Ultimately, this leads to the muscle pulling on a ligamentous or bony structure, resulting in movement. Thanks to the exquisite coordination of the motor nerve center, the timing and sequence in which muscle fibers are recruited allow for purposeful and effective motion. This is most elegantly evident to the sports physician who, typically, has the duty of providing care for individuals with very well developed neuromuscular systems, and the physiological support structure to allow muscle contraction to continue, often at a very high rate compared to nonathletic individuals.

The ability to provide for continuing muscular contraction ultimately depends on the availability of ATP within each sarcomere. This is provided for by three interlinked and overlapping *energy systems* that not only provide very rapid resynthesis of ATP for short bursts of activity but can also provide for low to moderate intensity activity to be continued almost indefinitely.

Energy Systems

There is a small storage reservoir of both ATP and a related compound, creatine phosphate (CP), in the cytoplasm of each sarcomere. These substances, collectively referred to as *phosphagens*, can provide for very rapid resynthesis of ATP on the myosin head, allowing for brief but very high-intensity bursts of muscular activity. However, the total quantity of phosphagens is very low. If other sources of ATP were not available, the duration of phosphagen-powered exercise would be only in the order of seconds. The second energy system is related to the anaerobic degradation of muscle glycogen to pyruvate. This not only yields pyruvate that can be oxidized (in the third [aerobic] energy system) but also directly provides ATP that becomes part of the cytoplasmic phosphagen pool. Because pyruvate can be produced more rapidly than it can be oxidized, and because pyruvate accumulation would stop the ATP production coming from this second energy system, pyruvate may be reversibly converted to lactate, which may then be transported out of the cell and used by other tissues. This provides not only for continued glycogen to pyruvate hydrolysis but (through the proton release correlated with lactate transport) also provides a negative feedback loop to limit the duration of high-intensity exercise (e.g., the metabolic acidosis induced by lactate contributes to both increases in ventilation and to perceptual responses such as local muscle discomfort that ultimately cause the individual to reduce the intensity of exercise). The third energy system depends on the oxidation in the mitochondria of either pyruvate, acetyl CoA formed directly from glucose, or free fatty acids. This is a low power but very high capacity energy system that is dependent on the availability of molecular O_2 within the cell.

The Oxygen Connection

Although the phosphagen and the glycogen to pyruvate energy systems are quite important (particularly at the beginning of exercise or during very high-intensity exercise), the oxidative energy system is quantitatively the most important. And, because it depends on the availability of O_2, which is plentiful in the room air but very scarce at the level of the sarcomere, much of the physiology of the body is organized to transport O_2 to the tissues. This requires the combined actions of the cardiorespiratory system to extract O_2 from the inhaled air and transport O_2 in the arteries, to deliver CO_2 (a prime waste product of oxidative metabolism) back to the lung, and then to selectively deliver O_2 to the active muscles, with active reductions of blood flow to less active tissues. The characteristic changes in heart rate, stroke volume, end diastolic volume, and ejection fraction that are hallmarks of the cardiovascular response to exercise are all designed to facilitate increasing the cardiac output to a level consistent with providing O_2 to the tissues. The cardiovascular response to exercise is well integrated by the Fick equation, which defines this response. Likewise, the characteristic changes in pulmonary tidal volume and respiratory frequency during exercise are designed to facilitate adequate alveolar O_2 and CO_2 concentrations so that delivery of blood to the lungs results in appropriate gas exchange. Lastly, coordinated vasodilation in the active tissues, often regulated by the metabolites of muscular contraction, is designed to allow selective delivery of blood to the active tissues. This allows for optimizing O_2 delivery to the tissues with the minimal increase in cardiac output.

Adaptations to Chronic Exercise

The other aspect of exercise physiology that is immediately obvious, and of particular importance for the sports physician is the adaptability of both the musculoskeletal system and the cardiorespiratory support system to regularly performed exercise. This is elegantly obvious in the legend of Milo of Crotona. Milo was a young farm boy who lifted a newly foaled bullock on his shoulders and walked around the barnyard. On successive days, Milo continued lifting the growing bullock, until he was capable of lifting a fully grown bull, becoming the strongest man in the world (and an Olympic champion in the ancient Games) in the process. This feat was actually reproduced in the early days of television for a show called "You Asked For It." Apparently, a farm boy lifted a growing cow for some months. The cow gained more than 200 lb although the boy gained only 3 lb. The adaptability of the exercise capacity is also elegantly demonstrated by the large number of normal individuals (and even cardiac patients) who can adapt well enough to exercise training to complete marathon length races without particular problems.

The adaptation to repetitive exercise can be understood in terms of several factors that can be recalled using the anagram P-ROIDS (a humorous word play on the fact that urine is the most common testing medium for anabolic steroid abuse). These principles are:

Progression
Reversibility
Overload
Individual differences
Specificity

Guidelines for, and the scientific rationale behind, each of these principles of the exercise training response are available in the literature (1,2).

EXERCISE STRESS TESTING

Physicians are often called on to perform evaluative procedures to determine the presence of pathological states that might influence participation in exercise and/or to provide guidance regarding increased levels of activity. At the outset it is critical to remember that exercise testing is simply an extension of the history and physical examination. Just as the physician might manipulate an injured limb to determine what motions lead to discomfort, and thereby evaluate the nature of the presenting complaint, a patient's responses during incremental exercise may allow the physician to observe the patient when he/she is symptomatic. In a general sense, there are several broad indications for exercise stress testing including the following:

Evaluation of exertional discomfort. Including provocation of exertional angina pectoris, dyspnea or exertional bronchospasm, claudication, palpitations, or hemodynamic abnormalities.

Provocation of occult pathology. Particularly, occult cardiovascular disease in which the first presentation is often fatal, particularly in males. Provocation of pathophysiology before the presentation of sudden death or acute myocardial infarction provides the physician with many more options for treating the patient.

Defining prognosis in known pathological states. This is particularly critical when deciding amongst several therapeutic options. Effectively, this can guide the physician regarding which patients might benefit from more aggressive or invasive therapy, and which may effectively be treated with less invasive therapies.

Evaluation of therapy. Improved exercise tolerance and disability evaluation.

Exercise prescription. Guidance regarding the appropriate Frequency, Intensity, and the Time and Mode (FIT'M) of exercise to achieve therapeutic goals. Accepted guidelines recommend at least 30 minutes of moderate-intensity exercise, performed in one or more sessions on most days of the week. However, for improving physical fitness and performance capacity, a likely goal amongst the patients of sports physicians, more strenuous training (particularly higher-intensity training) is usually critical to success.

Graded Cardiac Stress Testing

The most familiar form of exercise testing for most physicians is the cardiac stress test. This procedure is typically conducted either to evaluate exertional discomfort that might be consistent with cardiovascular disease or to reveal the presence of occult cardiovascular disease. Most typically, exercise is performed on either a treadmill or cycle ergometer, although other forms of exercise can be used effectively. There are a variety of exercise protocols. The most commonly used is the Bruce treadmill protocol (3) (see Table 3.1). Although this protocol starts at a fairly high energy requirement (approximately 5 times the average resting metabolic rate or 5 metabolic equivalents [METs]) and has relatively large increments between stages, it is still a well recognized and convenient way to conduct this aspect of the physical examination. We have created a convenient modification of the Bruce protocol, that allows for a lower-intensity start and smoother transition between stages (see Table 3.2). Although lagging slightly behind the Bruce protocol, on a METs/minute basis, the modified protocol is much better tolerated than the standard Bruce protocol.

During the exercise test, the exercise capacity is typically estimated from established prediction equations (4), and then interpreted in light of age and gender norms, for active individuals. Active individuals are arguably the proper reference group, rather than the "healthy sedentary" who has traditionally been used because there is adequate evidence that sedentary individuals are at risk for a number of disease states (see Table 3.3). Exercise capacities in the range of 85% to 115% of predicted are considered normal. Exercise capacities below 85% of predicted (mean—1 SD) or particularly below 70% of predicted (mean—2 SD) are considered abnormal and are consistent with a poor prognosis regardless of the presence or absence of pathophysiological findings (e.g., electrocardiographic [ECG] or hemodynamic abnormalities). It is critically important to account for the presence of handrail support, as *any* degree of handrail support will allow the patient to exercise longer and thereby have a higher predicted exercise capacity than truly present. This would give an incorrectly favorable prognosis for the patient. This problem is addressed in current prediction equations (Tables 3.1 and 3.2).

TABLE 3.1
BRUCE TREADMILL PROTOCOL

				METs Achieved	
Stage	**Time (min)**	**Speed (mph)**	**Grade (%)**	**Without HRS**	**With HRS**
1	1	1.7	0	3.0	2.8
	2	1.7	10	3.9	3.7
	3	1.7	10	4.6	4.4
2	4	2.5	12	5.2	5.0
	5	2.5	12	5.9	5.7
	6	2.5	12	6.6	6.4
3	7	3.4	14	7.2	7.0
	8	3.4	14	7.9	7.7
	9	3.4	14	8.6	8.3
4	10	4.2	16	9.7	9.0
	11	4.2	16	10.9	9.6
	12	4.2	16	12.1	10.3
5	13	5.0	18	13.3	10.9
	14	5.0	18	14.6	11.6
	15	5.0	18	15.7	12.2

MET = metabolic equivalent; HRS = hand rail support.
Estimated METs = multiples of the resting metabolic rate based on the longest time completed. If the patient starts without HRS, but concludes the test with HRS, use the lower value. To estimate VO_2max, multiply METs by 3.5.

TABLE 3.2
MODIFIED BRUCE TREADMILL PROTOCOL

Stage and Time (min)	Speed (mph)	Grade (%)	METs Achieved	
			Without HRS	With HRS
1	1.4	0	3.3	3.4
2	1.7	5	4.1	4.0
3	1.7	10	4.7	4.4
4	2.0	11	5.3	4.9
5	2.4	11	5.9	5.3
6	2.5	12	6.4	5.8
7	2.8	14	7.0	6.2
8	3.2	14	7.6	6.6
9	3.4	14	8.3	7.1
10	3.6	16	9.2	7.8
11	3.8	16	10.3	9.2
12	4.2	16	11.3	9.4
13	4.2	18	12.4	10.2
14	4.6	18	13.5	11.0
15	5.0	18	14.4	11.7

MET = metabolic equivalent; HRS = hand rail support.

Should a less formal exercise protocol be desired, there are predictive equations that allow the estimation of exercise capacity (5). Typically, the graded cardiac stress test is continued either until the patient develops signs or symptoms of cardiovascular pathology or until the patient is fatigued. General guidelines for the conduct and interpretation of exercise testing are available (6). During graded cardiac stress testing, the patient is monitored using both ECG and hemodynamic monitoring. Characteristic changes in the configuration of the ST segment of the ECG, particularly if correlated with the development of symptoms or hemodynamic abnormalities, are the diagnostic hallmark of exertional myocardial ischemia.

The sensitivity and specificity of ECG stress testing is at best modest, averaging approximately 75% each. Sensitivity and specificity may be augmented with either myocardial perfusion imaging or measures of left ventricular function using either radionuclides or ultrasound. However, recent data has demonstrated that long neglected hemodynamic markers including chronotropic incompetence, the pattern of heart rate recovery following exercise, the pattern of blood pressure changes during and following exercise, and the interaction of exercise capacity, symptoms, and ECG changes (the Duke Index) (7,8) can all contribute meaningfully to the interpretation of the exercise test, perhaps rivaling the diagnostic power of more technically demanding approaches (9). The most recent approach, which predominately focuses on prognosis, uses the combined results of exercise capacity-ECG findings-symptoms (e.g., Duke Index) and heart rate responses during and following exercise to achieve powerful indicators of prognosis (9).

Maximal Oxygen Uptake Testing

An extension of the normal graded exercise test involves the measurement of respiratory gas exchange either to improve the precision of evaluating exercise capacity, to discriminate between cardiovascular and pulmonary pathologies, or to evaluate chronic heart failure (10,11). It is also one of the gold standards for evaluating exercise training programs and athletes, as changes in the maximal oxygen uptake (Vo_2max) are highly predictable responses to the beginning of exercise training, and very high values are characteristic in elite endurance athletes. Vo_2max values of approximately double the age and gender reference values of 45 and 35 mL/minute/kg are typically observed in elite endurance athletes. Direct measurement of respiratory gas exchange can allow definition of not only the Vo_2max, which has been the traditional index of cardiorespiratory endurance (12,13), but also the ventilatory and respiratory compensation thresholds that may be superior markers of sustainable exercise capacity (14).

Recent studies have suggested that the gas exchange responses during free range exercise or competitive simulations may be somewhat different than during incremental exercise, which is the traditional way of exercise testing (15,16). Gas exchange testing is still not widely available in many clinical settings secondary to the expense of the technology required to measure gas exchange and to the lack of wide experience in the interpretation of gas exchange studies. This often limits the procedure to teaching hospitals or to liaisons between sports physicians and university exercise science departments. At the same time, respiratory gas analysis systems are becoming more user

TABLE 3.3
PREDICTED VALUES AND NORMAL RESPONSES

Predicted Treadmill METs
Males = 18.7 − 0.15 × age
Females = 14.8 − 0.10 × age
For predicted V_{O_2}, multiply METs by 3.5
For cycle exercise, multiply predicted treadmill by 0.90
Predicted Maximal HR
220—age
Chronotropic Incompetence
Achieving <80% of the difference between the pretest resting HR and the age-predicted HR
Normal HR Recovery
HR decreases ≥12 beats/min in the first minute of recovery
Normal BP Response
SBP increases 5–10 mm Hg/MET above the standing control (e.g., 1 MET)
Normal BP Recovery
SBP at 3 min post exercise <0.90 × peak SBP

MET = metabolic equivalent; HR = heart rate; BP = blood pressure; SBP = systolic blood pressure.

friendly and have become fully portable, even suitable for direct measurements during training and competition, and clinical interpretative algorithms have become simpler and easier to apply (11).

Lactate Testing

Because of the central role of pyruvate in two of the ATP-generating energy systems, because lactate can serve as a "safety value" during periods of high rates of pyruvate production, and because lactate is relatively easy to measure in peripheral blood, there has been a long standing interest in lactate as a marker of the relative metabolic status. Because lactate may also be involved in the disproportionate increase in ventilation during heavy submaximal exercise, and thereby may be a useful marker of sustainable exercise capacity, measurement of lactate during incremental exercise, or even at certain points during training or competition may provide significant information about the metabolic status during exercise (14).

Typically, capillary blood for lactate testing is obtained either from a fingertip or earlobe, and can be analyzed either with portable dry chemistry analyzers (such as those used for glucose monitoring by diabetic patients) or with comparatively simple wet chemistry analyzers. The procedure is relatively quick, inexpensive, and comparatively noninvasive. Although there are a number of interpretative approaches (14), and some controversy regarding the linkage between blood lactate concentrations, lactate production and removal rates, and regarding the linkage between blood lactate and exertional hypernea (17,18), the technique has achieved wide use, particularly in the sports population. Especially, among endurance athletes, heart rate or pace relationships between various lactate and/or ventilatory markers of different metabolic zones (e.g., thresholds) are thought to be highly useful in terms of defining training zones (19).

SUMMARY

Exercise physiology is about the contraction of skeletal muscles, and how the body provides for and regulates ATP production to support the energetic requirements of muscular contraction. Because of the quantitative importance of aerobic ATP generation, and the relative ease of measuring aerobic metabolism, this aspect of exercise physiology has received particular attention in the literature as an effective method for provocation of pathophysiological conditions. Further, because exercise and the physiological support structures of exercise are effective challenges to the integrity of a number of organ systems, exercise testing may serve as an effective method of revealing occult pathophysiology.

Exercise testing, which ultimately is an extension of the history and physical examination, is effective in accomplishing a number of tasks for the sports physician. There are a variety of protocols available for provoking the subject in a way appropriate to the clinical question posed by the physician. Although ECG stress testing is ordinarily the main approach to cardiac stress testing, recent studies have suggested that hemodynamic and exercise capacity information that have traditionally been considered to have less diagnostic power may, in fact, have remarkable value. The exercise test may be meaningfully augmented by the application of either respiratory gas exchange or blood lactate measuring technology. Although in their infancy in terms of clinical use, these technologies can significantly augment the value of exercise testing.

REFERENCES

1. American College of Sports Medicine. *Guidelines for graded exercise testing and exercise prescription*, 6th ed. Philadelphia: Lippincott Williams and Wilkins, 2000.
2. Foster C, Cadwell K, Crenshaw B, et al. Physical activity and exercise training prescriptions for patients. *Cardiol Clin* 2001;19:447–457.
3. Bruce RA, Kusumi F, Hosmer D. Maximal oxygen intake and the nomographic assessment of functional aerobic impairment in cardiovascular disease. *Am Heart J* 1973;85:546–562.
4. McConnell TR, Fosgter C, Conlin NC, et al. Prediction of functional capacity during exercise testing: effect of handrail support. *J Cardiopulm Rehabil* 1991;11:255–260.
5. Foster C, Crowe AJ, Daiones E. Predicting functional capacity during treadmill testing independent of exercise protocol. *Med Sci Sports Exerc* 1996;28:752–756.
6. Gibbons RJ, Balady GJ, Beasley JW, et al. AHA/ACC guidelines for exercise testing. *J Am Coll Cardiol* 1997;30:260–315.
7. Mark DB, Hlatky MA, Harell FE. Exercise treadmill score for predicting prognosis in coronary artery disease. *Ann Intern Med* 1987;106:793–800.
8. Mark DB, Shaw L, Harrell FE. Prognostic value of a treadmill exercise score in outpatients with suspected coronary artery disease. *N Engl J Med* 1991;325:849–853.

9. Lauer MS. Exercise electrocardiogram testing and prognosis: novel markers and predictive instruments. *Cardiol Clin* 2001;19:401–414.
10. Wasserman K. Diagnosing cardiovascular and lung pathophysiology from exercise gas exchange. *Chest* 1997;112:1091–1101.
11. Essenbacher WL, Mannina A. An algorithm for the interpretation of cardiopulmonary exercise tests. *Chest* 1990;97:263–267.
12. Noakes TD. Challenging beliefs: ex Africa semper aliquid novi. *Med Sci Sports Exerc* 1997;29:571–590.
13. Bassett DR, Howley ET. Maximal oxygen uptake: "classical" versus "contemporary" viewpoints. *Med Sci Sports Exerc* 1997;29:591–603.
14. Foster C. Cotter: blood lactate, respiratory measurement and heart rate markers of the capacity for sustained exercise. In: Maud PJ, Foster C, eds. *Physiological assessment of human fitness*, 2nd ed. Champaign, IL: Human Kinetics Publishers, 2006:63–76.
15. Foster C, Green M, Snyder AC, et al. Physiological responses during simulated competition. *Med Sci Sports Exerc* 1993;25:877–882.
16. Foster C, Coye RB, Crowe A, et al. Comparison of free range and graded exercise testing. *Med Sci Sports Exerc* 1997;29:1521–1526.
17. Brooks GA. Anaerobic threshold: review of the concept and directions for future research. *Med Sci Sports Exerc* 1985;17:22–31.
18. Davis JA. Anaerobic threshold: review of the concept and directions for future research. *Med Sci Sports Exerc* 1985;17:6–18.
19. Lucia A, Hoyos J, Carvajal A, et al. Heart rate response to professional road cycling: the tour de France. *Int J Sports Med* 1999;20:167–172.

Nutrition

4

Leslie Bonci

Nutrition is an essential, but often neglected component of performance. Optimal nutrition provides the energy substrates for exercise as well as promotes muscle growth, enhances recovery, prevents injury, and supports rehabilitation. Still, many athletes do not fuel adequately or appropriately for their sports. Many use the excuse that eating right is too hard, or takes too much time, or is too inconvenient. In addition, athletes may turn to the "quick fix" supplements mistakenly assuming that they are equivalent or better than proper fuel and hydration. It is essential for the sports medicine physician to have a solid understanding of the types, quantity, and timing of foods and fluid to help the athlete to optimize performance.

Athletes with medical concerns, such as diabetes, hypoglycemia, or gastrointestinal disorders present special challenges, but they too must be optimally fueled for performance. The challenge is to have the athletes perceive the value of fuel and hydration as providing the edge in sport. The sports medicine physician can collect useful nutrition information from athletes by using the nutrition screening form in Figure 4.1. This form can identify athletes who may be at risk of disordered eating behavior as well as those who may be more likely to succumb to dehydration on the basis of fluid intake. Asking each athlete to record what supplements he/she uses can serve as a springboard for education as well as prevent potential drug/supplement interactions.

GOALS OF SPORTS NUTRITION

The goals of sports nutrition can be outlined as follows:

- Achieve/maintain ideal body mass
- Maintain proper hydration and electrolyte balance
- Provide adequate carbohydrate to optimize respiratory metabolism
- Preserve lean body mass with essential amino acids
- Develop high density skeletal structure
- Maximize oxygen delivery systems and oxidative phosphorylation with trace elements
- Improve performance by increasing the speed of muscle fiber contraction and the number of muscle fibers that contract
- Promote recovery from training

It is important to note that although the macronutrient needs are similar among sports, there may be quantitative differences based upon the following variables: type of sport, gender, body composition, and age. In discussing the science of sports nutrition, it is important to understand the energy systems and energy substrates that fuel activity.

ENERGY SYSTEMS

In order for any muscle to do physical work, adenosine triphosphate (ATP) is required. ATP is the energy catalyst, formed from the storage forms of carbohydrate and fat, that is, glycogen and fatty acids, and must be continuously formed, used, and reformed during physical activity. The other storage form of energy that can be used to fuel activity is creatine phosphate or phosphocreatine. Creatine is manufactured in the liver, kidney, and pancreas, and is stored in muscle. When energy demand increases due to exercise, the body relies on different types of energy systems to transfer stored energy to ATP to enable physical work to continue. There are three energy systems that will be used, depending on the duration and intensity of exercise. The phosphagen system is the first one that will be used when energy demand increases. This is an anaerobic energy system dependent upon ATP and creatine phosphate for high intensity, maximal outburst activity lasting less than 1 minute, such as a power-lift, a 6-second sprint, or a slam-dunk. As the duration of activity increases, the anaerobic

Nutrition Screening Form for Atheletes

1. Name:______________________________
2. Male _____ Female ________
3. Sport:______________________________
4. Position:____________________________
5. Age: ______ years
6. How would you describe your eating habits? (Check one)

a. ____ Good b.____ Fair
c. ____ Poor

7. How many times a day do you eat?________ number of times per day
8. How often do you eat out?_________ number of times per week
9. When you go out to eat, what are the 3 most common places you go to eat?

a. ____________________________________
b. ____________________________________
c. ____________________________________

10. Do you avoid any of the following foods? (Check all that apply)

a. ____ Red meat b. ____ Poultry (Chicken, turkey)
c. ____ Fish d. ____ Dairy (milk, cheese)
e. ____ Vegetables f. ____ Fruits
g. ____ Fried foods h. ____ Breads
i. ____ Grains (Pasta, rice) j. ____ Fast foods
k. ____ Sweets (candy, desrts)
l. ____ Alcohol
m.____ Fats/oils (mayo, salad dressings, butter)

11. Do you currently take any dietary supplements?

____Yes ____No

12. If Yes, which ones? (Check all that apply)

a. ____ Creatine b. ____ Protein shakes
c. ____ Amino acids d. ____ HMB
e. ____ Vitamins f. ____ Minerals
g. ____ Herbs h. ____ "Andro" / DHEA
i. ____ Pyruvate
j. ____ Energy boosters (e.g. Ephedra, Ma Huang)
k. ____ Other, specify______________________________

13. Do you know which dietary supplements are banned or restricted by your sports organization?___ Yes ____No
14. In atypical workout, about how many cups of water, juice, sports drink, or non-caffeinated beverages do you drink before or during exercise? (Check one)

a. ____ none b.___ one or two cups
c. ____ three to five cups d.___ more than five cups

15. Overall, how satisfied are you with the physical appearance of your body? (Check one)

a. ____ very satisfied b.___ somewhat satisfied
c. ____ somewhat dissatisfied d. ___ very dissatisfied

16. How easy or difficult is it to for you to maintain your in-season weight? (Check one)

a. ____ very easy b.___ somewhat easy
c. ____ somewhat difficult d.___ very difficult

17. Do you have any personal goals for body composition?___ Yes ____No

If yes, which ones? (Check all that apply)

a. ____ Gain lean mass/weight gain
b. ____ Decrease body fat
c. ____ Lose weight
d. ____ Maintain current body composition
e. ____ None

Figure 4.1 Nutrition Screening Form for Athletes.

glycolysis system will allow ATP to be produced under anaerobic conditions for an additional 1 to 3 minutes after creatine phosphate levels diminish. This energy system will be used at the beginning of a road race; for a short duration, high-intensity event such as a 400-m sprint; in sports which are a combination of endurance and maximal outbursts, such as soccer, football, hockey, and basketball; and in the final sprint at the end of a road race. The aerobic system uses the three fuel substrates: carbohydrate, fat, and protein in the form of glucose, fatty acids, and amino acids for longer duration events such as distance cycling or a marathon.

ENERGY SUBSTRATES

To fuel the body optimally during activity, the body must have adequate stores of the macronutrients used for energy. Glycogen, the storage form of carbohydrate is stored in the muscle and liver. Most exercise is fueled by carbohydrate and fat, with protein providing a fuel source if carbohydrate stores are inadequate. Fuel usage is determined by the intensity and duration of activity as well as the level of training. During exercise, muscle glycogen is the major source, followed by liver glycogen and then blood glucose. Aerobic training and diet manipulation can significantly increase muscle glycogen stores (1). Muscle glycogen is used for intense, short duration activity and for endurance exercise. The rate of utilization of muscle glycogen is most rapid during the early part of exercise and is related to exercise intensity. Muscle glycogen declines with continued exercise, and is selectively depleted from the muscle(s) that are involved in physical work. As muscle glycogen stores decline, blood glucose and liver glycogen become important fuel sources. Plasma-free fatty acids will be used as a fuel source during endurance type activities through the process of adipose tissue lipolysis. Amino acids can be broken down to glucose to provide energy during activity, but only when carbohydrate stores are low.

Fatigue impairs performance. Subpar nutrition can be a significant cause of fatigue due to the following:

- Inadequate fluid intake
- Inadequate calorie intake
- Inadequate carbohydrate intake
- Inadequate protein intake
- Iron deficiency
- Vitamin/mineral deficiency

FLUID GUIDELINES

Fluid balance is essential for cardiovascular functioning, thermoregulation, injury prevention, optimal performance, and recovery from exercise. Fluid loss can be significant during exercise, in some cases up to 4 L/hour (2). In addition, exercise blunts the thirst mechanism, raising special challenges when encouraging the athlete to drink more. Fluid loss of more than 1.8% of total body weight can increase heart rate by 8 beats/minute thus impairing performance. In addition, mental functioning is impaired through a decrease in sustained attention, response time, and task accuracy, and an increase in error rate (3). Heat-related injuries increase with increased body water loss, as well as an increase in core body temperature. In addition, the perceived effort of exertion increases with dehydration, as does a difficulty in concentrating.

An athlete can become dehydrated due to changes in altitude, increases in training intensity and frequency, sudden climate changes, and long flights. The body cannot tolerate even slight dehydration, but unfortunately thirst sensation is dulled by exercise and voluntary fluid consumption is insufficient to meet fluid needs. Dehydration also reduces the gastric emptying rate, complicating the rehydration process (4). Curtailing fluid intake is a common practice in certain sports. The chronic dehydration that often accompanies weight class sports can impair the athlete's ability to optimally train and compete.

The goal of fluid intake is to prevent dehydration. The American College of Sports Medicine (ACSM) published a position stand on fluid replacement in 1996 providing rationale and guidelines for hydration (5). The National Athletic Trainer's Association published a similar position paper in 2000 (6). Athletes require a minimum fluid of 20 to 40 oz/hour of exercise, but most athletes consume only 8 oz/hour (5). A larger fluid intake during exercise leads to greater cardiac output, greater skin blood flow, lower core temperature, and reduced perceived effort of exertion (5). The overall goal is clear and copious urine as a sign that the body is well hydrated.

Athletes may ask for a recommendation for the types of fluid to consume. It is important to consider the sport, duration, calorie needs, and taste preferences. Water is a noncalorie fluid that works well for short duration activities, but it not as beneficial for exercise lasting longer than 60 minutes and/or shorter duration but more intense exercise. Juices can provide calories and carbohydrate but contain fructose, which has a decreased absorption rate and may cause gastrointestinal distress and are generally not advised before exercise. Carbonated beverages before activity may cause gastrointestinal distress, and oftentimes confer a feeling of fullness before fluid needs have been met. High levels of caffeine in the energy drinks may have a stimulatory effect, and the concentration of carbohydrate may slow gastric emptying. In addition, some of the protein powders contain diuretic herbs such as lovage, buchu, saw palmetto, and nettle. Alcoholic beverages have a diuretic effect, causing the body to lose valuable fluids before activity begins. Sports drinks can be an appropriate option for longer duration sports, and are certainly extremely popular with young athletes. Sports drinks contain a dilute glucose solution which stimulates water and sodium absorption so that more fluid is absorbed than from plain water (7,8). Because sports drinks have a fairly low carbohydrate content, they empty more rapidly from the stomach than a more concentrated beverage. With the flavor, athletes are also inclined to drink more than they would of plain water alone.

To achieve optimal gastric emptying, fluids should be cold or cool. A large volume of fluid empties more rapidly than smaller amounts. One liter of fluid empties from the stomach and will be absorbed by the intestine within 1 hour (5). This can be an advantage during exercise, when the athlete does not want to have a "full" feeling in the stomach while physically active. Athletes need to practice drinking during training to determine a comfort level, and to learn to drink proactively, instead of reactively. The recommended fluid intake is 2 to 3 quarts/day for basic needs plus 1 L of fluid for every 1,000 calories expended (5). Strategies for fluid replacement pre, during, and post exercise are listed here (8):

- *Pre-exercise* 500 mL (16 to 17 oz) of fluid 1 to 2 hours before exercise 8 to 16 oz (approximately 0.25 L–approximately 0.5 L) 15 minutes before exercise
- *During exercise* 4 to 16 oz every 15 to 20 minutes during exercise or (approximately 0.5 L–approximately 2 L/hour) with sports drink as a preferred beverage for optimal hydration and to decrease the risk of cramping
- *Post exercise* 24 oz of fluid (approximately 0.75 L) for every pound lost during exercise to achieve normal hydration within 6 hours of activity

For children younger than 10 years, the goal is to drink to satisfy thirst plus an additional 3 to 4 oz. Older children and adolescents should also drink to satisfy thirst plus an additional 8 oz of fluid (9).

Some athletes may inquire about the use of glycerol for hyperhydration. Glycerol is a three-carbon molecule which is the structural core of triglycerides and phospholipids. Glycerol ingestion increases blood osmolarity, decreasing urine production and increasing fluid retention. Although glycerol is easily absorbed, the increased weight may be a disadvantage, and glycerol loading can cause headaches, dizziness, bloating, and nausea (10,11). To encourage optimal hydration, coaches, athletic trainers, parents, and other health care professionals can assist the athlete in the following ways:

- Recommend that the athlete carry fluid with him/her. Dry mixes of sports drink, lemonade, or fruit punch are lightweight and easy to carry, and can be added to drinking water to provide fluid and carbohydrate.
- Reinforce the need to drink on schedule, not sporadically.
- Recommend that fluid breaks be a scheduled part of practice.
- Drink beyond thirst.
- Drink enough before exercise to have a full stomach. Gastric emptying is more rapid and efficient when the stomach is somewhat full rather than empty.
- Fluid is useful to the body only if swallowed, not poured over one's head.
- Encourage athletes to swallow, not spit fluids.
- Alcohol and caffeine are not optimal rehydration beverages due to their diuretic potential. Gently encourage other beverages before these are used.
- Educate athletes as to the disadvantages of using "energy" drinks such as *Red Bull, Lizard Fuel, Adrenaline Rush,* which contain large doses of caffeine which may not contribute to increased performance.
- Encourage athletes to weigh in and out to get an idea of the amount of fluid lost during exertion, and recommend 24 oz of fluid for every pound lost.
- Have players monitor the color of their urine, with the keywords being "light" in color and "lots" in amount as an indication of good hydration.

ELECTROLYTES

In addition to the fluid loss that accompanies exercise, electrolyte loss occurs as well. An athlete working out for 2 to 3 hours can lose up to 4 to 5 quarts of sweat. One pound of sweat contains 80 to 100 mg of potassium and 400 to 700 mg of sodium. In a 2- to 3-hour exercise session, an individual can lose up to 300 to 800 mg of potassium and 1,800 to 5,600 mg of sodium. The answer is not sodium or potassium tablets, but foods and fluids that provide the electrolytes (see Table 4.1). Encourage athletes to be more liberal with the use of salt or salty foods before working out, and to make an effort to include more high-potassium foods daily.

CALORIE REQUIREMENTS

If calorie needs are not met, the body will fatigue earlier and performance will be curtailed. Some athletes skimp on calories, increasing the likelihood of early fatigue and risk of injury. Others eat in excess of need, resulting in excess stores of adipose tissue, which can adversely affect performance. Calorie needs are higher for an athlete, than a nonexercising individual, and need to be individualized according to gender and weight. An athlete who has been injured may require additional calories early in the recovery process to aid tissue repair, but oftentimes will require fewer calories as the frequency and intensity of activity declines. Athletes who retire from their sport need to learn to eat less than in their playing days or suffer the consequences of carrying around excess weight. The Institutes of Medicine Food and Nutrition Board have recently revised calorie guidelines as follows (12):

For Male athletes 30 years and older:

$$\begin{aligned}\text{Total energy expenditure} &= 662 - 9.53 \times \text{age(yr)} + \text{PA} \\ &\quad \times (15.91 \times \text{weight([kg]} \\ &\quad + 539.6 \times \text{height[m])} \\ \text{PA} &= 1.48 \\ \text{kg} &= \text{weight (lb) divided by 2.2} \\ \text{m} &= \text{height (inches)} \\ &\quad \times 2.54 \text{ divided by } 100\end{aligned}$$

For Female athletes 30 years and older:

$$\begin{aligned}\text{Total energy expenditure} &= 354 - 6.91 \times \text{age(yr)} + \text{PA} \\ &\quad \times (9.36 \times \text{weight[kg]} + 726 \\ &\quad \times \text{height[m])} \\ \text{PA} &= 1.45 \\ \text{kg} &= \text{weight(lb) divided by 2.2} \\ \text{m} &= \text{height(in.)} \\ &\quad \times 2.54 \text{ divided by } 100\end{aligned}$$

For males and females between 19 and 30 years:

Add 7 kcal/day for women and 10 kcal/day for men for every year before 30

TABLE 4.1
POTASSIUM AND SODIUM SOURCES

Potassium Sources		
Food	**Amount**	**Potassium (mg)**
Gatorade	16 oz	60
Yogurt	8 oz	520
Grapefruit juice	8 oz	405
Banana	1 medium	451
Nectarine	1 medium	288
Orange	1	233
Sodium Sources		
Food	**Amount**	**Sodium (mg)**
Gatorade	16 oz	220
V8 juice	8 oz can	620
Pretzels	1 small handful	486
Nuts, dry roasted	1/4 cup	230
Cheese crackers (cheese on wheat)	6	252
Cheese pizza	1 slice	336
Dill pickle	1	1900
Soy sauce	1 tsp	305
Salt	1 tsp	2300

For males and females older than 30 years:

Subtract 7 kcal/day for women and 10 kcal/day for men for every year after 30

For children and teens younger than 19 years, use the following guidelines to estimate calories:

Boys/girls aged 7 to 10: 2,000 calories/day (13)
High school males: 3,000 to 6,000 calories/day (13)
High school females: 2,200 to 4,000 calories/day (14)

The goal is to achieve a balance in the diet through a mix of carbohydrate, protein, and fat. This has become especially challenging in light of the popular eating plans recommending that entire categories of foods be limited or avoided. Whereas endurance athletes are more apt to rely on carbohydrate as the mainstay of diet, strength-trained athletes may be more likely to have been advised to consume a high-protein diet. Although the overall amount of food consumed may vary, every athlete should aim to include protein, carbohydrate, and fat at every meal/snack.

CARBOHYDRATE REQUIREMENTS

Achieving and maintaining optimal carbohydrate intake is important for training intensity, preventing hypoglycemia during exercise, serving as a fuel substrate for working muscles, and assisting in postexercise recovery. Carbohydrate use increases with increased exercise intensity, but decreases with increased exercise duration. The goal of carbohydrate ingestion is to fill carbohydrate stores in the muscles and liver. The higher the initial glycogen the longer an athlete can exercise at a given intensity level. Eating increases glycogen stores whereas exercise depletes glycogen stores. Glycogen depletion can occur in sports requiring near maximal bursts of effort.

Athletes who do not optimally refuel may experience gradual and chronic glycogen depletion that can ultimately decrease endurance and performance. A tip-off is the athlete who experiences sudden weight loss, a consequence of training glycogen depletion. To maintain optimal glycogen stores, carbohydrate needs must be estimated on the basis of the number of hours the athlete trains daily. Carbohydrate requirements are always higher for training than for competition. Some athletes may consume inadequate amounts of carbohydrate due to calorie restriction, avoidance of certain foods such as sugar, fad diets, sporadic infrequent meals, and poor nutrition knowledge of good carbohydrate sources versus marginal choices. Needs can be estimated as per values shown in Table 4.2 (15):

There has been much discussion as to which type of carbohydrate is better for sports, simple versus complex. The distinction is not that clear, and what matters most is the total amount of carbohydrate consumed on a daily basis.

TABLE 4.2
ESTIMATION OF CARBOHYDRATE NEEDS

Number of Hours of Training	Grams Carbohydrate/ Pound Body Weight
1	2.7–3 gm
2	3.6 gm
3	4.5 gm
4	5.4–5.9 gm

Athletes can use the "Nutritional Facts" panel on a food label to quantify the amount of carbohydrate ingested. Some athletes are more comfortable ingesting carbohydrates in a liquid form, such as *Gatorade Energy Drink or UltraFuel.* Table 4.3 lists the carbohydrate content of common foods.

Recently, athletes have begun experimenting with manipulating the type of carbohydrate consumed at various points during exercise according to the glycemic index of the food (16). The glycemic index indicates the actual effects of carbohydrate-rich foods and fluids on blood glucose and insulin levels. The glycemic index ranks foods on the basis of the blood glucose response following ingestion of a test food that provides 50 gm of carbohydrate compared with the blood glucose response from a reference food. The response reflects the rate of digestion and absorption of a carbohydrate-rich food. Foods are classified into three categories—high, moderate, and low glycemic index foods as outlined in Table 4.4.

TABLE 4.3
CARBOHYDRATE CONTENT OF CERTAIN FOODS

Food	Amount	Carbohydrates (gm)
Bagel	2 oz	38
Bagel	4 oz	76
Cheerios	1 cup	23
Corn Pops	1 cup	28
Granola, low-fat	1 cup	82
Swedish fish	1 handful	39
Orange juice	8 oz	27
Coke	8 oz	27
Gatorade	8 oz	14
Sports gel	1 oz	28
Gatorade high-energy drink	12 oz	70
Yogurt and fruit	8 oz	42
Raisins	1/4 cup	31
Pretzels	1 handful	22

TABLE 4.4
HIGH, MODERATE, AND LOW GLYCEMIC INDEX FOODS

High Glycemic Index	Moderate Glycemic Index	Low Glycemic Index
Glucose	Rice cakes	Rice
Carrots	Vanilla wafers	Plums
White potatoes	Bagels	Dairy foods
Honey	Crackers	Apples
Corn flakes	Soda	Dried beans
White bread	Cakes/cookies	Pasta
Corn chips	Wheat bread	Peaches
Sports drinks	Sugar	Fructose
	Ice cream	Nuts
	Sweet potatoes	
	High-fiber cereal	
	Potato chips	

Although manipulating the meal choices based on the glycemic index may enhance carbohydrate availability and may improve athletic performance, the results will vary from athlete to athlete. Ingesting low glycemic index foods before competition may be used to allow for sustained availability of carbohydrates during exercise and to prevent an insulin surge and subsequent decrease in blood glucose. This may be most useful for the athlete who experiences hypoglycemia during competition or fatigue early. Athletes who are not thrilled with the food items on the low glycemic index list may opt to wait to consume carbohydrates a few minutes before exercise, in a liquid form. Once exercise begins, the rise in the hormones—epinephrine, norepinephrine, and growth hormone—inhibits insulin release and the blood glucose lowering effect of insulin. Athletes who are not sensitive to changes in blood glucose may benefit from consuming high glycemic index foods 1 hour before exercise, especially the athlete who has a morning event after an overnight fast; but this regime would not be beneficial for athletes participating solely in anaerobic events. Athletes will need to experiment to find out which foods work well, and more importantly do not cause gastrointestinal distress. Consuming dried beans or lentils before exercise may be fine for a cyclist, but may not be desirable for a runner.

Athletes have also experimented with the concept of carbohydrate loading or muscle glycogen supercompensation, which combines tapering of exercise with a high carbohydrate intake to top off muscle glycogen stores. The original method called for a depleting exercise protocol coupled with a low carbohydrate diet, followed by 3 days of rest with an extremely high carbohydrate diet. This often made the athlete feel exhausted during the low carbohydrate intake phase, and very heavy during the carbohydrate loading phase. Current guidelines recommend 3 to 5 days of carbohydrate loading to attain maximal glycogen levels and the exercise done to lower glycogen stores must be the same as the athlete's competitive event (17). Carbohydrate loading is advantageous only for endurance athletes whose event lasts longer than 90 minutes. Carbohydrate loading before a 10-K event is not helpful and may actually make the athlete feel heavier and stiff.

Carbohydrate needs for activity are divided into three distinct time periods: pre, during, and post exercise. The goal of pre-exercise carbohydrate is to provide energy for the athlete who exercises heavily in excess of 1 hour. Pre-exercise carbohydrate will also help prevent the feelings of hunger, which can be distracting, especially in a competition. The pre-exercise carbohydrate will also elevate blood glucose levels to provide energy for the exercising muscles. Current guidelines recommend 1.8 gm of carbohydrate/lb of body weight within 3 to 4 hours pre-exercise, and 0.5 gm/lb 1 hour pre-exercise (18,19). Examples are listed here.

Example

3 to 4 hours pre-exercise:

120-lb athlete would require 216 gm carbohydrate
12 oz glass of cranberry juice = 54 gm carbohydrate
8 oz yogurt, flavored with ½ cup granola = 96 gm carbohydrate
English muffin with 1 tbsp of peanut butter and 1 tbsp jelly = 46 gm
TOTAL: 196 gm of carbohydrate

0.5 gm carbohydrate 1 hour pre-exercise:

120-lb athlete: 60 gm carbohydrate
12 oz of Gatorade High Energy Drink = 90 gm

Carbohydrate consumption during exercise maintains the availability and oxidation of blood glucose late in exercise and improves endurance. During exercise, the ingestion of carbohydrate exerts a liver glycogen sparing effect resulting in delayed hypoglycemia. Ingesting carbohydrates may also be advantageous in stop and go sports, and should be encouraged during breaks in play. Guidelines recommend 30 to 60 gm of carbohydrate/hour during exercise in the form of:

5 to 10 oz of a sports drink every 15 to 20 minutes
2 gels/hour + water (average 20–28 gm carbohydrate/packet)
A handful of gummy type candy + water (20).

Postexercise fueling is vital for optimal recovery to enable an athlete to compete again in 2 or 24 hours. Exercise depletes muscle and liver glycogen stores and increases the likelihood of muscle damage; therefore, post exercise fuel in the right combination and at the appropriate time can assist in muscle tissue repair, resynthesis of muscle and liver glycogen stores, and restoration of normal hydration. It takes 20 to 24 hours post exercise for the body to replenish muscle glycogen stores maximally. Timing is an essential part of the recovery process, because the muscles are most receptive to fuel within 15 minutes of exercise, when the enzymes that produce glycogen are most active and can most effectively replace depleted glycogen stores. A delay in intake of post exercise fuel will slow the recovery rate. Because the energy demands of training exceed those of competition, post exercise eating needs to be a routine part of the athlete's training regimen and not just used in a competition situation. Refueling should be a priority for an athlete after workouts or competition. Because exhaustive, intense exercise can suppress appetite, an athlete may complain of an inability or lack of desire to eat after activity. Athletes should be encouraged to eat and/or drink foods/fluids that they enjoy, but most importantly, the food needs to be readily available and accessible. Table 4.5 lists some good postexercise foods/beverages.

The recommendations are 0.7 gm of carbohydrate/lb within 30 minutes of exercise and again 2 hours later for those training for more than 90 minutes at a time (21).

Example

For the 120 lb athlete, 84 gm of carbohydrate:

A 4 oz bagel with 1 tbsp jelly = 89 gm carbohydrate
16 oz *UltraFuel* = 100 gm carbohydrate
16 oz fruit punch and a cereal bar = 87 gm carbohydrate

Some studies have suggested that consuming protein and carbohydrate together post exercise can enhance muscle glycogen resynthesis by stimulating insulin. The

TABLE 4.5
POST EXERCISE FOODS/FLUIDS

Nonperishable Items
Sports bars
Peanut butter or cheese crackers
Dry cereal
Trail mix with cereal, nuts, and dried fruit
Granola or cereal bars
Graham crackers
Breakfast bars
Perishable Items
Yogurt
Pudding
Cans of a high-carbohydrate drink (Gatorade Nutrition Shake, Boost, Carnation Instant Breakfast)
Milk to which a chocolate powder, or Instant Breakfast could be added

recommended guidelines call for a 1:3 ratio of protein to carbohydrate (22–24).

Examples of this would include:

Gatorade Nutrition Shake (carbohydrate/protein sports supplement beverage)
Sports bars (not the high protein or low carbohydrate type)
Trail mix of 3 parts cereal to 1 part nuts
Yogurt and granola

PROTEIN REQUIREMENTS

Although most athletes are aware of the need for carbohydrate as part of a good training diet, protein intake tends to run the gamut from minimal to excessive intake, where the athletes who need it most consume the least and those who need it least consume the most. Protein is important for muscle growth and repair, and aids in recovery and repair following muscle damage. As a fuel source, protein will provide up to 15% of the fuel during activity when muscle glycogen stores are low, and only 5% when muscle glycogen stores are adequate (25). If training sessions are too frequent, and/or protein intake is insufficient to meet needs, protein catabolism will exceed anabolism resulting in reduced gains or loss of body protein (26). Achieving optimal protein nutriture can be challenging. Athletes who do not meet their needs are more likely to experience decreased muscle mass, a suppressed immune system, increased risk of injury, and chronic fatigue. Conversely, athletes who routinely exceed protein needs may experience increased risk of dehydration, increased body fat stores, calcium loss, and an unbalanced diet that is often deficient in carbohydrate. Protein requirements are outlined in Table 4.6 (26).

Traditionally, strength-training athletes have emphasized protein, sometimes to the exclusion of other essential nutrients; however, the maximum recommended protein intake is 1 gm/lb of body weight. On the other hand, endurance athletes require more protein in the early stages of training to increase aerobic enzymes in the muscle, for red blood cell and myoglobin formation, and to replace protein stores that are oxidized during exercise. Ideally, food sources of protein will comprise most protein in the diet, rather than protein powders or amino acid supplements. Table 4.7 lists various food sources of protein.

TABLE 4.6
PROTEIN REQUIREMENTS FOR VARIOUS TYPES OF ATHLETES

Type of Athlete	Protein Requirements (gm/lb body weight/d)
Recreational athlete	0.5–0.75
Competitive athlete	0.6–0.9
Athlete building mass	0.7–0.9
Teenage athlete	0.9–1.0
Athlete restricting intake	0.7–1.0
Maximum usable amount	1.0

TABLE 4.7
PROTEIN CONTENT OF SELECT FOODS

Food	Amount	Protein (gm)
Chicken breast	3 oz	21
Chicken thigh	3 oz	21
Cod	3 oz	21
Hamburger	3 oz	21
Steak	3 oz	21
Pork chop	3 oz	21
Egg	1	7
Soy burger		15–18
Nuts	1/4 cup	10
Peanut butter	2 tbsp	8
Cheese	1 slice	7
Refried beans	1/2 cup	7
Milk	8 oz	8
Yogurt	8 oz	9–11
Protein powders	per scoop	32–45
Nonfat dry milk powder	1/4 cup	8
Amino acid pills	1 serving	10

Many athletes are drawn to protein powders or amino acid supplements as a means to increase protein intake. No studies have shown benefits of amino acid supplements as an ergogenic aid, and gastrointestinal distress can be a problem (27). Protein powders can be fairly costly, require mixing, and palatability can be a problem. If an athlete wants to use a protein powder, nonfat dry milk powder is inexpensive, shelf-stable, tasteless, and an excellent source of calcium as well. The NCAA only permits institutions to provide non–muscle-building supplements, or products that contain no more than 30% of the total calories from protein, to student athletes; so meeting protein needs through food will be extremely important (27).

FAT REQUIREMENTS

Fat is an energy substrate for low-intensity, longer duration exercise. Fat provides a concentrated calorie source to provide energy for the athlete. A diet that is too low in fat may limit performance by inhibiting intramuscular triglyceride storage, thereby resulting in earlier fatigue during exercise (28). Excess fat intake can increase fat stores and cause gastrointestinal discomfort before exercise. Conversely, inadequate fat intake can decrease serum testosterone thereby decreasing muscle mass (29).

TABLE 4.8
FAT CONTENT OF SELECT FOODS

Food Item	Amount	Fat Content (gm)
Olive oil[a]	1 tbsp	14
Soft margarine[a]	1 tbsp	11
Mayonnaise	1 tbsp	11
Salad dressings:		
Italian[a]	1 tbsp	7
Ranch	1 tbsp	10
Blue cheese	1 tbsp	8
Nuts[a]	1/4 cup	32
Peanut butter[a]	2 tbsp	16
Cream cheese	2 tbsp	11
Bacon	2 slices	6
Chips	1 oz	10
French fries	Small	12
Ice cream	1 scoop	20
Prime rib	3 oz	23
Burger	1 regular	10
Big Mac	1	32
Drumstick, fried	1	11
Wing, fried	1	15

[a]Heart healthier choice.

TABLE 4.9
DIETARY REFERENCE INTAKES

Zinc: 15 mg
Vitamin C
  Women: 75 mg
  Men: 90 mg
Tolerable upper limit: 2,000 mg
Iron
  Women: 15 mg
  Men: 10 mg
Calcium: men and women
  9–13 yr: 1,300 mg
  19–50 yr: 1,000 mg
  >51 yr: 1,200 mg
Tolerable upper limit: 2,500 mg
For athletes who need to boost iron stores through food and/or supplemental iron, it is important to note that some foods/nutrients interfere with iron absorption:

- Phytates (bran, whole grains)
- Oxalates (spinach, beer, nuts)
- Polyphenols (coffee, tea)
- Excess intake of calcium and magnesium
- Consumption of guarana

Although recommendations for fat intake can vary from 20% to 40% of daily calories, a good rule of the thumb to estimate is as follows:

Weight(lb) × 0.45 = number of grams of fat per day (30).

Sources of fat are listed in Table 4.8.

The following tables provide guidelines for male and female athletes on the basis of body weight and number of servings per day. This can be an easy way to steer athletes toward achieving nutrient requirements.

Athlete's guide to proper fueling:

Appendix 4.2 give lists of carbohydrate, protein, and fat food choices.

Carbohydrate food choices contain 50 gm of carbohydrate
Protein food choices contain 20 gm of protein
Fat containing food choices have 10 gm of fat

MICRONUTRIENT REQUIREMENTS

Athletes will often inquire as to the need for vitamin–mineral supplementation. The needs for an athlete may be slightly higher than for someone who does not exercise regularly; but these requirements can be met through a multivitamin–mineral supplement, not a mega dose tablet. In 1998, the Food and Nutrition Board of the National Academy of Sciences established Dietary Reference Intakes for select vitamins and minerals (31). The recommendations for minerals are listed in Table 4.9.

Ways to Increase Iron Supply

- Include more lean red meat or dark meat of poultry (several times a week).
- Do not drink coffee or tea with meals—wait 1 hour.
- Add orange juice or other vitamin C–containing foods to meals.
- Consider a cast iron skillet for cooking acidic foods (spaghetti sauce, tomato soup).
- Eat more mixed meals (protein and carbohydrate together instead of just a bagel or salad).

  The iron in plant foods is better absorbed if eaten at the same meal with the iron in animal foods and a vitamin C source.
- Cook foods for a short amount of time in a minimal amount of water to maximize iron intake.
- Choose breads, cereals, pastas with the words *iron-enriched* or *fortified* on the label.

Table 4.10 lists animal (heme) and plant (non-heme) iron sources.

WEIGHT MANAGEMENT ISSUES

Every athlete has to face issues surrounding weight at some point in his/her career. The question is whether body fat or weight is the most important variable, and is dependent on the type of sport. Weight standards

TABLE 4.10
IRON SOURCES

Heme Iron	Nonheme Iron
Red meat (beef, pork, lamb)	Grains (cereals, whole grain or enriched breads)
Poultry (especially dark meat)	Dark green leafy vegetables
Fish	Dried beans and peas
Chicken or beef liver	
Oysters	
Plant-Based Iron-Rich Foods	
Dried fruit (apricots, prunes, dates)	
Beans	
Peas	
Tofu	
Kale	
Collard greens	
Cream of wheat	
Iron-fortified cereals	
Blackstrap molasses	
Oatmeal	
Sunflower seeds	
Almonds	
Enriched pasta or macaroni	
Wheat germ	
Refried beans	
Tomato juice	
Prune juice	

are used more in certain sports than others, such as the following:

- Sports based on skill (archery, bowling); weight is generally not an issue
- Sports with weight division (crew, wrestling, jockeys)
- Sports with low body fat for optimal performance (distance runners)
- Sports with appearance/aesthetic criteria (gymnastics, figure skating)

Body Composition Assessment Tools

The goals of body composition measurement are to assess fat mass and fat-free mass. Unfortunately, many athletes are traumatized by the reading, or chastised by coaches who believe in a certain magic number. As a health care provider, should an athlete need to have body composition measured, it is important to have an understanding of the various tools used.

1. *Hydrostatic Weighing Assesses body density to determine fat.* Leaner individuals weigh more under the water because of higher body density and lower percentage body fat. This method is established and has good accuracy. However, the subject needs to be submerged, and this method may underestimate percentage body fat in black athletes because of higher bone density.
2. *Displacement Plethysmography—Bod Pod.* Body volume is derived from the difference between the empty chamber air volume and air volume with the individual inside. This method hassimilar accuracy to underwater weighing, and is less stressful to the subject. However, the equipment is expensive and there is limited research on validation of body composition using this technique.
3. *Dual Energy X-ray Absorptiometry (DEXA).* The DEXA measures attenuation of two energies of x-rays through the body. This method is unique in that it can provide regional and whole body percentage fat estimates. It is very expensive and also requires a highly skilled technician.
4. *Anthropometry.* Anthropometric measurements include:
   - Height and weight measurements
   - Limbs and torso circumference
   - Skinfold thickness, which measures the thickness of subcutaneous tissue proportional to the total body fat mass to estimate the regional distribution of subcutaneous fat.

   Results can vary depending on the technician's skill, type of caliper used, and the prediction equation. This method is not as accurate for very underweight, or very muscular or overfat athletes.
5. *Body Mass Index (BMI).* BMI assesses weight relative to height but overestimates body fat in muscular individuals.
6. *Bioelectrical Impedance Analysis (BIA).* The BIA method passes a small electrical current through the body to measure the resistance encountered. Tissues with higher water content conduct electrical currents with less resistance. However, the accuracy of the results is affected by the subject's hydration status. BIA consistently overestimates body fat in very lean subjects and underestimates body fat in the obese. In addition, there is a lack of validation studies in populations other than white European and North American non-Hispanic whites.
7. *Near Infrared Interactance (Futrex).* This method uses near infrared spectroscopy to provide information about the chemical composition of the body. The limitations of this technique are that it estimates fatness over the biceps, not the whole body.

To get the most out of these tests, the subject should not exercise several hours before the assessment. In addition, adequate hydration is critical. The measurement of height and weight should be precise. To assess changes in body composition, the same measurer using the same technique should perform measurements. It is very important to use population-specific equations to determine body fat when appropriate.

TABLE 4.11
BODY FAT PERCENTAGES IN ATHLETES[a]

	% FAT	
Sport	**Men**	**Women**
Baseball/softball	8–14	12–18
Basketball	6–12	10–16
Bodybuilding	5–8	6–12
Canoe/kayaking	6–12	10–16
Cycling	5–11	8–15
Fencing	8–12	10–16
Football	6–18	—
Golf	10–16	12–20
Gymnastics	5–12	8–16
Horse racing	6–12	10–16
Ice/field hockey	8–16	12–18
Pentathlon	—	8–15
Racquetball	6–14	10–18
Rowing	6–14	8–16
Rugby	6–16	—
Skating	5–12	8–16
Skiing	7–15	10–18
Ski jumping	7–15	10–18
Soccer	6–14	10–18
Swimming	6–12	10–18
Synchronized swimming	—	10–18
Tennis	6–14	10–20
Track and field, running events	5–12	8–15
Track and field, field events	8–18	12–20
Triathlon	5–12	8–15
Volleyball	7–15	10–18
Weightlifting	5–12	10–18
Wrestling	5–16	—

[a]Based on several studies.

Table 4.11 lists body fat percentages in athletes.

Many athletes strive to attain the lowest body fat possible, jeopardizing health and performance in the process. Disordered eating behavior to reduce weight can decrease the metabolic rate, making the body less efficient at burning fat. Rapid weight loss reduces the plasma volume and blood distribution to active tissues and may adversely affect thermoregulation, which can impair performance. An athlete who is interested in losing or gaining weight should seek the expertise of a sports nutritionist who can customize a program to allow the athlete to meet his/her goals.

Because athletes often try fad diets for weight loss, which are often restricted in energy intake, the end result can be a tired, poorly nourished athlete who is overly hungry, and does not exercise or recover efficiently. It is important to note that achieving success with weight management is a minimal investment of 3 months to change the underlying habits that determine food choices. Here are some facts about weight loss worth sharing with athletes:

- Body fat loss does not happen overnight.
- Dieting is stressful to the body.
- For a weight loss program to be successful, the athlete must be ready to address his/her weight and put the time into working on weight loss goals.
- Weight loss typically occurs in steps, not a slide. Hitting a plateau is a very normal part of weight loss.
- Successful weight loss combines:
  - Physical activity
  - Eating habits/behaviors
  - Food choices
- The goal is to lose excess body fat, not muscle mass or fluid. Athletes who need or want to lose weight should have a body fat assessment, to more accurately set weight goals, so that the athlete does not end up losing lean mass.
- Losing weight has two components:
  - Weight loss
  - Keeping the weight off

Many athletes try the following misguided and incorrect techniques for weight loss:

- Assuming that dieting is all about will power
- Curtailing eating after 6 p.m. because of the misguided belief that eating later will put on the pounds
- Skipping meals
- Skimping on calories
- Excluding entire food groups
- Eliminating all foods that one likes
- Ignoring the importance of the portion size
- Forgetting about the calorie cost of beverages
- Setting unrealistic weight goals
- Opting for the fad diets or gimmicks

Those who are most successful with weight loss are monitoring their intake. We have to know what we eat, how much, and when to be able to modify our behaviors. A good starting place is to have your athletes keep a food log of everything that goes into the mouth, whether a food or beverage, meal or snack to get an idea of the following:

Food and beverage choices
Eating due to hunger or other reason
Amount eaten
Time of eating

Activities while eating—talking on the phone, eating in the car, working on the computer while eating, or watching television

Appendix 4.3 depicts an example of a food diary. Encourage your athletes to keep a food log for a few days to get an idea of what current eating is like.

TABLE 4.12
TECHNIQUES FOR WEIGHT GAIN

Aim for 500–1,000 additional calories daily
Eat on a schedule, more frequent meals and snacks
The goal is 1/2 lb of weight gain per week
Foods and beverages need to contain calories (juice instead of water)
Choose higher calorie items (nuts instead of pretzels)
Eat 1/4 more at each meal and snack
Eat more every day of the week
Eating needs to be a priority

It is very important to encourage athletes to include foods that they like, but perhaps in smaller amounts, and to make athletes aware that an occasional "cheat" is fine. Weight loss is a long term goal, not an overnight effort.

There are athletes who try as they can, seem unable to gain weight. Oftentimes, the problem is the erratic eating pattern, and the assumption that eating as much as one can at one time will rectify the problem. Consistency with number of meals per day is the most important variable for weight gain. Table 4.12 outlines techniques for weight gain.

Disordered Eating

Body image distortion and eating disorders are physically and psychologically damaging. Athletes with body image issues and/or eating issues need to be dealt with, preferably through a multidisciplinary approach including the physician, therapist, dietitian, and athletic trainer. For the best outcome, the individual who has the best rapport with the athlete should be the point person (32). Table 4.13 lists the characteristics of anorexia athletica (33).

TABLE 4.13
CHARACTERISTICS OF ANOREXIA ATHLETICA

Intense fear of weight gain in a person who is already lean
Restricted calorie intake coupled with excessive exercise
Energy intake is below that necessary for training
Binge eating may be present
Laxatives and diuretics may be used
Delayed puberty
Menstrual dysfunction
Gastrointestinal complaints

(33,34).

NUTRITIONAL ERGOGENIC AIDS

Those who work in the sports arena must be aware of products that athletes/clients choose to take, and offer guidelines for use as well as information regarding side effects. The goal of nutritional ergogenic aids is **performance enhancement**, but unfortunately, several supplements may have the opposite effect, or act as ergolytic substances. Nutritional supplements are big business, and the list of products is growing daily. Athletes will continue to look for the magic bullet, and as highly disciplined as one might be regarding training, the same degree of care and perseverance does not necessarily translate to supplement use.

The important points about supplement usage include the following:

- Supplements are not one size fits all
- Natural and safe are NOT synonymous terms
- Supplements may be age and gender specific
- Supplements can adversely interact with prescription medications
- Supplements are sports specific, and may be position specific
- The efficacy of supplements is contingent upon the underlying hydration, diet, and training
- The issue of "stacking" may create safety problems
- The Internet has increased the availability and accessibility of supplements

The efficacy of a product may be affected by fluid balance, meal composition, and training. In addition, athletes who are already at the peak of physical ability and consume an optimal diet will for the most part realize little, if any, benefit from supplement use. There is nothing wrong with the placebo effect, provided the supplement will not be harmful to the athlete. It is important to work with the athlete, not talk to them about supplement use. The Dietary Supplement and Health Education Act (DSHEA) of 1994 details labeling guidelines that were put into effect in March 1999. Labels must have a supplement facts panel detailing the contents and amount, and an ingredient list. This Act also allows companies to make claims about their products, which can cause consumer confusion.

Table 4.14 lists the most commonly cited reasons for use and Table 4.15 lists the most commonly used supplements.

The most frequently and widely used category of nutritional ergogenic aids are those with supposed anabolic effects, to mimic the benefits of steroids in a legal manner. Creatine is by far the most widely used supplement taken by both recreational and professional athletes. Creatine is synthesized in the kidney, pancreas, and liver from amino

TABLE 4.14
REASONS FOR SUPPLEMENT USE

The "Edge"
Alterations in body composition
Weight management
Injury prevention
Exercise recovery
Increased energy
Peer use

acid precursors, methionine, arginine, and glycine. It is also found in meat, fish, and poultry and is absorbed intact by the gut when ingested. The ergogenic effect of creatine is attributed to its ability to increase tissue creatine levels, resulting in increased work capacity for intense activity and expediting the exercise recovery rate. This effect is seen more with activities requiring maximal or near maximal effort, not those involving submaximal endurance exercise.

These benefits are most likely to be seen with a loading regimen of 20 to 25 gm of creatine over 5 to 7 days, divided into four, 5 gm doses, or 3 gm/day over a 30-day period. For optimal effect, each dose of creatine should be consumed with some carbohydrate, and without caffeine, which can counteract the ergogenic effect. Muscle hypertrophy and fluid retention can cause a weight gain of 4 to 7 lb during the loading phase. This increase may be advantageous for the strength athlete, but less so for the athlete who must move quickly. The extra weight may be more of a detriment than a benefit. Short-term studies do not show an increase in muscle strains, cramps, or muscle pulls with creatine, but encouraging the athlete to maintain optimal hydration status is crucial. Creatine loading is sufficient to achieve the ergogenic effect, as the creatine levels will fall to presupplementation levels 6 weeks post loading. Another appropriate loading dose is 3 gm/day over a 1-month period. Use should be discontinued with training cessation or injury. Because studies have not been conducted on high school athletes, it would be prudent to dissuade this group from supplementing with creatine; however, because this is not always possible, try to encourage young athletes to use only half the dose, and reinforce the need for adequate training, and fluid and fuel intake.

Other anabolic agents include HMB (beta-hydroxy-beta-methyl-butyrate), which in clinical studies has resulted in an increase in muscle mass, although the number of studies has been quite small. Boron is a trace mineral involved in cellular functions, but does not increase testosterone levels, as claims would suggest. It can suppress appetite and impair digestion in doses more than 50 mg/day. Yohimbe is derived from the tree bark of a South American plant, and confers a stimulant effect, not an anabolic effect. Ingestion of this product can cause dizziness, nervousness, headaches, nausea, vomiting, and increased blood pressure. It can also interact with blood pressure medication and can increase the toxicity of psychotherapeutic medications and may be harmful to the kidneys. Chromium is an essential mineral involved in blood glucose control, which can be taken in a dosage of 50 to 300 μg/day, but it does not have any anabolic effects.

The other supposed anabolic agents include dehydroepiandrosterone (DHEA), androstenedione, and tribulus terrestris (Tribestan). All of these are banned by the NCAA, NFL, USOC, and The American Tennis Federation. Recently, an article published in JAMA demonstrated the ineffectiveness of androstenedione as an anabolic substance or strength enhancer, but did demonstrate potential worrisome side effects including a decrease in serum high density lipoprotein (HDL) level and an increase in serum estrone and estradiol, increasing the likelihood of gynecomastia (breast enlargement). Several laboratory tests have shown that the amount of actual product in these supplements can vary dramatically, and some products contain 19-norandrostenedione, which can result in a positive drug test for nandrolone.

One of the newer products that has seen a rise in popularity and an increase in sales revenue is NO (nitric oxide) sold as NO stimulators such as NO XPlode. NO, or nitric oxide is formed from the amino acid arginine. NO stimulators such as *NO Xplode*. Advertised as a hemodilator with anabolic claims, the studies have not demonstrated an increase in muscle blood flow during exercise following NO ingestion.

Protein is certainly essential for muscle growth and development, but food sources will typically suffice to meet needs. If any supplements are used, protein powders will confer far more benefits than amino acid supplements; however, some protein powders are very high in protein, and are typically used in addition to protein-containing foods. The research on amino acid supplementation has not shown a consistent performance-enhancing effect, and has been associated with gastrointestinal side effects that may negate any potential ergogenic benefits. In addition, selective amino acid supplementation is a very inefficient

TABLE 4.15
MOST COMMONLY USED SUPPLEMENTS

Creatine
Ginseng
Ephedra
Protein supplements: powders/amino acids
Vitamin–mineral supplements
Anti-inflammatory supplements

way to provide protein to the body, and can create an amino acid imbalance.

Energy Boosters

Many athletes choose to take supplements to boost energy. The most common ingredients in these type of products are (a) ginseng, (b) ephedra, and (c) caffeine. Ginseng functions as an adaptogen, or immune system stimulant, but does not have an effect on performance. Athletes who choose to take ginseng should look for *Panax* ginseng standardized to 4% to 7% ginsenosides with the following dosing regimen: 100 to 200 mg/day for 2 to 3 weeks, then 1 to 2 weeks of no use.

Ephedra (Ma Huang) is a central nervous system stimulant that is found in many cold, cough, and antiasthmatic preparations. It is an extremely popular "fat-burning" supplement sold as *Metabolife, Xenadrine, Herbal Rush, Energy Rush, Thermoburn,* or *Thermofuel* among others. Ephedra may delay fatigue by sparing the body's glycogen reserves during exercise, BUT can also increase blood pressure, respiration rate, heart rate, anxiety, migraines, and irregular heartbeat and cause insomnia and nervousness. Oftentimes ephedra and caffeine will be in the same product, which can be detrimental to the heart. The maximum safe level of ephedra is 24 mg/day, but many of these products contain in excess of 300 mg/dose. This supplement is contraindicated in those with a history of heart disease or hypertension, kidney or thyroid disease, seizure disorder, or diabetes.

Synephrine (bitter orange, green orange, kijitsu, citrus aurantium) is also a central nervous system stimulant. Marketed as ephedra-free, many athletes turn to this product instead. *Xenadrine, HydroxyCut, MM4, ThermoAdvantage,* and *System Six* are some of the products on the market. Ephedra and synephrine are banned by the USOC, NFL, and NCAA.

Caffeine is a stimulant that may work in certain athletes by increasing free fatty acid availability to delay fatigue, improve reaction time, and reduce the perceived effort of exertion. It tends to be most effective in caffeine-naïve, trained endurance athletes with a dose of 200 to 300 mg of caffeine 1 hour before the event. The legal limit of caffeine is 800 mg, but this level can cause nervousness, anxiety, irritability, headaches, diarrhea, and increased urination. In addition to products such as Vivarin, No-Doz, and Excedrin, caffeine can be found in herbal forms: guarana, mate, and kola nut. Taroxotone is a caffeine supplement containing 450 mg of caffeine/dose.

Weight Loss Agents

The other category of supplements is weight loss agents. These products contain ingredients such as L-carnitine (may prevent lactic acid accumulation but does not promote fat loss), quercetin (an antioxidant important for the heart but not to lose body fat), hydroxycitrate (a diuretic), ephedra and caffeine, and senna and/or cascara (herbal laxatives). Chitin or chitosan is advertised as a fat trapper or fat blocker, and is the ground up shells of insects and shellfish that may lower cholesterol, but does not lower body fat. It can bind with calcium, iron, and magnesium, and interfere with the absorption of vitamins A, D, E, and K. Weight loss experienced with the use of these products is primarily due to water loss associated with the laxative/diuretic components, and not fat loss. There is some research looking at conjugated linoleic acid (CLA) for fat loss, but the studies have been small and are not conclusive.

Anti-inflammatory Supplements

Athletes are intrigued by the claims for products that say they will diminish pain, and/or aid in cartilage regeneration. The most popular supplements are listed here.

- *SAM-e (S-adenosylmethionine).* May increase cartilage thickness

  May relieve pain and improve joint mobility

  May be as effective as nonsteroidal anti-inflammatory drugs (NSAIDS) 200 to 400 mg thrice a day

  May cause nausea in large doses
- *Phosphatidylserine (PS).* May not be of benefit for injury prevention due to the effects on cortisol levels
- *Methylsulfonylmethane (MSM).* May relieve pain 2 gm/day or applied externally as a cream, gel, or lotion
- *Turmeric (Curcumin).* May work best for acute injuries 400 mg 3 times a day
- *Boswellia.* An herb in extract form with anti-inflammatory properties 300 to 500 mg/day to decrease inflammation and soreness
- *Glucosamine and chondroitin sulfate.* May reduce pain and stiffness

  May take 2 months to see results and can cause indigestion and nausea

  Glucosamine may be contraindicated for diabetics and chondroitin should not be used by hemophiliacs or those on aspirin or blood thinners

  The dosage is glucosamine 500 mg thrice a day and chondroitin sulfate 400 mg thrice a day

The following suggestions are applicable to health care providers working with athletes:

- Ask clients what they take as well as the dose and frequency
- Ask to see the label of the product
- Document the information in the medical record
- Inquire rehydration tactics and eating habits
- Encourage clients to try only one product at a time
- Advise the athlete to discontinue supplement use if he/she notices any unusual dizziness, stomach upset, or headaches
- Be familiar with supplements

Appendix 4.4 lists some reputable references for supplements.

SUMMARY

All athletes have a responsibility to be optimally nourished as part of their training and conditioning. Everyone involved in the athlete's care should stress the need for adequate fuel and fluid in addition to helping the athlete make informed choices regarding supplement use. The role of nutrition in maximizing performance, enhancing recovery and injury prevention, and rehabilitation can only help the athlete to perform at his/her peak, as well as improve the quality of life.

REFERENCES

1. William MH. *Nutrition for health, fitness and sport*, 5th ed. Boston: McGraw-Hill, 1999.
2. Sawka MN, Pandolf KB. Effects of body water loss on physiological function and exercise performance. In: Gisolfi CV, Lamb DR, eds. *Perspectives in exercise science and sports medicine: fluid homeostasis during exercise*. Indianapolis: Benchmark Press, 1990:1–38.
3. Murray R. Fluid needs in hot and cold environments. *Int J Sports Nutr* 1995;5:S62–S73.
4. Neufer PD, Young AJ, Sawka MN. Gastric emptying during exercise: effects of heat stress and dehydration. *Eur J Appl Physiol* 1989;58:433–439.
5. American College of Sports Medicine. Position stand on exercise and fluid replacement. *Med Sci Sports Exerc* 1996;28:i–vii.
6. National Athletic Trainer's Association. Position statement: fluid replacement for athletes. *J Athl Train* 2000;35:212–224.
7. Montain SJ, Coyle EF. The influence of graded dehydration on hyperthermia and cardiovascular drift during exercise. *J Appl Physiol* 1992;73(4): 1340–1350.
8. Murray R. Fluid, electrolytes, and exercise I. In: Dunford M, ed. *Sports nutrition: a practice manual for professionals*, 4th ed. Chicago: American Dietetic Association, 2006:94–115.
9. Maughan RJ, Shirreffs SM, Galloway DR, et al. Dehydration and fluid replacement in sports and exercise. *Sports Exerc Inj* 1995;1:148–153.
10. Bar-Or O. Children's responses to exercise in hot climates: implications for performance and health. *Sports Sci Exch* 1994;7(49):1–5.
11. Murray R. Nutrition for the marathon and other endurance sports: environmental stress and dehydration. *Med Sci Sports Exerc* 1992;24:S319–S323.
12. Wagner DR. Hyperhydrating with glycerol: implications for athletic performance. *J Am Diet Assoc* 1999;99:207–212.
13. Food and Nutrition Board. *Dietary reference intakes for energy, carbohydrate, fiber, fat, fatty acids, cholesterol, protein, and amino acids*. National Academy Press, 2002.
14. Food and Nutrition Board. *Recommended dietary allowances*, 10th ed. Washington. National Academy Press, 1989.
15. Walberg-Rankin J. Dietary carbohydrate as an ergogenic aid for prolonged and brief competition in sport. *Intl J Sports Nutr* 1995;5(suppl):S13–S28.
16. Coleman E. Carbohydrate and exercise. In: Rosenbloom C, ed. *Sports nutrition: a guide for the health professional working with active people*. Chicago: The American Dietetic Association, 2000.
17. Burke LM, Collier GR, Hargreaves M. The glycemic index: a new tool in sports nutrition? *Int J Sports Nutr* 1998;8:401–415.
18. Sherman WM, Costill DL, Fink WJ, et al. The effect of exercise and diet manipulation on muscle glycogen and its subsequent use during performance. *Int J Sports Med* 1981;2:114–118.
19. Sherman WM, Brodowicz G, Wright DA, et al. Effects of 4 hr pre-exercise carbohydrate feedings on cycling performance. *Med Sci Sports Exerc* 1989;12:598–604.
20. Sherman WM, Peden MC, Wright DA. Carbohydrate feeding 1 hr before exercise improves cycling performance. *Am J Clin Nutr* 1991;54:866–870.
21. Coyle EF, Montain SJ. Benefits of fluid replacement with carbohydrate during exercise. *Med Sci Sports Exerc* 1992;24(Suppl 9):S324–S330.
22. Ivy JL, Lee MC, Broznick JT, et al. Muscle glycogen storage after different amounts of carbohydrate ingestion. *J Appl Physiol* 1988;65:2018–2023.
23. Blom PCS, Hostmark AT, Vaage O, et al. Effects of different post exercise sugar diets on the rate of muscle glycogen synthesis. *Med Sci Sports Exerc* 1987;19:471–496.
24. Tarnopolsky MA. Influence of differing macronutrient intakes on muscle glycogen resynthesis after resistance exercise. *J Appl Physiol* 1998;84: 890–896.
25. Tarnopolsky MA, Bowman M, MacDonald JR, et al. Post exercise protein-carbohydrate supplementation increases muscle glycogen in men and women. *J Appl Physiol* 1997;83:1877–1883.
26. Lemon PWR. Effects of exercise on dietary protein requirements. *Int J Sports Nutr* 1998;8:426–447.
27. Clark N. *Nancy Clark's sports nutrition guidebook*, 2nd ed. Champaign: Human Kinetics, 1997.
28. *NCAA Bylaw* 16.5.2.2 Proposal 99–72, August 2000. Nutritional Supplements.
29. William C. Dietary macro and micronutrient requirements of endurance athletes. *Proc Nutr Soc* 1998;57:1–8.
30. Brownell KD, Nelson-Steen S, Wilmore JH. Weight regulation in athletes: analysis of metabolic and health effects. *Med Sci Sports Exerc* 1987;18: 546–556.
31. Murray R, Horswill CA. Nutrient requirements for competitive sports. In: Wolinsky I, ed. *Nutrition in exercise and sport*, 3rd ed. Boca Raton: CRC Press, 1998.
32. Food and Nutrition Board. National Academy of Sciences. *Dietary reference intakes*. 1998.
33. Anorexia Nervosa and Related Eating Disorders (ANRED). *Identifying the athlete with an eating disorder and the initial intervention*. http://www/anred.com/ath-id.html, 01/06.
34. Sundot-Borgen J. Risk and trigger factors for the development of eating disorders in elite female athletes. *Med Sci Sports Exerc* 1994;4:414–419.

APPENDIX 4.1
CALORIES AND MACRONUTRIENT REQUIREMENTS BY BODY WEIGHT

Weight	Calories	Carbohydrate Selections	Protein Selections	Fat Selections
100	2,000	6	4	5
110	2,200	7	4	6
120	2,400	7	4.5	7
130	2,600	8	5	7
140	2,800	8.5	5	8
150	3,000	9	5.5	8
160	3,200	9.5	6	9
170	3,400	10	6	9
180	3,600	11	7	10
190	3,800	11.5	7	10.5
200	4,000	12	7.5	11
210	4,200	12.5	8	11.5
220	4,400	13	8	12
230	4,600	13.5	8.5	12.5
240	4,800	14	8.5	13
250	5,000	14.5	9	13.5
260	5,200	15	9	14
270	5,400	15.5	9.5	14.5
280	5,600	16	9.5	15
290	5,800	16.5	10	15.5
300	6,000	17	10	16
310	6,200	17.5	10.5	16.5
320	6,400	18	10.5	17
330	6,600	18.5	11	17.5
340	6,800	19	11	18
350	7,000	19.5	11.5	18.5

APPENDIX 4.2

Food Group Choices		
Carbohydrate	**Protein**	**Fat**
A large bagel	A computer mouse size of:	A tablespoon of peanut butter
1 1/2 cups pasta	Piece of chicken	1/4 cup of nuts
A cup of rice	Piece of beef	Two pats of butter
A cup of Cheerios	Piece of fish	2 tsp of mayonnaise
A low-fat fruit muffin	A 3 oz can of tuna	2 tsp of oil
Two cups of oatmeal	3/4 cup of cottage cheese	Two strips of bacon
A cup of applesauce	One soy burger	2 tbsp cream cheese
A large baked potato	1 1/2 cups pinto beans	4 tbsp sour cream
A cup of corn	3 slices of cheese	1 tbsp of regular salad dressing
5 fig bars	3 thin slices of lunch meat	
1 1/2 cups of grapes	3 eggs	2 tbsp of light salad dressing
1 1/2 English muffins	A mayonnaise jar lid–sized hamburger or turkey burger	
Four 4-in. diameter pancakes		
1 cup pudding	3/4 cup egg substitute	
Two handfuls of pretzels	8 oz tofu	

APPENDIX 4.2
(continued)

Food Group Choices

Carbohydrate	Protein	Fat
2 cups of juice 1 1/2 cups frozen yogurt 32 oz sports drink 2 packets flavored oatmeal 25 animal crackers 2 bananas 2 cups of grapes 10 large marshmallows Licorice, 12 oz package 3/4 cup granola 2 cereal bars 20 jelly beans 16 oz lemonade/fruit punch 1 1/2 cups sweetened cereal 1/2 bag of microwave low-fat popcorn One Pop Tart 15 vanilla wafers 1/2 cup raisins **Double Duty Foods** Carbohydrate + protein Yogurt 8 oz container = 50 gm carbohydrate + 12 gm of protein Sports bars (Clif, PowerBar, Gatorbar) Certain beverage supplements: Gatorade Nutrition Shake, Boost Milk: 16 oz chocolate milk = 50 gm carbohydrate, 16 gm protein Cheese pizza (2 slices = 80 gm of carbohydrate, 16 gm of protein)	**High Fat Carbohydrate Foods** Try to limit! Not as performance boosting! Doughnuts Ice cream Most cookies Chocolate Chips French fries	

APPENDIX 4.3
FOOD DIARY

Time	Food/Beverages	Amount	Hunger (H) or Other Reason for Eating (O)	Activities While Eating

APPENDIX 4.4

Supplement References
www.consumerlab.com To test the purity of supplements
Dietary Supplements: An Advertising Guide for Industry
http://www.ftc.gov/bcp/guides/guides.htm
Dietary Supplements Quality Initiative: http://www.dsqi.org
Product Evaluation: Consumer Labs: www.consumerlabs.com
Office of Dietary Supplements (NIH) http://dietary-supplements.info.nih.gov
Gatorade Sports Science Institute: www.gssiweb.com
International Bibliographic Information on Dietary Supplements (IBIDS)
http://odp.od.nih.gov/ods/databases/ibids.html
National Center for Drug Free Sports:
(816) 474–8655 or info@drugfreesport.com
Natural Products Database: www.naturaldatabase.com

2
Preventive Sports Medicine

5 Preparticipation Screening

James L. Moeller   Douglas B. McKeag

INITIAL CONSIDERATIONS

Performance of the preparticipation physical examination (PPPE) has been part of the primary care physician's armamentarium for years. As more people participate in exercise and conditioning programs, the consistent advice from the medical establishment is "confirm your state of physical fitness before beginning an exercise program." That advice carries with it an unspoken implication that the PPPE should at least assess risk of injury or harm from anticipated exercise. Some say these evaluations are merely a specialized health screening and argue about what should constitute the PPPE. At the very least, consistency is of utmost importance. The examination should assess risk factors and detect disease/injury that might cause problems during subsequent physical activity. Once past this generalized goal, disagreement arises from the different philosophical and medical viewpoints. The purpose of this chapter is to outline what should be determined and assessed, and how, when, and where such an examination should be conducted. It will not address the question of whether PPPEs are worthwhile.

The American Academy of Family Physicians, American Academy of Pediatrics, American College of Sports Medicine, American Medical Society for Sports Medicine, American Orthopaedic Society for Sports Medicine, and American Osteopathic Academy of Sports Medicine published a joint monograph outlining the PPPE in 1992 and which they updated in 1997 and again in 2005 (1,2). The PPPE outlined in this monograph is currently considered the standard for school-aged and young adult competitive athletes. Recommendations for the older athlete are less clear. Perhaps the most important point to remember regarding the PPPE is that it does **NOT** take the place of a comprehensive physical and health appraisal examination (CPE) in any age-group.

ESSENTIALS

By nature, any exercise evaluation of an individual should involve an awareness of the stress the exercise places upon three major body systems—musculoskeletal, cardiovascular, and psychological. It is logical to emphasize these areas in the PPPE. The major question is, "Will this individual be at any greater risk of injury or illness given the anticipated exercise program?" Any evaluation should include clearly defined objectives (see Table 5.1). Failure to meet these objectives will do both the athlete and the physician a disservice. A final note: the number of PPPEs must not compromise the principles of efficacy and cost effectiveness.

Different situations and settings call for different types of evaluation. Flexibility in changing the PPPE is implicit in any of the subsequent recommendations in this chapter. The PPPE should also meet community and individual needs. Although there is no "right" way to perform the PPPE, the physician should look at who the prospective athletes are, what the contemplated exercise program is, and what the motivation to participate is.

PROSPECTIVE ATHLETE

Understanding the characteristics of the target population is essential in determining what is assessed. One way to develop an appropriate PPPE is to look at prospective athletes by maturational age.

TABLE 5.1
OBJECTIVES OF THE PREPARTICIPATION PHYSICAL EXAMINATION

Primary objectives	Screen for conditions that may be life threatening or disabling Screen for conditions that may predispose to injury or illness Meet administrative requirements
Secondary objectives	Determine general health Serve as an entry point to the health care system, for adolescents Provide opportunity to initiate discussion on health-related topics

Prepubescent Athlete (Approximate Age Range: 6–10 Years)

Youngsters have always been involved in spontaneous play but there is a trend toward increased organization. One consideration with this age-group is the manifestation of previously undiagnosed congenital abnormalities. Physicians should be well acquainted with all the common abnormalities of the age-group. The psychological makeup of young athletes is also important. At this age, the philosophy of the program the candidate is anticipating joining can be a major factor in predicting possible poor outcomes. The most common reasons for youth non-participation in sports (including those who started and stopped, as well as those who never began) in order of prevalence are (a) not getting to play, (b) negative reinforcement, (c) mismatching (d) psychological stress, (e) failure, and (f) overorganization. When asked about sports participation, 95% of youngsters felt the most important thing about sports was having fun, not winning (3) and recent reports note that up to 90% of children involved in sports would rather play on a losing team than sit on the bench on a winning team (4). Generally, this population is very healthy. The physician can exert a great deal of influence in the patient's education aspects because habits have not been established. For instance, after correct methods of warm-up and cool-down are explained, a high degree of compliance can be expected.

Pubescent Athlete (11–15 Years)

These athletes are undergoing rapid body growth and change with the advent of physical, psychological, and sexual maturation. This group will have many non–exercise-related concerns (sexual activity, drugs). Given the appropriate examination format (see "Implementation" in this chapter), most of their questions can be addressed. If ever there is a time to expand a focused screening examination, it would be in this age-group. Most participating athletes at this age are involved in organized sports activities. The effect of exercise on human maturation directly relates to them.

Postpubescent/Young Adult Athlete (16–30 Years)

This group includes athletes with many reasons for exercising. Most elite athletes in the country are in this age-group, and it is also the age where most recreational athletes continue to compete. The PPPE needs to take into account the athlete's skill level. Most of these athletes begin in organized sports and then become more involved in recreational and individual sports as they grow older. Important points to take into account when formulating the PPPE for this age-group include the past medical history (especially as it concerns previous injuries), and the need to make the examination sport-specific.

Adults (31–65 Years)

Most adults participate primarily in informal recreational sports. They may be categorized into roughly two types, the sporadic and the regularly exercising athlete. Participation of the first type is organized around team-oriented sports (softball, basketball) that are played or practiced one or two times during the week. Such an individual is prone to acute injury and should be informed of the importance of proper warm-up before participation. The regularly exercising athlete may participate in an individual or paired sport such as running, swimming, cycling, or racket sports. These individuals are more apt to suffer overuse syndromes and need to have the necessity for true exercise prescription stressed to them. This group of athletes rarely participates in any type of pre-exercise evaluation and usually surfaces for evaluation only after an injury has occurred. Yet, from a motivational standpoint, they tend to be the most adamant about their athletic participation, resulting in prevention or illness of disease. In this age-group, a CPE is recommended instead of a screening PPPE.

Elderly (66 Years and Older)

Exercise in the "old elderly" has been shown to lead to improved sense of well-being, postpone disability and increase the duration of independent living (5). Many

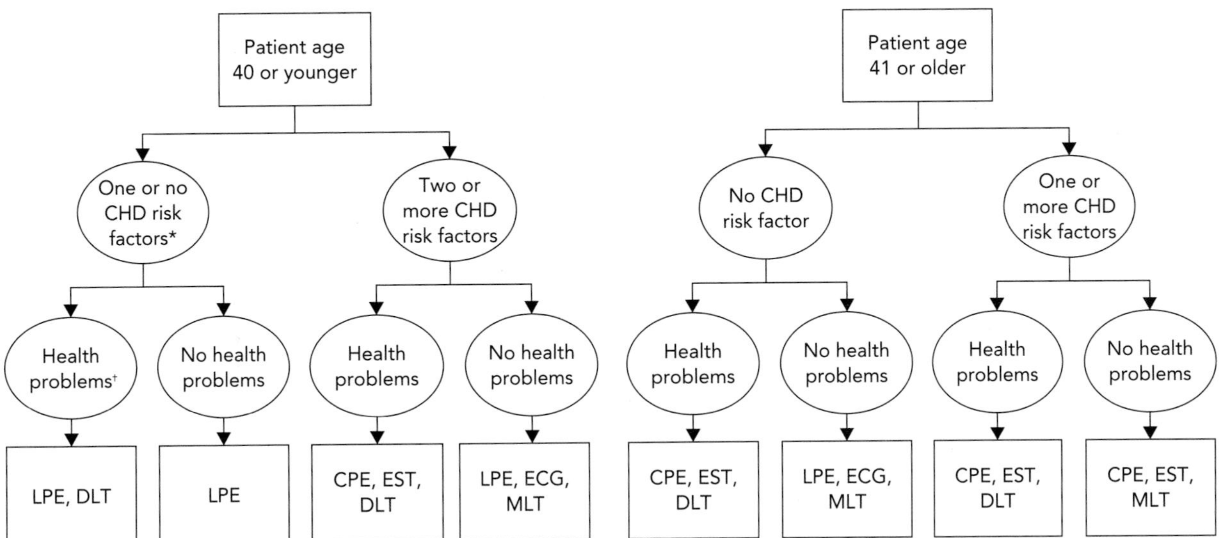

Figure 5.1 The office workup. LPE = limited physical exam; DLT = diagnostic laboratory; CPE = comprehensive physical exam; EST = exercise stress test; ECG = resting electrocardiogram; MLT = minimal laboratory testing.

elderly individuals enter exercise programs as a result of the well-recognized rehabilitation potential of exercise after a serious injury or illness. Exercise is now a major part of the therapeutic regimen for many injuries and illnesses such as myocardial infarction, coronary artery bypass, diabetes mellitus, asthma, and depression. These individuals often wish to continue exercising after their rehabilitation has ended. In most cases, the PPPE should merely be a part of the CPE called for in this age-group. The CPE is beyond the scope of this chapter, so when discussing this age-group we will only mention areas of the evaluation specific to athletic participation.

CONTEMPLATED EXERCISE PROGRAM

Not all exercises are the same. Depending upon the kind of exercise anticipated or wanted and what is discovered on the PPPE, several assessment options can be considered. There are three major types of exercise, aerobic, anaerobic, and combined (for an explanation of aerobic and anaerobic energy systems, see Chapter 3). Examples of aerobic exercise include repetitive endurance-type sports such as swimming, running, or biking. Examples of anaerobic exercise include sprinting and weight lifting. Most exercise tends to combine aerobic/anaerobic systems. Examples are soccer and basketball. Figure 5.1 portrays the type of office work-up that should be considered depending upon the patient's age and general health status.

MOTIVATION

Performing a PPPE begs the question, "why do you want to exercise?" Assessment of motivation is an extremely important part of the physical examination. In a prepubescent athlete, the answer may determine what comprises the remainder of the examination. In an adult athlete, overmotivation may predispose and predict future overuse problems. There are four major reasons (6) commonly given by older recreational athletes as their motivation to exercise:

1. Becoming healthy and gaining a feeling of self-satisfaction
2. Fear of dying
3. For the social components of exercise
4. As a part of a therapeutic regimen for illness or injury

IMPLEMENTATION

Formal, organized programs at any age (usually high school or college) involve enough athletes to warrant screenings. Conversely, physicians dealing with the informal recreational athlete should do so on an individual basis only. However, the objectives of the evaluations are similar, if not the same.

Implementation of the examination involves either the office-based or the station-based PPPE. The advantages and disadvantages of these PPPE formats are listed in Table 5.2. The required and optional components of the station-based PPPE are listed in Table 5.3. The locker room examination is still carried out in some instances but is not recommended. In this situation, one physician performs all aspects of each physical examination, usually in cramped quarters. There is little-to-no privacy for the individual athlete. It is done under rushed and noisy conditions and usually fails to address important questions.

TABLE 5.2

ADVANTAGES AND DISADVANTAGES TO OFFICE-BASED AND STATION-BASED PREPARTICIPATION PHYSICAL EXAMINATION FORMATS

	Office-Based PPPE	Station-Based PPPE
Advantages	Continuity of care • Establish patient–physician relationship • PMHx already known • Complete medical record available • Better continuity in event of injury Motivation can be better assessed If required, medical consultation can be quick with more complete follow-up	Many examinations can be performed in a short period of time • Uses a team approach (athletic trainers, school nurses, physician's assistants, coaches, etc.) under the direction of the team physician or PCP Cost effective Can encourage communication among the sports medicine team
Disadvantages	Many athletes do not have a personal or PCP Physician availability issues may lead to the examination taking place too early or too late Lack of consistency among physicians regarding interest and familiarity with sports and sport-related medical problems leading to inconsistency in judgments concerning qualification issues Not cost effective	Noisy and confusing when hundreds of athletes are in a fairly confined space • May make certain parts of the examination difficult (e.g., cardiac auscultation) Continuity of care may be compromised if the examining doctor is not the athlete's PCP • Coordinating consults may be difficult Examination is limited due to time constraints Privacy may be an issue depending on the set-up of the stations

PMHx = past medical history; PCP = primary care physician

TABLE 5.3

REQUIRED AND OPTIONAL COMPONENTS OF STATION-BASED PREPARTICIPATION PHYSICAL EXAMINATION

Required Stations	Personnel
Sign-in	Ancillary personnel (coach, nurse, medical assistant, community volunteer)
Height, weight	Ancillary personnel
Vital signs	Ancillary personnel
Vision	Ancillary personnel
Physical examination	Physician
History review, assessment, and clearance determination	Physician
Optional Stations	**Personnel**
Nutrition	Dietitian
Dental examination and mouth guard molding	Dentist
Injury evaluation	Physician
Flexibility	Athletic trainer, exercise physiologist, physical therapist
Body composition	Athletic trainer, exercise physiologist, physical therapist
Strength	Athletic trainer, exercise physiologist, physical therapist
Speed, agility, power, endurance, balance	Athletic trainer, coach, exercise physiologist

Adapted from Smith et al., 1997.

FREQUENCY

Many clinicians advocate the traditional yearly sports examination, and annual PPPEs for interscholastic sport participation are required by most States. Some consider evaluation necessary before each sport season (7). Most sports medicine physicians favor doing an examination before the beginning of any new level of competition in an athlete's career. For youngsters, this usually corresponds to school levels (grade school, junior high, high school, and college). We advocate an initial full-scale PPPE at the entrance to the particular level of participation, then the use of an intercurrent (or interval) review before the start of each sport season. This intercurrent review would include a full history and limited physical examination as directed by the history. It would allow for follow-up on rehabilitation of injuries incurred during the previous season or previous sport. Appendix 5.1 is a sample PPPE form that can be used for either the initial or intercurrent examination. For an intercurrent evaluation, the examining physician need only document the pertinent physical examination findings.

Basically, the optimal frequency of the PPPE has not been clearly established. Factors to consider when deciding on the frequency of PPPEs include (a) requirements of the school or the State, (b) cost to the athlete or family, (c) degree of risk of the sport, and (d) availability of qualified personnel.

It is important to keep two very important factors in mind: the age of the athlete in question, and the goals of the examination. Recommendations for each age-group are as follows:

1. *Prepubescent.* Initial examination should be done by the child's primary care practitioner (PCP) in the office setting. This first sports physical examination is most important because it may represent the first interaction the child has had with the health care system for perhaps 2 to 5 years. Follow-up intercurrent examinations should be held on a yearly basis with attention to vital signs, injuries incurred since the last examination, maturation and development, and the wearing of any new appliances (glasses, contact lenses, bridges).
2. *Pubescent/postpubescent.* The initial PPPE can be done with either the office-based or station-based technique. One screening examination for junior high school, high school, and college should be performed. Intercurrent examinations should focus on vital signs, observation for completion of physical development, recent injury, and non–sports-related health concerns (e.g., drug use, eating habits, sexual history).
3. *Adult (recreational).* Any adult 40 years of age or younger should undergo a physical evaluation by his/her PCP before beginning any exercise program of more than low intensity. Annual CPEs have otherwise become a thing of the past for healthy, asymptomatic adults.

TABLE 5.4

RISK ASSESSMENT CRITERIA FOR CONSIDERATION OF GRADED EXERCISE TESTING

- Age >35 years
- Type 2 diabetes of >10 years duration
- Type 1 diabetes of >15 years duration
- Presence of any additional risk factor for coronary artery disease
- Presence of microvascular disease (retinopathy or nephropathy, including microalbuminuria)
- Peripheral vascular disease
- Autonomic neuropathy

There is no evidence that a screening CPE in this population is needed. Periodic health evaluations have been shown to improve the delivery/receipt of specific, important screening tests, although they have not been shown to improve short-term or long-term clinical outcomes, nor do they affect long-term economic outcomes (8). Despite this, approximately two third of physicians feel that the annual CPE in this population is necessary, has proven benefit, and detects subclinical illness. Approximately 90% of PCPs routinely perform screening CPEs on asymptomatic adults (9). Any adult 40 years or older should have a periodic health evaluation to assist in delivery of proven preventive measures such as pap smears, cholesterol screening, and fecal occult blood testing. The timing of these evaluations should be based on age, gender, and disease risk and do not have to be part of a head-to-toe examination. This advice is independent of whether the person is an athlete. Cardiac stress testing should be considered for certain patients based on risk assessment for underlying cardiovascular disease as outlined by American College of Sports Medicine recommendations (see Table 5.4) (10). Recommendations vary based on age of the patient, intensity of the proposed exercise, and the presence/absence of cardiac risk factors.

TIMING

Only one principle should dictate the timing of the PPPE. Examinations should occur before a particular sport season with enough time to allow for adequate rehabilitation of injury, muscle imbalances, and other correctable problems, but not so far ahead as to make the passage of time an important factor in the development of new problems. Most sports medicine physicians recommend that the examination be performed approximately 6 weeks before the first preseason practice. If a longer time is taken, especially with the younger athlete, such factors as maturation and new injuries can decrease the comprehensiveness and effectiveness of the examination and decrease its preventive aspects.

CONTENT

History

A thorough history is the cornerstone of all medical evaluations. It is clearly the most sensitive and specific part of the PPPE process. Forms are preferable for a PPPE to insure that all essential information has been captured across various examiners. No one form could or should be advocated as being totally appropriate for a particular sports medicine program. However, recommended characteristics of that form can be found in Appendix 5.1. Any history form should be easy to complete, short (limited to one side of a piece of paper), self-administered, time efficient, and contain lay language easily understood by the athlete. Important highlights of any history include the following:

1. *Cardiovascular system history.* Used to rule out life-threatening cardiac abnormalities (e.g., hypertrophic cardiomyopathy [HCM], aberrant coronary arteries, arrhythmias). Table 5.5 lists the most common causes of nontraumatic sports death in high school and college athletes, and most causes are cardiac (11), highlighting the importance of the cardiovascular system history. Specific questions should include the following:
   a. *Have you ever passed out or nearly passed out during or after exercise?*
   b. *Have you ever had chest pain, discomfort or pressure during exercise?*
   c. *Have you ever had racing of your heart or skipped heartbeats during exercise?*
   d. *Have you had high blood pressure or high cholesterol?*

TABLE 5.5
MOST COMMON CAUSES OF NONTRAUMATIC SPORTS DEATH IN HIGH SCHOOL AND COLLEGE-AGED ATHLETES

Nontraumatic Sports Deaths	Total (n = 136)	Male (n = 124)	Female (n = 12)
Athletes with cardiovascular conditions	100	92	8
Hypertrophic cardiomyopathy	51	50	1
Probable HCM	5	5	0
Coronary artery anomaly	16	14	2
Myocarditis	7	7	0
Aortic stenosis	6	6	0
Dilated cardiomyopathy	5	5	0
Atherosclerotic coronary disease	3	2	1
Aortic rupture	2	2	0
Cardiomyopathy–NOS	2	2	0
Tunnel subaortic stenosis	2	2	0
Coronary artery aneurysm	1	0	1
Mitral valve prolapse	1	1	0
Right ventricular cardiomyopathy	1	0	1
Ruptured cerebellar AVM	1	0	1
Subarachnoid hemorrhage	1	0	1
Wolff-Parkinson-White syndrome	1	1	0
Athletes without cardiovascular conditions	30	27	3
Hyperthermia	13	12	1
Rhabdomyolysis and sickle trait	7	6	1
Status asthmaticus	4	3	1
Electrocution due to lightning	3	3	0
Arnold-Chiari II malformation	1	1	0
Aspiration-blood-GI bleed	1	1	0
Exercise-induced anaphylaxis	1	1	0
Athletes with cause of death undetermined	7	6	1

HCM = hypertrophic cardiomyopathy; NOS =; AVM = arteriovenous malformation; GI = gastrointestinal.
From van Camp et al. (11)

e. *Have you ever been told that you have a heart murmur or heart infection?*
f. *Has a doctor ever ordered a test for your heart (e.g., echocardiogram)?*
g. *Has anyone in your family died for no apparent reason?*
h. *Does anyone in your family have a heart problem?*
i. *Has any member of your family died from of heart problems before the age of 50?*
j. *Does anyone in your family have Marfan syndrome?*

A positive answer to any of these questions should raise a red flag to the possibility of a cardiac condition that could lead to sudden cardiac death. The presence of dizziness during or after exercise used to be considered a red-flag finding; however, a positive history of dizziness has low sensitivity and specificity for underlying cardiac disease.

2. *Neurological system history.* Used to assess the risk of recurrent or potentially permanent neurological injury. Questions should include the following:
   a. *Have you ever had a head injury or concussion?*
   b. *Have you ever been hit in the head and been confused or lost your memory?*
   c. *Have you ever been knocked out or become unconscious?*
   d. *Have you ever had a seizure?*
   e. *Do you have headaches with exercise?*
   f. *Have you ever had numbness or tingling in your arms or legs after being hit or falling?*
   g. *Have you ever been unable to move your arms or legs after being hit or falling?*
   h. *Have you ever had a stinger, burner, or pinched nerve?*

   A complete history of head trauma resulting from athletic competition is important to have when qualifying a potential athlete for a contact or collision sport. It is important to note and monitor cumulative, subtle, neurological loss of function. Athletes with a history of poorly controlled seizures should be disqualified from high-risk sports. A history of recurrent upper extremity paresthesias from contact sports may indicate the presence of cervical canal stenosis, an entity that puts an athlete at risk for permanent neurological injury.
3. *Respiratory system history.* Used primarily to identify exercise-induced bronchospasm. Questions include the following:
   a. *Do you cough, wheeze, or have trouble breathing during or after activity?*
   b. *Has a doctor ever told you that you have asthma or allergies?*
   c. *Is there anyone in your family who has asthma?*
   d. *Have you ever used an inhaler or taken asthma medicine?*
4. *Musculoskeletal system history.* Important questions include the following:
   a. *Have you ever had an injury such as a sprain, muscle or ligament tear, or tendinitis, which caused you to miss a practice or game?*
   b. *Have you broken or fractured any bones or dislocated any joints?*
   c. *Have you ever had a stress fracture?*
   d. *Have you ever had a bone or joint injury that required x-rays, magnetic resonance imaging, computed tomography scan, surgery, injections, rehabilitation, physical therapy, a brace, a cast, or crutches?*
   e. *Have you ever been told that you have or have you had an x-ray for neck instability?*
   f. *Do you regularly use a brace or assistive device?*
5. *Past medical history.* This should elicit information about chronic illnesses as well as any condition that may have led to limited sport participation or disqualification from participation. Questions should include inquiries regarding prior hospitalizations and surgeries. Responses to these questions may also explain functional abnormalities such as muscle imbalance, decreased respiratory volume, or below-normal exercise tolerance.
6. *Medications, drugs, and supplements.* The effect of medications and drugs on the exercising body can be serious. It is vital knowledge if an individual is injured or rendered unconscious. Otherwise, appropriate steps to treat an injured or ill athlete cannot be taken. Over-the-counter supplements (e.g., creatine) are used by many athletes of all ages for the purpose of performance enhancement. These substances are not regulated by the Food and Drug Administration and may contain a variety of other substances. There are anecdotal reports of various injuries associated with supplement use. Questions regarding medications should include prescription drugs, over-the-counter drugs and supplements.
7. *Allergies.* Common occurrences, such as allergies to bee stings, medications, foods, and other environmental substances need to be known so that prophylactic measures can be taken in case of exposure.
8. *Appliance use.* Information about mouth, eye, or ear appliances should be known in case an athlete is injured or unconscious. Such appliances can hinder resuscitation.
9. *Heat illness history.* Used to assess the risk of recurrent heat illness.
10. *Menstrual history.* Absence of menses may place young women at risk for fractures due to traumas or falls, or for stress fracture. Absence of menses may also be a red-flag sign of the female athlete triad.
11. *Additional history.* Other important areas of history include vision history, the loss or congenital absence of a paired organ, prior history of infectious mononucleosis, and a prior history of contagious skin lesions (particularly important in mat sport athletes). Questions regarding the history or family history of sickle trait and sickle cell disease should also be included. Nutritional history is very important, and may help to identify athletes at risk for developing eating disorders.

TABLE 5.6
PHYSICAL EXAMINATION EMPHASIS

Sport	Areas to Assess
Baseball	Shoulder, elbow, arm
Basketball	Ankles, knees
Football	Neck, head, knees, low back (linemen)
Gymnastics	Wrists, shoulders, low back
Handball	Wrist, hand, elbow, shoulder
Running	Back, hips, knees, ankles, feet
Soccer	Hips, pelvis, knee, feet
Swimming	Ears, nose, throat, shoulders
Wrestling	Body fat (%), neck, shoulders, skin

12. *"Are there any questions you'd like to ask the physician?"* This question allows the athlete to ask any question about any body system. The authors feel that the addition of this question to the PPPE history is very important.

Physical Examination

Whenever possible, a sport-specific physical examination, emphasizing those areas where injury and/or illness have the greatest epidemiological occurrence, is a primary goal (McKeag, 1985). Any examination assessing a sports candidate without an awareness of the demands of their specific sport suffers a major weakness (see Table 5.6).

Evaluation of a swimmer should be different from that of a football player. Regardless of age, sex, or situation, three areas of the PPPE should always be emphasized:

1. Cardiovascular system (including blood pressure determination)
2. Musculoskeletal system (including range of motion and strength assessment)
3. Psychological assessment (including motivation for exercise)

Because the prevalence of disqualifying conditions is so low among athletes and because few of these patients produce significant physical findings, the yield from the physical examination is very low (Runyan, 1983). The existing community sports medicine network, and specifically the office-based sports medicine practitioner, should take the time to study what is needed in the local environment.

Standard components of the physical examination should include the following:

1. *Height and weight.* Unusual variance in either of these vital signs should signal further investigation. Apart from some rare endocrine disorders, four common problems are:
   a. Eating disorders—abnormal eating or weight loss patterns are often seen in sports requiring strict adherence or emphasis on body weight such as wrestling, women's gymnastics, and cross-country or distance running.
   b. Exogenous hormone consumption—ingestion/injection of ergogenic aids for increased strength and power or suppression of puberty is unfortunately not an uncommon occurrence.
   c. Obesity—an athlete greater than 20% overweight for height, age, and stature has a relative cardiac and general health risk. Referral for dietary counseling is advised.
   d. Late maturation—occurring naturally or secondary to poor nutrition, delayed maturation can affect both height and weight measurements. Strenuous exercise before puberty may delay the maturation process.
2. *Vital signs*
   a. Blood pressure must be measured with a proper sized cuff to reduce the likelihood of false elevation or false reduction of blood pressure. Remember that in children, acceptable blood pressure varies with age, gender, and height (12) (see Table 5.7A and B). Many athletes weight train as part of their preseason training program. Sustained isometric activity (improper weight lifting) causes a marked and sometimes prolonged elevation in blood pressure that may lead to elevated blood pressure on the PPPE. Hypertension in the young athlete population should prompt consideration of secondary causes.
   b. Pulse should be obtained at the radial and femoral arteries. Radial artery pulse is adequate to determine heart rate and regularity. A nonpalpable, delayed, or reduced strength femoral pulse should raise the suspicion of coarctation of the aorta.
3. *Eyes*
   a. Visual acuity—the Snellen eye chart can be used to test correctable vision to better than 20/200. Such emphasis is necessary for detection of legal blindness, a major basis for disqualification, and impaired vision, a major factor in poor performance. Visual acuity should be 20/40 or better (with or without corrective lenses) in each eye.
   b. Pupils—pupil size is evaluated to look for anisocoria (unequal pupil size). The presence of anisocoria needs to be carefully documented and communicated to the athlete, parents, athletic trainer, and coach so the baseline difference is understood in the event of head injury. Pupillary response to direct and consensual light exposure is also evaluated.
4. *Ears, nose, and throat.* This portion of the PPPE is performed to document the general status of these areas.
5. *Cardiovascular examination.* Major emphasis in this area is necessary in any athletic screening examination. Sudden death in healthy athletes is uncommon but does occur and the primary mechanism usually

TABLE 5.7A
BLOOD PRESSURE LEVELS FOR BOYS BY AGE AND HEIGHT PERCENTILE

		Systolic BP (mm Hg)							Diastolic BP (mm Hg)						
		← Percentile of Height →							← Percentile of Height →						
Age (Year)	BP Percentile ↓	5th	10th	25th	50th	75th	90th	95th	5th	10th	25th	50th	75th	90th	95th
1	50th	80	81	83	85	87	88	89	34	35	36	37	38	39	39
	90th	94	95	97	99	100	102	103	49	50	51	52	53	53	54
	95th	98	99	101	103	104	106	106	54	54	55	56	57	58	58
	99th	105	106	108	110	112	113	114	61	62	63	64	65	66	66
2	50th	84	85	87	88	90	92	92	39	40	41	42	43	44	44
	90th	97	99	100	102	104	105	106	54	55	56	57	58	58	59
	95th	101	102	104	106	108	109	110	59	59	60	61	62	63	63
	99th	109	110	111	113	115	117	117	66	67	68	69	70	71	71
3	50th	86	87	89	91	93	94	95	44	44	45	46	47	48	48
	90th	100	101	103	105	107	108	109	59	59	60	61	62	63	63
	95th	104	105	107	109	110	112	113	63	63	64	65	66	67	67
	99th	111	112	114	116	118	119	120	71	71	72	73	74	75	75
4	50th	88	89	91	93	95	96	97	47	48	49	50	51	51	52
	90th	102	103	105	107	109	110	111	62	63	64	65	66	66	67
	95th	106	107	109	111	112	114	115	66	67	68	69	70	71	71
	99th	113	114	116	118	120	121	122	74	75	76	77	78	78	79
5	50th	90	91	93	95	96	98	98	50	51	52	53	54	55	55
	90th	104	105	106	108	110	111	112	65	66	67	68	69	69	70
	95th	108	109	110	112	114	115	116	69	70	71	72	73	74	74
	99th	115	116	118	120	121	123	123	77	78	79	80	81	81	82
6	50th	91	92	94	96	98	99	100	53	53	54	55	56	57	57
	90th	105	106	108	110	111	113	113	68	68	69	70	71	72	72
	95th	109	110	112	114	115	117	117	72	72	73	74	75	76	76
	99th	116	117	119	121	123	124	125	80	80	81	82	83	84	84
7	50th	92	94	95	97	99	100	101	55	55	56	57	58	59	59
	90th	106	107	109	111	113	114	115	70	70	71	72	73	74	74
	95th	110	111	113	115	117	118	119	74	74	75	76	77	78	78
	99th	117	118	120	122	124	125	126	82	82	83	84	85	86	86
8	50th	94	95	97	99	100	102	102	56	57	58	59	60	60	61
	90th	107	109	110	112	114	115	116	71	72	72	73	74	75	76
	95th	111	112	114	116	118	119	120	75	76	77	78	79	79	80
	99th	119	120	122	123	125	127	127	83	84	85	86	87	87	88
9	50th	95	96	98	100	102	103	104	57	58	59	60	61	61	62
	90th	109	110	112	114	115	117	118	72	73	74	75	76	76	77
	95th	113	114	116	118	119	121	121	76	77	78	79	80	81	81
	99th	120	121	123	125	127	128	129	84	85	86	87	88	88	89
10	50th	97	98	100	102	103	105	106	58	59	60	61	61	62	63
	90th	111	112	114	115	117	119	119	73	73	74	75	76	77	78
	95th	115	116	117	119	121	122	123	77	78	79	80	81	81	82
	99th	122	123	125	127	128	130	130	85	86	86	88	88	89	90
11	50th	99	100	102	104	105	107	107	59	59	60	61	62	63	63
	90th	113	114	115	117	119	120	121	74	74	75	76	77	78	78
	95th	117	118	119	121	123	124	125	78	78	79	80	81	82	82
	99th	124	125	127	129	130	132	132	86	86	87	88	89	90	90
12	50th	101	102	104	106	108	109	110	59	60	61	62	63	63	64
	90th	115	116	118	120	121	123	123	74	75	75	76	77	78	79
	95th	119	120	122	123	125	127	127	78	79	80	81	82	82	83
	99th	126	127	129	131	133	134	135	86	87	88	89	90	90	91
13	50th	104	105	106	108	110	111	112	60	60	61	62	63	64	64
	90th	117	118	120	122	124	125	126	75	75	76	77	78	79	79
	95th	121	122	124	126	128	129	130	79	79	80	81	82	83	83
	99th	128	130	131	133	135	136	137	87	87	88	89	90	91	91

(continued)

TABLE 5.7A
(continued)

		Systolic BP (mm Hg)							Diastolic BP (mm Hg)						
		← Percentile of Height →							← Percentile of Height →						
Age (Year)	BP Percentile ↓	5th	10th	25th	50th	75th	90th	95th	5th	10th	25th	50th	75th	90th	95th
14	50th	106	107	109	111	113	114	115	60	61	62	63	64	65	65
	90th	120	121	123	125	126	128	128	75	76	77	78	79	79	80
	95th	124	125	127	128	130	132	132	80	80	81	82	83	84	84
	99th	131	132	134	136	138	139	140	87	88	89	90	91	92	92
15	50th	109	110	112	113	115	117	117	61	62	63	64	65	66	66
	90th	122	124	125	127	129	130	131	76	77	78	79	80	80	81
	95th	126	127	129	131	133	134	135	81	81	82	83	84	85	85
	99th	134	135	136	138	140	142	142	88	89	90	91	92	93	93
16	50th	111	112	114	116	118	119	120	63	63	64	65	66	67	67
	90th	125	126	128	130	131	133	134	78	78	79	80	81	82	82
	95th	129	130	132	134	135	137	137	82	83	83	84	85	86	87
	99th	136	137	139	141	143	144	145	90	90	91	92	93	94	94
17	50th	114	115	116	118	120	121	122	65	66	66	67	68	69	70
	90th	127	128	130	132	134	135	136	80	80	81	82	83	84	84
	95th	131	132	134	136	138	139	140	84	85	86	87	87	88	89
	99th	139	140	141	143	145	146	147	92	93	93	94	95	96	97

BP = blood pressure.

TABLE 5.7B
BLOOD PRESSURE LEVELS FOR GIRLS BY AGE AND HEIGHT PERCENTILE

		Systolic BP (mm Hg)							Diastolic BP (mm Hg)						
		← Percentile of Height →							← Percentile of Height →						
Age (Year)	BP Percentile ↓	5th	10th	25th	50th	75th	90th	95th	5th	10th	25th	50th	75th	90th	95th
1	50th	83	84	85	86	88	89	90	38	39	39	40	41	41	42
	90th	97	97	98	100	101	102	103	52	53	53	54	55	55	56
	95th	100	101	102	104	105	106	107	56	57	57	58	59	59	60
	99th	108	108	109	111	112	113	114	64	64	65	65	66	67	67
2	50th	85	85	87	88	89	91	91	43	44	44	45	46	46	47
	90th	98	99	100	101	103	104	105	57	58	58	59	60	61	61
	95th	102	103	104	105	107	108	109	61	62	62	63	64	65	65
	99th	109	110	111	112	114	115	116	69	69	70	70	71	72	72
3	50th	86	87	88	89	91	92	93	47	48	48	49	50	50	51
	90th	100	100	102	103	104	106	106	61	62	62	63	64	64	65
	95th	104	104	105	107	108	109	110	65	66	66	67	68	68	69
	99th	111	111	113	114	115	116	117	73	73	74	74	75	76	76
4	50th	88	88	90	91	92	94	94	50	50	51	52	52	53	54
	90th	101	102	103	104	106	107	108	64	64	65	66	67	67	68
	95th	105	106	107	108	110	111	112	68	68	69	70	71	71	72
	99th	112	113	114	115	117	118	119	76	76	76	77	78	79	79

TABLE 5.7B
(continued)

Age (Year)	BP Percentile ↓	Systolic BP (mm Hg) ← Percentile of Height →							Diastolic BP (mm Hg) ← Percentile of Height →						
		5th	10th	25th	50th	75th	90th	95th	5th	10th	25th	50th	75th	90th	95th
5	50th	89	90	91	93	94	95	96	52	53	53	54	55	55	56
	90th	103	103	105	106	107	109	109	66	67	67	68	69	69	70
	95th	107	107	108	110	111	112	113	70	71	71	72	73	73	74
	99th	114	114	116	117	118	120	120	78	78	79	79	80	81	81
6	50th	91	92	93	94	96	97	98	54	54	55	56	56	57	58
	90th	104	105	106	108	109	110	111	68	68	69	70	70	71	72
	95th	108	109	110	111	113	114	115	72	72	73	74	74	75	76
	99th	115	116	117	119	120	121	122	80	80	80	81	82	83	83
7	50th	93	93	95	96	97	99	99	55	56	56	57	58	58	59
	90th	106	107	108	109	111	112	113	69	70	70	71	72	72	73
	95th	110	111	112	113	115	116	116	73	74	74	75	76	76	77
	99th	117	118	119	120	122	123	124	81	81	82	82	83	84	84
8	50th	95	95	96	98	99	100	101	57	57	57	58	59	60	60
	90th	108	109	110	111	113	114	114	71	71	71	72	73	74	74
	95th	112	112	114	115	116	118	118	75	75	75	76	77	78	78
	99th	119	120	121	122	123	125	125	82	82	83	83	84	85	86
9	50th	96	97	98	100	101	102	103	58	58	58	59	60	61	61
	90th	110	110	112	113	114	116	116	72	72	72	73	74	75	75
	95th	114	114	115	117	118	119	120	76	76	76	77	78	79	79
	99th	121	121	123	124	125	127	127	83	83	84	84	85	86	87
10	50th	98	99	100	102	103	104	105	59	59	59	60	61	62	62
	90th	112	112	114	115	116	118	118	73	73	73	74	75	76	76
	95th	116	116	117	119	120	121	122	77	77	77	78	79	80	80
	99th	123	123	125	126	127	129	129	84	84	85	86	86	87	88
11	50th	100	101	102	103	105	106	107	60	60	60	61	62	63	63
	90th	114	114	116	117	118	119	120	74	74	74	75	76	77	77
	95th	118	118	119	121	122	123	124	78	78	78	79	80	81	81
	99th	125	125	126	128	129	130	131	85	85	86	87	87	88	89
12	50th	102	103	104	105	107	108	109	61	61	61	62	63	64	64
	90th	116	116	117	119	120	121	122	75	75	75	76	77	78	78
	95th	119	120	121	123	124	125	126	79	79	79	80	81	82	82
	99th	127	127	128	130	131	132	133	86	86	87	88	88	89	90
13	50th	104	105	106	107	109	110	110	62	62	62	63	64	65	65
	90th	117	118	119	121	122	123	124	76	76	76	77	78	79	79
	95th	121	122	123	124	126	127	128	80	80	80	81	82	83	83
	99th	128	129	130	132	133	134	135	87	87	88	89	89	90	91
14	50th	106	106	107	109	110	111	112	63	63	63	64	65	66	66
	90th	119	120	121	122	124	125	125	77	77	77	78	79	80	80
	95th	123	123	125	126	127	129	129	81	81	81	82	83	84	84
	99th	130	131	132	133	135	136	136	88	88	89	90	90	91	92
15	50th	107	108	109	110	111	113	113	64	64	64	65	66	67	67
	90th	120	121	122	123	125	126	127	78	78	78	79	80	81	81
	95th	124	125	126	127	129	130	131	82	82	82	83	84	85	85
	99th	131	132	133	134	136	137	138	89	89	90	91	91	92	93

(continued)

TABLE 5.7B
(continued)

		Systolic BP (mm Hg)							Diastolic BP (mm Hg)						
		← Percentile of Height →							← Percentile of Height →						
Age (Year)	BP Percentile ↓	5th	10th	25th	50th	75th	90th	95th	5th	10th	25th	50th	75th	90th	95th
16	50th	108	108	110	111	112	114	114	64	64	65	66	66	67	68
	90th	121	122	123	124	126	127	128	78	78	79	80	81	81	82
	95th	125	126	127	128	130	131	132	82	82	83	84	85	85	86
	99th	132	133	134	135	137	138	139	90	90	90	91	92	93	93
17	50th	108	109	110	111	113	114	115	64	65	65	66	67	67	68
	90th	122	122	123	125	126	127	128	78	79	79	80	81	81	82
	95th	125	126	127	129	130	131	132	82	83	83	84	85	85	86
	99th	133	133	134	136	137	138	139	90	90	91	91	92	93	93

BP = blood pressure.

involves the cardiovascular system. The catastrophe is almost always totally unexpected, all the more tragic and alarming. Most young athletes suffering sudden death have underlying cardiovascular disease (Maron et al., 1986). The following important points about the cardiovascular examination should be remembered:

a. Murmurs
   (1) A normal, "functional" heart murmur may be audible in any child sometime during development.
   (2) Murmur intensity does not always correlate with the significance of the murmur.
   (3) The differential diagnosis of normal murmurs in young athletes, as outlined by Strong and Steed (1984), should be familiar to the examiner.

   The following guidelines to listening to heart murmurs in athletes are helpful:
   (1) If the S_1 can be heard easily, the murmur is not holosystolic—therefore ventricular septal defect (VSD) and mitral insufficiency can be ruled out.
   (2) If S_2 is normal—Tetralogy of Fallot, atrial septal defect (ASD), and pulmonary hypertension are ruled out.
   (3) If there is no ejection click—aortic and pulmonary stenosis can be excluded.
   (4) If a continuous diastolic murmur is absent—patent ductus arteriosus is not present.
   (5) If no early diastolic decrescendo murmur exists—aortic insufficiency can be ruled out.

   When a murmur is detected, maneuvers designed to provoke the murmur should be employed. These maneuvers include Valsalva, deep breath, and squat-to-stand. For example, in HCM, Valsalva will decrease venous return, causing the murmur to increase in intensity. Certain murmurs should always be considered suspicious until proved otherwise, and prompt appropriate workup. These include any systolic murmur with ≥3/6 intensity, any diastolic murmur, or any murmur that increases with Valsalva. In these situations, certification should be postponed until the murmur has been evaluated sufficiently.

   Generally speaking, mild defects do not prevent participation in normal competition or activity. Athletes with moderate defects that produce signs or symptomatology such as cardiomegaly, shortness or breath, or abnormal electrocardiograms (ECGs) should be screened with a graded exercise test. For the most part, these individuals need to be eliminated only from strenuous competitive athletics. Finally, severe defects causing significant symptomatology should render an individual ineligible for any competitive athletics. Full disqualification recommendations are based on the findings of the 26th Bethesda Conference report. A summary of common innocent murmurs found in adolescents are described in Table 5.8.

b. Arrhythmias—isolated premature ventricular contractions (PVCs) represent the single most common arrhythmia encountered in the PPPE. Occurring in youngsters, they are rarely of consequence, but

TABLE 5.8
COMMON INNOCENT MURMURS IN CHILDREN

Type	Characteristic	Etiology	Differential Diagnosis	Notes
Pulmonary flow murmur	Grade 1/6 to 3/6 ejection murmur; left upper sternal border	Flow across normal pulmonic valve	ASD Valvular PS	Most common innocent murmur
Still's murmur	Grade 1/6 to 3/6 vibratory systolic murmur; halfway between lower left sternal border and apex	Vibrations under aortic valve	Small VSD Subvalvar AS Mitral regurgitation	Very characteristic sound, sometimes musical
Venous hum	Grade 1/6 to 3/6 continuous murmur through the second sound; one or both upper sternal borders	Turbulent flow at confluence of veins; disappears when neck is turned or patient supine	PDA	Maneuvers mentioned make diagnosis easy
Carotid bruit	Grade 1/6 to 3/6 ejection murmur; in the neck	Turbulence in carotid blood flow; murmur fainter as approach upper sternal borders	Valvular stenosis	

ASD = atrial septal defect; PS = pulmonary stenosis; VSD = ventricular septal defect; AS = aortic stenosis; PDA = patent ductus arteriosus.

numerous factors come into play with the older individual. Caffeine, tobacco, and alcohol ingestion, as well as bronchodilator therapy, can result in PVCs.

Three major characteristics make most arrhythmias benign (a) unifocal in origin, (b) disappearance with exercise, and (c) no history of syncope with exercise. Coupling of PVCs or bigeminy may indicate myocarditis and should temporarily disqualify an athlete. A finding of paroxysmal supraventricular tachycardia should initiate a search for the cause but, once controlled with medication, should not be a reason for disqualification. Controlled Wolfe-Parkinson-White syndrome should not be reason for disqualification. It is important to remember that bradycardia and some irregular rhythms are more common among conditioned athletes than among the general population (Salem, 1980). Other observed athletic irregularities include first- or second-degree heart block, Wenckebach phenomena, and junctional rhythms.

6. *Lungs*. The most common finding in this portion of the evaluation is clear, full breath sounds. Any pathological findings (e.g., wheezes, rubs, rales) should be referred for further evaluation or appropriate management.
7. *Skin*. This portion of the examination is concerned with the detection of contagious cutaneous infections (herpes, impetigo, or louse infestation) that should be screened. Such conditions are promoted by skin-to-skin contact in sports such as wrestling. Participation should be allowed only after the problem is controlled. Search for abnormal nevi is beyond the scope of the PPPE.
8. *Abdomen*. Any significant organomegaly deserves further investigation, with participation qualification delayed.
9. *Genitourinary*. Male examination should include a testicular examination (to detect absence or undescended testicle in youngsters; in older individuals to detect scrotal masses). The setting of the examination (office based versus station based) may not allow for genital examination. Testicular cancer is the leading cause of cancer death in men between the ages of 15 to 35 years, so even if unable to perform the examination, the physician should take the opportunity to educate young males on testicular cancer; particularly the importance of early detection and self-examination.

TABLE 5.9
TANNER STAGING

BOYS

Stage	Pubic Hair	Penis	Testis
1	None	Preadolescent	
2	Slight, long, slight pigmentation	Slight enlargement	Enlarged scrotum, pink slight rugae
3	Darker, starts to curl small amount	Longer	Larger
4	Coarse, curly, adult type but less quantity	Increase in glans size and breadth of penis	Larger, scrotum darker
5	Adult—spread to inner thighs	Adult	Adult

GIRLS

Stage	Pubic Hair	Breasts
1	Preadolescent (none)	Preadolescent (no germinal button)
2	Sparse, lightly pigmented, straight medial border of labia	Breast and papilla elevated as small mound; areolar diameter increased
3	Darker, beginning to curl increased	Breast and areola enlarged; no contour separation
4	Coarse, curly, abundant, but less than adult	Areola and papilla form secondary mound
5	Adult—female triangle and spread to medial surface	Mature, nipple projects, areola part of general breast contour

From Tanner, 1962 (13)

TABLE 5.10
MUSCULOSKELETAL SCREENING PHYSICAL EXAMINATION

Instruction to Athlete	Physician Observations
1. Stand facing examiner	Acromioclavicular joints, general habitus
2. Look: at ceiling, floor, over both shoulders, touch ears to shoulders	Cervical spine motion
3. Shrug shoulders (examiner resists)	Trapezius strength
4. Abduct shoulders 90 degrees (examiner resists at 90 degrees)	Deltoid strength
5. Full internal and external rotation of shoulders	Shoulder motion
6. Flex and extend elbows	Elbow motion
7. Pronation and supination of the elbows	Elbow and wrist motion
8. Spread fingers; make fist	Hand/finger motion and deformities
9. Stand with back to examiner	Symmetry of trunk and upper extremities
10. Extend back with legs straight	Pain suggests spondylolysis or spondylolisthesis
11. Flex back with legs straight	Range of motion of thoracic and lumbar spine; spine curvature; hamstring flexibility
12. Contract and relax quadriceps	Symmetry and alignment of lower extremities
13. "Duck walk" four steps	Motion of hip, knee and ankle; strength; balance
14. Stand on toes, then heels	Calf symmetry and strength; balance

Evaluation for hernia should be performed on an individual basis based on history of inguinal pain or a lump/bulge in the inguinal region or scrotum.

In females, genitalia examination is not part of the PPPE. A history of menstrual abnormality, early sexual activity, or lack of recent PAP smear usually indicates a need for further historical information and possibly a pelvic examination.

Assessment of physical maturation by Tanner staging (see Table 5.9) is no longer recommended as part of the routine PPPE (14). Tanner staging may be helpful in adolescent boys as a guide to counseling regarding sports safety and steroid usage. Prospective studies (McKeag, 1991) indicate that inappropriate maturational matching of athletes is a major injury risk factor in youth contact and collision sports. Tanner staging may be difficult, if not impossible, in station-based examinations. Dominant hand grip strength has been correlated to sexual maturation (as determined by Tanner stage) in unpublished reports (Bellisario et al., 1999).

10. *Musculoskeletal.* Full attention should be given to the range-of-motion of major joints and the relative strength of opposing muscle groups, comparing gross strength bilaterally. Table 5.10 and Figure 5.2 summarize a recommended, 14-point musculoskeletal screening examination. Always examine the site of any old injury to determine the presence of any residual effects.

Laboratory

In an asymptomatic population of young athletes, screening tests such as urinalysis, complete blood count, blood

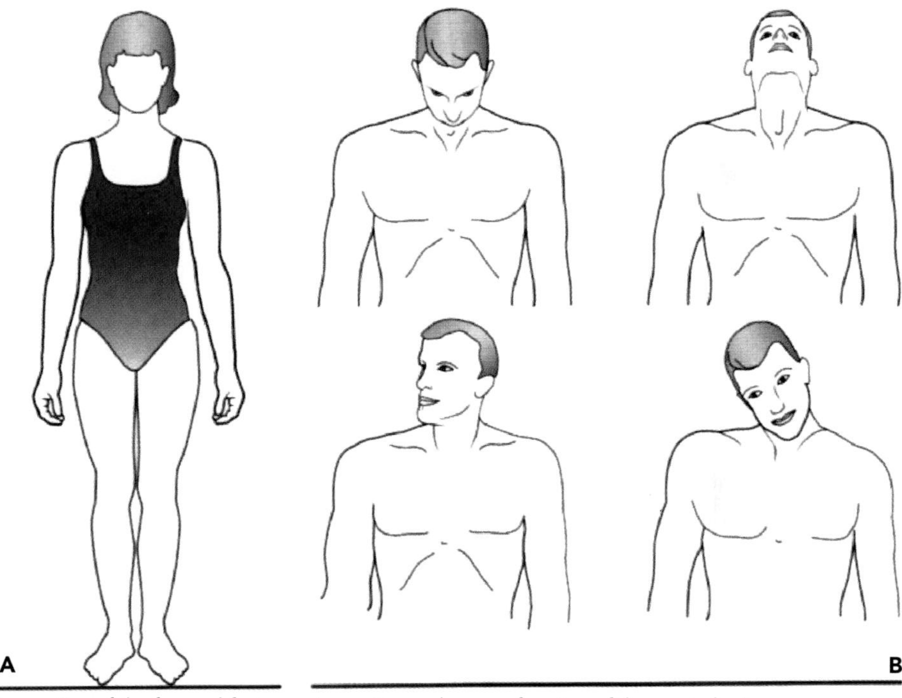

A
B
Inspection of the forward-facing athlete
Inspection and range of motion of the cervical spine

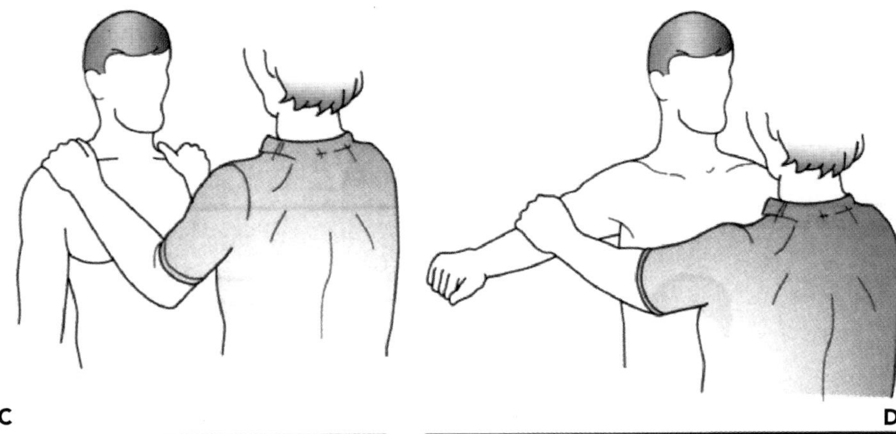

Figure 5.2 The 14-point musculoskeletal screening examination. (Reproduced with permission from American College of Sports Medicine, American Academy of Family Physicians, American Academy of Pediatrics, American Medical Society for Sports Medicine, American Medicine Society for Sports Medicine, American Orthopaedic Society for Sports Medicine, and American Osteopathic Academy of Sports Medicine. *Preparticipation physical evaluation,* 3rd ed. Minneapolis, New York: McGraw-Hill, 2005.)

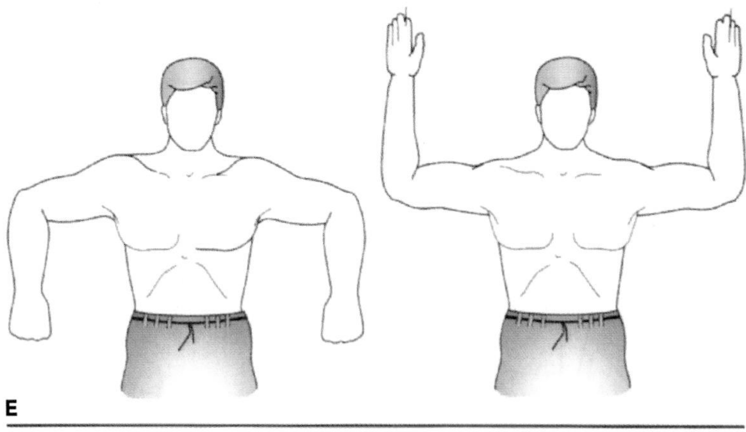

E

Internal and external rotation of the shoulder

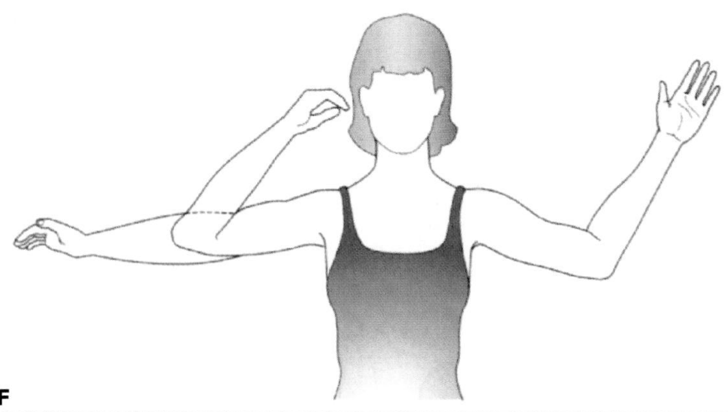

F

Flexion and extension of the elbows

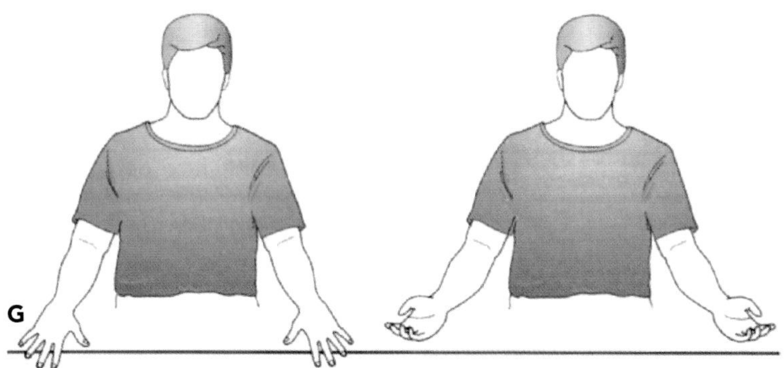

G

Pronation and supination of the elbows

Figure 5.2 *(continued)*

chemistries, and lipid profile are not cost effective and not recommended. For example, proteinuria in childhood is a benign event in all but 0.08% of cases (Peggs, 1986). The prevalence of benign proteinuria in adolescents makes the cost-benefit ratio of urinalysis inappropriate. Laboratory testing in this age-group should be based upon special circumstances. For the older recreational athlete, laboratory testing should be based on need as dictated by history and physical examination findings at the CPE.

Additional Screening Procedures

Any additional tests need to have adequate sensitivity, specificity, and predictive values to justify inclusion in a routine PPPE. There is no evidence that any additional screening procedure is cost effective in an asymptomatic population. Although not complete, a list of additional screening procedures follows. Any of these **may** be deemed necessary given the sport, age-group, or level of competition (but again, we do not recommend the tests as part of a routine PPPE):

1. *Audiometry/tympanometry*. Recommended if the patient complains of hearing loss, although findings of even profound hearing loss may not lead to disqualification from activities. May be recommended based on a positive finding on ear examination.
2. *Body composition testing*. Information on percent body fat and ideal body weight can be helpful and important

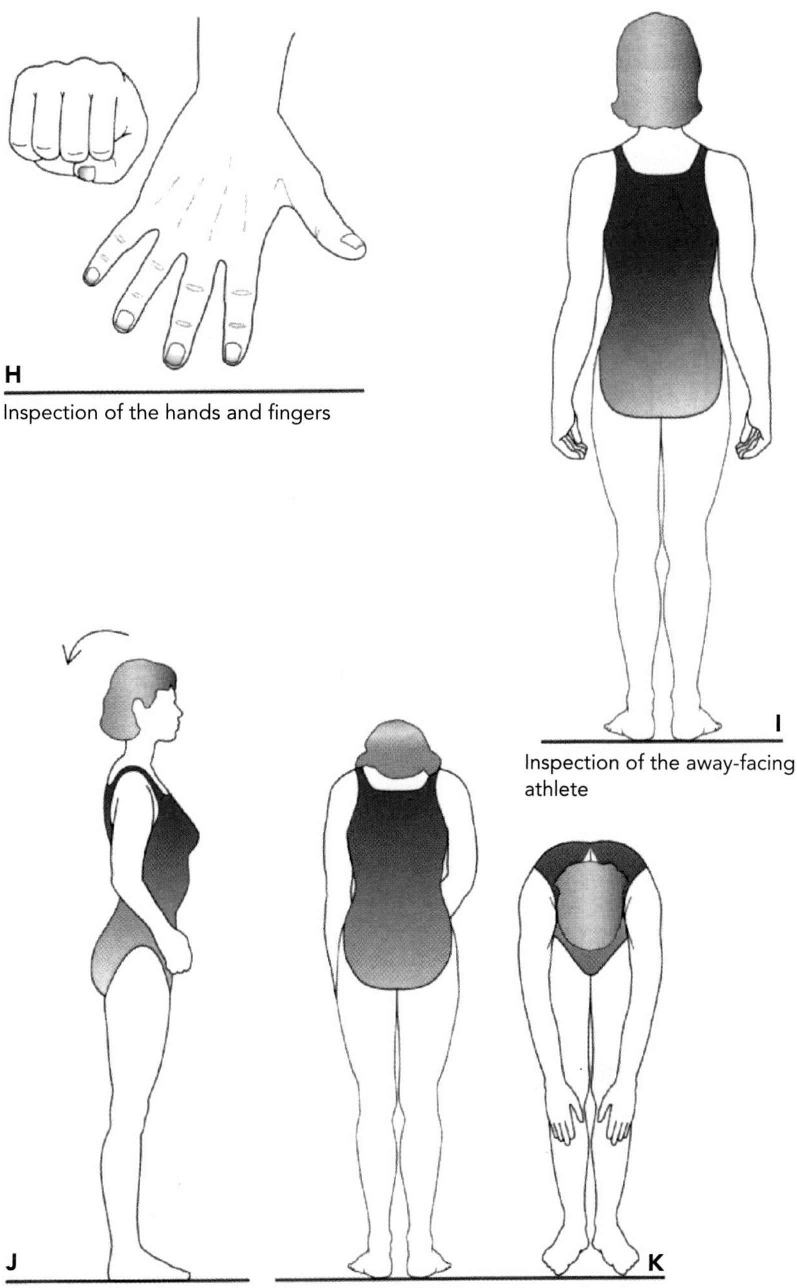

Figure 5.2 *(continued)*

in weight control sports such as wrestling. The most accurate means of such measurement is underwater immersion; however, skin fold measurements with calipers, using numerous regression equations to determine percent body fat, is a cheaper, albeit less accurate, method.

3. *Endurance and flexibility testing*. Although poor predictors of future injury, these tests can be included in an extended PPPE. Any unilateral laxity needs to be considered in light of the paired extremity, the age of the athlete, and the activity. This testing can be extremely useful in establishing a baseline for future monitoring of the effects of exercise, especially in the older athlete. Hyperlaxity of multiple joints may be a sign of a connective tissue disorder such as Marfan or Ehlers-Danlos syndrome.
4. *Hemoglobin/hematocrit*. May be important when the nutrition of a candidate is suspect or if there are complaints of fatigue, shortness of breath, or chest discomfort with exercise. A case can be made to screen athletes of African decent for sickle cell trait or disease, because these athletes appear vulnerable to heat illness, exertional rhabdomyolysis, and sudden death.
5. *Lipoprotein studies (fasting high density lipoprotein, cholesterol, and triglyceride levels)*. These studies are typically obtained as a part of the CPE in males older than 35 and

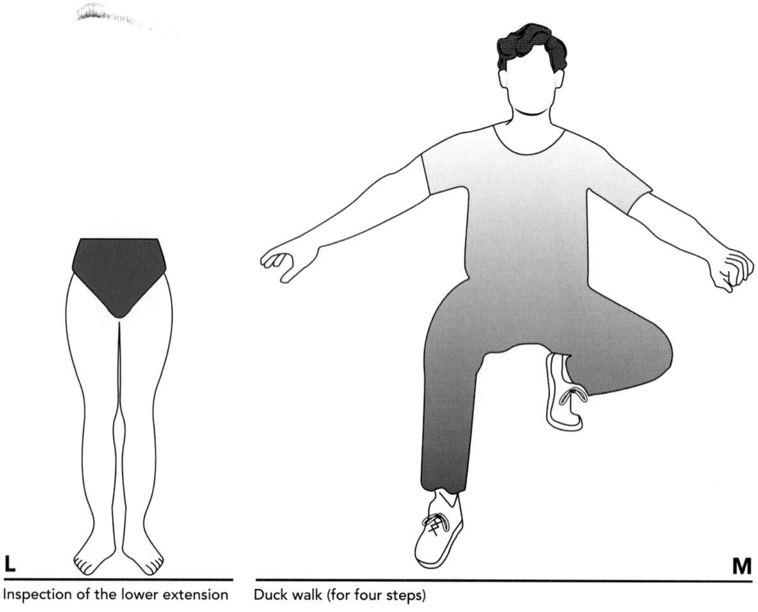

L
M
Inspection of the lower extension
Duck walk (for four steps)

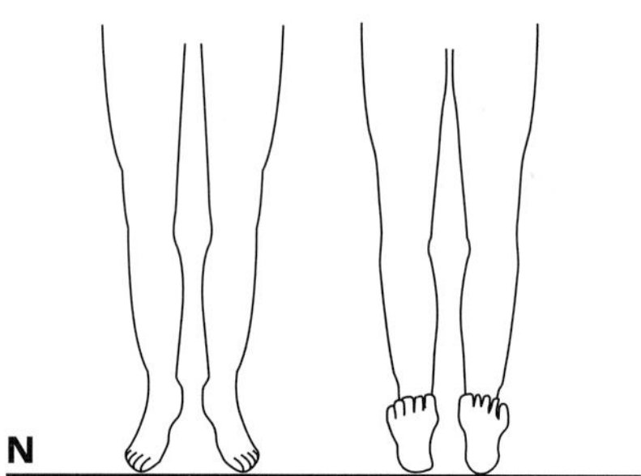

Figure 5.2 *(continued)*

females older than 45 years (or in younger patients with multiple risk factors or a strong family history of cardiac disease). Studies have shown that a large percentage of children have hypercholesterolemia, including many with no family history (15). The United States Preventive Services Task Force (USPSTF) currently does not recommend screening lipid testing in children (insufficient evidence for or against) (16).

6. *Drug testing.* Many colleges and elite level of sport organizations conduct random or reasonable suspicion drug testing, usually on an institutional basis. The timing of such a test may coincide with the PPPE.

TABLE 5.11
SUGGESTED SCREENING FORMAT FOR MARFAN'S SYNDROME

Screen all men over 6 ft and all women over 5 ft 10 in. on height with electrocardiogram and slit lamp examination when any two of the following are found:

1. Family history of Marfan's syndrome[a]
2. Cardiac murmur or midsystolic click
3. Kyphoscoliosis
4. Anterior thoracic deformity
5. Arm span greater than height
6. Upper to lower body ratio more than one standard deviation below the mean
7. Myopia
8. Ectopic lens

[a]finding *alone* should prompt further investigation.

Screening may encompass both ergogenic and recreational drugs. If a screening is done, counseling and rehabilitation programs are a necessary follow-up for any positive test result.

7. *Electrocardiogram (ECG).* Routine ECG testing in athletes is unwarranted because of the low prevalence of cardiac disease in young age-groups and the relative lack of specificity of the test. Because of the low specificity, false-positive results would likely outnumber true-positive results leading to inappropriate disqualification and/or an unnecessary, expensive workup. In a study of high school athletes screened with PPPE and ECG ($n = 5,615$), abnormal ECGs were noted in 2.6% and follow-up echocardiography was performed. These echocardiograms revealed no abnormalities in any of the athletes. In the same study 0.3% of athletes were disqualified from participation due to conduction abnormalities found on ECG. ECG is, however, appropriate as a natural extension if any cardiac abnormality is detected.
8. *Echocardiogram.* Screening cardiac echocardiography is perhaps the most controversial of additional tests for sport participation. At this time, screening echocardiography is not recommended due to practicality and cost efficiency issues. Considering the prevalence of HCM in the general U.S. population it would cost approximately $250,000 to detect one previously undiagnosed case. Echocardiogram is the test of choice for evaluating suspicious heart murmurs and to further evaluate the heart when the history raises red flags. Screening asymptomatic individuals at this time is not recommended.
9. *Pulmonary function testing (PFT).* Several studies have looked at routine PFTs or other pulmonary screens for exercise-induced bronchospasm. Although this condition is more common than previously suspected, there is no evidence that routine screening affects outcomes. Screening should be considered in those athletes whose history or performance suggests some component of bronchospasm. In these individuals, an exercise PFT should be performed rather than a static PFT, because the exercise test more closely approximates conditions which can produce bronchospasm. See Chapter 11 for full discussion of exercise induced bronchospasm (EIB) testing.
10. *Marfan syndrome.* Screening may be done where it seems appropriate in unusually tall men and women. A suggested screening format for this syndrome is given in Table 5.11.
11. *Sickle cell trait.* Sickle cell trait has been linked to an increased risk for heat illness and sudden cardiac death (see "Hemoglobin/hematocrit" earlier). Screening for sickle cell trait should be considered in athletes with a family history of sickle cell trait or in athletes of African descent and a history of exertional rhabdomyolysis.

ASSESSMENT

Assessment represents a clinical impression and conclusion, and is made after review of the medical history, the physical examination, and any necessary laboratory testing. The decision must take into account the athlete's type and level of sports involvement, not just a blanket approval to participate in any activity. The options available to the physician at the end of the PPPE are as follows:

1. Clearance without restriction for sport and level desired.
2. Clearance with recommendations for further evaluation or treatment includes medical recommendations for a sport or position.
3. Clearance deferred pending consultation, further evaluation, special treatments, special equipment fitting, or rehabilitation. This option implies that clearance must be obtained after remedial steps have been taken.
4. Disqualification—this option implies that the athlete has a condition that contraindicates his/her participation in certain types of sports or for any sport.

Decisions that involve clearance with limitation or disqualification should involve not only the physician, but the athlete, parents, and coach(es), as well as a representative of the organization or school system.

Any tables such as that reproduced as Table 5.12 should be considered only as guidelines for disqualifying conditions. All disqualifications or limitations in participation should be dealt with on an individual basis. Conditions that constitute absolute or relative contraindications for specific sports activity fall into six major categories (a) cardiopulmonary disorders, (b) neurological, (c) defects in paired organ systems, (d) organ enlargement, (e) active infection (with and without fever), and (f) musculoskeletal disorders. Once again, it is imperative to always weigh each case on its merits. Dogma has no place in the total disqualification of a potential athlete regardless of age. Any athlete who comes to a physician for a PPPE should leave with an appropriate idea of what he/she can or cannot do.

Copies of the PPPE should be made available to parents, primary care physician, team physician (if different), and school nurse. A copy should also be given to the team/school athletic trainer (or coach) that can be carried with the team to all practices and competitions so it is available in the event of injury or illness. Remember that the information documented in the PPPE is confidential medical information and should be treated as such.

INJURY PREDICTION

For years investigators have been attempting to identify conditions and factors that might predict injury in athletes. Most of the following have some proven value for this

TABLE 5.12
MEDICAL CONDITIONS AND SPORTS PARTICIPATION

Condition	May Participate
Atlantoaxial instability (instability of the joint between cervical vertebrae 1 and 2)	Qualified yes
Explanation: Athlete needs evaluation to assess risk of spinal cord injury during sports participation	
Bleeding disorder	Qualified yes
Explanation: Athlete needs evaluation	
Cardiovascular disease	
Carditis (inflammation of the heart)	No
Explanation: Carditis may result in sudden death with exertion	
Hypertension (high blood pressure)	Qualified yes
Explanation: Those with significant essential (unexplained) hypertension should avoid weight and power lifting, body building, and strength training. Those with secondary hypertension (hypertension caused by a previously identified disease) or severe essential hypertension need evaluation. The National High Blood Pressure Education Working group defined significant and severe hypertension	
Congenital heart disease (structural heart defects present at birth)	Qualified yes
Explanation: Those with mild forms may participate fully; those with moderate or severe forms or who have undergone surgery need evaluation. The 26th Bethesda Conference defined mild, moderate, and severe disease for common cardiac lesions	
Dysrhythmia (irregular heart rhythm)	Qualified yes
Explanation: Those with symptoms (chest pain, syncope, dizziness, shortness of breath, or other symptoms of possible dysrhythmia) or evidence of mitral regurgitation (leaking) on physical examination need evaluation. All others may participate fully	
Heart murmur	Qualified yes
Explanation: If the murmur is innocent (does not indicate heart disease), full participation is permitted. Otherwise, the athlete needs evaluation (see congenital heart disease and mitral valve prolapse)	
Cerebral palsy	Qualified yes
Explanation: Athlete needs evaluation	
Diabetes mellitus	Yes
Explanation: All sports can be played with proper attention to diet, blood glucose concentration, hydration, and insulin therapy. Blood glucose concentration should be monitored every 30 min during continuous exercise and 15 min after completion of exercise	
Diarrhea	Qualified no
Explanation: Unless disease is mild, no participation is permitted, because diarrhea may increase the risk of dehydration and heat illness. See fever	
Eating disorders	Qualified yes
Anorexia nervosa	
Bulimia nervosa	
Explanation: Patients with these disorders need medical and psychiatric assessment before participation	
Eyes	Qualified yes
Functionally one-eyed athlete	
Loss of an eye	
Detached retina	

TABLE 5.12
(continued)

Condition	May Participate
Previous eye surgery or serious eye injury *Explanation:* A functionally one-eyed athlete has a best-corrected visual acuity of <20/40 in the eye with worse acuity. These athletes would suffer significant disability if the better eye were seriously injured, as would those with loss of an eye. Some athletes who previously have undergone eye surgery or had a serious eye injury may have an increased risk of injury because of weakened eye tissue. Availability of eye guards approved by the American Society for Testing and Materials and other protective equipment may allow participation in most sports, but this must be judged on an individual basis	
Fever *Explanation:* Fever can increase cardiopulmonary effort, reduce maximum exercise capacity, make heat illness more likely, and increase orthostatic hypertension during exercise. Fever may rarely accompany myocarditis or other infections that may make exercise dangerous	No
Heat illness, history of *Explanation:* Because of the increased likelihood of recurrence, the athlete needs individual assessment to determine the presence of predisposing conditions and to arrange a prevention strategy	Qualified yes
Hepatitis *Explanation:* Because of the apparent minimal risk to others, all sports may be played that the athlete's state of health allows. In all athletes, skin lesions should be covered properly, and athletic personnel should use universal precautions when handling blood or body fluids with visible blood	Yes
Human immunodeficiency virus infection *Explanation:* Because of the apparent minimal risk to others, all sports may be played that the athlete's state of health allows. In all athletes, skin lesions should be covered properly, and athletic personnel should use universal precautions when handling blood or body fluids with visible blood	Yes
Kidney, absence of one *Explanation:* Athlete needs individual assessment for contact, collision, and limited-contact sports	Qualified yes
Liver, enlarged *Explanation:* If the liver is acutely enlarged, participation should be avoided because of risk of rupture. If the liver is chronically enlarged, individual assessment is needed before collision, contact, or limited-contact sports are played	Qualified yes
Malignant neoplasm *Explanation:* Athlete needs individual assessment	Qualified yes
Musculoskeletal disorders *Explanation:* Athlete needs individual assessment	Qualified yes
Neurological disorders	
History of serious head or spine trauma, severe or repeated concussions, or crainotomy *Explanation:* Athlete needs individual assessment for collision, contact, or limited-contact sports and also for noncontact sports if deficits in judgment or cognition are present. Research supports a conservative approach to management of concussion	Qualified yes
Seizure disorder, well-controlled *Explanation:* Risk of seizure during participation is minimal	Yes
Seizure disorder, poorly controlled *Explanation:* Athlete needs individual assessment for collision, contact, or limited-contact sports. The following noncontact sports should be avoided: archery, riflery, swimming, weight or power lifting, strength training, or sports involving heights. In these sports, occurrence of a seizure may pose a risk to self or others	Qualified yes
Obesity	Qualified yes

(continued)

TABLE 5.12
(continued)

Condition	May Participate
Explanation: Because of the risk of heat illness, obese persons need careful acclimatization and hydration	
Organ transplant recipient	Qualified yes
Explanation: Athlete needs individual assessment	
Ovary, absence of one	Yes
Explanation: Risk of severe injury to the remaining ovary is minimal	
Respiratory conditions	
Pulmonary compromise, including cystic fibrosis	Qualified yes
Explanation: Athlete needs individual assessment, but generally, all sports may be played if oxygenation remains satisfactory during a graded exercise test. Patients with cystic fibrosis need acclimatization and good hydration to reduce the risk of heat illness	
Asthma	Yes
Explanation: With proper medication and education, only athletes with the most severe asthma will need to modify their participation	
Acute upper respiratory infection	Qualified yes
Explanation: Upper respiratory obstruction may affect pulmonary function. Athlete needs individual assessment for all but mild disease. See fever	
Sickle cell disease	Qualified yes
Explanation: Athlete needs individual assessment. In general, if status of the illness permits, all but high exertion, collision, and contact sports may be played. Overheating, dehydration, and chilling must be avoided	
Sickle cell trait	Yes
Explanation: It is unlikely that persons with sickle cell trait have an increased risk of sudden death or other medical problems during athletic participation, except under the most extreme conditions of heat, humidity, and possibly increased altitude. These persons, like all athletes, should be carefully conditioned, acclimatized, and hydrated to reduce any possible risk	
Skin disorders (boils, herpes simplex, impetigo, scabies, molluscum contagiosum)	Qualified yes
Explanation: While the patient is contagious, participation in gymnastics with mats; martial arts; wrestling; or other collision, contact, or limited-contact sports is not allowed	
Spleen, enlarged	Qualified yes
Explanation: A patient with an acutely enlarged spleen should avoid all sports because of risk of rupture. A patient with a chronically enlarged spleen needs individual assessment before playing collision, contact, or limited-contact sports	
Testicle, undescended or absence of one	Yes
Explanation: Certain sports may require a protective cup	

From AAP policy statement, 2001 (17).

purpose. They are given here so the reader may further evaluate the literature as to the importance of each factor.

1. *Maturity staging.* Unbalanced competition between late and early maturing adolescents in contact sports such as football is a major factor in some serious injuries. This predictor is useful only with junior high school and early high school age athletes. Maturational staging is directly related to strength, power, and flexibility (Wilmore, 1979), but, by itself, is not a strong enough predictor of injury to qualify or disqualify any individual from competition. However, it is strong enough to base a recommendation for a delay in some types of sports participation.
2. *Flexibility.* The lack of body flexibility or (conversely) ligamentous laxity seen in many young athletes has been advocated as a predictor of future injury. Neither of these conditions has proved to be an effective predictor

and may simply represent a state of normalcy in the developing athlete.

3. *Family functioning.* An inadequate or poorly functioning family unit or acute crisis situations in the family have been linked to an increased rate of injury (Coddington, 1980).
4. *Cardiovascular fitness.* The unconditioned athlete is seen more often at the beginning of a season. A common assumption is that an individual should be conditioned for his or her sport before training; however, this is not the case most of the time. Cardiovascular unfitness leads to fatigue, which in turn leads to increased injury. Lack of conditioning is also a risk factor for heat illness.
5. *Lean body mass.* There is a misconception that the leaner the body, the better the performance. A study of high school wrestlers has shown that the most successful participants (State Tournament Champions) were not those with the lowest percentage of body fat. This has lead to unrealistic weight loss goals set by coaches in various sports. Some states have implemented a "minimum weight" program for sports such as wrestling in an attempt to decrease unhealthy weight loss practices. While obesity does slow down reaction time and decrease cardiovascular efficiency, extreme weight loss also results in major fatigue, loss of strength, and eventual injury.
6. *Muscular strength.* Detection of unilateral weakness in a muscle or a muscle group is a powerful indicator of future injury. All paired muscles should be tested, comparing sides as well as agonist-antagonist muscle groups. If any questionable results are seen in the clinical screening examination, isokinetic testing should be considered.

CONCLUSION

The PPPE for sports candidates of all ages represents one of several places where the office-based physician can prevent injury. Although such an examination is not cost effective, it can be justified if it is molded to the characteristics of the athlete and made as specific as possible. The PPPE should be a medical "chameleon," taking different forms as the need arises. Future PPPEs should have a higher level of sophistication that will include predictive factors in sport-specific examinations so as to lessen the number of injuries as well as assess general health.

REFERENCES

1. American Academy of Family Physicians, American Academy of Pediatrics, American Medical Society for Sports Medicine, American Medical Society for Sports Medicine, American Orthopaedic Society for Sports Medicine and American Osteopathic Academy of Sports Medicine. *Preparticipation physical evaluation*, 2nd ed. Minneapolis, New York: McGraw-Hill, 1997.
2. American Academy of Family Physicians, American Academy of Pediatrics, American Medical Society for Sports Medicine, American College of Sports Medicine, American Medicine Society for Sports Medicine, American Orthopaedic Society for Sports Medicine and American Osteopathic Academy of Sports Medicine. *Preparticipation physical evaluation*, 3rd ed. Minneapolis, New York: McGraw-Hill, 2005.
3. Henschen K, Griffin L. Parent egos take the fun out of Little League. *Psychol Today* 1977;3:18–22.
4. Matheson GO. editorial in The physician and sportsmedicine. 2001;29(9): 14–15.
5. Spirduso WW, Cronin DL. Exercise dose-response effects on quality of life and independent living in older adults. *Med Sci Sports Exerc* 2001;33(6):S598–S608.
6. McKeag DB. Preparticipation screening of the potential athlete. *Clin Sports Med* 1989;8(3):373–397.
7. Micheli LJ, Stone KR. The pre-sports physical: only the first step. *J Musculoskel Med* 1984;1(6)56–60.
8. United States Preventive Services Task Force. *Evidence report/technology assessment number 136: value of the periodic health evaluation.* AHRQ Publication No. 06-E011; April 2006.
9. Prochazka AV, Lundahl K, Pearson W, et al. Support of evidence-based guidelines for the annual physical examination: a survey of primary care providers. *Arch Intern Med* 2005;165(12):1347–1352.
10. American College of Sports Medicine (Position Statement). The recommended quantity and quality of exercise for developing and maintaining cardiorespiratory and muscular fitness in healthy adults. *Med Sci Sports Exerc* 1990;22:265–274.
11. Van Camp SP, Bloor CM, Mueller FO, et al. Nontraumatic sports death in high school and college athletes. *Med Sci Sports Exerc* 1995;27(5): 641–647.
12. National Heart, Lung and Blood Institute. The fourth report on the diagnosis, evaluation, and treatment of high blood pressure in children and adolescents. *Pediatrics* 2004;114:555–576. NIH Publication No. 05-5267.
13. Tanner JM. *Growth at adolescence*, 2nd ed. Oxford, England: Blackwell Science, 1962:28–39.
14. Carek PJ, Mainous A III. The preparticipation physical examination for athletics: a systematic review of current recommendations. *BMJ USA* 2003;2:661–664.
15. Garcia RE, Moodie DS. Routine cholesterol surveillance in childhood. *Pediatrics* 1989;84(5):751–755.
16. United States Preventive Services Task Force. *U.S. Preventive Services Task Force Guide: screening for high blood cholesterol and other lipid abnormalities.* AHCPR Publication No. 97–R004: July 1998.
17. American Academy of Pediatrics. Medical conditions affecting sports participation (RE0046). *Pediatrics* 2001;107(5):1205–1209.

SUGGESTED READINGS

36th Bethesda Conference. Eligibility recommendations for competitive athletes with cardiovascular abnormalities. *J Am Coll Cardiol* 2005;45(8):1313–1375.

Allman FL, McKeag DB, Bodner LM. Prevention and emergency care of sports injuries. *Fam Pract Recert* 1983;5:34–41.

American Medical Association. *Medical Evaluation of the athlete: a guide. Pamphlet #OP 209 Sports.* Chicago, Ill, 1979.

Bellisario RG, Rifat SF, Moeller JL. Dominant hand grip strength as an assessment of physical maturity in adolescents, poster presentation. *American Medical Society for Sports Medicine Annual Meeting.* Orlando, Florida, April 2002.

Delman A, Waugh T. School screening for scoliosis. *J Fam Med* 1983;31:6–12.

Fuller CM, McNulty CM, Spring DA, et al. Prospective screening of 5,615 high school athletes for risk of sudden cardiac death. *Med Sci Sports Exerc* 1997;29(9):1131–1138.

Goldberg B, Boiardo R. Profiling children for sports participation. *Clin Sports Med* 1984;3(1):153–169.

Hara JH, Puffer JC. The preparticipation physical examination. In: Mellion MB, ed. *Office management of sports injuries and athletic problems.* Chapter 1. Philadelphia: Harley and Belfus, 1988.

Maron BJ, Thompson PD, Puffer JC, et al. Cardiovascular preparticipation screening of competitive athletes: an addendum to a statement of health professional from the Sudden Death Committee (Council on Clinical Cardiology) and Congenital Cardiac Defects Committee (Council on Cardiovascular Disease in the Young), American Heart Association. *Circulation* 1998;97(22):2294.

Martens R. The uniqueness of the young athlete: psychologic considerations. *Am J Sports Med* 1980;8(5):382,385.

Monahan T. Sickle cell trait: a risk for sudden death during physical activity? *Phys Sportsmed* 1987;15(12):143–145.

Oppliger RA, Harms RD, Herrmann DE. et.al The Wisconsin wrestling minimum weight project: a model for weight control among high school wrestlers. *Med Sci Sports Exerc* 1995;27(8):1220–1224.

Shaffer TE. The adolescent athlete. *Pediatr Clin North Am* 1983;28:30–41.

Shaffer TE. The health examination for participation in sports. *Pediatr Ann* 1978;7(10):27–40.

Taylor RB. Pre-exercise evaluation: which procedures are really needed? *Consultant* 1983;4:94–101.

APPENDIX 5.1

PREPARTICIPATION PHYSICAL EXAMINATION (PPPE) HISTORY FORM

HISTORY FORM

Preparticipation Physical Evaluation

DATE OF EXAM

Name ______ **Sex** ____ **Age** ____ **Date of birth** ______

Grade___ **School** ______ **Sport(s)** ______

Address ______ **Phone** ______

Personal physician ______

In case of emergency, contact

Name ______ **Relationship** ______ **Phone(H)** ______ **(W)** ______

Explain "Yes" answers below.
Circle questions you don't know the answers to.

	Yes	No
1. Has a doctor ever denied or restricted your participation in sports for any reason?	☐	☐
2. Do you have an ongoing medical condition (like diabetes or asthma)?	☐	☐
3. Are you currently taking any prescription or nonprescription (over-the-counter) medicines or pills?	☐	☐
4. Do you have allergies to medicines, pollens, foods, or stinging insects?	☐	☐
5. Have you ever passed out or nearly passed out DURING exercise?	☐	☐
6. Have you ever passed out or nearly passed out AFTER exercise?	☐	☐
7. Have you over had discomfort, pain, or pressure in your chest during exercise?	☐	☐
8. Does your heart race or skip beats during exercise?	☐	☐
9. Has a doctor ever told you that you have (check all that apply): ☐ High blood pressure ☐ A heart murmur ☐ High cholesterol ☐ A heart infection		
10. Has a doctor ever ordered a test for your heart? (for example, ECG, echocardiogram)	☐	☐
11. Has anyone in your family died for no apparent reason?	☐	☐
12. Does anyone in your family have a heart problem?	☐	☐
13. Has any family member or relative died of heart problems or of sudden death before age 50?	☐	☐
14. Does anyone in your family have Marfan syndrome?	☐	☐
15. Have you ever spent the night in a hospital?	☐	☐
16. Have you ever had surgery?	☐	☐
17. Have you ever had an injury, like a sprain, muscle or ligament tear, or tendinitis, that caused you to miss a practice or game? If yes, circle affected area below:	☐	☐
18. Have you had any broken or fractured bones or dislocated joints? If yes, circle below:	☐	☐
19. Have you had a bone or joint injury that required x-rays, MRI, CT, surgery, injections, rehabilitation, physical therapy, a brace, a cast, or crutches? If yes, circle	☐	☐

Head	Head	Shoulder	Upper Arm	Elbow	Forearm	Hand/ fingers	Chest
Upper back	Lower back	Hip	Thigh	Knee	Calf/shin	Ankle	Foot/toes

	Yes	No
20. Have you ever had a stress fracture?	☐	☐
21. Have you been told that you have or have you had an x-ray for atlantoaxial (neck) instability?	☐	☐
22. Do you regularly use a brace or assistive device?	☐	☐
23. Has a doctor ever told you that you have asthma or allergies?	☐	☐
24. Do you cough, wheeze, or have difficulty breathing during or after exercise?	☐	☐
26. Have you ever used an inhaler or taken asthma medicine?	☐	☐
25. Is there anyone in your family who has asthma?	☐	☐
27. Were you born without or are you missing a kidney, an eye, a testicle, or any other organ?	☐	☐
28. Have you had infectious mononucleosis (mono) within the last month?	☐	☐
29. Do you have any rashes, pressure sores, or other skin problems?	☐	☐
30. Have you had a herpes skin infection?	☐	☐
31. Have you ever had a head injury or concussion?	☐	☐
32. Have you been hit in the head and been confused or lost your memory?	☐	☐
33. Have you ever had a seizure?	☐	☐
34. Do you have headaches with exercise?	☐	☐
35. Have you ever had numbness, tingling, or weakness in your arms or legs after being hit or falling?	☐	☐
36. Have you ever been unable to move your arms or legs after being hit or falling?	☐	☐
37. When exercising in the heat, do you have severe muscle cramps or become ill?	☐	☐
38. Has a doctor told you that you or someone in your family has sickle cell trait or sickle cell disease?	☐	☐
39. Have you had any problems with your eyes or vision?	☐	☐
40. Do you wear glasses or contact lenses?	☐	☐
41. Do you wear protective eyewear, such as goggles or a face shield?	☐	☐
42. Are you happy with your weight?	☐	☐
43. Are you trying to gain or lose weight?	☐	☐
44. Has anyone recommended you change your weight or eating habits?	☐	☐
45. Do you limit or carefully control what you eat?	☐	☐
46. Do you have any concerns that you would like to discuss with a doctor?	☐	☐
FEMALES ONLY		
47. Have you ever had a menstrual period?	☐	☐

48. How old were you when you had your first menstrual period? ____

49. How many periods have you had in the last 1 2 months?. ____

Explain "Yes" answers here: ______

I hereby state that, to the best of my knowledge, my answers to the above questions are complete and correct.

Signature of athlete ______ Signature of parant/guardian ______ Date ______

APPENDIX 5.2
PREPARTICIPATION PHYSICAL EXAMINATION FORM

Preparticipation Physical Evaluation

PHYSICAL EXAMINATION FORM

Name____ **Date of birth** __________________

Height_______ **Weight**_______ **% Body fat (optional)** _______ **Pulse**_____ **BP** ___ /___ (___ /___ ,___/___)

Height R 20/____ **L 20/** ____ **Corrected Y N** **Pupils: Equal** ____ **Unequal** ____

Follow-Up Questions on More Sensitive Issues	**Yes**	**No**
1. Do you fee stressed out or under a lot of pressure?		
2. Do you ever feel so sad or hopeless that you stop doing some of your usual activities for more than a few days?	☐	☐
3. Do you feel safe?	☐	☐
4. Have you ever tried cigarette smoking, even 1 or 2 puffs? Do you currently smoke?	☐	☐
5. During the past 30 days, did you use chewing tobacco, snuff, or dip?	☐	☐
6. During the past 30 days, have you had at least 1 drink of alcohol?	☐	☐
7. Have you ever taken steroids pills or shots without a doctor's prescription?	☐	☐
8. Have you even taken any supplements to help you gain or lose weight or improve your performance?	☐	☐
9. Questions from the Youth Risk Behavior Survey (http://www.cdc.gov/HealthyYouth/yrbs/index.htm) on guns, seatbelts, unprotected sex, domestic violence, drugs, etc.	☐	☐

Notes ____

	NORMAL	ABNORMAL FINDINGS	INITIALS*
MEDICAL			
Appearance			
Eyes/ears/nose/throat			
Hearing			
Lymph nodes			
Heart			
Murmurs			
Pulses			
Lungs			
Abdomen			
Genitourinary (males only)†			
Skin			
MUSCULOSKELETAL			
Neck			
Back			
Shoulder/arm			
Elbow/forearm			
Wrist/hand/fingers			
Hip/thigh			
Knee			
Leg/ankle			
Foot/toes			

*Multiple-examiner set-up only
†Having a third party present is recommended for the genitourinary examination

Notes ____

Name of physician (print/type)__________________________________ **Date** ____________

Address ______________________________________ **Phone** ________________

Signature of physician ____ **MD or DO**

Conditioning and Training Programs for Athletes/Nonathletes

6

Sally E. Nogle *Jeffrey S. Monroe*

SECTION A

GENERAL PRINCIPLES

The information outlined in this chapter comes from scientific application of theories and principles of exercise physiology, using both animal and human studies. The chapter begins with the adult male competitor: the type of participant used most often in studies done on training and conditioning. A discussion of the young athlete, the female athlete, and the older athlete follows.

METABOLIC SPECIFICITY

To maximize its beneficial effect, any training program must develop the specific physiological capabilities required to perform a given sport or activity (see Chapter 2). The most important physiological capability to be enhanced is the ability to supply energy (adenosine triphosphate [ATP] and the substrate phosphocreatine [PC]) to working muscles. ATP can be supplied in any of following three ways to the muscles:

1. ATP-PC system (anaerobic) used in maximum intensity exercises under ten seconds or less
2. Lactic Acid System (LA) (anaerobic) functions in high intensity exercise three minutes or less
3. Oxygen or aerobic system is utilized in activities greater than three minutes

As illustrated in Table 6A.1, the capacity and the rate at which energy (ATP) can be supplied by these three systems in the body differ. The rate of supply can be referred to as "power." The predominant energy source will be a function of the total amount and rate of energy demanded by that exercise (see Table 6A.2). When a training/conditioning program is constructed, such a regimen logically should specifically increase the capacity of the energy system used most often in that particular sport.

Factors to consider for achieving maximal benefits from a training program include the following:

- The mode of exercise used during training should be the mode used in the performance of the sports skill. For example—unless he is injured, an athlete should not train for running by swimming. However, training effects induced by running, although still specific, do appear to have beneficial cross-over effects for other sports.
- Training effects tend to be specific to muscle groups. The major objective of physical training is to cause specific and efficient biological adaptation to improve performance in specific events. Therefore the muscle groups used for these events must be trained.

Four major principles should be applied to any training/conditioning program:

- *Specificity.* Specific training elicits specific adaptations, enhancing specific actions.
- *Overload.* Overload refers to exercising at above normal levels, and is achieved by manipulating combinations of training frequency, intensity, duration, and type of

TABLE 6A.1
CAPACITY AND POWER OF THREE ENERGY SYSTEMS IN UNTRAINED MALE SUBJECTS

Energy System	ATP Production	
	Capacity (Total mol)	Power (mol/min)
ATP-PC	0.6	3.6
LA	1.2	1.6
O_2	∞	1.0

ATP = adenosine triphosphate; PC = phosphocreatine; LA = lactic acid; O_2 = oxygen.
Source: Fox EL. Physical training: methods and effects. *Orthop Clin North Am* 1977; 8:533–548, (1).

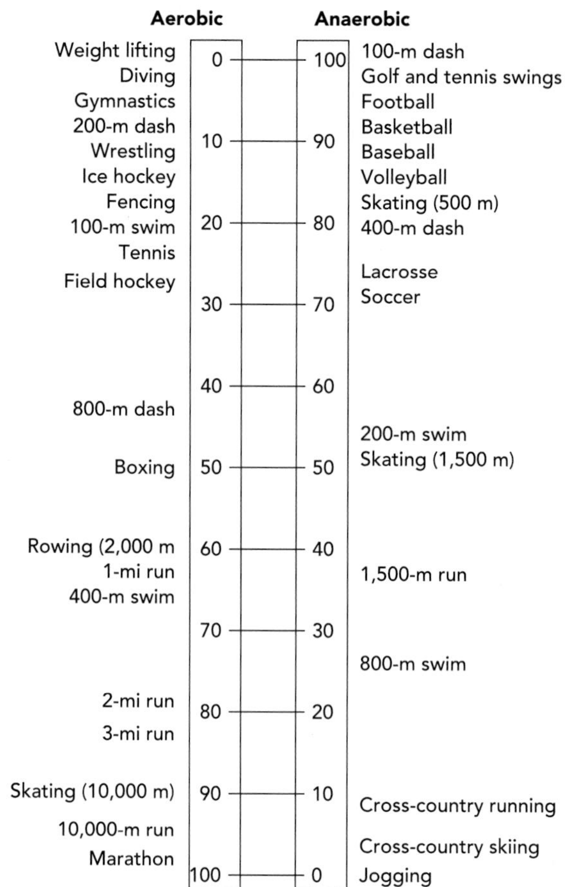

Figure 6A.1 A comparison of aerobic and anaerobic contributions of adenosine triphosphate (ATP) during the performance of various sports.

activity. This is also known as the *SAID Principle,* specific adaptations to imposed demands.

- *Individual differences.* People respond and perform differently to similar stimuli. Individual variations should be taken into account in the construction of any training program. A specific training program that works for one athlete may not for another.
- *Reversibility.* This refers to the principle of detraining. Unfortunately, the beneficial conditioning effects of exercise training are transient and reversible, so conditioning should be continuous in nature. A swift and significant detraining effect may be seen when a person stops exercising. After only 2 weeks of inactivity, significant reductions in work capacity can be measured (2).

Necessary steps in the construction of a conditioning program should include the following:

- Consider the predominant energy system used (see Table 6A.2 and Figure 6A.1).
- Select an appropriate training regimen (see Table 6A.3).
- Any training prescription and its content should include movement patterns specific to the sport and/or position to enhance motor unit recruitment patterns. Repetitive motor skill work will augment neuromuscular skills and enhance subsequent performance.
- To prevent boredom and overuse injuries, introduce variability into the training program. Overuse injury is a significant result of lack of training variability.

TABLE 6A.2
PERFORMANCE TIME AND ENERGY SYSTEMS

Performance Time	Predominant Energy System(s)
30 sec	ATP-PC
30 sec–1 ½ min	ATP-PC and LA
1 ½–3 min	LA and O_2
3 min	O_2

ATP = adenosine triphosphate; PC = phosphocreatine; LA = lactic acid; O_2 = oxygen.

EXERCISE PRESCRIPTION

For an in-depth justification of the recommendations given here, please refer to the American College of Sports Medicine (ACSM) statement on quality and quantity of exercise (Appendix 5A). As mentioned earlier, the four major training components of conditioning are frequency, intensity, duration, and mode of activity.

Frequency

Training should occur three to five times per week. In a primary care setting, the practitioner must clearly ask a patient to set aside time for an exercise program. This time must be sufficient for the complete workout and it should have a high priority on the individual's daily schedule.

TABLE 6A.3
DEFINITIONS OF VARIOUS TRAINING METHODS AND DEVELOPMENT OF THE ENERGY SYSTEMS

Training Method	Definition	ATP-PC	LA and O_2	O_2
Acceleration sprints	Gradual increases in running speed from jogging to striding to sprinting in 50-yd to 120-yd segments	90		5
Continuous fast running	Long-distance running (or swimming) at a fast pace	2	8	90
Continuous slow running	Long-distance running (or swimming) at a slow pace	2	5	93
Hollow sprints	Two sprints interrupted by periods of jogging or walking	20	10	5
Interval sprinting	Alternate sprints of 50 yd and jogs of 60 yd for distances of up to 3 mi	20	10	70
Jogging	Continuous walking or running at a slow pace over a moderate distance (e.g., 2 mi)	10–30	30–50	20–60
Repetition running	Similar to interval sprinting but longer work and relief intervals	10	50	40
Speed play (fartlek)	Alternating fast and slow running over natural terrain	20	40	40
Sprint training	Repeated sprints at maximal speed with complete recovery between repeats	90	6	4

ATP-PC = adenosine triphosphate phosphocreatine; LA = lactic acid.
Source: From Fox EL. Physical training: methods and effects. *Orthop Clin North Am* 1977;8:533–548.

Intensity

Intensity is the factor that varies the most when individuals first begin an exercise program. Consider the following when making recommendations about intensity of exercise:

1. Determine either the maximum aerobic capacity (Vo_{2max}) or maximum heart rate (MHR) (beats/minute). MHR levels adjusted to age and fitness have been estimated using graded exercise testing (see Table 6A.4). Another convenient, reasonably accurate method is MHR = 220—the age of the patient.
2. An appropriate training level should be established within these ranges:
   a. Vo_{2max}—Range—50% (beginners) to 85% (elite athletes).
   b. MHR—Range—60% (beginners) to 90% (elite athletes); average—70%.
3. Fine adjustments need to be made considering the following:
   a. Motivation.
   b. Musculoskeletal limiting factors.
   c. The body habitus—the more obese the individual is, the less intense and weight bearing a training program should be at the beginning.
4. Advise the patient to monitor pulse rate every 10 to 15 minutes through the course of activity. This can be done by educating the patient to take either carotid or radial pulse.

Duration

Fifteen to sixty minutes of continuous aerobic activity is recommended. The frequency of exercise is a factor with a wide and flexible range. An individual who exercises only three times a week needs a longer exercise period (usually 45–60 minutes) than someone who exercises five to six times a week, and who may only need 15 to 30 minutes of exercise. Consider the "F × I × D" product, frequency × intensity × duration, to get a rough idea of work done over a period. A desirable exercise program for the recreational noncompetitive adults will be of longer duration with low to moderate intensity because of better compliance and less chance of injury.

Mode of Activity

Improving aerobic capacity requires the use of large muscle groups, continuous exercise, rhythmic repetitive movement, and stimulation of the aerobic energy system. It should be mentioned that anaerobic exercise is usually static, very intense in nature, and only results in minimal beneficial effect on the cardiovascular system. Anaerobic exercise will increase muscular strength and endurance. This type of exercise is generally contraindicated for patients with heart disease and/or hypertension (see Table 6A.5). Consult Tables 6A.4 and 6A.5 for approximate sport-specific energy expenditures.

TABLE 6A.4

AGE-FITNESS ADJUSTED PREDICTED MAXIMUM HEART RATE (MHR) FOR THREE LEVELS OF FITNESS

	Predicted MHR, bpm		
Age	**Below Average**	**Average**	**Above Average**
20	201	201	196
21	199	200	196
22	198	199	195
23	197	198	195
24	196	198	194
25	195	197	194
26	194	196	193
27	193	196	193
28	192	195	192
29	191	193	192
30	190	193	191
31	189	193	191
32	188	192	190
33	187	191	189
34	186	191	189
35	184	190	188
36	183	189	188
37	182	189	187
38	181	188	187
39	180	187	186
40	179	186	186
41	178	186	185
42	177	185	185
43	176	184	184
44	177	184	184
45	174	183	183
46	173	182	183
47	172	181	182
48	171	181	182
49	170	180	181
50	168	179	180
51	167	179	180
52	166	178	179
53	165	177	179
54	164	176	178
55	163	176	178
56	162	175	177
57	161	174	177
58	160	174	176
59	159	173	176
60	158	172	175
61	167	172	175
62	156	171	174
63	155	170	174
64	154	169	173
65	152	169	173
66	151	168	172
67	160	167	171
68	149	167	171
69	148	166	170
70	147	165	170

MHR = maximum heart rate.

TABLE 6A.5

DISEASES THAT CONTRAINDICATE ANAEROBIC EXERCISING FOR RECREATIONAL ATHLETES

Cardiac	Vascular and Circulatory
Angina pectoris, uncontrolled or unstable	Anaemia, severe or of unknown cause
Aortic stenosis, severe	Aneurysm, large or dissecting
Cardiac arrhythmia, uncontrolled	Cerebrovascular accident, acute
Congestive heart failure, uncontrolled (class III or IV)	Embolism, pulmonary or systemic, acute
Myocardial infarction, acute	Hypertension, uncontrolled
Myocarditis or cardiomyopathy	Thrombophlebitis, acute
Valvular heart disease, severe	Transient ischemic attack, recent

Source: Adapted from Taylor RB. Pre-exercise evaluation: which procedures are really needed? *Consultant* 1983; 23:94–101, (3).

Additional Concepts

The primary care physician should also take into account the following considerations in prescribing an exercise program. They are not part of the five major factors normally considered in an exercise program, but they represent important additional information.

1. *Detraining.* A total loss of conditioning following rest or inactivity takes place between 10 and 34 weeks after training ceases. Stopping may be voluntary (vacations, other obligations) or involuntary (illness, injury).
2. *Epidemiological studies.* It appears that more injuries occur in weight-bearing activities than in non–weight-bearing ones. In addition, the only consistent biological characteristic associated with noncompliance or dropout from an exercise program is obesity (4). For this reason, we suggest foregoing most weight-bearing exercise until later in the program, especially for those patients who are obese.
3. *Energy equivalents.* These rough equivalents can give the prescribing physician some idea of possible "cross-over" training activities that can be used in the event of injury. The approximate formula is: **9 units biking = 4 units running = 1 unit swimming**. This formula is very useful for determining relative rest when treating overuse injuries.
4. Age should not be a deterrent to training. The major consideration of age is a need for a longer period of adaptation. Natural decreases in functional status that occur with age can be delayed or even reversed. Those decreases are outlined in Table 6A.6. The effect of a

TABLE 6A.6
AGE-RELATED DECREASES IN FUNCTIONAL STATUS

Cardiovascular system	↓Maximum heart rate	10 beats/min/decade
	↓Resting Stroke Volume	30% by 85 yr of age
	↓Maximum Cardiac Output	20%–30% by 65 yr of age
	↓Vessel compliance	↑Blood pressure 10–40 mm Hg
Respiratory system	↑Residual volume	30%–50% by 70 yr of age
	↓Vital capacity	40%–50% by 70 yr of age
Nervous system	↓Nerve conduction	10%–15% by 60 yr of age
	↓Proprioception and balance	35%–40% ↑ in falls by 60 years of age
Metabolism	↓Maximum O_2 uptake	9%/decade
Musculoskeletal system	↑Bone loss: male >35 female >55	l%/yr
	↓Muscle strength	20% by 65 yr of age
	↓Flexibility	Degenerative disease or inactivity

Source: Compiled from data: Fitzgerald PL. Exercise for the elderly. *Med Clin North Am* 1985;69(1):189.

chronic disease such as osteoarthritis may be reversed by the application of the right amount of exercise and movement for the affected joints.

5. A program that occurs fewer than 3 days a week, is less than 50% $V_{O_{2max}}$ levels in intensity, and has a duration of less than 10 minutes a day is inadequate to achieve a training effect.

MAJOR COMPONENTS OF A GOOD TRAINING PROGRAM

Preconditioning

Preconditioning is absolutely imperative at the beginning of exercise. Preconditioning gives the body time to adjust and provide a safer, more measured response to exercise. It is less taxing on the cardiovascular system and causes fewer injuries. Ten to 14 days at intensity levels lower than normal is advocated. For example, the use of the run-walk (run until tired, then walk, then run again) is appropriate as a preconditioning program for jogging. Another example is the use of low gear biking on level ground before adjusting to high gear cycling on hills.

Warm-Up

A warm-up lasting between 5 and 10 minutes should precede the beginning of every exercise program. The two components to any warm-up program are low intensity activity and stretching. The order is important. Warm-up should begin with 5 minutes of low intensity activity, preferably the same type that will be done during exercise, although jogging is a good all-purpose warm-up activity. The purpose of warm-up is to increase blood flow to major muscle groups, gradually increase the heart rate, reduce muscle stiffness, facilitate enzymatic activity, and ready the body for more strenuous effort. This should be followed by approximately 5 minutes of slow, gentle stretching (no bouncing) of major muscle groups, particularly those that will be heavily used during exercise. The warm-up period is not benign. Overstretching, "ballistic," and/or improper stretching have caused many acute soft tissue injuries (please refer to Chapter 8 for figures on poor stretching techniques). The period can be expanded to include 5 to 10 minutes of muscular strength and endurance exercises (push-ups, pull-ups, sit-ups, etc.). It should be noted that the warm-up phase should never be eliminated.

Exercise Period

Discussed earlier in this chapter.

Cooldown

This is another transition period and should consist of low intensity activity such as jogging and some light stretching. This important component should last 3 to 5 minutes. It covers an extremely dangerous physiological time in the course of a workout session. Just as the warm-up physiologically prepares an individual for the exercise stimulus, the cooldown allows for proper recovery from exercise. During the cooldown, there are rapid changes in peripheral vascular resistance and venous return so that the induction of life-threatening cardiac arrhythmias is most likely to occur. This part of the training program allows the body (specifically the cardiovascular system) to accommodate and adjust to the non–exercise mode.

Progression—Part 2

- If an increase is contemplated in an exercise program, it should be accomplished slowly over a period. There should be no pain or history of recent injury before an increase is undertaken.

- Never increase two of the three components of a training program simultaneously; (frequency, intensity, and duration). Only one component at a time should ever be increased, and that too on a gradual basis. For example, a patient on a jogging program should be advised to add no more than 10% to 15% at a time to the distance or time being run, with the increases coming no more often than every 2 weeks while the same frequency and intensity are maintained.

Return From Injury

- *Relative rest versus absolute rest.* Relative rest refers to decreasing the training regimen but allowing an athlete to train at a lower level. Absolute rest pulls an athlete completely off training. From a primary care perspective, we feel that patient compliance is easier to achieve and there is less muscle atrophy and detraining if the relative rest concept is advocated for most patients.
- *Alternative activity.* There are many times in the treatment of injuries when a particular mode of activity is contraindicated. An alternative activity is an option for some patients. The basic premise is to decrease the force load placed upon the body by the activity in question (see Table 6A.7).

Light Intensity Training Program

The objective of Light Intensity Training (LIT) is to steer away from dogma concerning a return to activity after injury, and allow an individual some self-determination in how quickly the return is accomplished. This program can be instituted when the individual is able to ambulate or perform "activities of daily living" without symptoms (pain, swelling). A specific activity is begun on an every other day basis and at a very low level without regard for duration or intensity. The three options to be considered during and after this trial return to activity are as follows:

- If pain and/or swelling develops during the activity—stop all activity immediately and decrease the following day's activity by 25% (at the start, less as distance or duration of activity increases).
- If pain and/or swelling develop after exercise is completed—continue the following day at the same level, but do not increase the level of activity.

TABLE 6A.7
EQUIVALENT FORCE LOADS

Jumping	10–14× body weight
Running	4–7× body weight
Walking	1× body weight
Biking	0.25–0.50× body weight
Swimming	0× body weight

- If pain and/or swelling are not present during or after activity—increase activity slightly (up to 25% at the start, less later).

This program allows an orderly stepwise return to a previous training regimen and incorporates the cooperation and help of the patient.

SECTION B
THE YOUNG ATHLETE

This section presents those aspects of conditioning/training programs for young athletes that might differ from what already has been discussed.

It is appropriate to discuss the role of exercise in adolescents and younger children. The leadership of a knowledgeable primary care physician who can lend assistance to a community organizing a youth sports program can be powerful and invaluable. It may well represent one of the most effective preventive medicine interventions a physician can undertake in his community. Childhood and adolescence are the most active periods of life, and interest in exercise and sports is at its peak. Unfortunately, medical science has yet to quantify, or even describe with any degree of accuracy, the major characteristics of growth and exercise and how they relate to each other. The effect of both long- and short-term exercise on physical training of youth remains a matter of speculation. It should come as no surprise that medical science has difficulty setting fitness guidelines for preadolescents and adolescents. Nevertheless, a summary of exercise prescription for the youth is useful even if difficult to execute.

THE PREPUBESCENT ATHLETE

Unique physiological characteristics of the young athlete include the following:

- *Physical growth.* Of the three growth spurts occurring in humans, the first (inuteral) is nutritionally and genetically determined, and the second (occurring at approximately 54–60 months of age) takes place before major athletic involvement begins. However, the third (rapid growth associated with puberty) is affected by the amount of exercise.
- *Exploration of new areas of interest.* Inquisitive youngsters often look upon sports activity as a new experience.
- *Maturation.* With the initiation of maturational changes during puberty, there is an augmentation of strength, endurance, and neuromuscular skills.
- *Body proportion changes.* During the adolescent growth spurt, approximately 15% of the adult height and 40% of the skeletal mass are achieved.
- *Body composition alterations.* Prepubertal boys and girls have approximately the same percent body fat, but

during pubertal growth male body fat decreases whereas female body fat increases. In addition, muscular body strength in the male increases more than in the female.

- *Other considerations.* In addition to the physical changes, massive psychological and sociological changes occur simultaneously, affecting to a great extent the developing child and his/her attitude to athletic activities.

A summary of pertinent questions that might be asked of a physician about prepubescent training regimens include the following:

1. *Is such training dangerous to the preadolescent epiphysis?* No. In a large study of athletes with epiphyseal injuries, 98% resulted in uneventful recovery with no major medical intervention needed once proper diagnosis was made (5).
2. *Are there any special nutritional or thermoregulatory considerations for children in training?* No. The nutritional requirements of this group vary little from those of nonathletes of the same age group. Heavy growth demands dictate the rate of nutritional uptake. Little in the way of special diet or supplements is needed for young athletes as long as they eat a normal, well-balanced diet (6,7). The only special consideration would be replacing those calories used in training with pure complex carbohydrates. The thermoregulatory mechanism of the young athlete is extremely efficient, although the amount of sweating is less than in an adult. The capacity to thermoregulate remains higher and more efficient in the prepubescent child (8).
3. *Do growth and development benefit from training or are they impeded by exercise?* There appears to be no data to accurately answer this question, but several studies have indicated that a "normal" amount of exercise is beneficial for growth and development. Excesses in exercise can have a harmful dampening effect on growth and development.
4. *Are there psychological effects or ramifications of participation at a young age?* People exercise for many reasons and children are no different. The major motivation to participate in exercise or enter competitive sports is a desire to have fun (9–11). One study has shown that 95% of the children polled believed that having fun while participating in a sport was more important than winning; 75% would rather play on a loosing team than "sit" on a winning team (12).

   Sports competition can produce severe stress and anxiety, and psychological trauma can occur when children are subjected to repeated episodes of failure in competition. Two groups of vulnerable children have been identified: those with a low level of athletic competence due to late maturation, inexperience, or genetic lack of ability, and those who perceive they are not meeting the expectations of their age/peer group, coach, or (most importantly) parents (10,13).

   Seefeldt (14) offers the following "Bill of Rights" for young athletes:
   a. The right to participate in sports.
   b. The right to participate at a level commensurate with maturity and ability.
   c. The right to have qualified adult leadership.
   d. The right to play as a child and not as an adult.
   e. The right to share in the leadership and decision-making of their particular sport.
   f. The right to participate in a safe and healthy environment.
   g. The right to proper preparation for participation in sport.
   h. The right to an equal opportunity to strive for success.
   i. The right to be treated with dignity.
   j. The right to have fun in sports.
5. *What are children's norms, and how far can they drive themselves or be driven by others?* This represents one of the least known and most potentially dangerous areas of sports medicine. It is an important question to ask even if it is unanswerable at present.
6. *Can children achieve a training effect?* To answer this question, we must look closely at the growth and maturation processes taking place in the pubescent individual. The "trigger hypothesis" has been used to explain specific changes and lack of changes in the physical conditioning of children. This hypothesis states that there is one critical period in a child's development (termed the *trigger point*), usually coinciding with puberty, before which the effects of physical conditioning from any mode are minimal, if they occur at all. It is felt that this phenomenon is the result of the modulating effects of hormones, the same hormones that initiate puberty and influence the functional development and subsequent organic adaptations seen in the mature adult. We must be careful not to imply that prepubertal changes in conditioning do not occur. On the contrary, functional changes and adaptations are apparently as a normal consequence of the growth-maturation process (15,16). Figure 6B.1 illustrates a schematic drawing compiling data on $\text{V}\text{O}_{2\text{max}}$ levels of various age groups.

It has long been suspected that the ultimate limit for physiological performance is set by genetic makeup. The contribution of genetic potential to the adaptation to conditioning is major. Heredity has been shown to account for anywhere between 81% and 93% of the observed differences in cardiorespiratory endurance. Researchers who have studied the phenomenon of puberty state that certain yet-to-be-known organic adaptations involving endocrine functions must be present for puberty to occur. The trigger hypothesis (see Figure 6B.2) represents a parallel assumption that for organic adaptations for training and conditioning to occur, certain necessary conditions must precede those adaptations. An increase in lean to fat body ratio, maturation of the neuromuscular system, and increase in the levels of endocrine function must precede any significant training effect in children (17).

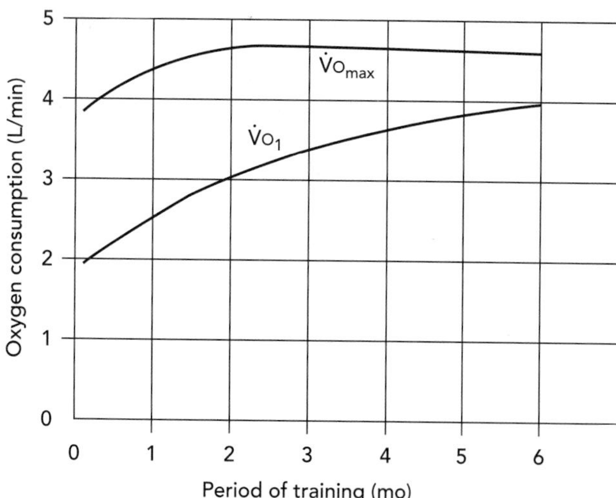

Figure 6B.1 Adaptation of body to training over time.

Both androgen and growth hormone are thought to play a part in the development of functional capacity in the pubescent individual. Androgen levels determine muscular response to resistance exercise. That response is minimal in a prepubertal youngster (18). Should a 9-year-old boy weight train? The risk (injury)–benefit (minimal muscle growth) ratio would say, "No." Because of its many functions throughout the body, growth hormone is believed to be the prime agent working in the presence of physical conditioning to induce organic adaptations. Prepubertal athletes and nonathletes differ little in their metabolic adaptation processes, yet they can be remarkably different in athletic performance. It appears that athletic performance in this age group is more dependent upon the level of skill development than on physiological conditioning. This principle should guide the practitioner in advising prepubertal athletes on constructing an athletic training program. Additionally, the primary care physician should be well versed in the clinical use of physical maturity staging to allow for accurate assessment of the stage of puberty before formulating any exercise program (see Chapter 4, Figure 4.3).

POSTPUBESCENT ATHLETE

Postpubertal children require physiological conditioning along with skill training for optimal athletic performance. There does not appear to be a definitive answer about whether conditioned prepubertal children will demonstrate greater physiological changes after puberty, but there is evidence to suggest that prepubertal conditioning may prime the body to accept changes occurring in the postpubertal individual because of training. Any postpubertal individual follows predictable adult patterns concerning exercise-induced adaptations from training and conditioning.

When working with a postpubertal individual, the concept of initial level of fitness at the beginning of an exercise program is important. An individual who starts at a low level of functioning should have room for considerable improvement. For many children who are beginning their first serious exercise training, the previous consideration is important. Aerobic fitness improvements of 5% to 25% can be expected from systematic training by postpubertal individuals. In strength training, it is not unusual to see 100% to 200% improvement during the adolescent years. Physiological adaptations to exercise in the postpubescent period may be dependent upon initial levels of strength and endurance, but they can be demonstrated within 1 to 2 weeks after starting a conditioning program if the intensity is sufficient. Optimal physical conditioning in the postpubescent individual also depends upon the frequency, intensity, and duration of exercise, just as it does with adults. Most changes seen in this group result from the intensity of the training overload. Wilmore (19) indicates

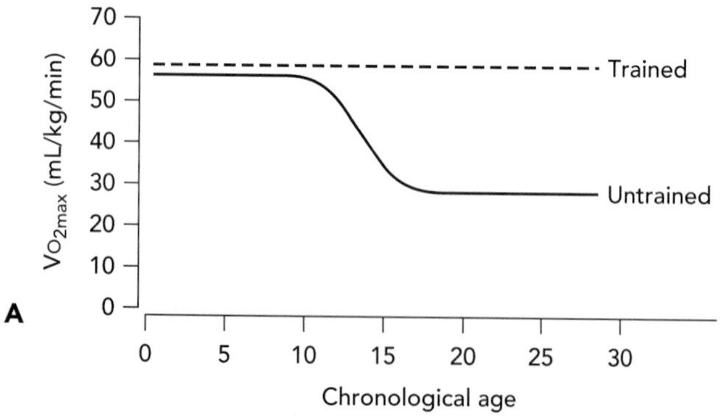

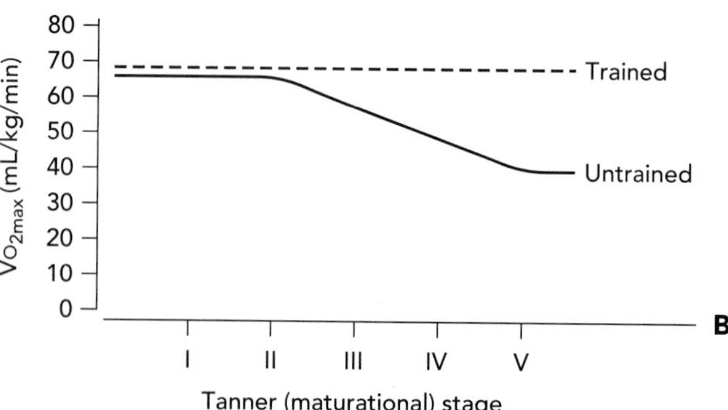

Figure 6B.2 Trigger hypothesis. **A:** Cardiorespiratory performance during childhood and adolescent years. Trained refers to individuals maximally trained by aerobic means, regardless of age or sex. Untrained refers to individuals whose exercise is limited to activities of daily living. **B:** Cardiorespiratory performance is related to maturational stage. Trained refers to individuals maximally trained by aerobic means, regardless of age or sex. Untrained refers to individuals whose exercise is limited to activities of daily living.

that the greater the relative training intensity, the greater the training adaptation. There probably is a "minimal" threshold intensity below which training effects will not occur, as well as a possible "ceiling" threshold above which there are no further gains in adaptation. Studies of the frequency of activity in the postpubertal individual have shown that training more than 3 to 4 days a week yields very little additional change in physiological function. It appears that rest between exercise sessions is an important component in producing biological adaptations in this age group. The duration of exercise to build endurance requires a minimum of 25 to 30 minutes and an approximate 300 kcal expenditure for adaptations to take place. Strength training workouts need not exceed 40 minutes at maximum intensity levels.

SECTION C
THE FEMALE ATHLETE

There has been a dramatic increase in the participation of women in physical activity in the past few decades. More women of all ages are exercising and training intensively for endurance events. More women of all ages can be seen in a variety of sports in the competitive and recreational setting. This surge in participation has raised a number of issues that pertain to the female athlete. Many relate to the female reproductive/endocrine function. Puberty may be delayed in young women involved in intensive training programs, and menstrual cycle abnormalities resulting from endurance training have been increasingly reported. These include shortened luteal phases, oligomenorrhea, amenorrhea, and anovulation. Concerns about future infertility and accelerated osteoporosis, in addition to the effects of active exercise programs on pregnancy, fetal growth retardation, and birth complications must be addressed.

It is important to look at the physical and mental makeup of the female athlete involved in exercise and sport. There are obvious physical differences between male and female athletes (see Table 6C.1) that may affect their potential for sports participation (20). However, the female can and should enjoy all the benefits of sports, exercise, and better health through active participation in a regular program.

The change in society's attitudes toward athletic participation by women during the early 1970s, along with opportunity for older women to become actively involved in exercising, has led more female athletes to seek advice about exercise. The physical skills and knowledge about sports by women born after 1960 is vastly different from those of older women who are entering the sports world as novices. The older woman may be enthusiastic in pursuing a regular exercise program, but she lacks the rudimentary knowledge of conditioning techniques, how to select appropriate equipment and clothing, and how to protect herself from overuse and acute injuries.

AEROBIC POWER

Habitual level of activity, not gender or age, is the primary determinant of an individual's cardiovascular fitness. Male and female athletes who participate in the same sport are more similar in aerobic power ($\dot{V}O_{2max}$) than athletes of the same sex in different sports. The elite male athlete has a higher $\dot{V}O_{2max}$ than the elite female athlete. The lower oxygen carrying capacity of a woman, a reflection of lower hemoglobin levels, is probably the major factor in this difference. Absolute levels of $\dot{V}O_{2max}$ usually are higher for men because males have a larger body mass than females and $\dot{V}O_{2max}$ is directly related to body size. This presents a problem for women only in the sports or activities in which both sexes must perform at the same absolute work rate.

One of the most important concepts in all descriptive research studies is the fact that female athletes can obtain high levels of cardiovascular fitness. They are physiologically capable of undergoing the physical stress of endurance sports and they do not, as many texts imply, reach their peak fitness levels at age 15 (20). Older female athletes generally possess cardiovascular fitness levels equivalent to those of sedentary women a decade younger, whereas older women trained specifically for endurance events, gain two decades or more in fitness levels. Women who were inactive during their early adult years but now are actively engaged in physical fitness programs show significant training effects, which may improve longevity and general fitness.

Gender per se is not the factor that must be considered when prescribing exercise for women. The female's initial level of fitness, her previous exercise experience, and her level of knowledge and skill are more important. The younger female with no previous experience in sports who wants to be in a regular exercise program will require much more guidance than a woman with prior competitive experience. The basic principles of exercise prescription outlined in this chapter apply equally to men and women. It is likely, however, that there will be greater variation in the background and experience of women seeking advice regarding exercise.

STRENGTH

The potential of female athletes to develop strength has been greatly underestimated. Women benefit from strength training and demonstrate improved athletic performance and prevention of injury. The female athlete can obtain approximately the same kind of increase in strength as men with only a fraction of the male athlete's increase in bulk. Increased muscle mass in men gives the male athletes a strength advantage that most women are unlikely to overcome. The anabolic properties of testosterone account for the major difference in muscle size between the sexes. In general, the overall strength of women is approximately 67% that of men. Upper body strength of the female

TABLE 6C.1

PHYSIOLOGICAL DIFFERENCES BETWEEN MEN AND WOMEN AND THEIR EFFECTS ON ATHLETIC PERFORMANCE

Body System	Men	Women
Musculoskeletal		
Ligaments	Joints are more taut; stronger ligamentous structure	Joints are usually more lax; more delicate ligamentous structure
Bones	Larger, longer bones; greater articular surface and larger structure produce a mechanical advantage; greater lever arm and more force in kicking, sticking, and hitting	Smaller, shorter, less dense bones; more susceptible to stress fractures
Pelvis	Narrower; must widen stance to achieve a woman's degree of balance	Wider; lower center of gravity produces excellent balance; increase valgus angulation at hip; greater incidence of inflammatory hip disorders, iliotibial tendinitis, and trochanteric bursitis
Knee	Less acute angle of femoral articulation; smaller valgus attitude (50–70); fewer knee injuries	Increased angle between the femur and tibia; wider pelvis and weaker quadriceps allow the patella to move laterally, leading to patella subluxation and chondromalacia; greater valgus attitude (90–100); vastus medialis is usually undeveloped; improper patella tracking
Foot	Less foot pronation; less likely to experience lower leg injuries	More foot pronation; more likely to have shin splints and chondromalacia develop
Muscle mass	Approximately 40% of total body weight; more power and speed	Approximately 23% of total body weight; less power and speed; more difficulty with lifting, throwing, and sprinting
Metabolic		
Body fat	Approximately 14% of total body weight; less efficient in energy utilization	Approximately 22%–25% of total body weight; better energy utilization
Endurance	Less efficient use of glycogen storage; more calories needed to sustain the same amount of muscular activity; often "hit the wall" (depletion of glycogen stores)	More efficient use of glycogen storage; equal or greater endurance; excel in long-distance sports; rarely "hit the wall"
Hematopoietic		
Blood	Greater iron supply and less depletion; less chance of having anemia and the resulting fatigue develop	Greater depletion of iron supply; more prone to iron deficiency anemia
Vo_{2max}	Greater; higher oxygen capacity; more hemoglobin; can reach maximum training peak earlier	Smaller; begin training with lower oxygen capacity and lower arterial oxygen; less hemoglobin; must train longer to reach maximum training peak

athletes averages approximately 65% of the male athletes, whereas leg strength is almost identical when expressed relative to body mass. The major gender differences lie in the size of the muscle fiber. Although fiber area can be increased with strength training, men still maintain an advantage in fiber size because of biological differences between the sexes.

Female athletes should not be discouraged from developing the muscular strength to meet the demands of their sport. Development of upper and lower body strength should be a priority for most female athletes. Female athletes should be encouraged to strengthen their quadriceps and hamstring muscles to prevent knee injuries.

BODY COMPOSITION

Generally, female athletes have a higher percent body fat than do male athletes. Endurance athletes such as runners and cross-country skiers may average 12% to 48% body fat, whereas some marathon runners will have 6% to 8%

body fat. Female athletes in team sports such as basketball, lacrosse, volleyball, swimming, and tennis average 18% to 24% body fat. These are average figures and there are wide variations. Also, they are estimates that are only one aspect of an athlete's physiological profile. Excessive body fat percentage, which is determined by appropriate techniques, may require dietary and exercise interventions to promote weight reduction. Education about nutrition is mandatory for all female athletes. Improper interpretation of body fat percentage may lead some female athletes toward pathological weight reduction techniques. The physician should be cautious when using body fat data alone to counsel athletes to lose weight. An older female athlete is likely to have 10% to 15% less body fat than sedentary women of the same age. An increase in percent body fat is not an inevitable consequence of aging in active women.

HEAT INTOLERANCE

When men and women are matched for exercise at the same percentage of Vo_{2max}, there are no differences in their ability to work in the heat. High intensity exercise, in combination with high ambient heat, is a dangerous combination no matter how well trained the athlete. Men and women matched for cardiovascular fitness, body surface area, and surface area to mass will acclimatize to the heat equally well. An erroneous past belief held that women sweat less than men and have difficulty coping with heat stress.

The sweating response is related to a need for heat loss through evaporation of sweat and is related to absolute, not relative, workload. Although a heavier male and lighter female run at the same percentage of Vo_{2max}, the male will produce more heat. Also, regardless of gender, the person who is acclimatized to heat and well-conditioned will sweat sooner and in greater quantity than the untrained person. In summary, numerous studies have failed to find any evidence that gender per se affects thermoregulatory response or that women are at greater risk of developing heat stress injury. Females who are beginning to exercise after years of sedentary living or who are obese should be warned of the potential hazards of exercising strenuously in hot weather. Beyond this, the same precautions for hot weather exercising apply equally to male and female athletes (20).

EFFECTS ON MENSTRUAL CYCLE

An increased incidence of menstrual abnormalities is associated with increased participation of women in regular exercise programs. Exercise-related menstrual problems are well recognized in women in endurance sports or professional dance. Studies have shown that exercise-induced menstrual dysfunction is difficult to induce with exercise alone. There are multiple risk factors, including low body weight, changes in nutrition, eating disorders, weight and body fat loss, history of late menarche, and previous menstrual irregularity (21–25). Compared with an incidence of 3% to 5% in the general population, 15% to 20% of exercising women and upwards of 50% of female endurance athletes experience menstrual abnormalities. Exercise alone does not delay the onset of puberty or affect future pregnancies. In fact, regular exercise can decrease dysmenorrhea and may help certain women attain more regularity in their menstrual cycle (26).

Amenorrhea is defined as follows: primary, no menses by age 18; secondary, no menses for 6 or more months after the initial onset of menarche. The average age of a menarche in the United States was 12.5 to 13.0 years in 1990, but continues to decline. However, a higher age for menarche is seen in ballerinas and gymnasts. Generally, linear growth is not affected during periods of amenorrhea, but it may be compromised if an eating disorder is present as well. It is important to note that longitudinal studies have shown a return of normal menstrual function in women who continue to train but gain body mass, and in those who decrease training intensity while maintaining low body fat (27,28).

Any female athlete presenting with amenorrhea or changes in her menstrual cycle should be medically evaluated. Women who exercise are susceptible to the same problems as other women who present with infertility or menstrual problems. The physician should determine that the athlete's menstrual abnormality is related to her sports participation and not due to other pathological etiologies.

A thorough history should be taken for each female athlete with amenorrhea, followed by a physical and the following laboratory tests: an initial complete blood count (CBC), thyroid-stimulating hormone (TSH), erythrocyte sedimentation rate (ESR), pregnancy test, and serum estradiol. If the Hgb is low then an iron/total iron binding capacity (TIBC) should be performed. If there is galactorrhea, then the prolactin level should be checked. If the TSH is abnormal then a T_3, T_4 and free T_4 should be undertaken. Any female athlete who has menstrual cycles should undergo documentation of basal body temperature for at least a 1-month period to assure that ovulation is taking place (26).

After the history, physical, and laboratory tests have been performed, a progesterone challenge is administered. If it is negative, follicle stimulating hormone (FSH), luteinizing hormone (LH), testosterone, and dehydroepiandrosterone sulfate (DHEA-S) levels should be measured. An increase in DHEA-S suggests an adrenal source of excess androgen production, whereas an elevated level of testosterone suggests ovarian origin. Plasma LH and FSH levels help rule out primary ovarian failure. An abnormal LH to FSH ratio supports the diagnosis of polycystic ovarian disease. In cases where there are these additional findings, it is very difficult to predict when the next ovulation will occur. Consequently, oral contraceptives are probably contraindicated and a barrier method of contraception should be used. If the estradiol level is normal, and there is a normal E1/E2 ratio <1, and withdrawal bleeding following a progesterone challenge, the physician should consider cycling the athlete with progesterone every 3 to 6 months to prevent endometrial hyperplasia.

Oral contraceptives carry a risk of cerebral vascular accident, especially in patients who smoke or who have a history of migraine headaches. The risk of thromboembolic complications is related to estrogen dosage and is less significant with current low dose contraceptives. Oral contraceptives can be considered in a female athlete aged less than 30 years who does not smoke or have hypertension or migraines. A history of fractures may also influence the decision to provide replacement hormones.

Although not proven, exercise-associated menstrual dysfunction is probably reversible. This theory is supported by findings of resumed menses after training is interrupted or decreased in amount or intensity. However, it is important not to assume that the female athlete has amenorrhea due to strenuous athletic activity. Other causes of amenorrhea include pregnancy, anorexia nervosa, chronic illness, and central nervous system (CNS) neoplasms, and should be considered and ruled out by history, physical examination, laboratory testing, CT scan, or magnetic resonance imaging (MRI). If amenorrhea is the result of strenuous athletic activity, the athlete should be advised to decrease her activity and perhaps seek nutritional counseling (see Figure 6C.1). Hormone replacement should be considered as an alternative.

The most effective physiological approach to amenorrhea is the encouragement of time off from intensive training. Two months appear to be enough for this purpose in most cases. An alternative action may be a 10% reduction in exercise frequency and intensity. This technique has been shown to be effective in restoring normal ovulatory function in adult athletes with amenorrhea (26,29,30).

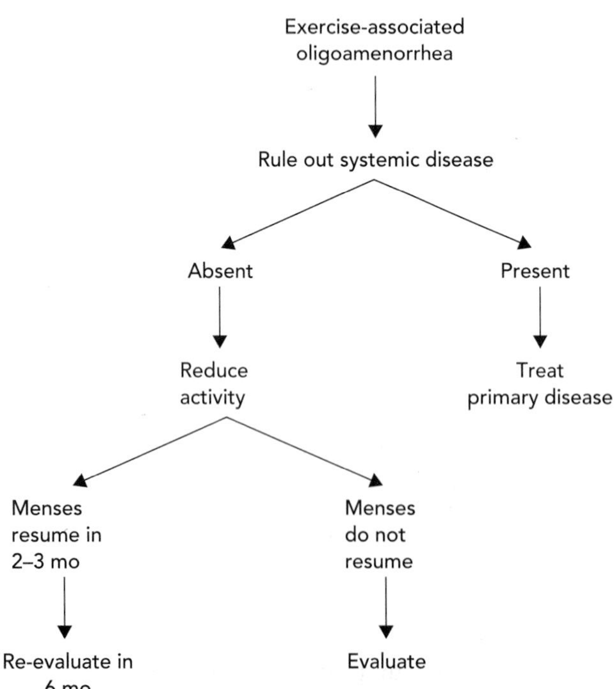

Figure 6C.1 Evaluation of exercise-associated oligomenorrhea.

OSTEOPOROSIS

Athletes of both sexes undergo decreases in bone mass with aging, beginning at age 30 to 35 in women and approximately age 50 in men. The loss in women occurs three times faster than in men. The perimenopausal female is at an even higher risk of accelerated bone loss for a 5-year period around the time of menopause (31–36).

EXERCISE IN PREGNANCY

Many patients remain active during pregnancy and there are physical and psychological benefits from exercise during that time. In fact, research has shown that if a woman continues to remain physically active during her pregnancy her aerobic fitness will decline very little (37). Multiple physiological changes occur during pregnancy to accommodate fetal development (38). Many women are concerned that exercise could lead to premature labor and delivery, miscarriage, or poor fetal outcome, so they ask their physicians for guidelines on exercise.

Physiological Changes in Pregnancy

Normal physiological changes of pregnancy may affect the total exercise capacity of the female athlete. Some of the common effects of pregnancy are a 40% to 50% increase in plasma volume with a 30% to 50% increase in cardiac output, decreased hematocrit and hemoglobin concentration, increased respiratory rate, increased lumbar lordosis, and softening of the joints by the hormone relaxin.

Cardiovascular

Pregnancy causes an increase in maternal blood volume, heart rate, cardiac stroke volume, and consequently, cardiac output. Blood volume and associated cardiac output start to rise at 6 to 8 weeks of gestation and reach a peak increase of 40% to 50% by the middle of the second trimester (39). Stroke volume and heart rate rise early in pregnancy and peak by mid-pregnancy, with stroke volume increasing by as much as 30% and heart rate by 15 to 20 beats/minute. The rise in cardiac output creates a marked cardiovascular reserve in early pregnancy when exercise is well tolerated by most patients. Some women reported an improved exercise tolerance then as compared with prepregnancy levels. Cardiovascular reserve generally decreases after 28 to 32 weeks of gestation.

The increase in blood volume is important because many complications of pregnancy, such as premature labor, hypertension, and growth retardation, are associated with maternal hypovolemia or failure of plasma volume expansion. Anemia is common in the second and third trimester of pregnancy and may be significant, but it most often reflects an expansion of plasma volume that exceeds the increases in red cell mass. It is important to help women understand that if they begin exercising before conception, it might improve their cardiac reserve and prevent complications from hypovolemia.

Resistance Exercise

Strength training and resistance exercises have become more prevalent for women as many, who were athletes, started utilizing these exercises when they were in high school or college. There is little research on the interaction between pregnancy and resistance training (40–43). Because of this paucity of research and no clear-cut guidelines, the American College of Obstetricians and Gynecologists (ACOG) does not address this issue in their guidelines. However, one recommendation that has been made by (44) is for pregnant women to avoid performing resistance exercises in the supine position.

Respiratory

As pregnancy progresses, effective maternal vertical chest height decreases by approximately 4 cm as the enlarging uterus pushes on the diaphragm. Chest diameter increases in a compensatory mechanism by as much as 10 cm. Consequently, vital capacity remains essentially unchanged, but functional residual volume is markedly reduced in late pregnancy, causing a decrease in oxygen reserve (45).

Weight Gain

The female athlete must overcome the added discomfort and increased work load that results from weight gain as the pregnancy progresses. Most women gain an average of 10 to 12 kg (22–26 lb) secondary to increased body fluid, increased uterine weight and contents, and breast enlargement. The increase in body mass has little effect on the performance of non–weight-bearing activities (swimming, cycling), but it significantly increases the energy costs and physical discomforts associated with weight-bearing activities (jogging, aerobics, tennis).

Musculoskeletal Changes

Pregnant women may be more susceptible to musculoskeletal injuries due to the changes that are occurring. Increased estrogen and relaxin levels cause softening of connective tissue in addition to relaxation of ligaments and joints. These changes may cause pain that interferes with movement and decreases the exercise tolerance. Specific joints, especially the interspinous and sacroiliac joints, pubic symphysis, and knees and ankles, become less stable and may be more prone to sprains. The expanding uterus moves the center of gravity more anteriorly, resulting in progressive lumbar lordosis and alterations in balance and the potential for low back pain. Because of these normal changes in pregnancy, the female athlete may need to vary or modify athletic activities later in the course of pregnancy.

Energy and Metabolism

The base line increase in energy expenditure due to pregnancy is estimated to be approximately 150 kcal a day during the first trimester and 350 kcal a day during the second and third trimesters. The World Health Organization advises that an average addition of 285 kcal/day over baseline requirements is adequate to meet the needs of most pregnant women (46). As the pregnancy progresses, the increased plasma insulin and fetal use of glucose predispose women to symptomatic hypoglycemia, which may be worsened by exercise (45).

POTENTIAL RISKS OF EXERCISE

Concerns about potential effects of exercise during pregnancy center on several major areas: acute fetal distress, hyperthermia, miscarriage or premature delivery, decreased fetal weight, and maternal musculoskeletal injuries. Many of these concerns have developed from animal research data, which differs from results obtained in recent human studies. Pregnancy is a normal occurrence, and both fetal and maternal outcome studies on athletes have shown good results for most women. In fact, labors are shorter with fewer complications, less medication is used, and there is a quicker return to activity. Most animal studies used untrained pregnant animals that were exercised to exhaustion. Most of the human studies were on physically fit women exercising at more moderate levels.

Acute Fetal Distress

Concerns for the fetus center around appropriate fetal oxygenation and the effects of exercise on creating fetal hypoxia. One issue is whether exercise-induced blood flow to the working muscles might lower placental blood flow. Human studies have reported fetal bradycardia when the mothers do moderate to strenuous exercise (47–49). Many researchers believe that the bradycardia is normal and that there is a return to baseline fetal heart rates within 10 to 15-minutes after exercise ceases. Prolonged fetal bradycardia and tachycardia are also believed to be signs of fetal hypoxia or stress. Studies have shown the fetal heart rate to increase when healthy women exercise submaximal levels (49,50). However, pregnant women who do exercise at these levels have had normal neonatal outcomes (51,52). Most guidelines for exercise during pregnancy use 140 to

160 beats/minute as a safe target range for the maternal heart rate. This approximates 70% to 80% of the MHR for the average pregnant woman and is a relatively safe level of exercise during pregnancy.

Hyperthermia

Hyperthermia has been reported to cause fetal damage and abortion in several animal species when maternal core temperatures reached or exceeded 102°F (33.88°C) during early gestation (53). In humans, an increase in temperature due to the use of hot tubs during pregnancy has shown an increase in neural tube defects (54). However, some research studies have shown that thermal balance is maintained during exercise by several thermoregulatory adaptive mechanisms that are present during pregnancy (55,56). Because there is limited research in this area due to various difficulties and the ethic in conducting this type of research, the concerns regarding increased temperature with strenuous exercise, especially in hot environments, remain. Therefore, pregnant women should be advised to avoid hot environments, to control the intensity and duration of exercise, and to remain well hydrated in order to limit core temperature increases.

Premature Delivery and Miscarriage

Despite early animal studies that showed fetal mortality when mothers exercised to exhaustion, human studies show that moderate exercise does not appear to increase the risk of fetal mortality where there is no history of premature delivery or miscarriage (41,57). A pregnant woman with an incompetent cervix or history of more than one premature delivery or miscarriage may be at greater risk for a recurrence of fetal death and should avoid exercise during pregnancy.

Decreased Fetal Weight

The literature has shown various results on the effect of exercise during pregnancy on fetal weight (38,58–64). However, there has not been any increase in the rate of neonatal complications (52,65). Overall, it appears that pregnant women who exercise more than 4.6 days/week will deliver lighter babies than those who exercise 3 to 4 days a week (60). However, it should be noted that term babies who are born at the lower end of normal weight do not appear to have any significant health risks (66).

TABLE 6C.2
CONTRAINDICATIONS TO EXERCISE DURING PREGNANCY

General Contraindications
Hemodynamically significant heart disease
Recurrent cervical incompetence
Current uterine bleeding
Current ruptured membranes
Intrauterine growth retardation
Fetal distress
Previous miscarriage (more than one)
Previous premature labor (more than one)
Uncontrolled hypertension
Uncontrolled diabetes mellitus
Uncontrolled renal disease
Hemodynamically significant anemia
Relative Contraindications
Essential hypertension
Controlled diabetes mellitus
Excessive obesity
Malnutrition
Multiple gestations
Thyroid disease
Anemia

RECOMMENDATIONS FOR THE PREGNANT FEMALE ATHLETE

In general, recommendations for exercise training during pregnancy should be individualized (67,68). Pregnancy is not the time to begin a new sport or conditioning program. It is important to know the prepregnancy fitness and activity levels. There are some relative contraindications to increased exercise during pregnancy, including diabetes, hypertension, anemia, infection, vaginal bleeding, any contractions that persist more than 1 hour after exercise, phlebitis, extreme fatigue, leaking amniotic fluid, or toxemia (see Table 6C.2).

The sedentary pregnant woman who wants to start exercising should begin with a gentle walking or swimming program. Easy-going muscle strengthening and pelvic floor strengthening exercises in prenatal classes are recommended. Water skiing, horseback riding, ice skating, weight lifting, anaerobic exercises, and strenuous racquet sports that increase core temperature, along with scuba diving (possible decompression sickness of the fetus), should be avoided by all pregnant female athletes.

Non–weight-bearing exercises such as biking or swimming are generally preferable. The pregnant woman should allow for changes in balance and timing over time. Body temperature should be monitored frequently during exercise and kept below 101°F (38.33°C) maximum. Overheating should be avoided and the pregnant female athlete should keep her MHR between 140 to 160 beats/minute (<85% of MHR) during exercise. She should consume adequate calories, calcium and iron, and maintain proper hydration. Exercise should be done three times a week at a moderate level of intensity and with adequate emphasis on flexibility.

General and relative contraindications to exercise during pregnancy are represented in Table 6C.2. Pregnant patients with heart disease may experience a marked decrease in cardiac output even in the early stages. They should see a cardiologist to determine the appropriate activity levels. Relative contraindications to exercise during pregnancy exist, but an exercise program can be designed that consider the specific needs of the patient. General guidelines for exercise in the pregnant athlete should take into account her level of aerobic training before conception. Well-trained women will handle the additional demands of exercise better during pregnancy than the untrained women. Sedentary women can begin some type of physical activity during pregnancy so long as they begin at low intensity and increase the exercise intensity gradually. The ACOG (69) has developed a set of guidelines for safe exercise during pregnancy that applies to most women. These guidelines have been well received by the public and by physicians and have become the legal standard in some states. These guidelines were originally very general and conservative and did not apply to the high-performance athlete who becomes pregnant (68). However, they have been revised as new research has demonstrated the ability of women to exercise during pregnancy without complications. In fact, they have recently supplemented their previous guidelines with updated information that includes their support for women staying active during pregnancy (70). They do stress the need for close medical supervision for those women who are involved in strenuous exercise. These guidelines should be considered as a framemark that should be modified by the physician according to his/her knowledge of the patient. Signals to stop exercising are shown in Table 6C.3 (71).

The ACSM guidelines on the frequency, intensity, and duration of exercise can be very useful in developing an exercise program for gestational women, although the guidelines were not developed specifically for pregnant women. Most pregnant patients can start exercising up to 75% of predicted MHR and increase their exercise intensity gradually. Women who have exercised before pregnancy can exercise up to 85% of the predicted MHR. Most authorities agree that the pregnant patient may easily perform three to five exercise sessions per week as long as the patient continues to gain weight adequately and increases caloric intake to account for the calories used during exercise. Weight-bearing activities may be alternated with non–weight-bearing activities to control any musculoskeletal symptoms that may occur during the exercise cycle.

The following recommendations can be made for the three trimesters of pregnancy. Hot baths, whirlpools, and saunas should be avoided during the first trimester. A new strenuous exercise program should not be started by a female athlete who knows she is pregnant. However, it is not necessary to make major changes in an ongoing exercise program. During the second trimester, female athletes should not resort to special diets except when hypertension or diabetes mellitus complicates the pregnancy. Foods high in energy content and low in nutritional value should be avoided. A well-balanced diet should be prescribed and followed. Exercise during pregnancy is not intended to control body mass but rather to control body tone. Strong muscles may shorten the labor period, make delivery easier for both mother and baby, and hasten the postpartum return to optimal fitness.

During the third trimester, exercises that compromise blood flow to the mother's vital organs and the fetus should be avoided. Long periods of standing or lifting heavy objects also should be avoided. Individuals vary considerably in their exercise tolerance during the final trimester and the exercise program may need to be restricted. If training is continued, it should be under close supervision by the physician. Safe exercises during pregnancy, which can normalize or improve fetal and maternal outcomes, are possible by adhering to these general guidelines and the specific recommendations that follow.

TABLE 6C.3
SIGNALS TO STOP EXERCISING

Breathlessness
Dizziness
Headache
Muscle weakness
Nausea
Chest pain or tightness
Back pain
Hip or pubic pain
Difficulty walking
Generalized edema
Decreased fetal activity
Uterine contractions
Vaginal bleeding
Amniotic fluid leakage

Specific Recommendations

Jogging. women should not start jogging during pregnancy if they have not been running before. If jogging is begun during pregnancy, it should be at low intensity and frequency levels, with monitoring for the symptoms listed in Table 6C.3. As the pregnancy progresses, speed and distance are gradually reduced so that the perceived level of exertion remains the same throughout the program.

Cycling. Cycling can be started during pregnancy; a stationary bike is generally safer than a standard bicycle. The serious cyclist may switch from a racing or touring bicycle to an upright model during the last trimester.

Aerobics. Generally, low to moderate impact aerobics should be well tolerated by pregnant women up through the third trimester. The ACOG guidelines suggest that there should be restrictions in the use of the supine position as well as bouncing movements after the fourth month of gestation.

Swimming. Swimming is an excellent aerobic exercise that can be safely initiated during pregnancy. Swimming in excessively cold or hot water should be avoided to minimize the potential effects of hypo- or hyperthermia on the fetus (72).

Weight lifting. Many pregnant athletes lift light weights throughout their pregnancy to maintain strength. Proper breathing techniques should be maintained throughout the lifting cycle. Lifting heavy weights, especially by patients with low back problems, or doing exercises that strain the lower back should be avoided.

Contact sports. Because of potential trauma to the abdomen and fetus, pregnant women should avoid collision sports and contact sports such as football, field hockey, basketball, volleyball, gymnastics, and horseback riding. Racquet sports such as tennis, racquetball, and squash are believed to be fairly safe. As the pregnancy progresses, the intensity of participation should be reduced to prevent injuries. Water-skiing should be avoided because of the possibility of high-speed falls and the potential for forceful entry of water into the uterus and subsequent miscarriage (73).

Scuba diving. Inexperienced divers should avoid scuba diving during pregnancy because of the potential for decompression sickness, maternal acid base and nitrogen imbalances, and intravascular air embolism in the fetus. Some researchers say that experienced pregnant divers may continue on a conservative basis, with dives not exceeding 33 ft in depth or lasting longer than 30 minutes (74).

Downhill and cross-country skiing. The experienced pregnant athlete can continue to ski cautiously during pregnancy. Downhill skiing may present a significant danger during the later stages of pregnancy, especially if the skier is inexperienced. Healthy women have been known to cross-country ski up to the day of delivery without problems.

Ice skating. Ice skating is likely to be more dangerous than snow skiing because of its potential for falls on hard ice. Skating should be pursued only with extreme caution and only by very experienced skaters (72).

There are many benefits of exercise for pregnancy. Exercise during pregnancy leads to shorter labors, easier deliveries, and increased self-esteem. Following a vaginal delivery, exercise may be started within 1 week and water sports can begin when all bleeding stops (75). After a cesarian section the general recommendation is to have 6 to 10 weeks of an exercise-free period. The scar following a cesarian section is maximally strong 21 days postsurgery, but should not be stressed before that time. After a dilation and curettage, weight training and aerobic exercise can be started within 2 days and water sports within 1 week.

POSTPARTUM EXERCISES

Depending on the type of delivery and its progress, exercise programs should be resumed as soon as possible within the comfort range of the patient. Even before leaving the hospital, the mother can begin restoring muscular tone to the abdomen and pelvis to reduce the likelihood of urinary incontinence or a prolapsed uterus. During the postpartum period, Kegel exercises to strengthen the muscles of the pelvic floor are recommended. Multiple exercises and stretching programs are outlined in other textbooks. Exercise promotes improved blood flow and may prevent the complications of varicose veins, cramps, edema, and thrombophlebitis.

SUMMARY OF EXERCISE PRESCRIPTION FOR THE FEMALE ATHLETE

Exercise can be prescribed for female athletes of all ages if the requirements of a properly designed program are followed. Specific information relative to the exercise needs and concerns of the female athlete have been outlined here and should be considered when a physician designs an exercise program. A properly designed program will prevent undue injury and lead to more successful, long-term, enjoyable exercise for female athletes (76).

SECTION D

THE OLDER ATHLETE

The number of older adults in United States has increased markedly over the past 15 years. More than 10% of the U.S. population is now aged 65 years or more, as compared with less than 5% at the turn of the century. The U.S. Census Bureau predicts that by 2030 approximately 20% to 21% of the population will be aged 65 or more.

The aging process represents a gradual decline in the ability of an individual to adapt to environmental changes. As the U.S. population ages, health care providers will be challenged to meet their special needs, especially helping them to remain functional. One way this goal may be met is through programs of regular exercise. Physical activity has more potential for promoting healthy aging than anything science or medicine has to offer today (77). Early retirement, more leisure time, and an increased awareness of the benefits of exercise have prompted many older people to increase their activities. The upsurge has meant more acute and chronic injuries in this age group. Some physicians tell their older patients with exercised-induced symptoms to stop their activity altogether, but this is not warranted. We will examine the importance and benefits of exercise in older people and evaluate the most common types of injuries. There is little evidence that the elderly are less physically active than younger people; in fact, exercise may increase longevity. The growing number of older people and their role in society makes it imperative that health professionals understand their needs and problems.

Before instituting an exercise program in an older person, consider the exercise goals of the patient, the availability of equipment and facilities, and cost of the program. Do a thorough assessment of the patient's health by reviewing the following: (a) appropriate history and physical, (b) assessment of nutritional status, present activity level, smoking habits, alcohol use, and weight, (c) diseases that lead to decreased exercise tolerance, (d) orthopedic problems and disabilities that produce physical limitations, (e) any prior injuries and rehabilitation, (f) the patient's current physical condition and training status, and (g) medications that may interfere with or alter the exercise response.

Physical changes that occur during aging include decreased cardiac output (decreased stroke volume, decreased heart rate), decreased ventilatory capacity, decreased pulmonary blood flow, decreased aerobic power, and decreased physical work capacity; decreased body muscle mass and strength, decreased nerve conduction, decreased elasticity of tissue, and progressive bone loss; hypertension (blood pressure >150/95) in 50% of patients aged above 80, and increased potential for developing heat stress (see Table 6D.1) (78).

Gerontologists distinguish three categories of senior citizens: "old-old" persons over 75 years of age, "young-old" persons under 75 years of age, and "athletic-old" persons who have maintained fitness throughout their lives. These older patients should be considered when looking at maximal oxygen uptake. Old-old persons can reach a maximal oxygen uptake of 2.4 METs (7–14 mL oxygen uptake/kg/body weight). Young-old persons can attain maximum oxygen uptake of 5.7 METs (17.5–24.5 mL/kg). The athletic-old can achieve maximal oxygen uptake greater than 10 METs (79).

Among the benefits of exercise for older adults are improved muscle tone, range of motion, posture, coordination, and physical work capacity; increased Vo_{2max}, decreased blood pressure; improved weight control and body image; a reduction in the amount of low back pain; an improvement in accident prevention; improved social contacts and sleep patterns and a decreased incidence of depression; and improved functional ability and independence (80).

Studies have demonstrated that elderly participants in regular exercise programs will show a gradual training effect, although the elderly need more time to adapt (81). The benefits of physical conditioning on cardiovascular systems in older patients are similar to those observed in younger patients even though the initial baseline in older patients is lower (82). Respiratory fitness does not appear to limit exercise capacity in normal individuals of any age. The ventilation changes that occur with aging do not preclude significant improvement in aerobic capacity with training (79). An active lifestyle appears to delay the natural lengthening of neurovascular reaction times that comes with aging.

TABLE 6D.1
BIOLOGICAL FUNCTIONAL CHANGES BETWEEN THE AGES OF 30 AND 70

Work capacity (%)	↓ 25–30
Cardiac output	↓ 30
Maximum heart rate (beats/min)	↓ 24
Blood pressure (mmHg)	
Systolic	↑ 10–40
Diastolic	↑ 5–10
Respiration (%)	
Vital capacity	↓ 40–50
Residual volume	↑ 30–50
Basal metabolic rate (%)	↓ 8–12
Musculature (%)	
Muscle mass	↓ 25–30
Hand grip strength	↓ 25–30
Nerve conduction velocity (%)	↓ 10–15
Flexibility (%)	↓ 20–30
Bone (%)	
Women	↓ 25–30
Men	↓ 15–20
Renal function (%)	↓ 30–50

Source: Smith EL, Gilligan C. Physical activity prescription for the older adult. *Phys Sportsmed* 1983;11:91.

Much of the early gains in strength elderly people achieve on a training program are due to increased neuronal activation rather than muscle hypertrophy (83). The expected improvement in strength from resistance training is difficult to assess, because strength increases are affected by the participant's initial level of strength and his potential for improvement, which is in turn affected by the presence of chronic disease. Elderly patients with arthritis can increase Vo_{2max}, flexibility, and muscle strength with low intensity exercise programs with no adverse effects on joints (84,85). Mean bone mineral content can increase 20% over controls with high intensity training. Studies also confirm that exercise is beneficial in increasing mineral content in the elderly with senile osteoporosis (86). Many of the benefits of exercise have been well documented in other textbooks.

The goals of the exercise evaluation are as follows: (a) to determine the appropriate exercise (type, frequency, intensity, and duration) for the patient; (b) to evaluate any chronic health problems that may compromise physical capacity; (c) to become aware of medical conditions that preclude vigorous activity; (d) to instruct the patient how to start his exercise gradually and increase the activity level appropriately; (e) to understand the absolute contraindications for exercise participation; (f) to perform a thorough history, physical examination, and appropriate laboratory tests, urinalysis, electrocardiograph (ECG), and graded exercise test (GXT). After age 65, 30% of the patients develop myocardial ischemia during exercise, so the use of a modified GXT protocol is imperative (87–90).

The goals of an exercise program for elders should include increasing cardiovascular fitness, endurance, flexibility, balance and strength through walking, jogging, swimming or biking. Caution should be exercised while running, staying within the aerobic limits established by the GXT or alternative evaluation and establishing a target heart rate of 60% to 75% of the MHR. Some other precautions are required with jumping rope and heavy weight lifting, and avoiding isometric exercise in hypertensive patients. In addition, patients with decreased visual or hearing acuity must be made aware of the dangers of exercising without special precautions.

Principles of injury treatment in the elderly athlete include a proper analysis of the specific movement or activity producing the injury and then modifying it, provision of an appropriate and aggressive rehabilitation program, and instruction in the maintenance of strength and as much normal muscle and tendon range of motion as possible through an appropriate flexibility program.

With these guidelines in mind, a safe and effective exercise program can be developed for the older patient who is interested in sports and exercise. The more competitive adult will pursue an active program with an increased focus on flexibility, strength training, agility, and neuromuscular skill attainment, in addition to a high level of cardiorespiratory fitness (91).

SECTION E
THE SEDENTARY ADULT

There have been many published studies on the effect of regular physical activity. Most sought to learn whether people who are active are healthier than less active or sedentary people (92). Not all studies support the hypothesis that active people are healthier, but most demonstrate that active individuals fare better, particularly with regard to chronic disease. Coronary artery disease is the major area for which we have evidence that active people are healthier and have substantially lower mortality rates.

Research studies have also demonstrated other potential benefits from regular activity. Paffenbarger et al. (93) studied some Harvard alumni and found a lower total mortality rate in active people. Such disorders as obesity, osteoporosis, and hypertension were less prevalent in the active group. The amount and type of activity that is beneficial seems to be well within the capacity of most adults. The risk for these diseases can be lowered by activities such as walking, stair climbing, hiking, and even the routine activities of everyday life. Healthy people should try to reduce other risk factors for heart disease by lowering dietary cholesterol, avoiding cigarettes, and treating hypertension if it is present. This should be routine advice for patients likely to develop heart disease. A comprehensive approach that includes these behavioral modifications, treatment techniques, and a regular exercise program can significantly change the long-term health of active individuals (91).

Before giving an exercise prescription to a sedentary adult, the physician should begin with a thorough history and physical and appropriate laboratory testing. Some type of stress test should be performed on patients with multiple primary risk factors and/or symptoms of coronary heart disease. Testing protocols that use constant treadmill speeds with gradual work increments and increases in grade are available and are suitable for the elderly (94,95). The goal of the exercise treadmill test should be to express the patient's full range of exercise performance over a reasonable period. A bicycle ergometer is another useful method of exercise testing in the elderly population. Grossly overweight patients and those in the coronary-prone age (men aged 40–49) should undergo stress testing (96). We strongly recommend that healthy patients undergo some form of submaximal exercise test to determine functional capacity in conjunction with a general fitness assessment.

Absolute contraindications for exercise training and testing have already been presented. Exercise testing is useful in those patients in whom the closer monitoring of the exercise programs may be needed. These patients should undergo a medically supervised test for functional capacity. Patients with the following conditions require supervised stress testing (97):

- Recent myocardial infarction or post–coronary artery bypass surgery
- Presence of a pace maker—fixed rate or demand
- Use of chronotropic or inotropic cardiac medications
- Presence of morbid obesity combined with multiple coronary risk factors
- Occurrence of ST-segment depression at rest
- Severe hypertension
- Intermittent claudication

Both medical and environmental conditions that require moderation of activity or caution in prescribing exercise are listed in Tables 6E.1 and 6E.2. All exercise programs for sedentary adults or beginning exercisers should follow the requirements of proper exercise prescription described earlier. A simple check list such as a Physical Activity Readiness Questionnaire (PARA) along with an updated version of the Cornell Medical Index can help identify individuals who need detailed clinical examination before a training program is initiated (98). Peripheral neuropathy, gait disturbance, impaired equilibrium, orthostatic hypertension,

TABLE 6E.1
CONDITIONS REQUIRING CAUTION IN EXERCISE PRESCRIPTION

Viral infection or cold
Chest pain
Irregular heart beat
Exercise-induced asthma
Prolonged, unaccustomed physical activity
Conduction disturbances (LBBB, complete AV block, or bifascicular block with or without first degree block)

LBBB = left bundle branch block; AV = atrioventricular.

or degenerative joint disease should alert the physician to the increased risk of falls or other injury. Joint stability and range of motion must be assessed before exercise so that activities can be adjusted if needed (79). All exercise programs should include warm-up, flexibility, and strength training exercises.

INTENSITY OF EXERCISE

The most important variable in any exercise prescription is intensity, but it is the most difficult factor to determine. Intensity is expressed as a percentage of MHR, heart rate reserve (HRR) (maximum HR–resting HR), or functional capacity (Vo_{2max} or METs). The intensity rate for training depends on the initial fitness level of the adult. Unconditioned individuals have a low threshold for improving functional capacity, whereas conditioned patients require a greater intensity level to increase their aerobic fitness.

Determining Intensity by Heart Rate

MHR is determined through a linear relation between the heart rate and Vo_{2max}. Intensity is expressed as a percentage of MHR (HR_{max}), where $HR_{max} = 220HR - age$. Intensity levels of 60% to 80% of MHR can induce training. These values correspond to approximately 60% to 80% of functional capacity. The predicted MHR in the above formula deviates by ±15 beats/minute from the actual value using standard deviation tests.

The Karvonen method of prescribing exercise intensity is based on the following formula using HRR: $HRR = (HR_{max} - HR_{rest})$.

The training heart rate (THR) is calculated as follows: $THR = ([0.60 to 0.85] \times [HR_{max} - HR_{rest}]) + HR_{rest}$, where (0.60 to 0.85) represents a potential range of training intensities from 60% to 85% of MHR. Intensity should begin at low levels and increase gradually as fitness improves. This method has an advantage over simple measures of MHR because variability in the athlete's resting heart rate is accounted for in the formula (96). Table 6E.3 shows average MHRs and THR for various age groups.

Exercise Prescription Using METs

Intensity of exercise may be prescribed in metabolic units (MET) units (1 MET = O_2 consumption of 3.5 mL/kg/minute/m^2) once the functional capacity has been determined. This method allows prescription of activity only where documented metabolic costs are available (see Table 6E.4). A range of 60% to 85% of maximum METs (MMET) corresponds to low and peak conditioning intensity levels. An average training intensity MET (TMET) is calculated as follows: $TMET = ([MMET \times 60] + MMET)/100$.

Concurrent measurements of heart rate and metabolic rate (METs) during a GXT allows for interpretation of functional capacity at any heart rate. Since 1 MET is equal to 4.2 kj/kg/hour/m^2, energy expenditure per session also can be determined (1 kcal = 4.18 kj).

DURATION

The exercise must last long enough to increase energy expenditure by at least 12,000 kj or 287 calories. Short periods of exercise (5–10 minutes) can induce cardiovascular training if performed at high intensity levels (90%–95% of functional capacity). The ideal duration of exercise for most athletes is 20 to 60 minutes of continuous aerobic activity performed at moderate intensity. Exercise sessions should be extended gradually from the initial 15 to 20 minutes as cardiovascular endurance improves. High intensity programs have poor compliance and account for a high incidence of musculoskeletal injuries. Because fat utilization increases significantly after approximately 20 minutes of light to moderate exercise, body fat reduction will be better during longer periods of aerobic exercise.

FREQUENCY

The threshold for improvement of aerobic power seems to be two sessions of exercise/week, but intensity must be relatively high if gains are to occur. The minimum

TABLE 6E.2
CONDITIONS REQUIRING MODERATION OF ACTIVITY

Extreme heat and high relative humidity
Extreme cold, especially when strong winds are present
Following heavy meals
Exposure to high altitudes (>1,700 m)
Significant musculoskeletal injuries

TABLE 6E.3

AVERAGE MAXIMUM HEART RATES BY AGE AND RECOMMENDED TRAINING HEART RATES (THR) FOR NORMAL ASYMPTOMATIC PARTICIPANTS DURING EXERCISE

Age (yr)	10–19	20–29	40–49	50–59	60–69
HR_{max}	185	190	180	170	160
Peak THR 0.9 (HR_{max}−75) +75	174	179	170	161	152
Lowest THR 0.6 (HR_{max}−75) +75	141	144	138	132	126
Average THR 0.7 (HR_{max}−75) +75	152	155	149	141	135

Source: Modified from the American College of Sports Medicine. *Guidelines for graded exercise testing and exercise prescription*, 2nd ed. Philadelphia: Lea & Febiger, 1980, (99). Reprinted from Fox E. *The physiological basis of physical education and athletics*, 3rd ed. Philadelphia: WB Saunders, 1981:412.

exercise frequency recommended for adults is three sessions a week. This is an optimal frequency for people who are beginning exercise programs and allows for sufficient rest to prevent musculoskeletal overuse syndromes. Obese adults or those with low functional capability (<3 METs) may do better with a program of repeated exercise sessions of 5 minutes each several times a day. When, functional capacity improves, one or two longer daily sessions may be undertaken.

As functional capacity improves, exercise sessions usually can be increased to three or more a week. The program should include easier days when both the duration and intensity of exercise are reduced. Five days of exercise/week is sufficient to obtain optimal fitness levels. Progression from 3 to 5 days a week should occur gradually over a 4-week period, and include no more than three intense sessions weekly. Exercising 7 days a week does not further improve aerobic power and cause overuse problems. The exception to this general rule is the obese adult who can profit from daily low intensity sessions aimed at making the energy expenditure necessary to reduce body fat.

Isotonic resistance training or other strength training methods should be incorporated into a regular aerobic program no more than 2 or 3 days a week. A minimum of 8 to 10 exercises involving the major muscle groups should be performed, with 8 to 12 repetitions to near fatigue for each exercise. A need for longer recuperative periods after performing heavy resistance work makes the rest period necessary.

EXERCISE MODE

The focus of any exercise program should be on components such as cardiorespiratory endurance, body composition, flexibility, muscular strength, and endurance. Reduced joint mobility is often secondary to arthritis and is a disabling condition for many elderly patients. An exercise program should be designed to maintain adequate levels of strength and dynamic flexibility in the major joints. Accidents are a major cause of injury and death in the elderly, and many of them can be linked to inadequate muscle strength. Strength deficits impair a person's ability to control body weight, handle external objects, or perform activities of daily living. Properly designed and graded resistance exercises promote maintenance of acceptable levels of muscle strength.

The most critical factor in an older person's ability to function independently is his/her ability to move without assistance. Those who maintain adequate levels of cardiorespiratory fitness and acceptable body composition are more apt to retain that ability longer than those who become obese or allow their muscular and cardiorespiratory systems to deteriorate. The preferred types of aerobic exercise are exercises that use large muscle groups in a rhythmic and continuous manner. Dissimilar activities affect the heart rate differently, so strict attention should be paid to the energy requirements for each specific exercise or sport (see Table 6E.4).

Similar cardiovascular training can be generated by jogging/running, swimming, bicycling, or cross-country skiing programs. Less intense activities such as golf, bowling, and archery offer little training stimulus because heart rates rarely exceed 100 beats/minute. Rope skipping has become popular but it can produce excessively high heart rates and should be avoided by people with restricted exercise intensity levels. Tennis and squash are adequate training stimuli if the skill level is high enough. Squash does involve rapid starting and stopping and it increases systolic blood pressure and myocardial oxygen demands. For those reasons, it should be prescribed only for healthy, risk-free patients.

Sustained isometric activities against heavy resistance are strongly discouraged in unconditioned, hypertensive, and coronary-prone patients. These activities provide little or no improvement in VO_{2max}. Weight training programs should have enough intensity to elicit a strength training effect while minimizing the risk of musculoskeletal injury or an elevation in blood pressure. Therefore, they should use low weights and high repetitions. The exercise should be enjoyable and the patient should be able to see improvement. This increases motivation and compliance.

TABLE 6E.4
APPROXIMATE METABOLIC COST OF ACTIVITIES[a]

Intensity (70-kg Person)	Endurance Promoting	Occupational	Recreational
1½–2 METs 4–7 mL/kg 2–2½ kcal/min	Too low in energy level	Desk work, driving auto, electrical calculating machine operation, light housework-polishing furniture or washing clothes	Standing, strolling (1 mph), flying, motorcycling, playing cards, sewing, knitting
2–3 METs 7–11 mL/kg/min 2½–4 kcal/min/	Too low in energy level unless capacity is very low	Auto repair, radio and television repair, janitorial work, bartending, riding lawn mower, light woodworking	Level walking (2 mph), level bicycling (5 mph), billiards, bowling, skeet shooting, shuffleboard, powerboat driving, golfing with power cart, canoeing, horseback riding at a walk
3–4 METs 11–14 mL/kg/min 4–5 kcal/min	Yes, if continuous and if training heart rate is reached	Brick laying, plastering, wheelbarrow (100-lb load), machine assembly, welding (moderate load), cleaning windows, mopping floors, vacuuming, pushing light power mower	Walking (3 mph), bicycling (6 mph), horseshoe pitching, volleyball (6 person, noncompetitive), golfing (pulling bag cart), archery, sailing (handling small boat), fly fishing (standing in waders), horseback riding (trotting), badminton (social doubles)
4–5 METs 14–18 mL/kg/min 5–6 kcal/min	Recreational activities promote endurance. Occupational activities must be continuous, lasting longer than 2 min	Painting, masonry, paperhanging, light carpentry, scrubbing floors, raking leaves, hoeing	Walking (3½ mph), bicycling (8 mph), table tennis, golfing (carrying clubs), dancing (foxtrot), badminton (singles), tennis (doubles), many calisthenics, ballet
5–6 METs 18–21 mL/kg/min 6–7 kcal/min	Yes	Digging garden, shoveling light earth	Walking (4 mph), bicycling (10 mph), canoeing (4 mph), horseback riding (posting to trotting), stream fishing (walking in light current in waders), ice or roller skating (9 mph)
6–7 METs 21–25 mL/kg/min 7–8 kcal/min	Yes	Shoveling ten times/min (4½ kg or 10 lb), splitting wood, snow shoveling, hand lawn mowing	Walking (5 mph), bicycling (11 mph), competitive badminton, tennis (singles), folk and square dancing, light downhill skiing, ski touring (2½ mph), water skiing, swimming (20 yards/min
7–8 METs 25–28 mL/kg/min 8–10 kcal/min	Yes	Digging ditches, carrying 36 kg or 80 lb, sawing hardwood	Jogging (5 mph), bicycling (12 mph), horseback riding (gallop), vigorous downhill skiing, basketball, mountain climbing, ice hockey, canoeing (5 mph), touch football, paddleball
8–9 METs 28–32 mL/kg/min 10–11 kcal/min	Yes	Shoveling 10 times/min (5½ kg or 14 lb)	Running (5½ mph), bicycling (13 mph), ski touring (4 mph), squash (social), handball (social), fencing, basketball (vigorous), swimming (30 yd/min), rope skipping
10+ METs 32+ mL/kg/min 11+ kcal/min	Yes	Shoveling 10 times (7½ kg or 16 lb)	Running (6 mph = 10 METs, 7 mph = 1½ METs, 8 mph = 13½ METs, 9 mph = 15 METs, 10 mph = 17 METs), ski touring (5+ mph), handball (competitive), squash competitive), swimming (>40 yd/min)

[a]Energy range will vary depending on skill of exerciser, pattern of rest pauses, environmental temperature, etc. Caloric values depend on body size (more for larger person). Table provides reasonable relative strenuousness values, however.

Source: (From Gibson SB, Gerberich SG, Leon AS. Writing the exercise prescription: an individulized approach. *Phys Sportsmed* 1983;11(7):88–89.) (Table modified with permission from Fox SM III, Naughton JP, Gorman PA. Physical activity and cardiovascular health, 3. The exercise prescription: frequency and type of activity. *Mod Concepts Cardiovasc Dis* 1972;41:25–30.)

Aerobic Activities

Continuous and intermittent (interval) exercise can elicit a training response (77). Interval training (high intensity, short duration, with rest periods) is widely recognized and is a form of training practiced by most endurance athletes. High intensity exercise may be performed without significant accumulations of LA. The high-speed training should result in faster performance times. A sedentary adult can accomplish more total work with less physiological stress by doing interval training.

We recommend prescribing exercise on a run-walk basis initially. As functional capacity improves, a higher energy output may be performed more continuously (see Table 6E.5). Activities that yield a constant heart rate response (walking/jogging, jogging/running, cross-country skiing, swimming, cycling) are preferred, as close control of both duration and intensity of exercise is desired. More intense interval activities are recommended only after an adequate period of continuous training (usually 6 to 10 weeks).

Flexibility exercises and calisthenics should be performed during the warm-up and cooldown periods. They should be done slowly, utilizing static stretching techniques (reach and hold). Bounce-stretching beyond the normal range of motion of the muscle is ill-advised and may lead to acute soft tissue injury.

Building muscular strength through dynamic, high resistance, low repetition exercises should be strongly discouraged in patients who are poorly conditioned, hypertensive, or at risk of cardiovascular disease. Dynamic and static strength exercises, especially when combined with a Valsalva maneuver, may cause an excessive rise in systemic blood pressure, reduce venous return, and increase the after-load of the heart. Low resistance, high repetition strength exercises without breath-holding are a better alternative.

Reduced muscle strength and degenerative changes in bones and joints because of aging may result in higher injury rates in certain activities. Non–weight-bearing activities such as swimming and cycling have many advantages for sustaining aerobic activity while decreasing the effects of gravity on the joints of the lower extremity. Road hazards and falls on the pool deck are the potential sources of injury for these activities. Stationary cycling is recommended for the less healthy adult. Cross-country skiing on flat, well-groomed trails is an excellent athletic activity for the elderly. Impaired coordination and osteoporosis increase the risk of injury, and alternate forms of exercise should be considered in icy conditions. Rhythmic calisthenics and low impact aerobics can provide both sustained activity and opportunities for gentle warm-up and cooldown periods.

Proper counseling is essential to avoid overuse or sudden twisting injuries. Access to aerobic machines such as Nordic Track, Stair Climber, Elliptical, and Concept Rowing may add to the aerobic fitness potential for the elderly. However, lack of access to these machines may limit continued participation. The exercise potential in daily living activities should be used to supplement formal exercise. Walking to the store, vacuuming, hedge trimming, painting, and gardening assist in improving fitness. Many stairways are available and can provide valuable sources for physical training if the individual's vision and balance are good.

All exercise sessions should include a warm-up period, the endurance phase, and a cooldown period. The warm-up period should last 5 to 10 minutes and consists of calisthenics, stretching exercises, and slow jogging or

TABLE 6E.5

AVERAGE WORK INTENSITIES FOR ACTIVITIES SUITABLE FOR EXERCISE PRESCRIPTION

	Average Work Intensity	
Activity	**METs**	**Kcal/hr (75 kg)**
Walking, 0% grade		
2.5 mph	3.0	225
3.0 mph	3.3	240
3.5 mph	3.5	262
4.0 mph	4.6	345
Jogging-running		
4.5 mph	5.7[a]	375–490
5.0 mph	8.4	630
6.0 mph	10.0	750
7.0 mph	11.4	855
8.0 mph	12.8	960
Cycling (ergometer)		
300 kpm	3.7	278
450 kpm	5.0	375
600 kpm	6.0	450
750 kpm	7.0	525
900 kpm	8.5	630
1,050 kpm	10.0	750
1,200 kpm	11.0	825
1,500 kpm	13.5	1,010
Swimming, crawl[b]		
20 yr/min	6.0	420
30 yr/min	9.0	675
40 yr/min	12.0	900
Games (average intensity)		
Basketball	7–15	525–1,125
Volleyball	5–12	375–900
Soccer	7–15	525–1,125
Handball	8–12	600–900
Tennis	6–10	450–750

[a]Metabolic cost of jogging at 4 to 5 mph is variable owing to the transition between fast walk and slow jog.
[b]Metabolic cost of swimming is highly variable owing to efficiency, buoyancy, and technique; values may vary by 25%.
Source: From Hanson PG, Giese MD, Corliss RJ. Clinical guidelines for exercise training. *Postgrad Med* 1980;67:120, (100).

walking. The endurance phase involves exercising at the prescribed duration and intensity level. A gradual cooldown phase lasts 5 to 10 minutes and consists of exercises similar to those used during warm-up. Abrupt cessation of exercise, especially in warm, humid temperatures, may cause venous pooling, circulatory collapse with syncope, vertigo, nausea, and possibly myocardial ischemia. Hot showers, saunas, and whirlpools should be avoided until well after the cooldown period and they are contraindicated in patients with coronary heart disease.

MONITORING EXERCISE

Palpation of the carotid or radial pulse is the easiest method to monitor intensity and progression of exercise. This method can be as accurate as telemetry. Wrist palpation avoids the possibility of reflex hypotension that can occur with overly vigorous carotid massage. During the first sessions of exercise, patients should stop after 3 to 5 minutes of exercise and locate the radial pulse. The pulse is counted for 6 seconds and this number is multiplied by 10 to yield a per-minute rate. Pulse counting should begin immediately because the heart rate decreases rapidly after exercise ends.

PROGRESSION OF THE EXERCISE PROGRAM

Increases in intensity, frequency, and duration of exercise can be made as the athlete becomes more cardiovascularly fit. The rate of progression is difficult to predict because it depends on the individual athlete and his exercise goals, and upon the training environment. The ACSM has recommended a three-phase exercise progression that will allow an individual to attain optimal fitness without undue risk of musculoskeletal injuries.

The initial stage of exercise includes the first 5 weeks of the program. Stretching, light calisthenics, and low intensity aerobics are introduced so as to avoid undue discomfort that might be discouraging. The aerobic phase should be started at a lower intensity level than the ultimate goal. The athlete is ready to progress when the following objectives are met: a 3 to 8 beat/minute decrease in heart rate during the aerobic exercise phase, voluntary adoption of a slightly faster jogging/walking pace, and an improvement in functional capacity demonstrated by exercise testing.

Objective measurements can provide useful indications for exercise progression, as can the athlete's level of fatigue, facial expression, breathing pattern, perceived exertion, and movement patterns.

When the program first begins, the aerobic sessions should last 12 to 15 minutes. The athlete should attempt to expend 800 kj/session (approximately 200 kcal) during the first week of training, and try to reach the recommended 1,200 kj (approximately 300 kcal)/session by the end of the first phase. The second phase of the program commonly lasts from week 6 to week 27. Exercise duration is extended and intensity is gradually raised from 60% to a range of 70% to 90%. If the patient's functional capacity is low, the transition from walking to jogging is best accomplished by first using a discontinuous walk/run pattern and gradually progressing to a more steady and continuous pattern.

The third or maintenance phase of exercise is reached after 6 months of regular activity. At this point, the athlete is exercising at 70% to 90% of the estimated functional capacity for at least 45 to 60 minutes, four to five times per week. Compliance is important, as are the exercise goals of the athlete, if the program is to continue to satisfy the participant's needs over long periods. Other aerobic activities should be introduced during this period, not only for variety but also to avoid overtraining of selected muscles and to diminish the potential for overuse injuries.

SUMMARY

It is important to encourage sedentary adults to enter regular exercise programs. Individual patients/athletes respond in different ways to any exercise program, so the exercise prescription should be set up with a specific individual in mind. The program should appeal to the patient and conform to family leisure and business schedules. Availability of equipment and costs of the program should be considered. The use of training diaries and follow-up tests to monitor progress provides external feedback along with the usual rewards of improved well-being and vigor experienced by the athlete. Physician support and encouragement improve compliance and help determine the effectiveness of the program.

Older athletes should be told that the early stages of exercise are most uncomfortable, that initial improvements in fitness levels are rapid, but that further improvements occur much more slowly. The athlete should be well aware of the potential problems associated with increasing any of the variables of intensity, duration, or frequency too rapidly. The concept of maintaining optimal fitness should be stressed. Most adult athletes will find it difficult to show continued improvement in fitness as they did during the early stages of their exercise program. The musculoskeletal system is prone to overuse injuries when training progresses too fast. Adequate rest periods between exercise bouts should be stressed to avoid overuse injuries caused by errors in the training regimen.

Appropriate exercise prescription for the sedentary adult is easy to provide. The primary care physician can use the principles outlined here and encourage safe and effective exercise for all adult patients.

REFERENCES

1. Fox EL. Physical training: methods and effects. *Orthop Clin North Am* 1977;8:533–548.
2. McArdle WD, Katch FI, Katch VL. *Exercise physiology*, 5th ed. Lippincott Williams & Wilkins, 2001.

3. Taylor RB. Pre-exercise evaluation: which procedures are really needed? *Consultant* 1983;23:94–101.
4. Dishman RK. Biologic influences on exercise adherence. *Res Q Exerc Sport* 1981;52:143–159.
5. Larson RL, McMahan RO. The epiphyses and the childhood athlete. *JAMA* 1966;196:607–612.
6. Harvey JS. Nutritional management of the adolescent athlete. *Clin Sports Med* 1984;3:671–678.
7. Marino DD, King JC. Nutritional concerns during adolescence. *Pediatr Clin North Am* 1980;27:125–139.
8. Lamb DR. Proper nutrition and hydration in athletics. *Read before the 1985 Sports Medicine Congress/Exposition*. Indianapolis, IN, July 1985.
9. Gill D, Gross J, Huddleston S. Participation motivation in youth sports. *Int J Sport Psychol* 1983;14:1–14.
10. Gould D. Promoting positive sport experiences for children. In: May JR, Asken MJ. *Sport psychology: the psychological health of the athlete*. Champaign: Human Kinetics, 1987:77–98.
11. Gould D, Feltz D, Weiss M. Motives for participating in competitive youth swimming. *Int J Sport Psychol* 1985;16:126–140.
12. Henschen KP, Straub WF. Sport psychology: an analysis of athlete behavior. Ithaca Mouvement Publications, 1995.
13. Roberts GC, Kleiber DA, Duda JL. An analysis of motivation in children's sport: The role of perceived competence in participation. *J Sport Psychol* 1981;3:206–216.
14. Seefeldt V. Physical fitness guidelines for preschool children. *Proceedings of the National Conference on Physical Fitness and Sports for All*. Washington, DC, February 1980.
15. Hamilton P, Andrew GM. Influence of growth and athletic training on heart and lung functions. *Eur J Appl Physiol* 1976;36:27–38.
16. McKeag DB. Adolescents and exercise. *J Adolesc Health Care* 1986;7:121s.
17. Gilliam TB, Freedson PS. Effects of a 12-week school fitness program on peak VO_2 body composition, and blood lipids in 7 to 9 year old children. *Int J Sports Med* 1980;1:73–78.
18. Vrijens J. Muscle strength development in the pre- and post-pubescent age. *Med Sport* 1978;11:152–158.
19. Wilmore JH. Physical conditioning of the young athlete. In: Smith NJ, ed. *Sports medicine for children and youth*. Columbus, Ohio: 10th Ross Roundtable, 1979:63.
20. Drinkwater BL. Physiological characteristics of female athletes. In: Welsh RP, Shephard RJ, eds. *Current therapy sports medicine*. St. Louis: CV Mosby, 130–134.
21. Bonen A, Keizer HA. Athletic menstrual cycle irregularity: endocrine response to exercise and training. *Phys Sportsmed* 1984;12(8):78–94.
22. Brooks-Gunn J, Warren MP, Hamilton H. The relationship of eating disorders to amenorrhea in ballet dancers. *Med Sci Sports Exerc* 1987;19(1): 41.
23. Cummings DC, Vickovic MD, Wall SR, et al. The effect of acute exercise on pulsatile release of luteinizing hormone in women runners. *Am J Obstet Gynecol* 1985;153:482.
24. Duester PA, Kyle SB, Moser PB, et al. Nutritional intakes and status of highly trained amenorrheic and eumenorrheic women runners. *Fertil Steril* 1986;46:636.
25. Frisch RE, McArthur JW. Menstrual cycles: fatness as a determinant of minimum weight for height necessary for their maintenance or onset. *Science* 1974;185(4155):949–951.
26. Shangold MM. How I manage exercise-related menstrual disturbances. *Phys Sportsmed* 1986;14(3):113–120.
27. DeSouza MJ, Maresh CM, Abraham A, et al. Body compositions of eumenorrheic, oligomenorrheic and amenorrheic runners. *J Appl Sport Sci Res* 1987;2(1):13.
28. Sanborn CF, Albrecht BH, Wagner W Jr. Athletic amenorrhea: lack of association with body fat. *Med Sci Sports Exerc* 1987;19(3):207.
29. Killinger DW Athletes with menstrual irregularities. In: Welsh RP, Shephard RJ, eds. *Current therapy sports medicine*. St. Louis: CV Mosby, 1985–86:121–122.
30. Lutter JM, Cushman S. Menstrual patterns in female runners. *Phys Sportsmed* 1982;10(9):60–72.
31. Cann CE, Martin MC, Genant HK, et al. Decreased spinal mineral content in ammenorrhic women. *JAMA* 1984;251:626.
32. Cummings SR, Black D. Should perimenopausal women be screened for osteoporosis. *Ann Intern Med* 1986;104:817–823.
33. Drinkwater BD, Nilson KL, Chesnut CS III. Bone mineral content of ammenorrheic and eumenorrhoic athletes. *N Engl J Med* 1984;311:277.
34. Gonzales ER. Premature bone loss found in some non-menstruating sportswomen. *JAMA* 1982;248:513.
35. Markus R, Cann C, Madvig P, et al. Menstrual function and bone mass in elite women distance runners: endocrine and metabolic features. *Ann Intern Med* 1985;102(2):158–163.
36. Smith DM, Khairri MR, Norton J. Age and activity effects on bone and mineral loss. *J Clin Invest* 1976;58:716.
37. Pivarnik JM, Ayres NA, Mauer MB, et al. Effects of maternal aerobic fitness on cardiorespiratory responses to exercise. *Med Sci Sports Exerc* 1993;25:993–998.
38. Clapp J. Oxygen consumption during treadmill exercise, before, during and after pregnancy. *Am J Obstet Gynecol* 1989a;161:1458.
39. Romen Y, Hartel R. Physiologic and endocrine adjustments to pregnancy. In: Hartel R, Siswell RA, eds. *Exercise in pregnancy*. Baltimore: Williams & Wilkins, 1986:59–82.
40. Avery ND, Stocking KD, Tranmer JE, et al. Fetal responses to maternal strength conditioning exercises in late gestation. *Can J Appl Physiol* 1999;24:362–376.
41. Hall DC, Kaufmann DA. Effects of aerobic and strength conditioning on pregnancy outcomes. *Am J Obstet Gynaecol* 1987;157:1199–1203.
42. Lotgering FK, van den Berg A, Struijk PC, et al. Arterial pressure response to maximal isometric exercise in pregnant women. *Am J Obstet Gynecol* 1992;166:538–542.
43. Nisell H, Hjemdahl P, Linde B, et al. Sympatho-adrenal and cardiovascular reactivity in pregnancy-induced hypertension I. Responses to isometric exercise and a cold pressor test. *Br J Obstet Gynecol* 1985;92:722–731.
44. Pivarnik JM, Rivera JM. Exercise in pregnancy. In: Ransom SB, Dombrowski MP, Evans MI et al. eds. *Contemporary therapy in obstetrics and gynecology: issues and controversies 2000/2001*. Philadelphia: WB Saunders, 2002:85–89.
45. Goodlin RC, Buckley KK. Maternal exercise. *Clin Sports Med* 1984;3:881–894.
46. Joint FHO/WHO/UNU Expert Consultation. *Energy and protein requirements*. Albany, NY. World Health Organization, 1985.
47. Carpenter MW, Sady SP, Hoegsberg B, et al. Fetal heart rate response to maternal exertion. *JAMA* 1988;259:3006–3009.
48. Dale E, Mullinex KM, Bryan DH. Exercise during pregnancy: effects on the fetus. *Can J Sports Sci* 1982;7:98.
49. Wolfe LA, Brenner IKM, Mottola MF. Maternal exercise, fetal well-being and pregnancy outcome. *Exerc Sport Sci Rev* 1994;22:145–194.
50. Clapp JF III, Little KD, Capeless EL. Fetal heart rate response to sustained recreational exercise. *Am J Obstet Gynecol* 1993;168:198–206.
51. Beller JM, Dolmy EG. Effect of an aerobic endurance exercise program on maternal and fetal heart rate during the second and third trimester. *Med Sci Sports Exerc* 1987;19:S5.
52. Collings C, Curet LB. Fetal heart rate response to maternal exercise. *Am J Obstet Gynaecol* 1985;151:495–501.
53. Henswal and Scientific Affairs. AMA Effects of physical forces in the reproductive cycle. *JAMA* 1984;251:247–251.
54. Milunsky A, Ulcickas M, Rothman KJ, et al. Maternal heat exposure and neural tube defects. *JAMA* 1992;268:882–885.
55. Clapp JF. The changing thermal response to endurance exercise during pregnancy. *Am J Obstet Gynecol* 1991;165:1684–1689.
56. Clapp JF, Bathay ER, Wesley M, et al. Thermoregulatory and metabolic responses to jogging prior to and during pregnancy. *Med Sci Sports Exerc* 1987;19:124–130.
57. Clapp JF III. The effects of maternal exercise on early pregnancy outcome. *Am J Obstet Gynecol* 1989b;161:1453–1457.
58. Bell RJ, Palma SM, Lumley JM. The effect of vigorous exercise during pregnancy on birth-weight. *Aust N Z J Obstet Gynaecol* 1995;35:46–51.
59. Berkowitz GS, Kelsey JL, Holford TR, et al. Physical activity and the risk of spontaneous preterm birth. *Epidemiol Prev* 1993;15:414–443.
60. Campbell MK, Mottola MF. Recreational exercise and occupational activity during pregnancy and birth weight. A case-control study. *Am J Obstet Gynecol* 2001;184:403–408.
61. Clapp JF III, Dickstein S. Endurance exercise and pregnancy outcome. *Med Sci Sports Exerc* 1984;16:556–562.
62. Clapp JF III. The course of labor after endurance exercise during pregnancy. *Am J Obstet Gynecol* 1990;163:1799–1805.
63. Clapp JF III, Capeless EL. Neonatal morphometrics after endurance exercise during pregnancy. *Am J Obstet Gynecol* 1990;163:1805–1811.
64. Pivarnik JM. Potential effects of maternal physical activity on birth weight: brief review. *Med Sci Sports Exerc* 1998;30:400–406.
65. Kolpa PH, White BM, Visscher R. Aerobic exercise in pregnancy. *Am J Obstet Gynecol* 1987;156:1395–1403.
66. Pivarnik JM, Perkins CD, Moyerbrailean TB. Athletes and pregnancy. *Clin Obstet Gynecol* 2003;46(2):403–414.
67. Dale E, Maharam LG. Exercise and pregnancy. In: Welsh RP, Shephard RJ, eds. *Current therapy sports medicine 1985–86*. 1986:122–125.
68. Gauthier MM. Guidelines for exercise during pregnancy: too little or too much? *Phys Sportsmed* 1986;14(4):162–169.
69. American College of Obstetricians and Gynecologists. *Technical bulletin no. 173. Women and exercise*. Washington, DC: American College of Obstetricians and Gynecologists, 1994.
70. American College of Obstetricians and Gynecologists. Exercise during pregnancy and the postpartum period. ACOG Committee Opinion 267. *Obstet Gynecol* 2002;99:171–173.
71. Paisley JE, Mellion MB. Exercise during pregnancy. *Am Fam Physician* 1988;38(5):143–150.
72. St John Repovich WE, Wiswell RA, Artal R. Sports activities and aerobic exercise during pregnancy. In: Artal R, Wiswell RA, eds. *Exercise and pregnancy*. Baltimore: Williams & Wilkins, 1986:205–214.
73. Mullinax KM, Dale E. Some considerations of exercise during pregnancy. *Clin Sports Med* 1986;5:559–570.
74. Bergfeld JA, Martin MC, Shangold MM, et al. Women in athletics: five management problems. *Patient Care* 1987;21:60–64,73–74,76–80,82.

75. Leaf DA. Exercise during pregnancy: guidelines and controversies. *Post-Grad Med* 1989;85:233.
76. Warren MP. Exercise in women—effects on reproductive system and pregnancy. In: DiNubile NA, ed. *Clinics in sports medicine*. Philadelphia, PA: WB Saunders, 1991:131.
77. Shephard RJ. *Prescribing exercise for the senior citizen: some simple guidelines*. Chicago Year Book, 1989.
78. Clarke HH. Exercise and aging. President's council on physical fitness and sports. *Phys Fitness Res Dig* 1977;7(2):1–27.
79. Fitzgerald PL. Exercise for the elderly. *Med Clin North Am* 1985;69(1):189.
80. Williams RS. How beneficial is regular exercise? *J Cardiovasc Med* 1982;119:1112–1120.
81. Fiatarone MA, Marks EC, Ryan ND, et al. High intensity strength training in non nonagenarians. *JAMA* 1990;263:3029.
82. Ninimaa V, Shepard RJ. Training and oxygen conductance in the elderly: the cardiovascular system. *J Gerontol* 1978;33:362.
83. Elia EA. Exercise in the elderly. In: DiNubile MA, ed. *Clinics in sports medicine*, Vol. 10(1). Philadelphia PA: WB Saunders, 1991:141.
84. Ike RW, Lambman RM, Castor CW. Arthritis and aerobic exercise. *Phys Sportsmed* 1989;17:128.
85. Minor MA, Hewett JE, Webel RR, et al. Efficacy of physical condition exercise in patients with rheumatoid arthritis and osteoarthritis. *Arthritis Rheumatol* 1989;32:1396.
86. Aloia JF, Cohn SH, Ostuni JD, et al. Prevention of involutional bone loss by exercise. *Ann Intern Med* 1978;89:356.
87. Barry HC. Exercise prescriptions for the elderly. *Am Fam Physician* 1986;34(3):155–162.
88. Elkowitz EB, Elkowitz A. Prescribing exercise for the elderly. *J Fam Prac Recert* 1986;8(1):117–130.
89. Laslett LJ, Amsterdam EA, Mason DT. Exercise testing in the geriatric patient. *Ann Intern Med* 1980;112:56.
90. Mean WF, Hartwig R. Fitness evaluation and exercise prescription. *J FamPract* 1981;13:1039–1050.
91. Simons-Morton BG, Pate RR, Simons-Morton DS. Prescribing physical activity to prevent disease. *Postgrad Med* 1988;83(1):165.
92. Laporte RE, Blair SN. Physical activity or cardiovascular fitness: which is more important for health? A pro and con. *Phys Sportsmed* 1985;13:145–157.
93. Paffenbarger RS, Hyde RT, Wing AL, et al. Physical activity—all cause mortality and longevity of college alumni. *N Engl J Med* 1986;314:605–613.
94. Smith EL, Gilligan C. Physical activity prescription for the older adult. *Phys Sportsmed* 1983;11:91.
95. Ciscovick DS, Weiss MS, Fletcher RH, et al. The incidence of primary cardiac arrest during vigorous exercise. *N Engl J Med* 1984;311:874.
96. Goodman JM, Goodman LS. Exercise prescription for the sedentary adult. In: Welsh RP, Shephard RJ, eds. *Current therapy in sports medicine*. Toronto: PC Decker Inc, 1985:17–24.
97. Smith LK. Medical clearance for vigorous exercise. *Postgrad Med* 1988;83(1):146.
98. Shephard RJ. Physical training for the elderly. *Clin Sports Med* 1986;5:515.
99. American College of Sports Medicine. *Guidelines for graded exercise testing and exercise prescription*, 2nd ed. Philadelphia: Lea & Febiger, 1980.
100. Hanson PG, Giese MD, Corliss RJ. CLinical guidelines for exercise training. *Postgrad Med* 1980;67:120–138.

7

Exercise as Medicine: The Role of Exercise in Treating Chronic Disease

Eric J. Anish *Chris A. Klenck*

Regular physical activity is considered an important component of a healthy lifestyle. Epidemiological studies have demonstrated that a sedentary lifestyle or comparatively low levels of habitual physical activity is associated with increased all-cause mortality rates (1). Alternatively, routine physical activity at higher levels is associated with decreased overall mortality and has also been shown to play a beneficial role in the primary prevention of a variety of medical conditions (see Table 7.1). Consequently, health care providers are encouraging individuals of all ages to participate in greater amounts of physical activity. Several public health recommendations have been published detailing the types and amounts of physical activity that are required for health promotion and disease prevention (1–3). In addition to its role as a preventative health strategy, regular physical activity, including formal exercise training, has been shown to be of benefit in the treatment of numerous common, chronic medical problems including diabetes mellitus (DM), hypertension, dyslipidemia, obesity, osteoporosis and depression. This chapter will focus on the use of exercise as a therapeutic modality in the management of these chronic medical conditions.

SECTION A
DIABETES MELLITUS

DM is a group of metabolic diseases characterized by hyperglycemia resulting from defects in insulin secretion, insulin action, or both (5). The chronic hyperglycemia of diabetes is associated with the development of several adverse medical conditions including retinopathy, nephropathy, and neuropathy. Individuals with DM are also at an increased risk for developing cardiovascular disease, which remains a major cause of morbidity and mortality in this population.

There are several types of DM. Most cases of DM fall into two broad categories. In one category (type 1 DM), the cause is an absolute deficiency of insulin secretion, often related to pancreatic beta-cell destruction. In the absence of exogenous insulin, individuals with type 1 DM are prone to develop ketoacidosis. In the other much more common category (type 2 DM), the etiology is a combination of resistance to insulin action and inadequate compensatory insulin secretory response (5). Other major categories of DM include gestational diabetes and diabetes that develops secondary to other disease states (e.g., Cushing's syndrome, hyperthyroidism, hemochromatosis) or as a result of drug-use (e.g., glucocorticoids, pentamidine, interferon alpha).

The diagnosis of DM can be made based on one or more of the following criteria: (a) symptoms of diabetes plus a random plasma glucose concentration of 200 mg/dL or more; (b) fasting plasma glucose of 126 mg/dL or more; (c) 2-hour postprandial glucose of 200 or more following a 75-g glucose load during an oral glucose tolerance test. Each criteria must be repeated on a different day in the absence of unequivocal hyperglycemia to confirm the diagnosis (5).

In the United States alone, it is estimated that 20.8 million people (7% of the population) currently have been diagnosed with DM. The estimated direct and indirect cost

TABLE 7.1

BENEFICIAL EFFECTS OF REGULAR PHYSICAL ACTIVITY (PRIMARY PREVENTION OF CHRONIC DISEASE)

- Type 2 diabetes mellitus
- Hypertension
- Dyslipidemia
- Obesity
- Osteoporosis
- Depression
- Coronary heart disease
- Cerebrovascular disease
- Colon cancer

Source: From Kesaniemi YA, Danforth E, Jensen MD, et al. Dose-response issues concerning physical activity and health: an evidence-based symposium. *Med Sci Sports Exerc* 2001;33:S351–S358, (4).

of caring for this population is approximately $132 billion annually (6). An increasing prevalence of DM is not only occurring in the United States, but also being witnessed around the world. By 2025, approximately 300 million people worldwide will be diagnosed with DM. As a result, diabetes and its complications will result in an increasing burden on health care costs in the United States and abroad (7).

THE ROLE OF EXERCISE IN TREATING DIABETES MELLITUS

For years, the traditional cornerstones of therapy for patients with DM have been dietary modification and medication. Exercise also has been encouraged in patients with DM because regular physical activity may help to control hyperglycemia through improved glucose utilization. However, a variety of factors can influence the effect that exercise can have on blood glucose. Variables that should be considered include the type of diabetes involved (type 1 versus type 2), the type of exercise performed (aerobic versus anaerobic), the duration and intensity of physical activity, concurrent use of medications (e.g., sulfonylureas, insulin), and the patient's baseline cardiorespiratory fitness level (8).

In order to better understand the effect that exercise can have on glycemic control, it is important to appreciate the relation between exercise and glucose utilization. In normal human metabolism, during a single episode of exercise, the muscles initially utilize glucose in the muscle and later convert muscle glycogen to glucose to provide energy. Exercise then stimulates an insulin-independent transport of glucose from the circulation into the exercising muscle. As the blood glucose concentration drops, insulin secretion decreases and the release of glucagon increases. These hormonal changes result in enhanced hepatic glucose production secondary to increased glycogenolysis and to gluconeogenesis. With further exercise, other counter-regulatory hormones (e.g., epinephrine, norepinephrine, growth hormone, and cortisol) begin to play a role in maintaining adequate blood glucose levels (9).

With regular moderate-intensity physical activity, training-effects occur that result in more efficient use of energy by muscle. These changes include the development of new muscle capillaries and increases in the quantity of mitochondrial enzymes (9). Studies have also demonstrated that regular endurance exercise training increases the concentration of GLUT4 mRNA and protein in skeletal muscle. GLUT4 is a protein that serves as a glucose transporter. The exercise-related increase in muscle GLUT4 is physiologically important because elevated GLUT4 augments muscle glucose transport and enhances whole-body glucose tolerance (10).

GLUT4 is predominantly found in association with intracellular vesicles that translocate to the cell membrane in order to increase glucose transport. The maximal rate of muscle glucose transport is determined by both the total number of GLUT4 molecules and the proportion of these molecules that are translocated to the cell membrane in response to insulin and/or muscle contraction (10). It has been demonstrated that in type 2 diabetes, impairment of insulin-stimulated GLUT4 translocation exists. This defect is felt to be one of the primary contributors to diabetes-related insulin resistance. In contrast, there does not appear to be any decrement in muscle contraction-induced translocation of GLUT4 during exercise (11).

In patients with DM, several physiological responses to exercise are altered based upon the plasma insulin concentration at the time of exercise and the degree of pre-exercise glycemic control. Additionally, the use of exogenous insulin can have a profound effect on glucose concentrations during exercise. Well-controlled diabetic patients on insulin therapy often will have a much larger drop in blood glucose concentrations than that seen in non–insulin dependent diabetic patients or individuals without diabetes. Because the effects of exogenous insulin cannot be turned off, muscle glucose uptake and the inhibition of hepatic glucose production may continue to occur despite dropping levels of blood glucose (9).

In patients with poor glucose control, exercise can actually result in blood glucose elevations. This occurs when inadequate amounts of insulin result in impaired glucose uptake by muscle and when hormones such as epinephrine, cortisol, and growth hormone, which are released during exercise, cause increased hepatic glucose production (9).

EXERCISE AND LONG-TERM GLYCEMIC CONTROL

With regard to the long-term effects of routine exercise on glucose control, the effects differ between patients with type 1 DM and those with type 2 DM. The results of several studies have found that exercise interventions can reduce glycosylated hemoglobin levels (HbA_{Ic}) in people with type 2 DM. Many of the studies demonstrating a beneficial effect of regular aerobic exercise on long-term glucose control in type 2 DM have utilized physical activity performed for 30 to 60 minutes, at 50% to 80% of maximal oxygen uptake (Vo_{2max}), three to four sessions per week. With this type of exercise program, reductions in HbA_{Ic} of 10% to 20% from baseline could be achieved (12).

Studies utilizing resistance training have also demonstrated a beneficial effect on long-term glucose control in type 2 DM. Eriksson et al. (13) examined the effects of an individualized progressive resistance-training program. Subjects performed circuit-type resistance exercises two times per week. After 3 months of training, the average HbA_{Ic} dropped from 8.8% to 8.2% ($p < 0.05$). The investigators found that glycemic control correlated strongly with changes in muscle size, quantified using magnetic resonance imaging. More recently, Castaneda et al. (14) evaluated the use of a high-intensity progressive resistance-training program on glycemic control in type 2 diabetic patients with a mean age of 66 years. The investigators performed a 16-week randomized controlled trial using multiple exercises, performing three sets, three times per week. The results showed a statistically significant reduction in HbA_{Ic} levels from 8.7% to 7.6%, increase in muscle glycogen stores, and decrease in dosages of prescribed diabetes medication in 72% of the exercisers ($p = 0.004 - 0.05$) compared to a control group.

In 2001, Boule et al. (15) published a meta-analysis of controlled trials that evaluated the effects of exercise interventions (duration >8 weeks) on glycemic control in patients with type 2 DM. Twelve aerobic training studies and two resistance-training studies were included in the analysis. The investigators found that the weighted mean postintervention HbA_{Ic} was lower in the exercise groups compared with control groups (7.65% versus 8.31%, $p < 0.001$). It is important to note that the difference in postintervention body mass between exercise groups and control groups was not statistically significant. The same authors published a subsequent meta-analysis in 2003 showing that exercise intensity predicted a greater postintervention weighted mean difference in HbA_{Ic} ($r = -0.91$, $p = 0.002$) than exercise volume ($r = -0.46$, $p = 0.26$) (16). These results suggest that increasing exercise intensity may achieve even greater benefits in glycemic control. The weighted mean difference in HbA_{Ic} of −0.66 demonstrated between the exercise and control groups in the first study, and −0.91 in the high intensity group in the second, has important clinical implications. This degree of improvement in glycemic control is associated with significant reductions in diabetic complications. Results of the United Kingdom Prospective Diabetes Study (UKPDS) published in 1998 (17,18) demonstrated a continuous relation between the risks of microvascular and cardiovascular complications and glycemia. For every percentage point decrease in HbA_{Ic} (e.g., 9%–8%) there was a 35% reduction in the risk of microvascular complications, a 25% reduction in diabetes-related deaths, an 18% reduction in combined fatal and nonfatal myocardial infarction, and a 7% reduction in all-cause mortality.

In contrast to the response in type 2 DM, improvement in long-term glucose control through exercise training in type 1 DM has not been demonstrated as clearly (19). Presumably this is due to the lesser importance of insulin resistance in these patients (9). Studies have demonstrated that in patients with type 1 DM a single bout of exercise can have a blood glucose lowering effect. As determined by HbA_{Ic} values, these effects of exercise, in isolation, have not typically been shown to result in long-term improvement in glucose control (12,20,21). However, a recent study by Herbst et al. (22) evaluated the effect of regular physical activity on glycemic control in type 1 diabetic patients aged 3 to 20 years. In this cross-sectional analysis of data for 19,143 patients, the authors grouped subjects by the frequency of regular physical activity (none versus one to two times per week versus three or more times per week). They found that HbA_{Ic} values were greater in the groups without regular physical activity compared to those with regular physical activity of three or more times per week (8.4% versus 8.1% respectively, $p < 0.001$). Multiple regression analysis showed that regular physical activity was one of the most important factors influencing HbA_{Ic}. Despite these results, intensive insulin therapy and/or dietary restriction still need to be implemented to achieve adequate glycemic control (23).

EXERCISE, DIABETES, AND MORTALITY

Despite the apparent inadequacy of exercise to improve long-term glycemic control in patients with type 1 DM, physical activity is associated with a decreased risk of overall-mortality in this population. The benefits of physical activity on overall-mortality were demonstrated in a cohort of 548 type 1 diabetic patients enrolled in the Pittsburgh Insulin-Dependent Diabetes Mellitus Morbidity and Mortality Study (24). Physical activity was measured by survey in 1981, and mortality was ascertained through 1988. After controlling for numerous potential confounders (e.g., age, body mass index [BMI], tobacco use, etc.), the investigators found that overall activity level was inversely related to mortality risk. Sedentary males (energy expenditure <1,000 kcal/week) were three times more likely to die than active males (energy expenditure <1,000 kcal/week).

The beneficial effect of physical activity on overall-mortality has also been demonstrated in type 2 diabetics. Wei et al. (25) performed a prospective cohort study of over 1,200 men with type 2 DM. The subjects completed a maximal exercise treadmill test to determine cardiopulmonary fitness. Based on performance, subjects were categorized as "low fit, moderately fit, or high fit."

Participants also completed an extensive self-report of personal and family history, including physical activity patterns. These individuals were followed-up for an average of 11.7 years. Adjustments were made for a variety of factors that might affect overall mortality (e.g., age, tobacco use, hypercholesterolemia, hypertension, etc.). The investigators found that the low-fitness group had an adjusted risk for all-cause mortality of 2.1 (95% CI, 1.5–2.9) compared with fit men. Additionally, men who reported being physically inactive had an adjusted risk for all-cause mortality of 1.7 (95% CI, 1.2–2.3) compared with men who reported being physically active. Another recent study showed diabetic men in the lowest, second, and third quartiles of cardiorespiratory fitness to have an overall mortality risk, that is, 4.5, 2.8, and 1.6-fold, respectively, greater than men in the highest quartile for fitness (26).

ADDITIONAL BENEFITS OF EXERCISE IN DIABETES MELLITUS

Independent of its action of blood glucose control, regular exercise can have several beneficial effects for patients with DM. One area in which exercise can have a significant impact is in cardiovascular disease risk reduction. In patients with both type 1 and type 2 DM, routine exercise can decrease risk factors for cardiovascular diseases such as dyslipidemia, hypertension, and coagulation abnormalities (21). Additionally, participation in regular physical activity may help promote reductions in tobacco use and alcohol consumption (21). Regular exercise has also been shown to have mental health benefits for diabetic patients. Although difficult to determine, routine exercise has been associated with an elevated "sense of well-being," increased "self-esteem," and an enhanced "quality of life" (21). Some of these psychological benefits may be derived from the ability of active participation in exercise and organized sports activities to promote socialization and peer acceptance (27). As a result, the American Diabetes Association (ADA) concludes its position statement on diabetes and exercise (12) by stating, "all patients with diabetes should have the opportunity to benefit from the many valuable effects of physical activity."

EXERCISE RISKS IN DIABETES MELLITUS

Although exercise can be highly beneficial for patients with DM, at the same time, it can pose certain risks (see Table 7A.1). Before initiating an exercise program, individuals with diabetes should undergo a medical evaluation to screen for microvascular and macrovascular complications that may be exacerbated by exercise (12). A complete discussion of all the exercise-associated risks for diabetic patients and the specific recommendations regarding the preparticipation medical evaluation of these individuals is beyond the scope of this chapter. This information can be found in several recent publications (7, 12,27). However, this section will review two of the major complications, hypoglycemia and myocardial ischemia, which are seen in diabetic patients who exercise.

TABLE 7A.1
RISKS OF EXERCISE FOR PATIENTS WITH DIABETES MELLITUS

Organ System	Potential Adverse Event
Metabolic	Hyperglycemia
	Hypoglycemia
Cardiovascular	Coronary artery disease
	Myocardial ischemia
	Cardiac arrest
	Sudden cardiac death
	Arrhythmia
	Abnormal blood pressure response
	Peripheral vascular disease (claudication)
Kidneys	Proteinuria
Eyes	Retinal hemorrhage
Musculoskeletal	Ulcerations
	Degenerative joint disease

Source: From (7,12,27,28)

Hypoglycemia remains the most common risk encountered for diabetic patients who exercise. Although this can occur in patients with type 2 DM, particularly those taking sulfonylureas, it is of greater concern in patients taking exogenous insulin. Because the effects of exogenous insulin continue despite declining blood glucose levels, muscle glucose uptake and the inhibition of hepatic glucose production may continue, resulting in profound hypoglycemia. Additionally, many diabetic patients, particularly those that have had the disease for 5 years or more, have impaired counter-regulatory mechanisms for combating hypoglycemia (27). Exercise can also enhance the absorption of exogenous insulin, particularly if it has been injected into an exercising extremity. This can further increase the risk of exercise-related hypoglycemia (27).

Even if blood glucose levels remain stable during exercise, patients with diabetes may subsequently develop delayed hypoglycemia. This often occurs at night, 6 to 15 hours after exercise, but may develop as late as 28 hours after exercise. This insidious drop in blood glucose results from the residual effect of exercise-enhanced insulin sensitivity. Additionally, hepatic glycogen synthesis to replenish stores depleted by exercise may also contribute to delayed hypoglycemia. Because liver glycogen is replaced more slowly than muscle glycogen, carbohydrate requirements may be increased for up to 24 hours after prolonged exercise (27). Strategies to help reduce the risk of exercise-related hypoglycemia are outlined in Table 7A.2.

TABLE 7A.2
RISK REDUCTION STRATEGIES FOR EXERCISE-RELATED HYPOGLYCEMIA IN PATIENTS WITH DIABETES MELLITUS

Close monitoring of glucose levels before, during, and after activity
Adjust medication dose and/or food intake before exercise
Perform daily, rather than sporadic, exercise done at the same time in order to facilitate diet and medication adjustments
Morning exercise recommended
Multidose insulin regimens make it easier to adjust dosage when exercise is anticipated
Consider use of lispro (Humalog) insulin (faster onset and shorter half-life)
If pre-exercise blood glucose <100, take a carbohydrate snack (15 g of carbohydrate will raise blood glucose approximately 50 mg/dL)
Avoid exercise when insulin is at its peak activity
Inject insulin in abdomen, not exercising extremities
Eat a well-balanced meal 2–3 hr before a planned bout of exercise
Ingest carbohydrate containing foods/beverages during sustained activity (30–60 g/hr if activity lasts >1 hr)
Replete glycogen stores immediately postexercise
Have easy access to carbohydrate containing foods should hypoglycemia begin to develop
Have easy access to glucagon (1 mg) for SQ/IM injection
Train coaches, athletic trainers, fellow athletes to recognize the early warning signs of hypoglycemia

Source: From American Diabetes Association. Physical activity/exercise and diabetes. *Diabetes Care* 2004;27(Suppl 1): S58–S62; Colberg SR, Swain DP. Exercise and diabetes control: a winning combination. *Phys Sportsmed* 2000;28:63–81; White RD, Sherman C. Exercise in diabetes management: maximizing benefits, controlling risks. *Phys Sportmed* 1999;27:63–76.

Another concern for diabetic patients who exercise is the development of myocardial ischemia or sudden death. These adverse events are related to underlying atherosclerotic coronary artery disease. In many diabetic patients, atherosclerosis is more extensive and develops earlier than in the general, nondiabetic population. Although routine exercise can help improve many of the risk factors for coronary artery disease and decrease the long-term risk of developing cardiovascular disease, there is an actual transient increased risk for myocardial infarction, cardiac arrest, and sudden death during vigorous physical activity (29).

The ADA has recommended a graded exercise stress test if a patient, about to embark on a moderate- to high-intensity exercise program, is at high risk for underlying cardiovascular disease based on specific criteria (see Table 7A.3). If patients will only be participating in low-intensity physical activities (<60% maximal heart rate), formal exercise stress testing may not be necessary, although appropriate clinical judgment needs to be executed (12).

TABLE 7A.3
CRITERIA THAT SHOULD PROMPT CONSIDERATION FOR EXERCISE STRESS TESTING IN DIABETICS BEFORE MODERATE- OR HIGH-INTENSITY EXERCISE

Type 2 DM >10 yr duration
Type 1 DM >15 yr duration
Age >35 years
Presence of any additional risk factors for coronary artery disease (see Table 7B.5)
Presence of microvascular disease
Peripheral vascular disease
Autonomic neuropathy

DM = diabetes mellitus.
Source: From American Diabetes Association. Physical activity/exercise and diabetes. *Diabetes Care* 2004;27(Suppl 1): S58–S62.

Additionally, in patients with known coronary artery disease, the ADA recommends that these individuals undergo a supervised evaluation of the ischemic response to exercise, ischemic threshold, and the propensity to arrhythmia during exercise (12). It is important to remember that even patients who are identified as low risk for exercise-related complications and are participating in low- to moderate-intensity activities cannot be completely assured that such activity will not acutely increase the risk of an adverse cardiac event. Nevertheless, it does appear that the long-term health benefits of regular exercise outweigh the acute cardiovascular risks. Therefore, regular exercise should be encouraged in this population of diabetic patients.

SECTION B
HYPERTENSION

According to the Seventh Report of the Joint National Committee (JNC 7) on Prevention, Detection, Evaluation, and Treatment of High Blood Pressure (30), hypertension is defined as a *systolic blood pressure* (SBP) of 140 mm Hg or greater, a diastolic blood pressure (DBP) of 90 mm Hg or greater, or the use of an antihypertensive medication. In addition, individuals with SBP of 120 to 139 or DBP of 80 to 89 are defined as having prehypertension. According to these criteria, approximately 50 million adults have hypertension in the United States alone, making it the most common primary diagnosis in America. Only 34% of these individuals have their blood pressure (BP) controlled below 140/90. The extremely high prevalence of hypertension and

TABLE 7B.1
LIFESTYLE MODIFICATIONS FOR HYPERTENSION MANAGEMENT

Weight loss if overweight (BMI ≥25 kg/m^2)
Limit alcohol intake to no more than 1 oz of ethanol/d for men or 0.5 oz of ethanol/d for women and lighter-weight people
Reduce sodium intake to no more than 100 mEq/L (2.4 g of sodium or 6 g of sodium chloride)
Institute a DASH (Dietary Approaches to Stop Hypertension) eating plan with diet rich in fruits, vegetables, and low-fat diary products with a reduced content of saturated and total fats
Increase aerobic physical activity (at least 30 min/d most days of the week)

BMI = body mass index.
Source: From Joint National Committee on Detection, Evaluation, and Treatment Of High Blood Pressure. The seventh report of the joint national committee on prevention, detection, evaluation, and treatment of high blood pressure. *JAMA* 2003;289:2560–2572.

hypertension-related complications such as stroke, heart failure, and end-stage renal disease imposes a tremendous financial and social burden on our society (30).

One of the primary objectives of treating hypertension is to reduce morbidity and mortality by the least intrusive measures possible (30). This goal may be achieved through lifestyle modification alone or in combination with pharmacotherapy. Lifestyle modifications (see Table 7B.1) have been shown to be effective in lowering BP, with little cost or health risk to those who implement these changes. One of the recommended lifestyle changes included in the JNC 7 guidelines is participation in regular aerobic physical activity, enough to achieve at least a moderate level of physical fitness. The following section will examine the relationship between regular exercise and BP reduction in hypertensive patients.

PHYSICAL ACTIVITY AND BLOOD PRESSURE REDUCTION

The rationale for using exercise to help reduce BP in hypertensive patients is based on the results of population studies. Several cross-sectional studies have demonstrated that BP tends to be significantly lower in active individuals compared with groups of sedentary peers (31). The results of several prospective observational studies provide further support for the use of physical activity to help reduce BP. Blair et al. (32) investigated the association between baseline cardiorespiratory fitness (as determined by a maximal, graded exercise treadmill test) and the subsequent development of hypertension in a group of 4,820 men and 1,219 women aged 20 to 65 years at time of entry into the study. During the 1 to 12 year follow-up interval (median 4 years) there were 240 new cases of hypertension detected. After adjustments were made for a number of potential confounding variables (e.g., age, baseline BP, BMI, etc.), the investigators found that the relative risk of developing hypertension in the low-fitness group was 1.52 times the risk of a person in the high-fitness group (95% CI, 1.08–2.15, $p = 0.02$).

Although the results of such observational studies support the role of regular physical activity in the prevention of hypertension, they do not answer the question of whether exercise can be used to treat hypertension. Several prospective, interventional studies have addressed this issue and provide compelling evidence of the therapeutic effects of exercise on hypertension. Many of these studies have found exercise to be beneficial in reducing BP in hypertensive patients, independent of any changes in weight or body composition that may have occurred (33). However, it is important to note that tremendous heterogeneity is found in the hypotensive efficacy reported in various studies. This relates to the variability of the subjects enrolled (age, gender, ethnicity, baseline level of BP), the characteristics of the physical activity intervention (aerobic versus resistance training, exercise modality, intensity, frequency, duration), the length of the intervention, and the duration of long-term follow-up.

AEROBIC EXERCISE TRAINING IN HYPERTENSION

In 2004, the American College of Sports Medicine (ACSM) updated its position stand on exercise and hypertension (34). In this work, the authors examined the effect of endurance training on resting, ambulatory, and exercise BP. Meta-analyses of randomized controlled trials showed resting BP was reduced significantly in response to exercise. More specifically, recent meta-analyses involving 127 randomized controlled trials irrespective of baseline BP showed reductions of SBP/DBP ranging from 3.4 to 4.7/2.4 to 3.1 mm Hg. In those studies in which average baseline BP was in the hypertensive range (SBP ≥140 mm Hg or DBP ≥90 mm Hg), average BP reduction was 7.4/5.8 mm Hg (34). Furthermore, studies comparing hypertensive subjects to normotensive counterparts found significantly greater reductions in resting SBP/DBP in those with hypertension (6/5 mm Hg) versus those without (2/1 mm Hg) (34), suggesting a more pronounced reduction in hypertensive patients. In addition, ambulatory BP monitoring was utilized in 11 randomized controlled trials in assessing exercise-induced reductions of BP. The baseline SBP/DBP for these studies averaged 135/86. Results showed that the weighted net reduction in BP as a result of exercise averaged 3.0/3.2 mm Hg (34). Finally, exercise BP was evaluated in eight randomized controlled trials using cycle ergometer exercise at a median workload of 100 W and two studies using treadmill exercise at an energy expenditure of 4 metabolic equivalents (METs). Pre-exercise training SBP averaged 180 mm Hg and heart rate 124 bpm. The results showed a significant weighted net training-mediated decrease in SBP of 7.0 mm Hg and in heart rate of 6 bpm (34).

The updated ACSM position paper also discusses the phenomenon of postexercise hypotension (PEH) (34). PEH is described as "the decrease in arterial BP below control levels after a session of dynamic exercise." Multiple studies have evaluated the occurrence of PEH in both normotensive and hypertensive subjects. These studies have shown that BP is reduced up to 22 hours after an endurance exercise bout. The greatest decreases in BP are seen in those patients with the highest baseline BP values (34).

This reduction in BP can have a significant impact on hypertensive-related medical complications. Modest reductions in SBP and DBP of 2 mm Hg has been shown to reduce the risk of stroke by 14% and 17% respectively. The risk of coronary artery disease has been shown to be reduced by 9% and 6% for the same 2 mm Hg reduction in SBP and DBP respectively (34). Data from studies utilizing pharmacological treatment of hypertension have demonstrated that a decrease in DBP of 5 to 6 mm Hg is associated with an approximate 35% to 40% reduction in stroke, and a 20% to 25% reduction in coronary heart disease (35).

Other important features of the ACSM position paper with respect to the BP lowering effects of exercise include the following: (a) benefits were seen across a wide range of ages, but there is insufficient evidence to support using exercise as a treatment modality for reducing BP in children or adolescents; (b) there were no gender related differences in BP reduction elicited with endurance exercise training; (c) no evidence exists to support ethnic differences in the BP response to acute or chronic exercise; (e) training at moderate intensity (40%–70% $\dot{V}O_{2max}$) had the same, or greater, BP lowering effect as higher-intensity training programs. This final point is particularly important when prescribing exercise for hypertensive patients who are frail, elderly, sedentary, or who have other concurrent chronic illnesses. These individuals may be at increased risk of exercise-related orthopedic or cardiovascular complications if higher intensity physical activity is attempted (34).

In summary, there is convincing evidence that regular aerobic exercise training can lower BP in hypertensive patients. Low- to moderate-intensity exercise (<70% $\dot{V}O_{2max}$) utilizing large muscle groups, performed on most, preferably all, days of the week for 30 minutes or more per session can help achieve BP reduction (34,36). In addition, resistance exercise can supplement aerobic activity for further BP reduction (34). The duration of the exercise program should be at least 1 to 3 months to reach a stable level of training, and the regimen should be continued indefinitely because the hypotensive effect of exercise training dissipates quickly after the training program is discontinued (37).

RESISTANCE TRAINING IN HYPERTENSION

Although most of the studies examining the effects of exercise on BP have used endurance (aerobic) training, some investigators have looked at the impact of resistance training. Traditionally, hypertensive patients have been discouraged from performing resistance training because of concerns about precipitating a cerebrovascular event or myocardial ischemia. These fears were based on the results of studies that demonstrated dramatic, acute elevations in BP during a single episode of heavy resistance training (38) and the publication of case-reports describing isolated adverse events (39). However, studies investigating the impact of long-term participation in resistance training have failed to document a deleterious effect (40–42). In fact, regular strength training has been shown to blunt the acute BP response to static exercise in both normotensive and hypertensive subjects (34,37).

In 1997, Kelly (43) published a meta-analysis of nine studies examining the effects of dynamic resistance exercise (i.e., weight training) on BP in adults. The results of this study demonstrate that dynamic resistance exercise reduces systolic and diastolic BP by 3% and 4%, respectively. More recently, Cornelissen and Fagard (44) published a meta-analysis of nine studies, also evaluating the effect of resistance training on BP. This study showed similar results with a reduction in SBP of 3.2 mm Hg ($p = 0.10$) and DBP of 3.5 mm Hg ($p < 0.05$). However, these results must be viewed with regard to certain limitations : (a) small sample size (only three of the nine studies included hypertensive patients); (b) absence of data for selected variables (e.g., timing of BP measurement following the exercise sessions); and (c) lack of information on the dynamic resistance training protocol used. This last point is extremely important because without this information one cannot accurately identify or quantify the actual training stimulus. Different forms of weight training can result in dissimilar physiological responses. For example, compared with conventional weight training (see Table 7B.2), circuit weight training, which combines features of both dynamic and resistance exercise will engage aerobic metabolism and have the capacity to improve aerobic capacity as well as strength. Studies examining the effects of weight training on BP have consistently found circuit weight training to be more effective in reducing BP than conventional weight training strategies (45). It may be concluded, then, that traditional weight training ideally should be paired with aerobic exercise for optimal benefits in treating hypertension (46).

MECHANISMS OF BLOOD PRESSURE REDUCTION WITH EXERCISE

Several theories have been proposed to help explain the effect that regular exercise can have on BP (see Table 7B.3). However, many of the studies performed to test these

TABLE 7B.2

COMPARISON OF CONVENTIONAL WEIGHT TRAINING WITH CIRCUIT WEIGHT TRAINING

Conventional Weight Training	Circuit Weight Training
Primarily anaerobic	Engages aerobic metabolism
Develops strength only	Develops strength and aerobic capacity
High weight loads	Mild to moderate weight loads
High static component	Moderate static component
Few repetitions	Frequent repetitions

Source: From Stewart KJ. Weight training in coronary artery disease and hypertension. *Prog Cardiovasc Dis* 1992;35:159–168, (47).

theories and to try to establish the mechanisms involved in the antihypertensive effects of exercise training have yielded conflicting results (40). One theory that has gained widespread acceptance centers on the ability of regular exercise to reduce sympathetic nervous system tone. This is supported by studies that have demonstrated reduced levels of plasma norepinephrine with exercise training and a correlation between the degree of norepinephrine reduction and the magnitude of BP improvement. A comprehensive review of the literature related to the antihypertensive effects of regular exercise is beyond the scope of this chapter and can be found in other publications (40,48–50).

For many patients, the initiation and continuation of a regular exercise program is often accompanied by other lifestyle changes such as diet modification, weight loss, smoking cessation, and decreased alcohol consumption, all of which may result in BP reduction independent of the direct effects of exercise. In general, for many people, regular exercise promotes a healthier overall lifestyle that can reduce multiple risk factors for the development of high BP.

TABLE 7B.3

PROPOSED MECHANISMS OF BLOOD PRESSURE REDUCTION WITH EXERCISE

- Decreased sympathetic nervous system tone
- Decreased sensitivity of adrenoreceptors
- Increased levels of atrial natriuretic factor
- Alterations in insulin metabolism
- Altered renal sodium metabolism
- Changes in renin–angiotensin axis

Source: From (31,36,37,40).

ANTIHYPERTENSIVE MEDICATION AND EXERCISE

Whether secondary to an inadequate response to lifestyle modification alone or due to the severity of the BP elevation, many patients will require antihypertensive medication. In addition to achieving adequate control of BP, other goals of pharmacotherapy include avoiding impairment of exercise performance or the development of additional exercise-related complications. Listed below are the common classes of antihypertensives with some of their individual characteristics related to exercise participation and performance (31,33,51–63).

Diuretics

- Reduce plasma volume (may counteract plasma volume expansion that can occur with endurance training)
- Decrease stroke volume
- Cause reflex increase in total peripheral resistance (may decrease muscle blood flow)
- May impair thermoregulation and exacerbate dehydration (related to decreased plasma volume)
- Associated with hypokalemia and hypomagnesemia
- May cause muscle cramping in the setting of normal serum electrolyte concentrations
- Banned by the International Olympic Committee (IOC) and the National Collegiate Athletic Association (NCAA) because of their use as urinary masking agents to hide doping agents like anabolic steroids.

Beta-Blockers

- Decrease the normal exercise-induced rise in BP, heart rate, and myocardial oxygen consumption.
- May be a good drug choice for patients with coronary heart disease or hypertensive patients with an exaggerated rise in BP during exercise
- Increase exercise tolerance in the setting of coronary heart disease
- Decrease the duration and intensity of maximal exercise sessions in patients without underlying coronary heart disease (effects are greater with nonselective $beta_1$- and $beta_2$-blockers than with selective $beta_1$-blocking agents)
- Reduce blood flow to muscles resulting in more rapid muscle fatigue during exercise (more prominent during the first few weeks of treatment)
- Decrease lipolysis and glycogenolysis (results in less energy substrate available during exercise)
- May impair thermoregulation
- Associated with an increased incidence of hyperkalemia
- May mask hypoglycemic response in diabetic patients
- May worsen asthma or trigger or exacerbate exercise-induced bronchospasm

- Banned by the IOC and NCAA because of ability to reduce tremor and performance anxiety and improve accuracy in skill events such as archery and riflery

Angiotensin Converting Enzyme (ACE) Inhibitors

- Have a good hemodynamic profile during exercise (e.g., increase stroke volume, decrease total peripheral resistance, no decrease in $\dot{V}O_{2max}$ or rate of perceived exertion)
- May increase risk of postural hypotension secondary to venous pooling of blood in athletes who stop abruptly after vigorous endurance exercise
- Associated with a theoretical increased risk of exercise-induced anaphylaxis
- Considered by many to be the drugs of choice for most athletes with hypertension because of the favorable hemodynamic profile and low incidence of side effects

Angiotensin II Receptor Blockers (ARBs)

- Although no studies have looked at the effects of ARBs on athletic performance, they would seem to be similar to the ACE inhibitors in terms of hemodynamic effects
- No build-up of bradykinins which are associated with EIA

Calcium Channel Blockers (CCBs)

- The three classes of CCBs have different hemodynamic effects.
  1. Phenylalkylamines (e.g., verapamil) decrease left ventricular contractility, restrict heart rate, and cause mild arterial dilatation
  2. Dihydropyridines (e.g., nifedipine) have minimal effect on contractility, no heart rate slowing effect, and are potent vasodilators
  3. Benzothiazepines (e.g., diltiazem) have effects on both the conducting system (dihydropyridines < benzothiazepines < phenylalkylamines) and the arterial tree (phenylalkylamines < benzothiazepines < dihydropyridines)
- No decrease in $\dot{V}O_{2max}$ (all three classes of CCBs)
- No studies have documented a significantly negative impact on functional capacity during exercise.
- May increase risk of postural hypotension secondary to venous pooling of blood in athletes who stop abruptly after vigorous endurance exercise
- Can increase exercise-related gastroesophageal reflux (secondary to lower esophageal sphincter relaxation)

Alpha$_1$ Antagonists

- Decrease mean arterial pressure and total peripheral resistance with dynamic exercise
- Do not suppress cardiac output
- No impairment of exercise capacity
- May increase risk of postural hypotension secondary to venous pooling of blood in athletes who stop abruptly after vigorous endurance exercise
- Considered to be a good choice for use in athletes

Central Alpha Agonists

- No adverse effects on exercise from a hemodynamic standpoint
- May cause fatigue and sedation that could impair exercise performance
- May increase risk of exercise-associated collapse secondary to orthostatic hypotension

EXERCISE-RELATED RISKS IN HYPERTENSION

Although routine exercise can help improve many of the risk factors for coronary artery disease and decrease the long-term risk of developing cardiovascular disease, vigorous physical activity can actually precipitate sudden death. In an adult population over the age of 35, this results largely from the presence of underlying coronary artery disease (64). Because even mild hypertension is a risk factor for the development of coronary artery disease, certain steps should be taken to help minimize the risk of exercise-related cardiovascular complications in hypertensive patients about to embark on an exercise program.

One measure that may be beneficial is a formal, pre-exercise medical evaluation. The extent of this assessment will vary based on a variety of factors, including the patient's age, the presence of underlying medical problems, and the exercise intensity to be performed. It may be advised that certain patients with hypertension undergo a formal exercise stress test as a component of the preparticipation evaluation. This is often recommended in an attempt to detect underlying coronary artery disease and to help assure safety of participation in exercise (46). However, the role of preparticipation testing exercise remains somewhat controversial.

Exercise testing can identify individuals at increased risk of symptomatic or silent cardiac ischemia and/or malignant ventricular arrhythmias, with the greatest diagnostic yield occurring in symptomatic individuals or those with an intermediate pretest probability (i.e., 10%–90%) of coronary artery disease. However, in asymptomatic adults, exercise stress testing has been shown to be a poor predictor of major cardiac complications during exercise (e.g., acute myocardial infarction and sudden cardiac death) (29).

Guidelines have been published to assist health care professionals in deciding which individuals should undergo pre-exercise stress testing. The ACSM (46) stratifies individuals into low-, moderate-, and high-risk groups (see Tables 7B.4, 7B.5, and 7B.6) and recommends exercise testing for individuals based on their level of risk and the intensity of activity to be performed (see Table 7B.7). Additionally, the American Heart Association and other working groups (65,66) have recommended exercise testing for the following individuals who are planning on participating in regular physical training and competitive sports: (a) men

TABLE 7B.4
INITIAL AMERICAN COLLEGE OF SPORTS MEDICINE'S RISK STRATIFICATION

Low Risk
Men <45 yr of age and women <55 yr of age who are asymptomatic and meet no more than one risk factor threshold from Table 7B.5
Moderate Risk
Men >45 years of age and women >55 years of age or those individuals who meet the threshold for two or more risk factors from Table 7B.5
High Risk
Individuals with one or more signs/symptoms listed in Table 7B.6 or known cardiovascular (cardiac, peripheral vascular, or cerebrovascular disease), pulmonary (chronic obstructive pulmonary disease, asthma, interstitial lung disease, or cystic fibrosis), or metabolic (diabetes mellitus, thyroid disorders, renal or hepatic disease) disease

Source: Modified from Box 2-2, American College of Sports Medicine. *ACSM's guidelines for exercise testing and prescription*, 6th ed. Philadelphia: Lippincott Williams & Wilkins, 2000.

older than 40 to 45 years of age; (b) women older than 50 to 55 years of age (or postmenopausal); (c) those with one or more independent coronary risk factors. These factors include dyslipidemia, hypertension, current or recent cigarette smoking, DM, or history of myocardial infarction or sudden cardiac death in a first-degree relative aged less than 60 years. In addition, all athletes aged 65 years or more should undergo exercise testing even in the absence of risk factors or symptoms.

SECTION C
DYSLIPIDEMIA

Lipoproteins are macromolecular complexes that carry hydrophobic plasma lipids, particularly cholesterol and triglyceride (TG), in the plasma. Based on their densities, lipoproteins have been classified into five major classes: (a) chylomicrons; (b) very low density lipoproteins (VLDL); (c) intermediate density lipoproteins (IDL); (d) low density lipoproteins (LDL); and (e) high density lipoproteins (HDL) (67). Each lipoprotein contains characteristic proportions of lipids and type-specific apoproteins. With increasing lipoprotein density, the relative amount of lipid decreases and the amount of apoprotein increases. Therefore, TG is the major lipid component of chylomicrons and VLDL, whereas cholesterol is the major component of LDL.

A variety of environmental, genetic, and pathological factors can influence the metabolism of cholesterol and TG (see Table 7C.1). When these factors combine to create elevated blood lipid and lipoprotein concentrations, the condition is referred to as dyslipidemia. The diagnosis of dyslipidemia is sometimes based on plasma levels of lipids or lipoproteins above the 90th or 95th percentile of those found in a reference population (68).

Epidemiological data have documented a continuous, graded relationship between serum total cholesterol (TC) concentration and risk of coronary heart disease. Additionally, a low level of HDL has been identified as an important risk factor for coronary atherosclerosis. In contrast, an elevated serum HDL (above 60 mg/dL) is considered protective against coronary heart disease (69).

The relation between hypertriglyceridemia and cardiovascular disease is more complex. Numerous population studies have shown a dose-response relation between increasing TGs and heart disease. However, in multivariate analyses controlling for other risk factors (such as hypertension, physical inactivity, and obesity) the effect of hypertriglyceridemia is diminished (46). Many argue that TGs *per se* are not atherogenic, instead it is coexistent lipoproteins such as small, dense LDL (LDL subclass pattern B) and other cardiovascular risk factors such as hyperinsulinemia and increased visceral adipose tissue (which often accompany hypertriglyceridemia) that increase risk for coronary heart disease (46,70).

The treatment of dyslipidemia typically relies upon the combination of diet, weight loss, exercise, and drug therapy. A summary of the Third Report of the National Cholesterol Education Program (NCEP) Expert Panel on Detection, Evaluation, and Treatment of High Cholesterol in Adults (71) recommends a multifaceted lifestyle approach to reducing LDL and subsequent risk for coronary heart disease. Included in these recommendations are a reduced intake of total and saturated fat and dietary cholesterol. Weight loss, in order to achieve a normal body weight (BMI 18.5–24.9), is also encouraged for overweight patients. Additionally, it is recommended that regular, moderate-intensity physical activity be performed as a routine component in the management of dyslipidemia. In addition to modifying LDL cholesterol goals, lifestyle modifications were further emphasized in a 2004 update of the Third Report of the NCEP guidelines (72). If physical activity is to be used as a therapeutic modality in the management of dyslipidemia, health care providers must appreciate the metabolic effects of regular physical activity and be able to provide patients with specific recommendations to help promote safe and effective physical activity regimens.

AEROBIC EXERCISE AND LIPID METABOLISM

Evaluating the impact of exercise on lipids and lipoprotein concentrations can be complicated. Many of the changes

TABLE 7B.5

CORONARY ARTERY DISEASE RISK FACTOR THRESHOLDS FOR AMERICAN COLLEGE OF SPORTS MEDICINE'S RISK STRATIFICATION

Risk Factor	Defining Criteria
	Positive
Family history	Myocardial infarction, coronary revascularization, or sudden death before 55 yr of age in father or other male first-degree relative, or before 65 yr of age in mother or other female first-degree relative
Cigarette smoking	Current cigarette smoker or those who quit within the previous 6 mo
Hypertension	Systolic blood pressure of ≥140 mm Hg or diastolic ≥90 mm Hg, confirmed by measurements on at least two separate occasions, or on antihypertensive medication
Hypercholesterolemia	Total serum cholesterol of >200 mg/dL or HDL cholesterol of <35 mg/dL, or on lipid-lowering medication. If low-density lipoprotein cholesterol is available, use >130 mg/dL rather than total cholesterol of >200 mg/dL
Impaired fasting glucose	Fasting blood glucose of >110 mg/dL confirmed by measurements on at least two separate occasions
Obesity	Body mass index of >30 kg/m^2 or waist circumference of >100 cm
Sedentary lifestyle	Persons not participating in a regular exercise program or meeting the minimal physical activity recommendations from the U.S. Surgeon General's report (i.e., accumulating ≥30 min of moderate intensity physical activity most days of the week)
	Negative
High serum HDL cholesterol	>60 mg/dL

HDL = high-density lipoprotein.
Source: Modified from Table 2-1, American College of Sports Medicine. *ACSM's guidelines for exercise testing and prescription*, 6th ed. Philadelphia: Lippincott Williams & Wilkins, 2000.

in blood lipids that occur with physical activity have both an acute and a chronic component (73,74). Isolated bouts of physical activity can elicit acute, transient effects on blood lipids and lipoproteins. Additionally, a variety of factors can affect an individual's acute metabolic response to exercise, including baseline cardiorespiratory fitness, pre-exercise lipid levels, intensity and duration of the exercise session, timing of blood samples following exercise, change in dietary composition, and lack of and/or incomplete estimation of changes in plasma volume (plasma volume can contract during an exercise session or expand in the days after exercise by 10% or more) (73,74). Furthermore, when evaluating women, factors such as the use of oral contraceptives and the woman's position in her menstrual cycle must be considered (73).

It has also been demonstrated that, over time, regular exercise can have chronic effects on lipid metabolism. The frequent repetition of isolated exercise sessions may result in more permanent adaptations, referred to as the exercise training response (74). Just as demonstrated in research examining the acute effects of exercise on lipids and lipoproteins, a variety of confounding variables also can affect the results of studies examining the relation between long-term exercise adherence and lipid metabolism. Factors that must be considered when evaluating these results include pretraining lipoprotein levels, the volume of exercise performed, the type of exercise performed (e.g., aerobic versus resistance training), the duration of the training program, concomitant dietary changes, or changes in body weight or composition. It is also important to remember that certain congenital deficiencies in lipid transport can result in dyslipidemia and that these individuals may have a significantly different response in terms of lipid metabolism compared with healthy individuals. For example, exercise is unable to augment the effects of lipoprotein lipase (LPL) in patients with LPL deficiency, nor can exercise increase HDL concentrations in individuals with low HDL secondary to hypoalphalipoprotein syndrome (75).

Triglycerides. Studies dating back to the 1960s (76,77) have demonstrated that a single session of endurance exercise training involving aerobic physical activity can result in significant reductions in serum TG levels. The most reproducible results have been obtained in studies utilizing fit subjects performing prolonged endurance events. The reduction in TG values with exercise is not immediate, but tends to occur 18 to 24 hours after activity and tends to be most pronounced in those individuals with higher pre-exercise TG values (74). In contrast, TG levels are usually not

TABLE 7B.6

SIGNS AND SYMPTOMS SUGGESTIVE OF CARDIOVASCULAR OR PULMONARY DISEASE

Pain, discomfort (or other anginal equivalent) in the chest, neck, jaw, arms, or other areas that may be due to cardiac ischemia
Shortness of breath at rest or with mild exertion
Dizziness or syncope
Orthopnea or paroxysmal nocturnal dyspnea
Ankle edema
Palpitations or tachycardia
Intermittent claudication
Known heart murmur
Unusual fatigue or shortness of breath with usual activities

Source: From Box 2-1, American College of Sports Medicine. *ACSM's guidelines for exercise testing and prescription*, 6th ed. Philadelphia: Lippincott Williams & Wilkins, 2000.

altered in response to an acute session of exercise that is low in intensity and short in duration (73,78). In terms of the long-term effects of physical activity, both cross-sectional and exercise training studies have shown that endurance exercise training may decrease plasma TG levels. Several studies that enrolled previously inactive patients with elevated TG levels into exercise training programs, ranging from 3 to 12 months, have demonstrated an approximate 10% to 20% reduction in TG concentration (79). Often, the best response was seen in those individuals with the highest baseline TG levels (73,79). Greater reduction also tends to be seen with higher volume endurance exercise training. Importantly, the decrease in TG levels seen with exercise is independent of changes in weight or body composition (73).

Total Cholesterol and Low Density Lipoprotein. Acute sessions of endurance exercise generally result in small reductions in TC and LDL. The impact of acute exercise on TC is the result of changes in the various lipoprotein subfractions. Therefore, change in TC alone has little physiological significance. Studies have reported acute decreases in LDL from 5% to 8% following prolonged aerobic exercise in hypercholesterolemic men (80–82). However, it should be noted that rather large amounts of energy expenditure were required in order to achieve such reductions (73). Additionally, some of this reduction may be attributable to plasma volume expansion that may occur with acute exercise. One study showed that in a group of consistently active endurance athletes there was an increase in LDL-C of 10% after stopping their training for only 2 days. Further rest did not augment this increase and it was accompanied by an acute decrease in plasma volume (83).

The results of long-term exercise training programs on TC and LDL have yielded results similar to those seen in acute exercise trials. In 2001, Leon and Sanchez (84) published a review of studies over the preceding three decades pertaining to intervention trials on the effects of ≥12 weeks of aerobic exercise training on blood lipids and lipoprotein outcomes in adult men and women. In the absence of simultaneous dietary interventions, mean reductions in LDL of approximately 5% ($p < 0.05$) were seen across these studies. Concurrent reductions in dietary fat intake and/or a hypocaloric diet augmented the reduction in LDL. Meanwhile, results from most cross-sectional and endurance-training studies have failed to demonstrate any significant reduction in TC. The few studies that did show a beneficial effect

TABLE 7B.7

AMERICAN COLLEGE OF SPORTS MEDICINE RECOMMENDATIONS FOR EXERCISE TESTING PRIOR TO PARTICIPATION IN A MODERATE- TO VIGOROUS-EXERCISE PROGRAM

	Low Risk	Moderate Risk	High Risk
Moderate exercise[a]	Not necessary	Not necessary	Recommended
Vigorous exercise[b]	Not necessary	Recommended	Recommended

[a] Moderate exercise is defined as activities that are approximately 3–6 METs. Moderate exercise may alternatively be defined as an intensity well within the individual's capacity, one that can be comfortably sustained for a prolonged period of time (~45 min), which has a gradual initiation and progression, and is generally noncompetitive. If an individual's exercise capacity is known, relative moderate exercise may be defined by the range 40%–60% $\dot{V}O_{2max}$.
[b] Vigorous exercise is defined as activities >6 METs. It may also be defined as exercise intense enough to represent a substantial cardiorespiratory challenge. If an individual's exercise capacity is known, vigorous exercise may be defined as an intensity of >60% $\dot{V}O_{2max}$.
Source: Modified from Table 2-2, American College of Sports Medicine. *ACSM's guidelines for exercise testing and prescription*, 6th ed. Philadelphia: Lippincott Williams & Wilkins, 2000.

TABLE 7C.1
FACTORS INFLUENCING LIPID METABOLISM

Gender
Age
Body fat distribution
Dietary composition
Tobacco use
Alcohol use
Genetic inheritance
Physical activity level
Medication use: oral contraceptive pills, corticosteroids, diuretics, beta-blockers
Endocrine–metabolic disease: diabetes mellitus, hypothyroidism, Cushing's disease, Addison's disease, acromegaly
Hepatic disease: obstruction, parenchymal disease
Renal disease: nephrotic syndrome, chronic renal failure

Source: From Busby-Whitehead MJ, Blackman MR. Clinical implications of abnormal lipoprotein metabolism. In: Barker LR, Burton JR, Zieve PD, eds. *Principles of ambulatory medicine.* Baltimore: Lippincott Williams & Wilkins, 1999:1127–1129; Durstine JL, Moore GE. Hyperlipidemia. In: Durstine JL, ed. *American College of Sports Medicine's exercise management for persons with chronic diseases and disabilities.* Champaign, IL: Human Kinetics, 1997:101–105.

had methodological flaws such as not including an inactive control group or failing to account for confounding variables such as weight loss or changes in body composition (73,79).

High Density Lipoprotein. The one lipoprotein that seems to respond most favorably to aerobic exercise is HDL (73,78,79,84–87). HDL values often increase with an acute bout of exercise. However, the degree of elevation can be quite variable. Increases ranging from 4% to 43% have been reported (74). The degree of HDL elevation tends to parallel a concomitant decline in TG levels, suggesting mediation by comparable metabolic effects.

The minimum energy expenditure required to increase HDL has not been clearly defined. It appears that there may be a threshold for the volume of work completed that is necessary to induce consistent increases in HDL (73). Additionally, baseline cardiorespiratory fitness may strongly influence the HDL response to exercise. Moderately fit subjects have experienced acute elevations in HDL after expenditure of 350 to 400 calories (80,88), whereas more highly trained individuals have required energy expenditure closer to 1,000 calories in order to achieve an increase in HDL (89).

In terms of longitudinal physical activity programs, some exercise intervention studies have not shown a significant response, whereas several others have demonstrated that HDL rises with regular physical activity or exercise participation. Exercise-induced changes in HDL ranging from 4% to 25% have been reported. Studies have observed correlations between the amount of time engaged in exercise training and the degree of elevation of HDL (79). Therefore, it appears that HDL often increases in a dose-dependent manner with increasing energy expenditure (79,84).

RESISTANCE TRAINING AND LIPID METABOLISM

Compared with studies investigating the effects of aerobic exercise on lipid metabolism, those examining the impact of resistance training have yielded more inconsistent results. For example, several interventional studies have demonstrated no significant change in serum TG levels with resistance exercise training (90–93). In contrast, Goldberg et al. (94) did find lower TG concentrations in women after 16 weeks of resistance training.

Studies have demonstrated decreased TC and LDL in response to resistance training. However, when these changes were observed, they were often associated with a concurrent decrease in body fat and an increase in lean body mass. In contrast, when body composition remains unchanged, longitudinal studies generally do not demonstrate any significant alterations in TC or LDL concentrations (74,95).

Data from studies examining the influence of resistance exercise on HDL have also yielded conflicting results. Hurley et al. (96) conducted a longitudinal resistance-training study that did reveal an increase in HDL in men. However, no changes were noted in women. Other studies conducted in both men (90–94) and women (90,94,97) have found no influence of resistance training on HDL concentrations.

MECHANISMS OF EXERCISE-INDUCED CHANGES IN LIPID METABOLISM

The precise mechanisms by which acute and long-term exercise training can alter blood lipid and lipoprotein concentrations are not completely understood. Certain types of physical activity have been shown to alter the rates of synthesis, transport, and clearance of lipid and lipoproteins from the circulation (73). Exercise exerts its effects by enhancing the activity of several enzymes that play critical roles in lipoprotein metabolism. LPL, lecithin:cholesterol acyltransferase, and cholesteryl ester transfer protein activity have all been shown to be increased with either a single exercise session or with regular exercise participation (73,79).

EXERCISE PRESCRIPTION FOR DYSLIPIDEMIA

Because the impact of exercise on dyslipidemia is dependent on a number of variables related to both the baseline characteristics of the individual and to the nature of the physical activity performed, specific recommendations regarding the use of exercise, as adjuvant therapy to help treat dyslipidemia, must be individualized. Given this caveat, the primary goal for an exercise training program being utilized to address dyslipidemia appears to be caloric expenditure through aerobic exercise training utilizing large muscle groups. To achieve optimal efficacy, this activity should be performed for at least 40 minutes at moderate intensity (40%–70% $\dot{V}O_{2max}$), 5 to 7 days/week (75). However, studies do suggest that different energy expenditure thresholds may exist in order to achieve improvements in lipid and lipoprotein concentrations through exercise. For example, improvements in serum TGs can be seen after 2 weeks of aerobic training (45 minutes/day), whereas improvements in TC may not be seen for approximately one year after initiating a consistent aerobic exercise-training program (75). Additionally, resistance exercise may have a role in treating dyslipidemia, although, based upon the conflicting results of longitudinal intervention studies, weight training should not be used exclusively as an exercise modality to achieve lipid-lowering effects.

Despite measures such as dietary modification, weight loss, and regular exercise, many individuals with dyslipdemia will still require drug therapy in order to achieve adequate control. Commonly used agents include nicotinic acid (niacin), bile acid-binding resins (e.g., cholestyramine and colestipol), fibric acid derivatives, (e.g., gemfibrozil and fenofibrate), and the hydroxymethylglutaryl coenzyme A (HMG CoA) reductase inhibitors (e.g., atorvastatin, lovastatin, and pravastatin). These medications have few hemodynamic effects and therefore should not directly affect exercise performance. However, there is some data suggesting that exercise may potentiate the risk of developing drug-induced muscle injury that can be seen with certain lipid-lowering agents such as the HMG CoA reductase inhibitors, the fibric acid derivatives, and nicotinic acid (75).

In general, dyslipidemia does not affect the exercise response to a single exercise session. However, if this condition has been long-standing and has contributed to the development of cardiovascular disease, then the secondary disease process may indeed limit one's exercise capacity (75). Additionally, the possibility of underlying cardiovascular disease must be considered when prescribing an exercise regimen as part of a treatment program for dyslipidemia. Based on a variety of factors including the patient's age, the presence of additional risk factors for coronary artery disease, or major signs or symptoms suggestive of cardiopulmonary disease, the presence of elevated lipoproteins may necessitate the performance of a preparticipation exercise stress test (46,75).

TABLE 7D.1

DISEASE STATES ASSOCIATED WITH BEING OVERWEIGHT OR OBESE

High blood pressure
Dyslipidemia
Type 2 diabetes mellitus
Coronary heart disease
Gallbladder disease
Osteoarthritis
Sleep apnea
Cancer of the endometrium, breast, prostate, and colon

Source: From American College of Sports Medicine Position Stand. Appropriate intervention strategies for weight loss and prevention of weight regain for adults. *Med Sci Sports Exerc* 2001;33(12):2145–2156; Executive summary of the clinical guidelines on the identification, evaluation, and treatment of overweight and obesity in adults. *Arch Int Med* 1998;158:1855–1867; McInnis KJ. Exercise and obesity. *Coron Artery Dis* 2000;11:111–116.

SECTION D
OBESITY

According to the 1999 to 2000 National Health and Nutrition Examination Survey (NHANES), approximately 65% of adults in the United States are overweight or obese. This number reflects a 16% increase over the number of overweight or obese adults reported in the NHANES III data. Furthermore, nearly one third of these adults are considered to be obese (over 60 million) (98). During the last decade of the twentieth century, the number of overweight individuals rose substantially across all ages, sexes, and racial and ethnic groups (99,100). Higher body weights are associated with increased morbidity from a number of medical conditions (see Table 7D.1). Overweight and obesity is also associated with an increase in all-cause mortality. Additionally, obese individuals may suffer from social stigmatization and discrimination (101).

In the past, the terms *overweight* and *obese* have been defined in a variety of ways. Recently, definitions based on BMI have become quite popular (see Table 7D.2). Epidemiological and observational studies have demonstrated, that for most individuals, BMI provides an acceptable approximation of total body fat (100). Taking a person's weight in kilograms and dividing this by the square of the subject's height in meters calculates BMI. Tables are readily available to help calculate BMI (web link: http://www.nhlbi.nih.gov/guidelines/obesity/bmi_tbl.htm).

PHYSICAL ACTIVITY AND OBESITY

Obesity is a complex multifactorial disease that results from an interaction of genotype and the environment. Social, behavioral, cultural, physiological, metabolic, and genetic factors may all play a role. The extent to which each of these factors contributes to the development of obesity is not yet fully understood. Although several variables may influence body weight and body composition, one of the

TABLE 7D.2
CLASSIFICATION OF OVERWEIGHT AND OBESITY BY BODY MASS INDEX (BMI)

Classification	BMI, kg/m^2
Underweight	<18.5
Normal	18.5–24.9
Overweight	25.0–29.9
Obesity, class	
I	30.0–34.9
II	35.0–39.9
III	≥40

Source: From Executive summary of the clinical guidelines on the identification, evaluation, and treatment of overweight and obesity in adults. *Arch Int Med* 1998;158:1855–1867.

principle determinants is clearly caloric balance (101). Caloric balance refers to the difference between caloric intake (the energy equivalent of food ingested) and caloric expenditure (the energy equivalent of resting metabolic rate, physical activity, and the thermic effect of food) (46). On a very basic level, the principles of thermodynamics dictate that increased caloric intake, decreased caloric expenditure, or both must be contributing factors to weight gain (102).

Studies suggest that there has been little change in total caloric intake per capita during the past few decades (102). There are no direct data on population levels of energy expenditure, although a general decline in physical activity in our society has been observed (103). Some of this decrease in overall energy expenditure is believed to be secondary to less participation in household work and daily routine physical activity (104). Additionally, data have shown that almost one in every four U.S. adults engages in no leisure-time physical activity (1). Therefore, it has been proposed that one way to address the worsening problem of obesity is to reduce sedentary behavior by participating in greater amounts of voluntary and spontaneous physical activity.

TRADITIONAL EXERCISE AND WEIGHT LOSS

For those individuals who are overweight or obese, increasing physical activity can help establish the negative caloric balance required for weight loss. This concept is supported by several longitudinal and cross-sectional studies that have consistently found that physical activity is inversely related to weight (103). Therefore, exercise is often recommended along with other strategies, such as dietary changes, behavior therapy techniques, drugs, and surgery, to help people lose weight and maintain weight loss over time.

It has been suggested that exercise alone is an ineffective way to lose weight (103,105,106). However, many of the studies from which this conclusion was drawn suffer from important limitations that confound their results (107). Most of the studies reporting that exercise alone did not result in substantial weight loss had subjects performing physical activity that would result in only modest caloric expenditure. Given the amount of exercise-related energy expenditure, one would not expect to see substantial weight loss in these subjects.

Bouchard et al. (108) were able to demonstrate the impact of exercise alone on weight loss in a group of five young (average age 25 years), overweight men (average BMI 27.5). The study was conducted at a residential facility where caloric intake and daily energy expenditure could be held constant. The participants exercised on a stationary bicycle twice a day for 53 minutes each session, at 55% of $\dot{V}O_{2max}$, 6 days/week, for a 100-day study period. The exercise program was designed to induce a 1,000 kcal energy deficit. On average, the subjects lost close to 18 lb. Greater than 80% of this weight loss was accounted for by reductions in fat mass. Although the total number of subjects in this study was small, it provides support for the conclusion that exercise alone can produce weight loss. However, from a practical standpoint, one must realize that many overweight adults have poor baseline cardiorespiratory fitness levels and would not be able to tolerate the volume of physical activity performed in Bouchard's study.

In weight loss studies comparing the effectiveness of diet (decreasing caloric intake) versus exercise (increasing caloric expenditure), often the energy deficit prescribed by exercise was much less than the corresponding deficit prescribed by caloric restriction (107). It is therefore, not surprising that these studies found that the weight loss achieved through diet was greater than that seen with exercise. These observations emphasize the importance of matching the energy deficits achieved through caloric restriction and physical activity when these two weight loss strategies are being compared in controlled studies. When this measure has been taken, studies do in fact demonstrate that exercise alone can achieve similar degrees of weight loss (109,110). However, it should be noted that, for many people who are overweight or obese, achieving a significant energy deficit may be more easily achieved through dieting than exercise, particularly if an individual's caloric intake is quite high (100).

THE COMBINATION OF DIET AND EXERCISE FOR WEIGHT LOSS

Many investigators have examined the effects of combining exercise with caloric restriction. Some researchers have found diet plus exercise to result in more weight loss than diet alone, whereas others have found no difference (111). In 1997, Miller et al. (112) published a meta-analysis of the preceding 25 years of weight loss research that included data on the effects of diet plus exercise as a treatment strategy. The authors reported that average weight loss in diet alone and diet plus exercise were similar (10.7 kg and 11.0 kg, respectively). Additionally, Wing (113) reviewed the results from 13 randomized trials comparing diet alone versus diet and exercise. Only two of the studies showed a statistically significant difference in the weight loss achieved utilizing diet plus exercise compared with diet alone. Of these two studies, one showed a significant difference in men only and the other trial demonstrated only a modest difference between the two groups (diet and exercise group lost an average of 1.7 kg more than the diet only group after 6 months).

These results may seem somewhat surprising because one might presume that the additional energy expenditure related to exercise would result in more substantial weight loss than that achieved through diet alone. There are, however, some plausible explanations for why the effect of exercise was unimpressive. First, many of these studies were of short duration. If caloric intake was held constant and study participants were asked to increase their physical activity by 1,000 kcal/week, and the study were to last only 4 to 6 months, then a weight loss of only 2 to 3 kg would be expected. In many of the studies performed comparing diet with diet plus exercise, this was close to the degree of weight loss that was observed (113). Additionally, the results of other studies demonstrating no significant benefit of exercise and diet over diet alone are confounded by the issue of whether subjects in the diet plus exercise programs compensated for the energy expended through exercise by reducing physical activity at other times during the day or by consuming more calories (113).

EXERCISE AND WEIGHT LOSS MAINTENANCE

Perhaps the most important role that physical activity plays in weight loss therapy is its ability to help maintain weight loss after it has been achieved (111). Continued participation in regular exercise appears to be one of the best predictors of successful weight management (100). The importance of physical activity in maintaining weight loss is demonstrated in data from the National Weight Control Registry, a group of men and women who had lost at least 30 lb (mean = 66 lb) and maintained this weight loss for at least one year (mean = 6.9 years). One of the characteristics of this group of weight loss maintainers was their involvement in regular physical activity. On average, those individuals who successfully maintained their weight loss averaged an hour or more of physical activity per day (114). Other studies have shown that unless people remain physically active after weight loss is achieved, most of this lost weight is regained over 1 or 2 years (102,115).

ADDITIONAL BENEFITS OF EXERCISE IN OBESITY

Whether used alone or in combination with caloric restriction, exercise provides many health and fitness benefits for overweight individuals beyond weight loss itself. One advantage that exercise-induced weight reduction has over diet-induced weight loss is its effect on body composition. Studies have shown that exercise can result in greater reductions of fat compared to diet-induced weight loss. Exercise is capable of attenuating the loss of lean tissue that occurs with weight loss (109,110,116,117). This is important given the role that lean tissue plays in resting metabolic rate (103).

Even if weight loss is minimal or not achieved altogether, regular exercise can still result in significant health benefits for overweight and obese individuals. Consistent exercise can improve both the metabolic and cardiovascular risk profiles of these individuals, irrespective of any change in body composition or weight loss (118). In an overweight population, regular exercise may result in a reduction of blood lipids, improvement in insulin sensitivity and glucose tolerance, and a reduction in abdominal and visceral fat (111,119).

Additionally, higher levels of cardiorespiratory fitness appear to improve all-cause mortality in overweight and obese individuals independent of age and other potential confounders (102). Investigators at the Cooper Clinic followed 21,925 men between the ages of 30 and 83 who underwent assessments of body composition and cardiorespiratory fitness. This study (120) found that percent body fat was directly associated with all-cause mortality. However, this direct trend of increasing mortality with increasing body fatness was attenuated by improved cardiorespiratory fitness. This study demonstrated that fit men had a lower risk of all-cause mortality compared to unfit men in each stratum of body fatness. Additionally, this study found that obese men who were fit had a much lower risk of all-cause mortality than unfit men in the lowest body fat group.

NONTRADITIONAL EXERCISE AND WEIGHT LOSS

Regular exercise can clearly help with weight control and contribute to overall health by delaying and preventing morbidity and mortality. However, promoting the initiation and maintenance of an exercise program can be extremely challenging. A traditional, structured exercise program may pose certain challenges for some people who are overweight. For these individuals, vigorous exercise may be uncomfortable or even painful. Also, the overweight and obese may not feel comfortable going to an exercise facility where they are among thin, fit individuals. As a result, it has been suggested that encouraging lifestyle activity that can be accumulated during the day, both at home and at work, may be a better approach to increasing physical

TABLE 7D.3
EXAMPLES OF LIFESTYLE ACTIVITIES

Climbing stairs instead of riding elevators and escalators
Walking instead of driving/riding short distances
Parking some distance from your final destination and walking the remainder
Playing actively with children
Being physically active around the home (e.g., gardening, raking leaves, mowing the lawn, vacuuming, etc.)
Using fewer labor-saving devices such as remote controls

Source: From Anderson RE. Exercise, an active lifestyle, and obesity: making the exercise prescription work. *Phys Sportsmed* 1999;27:41–50; Executive summary of the clinical guidelines on the identification, evaluation, and treatment of overweight and obesity in adults. *Arch Int Med* 1998;158:1855–1867; Pate RR, Pratt M, Blair SN, et al. Physical activity and public health: a recommendation from the Centers for Disease Control and Prevention and the American College of Sports Medicine. *JAMA* 1995;273:402–407.

activity and promoting weight loss (102,121). Examples of lifestyle activities are found in Table 7D.3.

Studies have demonstrated that increasing lifestyle activity can be just as efficacious as a formal exercise program to help with weight control. In 1999, Anderson et al. published an important study (122) demonstrating the benefits of lifestyle activity. These investigators randomized 40 obese women (mean BMI = 32.9 kg/m^2) to a 16-week program of dietary modification (1,200 calorie low-fat diet) combined with either a structured aerobic exercise program or moderate-intensity lifestyle activity. All participants also received a comparable cognitive behavioral weight loss program. In the diet plus structured aerobic exercise group, subjects attended three step-aerobics classes per week. The total duration of aerobic exercise reached 45 minutes by week 8. It was estimated that approximately 450 to 500 kcal were expended during each 45-minute session. Participants in the lifestyle group were advised to increase their levels of moderate-intensity physical activity by 30 minutes/day on most days of the week. This group was taught to incorporate short bouts of activity into their daily schedules (e.g., walk instead of drive short distances and take stairs instead of the elevator). At 16 weeks, weight loss averaged 7.9 kg in the lifestyle group and 8.3 kg in the aerobic group. This difference was not statistically significant. After the 16-week program, participants attended four quarterly follow-up sessions, during which strategies for weight maintenance were reviewed. When the subjects were assessed at the 1-year follow-up point, subjects in the lifestyle group had regained a mean weight of 0.08 kg from the end of the 16-week program, whereas the aerobic group had regained a mean of 1.6 kg. Again, this difference between groups was not statistically significant. Also at the 1-year follow-up, subjects were asked to report the percentage of weeks that they accumulated 30 minutes or more of moderate-intensity activity on at least 5 days of the week during the 12 months after completing the 16-week intervention. The data from both the aerobic exercise and lifestyle group was collapsed together and the participants were divided into tertiles of physical activity. This revealed that the least active group had regained significantly more of their lost weight than the middle or the most active groups. In summary, this study demonstrated that a program of diet plus lifestyle activity may result in the same benefits in terms of weight control that a combined program of diet and more vigorous, structured exercise may offer.

Studies demonstrating the benefits of lifestyle physical activity on weight control are important because, outside of research settings, traditional structured exercise programs utilizing the recommendations often prescribed to achieve physical fitness (20–60 minutes of continuous aerobic exercise performed 3–5 days/week at 60%–85% $\dot{V}O_{2max}$) have been unsuccessful in motivating most adults to become habitually physically active (104). Therefore, lifestyle activity may improve long-term adherence to increased physical activity.

EXERCISE RISKS ASSOCIATED WITH OBESITY

Another potential advantage of lifestyle physical activity over more traditional forms of exercise relates to safety. Although energy expenditure remains the primary objective of increasing physical activity in the treatment of obesity, this must be balanced against the risk of physical injury. Injury prevention is critical for overweight and obese individuals who are attempting to increase their physical activity. Physical injury may be an important factor in the discontinuation of an exercise program.

Overweight and obese individuals are at an increased relative risk for orthopedic injuries (46). Excess body weight can place substantial stress on weight-bearing joints (e.g., knees), resulting in various overuse syndromes (Chapter 23). Low-impact or non–weight-bearing activities may be necessary in order to avoid musculoskeletal injury. Additionally, physical activity should be initiated slowly and advanced gradually in terms of time and effort.

Another concern for overweight or obese individuals who exercise is thermoregulation. Excess body weight can influence one's adaptability to physical activity in a warm environment. Risk of heat-related illness may be reduced by: (a) exercising during cooler times in the day, (b) maintaining adequate hydration, and (c) wearing loose-fitting clothing (123).

It is well established that obesity can enhance risk factors for coronary heart disease, such as high BP, high blood cholesterol and TG levels, low HDL cholesterol, and insulin resistance with hyperinsulinemia. However, there is now a growing body of evidence that supports the role of obesity as an independent risk factor for the development of coronary heart disease (100). In

TABLE 7D.4
BENEFITS OF A FORMAL MEDICAL EVALUATION PRIOR TO INITIATING A WEIGHT-LOSS PROGRAM

Overweight/obesity-related disease identification
Assessment for potential musculoskeletal injury
Body composition assessment
Nutrition counseling
Discussion of behavior modification techniques
Individualized exercise prescription
Establish a reasonable target weight

Source: From McInnis KJ. Exercise and obesity. *Coron Artery Dis* 2000;11:111–116; Wallace JP. Obesity. In: Durstine JL, ed. *American College of Sports Medicine's exercise management for person's with chronic disease and disabilities*. Champaign, IL: Human Kinetics, 1997:106–111.

fact, in 1998, the American Heart Association reclassified obesity as a major cardiovascular risk factor (124). Also, the Executive Summary of the Third Report of the NCEP Expert Panel on Detection, Evaluation, and Treatment of High Blood Cholesterol in Adults recognizes overweight and obesity as major underlying risk factors for coronary heart disease (71). Therefore, when exercise is recommended as a component of weight loss therapy, one must consider the possibility of underlying coronary heart disease. This is important to assess because vigorous physical activity is associated with a transient increased risk for myocardial infarction, cardiac arrest, and sudden death (29). The risk of such serious cardiovascular complications may be minimized by having overweight individuals undergo a careful preparticipation medical evaluation and by receiving appropriate guidelines for exercise participation from an appropriately trained health care professional (100).

Given that exercise may pose certain health risks for people who are overweight, it may be prudent for these individuals to undergo a formal preparticipation medical evaluation. Certainly, if one has medical problems related to excess weight or other chronic medical conditions, or if one is considering engaging in vigorous physical activity, then one should first consult a physician (1,123). Even if these conditions do not apply, there may still be several advantages for overweight individuals to see a physician before initiating an exercise program (see Table 7D.4).

SECTION E
OSTEOPOROSIS

Osteoporosis is a common human bone disease characterized by a reduction of bone mass (or density) or the presence of a fragility fracture. Bone mineral density (BMD) is commonly measured using dual energy x-ray absorptiometry (DEXA). BMD is reported as the number of standard deviations from the mean for normal young adults of the same sex (T-score) and as the number of standard deviations from the mean for persons of the same sex and age (Z-score). The World Health Organization defines osteoporosis as a T-score of less than −2.5. Osteopenia is defined as a T-score between −1.0 and −2.5 (125). It is estimated that approximately 44 million people have either osteoporosis or low bone mass, with 8 million women and 2 million men in the United States having osteoporosis (T-score < −2.5). The number of people with osteoporosis is expected to rise to 12 million by 2010 and 14 million by 2020 (126).

One of the major concerns related to osteoporosis is the subsequent risk of developing an osteoporotic fracture. A loss of one standard deviation of bone mass may give rise to a twofold risk of spine fracture or a 2.5-fold risk of hip fracture (127). Osteoporotic fractures represent a major health problem in the United States. Mortality rates as high as 15% to 20% in the first year following a hip fracture have been reported in elderly patients (128). Current expenditures for osteoporotic fractures and their sequelae are in excess of $15 billion annually. These costs are expected to escalate with the increasing age of the general population (125).

TREATMENT OF OSTEOPOROSIS

Several treatment options are available to help combat osteoporosis. Both pharmacological and nonpharmacological strategies may be utilized. Commonly used drugs include estrogens, bisphosphonates (e.g., alendronate, risendronate), calcitonin, selective estrogen receptor modulators (e.g., raloxifene), and more recently recombinate human parathyroid hormone (teriparatide). Nonpharmacological measures include smoking cessation (in smokers), dietary modification (assuring adequate intake of calories, calcium, and vitamin D), and physical activity. Although all of these modalities have the capacity to maintain or slow the loss of bone, exercise training is the only one that has the ability to simultaneously influence multiple risk factors for osteoporotic fractures. Strength training in particular has been shown to improve balance, strength, muscle mass, and overall physical activity, all of which help to reduce the risk of falls in the elderly (129).

With regard to BMD, physical activity is important because bone is very responsive to mechanical loading. According to the principle known as *Wolf's law*, bone accommodates the loads imposed on it by altering its mass and distribution of mass. When habitual loading increases, bone is gained; when loading decreases, bone is lost. The relation between mechanical loading and bone mass is curvilinear, with the effect of immobility on bone mass being substantially greater than the effect additional walking has on an already ambulatory individual (130).

Studies suggest that bone's adaptation to loading is determined by three basic rules: (a) dynamic rather than static loading is effective; (b) only a short duration of mechanical loading is necessary to initiate an adaptive response, and the capacity of bone tissue to respond to the stimulus at one time is saturated by few loading cycles; and (c) bone cells accommodate to customary loading, making them less responsive to routine loading signals (131). If one applies these basic rules to exercise regimens designed to help prevent or reverse osteoporosis, then certain requirements should be met. First, each exercise session should incorporate movements resulting in high loads at high rates and they should load the bone from multiple directions. However, the number of movements does not need to be great and the loading can result from the force of gravity or by muscular contractions. Next, these forces must focus specifically on the target bone area to be effective. Loading must repeat frequently and continuously in order to maintain BMD, and loading should increase periodically if a further increase in bone mass is to be achieved (131).

PHYSICAL ACTIVITY AND BONE MASS

Whether an individual develops osteoporosis is dependent on peak bone mass accumulated in youth and the subsequent rate of bone loss that occurs as one ages. Cross-sectional studies in both athletes and the general population, several longitudinal studies, and numerous randomized controlled trials have demonstrated that physical activity in youth can contribute to increased peak bone mass (128,131).

Data from cross-sectional studies support a positive correlation between physical activity and BMD in both men and women (132–134). Additionally, prospective, interventional studies have demonstrated that both aerobic and resistance exercise training can have a beneficial effect on bone. The positive effects of exercise on bone have been demonstrated in both postmenopausal (129) and premenopausal women (135), as well as in older men (136).

Nelson et al. (129) conducted a randomized controlled trial of 1-year duration, involving 40 postmenopausal women. At baseline, these women did not engage in any regular exercise program, had not taken estrogen or other medications known to affect bone over the preceding 12 months, and were similar in terms of average BMI and BMD at the femoral neck and lumbar spine. Twenty-one women were randomized to a high-intensity strength-training program performed 2 days/week, with each session lasting 45 minutes. The women in the control group were asked to maintain their current level of activity. After 1 year, the women in the resistance-training group gained an average of 1% BMD of the femoral neck and lumbar spine. In contrast, the control group lost 2.5% and 1.8% at these sites, respectively. Furthermore, the resistance-trained women had a 35% to 76% increase in strength, a 14% improvement in dynamic balance, a 1.2 kg increase in total body muscle mass, and a 27% increase in overall physical activity, whereas the control group showed declines in all of these parameters. These additional outcomes may help to further influence a reduction in overall risk of osteoporotic fractures.

Subsequently, Friedlander et al. (135) investigated the effects of exercise on peak bone mass in 127 premenopausal women (ages 20–35 years). The subjects were randomized to either a combined aerobics and weight training program or to a stretching program. In the exercise group, subjects attended three 1-hour exercise classes per week. These classes incorporated a variety of strengthening exercises and both low- and high-impact aerobic exercises. During the aerobic components, an attempt was made to maintain heart rates between 70% to 85% of maximum. The participants in the stretching group served as controls and attended twice weekly stretching classes. After 2 years, subjects in the exercise group experienced significant increases in BMD in the spine (2.5%), femoral neck (2.4%), trochanter (2.3%), and calcaneus (6.4%). In comparison, those individuals randomized to the stretching group experienced no significant changes in BMD at any site.

In 2000, Maddalozzo and Snow (136) published results of a trial comparing the effects of a moderate-intensity seated resistance-training program with a high-intensity standing free weight exercise program on bone mass in healthy older men. Twenty-eight men (54 ± 3.2 years) served as their own controls for 12 weeks, and then were randomly assigned to a moderate- or high-intensity training group. Prior to and after the control period and at the end of training, bone mass was assessed by DEXA. The training sessions were conducted for 24 weeks with a frequency of three times per week for approximately 75 minutes under close supervision of a personal trainer. Subjects in both the high- and moderate-intensity groups followed a training program that activated all major muscle groups. The moderate-intensity weight-training group performed three sets of 10 to 13 repetitions at 40% to 60% of 1 repetition maximum (RM) with 20 to 40 seconds rest between sessions. The high-intensity program consisted predominantly of a schedule of three sets of eight repetitions at 70% of 1 RM. At the end of the study period, the investigators found that high-intensity training resulted in a gain in BMD at the spine (1.9%, $p < 0.05$), whereas moderate-intensity training produced no changes at this site. Trochanteric BMD improved as a result of both high and moderate intensity training, 1.24% and 1.02%, respectively ($p < 0.05$).

Interestingly, the amount of weight lifted in a resistance training program may further increase BMD. In 2003, Cussler et al. (137) studied 140 calcium-supplemented women aged 44 to 66 years enrolled in a 1-year progressive strength-training program. They found that improvement in femoral trochanter BMD was linearly related to the total amount of weight lifted ($p < 0.01$). However, the association between weight lifted and BMD for femur neck or lumbar spine was not significant.

ACQUISITION AND MAINTENANCE OF BONE MASS

Mechanical loading through exercise is just one of several factors known to influence the acquisition and maintenance of bone mass. However, its impact is relatively small in comparison to genetic endowment, which is estimated to contribute at least 70% to the variation in peak bone mass. Therefore, although certain forms of exercise can enhance BMD, rather narrow limitations seem to exist in terms of the degree of improvement that can be achieved (133).

Other variables that play critical roles in bone remodeling include reproductive hormone status and nutrient intake (130). Deficits in either of these areas can result in the development of osteopenia or osteoporosis. For example, even if a female athlete consumes adequate dietary calcium and vitamin D and participates in sports involving mechanical loading of the skeleton, she may experience significant bone loss if she develops exercise-related amenorrhea.

Drinkwater et al. (138) reported that the hypoestrogenic status of 14 amenorrheic athletes was associated with a decrease in regional bone mass compared to 14 eumenorrheic peers. The two groups were similar in terms of nutritional intake, including calcium. They were also comparable with regard to percentage body fat, age at menarche, years of athletic participation, and frequency and duration of training. The two groups did differ in terms of number of miles run per week (amenorrheic group 41.8 mi; eumenorrheic group 24.9 mi). When bone mass was measured using dual-photon and single-photon absorptiometry, vertebral mineral density was found to be significantly lower in the amenorrheic group (mean, 1.12 g/cm^2) than in the eumenorrheic group (mean, 1.30 g/cm^2). Please note the change in value. The results of this study demonstrate that although exercise may improve the skeletal health of many young women, over-exercise leading to amenorrhea may have deleterious effects on bone mineral density.

The ACSM's position stand published in 2004 provides recommendations for the preservation of bone health during adulthood (128). The authors suggest weight-bearing endurance activities (i.e., tennis, jogging), activities that involve jumping (i.e., volleyball, basketball), and resistance exercise (i.e., weight lifting). The intensity should be moderate to high with weight-bearing endurance activities done three to five times per week and resistance exercise two to three times per week. Each session should ideally last 30 to 60 minutes of these combined activities.

EXERCISE RISKS FOR INDIVIDUALS WITH OSTEOPOROSIS

There are a number of special considerations for patients who are using exercise as a treatment modality for osteoporosis. Exercise programs for patients with osteoporosis should help increase their ability to perform activities of daily living, minimize their risk for subsequent fractures, and, hopefully, lead to a reduction in the risk for falls (130). Most importantly, the program must be safe. For patients with established osteoporosis, certain precautions should be considered when implementing an exercise program. Many patients with osteoporosis may have poor cardiorespiratory fitness because of decreased mobility. Additionally, severe kyphosis secondary to osteoporotic vertebral fractures can also impair pulmonary function (decreased vital capacity). This may result in increased fatigability. Therefore, when exercise training is implemented, it should be low-intensity and the progression of physical activity should be slow (139).

To help minimize the risk associated with exercise, other orthopedic limitations related to osteoporosis must be considered. For example, in patients with vertebral osteoporosis, exercises involving back flexion place an anterior load on vertebral bodies. This additional stress can increase the relative risk of suffering a vertebral fracture (130). Patients with extreme kyphosis related to osteoporotic vertebral fractures may be at increased risk for falls. The kyphotic deformity alters center of gravity and can affect gait and balance (139).

When recommending exercise to an individual with osteoporosis, one must also consider the possibility that this person may have anxiety about falls and subsequent fractures. Initiating a program under the supervision of a trained professional, such as a physical therapist, who is experienced in working with osteoporotic clients may be advised. If exercise is to be performed at home, then careful attention must be paid to minimizing environmental risks. The exercise area should be free of hazards such as loose floor tiles or rugs, buckled carpeting, and poorly placed exercise equipment that might serve as obstacles over which a patient might stumble. Wall railings in exercise areas may also be beneficial in areas where exercise is performed while standing (139).

SECTION F
DEPRESSION

Depression is a major public health problem. According to the World Health Organization (140), an estimated 121 million people currently suffer from depression. Additionally, 5.8% of men and 9.5% of women will experience a depressive episode in any given year. The essential feature of a major depressive episode is a period of at least 2 weeks during which there is either depressed mood or the loss of interest or pleasure in nearly all activities. The individual must also experience at least four of the following symptoms: changes in appetite or weight, sleep, and psychomotor activity; decreased energy; feelings of worthlessness or guilt; difficulty thinking, concentrating, or making decisions; or recurrent thoughts of death or suicidal ideation, plans, or attempts (141).

Treatment for depression often involves psychotherapy, medication, or a combination of the two. Commonly utilized forms of psychotherapy include cognitive therapy, behavioral therapy, and interpersonal therapy. The major classes of drugs used to treat depression are the tricyclic antidepressants (TCAs, e.g., amitriptyline, nortriptyline), selective serotonin reuptake inhibitors (SSRIs, e.g., fluoxetine, paroxetine), heterocyclics (e.g., bupropion, deseryl), monoamine oxidase inhibitors (e.g., phenelzine, tranylcypromine), and agents such as venlafaxine that inhibit the reuptake of both serotonin and norepinephrine (142). An often-underutilized adjunct to traditional pharmacological and psychological treatment modalities for depression is regular physical activity (143). Numerous cross-sectional and longitudinal studies have demonstrated the beneficial effects of regular exercise on the clinical course of several depressive disorders, including major depressive disorders and minor depression (144).

EFFECTS OF EXERCISE ON DEPRESSION

Interest in the use of exercise to treat depression grew after it was noted that depressed patients tended to be less physically active and more deconditioned than nonpsychiatric controls (145–148). Additionally, several prospective studies demonstrated that a low level of baseline physical activity was predictive of an increased risk of developing depression. This strong inverse relationship remained after adjusting for other potential confounders such as age, concurrent chronic illnesses, education, employment, and income (145).

In 1979, Greist et al. (149) performed one of the first interventional studies designed to examine the therapeutic effect of exercise on depressed patients. In this study, 28 outpatients meeting the Research Diagnostic Criteria (RDC) for minor depression were randomized either to running (1 hour three to four times per week) or to one or two types of psychotherapy (one session per week) for a total of 12 weeks. Reductions in depression scores were seen in all the three treatment groups. Outcome comparisons demonstrated that the running treatment was as equally effective as the two forms of psychotherapy. Although this study had several methodological flaws, many of which the authors acknowledged in their publication, these results seemed to indicate that exercise might be a promising approach in the treatment of depression.

In 1984, McCann and Holmes (150) published a study in which 43 women with Beck Depression Inventory (BDI) scores above the cut-off for mild depression were randomized to either aerobic exercise (an aerobics class that met for 1 hour twice per week plus additional exercise on those days when the class did not meet), relaxation training (20 minutes four times per week), or a waiting list control group. After 12 weeks, depression scores decreased in all three groups, but a statistically significant greater improvement was seen in the aerobic exercise group.

The following year, Martinsen et al. (151) published an interventional study examining the effects of systematic aerobic exercise on depression. The study involved a group of 43 hospitalized patients who satisfied the DSM criteria for major depression and were receiving individual psychotherapy. Fourteen subjects in the control group and nine people in the training group were using tricyclic antidepressants. Based on assessment using the BDI, 9 weeks of moderate-intensity aerobic training performed for 1 hour three times per week resulted in significant reductions in depressive symptoms. The greatest antidepressant effect was seen in those individuals who experienced the largest training-induced increase in $\dot{V}O_{2max}$. However, additional studies have demonstrated that improvement in cardiorespiratory fitness is not necessary for exercise to have beneficial effects on mental health (145,147).

In addition to evaluating the effects of aerobic exercise on depressive symptoms, some investigators have evaluated the role of nonaerobic exercise training. In 1987, Doyne et al. (152) compared the effectiveness of aerobic and nonaerobic exercise in 40 women diagnosed as having a major or minor depressive disorder using the RDC. The subjects were randomly assigned to an 8-week exercise program performed four times per week, consisting of either walking/running at 80% of estimated maximal heart rate or weight training utilizing a standard 10-station program paced to keep heart rate at or below a 50% to 60% estimated maximum. An inactive wait-list control group had similar baseline characteristics. Utilizing several measures of depression, including the BDI, it was found that both the aerobic and resistance-training programs resulted in significant improvement in depressive symptoms compared with the control group. No significant between-group fitness changes were noted, indicating that the beneficial effects of exercise on psychological function were not dependent on improving cardiovascular fitness. These findings are supported by the results of a later study published in 1989 by Martinsen et al. (153). In this study, 99 hospitalized patients who met the DSM-III criteria major depression, dysthymic disorder, or depressive disorder not otherwise specified, were randomized to an 8-week program consisting of either aerobic (walking/running) or nonaerobic (strength, flexibility, coordination, relaxation training) exercise performed for 1 hour three times per week. Both groups achieved significant reductions in depressive scores on the Montgomery and Asberg Depression Rating Scale (MADRS). The difference in treatment outcome between the two groups was not statistically different. A significant improvement in maximal oxygen uptake occurred in the aerobic exercise group, whereas no improvement in cardiovascular fitness was seen with nonaerobic training. Consistent with the results from Doyne's study (152) performed 2 years earlier, aerobic fitness does not need to be achieved in order for exercise to have an antidepressant effect. It appears that it is the participation in exercise itself and not the acquisition of cardiovascular fitness that results in beneficial psychological effects (147).

Subsequently published meta-analyses (154,155) examining the effects of exercise on depression have concluded that both aerobic and anaerobic exercise can improve depressive symptoms in men and women. These studies have also demonstrated that individuals with the greatest degree of depression benefit the most from exercise training and that exercise was as effective in decreasing depression as psychotherapy.

EXERCISE AND RECURRENT DEPRESSION

Depressive disorders have a high rate of relapse. Keller et al. (156) found that 23% of outpatients with major depression who initially responded to pharmacotherapy subsequently developed disease recurrence within 18 months of stopping drug treatment. Continuation of antidepressant therapy (defined as the 4–9 months of treatment immediately following acute treatment response) is now considered the standard of care to prevent relapse (156). Therefore, one might speculate that the long-term value of exercise in the management of depression may be dependent upon whether patients remain physically active after completing a formal training program.

Studies examining whether exercise adherence correlates with depression scores have had variable results. Some investigators (147) have found that individuals who continue with regular exercise tend to have lower depression scores than sedentary ones, but the strength of this correlation is not clear. Studies have demonstrated that exercise adherence rates in psychiatric populations rival those seen in nonpsychiatric groups. Studies have reported that over 50% of depressed patients continued with regular exercise 1 year after termination of their formal exercise training programs (147).

MECHANISMS UNDERLYING THE ANTIDEPRESSANT EFFECT OF EXERCISE

Several hypotheses have been developed to explain the mechanisms by which exercise can exert beneficial effects on depressive disorders. Both biological and psychological mechanisms have been proposed. However, none of these theories have been confirmed through rigorous scientific study. Given the complexity of the interaction between exercise and psychological function, an integrative biopsychosocial model that incorporates several mechanisms will likely provide the best explanation (143).

Biological Mechanisms (From references [152,157,158]):

- Increases in body temperature with exercise result in a short-term tranquilizing effect.
- Regular exercise improves stress adaptation because the increase in adrenal activity with regular exercise increases steroid reserves that are then available to counter stress.
- As a result of improved fitness through exercise training, the cardiovascular response to stress is reduced. Protection against some of the physiological response to stress may result in fewer physical cues to which depressed attributions may be made.
- Reduction in resting muscle activity potential following exercise leads to tension release.
- Exercise enhances the neurotransmission of norepinephrine, serotonin, and dopamine.
- Exercise results in an increase in circulating beta endorphins.

Psychological Mechanisms (From references [152,157, 158]):

- Exercise resembles a graded-task assignment resulting in a sense of mastery as distinct achievements are noted.
- Exercise serves as a form of meditation that triggers an altered and more relaxed state of consciousness.
- Exercise is a form of biofeedback that teaches participants how to regulate their own autonomic arousal.
- Exercise provides distraction, diversion, or time away from unpleasant cognition, emotions, and behavior.
- Social reinforcement among exercisers may result in improved psychological states.

EXERCISE PRESCRIPTION FOR DEPRESSION

Many of the research studies in the area of exercise and depression suffer from methodological deficiencies. Lack of control groups, small sample sizes, inconsistent definitions of depression, nonrandom allocation of subjects to experimental conditions, short duration of exercise programs, and lack of long-term follow-up are examples of the weaknesses encountered (158). Nevertheless, it is remarkable that the results from most studies demonstrate that both aerobic and nonaerobic exercise training is associated with an antidepressant effect that does not differ significantly from other forms of treatment, including various forms of psychotherapy (147). Because of the methodological inconsistencies across studies, it is difficult to establish specific guidelines regarding the intensity, duration, and frequency of physical activity required to achieve beneficial psychological effects (159). The ACSM (160) has recommended that exercise prescription for individuals with depression should follow standard protocol regarding frequency and duration (i.e., 20 to 60 minutes of continuous or intermittent [minimum of 10 minute bouts] physical activity accumulated throughout the day, performed 3–5 days/week). The ACSM suggests that a more conservative approach may be necessary with regard to physical activity intensity (i.e., low to moderate).

Depression *per se* does not affect the physiological response to exercise as measured by cardiopulmonary exercise testing (160). However, several clinical manifestations of depression, such as fatigue, lassitude, low self-esteem, lack of motivation, and psychomotor retardation, may make exercising more challenging. As a result, many depressed patients may require additional support and encouragement to help them initiate an exercise-training program. It is also important to remember that those individuals receiving tricyclic antidepressants may experience dry mouth, weight gain, drowsiness, and increased heart rate, which may create additional problems during exercise (147).

Additionally, because many patients with psychiatric disease have low baseline fitness levels, the choice of training methods should be carefully evaluated (144). In particular, a slow increase in the volume of training may be beneficial. It has been proposed that, in a depressed population, a structured, supervised exercise program should be initially utilized in order to reinforce the elements of the exercise prescription and to provide more comprehensive education regarding exercise training (160). If such measures are taken, it is indeed possible to help a large proportion of depressed patients start and remain actively involved in regular exercise (147).

REFERENCES

1. Pate RR, Pratt M, Blair SN, et al. Physical activity and public health: a recommendation from the Centers for Disease Control and Prevention and the American College of Sports Medicine. *JAMA* 1995;273:402–407.
2. National Institute of Health Consensus Development Panel. Physical activity and cardiovascular health. *JAMA* 1996;276:241–246.
3. *Physical activity and health: a report of the surgeon general.* Atlanta: US Departments of Health and Human Services Centers for Disease Control and Prevention, 1996.
4. Kesaniemi YA, Danforth E, Jensen MD, et al. Dose-response issues concerning physical activity and health: an evidence-based symposium. *Med Sci Sports Exerc* 2001;33:S351–S358.
5. Report of the expert committee on the diagnosis and classification of diabetes mellitus. *Diabetes Care* 1997;20:1183–1197.
6. National Institute of Diabetes and Digestive and Kidney Diseases. *National Diabetes Statistics fact sheet: general information and national estimates on diabetes in the United States, 2005.* Bethesda, MD: U.S. Department of Health and Human Services, National Institute of Health, 2005.
7. Peirce NS. Diabetes and exercise. *Br J Sports Med* 1999;33:161–173.
8. Colberg SR, Swain DP. Exercise and diabetes control: a winning combination. *Phys Sportsmed* 2000;28:63–81.
9. McCulloch DK. *Effects of exercise in diabetes mellitus.* UpToDate Online 9.3, Available: http://www.uptodate.com. 2001.
10. MacLean PS, Zheng D, Dohm GL. Muscle glucose transporter (GLUT 4) gene expression during exercise. *Exerc Sport Sci Rev* 2000;28:148–152.
11. Goodpaster BH, Kelley DE. Exercise and diabetes. In: Thompson PD, ed. *Exercise and sports cardiology.* New York: McGraw-Hill, 2001:430–451.
12. American Diabetes Association. Physical activity/exercise and diabetes. *Diabetes Care* 2004;27(Suppl 1):S58–S62.
13. Eriksson J, Taimela S, Eriksson K, et al. Resistance training in the treatment of non-insulin-dependent diabetes mellitus. *Int J Sports Med* 1997;18:242–246.
14. Castaneda C, Layne JE, Munoz-Orians L, et al. A randomized controlled trial of resistance exercise training to improve glycemic control in older adults with type 2 diabetes. *Diabetes Care* 2002;25(12):2335–2341.
15. Boule NG, Haddad E, Kenny GP, et al. Effects of exercise on glycemic control and body mass in type 2 diabetes mellitus: a meta-analysis of controlled clinical trials. *JAMA* 2001;286:1218–1227.
16. Boule NG, Kenny GP, Haddad E, et al. Meta-analysis of the effect of structured exercise training on cardiorespiratory fitness in Type 2 diabetes mellitus. *Diabetologia* 2003;46(8):1071–1081.
17. UK Prospective Diabetes Study Group. Effect of intensive blood-glucose control with metformin on complications in overweight patients with type 2 diabetes mellitus. *Lancet* 1998;352:854–865.
18. UK Prospective Diabetes Study Group. Intensive blood-glucose control with sulphonylureas or insulin compared with conventional treatment and risk of complications in patients with type 2 diabetes. *Lancet* 1998;352:837–853.
19. Metcalf-McCambridge T, Colby R. Exercising with type 1 diabetes: guidelines for safe and healthy activity. *Your Patient Fit* 2000;14:22–27.
20. Landt KW, Campaign BN, James FW, et al. Effects of exercise training on insulin sensitivity in adolescents with type 1 diabetes. *Diabetes Care* 1985;8:461–465.
21. Zinker BA. Nutrition and exercise in individuals with diabetes. *Clin Sports Med* 1999;18:585–606.
22. Herbst A, Bachran R, Kapellen T, et al. Effects of regular physical activity on control of glycemia in pediatric patients with type 1 diabetes mellitus. *Arch Pediatr Adolesc Med* 2006;160:573–577.
23. Perry TL, Mann JI, Lewis-Barned NJ. Lifestyle intervention in people with insulin-dependent diabetes mellitus. *Eur J Clin Nutr* 1997;51:757–763.
24. Moy CS, Songer TJ, LaPorte RE, et al. Insulin-dependent diabetes mellitus, physical activity, and death. *Am J Epidemiol* 1993;137:74–81.
25. Wei M, Gibbons LW, Kampert JB. Low cardiorespiratory fitness and physical inactivity as predictors of mortality in men with type 2 diabetes. *Ann Intern Med* 2000;132:605–611.
26. Church TS, Cheng YJ, Earnest CP, et al. Exercise capacity and body composition as predictors of mortality among men with diabetes. *Diabetes Care* 2004;27(1):83–88.
27. White RD, Sherman C. Exercise in diabetes management: maximizing benefits, controlling risks. *Phys Sportmed* 1999;27:63–76.
28. Albright AL. Diabetes. In: Durstine JL, ed. *American College of Sports Medicine's exercise management for person's with chronic disease and disabilities.* Champaign, IL: Human Kinetics, 1997:94–100.
29. Thompson PD. The cardiovascular complications of vigorous physical activity. *Arch Intern Med* 1996;156:2297–2302.
30. Joint National Committee on Detection, Evaluation, and Treatment Of High Blood Pressure. The seventh report of the joint national committee on prevention, detection, evaluation, and treatment of high blood pressure. *JAMA* 2003;289:2560–2572.
31. Bove AA, Sherman C. Active control of hypertension. *Phys Sportsmed* 1998;26:45–53.
32. Blair SN, Goodyear NN, Gibbons LW, et al. Physical fitness and incidence of hypertension in healthy normotensive men and women. *JAMA* 1984;252:487–490.
33. Klaus D. Management of hypertension in actively exercising patients: implications for drug selection. *Drugs* 1989;37:212–218.
34. American College of Sports Medicine Position Stand. Exercise and hypertension. *Med Sci Sports Exerc* 2004;36(3):533–553.
35. Collins R, Peto R, MacMahon S, et al. Blood pressure, stroke, and coronary heart disease. Part 2: Short-term reductions in blood pressure; overview of randomised drug trials in their epidemiological context. *Lancet* 1990;335:827–838.
36. Gordon NF. Hypertension. In: Durstine JL, ed. *American College of Sports Medicine's exercise management for persons with chronic diseases and disabilities.* Champaign, IL: Human Kinetics, 1997:59–63.
37. Chintanadilok J, Lowenthal DT. Exercise in the prevention and treatment of hypertension. In: Thompson PD, ed. *Exercise and sports cardiology.* New York: McGraw-Hill, 2001:402–429.
38. MacDougall JD, Tuxen D, Sale J, et al. Arterial blood pressure response to heavy exercise. *J Appl Physiol* 1985;58:785–790.
39. Haykowsky MJ, Findlay JM, Ignaszewski AP. Aneurysmal subarachnoid hemorrhage associated with weight training: three case reports. *Clin J Sport Med* 1996;6:52–55.
40. Gordon NF, Scott CB, Wilkinson WJ, et al. Exercise and mild essential hypertension: recommendations for adults. *Sports Med* 1990;10:390–404.
41. Hagberg JM, Ehsani AA, Goldring D, et al. Effects of weight training on blood pressure and hemodynamics in hypertensive adolescents. *J Pediatr* 1984;104(1):147–151.
42. Kiveloff B. Huber 0: brief maximal isometric exercise in hypertension. *J Am Geriatr Soc* 1971;19:1006–1012.
43. Kelley G. Dynamic resistance exercise and resting blood pressure in adults: a meta-analysis. *J Appl Physiol* 1997;82:1559–1565.
44. Cornelissen VA, Fagard RH. Effect of resistance training on resting blood pressure: a meta-analysis of randomized controlled trials. *J Hypertens* 2005;23(2):251–259.
45. Harris KA, Holly RG. Physiological responses to circuit weight training in borderline hypertensive subjects. *Med Sci Sports Exerc* 1987;19:246–252.
46. American College of Sports Medicine. *ACSM's guidelines for exercise testing and prescription,* 6th ed. Philadelphia: Lippincott Williams & Wilkins, 2000.
47. Stewart KJ. Weight training in coronary artery disease and hypertension. *Prog Cardiovasc Dis* 1992;35:159–168.
48. Arakawa K. Antihypertensive mechanisms of exercise. *J Hypertens* 1993;11:223–229.
49. Duncan JJ, Farr JE, Upton SJ, et al. The effect of aerobic exercise on plasma catecholamine and blood pressure in patients with mild essential hypertension. *JAMA* 1985;254:2609–2613.
50. Grassi G, Seravalle G, Calhoun D, et al. Physical exercise in essential hypertension. *Chest* 1992;101:S312–S314.
51. Ades PA, Gunther PG, Meachem CP, et al. Hypertension, exercise, and beta-adrenergic blockade. *Ann Intern Med* 1998;109:629–634.
52. Derman WE, Sims R, Noakes TD. The effects of antihypertensive medications on the physiological response to maximal exercise testing. *J Cardiovasc Pharmacol* 1992;19:S122–S127.

53. Gillin AG, Fletcher PJ, Horvath JS, et al. Comparison of doxazosin and atenolol in mild hypertension, and effects on exercise capacity, hemodynamics and left ventricular function. *Am J Cardiol* 1989;63:950–954.
54. Gordon NF. Effect of selective and nonselective beta-adrenoceptor blockade on thermoregulation during prolonged exercise in heat. *Am J Cardiol* 1985;55:74D–78D.
55. Gordon NF, Scott CB, Duncan JJ. Effects of atenolol versus enalapril on cardiovascular fitness and serum lipids in physically active hypertensive men. *Am J Cardiol* 1997;79:1065–1069.
56. Lundborg P, Astrom H, Bengtsson C, et al. Effect of beta-adrenoceptor blockade on exercise performance and metabolism. *Clin Sci* 1981;61:299–305.
57. Omvik P, Lund-Johansen P. Long-term hemodynamic effects at rest and during exercise of newer antihypertensive agents and salt restriction in essential hypertension: review of epanolol, doxazosin, amlodipine, felodipine, diltiazem, lisinopril, dilevalol, carvedilol, and ketanserin. *Cardiovasc Drugs Ther* 1993;7:193–206.
58. Palatini P, Bongiovi S, Mario L, et al. Effects of ACE inhibition on endurance exercise haemodynamics in trained subjects with mild hypertension. *Eur J Clin Pharmacol* 1995;48:435–439.
59. Swain R, Kaplan B. Treating hypertension in active patients: which agents work best with exercise? *Phys Sportsmed* 1997;25:47–64.
60. Tanji JL. Exercise and the hypertensive athlete. *Clin Sports Med* 1992;11:291–302.
61. Tanji JL, Batt ME. Management of hypertension: adapting new guidelines for active patients. *Phys Sportsmed* 1995;23:47–55.
62. Ullrich IH, Reid CM, Yeater RA, et al. Increased HDL-cholesterol levels with a weight lifting program. *South Med J* 1987;80:328–331.
63. Vanhees L, Fagard R, Lijnen P, et al. Effect of antihypertensive medication on endurance exercise capacity in hypertensive sportsmen. *J Hypertens,* 1991;9:1063–1068.
64. Maron BJ, Epstein SE, Roberts WC. Causes of sudden death in competitive athletes. *J Am Coll Cardiol* 1986;7:204–214.
65. Maron BJ, Araujo CGS, Thompson PD, et al. Recommendations for preparticipation screening and the assessment of cardiovascular disease in masters athletes: an advisory for healthcare professionals from the working groups of the World Heart Federation, the International Federation of Sports Medicine, and the American Heart Association Committee on Exercise, Cardiac Rehabilitation, and Prevention. *Circulation* 2001;103:327–334.
66. Maron BJ, Thompson PD, Puffer JC, et al. American Heart Association scientific statement: cardiovascular preparticipation screening of competitive athletes. *Med Sci Sports Exerc* 1996;28:1445–1452.
67. Ginsberg HN, Goldberg IJ. Disorders of lipoprotein metabolism. In: Braunwald E, Fauci AS, Kasper DL, et al. eds. *Harrison's principles of internal medicine.* New York: McGraw-Hill, 2001:2245–2246.
68. Busby-Whitehead MJ, Blackman MR. Clinical implications of abnormal lipoprotein metabolism. In: Barker LR, Burton JR, Zieve PD, eds. *Principles of ambulatory medicine.* Baltimore: Lippincott Williams & Wilkins, 1999:1127–1129.
69. Rosenson RS. *Screening guidelines for dyslipidemia.* UpToDate Online 9.3, Available: http://www.uptodate.com. 2001.
70. Donahoo WT, Eckel RH. Evaluation, treatment, and implications of hypertriglyceridemia. *Prim Care Case Rev* 2001;4:53–61.
71. Executive summary of the third report of the National Cholesterol Education Program (NCEP) expert panel on detection, evaluation, and treatment of high blood cholesterol in adults (Adult Treatment Panel III). *JAMA* 2001;285:2486–2497.
72. Gundy SM, Cleeman JI, Merz CN, et al. Implications of recent clinical trials for the National Cholesterol Education Program Adult Treatment Panel III Guidelines. *Circulation* 2004;110:227–239.
73. Durstine JL, Haskell WL. Effects of exercise training on plasma lipids and lipoproteins. *Exerc Sport Sci Rev* 1994;22:477–521.
74. Thompson PD, Crouse SF, Goodpasture B, et al. The acute versus the chronic response to exercise. *Med Sci Sports Exerc* 2001;33:S438–S445.
75. Durstine JL, Moore GE. Hyperlipidemia. In: Durstine JL, ed. *American College of Sports Medicine's exercise management for persons with chronic diseases and disabilities.* Champaign, IL: Human Kinetics, 1997:101–105.
76. Carlson LA, Mossfeldt F. Acute effects of prolonged, heavy exercise on the concentration of plasma lipids and lipoproteins in man. *Acta Physiol Scand* 1964;62:51–59.
77. Holloszy JO, Skinner JS, Toro G. Effects of a six month program of endurance exercise on lipids of middle-aged men. *Am J Cardiol* 1964;14:753–760.
78. Altena TS, Michaelson JL, Ball SD, et al. Lipoprotein subfraction changes after continuous or intermittent exercise training. *Med Sci Sports Exerc* 2006;38(2):367–372.
79. Durstine JL. Exercise and lipid disorders. In: Thompson PD, ed. *Exercise and sports cardiology.* New York: McGraw-Hill, 2001:452–479.
80. Crouse SF, O'Brien BC, Grandjean PW. Effects of training and a single session of exercise on lipids and apolipoproteins in hypercholesterolemic men. *J Appl Physiol* 1997;83:2019–2028.
81. Crouse SF, O'Brien BC, Rohack JJ. Changes in serum lipids and apolipoproteins after exercise in men with high cholesterol: influence of intensity. *J Appl Physiol* 1995;79:279–286.
82. Grandjean PW, Crouse SF, Rohack JJ. Influence of cholesterol status on blood lipid and lipoprotein enzyme responses to aerobic exercise. *J Appl Physiol* 2000;89:472–480.
83. Thompson PD, Cullinane R, Eshleman SP, et al. The effects of caloric restriction or exercise cessation on the serum lipid and lipoprotein concentrations of endurance athletes. *Metabolism* 1984;33:943–950.
84. Leon AS, Sanchez OA. Response of blood lipids to exercise training alone or combined with dietary intervention. *Med Sci Sports Exerc* 2001;33:S502–S515.
85. Kokkinos PF, Fernhall B. Physical activity and high density lipoprotein cholesterol levels. *Sports Med* 1999;5:307–314.
86. Thompson PD, Yurgalevitch SM, Flynn MM. Effect of prolonged exercise training without weight loss on high-density lipoprotein metabolism in overweight men. *Metabolism* 1997;46:217–223.
87. Varady KA, Ebine N, Vanstone CA, et al. Plant sterols and endurance training combine to favorably alter plasma lipid profiles in previously sedentary hypercholesterolemic adults after 8 weeks. *Am J Clin Nutr* 2004;80(5):1159–1166.
88. Visich PS, Gross FL, Gordon PM, et al. Effects of exercise with varying energy expenditure on high-density lipoprotein-cholesterol. *Eur J Physiol* 1996;72:242–248.
89. Ferguson MA, Alderson NL, Trost SG, et al. Effects of 4 different single exercise sessions on lipids, lipoproteins, and lipoprotein lipase. *J Appl Physiol* 1998;85:1169–1174.
90. Braith RW. Resistance exercise training: its role in the prevention of cardiovascular disease. *Circulation* 2006;113(22):2642–2650.
91. Kokkinos PF, Hurley BF, Smutok MA, et al. Strength training does not improve lipoprotein-lipid profiles in men at risk for CHD. *Med Sci Sports Exerc* 1991;23:11341139.
92. Kokkinos PF, Hurley BF, Vaccaro P, et al: Effects of low- and high-repetition resistive training on lipoprotein-lipid profiles. *Med Sci Sports Exerc,* 1988;20:50–54.
93. Smutok MA, Reece C, Kokkinos PF, et al. Aerobic versus strength training for risk factor intervention in middle-aged men at high risk for coronary heart disease. *Metabolism* 1993;42:177–184.
94. Goldberg L, Elliot DL, Schutz RW, et al. Changes in lipid and lipoprotein levels after weight training. *JAMA* 1984;252:504–506.
95. Johnson CC, Stone MH, Lopez SA, et al. Diet and exercise in middle-aged men. *J Am Diet Assoc* 1982;81:695–701.
96. Hurley BF, Hagberg JM, Goldberg AP, et al. Resistive training can reduce coronary risk factors without altering VO2 max or percent body fat. *Med Sci Sports Exerc* 1988;20:150–154.
97. Manning JM, Dooly-Manning CR, White K, et al. Effects of a resistive training program on lipoprotein-lipid levels in obese women. *Med Sci Sports Exerc* 1991;23:1222–1226.
98. Hedley AA, Ogden CL, Johnson CL, et al. Prevalence of overweight and obesity among U.S. children, adolescents, and adults, 1999–2002. *JAMA* 2004;291(23):2847–2850.
99. Kuczmarski RJ, Carrol MD, Flegal KM, et al. Varying body mass index cutoff points to describe overweight prevalence among US adults: NHANES III (1988–1994). *Obes Res* 1997;5:542–548.
100. McInnis KJ. Exercise and obesity. *Coron Artery Dis* 2000;11:111–116.
101. Executive summary of the clinical guidelines on the identification, evaluation, and treatment of overweight and obesity in adults. *Arch Int Med* 1998;158:1855–1867.
102. Leermakers EA, Dunn AL, Blair SN. Exercise management of obesity. *Med Clin North Am* 2000;84:419–440.
103. Anderson RE. Exercise, an active lifestyle, and obesity: making the exercise prescription work. *Phys Sportsmed* 1999;27:41–50.
104. Pescatello LS, VanHeest JL. Physical activity mediates a healthier body weight in the presence of obesity. *Br J Sports Med* 2000;34:86–93.
105. American College of Sports Medicine Position Stand. Appropriate intervention strategies for weight loss and prevention of weight regain for adults. *Med Sci Sports Exerc* 2001;33(12):2145–2156.
106. Grundy SM, Blackburn G, Higgins M, et al. Roundtable consensus statement: physical activity in the prevention and treatment of obesity and its comorbidities. *Med Sci Sports Exerc* 1998;31:S502–S508.
107. Ross R, Freeman JA, Jansen I. Exercise alone is an effective strategy for reducing obesity and related comorbidities. *Exerc Sport Sci Rev* 2000;28:165–170.
108. Bouchard C, Tremblay A, Nadeau A, et al. Long-term exercise training with constant energy intake: effect on body composition and selected metabolic variables. *Int J Obes* 1990;14:57–73.
109. Ross R, Dagnone D, Jones PJ, et al. Reduction in obesity and related comorbid conditions after diet-induced weight loss or exercise-induced weight loss in men. *Ann Intern Med* 2000;133:92–103.
110. Sopko G, Leon AS, Jacobs DR, et al. The effects of exercise and weight loss on plasma lipids in young obese men. *Metabolism* 1985;34:227–236.
111. Votruba SB, Horvitz MA, Schoeller DA. The role of exercise in the treatment of obesity. *Nutrition* 2000;16:179–188.
112. Miller WC, Koceja DM, Hamilton EJ. A meta-analysis of the past 25 years of weight loss research using diet, exercise or diet plus exercise intervention. *Int J Obes* 1997;21:941–947.

113. Wing RR. Physical activity in the treatment of the adult overweight and obesity: current evidence and research issues. *Med Sci Sports Exerc* 1999;31:S547–S552.
114. McGuire MT, Wing RR, Klem ML, et al. Long-term maintenance of weight loss. Do people who lose weight through various weight loss methods use different behaviors to maintain their weight? *Int J Obes Relat Metab Disord* 1998;22:572–577.
115. Kayman S, Bruvold W, Stern JS. Maintenance and relapse after weight loss in women: behavioral aspects. *Am J Clin Nutr* 1990;52:800–807.
116. Ballor DL, Poehlman ET. A meta-analysis of the effects of exercise and/or dietary restriction on resting metabolic rate. *Eur J Appl Physiol Occup Physiol* 1995;71:535–542.
117. Kempen KP, Saris WH, Westerterp KR. Energy balance during an 8-week energy-restricted diet with and without exercise in obese women. *Am J Clin Nutr* 1995;62:722–729.
118. Miller WC. How effective are traditional dietary and exercise interventions for weight loss? *Med Sci Sports Exerc* 1999;31:1129–1134.
119. Ross R, Janssen I. Physical activity, total and regional obesity: dose-response considerations. *Med Sci Sports Exerc* 2001;33:S521–S527.
120. Lee CD, Blair SN, Jackson AS. Cardiorespiratory fitness, body composition, and all-cause and cardiovascular disease mortality in men. *Am J Clin Nutr* 1999;69:373–380.
121. King AC, Kierman M, Oman RF, et al. Can we identify who will adhere to long-term physical activity? Signal detection methodology as a potential aid to clinical decision making. *Health Psychol* 1997;16:380–389.
122. Anderson RE, Wadden TA, Bartlett SJ, et al. Effects of lifestyle activity vs structured aerobic exercise in obese women. *JAMA* 1999;281: 335–340.
123. Wallace JP. Obesity. In: Durstine JL, ed. *American College of Sports Medicine's exercise management for person's with chronic disease and disabilities*. Champaign, IL: Human Kinetics, 1997:106–111.
124. Eckel R, Krauss RM. American Heart Association call to action: obesity as a major risk factor for coronary heart disease. *Circulation* 1998;97:2099–2100.
125. Goroll AH, Mulley AG, eds. Screening for osteoporosis. In: *Primary care medicine: office evaluation and management of the adult patient*. Philadelphia: Lippincott Williams & Wilkins, 2000:821–823.
126. America's bone health. *The state of osteoporosis and low bone mass*. www.nof.org/advocacy/prevalence/index.htm. Accessed July 25, 2006.
127. Lane JM, Russel L, Khan S. Osteoporosis. *Med Sci Sports Exerc* 2000;372:139–150.
128. American College of Sports Medicine Position Stand. Physical activity and bone health. *Med Sci Sports Exerc* 2004;36(11):1985–1996.
129. Nelson ME, Fiatarone MA, Morganti CM, et al. Effects of high-intensity strength training on multiple risk factors for osteoporotic fractures: a randomized controlled trial. *JAMA* 1994;272:1909–1914.
130. Marcus R. Role of exercise in preventing and treating osteoporosis. *Rheum Dis Clin North Am* 2001;27:131–141.
131. Vuori IM. Dose-response of physical activity and low back pain, osteoarthritis, and osteoporosis. *Med Sci Sports Exerc* 2001;33:S551–S586.
132. Layne JE, Nelson ME. The effects of progressive resistance training on bone density: a review. *Med Sci Sports Exerc* 1999;31:25–30.
133. Snow-Harter C, Marcus R. Exercise, bone mineral density, and osteoporosis. *Exert Sport Sci Rev* 1991;19:351–388.
134. Recker RR, Davies M, Hinders SM, et al. Bone gain in young adult women. *JAMA* 1992;268:2403–2408.
135. Friedlander AL, Genant HK, Sadowsky S, et al. A two-year program of aerobics and weight-training enhances bone mineral density of young women. *J Bone Miner Res* 1995;10:574–585.
136. Maddalozzo GF, Snow CM. High intensity resistance training: effects on bone in older men and women. *Calcif Tissue Int* 2000;66:399–404.
137. Cussler EC, Lohman TG, Going SB, et al. Weight lifted in strength training predicts bone change in postmenopausal women. *Med Sci Sports Exerc* 2003;35(1):10–17.
138. Drinkwater BL, Nilson K, Chesnut CH, et al. Bone mineral content of amenorrheic and eumenorrheic athletes. *N Engl J Med* 1984;311:277–281.
139. Bloomfield SA. Osteoporosis. In: Durstine JL, ed. *American College of Sports Medicine's exercise management for person's with chronic disease and disabilities*. Champaign, IL: Human Kinetics, 1997:161–166.
140. World Health Organization. *Mental and neurological disorders*. www.who.int/mediacentre/factsheets/fs265/en/. Accessed on July 25, 2006.
141. American Psychiatric Association. *Diagnostic and statistical manual of mental disorders*, 4th ed. Washington, DC: American Psychiatric Association, 1994.
142. Paulsen RH. *Treatment of depression*. UpToDate Online 9.3, Available: http://www.uptodate.com. 2001.
143. Paluska SA, Schwenk TL. Physical activity and mental health. *Sports Med* 2000;3:167–180.
144. Meyer T. Broocks: therapeutic impact of exercise on psychiatric diseases: guidelines for exercise testing and prescription. *Sports Med* 2000;4:269–279.
145. Dunn AL, Trivedi MH, O'Neal HA. Physical activity dose-response effects on outcomes of depression and anxiety. *Med Sci Sports Exerc* 2001;33:S587–S597.
146. Farmer ME, Locke BZ, moscicki EK, et al. Physical activity and depressive symptoms: the NHANES I epidemiologic follow-up study. *Am J Epidemiol* 1988;128:1340–1351.
147. Martinsen EW. Benefits of exercise for the treatment of depression. *Sports Med* 1990;9:380–389.
148. Paffenbarger RS, Lee I-M, Leung R. Physical activity and personal characteristics associated with depression and suicide in American college men. *Acta Psychiatr Scand* 1994;377:S16–S22.
149. Greist JH, Klein MH, Eischens RR, et al. Running as treatment for depression. *Compr Psychiatry* 1979;20:41–54.
150. McCann IL, Holmes DS. Influence of aerobic exercise on depression. *J Pers Soc Psychol* 1984;46:1143–1147.
151. Martinsen EW, Medhaus A, Sandvik L. Effects of exercise on depression: a controlled study. *Br Med J* 1985;291:109.
152. Doyne EJ, Ossip-Klein DJ, Bowman ED. Running versus weight lifting in the treatment of depression. *J Consult Clin Psychol* 1987;55:748–754.
153. Martinsen EW, Hoffart A, Solberg O. Comparing aerobic and nonaerobic forms of exercise in the treatment of clinical depression: a randomized trial. *Compr Psychiatry* 1989;30:324–331.
154. Craft LL, Landers DM. The effect of exercise on clinical depression: a meta-analysis (abstract). *Med Sci Sports Exerc* 1998;30:S117.
155. North TC, McCullagh P, Tran ZV. Effect of exercise on depression. *Exerc Sport Sci Rev* 1990;18:379–415.
156. Keller MB, Kocsis JH, Thase ME, et al. Maintenance phase efficacy of sertraline for chronic depression: a randomized controlled trial. *JAMA* 1998;280:1665–1672.
157. Plante TG, Rodin J. Physical fitness and enhanced psychological health. *Curr Psychol : Res Rev* 1990;9:3–24.
158. Weyerer S, Kupfer B. Physical exercise and psychological health. *Sports Med* 1994;17:108–116.
159. Scully D, Kremer J, Meade M, et al. Physical exercise and psychological well being: a critical review. *Br J Sports Med* 1998;32:111–120.
160. Skinar GS. Mental illness. In: Durstine JL, ed. *American College of Sports Medicine's exercise management for persons with chronic diseases and disabilities*. Champaign, IL: Human Kinetics, 1997:230–232.

Injury Prevention

8

Michael P. Montico *Joanne Nguyen*
Scott W. Eathorne *Martha A. Steele*

Injury prevention is a concept that should serve as a foundation for building any quality sports medicine program servicing the athletic community. Unfortunately, many networks caring for active and athletic individuals focus primarily on injury treatment. The primary care sports medicine physician, as part of a multidisciplinary team, is perhaps best suited to help refocus sports medicine services to include a greater emphasis on injury prevention. To this end, it is important to recognize the role that each of the following factors play:

- Epidemiology of injuries
- Areas of preventive impact
  - Preparticipation evaluation (PPE)
  - Control of the sports environment

Through close examination and understanding of these factors, providers can better understand and anticipate certain injuries in the athlete and make efforts to avoid them.

Clinical epidemiology can provide a great deal of practical information for the sports medicine physician. Acquiring knowledge about the frequency and severity of injuries in a specific sport can aid the sports medicine physician in gauging what may happen, based upon what has happened. Epidemiology of injuries is also an important factor in guiding the focus of the PPE. The PPE, as a screening device, should provide the team physician with an assessment of the athlete's ability to participate in a specific sport. Both epidemiology of injuries (Chapter 2) and the PPE (Chapter 5) are fundamental principles to the concept of injury prevention and are discussed in more detail elsewhere in this text.

This chapter will concentrate on the other areas of potential preventive impact, which can be divided into external and internal factors (see Table 8.1).

TABLE 8.1
LIST OF INTERNAL (ATHLETE DEPENDENT) AND EXTERNAL (SPORTS MEDICINE ENVIRONMENT) FACTORS FOR POTENTIAL INJURY PREVENTION IMPACT

Internal Factors	External Factors
General health	Equipment
Conditioning	Weather conditions
Rehabilitation	Field conditions
Psychological status	Coaching
Nutritional status	Officiating/rule enforcement
Education	Balancing competition

INTERNAL FACTORS

Many factors that have a bearing on injury rates are the direct responsibility of the athlete. The athlete should be aware of the factors that are under their control, which include the following: general health, conditioning, adequate recovery, proper rehabilitation of old injuries, psychological stressors, appropriate nutrition, and education. With an understanding of these factors, the athlete can take an active role, with the help of the team physician, trainer, and/or coach, to correct and enhance areas of opportunity.

GENERAL HEALTH

Any athlete who wishes to participate in organized sports should be required to go through a PPE. The primary goal of this PPE is to help maintain the health and safety of the athlete during athletic participation. The medical history is the key element of the PPE, as it can identify most problems that may affect the athlete. For this reason, it is important that the athlete completes the historical questionnaire accurately, with a parent's review for a minor, before the examination.

Any preparticipation screening should answer these questions: (a) Is this candidate *mature enough* to compete in the sport or sports for which the screening is being done? (b) Is this person in *adequate physical condition* to compete in the sport? (c) Does this candidate have any *increased potential* for injury? (d) Does this person have *medical problems* that may be a cause has disqualification from competition? The team physician is doing him/herself? and the athlete an **injustice** if all of these questions cannot be answered following the examination.

CONDITIONING

It is the athlete's responsibility to be physically fit to begin competition or training. Being "in condition" means the athlete is equal to the neuromuscular demands and has the necessary strength and stamina for his/her sport (1).

Percent body fat and lean body mass can help determine an athlete's level of conditioning and can be determined in any number of ways (2). Skinfold analysis, which is performed with a hand held caliper, is a simplistic way to measure body fat. It provides a reasonable estimate of body composition. Hydrostatic (under water) weighing is one of the most accurate ways to determine body composition (3), but is more involved, requiring a tank, weighing scale, and the ability of the athletes to perform a maximal expiration and hold their breath under water while the weight is being recorded (4,5). Most coaches and trainers will use the skinfold analysis to establish the athlete's body composition. Those figures, along with periodic weighing, should be used to guide weight loss practices or weight maintenance.

WARM-UP

Warm-up exercises are designed to prepare the body for exercise, prevent injury, and enhance the athlete's performance (6,7). A good warm-up program consists of both general exercises that should be performed by all athletes and specific exercises that are targeted for the specific sport of the athlete, as well as specific position exercises (e.g., goalkeeper as opposed to field player warm-up in soccer).

General warm-up exercises should begin with large muscle groups, such as the quadriceps and hamstrings, as these are the main areas to which blood flow will be redistributed. Jogging and stationary biking are two such exercises often used. After the general warm-up, the athlete can begin more specific exercises for the particular activity they will soon undertake. For example, a swimmer should concentrate on further warming up the muscles, joints, tendons, and ligaments of the upper extremities, particularly the shoulder. A soccer player should concentrate on the lower extremities. Table 8.2 outlines some of the benefits of warm-up exercises. The whole warm-up session should last anywhere from 15 to 30 minutes, but may vary depending on the sport involved. The intensity may also vary, but at minimum it should produce an increase in heart rate and mild sweating. It is important not to warm up too early. There should be no more than 5 to 10 minutes between the end of warm-up and the beginning of the competition.

TABLE 8.2
WAYS IN WHICH WARM-UP EXERCISES PREPARE AN ATHLETE FOR A SPORTING EVENT

Increase blood flow to the muscles, which in turn increase oxygen delivery to the muscle
Increase circulation leading to decreased vascular resistance
Increase mechanical efficiency
Increase nerve impulse speed
Increase nerve receptor sensitivity
Increase range of motion
Decrease stiffness
Increase general alertness
Increase concentration with psychological preparation for the upcoming event

FLEXIBILITY AND MOBILITY TRAINING

Flexibility refers to the ability to move a specific joint through a full range of motion and is an important component in any good conditioning program. The flexibility of a joint is limited by the tightness of its connective tissue. Therefore, the goal of improving flexibility through stretching is to improve joint mobility.

There are several forms of stretching: static, dynamic, ballistic, and proprioceptive neuromuscular facilitation (PNF). Static stretching is performed by slowly moving into a stretched position and holding the pose for 15 to 30 seconds. Each stretch should be performed three to four times/session. The athlete should assume a pose that will allow him/her to feel the tissue elongation and not feel pain or discomfort.

Dynamic stretching involves maximal joint motion secondary to muscle contraction. It involves controlled swinging of the limb with the athlete gradually increasing the distance, speed, or intensity without going past his/her range of motion. Ballistic stretching involves quick bouncing movements where momentum is used to achieve greater range of motion. This type of stretching does not allow the muscle tendon unit enough time to fully adapt to its stretched pose and can increase the chance of injury (8). Therefore, this technique is NOT recommended.

TABLE 8.3
BASIC GUIDELINES FOR STRETCHING

Always precede stretching with a 5–10 min warm-up
Move slowly and gently into and out of each position
Do not bounce while stretching
Continue to breathe normally while stretching
Stretch to the point of tension, not to the point of pain or discomfort
Stretch before and after sporting activity
Hold the stretched position for 15–30 sec
Perform each stretch three to four times

Interestingly, there are multiple studies showing that static, dynamic, and ballistic stretching may all aid in improving performance measures such as range of motion and muscle strength (9).

PNF stretching combines passive stretching with isometric contraction to attain increased flexibility. It is performed by alternating contraction and relaxation of the agonist and antagonist muscles. For example, if the hamstring is the target muscle, it is gently stretched by a partner, contracted isometrically against resistance (usually the partner), relaxed and then stretched further in the same range of motion. The disadvantage of PNF is that it requires a partner and there is a tendency to overstretch. Some basic stretching guidelines are listed in Table 8.3. Of note, there are reports of acute stretch injury wherein specific mechanisms of stretching may be associated with muscle strain and discomfort (8). Knowledge of proper stretching techniques and awareness of an athlete's level of conditioning may decrease the incidence of such injury.

For a guide to inappropriate stretches, please consult Figure 8.1. In addition, there are multiple studies that find that static, dynamic, and ballistic stretching may all aid in improving performance measures such as range of motion, muscle strength, etc. (10).

STRENGTH AND POWER TRAINING

Strength is the ability to produce maximal force in a single muscular contraction. Power (P) is the ability to exert maximal amount of work (w) rapidly over time (t). Both of these elements are key in enhancing performance, preventing injuries, and recovering from injuries.

There are 3 types of resistance training that can be utilized to enhance strength and power: concentric (positive work), eccentric (negative work), and isometric (static work) (11,12). In concentric training, the muscle contracts as it shortens in length against a resisting force. The resistance can be in the form of the athlete's own body weight, free weights, weight machines, or rubber bands. Concentric exercises can be either isotonic or isokinetic. Isotonic exercises are those in which the resistance load is constant, thereby providing constant muscle tension throughout the range of motion of the exercise. Isokinetic exercises are performed on specialized machines, which are set at a fixed speed but variable resistance to accommodate the athlete.

Because isokinetic exercises require the use of specialized machines, isotonic concentric exercises are most commonly used in strength and power training. Examples of isotonic concentric exercises include dumbbell curls, machine leg extension exercises, and bench press.

In eccentric training, the muscle lengthens as the origin and insertion of the muscle separate during isotonic contraction. Eccentric training can be used to prevent musculotendinous injuries as well as to rehabilitate old injuries (13). Proper use of eccentric exercises is advocated, as misuse can cause delayed muscle soreness and tendinosis (14). An example of an eccentric exercise is slowly lowering the arm during the negative phase of a biceps curl.

COORDINATION AND PROPRIOCEPTIVE TRAINING

Proprioceptive training is especially important following an injury, and assists in preventing injury recurrence (15). It involves interaction between the musculoskeletal, musculotendinous, and central nervous system in order to provide the athlete with information about joint position, motion, pressure, and vibration. Proprioceptive training should begin as soon as possible during injury rehabilitation, as it can take weeks for the athlete to regain normal coordination (16). Examples of such exercises for the lower extremity include single leg knee bend, hopping, and jumping. Proprioceptive aids such as a mini-trampoline or a rocker board can also be used.

SPORT SPECIFIC TRAINING

Sport specific training is important to achieve maximum efficiency and prevent injuries. Most sport specific training can take place within the sport. For example, a runner can practice on the track while a soccer player can practice drills on the field. Speed and agility drills are often seen in training and are specific to the sporting event. After an injury, this type of training is necessary to get the athlete back to his/her sporting event and prevent injury recurrence.

RECOVERY

Equally important as training is the recovery period. An adequate recovery period is necessary to allow the athlete to recuperate from strenuous activity as well as benefit from the training and prevent injury. Overtraining and not allowing for an adequate recovery cause muscle soreness, fatigue, and lethargy, which will ultimately hinder the athlete's performance. It is necessary to provide recovery time when planning the athlete's training program (6). The athlete should have 1 to 2 recovery days or rest days incorporated into the weekly training schedule. If the training period is long, low-intensity training weeks should be included.

There are a number of things that the athlete can do to enhance the recovery process: an adequate cooldown period after exercise, whirlpool therapy, massage treatment, and adequate sleep. A cooldown period is essential after any sporting activity. It involves a less intense activity that allows the heart rate to progressively decelerate, and should include stretches for the muscle groups involved. The cooldown period can vary from 10 to 15 minutes. Whirlpool and massage appears to help in the recovery process by decreasing the muscle tone after exercise and relaxing the athlete. It also enhances increased blood flow to the muscles

A

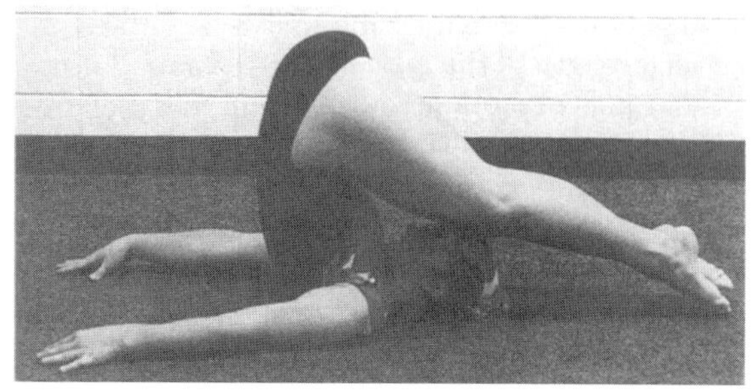

Yoga Plow
— interruption of circulation to the vertebral artery
— ↑ pressure to intervertebral discs in neck and lower back
— stretching of sciatic nerve

B

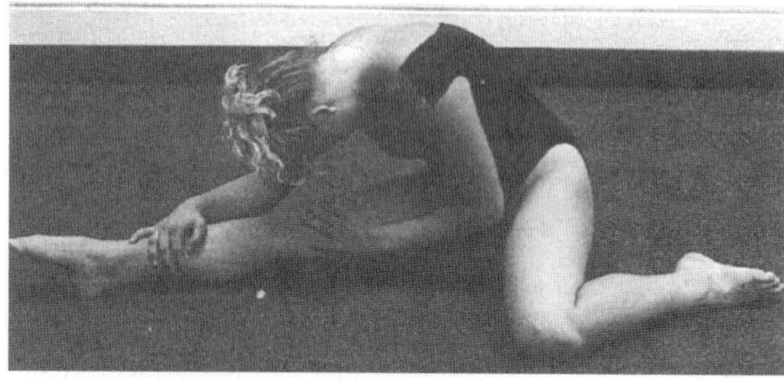

Hurdler's Stretch
— overstretching of groin muscles and ligaments
— meniscal injury
— medial collateral ligament injury
— sciatic nerve stretch

C

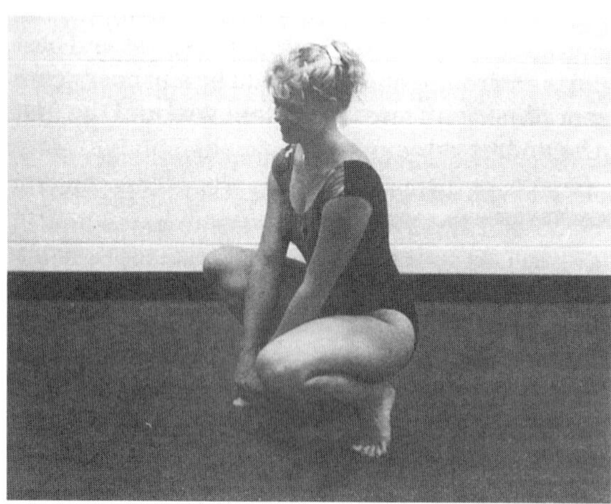

D

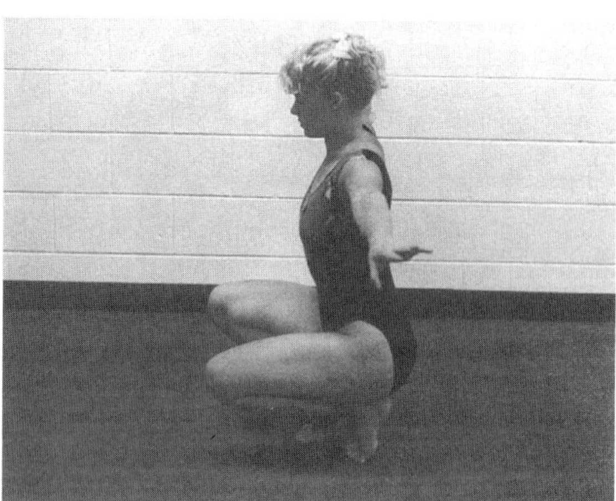

Duck Walk and Deep Knee Bend
— lateral meniscal damage (can be done briefly during a preparticipation musculoskeletal examination)

E

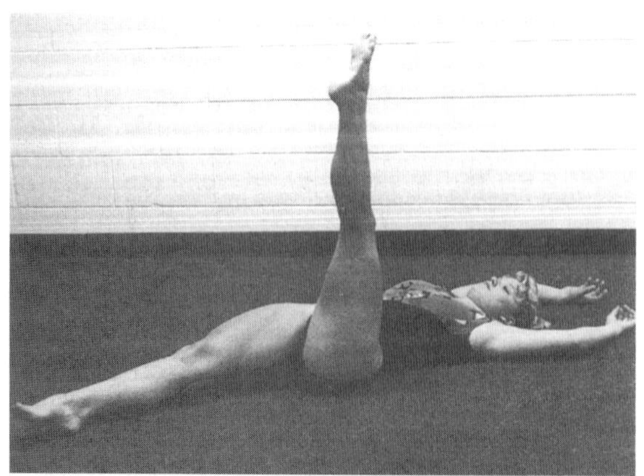

Still Leg Raises — Overstretching sciatic nerve

F

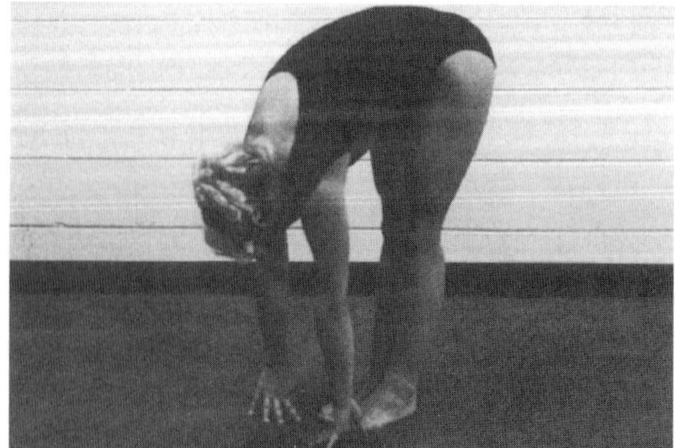

Toe Touching
— posterior longitudinal ligament involvement
— sciatic nerve damage

Figure 8.1 Inappropriate stretches and their possible injuries.

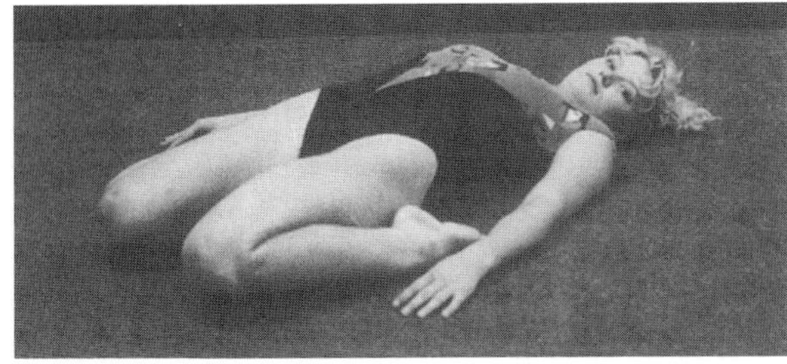

G

Knee Stretch
— involvement of patellar ligament, quadriceps tendon and both collateral knee ligaments

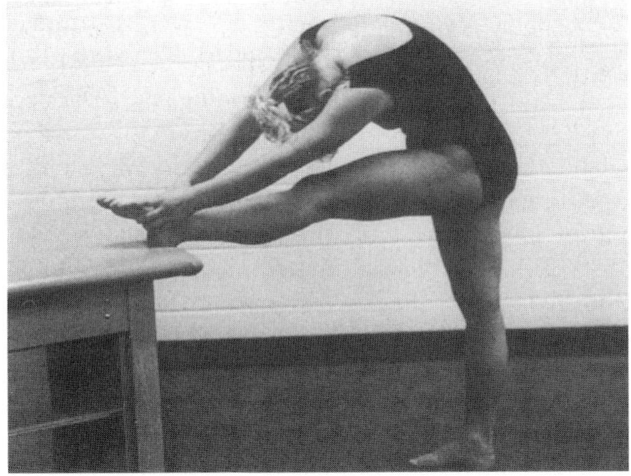

H

Ballet Stretches
— overstretching the sciatic nerve
— low back ligaments
— intervertebral discs

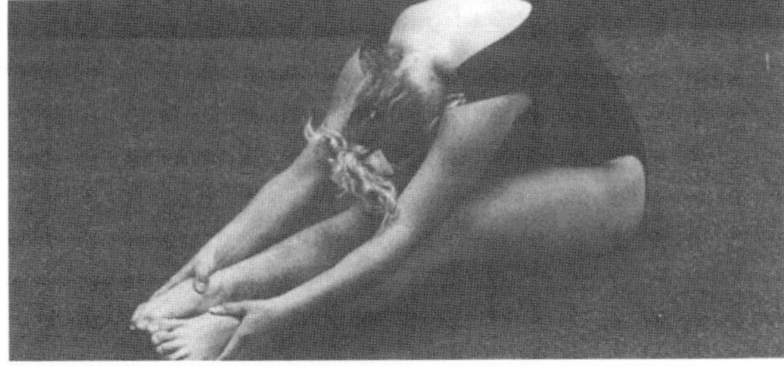

I

Full Sit-Ups
— greater than 30° hip flexion does not affect abdominal muscles
— overstretching of the lower back

Figure 8.1 *(continued)*

to promote clearance of metabolic products, that is, lactic acid (17). A massage therapist who is trained in deep muscle sport massage can help alleviate any symptomatic trigger points as well as improve soft tissue function (18). Adequate sleep is essential for recuperation after strenuous activity. An athlete should strive to get 8 hours of sleep each night, but may require as much as 12 hours, depending on the intensity and duration of training. Some athletes who are also involved in academics and work may require more rest, or risk succumbing to chronic fatigue and poor performance.

REHABILITATION OF OLD INJURIES

Rehabilitation is covered in detail in Chapter 35 and is mentioned here only as the most important factor in the return of an athlete to activity following injury. Reinjury can be minimized if rehabilitation is closely monitored by a team physician, physical therapist, or a trainer familiar with the injury and the demands of the sport and position played. Moving too slowly can result in an unnecessary loss of conditioning, whereas progressing too quickly may prevent proper healing. Full competitive activity must not be resumed until the athlete has met the following:

- No pain with activity
- Full strength of the injured area
- Full range of motion
- Proper mental attitude

The last requirement recognizes that each athlete responds differently to injury. Attention to all these criteria will give the best results. Progression from one rehabilitation phase to another may include some overlap in subjective and objective outcomes (i.e., pain and swelling may not be completely resolved before strengthening and flexibility). The athlete may still have some swelling from the acute phase but may be pain free and feel strong enough to progress to the subacute phase of rehabilitation.

PSYCHOLOGICAL STATUS

A healthy mental attitude is an essential component of sport participation. Athletes who participate in sports should compete because they enjoy the activity and want to improve their skills, general health, and self-esteem. If sport involvement is only secondary to parental or peer pressure, it can potentially be harmful to the athlete. This harm can come in the form of decreased self-esteem and impaired sporting performance, which can put the athlete at increased risk of injury.

Athletes with high self-esteem, positive mental attitude, good coping skills, good concentration, and a good social support structure tend to cope better with the stress and pressure that are associated with sport participation (19). Also, they tend to do better in rehabilitation and recover from the injury faster because they are able to cope well with the external pressures (i.e., pressure from the coach or teammates or the risk of being replaced) (20). A detailed discussion can be found in Chapter 36.

NUTRITION

What an athlete eats and drinks can affect general health as well as athletic performance. Nutrition is covered elsewhere (Chapter 4), but is mentioned here to underscore its importance. Optimum nutrition may enhance the athlete's performance whereas inadequate nutrition may hinder it. The nutritional aspects of training are vitally important, as proper diet fuels the body for vigorous physical training and competition. Athlete education should include appropriate selection of food and fluid, the timing of intake, and the role that supplements may have in optimal health and sport performance.

Adequate hydration is as vitally important as adequate nutrition. The athletes can optimize their performance when they maintain fluid balance during exercise, and, conversely, can hinder their performance with inadequate fluid intake (21,22). More serious consequences of dehydration are heat-related illnesses (i.e., heat stroke). Therefore, athletes should maintain adequate hydration before and during sporting events.

Ergogenic aids, diet aids, and supplements, many of which make claims to enhance sport performance, are "big business" (23). Athletes should be counseled about the use of these supplements and cautioned that they may not be safe, effective, or legal in the sports arena. Full discussion of this and an explanation of the team physician's role in drug use can be found in Chapter 37.

EDUCATION

As is true with all patients, the more knowledgeable, the less likely the athlete will become injured or ill. Athlete education is a positive action against most injury factors and a tool for enhancing athletic performance. Any athlete who participates should seek to learn more about the sport in which he/she is involved in, common injuries in that sport and how he/she can go about preventing such injuries, and proper employment of nutrition, hydration, and supplements in order to enhance and maintain performance. Knowledge is a tool that the athlete can use to ensure an enjoyable and, hopefully, a successful sport season.

EXTERNAL FACTORS

External factors in injury prevention are those that pertain to the sports medicine environment, and these factors can be closely related to injury rates. Equipment, weather conditions, and field conditions are important areas in which sports medicine physicians can have a significant impact on the sporting environment. With the cooperation of coaches and officials, the sports medicine physician can establish protocol and procedures that lead directly to a greater level of injury prevention.

EQUIPMENT

Equipment is a necessary component of athletic competition, and has many applications. Equipment can be utilized for the following:

- Protect the athlete from potential injury—use of helmets, mouthguards,
- Protect a pre-existing injury—bracing of joints, splinting,
- Alter biomechanics to avoid injuries—taping, arch supports,
- Protect the athlete from the environment—appropriate clothing/uniforms.

Regardless of its purpose, the sports medicine physician must ensure that equipment be used properly to promote injury prevention. Specific sports have special protective equipment, some of which may be mandatory. Safety standards are in place for some equipment, but a great deal of equipment used by athletes is not standardized or certified. In football, helmets and shoulder pads must be certified by National Operating Committee on Standards for Athletic Equipment (NOCSAE). It is recommended that helmets and shoulder pads be sent back to the manufacturer yearly for reconditioning (24). The periodic cleaning of sports equipment is important to ensure athlete safety, and prevent the spread of communicable disease. Wrestling mats must be cleaned with a disinfectant before and after each practice/competition (25). Any blood on the wrestling mat should be cleaned immediately with a chlorine/bleach solution. During competition the uniform may become saturated with blood, at which time it must be removed. If not saturated, bloodstains can be removed using a commercial product. Any contaminated laundry should be handled with gloves, double bagged, labeled as BIOHAZARD, and laundered appropriately (26). Use of community water bottles should be avoided whenever possible, and the practice of labeling water bottles for athletes with an illness is recommended (27). It is important to continually monitor both mandatory and personal equipment to ensure safety and appropriateness of all equipment. Equipment must fit properly and be used appropriately to ensure injury prevention. There are many examples of equipment contributing to increased injury rates:

- Overworn running shoes—overuse injuries, stress fractures (28)
- Loose fitting helmets—increased head and neck injuries (29)
- Improperly fit shoulder pads—increase in shoulder injuries (30)
- Prophylactic knee bracing—may lead to an increase in knee injuries (31)

Equipment can play a pivotal role in reduction and prevention of injuries. A study conducted on the effect of protective equipment in in-line skating injuries was revealing: the injury rates for wrist and elbow injuries was approximately 10 times greater in those who did not wear appropriate protective equipment (32). Sports medicine providers can contribute to athlete safety by promoting changes in equipment and competition, which may lead to injury prevention. In a recent study of over 29,000 Little League baseball injuries, it was found that approximately one third of these injuries could be prevented if changes in equipment were made. Proposed changes include reduced-impact balls, face guards, and break away safety bases (33).

In a study of college and minor league players, an 80% reduction in the number of sliding injuries was found when breakaway bases were used (34).

PLAYING CONDITIONS—HEAT

The prevention of injuries caused by the effects of heat is based on the practice of the following principles:

- Assessing the potential for heat injury
- Thermal acclimation
- Adequate hydration

In assessing potential for heat injury, it is important to avoid dangerous conditions. Table 8.1 can be used as a guide. Coaches and trainers must work in conjunction with the team physician to make appropriate adjustments to training schedules:

- Reschedule workouts to avoid extreme heat conditions
- Shorten duration of workouts
- Decrease intensity of training
- Allow athletes open access to hydration

Along with weather conditions, risk factors such as obesity, sleep deprivation, poor nutrition, and lack of conditioning should be screened for.

Avoiding dangerous conditions is important, but the sports medicine team should not overlook the role thermal acclimation plays in the athlete's conditioning program. Heat acclimation normally takes approximately 7 to 10 days for a given level of exercise (35). Allowing athletes to acclimate to the heat leads to the following results:

- More efficient sweating
- Lower skin temperatures
- Maintenance of lower overall core body temperature

Adequate hydration is critical in avoiding heat related injuries (36). The athletes, trainers, coaches, and administration must all be educated with regard to appropriate hydration practices. Pre- and postexercise body weight assessment can be a valuable tool in assessing hydration status. Athletes can take action to maximize their body's evaporative potential:

- Maintain maximal skin exposure—with loose fitting clothing
- Wear clothing with breathability, such as mesh or synthetic blends
- Periodic removal of headgear and toweling of face and head

The entire sports medicine team must remain alert in assessing for heat related illnesses. Many of the principles mentioned here can be utilized to avoid such injuries.

PLAYING CONDITIONS—COLD

Physical well being and proper attire are the two main principles of injury prevention in a cold environment. The potential for frostbite and other cold induced injuries can be directly related to wind chill. The important factors relating to physical well-being include proper nutrition, adequate hydration, and optimal conditioning. Optimal physical conditioning allows for more efficient thermoregulation by enabling athletes to derive more energy from fats while conserving carbohydrates.

The human body adapts poorly to cold environments, therefore proper attire is the basis of injury prevention in cold weather (37). Wearing clothing in multiple layers is the best way to defend the body against extreme temperatures (38). Multiple layers not only provide important insulation for the athlete, but also afford the athletes the ability to fine-tune their environment by adjusting the different layers. The base layer should keep the skin dry and warm, with clothing made of polypropylene being ideal due to its wicking properties. An insulation layer is used to trap warm air close to the athlete's body. This layer should be relatively loose fitting, and be designed to allow for proper ventilation. Finally an outer protective layer provides the athlete defense from the elements of wind and precipitation. While exercising in the cold, athletes can remain dry and protected by adjusting their attire and exercise level according to the given condition (38).

The following are some basic tips for athletes to follow when exercising in cold environments:

- Dress in multiple layers
- Stay dry—avoid perspiration and precipitation
- Protect your head—70% of heat loss occurs here
- Mittens are preferable to gloves
- Goggles may be necessary for eye protection
- Avoid the use of tobacco, alcohol, and caffeine in cold environments
- Never train alone

PLAYING CONDITIONS—AREA OF PLAY

The team physician should make it a practice to inspect the area of play before competition to ensure the safety of the athletes. Because most injuries occur on the field of play, it is important to remove any potential injury-causing obstacles before competition. Some possible hazards to consider are as follows:

- Irregularities in the field, uncovered drains—soccer, football
- Water on the court—basketball
- Unlatched doors—hockey
- Unbanked tracks—running
- Appropriate landing areas—field events
- Necessary buffer zone surrounding the field of play—all sports

The type of playing surface affects the quality of performance, and can be directly related to the occurrence of injuries. Review of the research suggests there may be a higher injury rate on artificial turf (39,40). The type of playing surface used is based on multiple factors that include the sport, safety, cost, durability, maintenance, climate, and amount and multiplicity of use. With the development of new synthetic surfaces, it is becoming more common to see the use of these surfaces in place of natural turf. Natural turf has long been regarded as safe for competition, and affordable to install and maintain. With the continued increase in the number of athletic events, maintenance of natural turf fields is becoming more challenging and expensive. This has lead to the installment of many artificial surfaces, which have the following advantages: efficient use of available space, minimal maintenance, uniform surface, and greater uniformity under heavy usage. The team physician should be aware of the playing surface as well as the area of play, to know knowing how these factors may predispose to injury.

COACHING

Having full support from the coaching staff is fundamental to developing a strong sports medicine program. The coaching staff should understand both the physical and psychological ramifications of athletic program design, and how these relate to injury prevention. Coaches can have a significant impact on injury prevention in many ways:

- Support of preparticipation screening
- Teaching of appropriate sport techniques
- Development of appropriate off-season and pre-season conditioning programs
- Adjustments of practices/competition based on weather and field conditions
- Support of proper hydration and nutrition principles
- Good working relationship with training staff and team physician

The coaching staff may be the single most important factor in promoting the confidence of athletes in the training staff and sports medicine team. The coaching staff can provide support of the sports medicine team by allowing for appropriate on-field and sideline evaluation and in supporting decisions made by the sports medicine team on return to play issues.

OFFICIATING/RULE ENFORCEMENT

Rules are developed to aid in the natural progression of athletic contests. Officials are responsible for administering the rules of a specific sport and ensuring a safe and equitable athletic environment. Officials should execute a pregame evaluation to ensure the overall safety of the competition. The pregame evaluation should include the following:

- Meeting with fellow officials
- Inspection of game and player equipment
- Inspecting the area of play
- Meeting with coaches and trainers to verify compliance with rules on specific equipment

Officials must ensure the safety of athletes by enforcing rules related to appropriate athletic techniques and execution. Injuries can result from improper athletic techniques such as spearing in football, high-sticking in hockey, and illegal holds in wrestling. It is the officials' responsibility to monitor for any improper techniques and enforce the rules accordingly. Officials can also promote safety for athletes in calling injury timeouts when appropriate, and allowing for stoppage of play for water breaks.

BALANCING COMPETITION

The concept of balancing competition can be of increased importance in the early adolescent age group. Differences in size, maturity, and skill level can lead to imbalanced competition, which can result in negative physical and psychological impact on the athlete. In high school athletics, there are different levels of competition available to athletes on the basis of age and ability. There are other examples of how to balance competition:

- Weight classes in wrestling
- Games pitched by coaches in little league baseball
- Running clocks or mercy rules in place when scores are one-sided
- Weight limit in youth football
- Administration of rules by officials to keep competition in balance

SUMMARY

Although injuries in sport are inevitable, they can be minimized in frequency and severity through a better understanding of their causes and occurrence, and application of the principles aimed at modifying those factors. The primary care sports medicine physician, as a key member of the multidisciplinary sports medicine team, is well positioned to champion an emphasis on injury prevention to ensure that athletes of all ages and disciplines participate in a safe and enjoyable environment.

REFERENCES

1. Hirata I. *The doctor and the athlete*. Philadelphia: JB Lippincott Co, 1974.
2. Heyward VH, Wagner DR. Body composition and athletes. In: *Applied body composition assessment*. Champaign, IL: Human Kinetics, 2004:159–173.
3. Terbizan DJ, Staiger S, DeBlauw C, et al. Driscoll, Sherri body composition measurement in college-age students: 1586 board #41 9:30 AM - 11:00 AM. *Med Sci Sports Exerc* 2005;37(Suppl. 5):S303.
4. Stransky FW. *The good news about nutrition, exercise and weight control*. Michigan: Momentum Books, Ltd., 2001.
5. McAdaragh GD, Janot JM, Vukovich MD. Accuracy of body composition methods in relation to hydrostatic weighing: a meta-analysis. *Med Sci Sports Exerc* 2004;36(Suppl. 5):S68–S69.
6. Brukner P, Khan K. *Clinical sports medicine*, 2nd ed. Australia: McGraw-Hill, 2000.
7. Reisman S, Walsh LD, Proske U. Warm-up stretches reduce sensations of stiffness and soreness after eccentric exercise. *Med Sci Sports Exerc* 2005;37(6):929–936.
8. Best TM, McCabe RP, Corr D Jr, et al. Evaluation of a new method to create a standardized muscle stretch injury. *Med Sci Sports Exerc* 1998;30(2):200–205.
9. Shrier I. Does stretching improve performance? A systematic and critical review of the literature. *Clin J Sport Med* 2004;14(5):267–273.

10. Hergenroeder AC. Prevention of sports injuries. *Pediatric* 1998;101:1057–1063.
11. Renstrom P, Kannus P. Prevention of sports injuries. In: Strauss RH, ed. *Sports medicine*, 2nd ed. Philadelphia: WB Saunders, 1991.
12. Kraemer WJ, Adams K, Cafarelli E, et al. Progression models in resistance training for healthy adults. *Med Sci Sports Exerc* 2002;34(2):364–380.
13. Kraemer WJ, Ratamess NA. Fundamentals of resistance training: progression and exercise prescription. *Med Sci Sports Exerc* 2004;36(4):674–688.
14. Gleeson N, Eston R, Marginson V, et al. Effects of prior concentric training on eccentric exercise induced muscle damage. *Br J Sports Med* 2003;37:119–125.
15. Crites BM. Ankle sprains. *Curr Opin Orthop* 2005;16(2):117–119.
16. Lephart SM, Pincivero DM, Giraldo JL, et al. The role of proprioception in the management and rehabilitation of athletic injuries. *Am J Sports Med* 1997;25:130–137.
17. Kokkonen J. Performance massage: muscle care for physically active people. *Human Kinet* 1993;17:53–83.
18. Kokkonen B. *The effects of sports massage on selected sports events*. Southwest Chapter of ACSM Conference Publication. November 15, 1996.
19. Marsh JS. Daigneault, John P. MD the young athlete. *Curr Opin Orthop* 2000;11(2):145–149.
20. Bauman J. Returning to play: the mind does matter. *Clin J Sports Med* 2005;15(6):432–435.
21. American College of Sports Medicine, American Dietetic Association, Dietitian of Canada. Joint position statement: nutrition and athletic performance. *Med Sci Sports Exerc* 2000;32:2130–2145.
22. Hew-Butler T, Verbalis JG, Noakes TD. Updated fluid recommendation: position statement from the International Marathon Medical Directors Association (IMMDA). *Clin J Sport Med* 2006;16(4):283–292.
23. Lombardo JA. Supplements and athletes. *South Med J* 2004;97(9):877–879.
24. NOCSAE. *Standard performance specification for recertified football helmets*. From http://www.nocsae.org/standards/documents.html.
25. Infection Control in Collegiate Wrestling. From www1.ncaa.org/ed_outre/health- safety.pdf, 06/06.
26. Kwikkel MA. Team hygiene and personal equipment. In: Mellion MB, Walsh WM, Shelton GL, eds. *The team physician's handbook*. St. Louis: Mosby, 1997.
27. Oliphant JA, Ryan MC, Chu A. Bacterial water quality in the personal water bottles of elementary students. *Can J Public Health* 2002;93(5):366–367.
28. Ballas MT, Tytko J, Cookson D. Common overuse running injuries: diagnosis and management. *Am Fam Physician* 1997;55(7):2473–2484.
29. National Safety Council. *Protect yourself: wear a helmet*. From http://www.nsc.org/library/facts/helmets.htm, 2004.
30. Roberts J. A program for fitting football shoulder pads. *Athl Purch Facil* 1982;6:16–20.
31. Teitz CC, Hermanson BK, Kronmal RA, et al. Evaluation of the use of braces to prevent injury to the knee in collegiate football players. *J Bone Joint Surg* 1987;69:2–9.
32. Frankovich RJ, Petrella RJ, Lattanzio CN. In-line skating injuries. Patterns and protective equipment use. *Phys Sportsmed* 2001;29:57–62.
33. Janda DH. The prevention of baseball and softball injuries. *Clin Orthop Relat Res* 2003;409:20–28.
34. Meuller FO, Marshall SW, Kirby DP. Injuries in little league baseball from 1987 through 1996. *Phys Sportsmed* 2001;29:41–48.
35. Theresa Pluth MSN, MPH, CRNP Heat Stroke. A comprehensive review. *AACN Clin Iss: Adv Pract Acute Crit Care* 2004;15(2):280–293.
36. American College of Sports Medicine position stand. Exercise and fluid replacement. *Med Sci Sports Exerc* 1996;28:i–vii.
37. Armstrong LE, Epstein Y, Greenleaf JE, et al. American College of Sports Medicine position stand. Heat and cold illnesses during distance running. *Med Sci Sports Exerc* 1996;25:i–x.
38. Stamford B. Smart dressing for cold weather workouts. *Phys Sportsmed* 1995;23:105–106.
39. Flynn RB. Sports surfaces. In: Mellion MB, Walsh WM, Shelton GL, eds. *The team physician's handbook*. St. Louis: Mosby, 1997.
40. Hart LE. Injury risk in men's university football. *Clin J Sport Med* 2003;13(6):386–387.

Covering Athletic Competition

9

Thomas R. Terrell James L. Moeller

Covering athletic events is one of the most enjoyable and important duties for a team physician. Most often this involves being on the sideline of an athletic event, be it a football game, swim meet, or basketball practice. Coach John Wooden of UCLA once said, "without adequate preparation, you prepare for failure." The same may be said for covering the sideline. Physicians must anticipate on-field emergencies and care for injuries on the sideline, while directing the appropriate transport of athletes.

Preparation for athletic event coverage begins long before the actual event, through meticulous planning and defining the roles of members of the sports medicine team. Coverage of events and competition will vary widely with different age groups, type of sports, and ability levels (recreational, high school, collegiate, professional, or international elite [Olympic level]). Sideline preparedness should anticipate the medical needs of the participating athletes, as well as provide on-site services and protocols for urgent and emergent medical care.

This chapter will focus on sideline/court coverage of contact and collision sports at the high school or collegiate level, as most team physicians function in this capacity. Essential elements required to promote athlete safety, provide excellent care at the competition site, and limit injury are reviewed. The critical interdependent roles of the sports medicine team—athletic trainer, team physician, emergency medical services (EMS) provider, coach, and consultants—are discussed in detail.

THE SPORTS MEDICINE TEAM

The sports medicine team includes both medically trained personnel and laypersons. The team physician is typically considered the leader of this team and is often ultimately responsible for the development of medical protocols and policies for the athletic organization. The athletic trainer perhaps serves the most pivotal role due to their consistent interaction with the athletes and other sports medicine team members. The roles of the various team members will be reviewed as well.

Role of the Athletic Trainer

A certified athletic trainer (ATC) is specially trained in the diagnosis, management, and rehabilitation of common musculoskeletal injuries in athletics. Owing to daily interaction with athletes and coaches, and regular communication with team doctors, consultants and team administrators, ATCs are central members of the sports medicine team. They continue to play a critical role in the initial on-the-field evaluation of the injured athlete at practice and games (1,2). They also facilitate communication between the other sports medicine team members.

ATCs manage musculoskeletal injuries, from initial diagnosis through treatment and rehabilitation. They are uniquely qualified in the use of modalities such as ice, ultrasound, electrical stimulation, as well as more advanced techniques such as proprioceptive neuromuscular facilitation or manual muscle therapy skills. In addition, ATCs provide general advice for treatment of common medical conditions, for example, "colds," viral upper respiratory infections, and so on. The ATC may counsel athletes on a number of important issues (3). A critical role played by the athletic trainer is in the area of injury prevention. ATCs also participate in screening for medical and orthopedic problems through the preparticipation examination (PPE) typically coordinated with the team physician.

Owing to the extensive time they spend working with athletes, ATCs are the most knowledgeable members of the sports medicine team regarding the personalities of athletes. The relationships they forge with athletes bolster the overall care and efficacy of a tailored rehabilitation plan. They are in an excellent position to informally counsel athletes about alcohol and drug issues, sexual activity, injury prevention and rehabilitation, nutrition, and eating disorders (3). More formal counseling is usually handled by the psychological consultant (4).

The ATC directs the medical coverage on the athletic playing field in most settings. It is important for the team physician and coach to support this role (2,5). Although it is true that the physician oversees most decisions off the field, the ATC is trained to evaluate and treat a plethora of conditions and injuries on the sideline and at practice.

In cases where inexperienced ATCs are covering an event, the physician may need to take a more proactive role in sideline coverage than is typically provided. Because the physician has the most expertise and training in the management of medical emergencies, the ATC should defer to the physician in emergency situations.

In summary, ATCs provide an invaluable resource for the total care of the athlete and functioning of the sports medicine team. We encourage institutions, beginning at least at the high school level, to have an ATC present at collision sporting events (e.g., football, soccer, wrestling). An ATC–team physician tandem provides the highest quality medical care for sports participants.

Role of the Team Physician

The team physician's role is critical to the overall success of the sports medicine team. The "Team Physician Consensus Statement" (6) describes the requirements for being a team physician. In addition the "Appropriate Sideline Medical Coverage," consensus statement (7) recommends an element of standardization of training and background for the budding team physician. Organizations and institutions seeking appropriate medical coverage can confidently refer to these documents for guidance on suitable qualifications for a team physician.

First of all, one must define the term *team physician* and delineate this role further. *"The team physician must have an unrestricted medical license and be an M.D. or D.O. who is responsible for treating and coordinating the medical care of athletic team members. The principal responsibility of the team physician is to provide for the well-being of individual athletes, enabling each to reach his/her full potential. The team physician should possess special proficiency in the care of musculoskeletal injuries and medical conditions encountered in sports. The team physician also must actively integrate medical expertise with other health care providers, including medical specialists, athletic trainers, and allied health professionals. The team physician must ultimately assume responsibility within the team structure for making medical decisions that affect the athlete's safe participation"* (6).

The many roles of the team physician are facilitated through building rapport with other members of the sports medicine team (5). It is vital that the team physician review the roles of the various team members with the entire team, so everyone understands their important position in the team. Attendance at practice and in the athletic training room helps to complete the role of the physician. Astute physicians understand the interplay of the different members of the sports medicine team and how to promote collaboration and synergy. Athletic team members are more comfortable sharing personal matters and feel more confident in the team physician's recommendations if he/she is seen as another "member of the team." By stepping away from the formal physician–patient interaction, white coat included, the physician actually integrates more effectively into the overall fabric of the athletic team.

The role of the team physician varies with the competitive level being covered, be it junior high school, high school, collegiate, professional, or elite. In addition, coverage of mass events such as marathons (8), triathlons (9), distance running events, or Special Olympic events requires different roles and responsibilities.

Role of the Coach

The role of the coach as part of the coverage team is significant as the team physician is not present at practice most of the time. Recent events such as the highly publicized heat stroke deaths of athletes have pushed coaches to the forefront of prevention of heat injuries (10). At the middle school or junior high school level, coaches are often the first to evaluate an athletic injury.

The coaches of most sports at the high school and college levels have a powerful influence over the behavior of the athletes and their motivation to pursue healthy lifestyle behaviors (11). A coach can make huge inroads on ensuring proper nutrition for their players. Core requirements for coaching include certification in basic cardiac life support (BCLS), sports nutrition, proper training and conditioning methods, prevention and basic recognition of heat illness, and the potential hazards of dietary and nutritional supplements. Formal first aid training is certainly recommended. If an athletic trainer is not at practice and an athlete has a history of anaphylaxis to insect venom, the coach should be appropriately trained in the proper use of an EpiPen.

The team physician or local community physician may educate coaches through presentations on topics relevant to their particular sport. For instance, education of coaches on the signs and symptoms of eating disorders in sports such as gymnastics is critical to achieve early detection of this enigmatic problem. The coach needs to appreciate the adverse role that subtle messages, often sent by the coaching staff, concerning the perceived relation between performance and body weight, can have. This can facilitate or spawn the development of eating disorders. By providing educational conferences on topics that coaches find relevant, the physician builds rapport in a less intense environment.

The coach should have a close working relationship with the athletic trainer at the high school, collegiate, or professional level. Communication between these parties is imperative, and respect for the decision making of the athletic trainer and physician on medical issues must be maintained. Under no circumstance is a coach to make isolated medical decisions for athletes or shop for other more desired opinions on care. The coach must understand the "return to play (RTP)" philosophy of the physician and respect it.

Ultimate decisions on RTP after injury or illness always reside with the physician, and part of this duty is to share the diagnosis and RTP considerations with the ATC and coach. Communication with the coach about an athlete's progress, current limitations in his/her play, and the expected time course to partial and full recovery provides the necessary information for the coach to plan his/her practice and game strategy. It is advisable for the physician to discuss recommendations with the ATC, administrator (athletic director [AD] or school principal in high school) and, when age appropriate, parent.

Role of Emergency Medical Services

In many states, it is required for EMS personnel to be present for high school collision sporting events such as football. In states where this is not required, many schools still opt to have EMS on-site for these events. In situations where there is no ATC or team physician present, EMS serves as the on-field responder to injuries. The role of EMS in this situation is to provide first aid care in the case of minor injury, and to stabilize and transport patients in the case of severe injury. There is much debate as to whether EMS personnel should make RTP decisions in this situation.

The role of EMS is significantly different when an ATC and/or team physician is present for the athletic contest. In this situation, EMS is present to provide support to the ATC and team doctor, and to transport injured players to appropriate medical facilities when called to do so. In most cases, they are also the primary responder to spectator medical issues. In this situation, EMS personnel should not respond to on-field injuries unless requested to do so by the ATC or team physician. These protocols must be reviewed so all members of the medical team understand and perform their roles appropriately. When these roles are not defined and understood, the care of the injured athlete suffers.

Role of the Athletic Director

The AD represents the central administration within the sports medicine team. It is imperative that the sideline physician have a professional working relationship with the AD, which reinforces the overall directive of the sports medicine team: to care for student-athletes at all phases of their participation and to make the preservation of the health and safety of all participants the primary goal of this team.

At all interscholastic and intercollegiate levels, the AD shares the responsibility of overseeing the sports medicine program in collaboration with a team physician and athletic trainer. Regardless of the level of participation, the AD should not attempt to pressure, directly or indirectly, the sideline physician into making medical judgments that benefit the school or organization and put the athlete at risk. Conversely, the team physician must appreciate the vulnerability of the institution to potential medicolegal damage through the unwarranted participation of an athlete at increased risk for injury, illness, or death due to athletic participation.

RECOMMENDED "EQUIPMENT" FOR THE TEAM PHYSICIAN

The necessary equipment for the team physician includes far more than a stethoscope. This section will discuss the educational training needs of a team doctor and will also discuss recommendations for the medical team "game bag."

A team physician must possess a fundamental knowledge of emergency care regarding sporting events and have a working knowledge of trauma, musculoskeletal injuries, and medical conditions that affect the athlete (5). Primary care physicians are uniquely qualified to serve as team physicians because of this. Many primary care trained physicians continue their medical training by completing accredited sports medicine fellowships upon completion of their primary training (12). After successful completion of a fellowship, the physician is eligible to test for and receive a Certificate of Added Qualification (CAQ) in Sports Medicine. The American Medical Association essentially considers this CAQ to be a subspecialty certification.

A team physician, however, need not be a fellowship trained sports medicine specialist. He/she needs to be interested in helping the community, enthusiastic, available, and knowledgeable. In fact, most community-based team physicians have no formal sports medicine training.

The "Medical Bag" and Sideline Supplies

The sideline physicians should always carry their own set of supplies—the "medical bag"—when covering an event (4,7,13–18). Different schools of thought exist on the amount and type of medical supplies, equipment and medication the team physician should have available in the team physician's bag (4,7,14–17).

The contents of the team physician bag may be altered as needed, based on the sport, age of participants, location, presence of ancillary personnel at an event, weather conditions, and whether spectator coverage is part of the physician's coverage duties. In many cases,

TABLE 9.1

RECOMMENDED MEDICAL SUPPLIES FOR CONTACT/COLLISION SPORT COVERAGE AND THE PARTY THAT COMMONLY PROVIDES THE VARIOUS ITEMS

Physician	ATC	Facility/School
Stethoscope	Trainer's Angel (Riverside, CA)	AED
Thermometer (digital) tympanic with an extra battery	Tape (cloth paper tape, athletic tape)	Spine board
Sphygmomanometer with appropriate size cuffs	Bandage scissors	Cervical collars
Oto/ophthalmoscope	Intravenous fluids (D5 LR or D5 1/2 NS—several bags of LR or NS)	Communication devices
Reflex hammer	IV fluid set-up kits	Emergency airway equipment
Penlight with cobalt blue filter	Angiocaths (18, 20, and 22 gauge)	Transport vehicle (e.g., extended golf cart)
Scissors	Sharps container	
Bandages	Biohazard bags	
Sterile/nonsterile gloves	Splints	
Syringes and needles	Digits	
Sharps container	Full and partial extremity	
Isopropyl alcohol	Crutches	
Betadine		
Sterile gauze		
Sterile saline		
Eye injury kit		
Eye irrigating solution (saline)		
Fluoroscein strips		
Hard eye shield for globe injury		
Eyepatches		
Skin injury kit		
suture kits and suture removal kits		
Steri-strips		
Dermabond laceration treatment		
Antibiotic ointment		

ATC = certified athletic trainer; AED = automatic external defibrillators; LR = lactated ringers; NS = normal saline.

ATCs, institutions, and specific facilities provide many of the recommended supplies for the coverage of various events. The team physician is not responsible for providing all medical supplies. For collision sports, the supplies recommended are detailed in Table 9.1. This list is merely a suggested set of supplies and equipment and is not meant to be a fixed requirement (7,15).

The ideal bag would be divided into individual compartments for organized storage and quick access to needed items (see Figure 9.1). Organization of the bag with labels, and perhaps a list of contents attached to the top, inside cover of the bag, assists individuals less familiar with its contents. A lock may be helpful, particularly if medications are stored. A copy of the medical license and DEA certificate of the doctor is advised if narcotic pain medications are carried. Because of the increased risk of theft of narcotic medications, we do not recommend carrying them in the bag.

In short, the physician should stock his/her bag with any piece of medical equipment he/she feels might be needed to treat common injuries or medical conditions encountered on the field of play. Many physicians and trainers will not only carry a large medical bag, but will stock a small shoulder bag or fanny pack with commonly used items such as gauze, tape, scissors, and bandages.

Emergency equipment should also be available, such as spine boards and cervical immobilization equipment, airway supplies, automated external defibrillators, and large splints for extremity injuries. Because of the size and expense of much of the emergency equipment, this equipment should be kept permanently at the sports venue and should be supplied by the institution or sports organization. Together, the team physician, ATC, and the institution should provide the needed equipment and supplies to respond to almost any emergency situation.

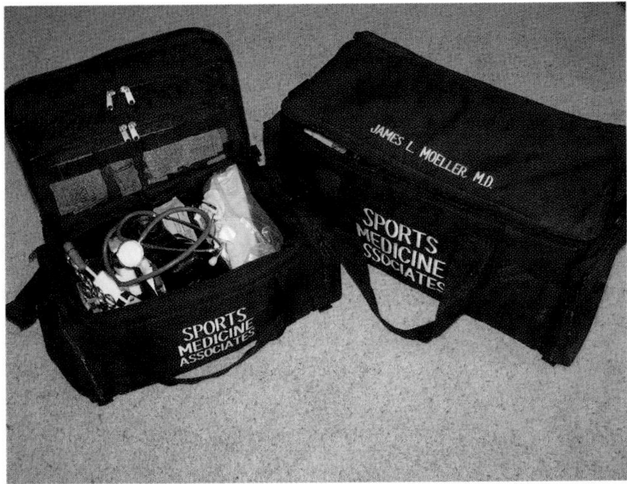

Figure 9.1 The inside and outside of a team medical bag.

Medications for Physician's Bag

Carrying any medications in the team physician's bag is a matter of great debate (7,16,17). The sideline treatment of a high school athlete is limited by the fact that the athlete usually is a minor and parental consent is required for administration of medications. This may create challenging situations because the parents must consent to administration of medications (15). Many physicians who cover high school events choose not to stock prescription medications for this reason (17). The issue of parental consent for administration of medications exists infrequently at the collegiate, professional, and elite levels, so team physicians in this setting are more likely to stock medications in their game bags.

When traveling domestically or internationally with a team, it is helpful to carry a more extensive supply of medications. Each practitioner should choose the medications with which he/she is comfortable. It is critically important that the physician not assume that the first aid kit available at the home, school, or travel destination will have adequate medications and supplies (16–18).

Certain guidelines should be followed in administering medications on the sideline. Physicians must appropriately follow federal and state regulatory guidelines.

Pharmacists are often affiliated with university sports programs to oversee this process (17). Accurate documentation of dispensed medications, both prescription and over the counter, provides an important historical record of medications administered. The list of medications in Table 9.2 provides guidelines for the reader, but by no means represents an all-inclusive list.

Medications commonly used to treat medical conditions may be banned by sports organizations such as the National Collegiate Athletic Association or International Olympic Committee (4,15). Physicians must take great care not to provide any substance to athletes that may lead to their disqualification. The U.S. Anti-Doping Agency provides a telephone hotline and helpful website (www.usantidoping.org).

TABLE 9.2
MEDICATION CLASSES THAT A TEAM PHYSICIAN SHOULD CONSIDER CARRYING IN THE "GAME BAG"

Oral decongestants
Antihistamines
Nasal decongestants
Nasal steroid preparations (e.g., fluticasone)
Non narcotic cough medications (e.g., Robitussin DM, Benzoate Perles)
Guaifenesin
Narcotic cough medications (e.g., codeine phosphate 10 mg, Tussionex, Robitussin DAC)
Inhaled bronchodilators
Inhaled steroid preparations
Other inhaled medications (e.g., cromolyn sodium)
Eye preparations—antibiotic eye drops and ointments, cycloplegics (e.g., cyclopentolate), anesthetic eye drop
EpiPen (two)
Gastrointestinal preparations—loperamide, Imodium, magnesium hydroxide, Pepto-Bismol, H_2 blocker; possibly proton pump inhibitors
Topical antibiotic creams (mupirocin 2% (Bactroban), neosporin) and cortisone creams (hydrocortisone 2.5%, triamcinolone 0.025% and 0/1%; high potency steroid cream), nystatin cream, lamisil cream
Ear medications—antibiotic drops (e.g., Tobrex, Cortisporin otic suspension) and anesthetic drops (e.g., Otocaine drops)
Broad spectrum antibiotics to cover standard infections, mostly respiratory (clarithromycin, azithromycin, ciprofloxacin, doxycycline, amoxicillin, cephalexin, amoxicillin-clavulanate)
Nonsteroidal anti-inflammatory medications
Acetaminophen
Lidocaine 1% with and without epinephrine for injections
Short acting glucocorticoid steroid for injections
Glucose gel or ampule of glucagon, (ampule of D50 in Banyan kit)
Bioterrorism preparation kit (ciprofloxacillin 500 mg 10 d supply and doxycycline 100 mg 60-d supply) syringe of atropine

ATC = certified athletic trainer; AED = automatic external defibrillators.
Source: Adapted from Buettner CM. The team physician's bag. *Clin Sports Med* 1998;2:365–373.

Automatic external defibrillators (AEDs) deserve special mention as their role in sports medicine coverage has increased. No mandatory recommendation for AEDs has been issued to date. Early studies on AED use in the college setting showed that resuscitation of college-aged athletes who experienced sudden cardiac arrest (SCA) was unlikely (none successful out of nine attempts) compared to the resuscitation of coaches, officials, or adult spectators (19,20). An NCAA-sponsored study on the utility and benefit of AEDs in treating SCA in athletes is ongoing. An AED remains a recommended piece of equipment for high school, collegiate, and professional sporting event coverage (21). For coverage of a mass event such as a marathon, AED access should be standard equipment.

In 2006, an inter-association task force issued a consensus statement regarding emergency preparedness and management of SCA in high school and college athletic programs (21). The goal of the statement is to assist programs in preparing for this emergency and in becoming familiar with the standardized treatment protocols. The recommendations of this task force are summarized in Table 9.3 (21).

PREPARATION FOR SIDELINE COVERAGE

"Sideline preparedness is the identification of and planning for medical services to promote the safety of the athlete, to limit injury, and to provide medical care at the site of practice or competition" (7). It is critically important

TABLE 9.3

RECOMMENDATIONS OF THE INTER-ASSOCIATION TASK FORCE ON EMERGENCY PREPAREDNESS AND MANAGEMENT OF SUDDEN CARDIAC ARREST IN HIGH SCHOOL AND COLLEGE ATHLETIC PROGRAMS

Emergency preparedness

- Every school or institution that sponsors athletic activities should have a written and structured EAP
- The EAP should be developed and coordinated in consultation with local EMS personnel, school public safety officials, on-site first responders, and school administrators
- The EAP should be specific to each athletic venue and encompass emergency communication, personnel, equipment, and transportation to appropriate emergency facilities
- The EAP should be reviewed and practiced at least annually with certified athletic trainers, team and attending physicians, athletic training students, school and institutional safety personnel, administrators, and coaches (6)
- Targeted first responders should receive certified training in CPR and AED use
- Access to early defibrillation is essential and a target goal of <3–5 min from the time of collapse to the first shock is strongly recommended (5,7)
- Review of equipment readiness and the EAP by on-site event personnel for each athletic event is desirable

Management of sudden cardiac arrest

- Management begins with appropriate emergency preparedness, CPR, and AED training for all likely first responders, and access to early defibrillation
- Essential components of SCA management include early activation of EMS, early CPR, early defibrillation, and rapid transition to advanced cardiac life support
- High suspicion of SCA should be maintained for any collapsed and unresponsive athlete
- SCA in athletes can be mistaken for other causes of collapse and rescuers should be trained to recognize SCA in athletes, with special focus on potential barriers to recognizing SCA, including inaccurate rescuer assessment of pulse or respirations, occasional or agonal gasping, and myoclonic or seizure-like activity
- Young athletes who collapse shortly after being struck in the chest by a firm projectile or by contact with another player should be suspected of having SCA from commotio cordis
- Any collapsed and unresponsive athlete should be managed as a SCA with application of an AED as soon as possible for rhythm analysis and defibrillation if indicated
- CPR should be provided while waiting for an AED
- Interruptions in chest compressions should be minimized and CPR stopped only for rhythm analysis and shock
- CPR should be resumed immediately after the first shock, beginning with chest compressions, with repeat rhythm analysis following 2 min or five cycles of CPR, or until advanced life support providers take over or the victim starts to move
- Rapid access to the SCA victim should be facilitated for EMS personnel

EAP = emergency action plan; AED = automatic external defibrillators; SCA = sudden cardiac arrest; CPR = cardiopulmonary resuscitation; EMS = emergency medical services.

Source: Adapted from Mellion M, Walsh MW. Medical supervision of the athlete: the team physician. In: Mellion M, Walsh MW, Shelton GL, eds. *The team physician's handbook,* 2nd ed. Philadelphia: Hanley and Belfus, 1997;1–7.

Courson R, Drezner J. *Inter-association task force recommendations on emergency preparedness and management of sudden cardiac arrest in high school and college athletic programs: consensus statement. Executive summary.* National Athletic Training Association, http://www.nata.org/statements/consensus/sca_executive_summary.pdf. 2006.)

to discuss and establish emergency medical protocols for management of life-threatening orthopedic and medical problems far in advance of game day (4,5,7,17,22–25). Preparation can be divided into two broad categories: "preseason" and "game day."

Pre-season is the ideal time to have the medical team meet and review individual and team roles as well as review and practice emergency protocols. This can help identify problems that should be resolved before the start of the season and/or actual emergency. This is also an appropriate time for the team physician and trainer to communicate with the entire coaching staff, team members, and parents, and review the goals of the sports medical team. A list of preseason preparation recommendations is included in Table 9.4 (26).

Game day preparations vary from checking field and environmental conditions to evaluating athletes for clearance before competition. Recommended game-day preparations are noted in Table 9.5. Other game day duties of the ATC and team physician include evaluation and management of illnesses and injuries on game day.

Response to in-game injuries requires that a "chain of command" be established for response to the injured athlete. In most high school, collegiate, or professional sports settings, the chain of command dictates that the injured player is first evaluated by the ATC (2,5,25). This practice helps keep order in the delivery of sports medicine care (2). If the trainer requires assistance, he/she should summon the physician either to come onto the playing field or to the team bench to assist with evaluation. In most instances, it is standard practice for the physician to stand ready to assist until summoned by the ATC. This approach will vary depending on the level of experience of the ATC and medical situation or injury. For instance, a student trainer may require more immediate assistance. There are certain circumstances in which the physician would be

TABLE 9.4

PRESEASON PREPARATION CHECKLIST FOR THE TEAM PHYSICIAN

Establish and coordinate a group of medical personnel and administrators devoted to preseason planning and preparticipation examinations
Establish a chain of command for handling of emergencies "on" and "off" the field
Rehearse the management of the common emergency situations and review medical and administrative protocols
Develop and post a written emergency plan in the training room and game site to assist in the speedy transport of critically injured/ill athletes to an identified emergency facility. This plan should include the following information:
Physical location (street address and cross-streets) of the school or venue
Floor, field (e.g., baseball diamond, football field, gymnasium, etc.)
Building name
Telephone number (with any prefix) to activate "911"
Regularly rehearse the emergency management plan
Establish a network of health care providers and facilities to function with the sports medicine team
Prepare a physician "medical bag" stocked with appropriate supplies and equipment for sideline coverage (may or may not include medications)
Meet with coaching staffs and administrators to review the roles of the various members of the sports medicine team

Source: Adapted from Anderson J, Courson RW, Kleiner DM, McLoda TA. National Athletic Trainer's Association position statement: emergency planning in athletics. *J Athl Train* 2002; 37:99–104.

TABLE 9.5

GAME DAY PREPARATION CHECK LIST FOR THE TEAM PHYSICIAN

Arrive at venue with sufficient time for all pregame preparations
Assess playing conditions including conditions of the venue and field of play itself, along with environmental conditions
Introduce self to the medical staff of the opposing team and review emergency protocols
Introduce self to game officials
Review of the emergency medical response plan with your medical team
Check and confirm functionality of medical and communication equipment
Identify examination and treatment sites
Meet with ambulance personnel and access their capabilities and equipment as well as your expectations regarding on-field chain of command
Provide final clearance for participation of injured or ill athletes on game day before competition (this may need to be done several hours before the game)
Choose a sideline location that gives clear visibility of the game action with quick ready access to the field of play
Assess game-day injuries and medical problems
Document care provided
Determine same-game return to play status of injured or ill athletes
Perform postgame review and make necessary modifications of medical and administrative protocols

Source: Adapted from the Sideline Preparedness Consensus Statement, American Medical Society for Sports Medicine, American Academy of Orthopaedic Surgeons, American Academy of Osteopathic Sports Medicine, American Academy of Pediatrics, American College of Sports Medicine. Sideline Preparedness for the Team Physician-A Consensus Statement. *Am J Sports Med* 2000;3:440–441.

remiss in not playing a more assertive role in the care of a severely injured athlete on the field.

At the conclusion of the season, the physician should meet with the medical team and evaluate all facets of sideline coverage and preparedness, particularly the administrative and clinical protocols. This post-season assessment serves to improve the performance of the sports medicine team in future seasons.

SPECIAL SPORTS COVERAGE SETTINGS

International Events

Traveling with a team to an international event presents unique challenges for a team physician (27). Each international event requires a great deal of preparation by the physician for the coverage to be successful. It requires more disciplined research into the medical facilities and capabilities of the host country and competition site. The physician and ATC should not assume that the host country will provide the necessary equipment and supplies for adequate medical coverage of the event (27). The physician must maintain a positive attitude and strong working interaction with the players and other members of the team.

Mass Participation Events

Sports medicine physicians participate in the coverage of mass events such as marathons or triathlons (9,28). Owing to the physical layout of the course and length of the event, the coverage of endurance events presents many logistical challenges to the sports doctor. The nature of medical care provided at an endurance event varies on the basis of the type of activity, scale of race, terrain, intensity of activity, and physical condition of the participants. For mass participation events, additional roles such as safety, disaster management for spectators and racers (29), and injury prevention can be part of the duties of the medical management team (30,31). A list of "essential" and "desired" medical care delivery and hydration/energy replacement needs are summarized in Table 9.6 (8).

Ideally, the medical director serves on the executive board of the race committee. For these events, excellent planning and preparation is critical for successful coverage. From this position, the medical director can best serve as an advocate for the health and safety of the participants. The chain of authority for medical and health decisions for pre-event planning and race day must be clearly established. The medical director should be allowed to make this decision

TABLE 9.6
ESSENTIAL AND DESIRED MEDICAL CARE AND HYDRATION/ENERGY REPLACEMENT NEEDS FOR MASS PARTICIPATION EVENTS

	Essential	Desired
Medical care delivery needs	Basic first aid	Early defibrillation
	CPR	Advanced cardiac and trauma life support
	Event specific medical care	IV fluid administration for non life-threatening illness
	Event specific musculoskeletal care	Hyper- and hypothermia evaluation and initial care
		Hyponatremia evaluation and initial care
Hydration/energy replacement needs	Provide fluids for competitors, medical team, and support staff	Cool fluids to 59°F–72°F (15°C–22.22°C) for optimal palatability and absorption
	Provide additional fluid choices containing carbohydrates and sodium for events involving continuous activity lasting >1 hr	Publish the fluid types and location before the event
	Encourage participants to replace sweat losses during activity and replace weight loss postevent	Utilize carbohydrate and salt solutions containing the following for optimal palatability and absorption:
		25–50 mmol/L sodium, 2%–8% carbohydrate for pre-event and event
		50–100 mmol/L sodium postevent (with normal diet)

CPR = cardiopulmonary resuscitation.
Source: Adapted from Herring SA, Bergfeld JA, Boyajian-O'Neill LA, et al. Mass participation event management for the team physician: a consensus statement. *Med Sci Sports Exerc* 2004;36:2004–2008.

TABLE 9.7

ADMINISTRATIVE DUTIES OF THE MEDICAL DIRECTOR OF A MASS PARTICIPATION EVENT

Essential Duties	Desirable Additional Duties
Develop an agreement concerning medical care and administrative responsibilities between the medical team and the organizing body	Organize the medical team at least 6 mo before the event
Assess potential environmental conditions and site and event risk factors	Schedule the event when historical environmental conditions are the most favorable
Organize the medical team before the event	Schedule the start time to accommodate the safest start and finish times for elite through novice competitors
Notify police, fire and rescue departments, and emergency medical facilities regarding the time, location, and access to the event and the expected number of casualties	Develop a tracking system so family members can find injured or ill participants
Develop and communicate medical protocols to include directing acute on-site care, determining who needs to be transported, as well as limits to participation or return to play	Conduct a postevent review of the medical care, administrative plan, and budget
Plan for operations, transportation, communication, and command and control	Review and analyze event injury, illness, and environmental data
Develop an adverse event protocol for deaths or catastrophic illness or injuries that addresses confidentiality, medical reporting, and public disclosure	Prepare a summary report
Adhere to the principles of Health Insurance Portability and Accountability Act (HIPAA)	
Develop and maintain medical and event records	
Follow modified universal precautions protocol for the handling and disposal of body fluids and contaminated medical waste and all other principles of OSHA standards	
Confirm and adhere to medical policies of applicable governing bodies	
Provide all-area access credentials to the medical team	

OSHA = occupational safety and health administration.

without undue influence or pressure from corporate sponsors or race directors. Other administrative duties of the medical director are listed in Table 9.7.

CONCLUSION

Coverage of sporting events presents a unique challenge and great responsibility to the physician. Preparation for the administrative issues and medical care begins much before game day. In addition, development of medical protocols and coordination of the medical team significantly increases the likelihood of successful sports coverage. The coach, team or school administration, athletic trainer, and physician work synergistically to improve athlete safety and reduce the risk of injury. Game day protocols involve the development of a well-stocked medical bag with appropriate sideline medical equipment, as well as thoughtful and efficient evaluation of injured and ill athletes.

REFERENCES

1. Howard K. The role of the athletic trainer. In: Baker C, Flandry F, Henderson JM, eds. *The Hughston clinic sportsmedicine book*. Baltimore: Williams & Wilkins, 1995:5–6.
2. Hunter SC. Coverage of games and events. In: Baker C, Flandry F, Henderson JM, eds. *The Hughston clinic sportsmedicine book*. Baltimore: Williams & Wilkins, 1995:9–11.
3. Ray R, Terrell T, Hough DO. Introduction to the counseling role: the role of the sports medicine professional in counseling athletes. In: Ray R, Wiese-Bjornstal DM, eds. *Counseling in sports medicine*. Champaign, IL: Human Kinetics Press, 1999:1–20.
4. Terrell T, Leski M. Sports medicine. In: Rakel R, ed. *Textbook of family medicine*, 5th ed. Philadelphia: WB Saunders Co, 2002:845–890.
5. Mellion M, Walsh MW. Medical supervision of the athlete: the team physician. In: Mellion M, Walsh MW, Shelton GL, eds. *The team physician's handbook*, 2nd ed. Philadelphia: Hanley and Belfus, 1997:1–7.
6. American Medical Society for Sports Medicine, American Academy of Orthopaedic Surgeons, American Academy of Osteopathic Sports Medicine, American Academy of Pediatrics, American College of Sports Medicine. Team physician consensus statement. *Am J Sports Med* 2000;3:440–441. Also at http://www.amssm.org.
7. American Medical Society for Sports Medicine, American Academy of Orthopaedic Surgeons, American Academy of Osteopathic Sports Medicine, American Academy of Pediatrics, American College of Sports Medicine. Sideline preparedness for the team physician-a consensus statement. *Am J Sports Med* 2000;3:440–441.
8. Herring SA, Bergfeld JA, Boyajian-O'Neill LA, et al. Mass participation event management for the team physician: a consensus statement. *Med Sci Sports Exerc* 2004;36:2004–2008.

9. Martinez JA, Laird R. Managing triathlon competition. *Curr Sports Med Rep* 2003;2:142–146.
10. Bergeron M, McKeag D, Casa DJ, et al. American College of Sports Medicine scientific roundtable. Youth football: heat stress and injury risk. *Med Sci Sports Exerc* 2005;37:1421–1430.
11. Gallaspy JB Jr, May JD. Coaching and its role in injury prevention. In: Mellion M, Walsh MW, Shelton GL, eds. *The team physician's handbook*, 2nd ed. Philadelphia: Hanley and Belfus, 1997; 10–12.
12. American Medical Society for Sports Medicine. *What is a sports medicine physician?* Overland Park, Kansas: http://http://www.newamssm.org/whatis.pdf. Accessed on August 15, 2006.
13. Rubin A. Emergency equipment: what to keep on the sidelines. *Phys Sportsmed* 1993;9:47–54.
14. Araujo D, Rubin A. Instituting the updated CPR protocol:the team physician's role. *Phys Sportsmed* 1994;22:51–56.
15. Buettner CM. The team physician's bag. *Clin Sports Med* 1998;2:365–373.
16. Daniels JM, Kary J, Lane JA. Optimizing the sideline medical bag. *Phys Sportsmed* 2005;12.
17. Yan CB, Rubin AL. Equipment and supplies for sports and event medicine. *Curr Sports Med Rep* 2005;4:131–136.
18. Leonard JC, Townsend HE. Ready, set, go!; Sports medicine on and off the field. *Postgrad Med* 1996;5:237–243.
19. Drezner JA, Rogers KJ. Sudden cardiac arrest in intercollegiate athletes: detailed analysis and outcomes of resuscitation in nine cases. *Heart Rhythm* 2006;7:755–759.
20. Drezner JA. Practical guidelines for automated external defibrillators in the athletics setting. *Clin J Sp Med* 2005;5:367–369.
21. Courson R, Drezner J. *Inter-Association Task Force Recommendations on emergency preparedness and management of sudden cardiac arrest in high school and college athletic programs: consensus statement. Executive Summary*. National Athletic Training Association, http://www.nata.org/statements/consensus/sca_executive_summary.pdf. 2006.
22. Howe WB. The team physician. *Prim Care* 1991;4:763–775.
23. Allman FL, Crow RW. On-field evaluation of sports injuries. In: Griffin LY, ed. *Orthopaedic knowledge update: sports medicine*, Rosemont, IL: American Academy of Orthopaedic Surgeons, 1994:141–149.
24. Brown DW. Medical issues associated with international competition. Guidelines for the traveling physician. *Clin Sports Med* 1998;17:739–754, vi.
25. Shah S, Luftman JP, Vigil DV. Football: sideline management of injuries. *Curr Sports Med Rep* 2004;1:145–153.
26. Anderson J, Courson RW, Kleiner DM, et al. National Athletic Trainer's Association position statement: emergency planning in athletics. *J Athl Train* 2002;37:99–104.
27. Cook J, Harcourt P. Traveling with a team. In: Brukner P, Khan K, eds. *Clinical sports medicine*. New York: McGraw-Hill, 2000:855–864.
28. Grange JT. Sideline and event management: planning for large events. *Curr Sports Med Rep* 2002;3:156–161.
29. Rubin AL. Safety, security, and preparing for disaster at sporting events. *Curr Sports Med Rep* 2004;3:141–145.
30. Noakes T. Medical coverage of endurance events. In: Brukner P, Kahn K, eds. *Clinical sports medicine*, 2nd ed. New York: McGraw-Hill, 2000:865–871.
31. Scott WA, Roberts WO. Medical coverage of endurance events. In: Garrett WE Jr, Kirkendall DT, Squire DL, eds. *Principles and practice of primary care sports medicine*. Philadelphia: Lippincott Williams & Wilkins, 2001:33–46.

SUGGESTED ADDITIONAL READINGS

Individual coverage of different types of sporting events are described in each of the following articles below.

Bugbee S, Knopp WD. Medical coverage of tennis events. *Curr Sports Med Rep* 2006;5:131–134.

Grange JT, Cotton A. Motorsports medicine. *Curr Sports Med Rep* 2004;3:134–140.

Honsik K, Boyd A, Rubin AL. Sideline splinting, bracing, and casting of extremity injuries. *Curr Sports Med Rep* 2003;2:147–154.

Jaworkski C. Medical concerns of marathons. *Curr Sports Med Rep* 2005;3:137–143.

Khalilli-Borna D, Honsik K. Wrestling and Sports Medicine. *Curr Sports Med Rep* 2005;3:144–149.

Meredith R, Butcher J. Field splinting of suspected fractures: preparation, assessment, and application. *Phys Sportsmed* 1997;10:29–42.

Pendergraph B, Ko B, Zamora J, et al. Medical coverage for track and field events. *Curr Sports Med Rep* 2005;4:150–153.

Stovitz SD, Satin DJ. Professionalism and ethics of the sideline physician. *Curr Sports Med Rep* 2006;5:120–124.

Stuart MJ. On-field examination and care: an emergency checklist. *Phy Sp Med* 1998;11:51–55.

Tucker A. Ethics and the professional team physician. *Clin Sports Med* 2004;23:227–241.

3
Clinical Sports Medicine

Management of On-site Emergencies

10

Brent S.E. Rich *Benjamin B. Betteridge* *Spencer E. Richards*

EMERGENCIES!!! By the very nature of the word, these are events that are "unexpected." Although unexpected, they should not be *unanticipated.* Anticipation of potential emergencies is the responsibility of the Sports Medicine Team. Preseason and preparticipation preparation is the time to identify the potential emergencies that may affect the involved sport and to plan accordingly. Although crippling or fatal events in sports are rare, this does not lessen the need for preparation and development of an emergency action plan.

Initial evaluation and triage is the first principle in emergency treatment. Rapid recognition will determine the need for either emergency response or routine management. Often, this initial management decides the ultimate outcome. If the Sports Medicine Team rehearses roles and responsibilities, it will go a long way to develop comfort and control in the chaotic moments of an emergency.

Included in the preparation for emergencies is the development of specific written emergency protocols. These include roles and responsibilities of the various members of the Sports Medicine Team, obtaining contact numbers for each member, and understanding how to mobilize the Emergency Medical System (EMS) in your area. Working with the local EMS providers and emergency room staffs in standardizing protocols is crucial to the systematic management of emergencies in sport. We must be cautious not to assume that emergency procedures will go smoothly when the time arises, but foresee and minimize the potential logistical problems that may impair proper treatment.

In this chapter, initial evaluation of the collapsed athlete will be presented, followed by a review of on-site emergencies from an organ system perspective (i.e., head and neck, musculoskeletal, cardiac, respiratory) and a discussion of life-threatening heat stroke. Additional non-emergent conditions in each of these areas will be reviewed in more detail in subsequent chapters. Finally, an outline for an emergency action plan will be presented.

ON-SITE MANAGEMENT OF THE COLLAPSED ATHLETE

The purpose of being an on-site or sideline member of the Sports Medicine team is to witness the mechanism of injury or trauma and implement the appropriate management steps. *Was contact or collision involved in the collapse? Did the collapse occur during activity or after the play was over? Does this emergency require additional providers or transport to appropriately manage the event?*

The on-site physician is responsible for the management of the athletic contest, although the athletic trainer is often the first person to triage and interact with the downed athlete. If the team physician is absent, the athletic trainer or the most qualified person present takes charge of the emergency. Mobilization of the EMS system by dialing 911 may be necessitated based on the situation. The initial evaluation includes a primary and secondary ABCD survey and can be done within the first few seconds of arriving on the scene. Stopping play and removing the athlete or other participants from ongoing danger is the next immediate responsibility.

The Primary Survey is performed quickly and in the following order:

1. Level of responsiveness (AVPU)
   a. A = alert
   b. V = responds to verbal stimuli
   c. P = responds to painful stimuli

d. U = unresponsive
e. If the patient is unresponsive, call for help or call 911
2. A = Airway
3. B = Breathing
4. C = Circulation
5. For a cardiopulmonary emergency, the fifth step is D = Defibrillation
6. E = Exposure

The Secondary Survey includes the following:

1. A = Advanced airway
2. B = Breathing
3. C = Circulation
4. D = Differential diagnosis

THE PRIMARY ABCD SURVEY

The initial assessment must follow an organized system of review. The **ABCD** mnemonic is the recommended triage assessment tool. (The 2005 Revised basic life support [BLS] guidelines are provided in Table 10.1)

AIRWAY AND CERVICAL SPINE

1. Look and listen for spontaneous breathing. If the patient is face-down and spontaneous breathing cannot be assessed, logroll the patient onto his/her back while immobilizing the cervical spine by gentle in-line traction. Competent assistance is crucial to keep the head and neck in proper alignment. If the neck is not in line with the body, gentle traction should be instituted to place in a neutral position. If this increases pain or causes neurological or circulatory compromise or resistance is detected, maintaining in the position found is acceptable until hospital evaluation. Exceptions are in the inability to establish an airway.
2. Establish airway access. If necessary, remove the face mask using appropriate tools. Be careful not to disrupt the neck.
3. Institute the *head-tilt, chin-lift,* or *jaw-thrust* maneuver. These maneuvers open the airway. The jaw-thrust maneuver is the safest method inasmuch as it does

TABLE 10.1
SUMMARY OF BLS ABCD MANEUVERS FOR INFANTS, CHILDREN, AND ADULTS

Maneuver	Adult Lay Rescuer: 8 yr HCP: Adolescent and Older	Child Lay Rescuers: 1–8 yr HCP: 1 Year to Adolescent	Infant Under 1 yr of Age
Airway	Head tilt–chin lift (HCP: suspected trauma, use jaw thrust)		
Breathing Initial	Two breaths at 1 sec/breath	Two effective breaths at 1 sec/breath	
HCP: rescue breathing without chest compressions	10–12 breaths/min (approximate)	12–20 breaths/min (approximate)	
HCP: rescue breaths for CPR with advanced airway	8 to 10 breaths/min (approximately)		
Foreign-body airway obstruction	Abdominal thrusts		Back slaps and chest thrusts
Circulation HCP: pulse check (10 sec)	Carotid		Brachial or femoral
Compression landmarks	Lower half of sternum, between nipples		Just below nipple line (lower half of sternum)
Compression method Push hard and fast Allow complete recoil	Heel of one hand, other hand on top	Heel of one hand or as for adults	Two or three fingers HCP (Two rescuers): Two thumb–encircling hands
Compression depth	1 ½–2 inches	Approximately one third to one half the depth of the chest	
Compression rate	Approximately 100/min		
Compression-ventilation ratio	30:2 (one or two rescuers)	30:2 (single rescuer) HCP: 15:2 (two rescuers)	
Defibrillation AED	Use adult pads. Do not use child pads Use pediatric system for child 1–8 yr if available	Use AED after five cycles of CPR (out of hospital) **HCP: for sudden collapse (out of hospital) or in-hospital arrest use AED as soon as available.**	No recommendation for infants <1 yr of age

BLS = basic life support; HCP = health care professional; CPR = cardiopulmonary resuscitation; AED = automatic external defibrillators not involve extending the neck, and is the preferred method if a cervical spine injury is suspected.

4. Clear the airway. Observation and removal of foreign matter or the mouthpiece with a finger sweep or suction device may be necessary if it is obstructing the airway.
5. If a clear and unobstructed airway is not accomplished by the jaw thrust, insert a nasal or oral airway. An oral airway should only be used in the unconscious person.
6. Supplemental oxygen may be used with or without an airway in place.

Process in Suspected Cervical Spine Injury

1. In an unconscious or altered conscious patient, a cervical spine injury must be assumed.
2. The head and neck must be maintained in a neutral position with slight in-line traction. Initial on-field evaluation requires one rescuer to maintain neck stabilization until the patient is adequately secured to a spine board.
3. Removal of the helmet is **not** recommended on the field of play.
4. The use of ammonia capsules or sudden movement is contraindicated in the unconscious patient.
5. Please see diagrams demonstrating the appropriate management of an athlete (see Figures 10.1–10.3).

BREATHING

1. Place the side of your face directly over the patient's mouth and nose, looking down the body axis. Look, listen, and feel for normal breathing by observing the rise and fall of the chest for 5 to 10 seconds, and feel for air movement. Estimate the respiratory rate.
2. Note signs of difficulty in breathing (pursed lip breathing, nasal flaring, retractions, leaning forward, used of accessory muscles, etc.). Observe the rhythm of respiration— prolonged inspiration suggesting upper airway obstruction or prolonged expiration suggesting lower airway obstruction. Listen for air movement (stridor, wheezing, snoring, gurgling, etc.).
3. Look in the mouth for a foreign object, if you see one, remove it with a finger sweep.
4. If breathing is absent, inflate the lungs with two slow breaths. Each breath should last approximately 2 seconds.
5. If after the airway is secured there are no spontaneous respirations, artificial ventilation is necessary. These methods include (a) mouth to mask, (b) bag-valve to mask, and (c) mouth to mouth.
6. Suction may be necessary if the patient vomits. Requirement of an appropriate suction device must be anticipated. Suction should be no longer than 15 seconds at a time. Logroll with the cervical spine stabilized to minimize aspiration risk.

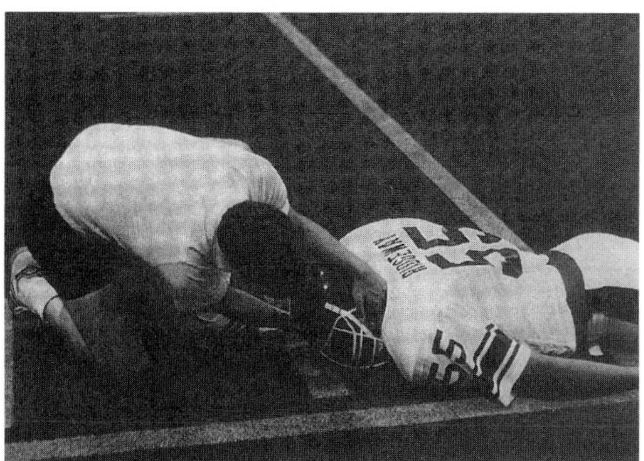

Figure 10.1 When an athlete has a suspected injury to the cervical spine, maintain the position of the head while checking for breathing.

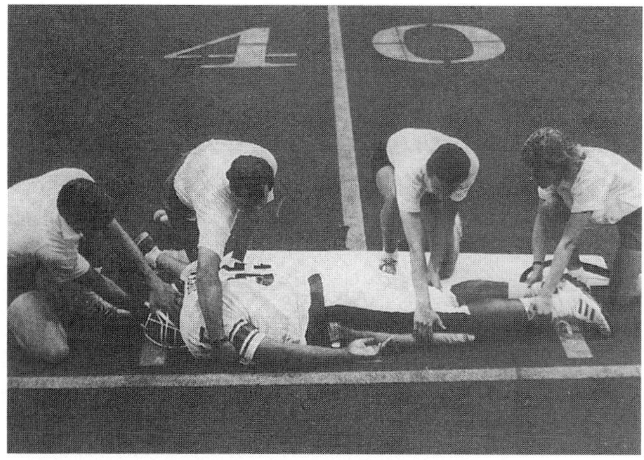

Figure 10.2 With assistance, place arms and legs in axial alignment with the torso, then "logroll" the athlete onto a spine board. The leader is always responsible for protecting the head and neck during transfer taking, taking care to prevent head movement not relative to the torso. The leader is also responsible for all movement commands of the injured athlete by the rescue team.

CIRCULATION

1. Assess for the presence of a pulse or other signs of circulation. In the emergency setting, feel for the carotid pulse to determine if the heart is beating. Check for circulation for 5 to 10 seconds. One can easily determine rate and regularity by palpation.
2. If the carotid pulse is present the systolic blood pressure is at least 60. If a radial pulse is present the systolic blood pressure is at least 80.
3. If circulation is present, but there is no normal breathing, rescue breaths should be applied at one breath every 6 to 8 seconds at a rate of 8 to 10/minute (1).
4. If a circulation is absent, cardiopulmonary resuscitation (CPR) should be started. A chest compression rate of

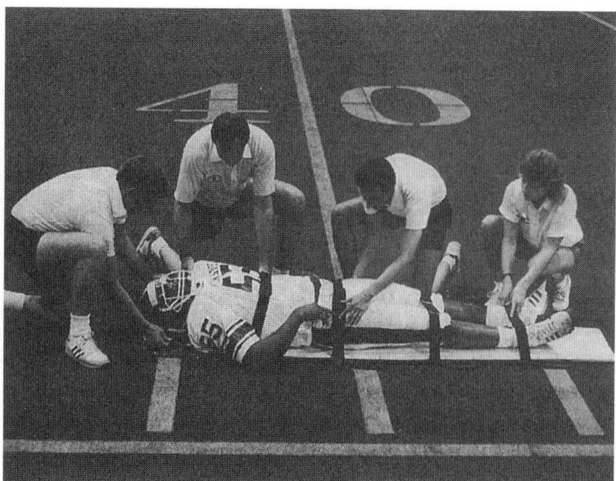

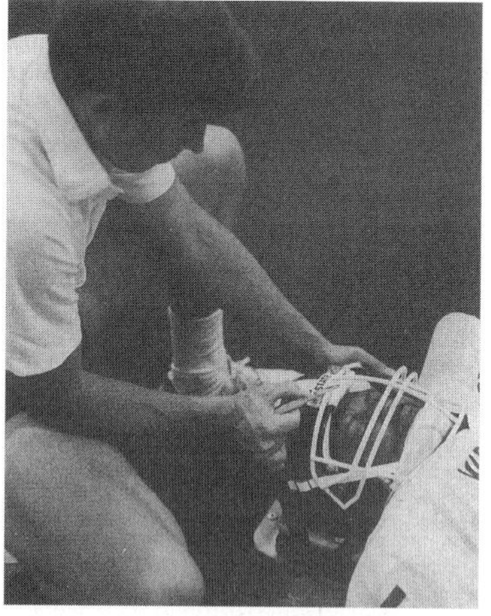

Figure 10.3 A: Once the athlete is on the spineboard, the head and neck continue to be protected until immobilization through straps is satisfactorily achieved. The leader remains at the athlete's head until transfer to emergency vehicle is complete. B: If breathing is compromised, the football face mask is attached to the helmet so that it can be removed easily with the use of a sharp pocket knife cutting plastic support clips. A respiratory airway then ca be achieved without any need to remove the helmet.

100/minute and a compression-to-ventilation ratio of 30:2 are appropriate for the adult victim.

DEFIBRILLATION

1. In adult cardiac arrest, early defibrillation has the greatest impact on survival. Automatic external defibrillators (AEDs) operated by non-paramedics are easy to use. After the pads are applied to the sternum and left chest, the unit will recognize ventricular fibrillation if present and provide the appropriate shock as instructed by the AED.

EXPOSURE

1. Inspect extremities and other body parts for fractures, bleeding, contusions, or evidence of deformity or disability.
2. Utilize a neurological grading system: the Glascow Coma Scale assesses eye opening, verbal, and motor responses. A score of less than 7 indicates coma (see Table 10.2).

SECONDARY ABCD SURVEY

Advanced Airway

1. Reassess the effectiveness of initial airway maneuvers and intervention.
2. Perform endotracheal intubation if indicated.

Breathing

1. Provide ventilation at 12 to 20 times/minute.
2. Confirm endotracheal tube placement (or other device) by at least two methods.
3. Provide positive pressure ventilation with 100% oxygen.

Circulation

1. Attach the patient to an electrocardiograph (ECG) monitor *as soon as possible* to allow continuous recording and reassessment of the cardiac rhythm.

TABLE 10.2
THE GLASCOW COMA SCALE

	Eyes	
Open	Spontaneously	4
	To verbal command	3
	To painful stimulus	2
No response		1
	Best Motor Response	
To verbal command	Obeys	6
To painful stimulus	Localizes pain	5
	Flexion-withdraws	4
	Flexion-abnormal (decorticate posture)	3
	Extension (decerebrate posture)	2
	No response	1
	Best Verbal Response	
Arouse patient (use painful stimulus if necessary)	Oriented and converses	5
	Disoriented and converses	4
	Inappropriate words	3
	Incomprehensible sounds	2
	No response	
TOTAL		***3–15***

2. Establish vascular access with the use of a large bore intravenous catheter and infuse with normal saline or lactated ringer's solution.
3. Administer medications appropriate to the clinical situation or cardiac rhythm.

Differential Diagnosis

1. Determine the cause of the clinical situation.

SYSTEM EVALUATION

The purpose behind system evaluation is to identify the conditions that may lead to death or significant morbidity. This list contains the most common conditions, but is not all-inclusive. Additional information will be presented in subsequent chapters.

HEAD AND NECK

Head and cervical spine injuries are among the most devastating and frightening injuries that can occur in sport (2). The most effective manner in caring for these injuries is to prevent their occurrence. Proper equipment, including protective helmets and mouth guards, are designed to protect the head from injury. Strengthening of the cervical and shoulder musculature will aid but cannot protect from all injuries. Proper tackling techniques and appropriate coaching will also decrease injury risk. Rule changes and penalties for improper use of helmets, hands, sticks, and so on. are also instituted to protect the head and neck. Despite all of these protective measures, injuries will occur.

Head and neck injuries account for 70% of traumatic deaths in sport and 20% of permanent disability (3). In children, 30% to 50% of cervical spinal cord injuries result in quadriplegia (4,5). Widespread media attention is given when a prominent athlete suffers a catastrophic injury to the head or neck, but the true incidence of such injuries from sports participation is unknown because of poor reporting measurements (6). However, of the 500,000 hospital admissions for traumatic brain injury in 1984, sporting injuries accounted for 3% to 10% (7). Although most of these injuries occur in contact or collision sports, the head and cervical spine are vulnerable in any sport and even during routine play (2,8).

Brain Injury

The brain is surrounded by cerebrospinal fluid (CSF) that acts to cushion or absorb externally applied stresses. Additionally, the scalp absorbs shock with thick skin and a layer of fat and muscle over the bony skull. The neck muscles also absorb stress and it is known that if an athletes neck muscles are tensed at the moment of impact, the athlete's head can sustain greater forces without injury.

Injuries to the brain occur by a number of methods:

1. A *coup* injury produces maximal brain trauma beneath the point of impact to the resting skull by a forceful blow.
2. If the moving head contacts an object, a *countracoup* injury may occur. This is a "rebound" injury as the brain strikes the opposite side of the skull from the point of impact due to movement of the brain through the CSF.
3. A skull fracture may result from a blow to the scalp resulting in a depressed or linear fracture, depending on the degree of force and the displacement that occurs at the moment of impact. The brain can be bruised or damaged.
4. Compressive or shearing forces can occur to brain tissue. The brain adapts relatively well to compressive forces whereas shearing forces cause more damage to vascular structures. Shearing forces are more common with rotational movement.

Intracranial Hemorrhage

The leading cause of death from athletic head injury is intracranial hemorrhage. There are four types of intracranial hemorrhage that can cause rapid death: epidural hematoma, subdural hematoma, intracerebral hematoma, and subarachnoid hematoma.

Epidural Hematoma

An epidural hematoma may reach a fatal size in 30 to 60 minutes after trauma. It is the most rapidly progressive intracranial hemorrhage. It results from a tear of the middle meningeal artery that supplies the dura or thick covering over the brain. It is frequently associated with a fracture of the temporal bone above the ear. The injured athlete may initially appear unconscious or stunned or remain conscious. Often there is a lucid interval followed by progressive decline in the level of consciousness. This emphasizes the need for serial neurological examinations after head trauma. The athlete will develop a progressive headache as blood accumulates and intracranial pressure rises. Because the brain injury involves compression from the bleeding artery, prompt evacuation of the clot commonly results in full recovery. There is often no permanent damage to the brain itself, however, all brain injuries should be observed for at least 24 hours post-injury.

Subdural Hematoma

A subdural hematoma involves the space between the dura and the brain tissue. This injury is the most common fatal athletic head injury (9). The damage is done by a diffuse injury to the surface of the brain or to vessels that connect the two structures. Differing from an epidural hematoma, brain tissue is often damaged with this injury, which may result in some impairment if the hematoma is not evacuated appropriately. Because the athlete may not regain consciousness after injury, emergent neurosurgical evaluation in mandated.

A subdural hematoma may develop slowly over a period of days to weeks. The athlete will present with a headache and mental "fogginess," which may be misconstrued to be a post-concussive syndrome. A computed tomography (CT) or an magnetic resonance imaging (MRI) may be indicated if the symptoms persist and the athlete is not able to return to full function in a timely manner.

Intracerebral Hematoma

An intracerebral hematoma develops from bleeding within the brain tissue itself. This is often due to a torn vessel and is often associated with a congenital and unsuspected vascular lesion (i.e., arteriovenous malformation or aneurysm). Death occurs rapidly, often before the athlete can reach the hospital.

Subarachnoid Hematoma

The fourth type of intracranial bleeding involves the subarachnoid space along the surface of the brain. Tiny surface vessels are damaged similar to a bruise. There is brain swelling, but because this injury is superficial, surgery is often not required. Monitoring for post-concussive symptoms such as headache, fatigue, confusion, lethargy, irritability, and difficulty concentrating should be performed. If these symptoms are present, participation is not allowed. The possibility for post-traumatic seizure should be recognized.

Cervical Spine Fractures/Dislocations

Cervical spine fractures/dislocations must be assumed when a downed athlete is found on the field. The main concern in bony injury is the possible end-result of quadriplegia. Because fracture or dislocation cannot be determined on the field of play, this injury must always be suspected and treated appropriately with head and neck immobilization and transport by spine board to the nearest medical facility. If the athlete is unconscious, there is no question but to stabilize and transport the athlete. Only after appropriate radiographs have been performed should neck manipulation be attempted. Up to 20% of unstable cervical spine injuries are missed when only a single cross-table lateral cervical spine radiograph alone is used (10). Therefore, a complete cervical series (including an odontoid, anterior posterior, lateral, oblique, and flexion-extension) is required after the cross-table lateral is negative. If circumstances suggest, advanced imaging of the cervical spine may be indicated for further evaluation.

Injuries to the cervical spine can also occur by unique mechanisms.

1. Compressive injuries may damage the bone (compression fracture) or disc (annular tear or herniation) by axial loading of the spine. This occurs from a blow to the top of the head and the force applied down the spine.
2. Flexion injuries compress the anterior portion of the vertebral body resulting in a wedge fracture, chip fracture or anterior dislocation. The posterior ligaments may be stretched or ruptured.
3. Extension or whiplash injuries compress the posterior elements and stretch the anterior ones. The spinous process or facets may be damaged and the anterior ligament may be torn.
4. Flexion-rotation injuries may result in subluxation of one vertebra on the adjacent one.

Laryngeal Fracture

Blunt trauma to the anterior neck may result in a laryngeal fracture. The fracture may impair the ability to breath. Orotracheal intubation may be difficult resulting in difficulty in bag-valve ventilation and requiring surgical cricothyrotomy. Subcutaneous emphysema may also be manifest in the patient, as well as other complications such as pneumomediastinum, pneumothorax, or pneumoperitoneum (11). This injury requires prompt evaluation in the emergency room by a trauma surgeon.

CARDIAC

Sudden cardiac death (SCD) is a rare entity. Unfortunately, when it occurs to a young, healthy, vibrant athletic individual, it becomes well publicized and the incidence of SCD is consequently perceived to be more common than it truly is. One study estimated that there are four cases of SCD per 1 million athletes/year (12). The causes of SCD can be subdivided by age group. Young athletes (aged 30 and less) die from structural cardiovascular disease, which is congenital in nature and manifest by exertional activities. These include hypertrophic cardiomyopathy, congenital coronary artery anomalies, pathology of the conduction system, annular heart disease, Marfan's syndrome, and myocarditis. In mature athletes (over age 30), atherosclerotic coronary artery disease is the most prevalent etiology. Cardiac risk factors include hypertension, diabetes, hypercholesterolemia, smoking, obesity, male gender, and positive family history. A complete discussion of all the causes of SCD is beyond the scope of this chapter, but emergency management of cardiac arrest will be discussed.

Chest pain has both cardiac and noncardiac causes in the differential diagnosis. Noncardiac causes include pneumonia, pulmonary embolism, esophageal reflux or spasm, gastritis, gastric ulcer, cervical radiculopathy, and Munchausen's syndrome. True cardiac chest pain representing cardiac arrest occurs approximately 300,000 times/year and is the initial manifestation of coronary disease in 20% to 25% of patients with coronary artery disease (13). In the athletic population, cardiac arrest from myocardial infarction is more common among the coaching staff and officials than among the athletes.

BLS includes assessing responsiveness, activating the EMS, assessing airway, breathing, and circulation, and initiating CPR if necessary. Advanced cardiac life support includes the use of automated defibrillators that determine the rhythm and the need for prompt defibrillation for ventricular fibrillation and pulseless ventricular tachycardia. The placement of AEDs in the hands of large numbers of people who are trained in their use may be the key intervention to increase the survival chances of out-of-hospital cardiac arrest (14). Use of AEDs in the athletic setting is determined by the availability and access of the AED and its trained use by medical personnel. AED use in the collegiate setting is more likely to save the life of a coach, official, or fan than an athlete (15).

Commotio cordis is another cause of SCD specific to the young athlete. This occurs after a blunt, low-impact chest wall blow, most commonly with a baseball. Ventricular fibrillation is the arrhythmia that causes SCD in commotio cordis, which occurs in the absence of structural cardiac abnormalities. Survival rates are low even with CPR and prompt defibrillation. The incidence of commotio cordis is unknown because of poor reporting, but the literature reveals 70 reported cases as of July 1998, with 50% occurring in organized sports and 50% occurring outside organized sports (16). The most common proposed mechanism for death is chest wall trauma that coincides with the 15 to 30 msec period of cardiac repolarization. The increased compliance of the chest wall in the immature frame of the young athlete transmits this force to the underlying heart resulting in cardiac arrest. Only 10% of the 70 patients in the literature review survived their event and only 2 of the 70 went on to full recovery (17). Proposed strategies to eliminate the possibility of commotio cordis include the use of softer baseballs and chest protection during sporting activity, although at present a consensus has not been reached.

RESPIRATORY

Respiratory distress in athletes includes the common respiratory conditions that occur to the general population: upper respiratory infections, sinusitis, asthma, bronchitis, pneumonia, and acute allergic reactions. General good hygiene, appropriate rest, and good nutrition are the commonsense approaches to prevent these conditions. Unfortunately, despite all of the appropriate measures, athletes still become ill.

Acute respiratory distress in the athletic population is most commonly caused by an asthma exacerbation. Asthma may be subdivided into intrinsic (caused by sinusitis, upper respiratory tract infections, or psychological stress), extrinsic (caused by exposure to an allergen), drug-induced asthma (hypersensitivity to medicinal or nonmedicinal substances), or exercise-induced asthma (caused by bronchospasm associated with exercise or exposure to cold). Dyspnea, cough, or wheezing are key symptoms and severity can range from mild to severe. Occasionally, an asthma attack may require assisted ventilation and use of intravenous steroids if conservative measures of rest, inhaled bronchodilators, or inhaled steroids are not effective.

Acute respiratory distress from exposure to an allergen (i.e., bee sting) may necessitate the availability of injectable catecholamine (i.e., EpiPen), which has a rapid onset of action (1–2 minutes after subcutaneous injection) and is short acting. The result is effective bronchodilation, but carries the side effect of raising blood pressure. Its alpha-adrenergic effect results in vasoconstriction relieving mucosal edema and congestion. If anaphylaxis develops, prompt transport to the emergency department and administration of injectable steroids or diphenhydramine is indicated.

A pneumothorax occurs when air enters the potential space between the parietal pleura and the visceral pleura. The air in the potential space collapses lung tissue resulting in a loss of oxygen exchange. A ventilation perfusion defect occurs because the nonventilated space is not oxygenated when blood is circulated. The most common cause is a laceration to the lung and this can occur in contact sports such as football, hockey, or lacrosse. The typical presentation involves acute shortness of breath with hyperresonance to chest percussion over the involved area. Chest x-ray reveals the lung collapse and pneumothorax. Transport to the emergency room and evaluation for chest tube placement is warranted. The chest tube should be placed in the fourth or fifth intercostals space anterior to the midaxillary line.

A tension pneumothorax is life-threatening medical emergency because with each inspiration air is drawn into the pleural cavity and does not escape with expiration. This leads to progressive enlargement of the pneumothorax. The presentation and physical examination includes progressive dyspnea, tachypnea, asymmetry of respiration, hypotension, distended neck veins, cyanosis, tracheal deviation to the opposite side of the pneumothorax, absent breath sounds on the affected side, and tachycardia. Treatment necessitates oxygenation and prompt recognition of the condition. Air tension is released by placing a large bore needle (14–16 gauge) into the second or third intercostal space just over the superior aspect of the rib in the midclavicular line of the involved side. Definitive treatment includes hospital transport and chest tube placement.

ORTHOPEDIC

Musculoskeletal injuries occur frequently in sports, but true life-threatening musculoskeletal emergencies are relatively rare. The purpose of this section is to describe the life or limb threatening emergencies that occur in sport.

Posterior Sternoclavicular Dislocation

The sternoclavicular joint is directly anterior to the superior mediastinum. As such, this articulation is in close proximity to several vital structures, including the brachiocephalic and subclavian veins and arteries, the phrenic, vagus and recurrent laryngeal nerves, the trachea and esophagus. If posterior displacement of the proximal end of the clavicle occurs in a traumatic event, it may lodge under the sternum and compress the trachea. In addition to significant pain that radiates toward the neck, the athlete may experience respiratory distress, shortness of breath, a feeling of suffocation or hoarseness. Esophageal compression may be expressed by difficulty swallowing or tightness in the throat. Closed reduction by using a *towel clip* may be indicated on the field of play, combined with abduction and extension of the shoulder. For the latter technique, the athlete is placed in a supine position with a bump or sandbag between the shoulder blades, and the affected shoulder is extended over the edge of the table. Traction is applied to the arm while countertraction is applied to the trunk. An audible snap or visible realignment is the result of a successful reduction. Evaluation and reduction may need to be done in the operating room under sedation (18,19).

Fat Embolism—Long Bone Fracture

Fat embolism syndrome is rare (<1% in retrospective reviews) but can be fatal (20,21). Although the etiology is poorly understood, the presumption is that marrow fat embolizes into the blood stream potentially causing end organ damage. Fat embolism is more common with polytrauma. Clinical evaluation may reveal respiratory distress, altered mental status, tachycardia, or fever. Treatment is supportive with appropriate respiratory assistance after prompt recognition. The Sports Medicine Team must be aware that the condition may exist. With appropriate on-field stabilization and prompt transport to the hospital for definitive care of long bone fracture, this condition may be prevented.

Hip Dislocations

Dislocations or fracture-dislocation of the proximal femur is a true orthopedic emergency. Significant force is required to cause the dislocation, and although they are rare in athletic activities, they do exist. Dislocations primarily occur posteriorly. Avascular necrosis of the proximal femur and post-traumatic arthritis are the main complications.

The classic presentation of the posterior dislocated hip can be remembered using the pneumonic PID, which stands for posterior, internally rotated, and adducted. In addition, the affected extremity is shortened. The treatment of hip dislocations is immediate reduction. Closed reduction can be attempted with conscious sedation if there is not an associated femoral neck or shaft fracture. When this injury occurs on the playing field, the circumstances typically dictate immediate transport to the emergency department for radiography and sedation before attempting a reduction maneuver. If an associated fracture is identified, open reduction with internal fixation is indicated (22).

Knee Dislocation

Like many other emergencies in sport, the true incidence of knee dislocations is unknown due to poor reporting. Suffice it to say, they are rare or uncommon injuries. Yet, the rarity of these injuries does not lessen the severity when they do occur. The knee can dislocate in multiple directions: anterior (40%), posterior (33%), lateral (18%), medial (4%), and rotational (5%) (23). Forced hyperextension is the mechanism causing anterior dislocation. At 30 degrees of hyperextension, the posterior capsule tears followed by the cruciate ligaments. At 50 degrees the popliteal artery is found to stretch causing intimal tears or thrombosis, before rupturing. Therefore, clinical suspicion for vascular injury is paramount. The collateral ligaments may be damaged in an anterior dislocation, but this must involve rotational stress. In sporting activity, the mechanism of injury of an anterior dislocation is an anterior blow to the knee or tibia with the foot fixed.

Limb salvage requires prompt identification of all of the involved structures and repair of the vascular supply (i.e., popliteal artery). Arteriography is required to identify and document patent blood supply and obtain vascular surgery consult as indicated. Nerve injuries are not as well understood, but the peroneal nerve can be damaged. Thorough evaluation of the neurological status before surgical repair is very important.

Complications of knee dislocations can be separated into non-operative and operative categories. Non-operative complications include vascular injury, neurological damage to the peroneal or tibial nerves, compartment syndrome, infection, and delayed wound healing. Operative complications include iatrogenic vascular injury, iatrogenic nerve injury, fluid extravasation leading to compartment syndrome, tourniquet ischemia, wound infections and delayed healing necessitating debridement and prolonged antibiotic use, complex regional pain syndrome, and loss of motion due to contractures and residual laxity (24). Clearly, these injuries require evaluation by an orthopedic surgeon experienced in treating this type of trauma.

ENVIRONMENTAL

A complete discussion of exertional heat illness will be discussed in Chapter 21. Heat stroke may result in significant mortality or morbidity (25). The human body maintains a balance between metabolic heat production and the four methods of heat dissipation: evaporation, radiation, convection, and conduction. Gender, age, hydration status, acclimation, and the sweating response also affect heat accommodation. However, environmental conditions may overwhelm the ability of the body to effectively dissipate excess heat. The most severe condition due to the inability to remove excess heat is heat stroke.

Heat stroke, or hyperpyrexia, results when the homeostatic and thermoregulatory mechanisms fail to dissipate excess heat resulting in core temperatures higher than 40°C (105°F). Exertional heat stroke effects can be subdivided into acute (within 1–12 hours) and late (>12 hours) phases. Acute phase reactions are hallmarked by central nervous system (CNS) dysfunction: altered consciousness, irrational behavior, stupor, irritability, convulsions, delirium, agitation, and progression to coma. Altered metabolic or electrolyte abnormalities include hyperkalemia or hypokalemia, hypernatremia or hyponatremia, hypocalcemia, hyperphosphatemia, hypoglycemia, lactic acidosis, uremia, leukocytosis, and elevated liver transaminases. Late effects primarily involve liver and kidney dysfunction. Acute renal failure, disseminated intravascular coagulation (DIC), rhabdomyolysis, and metabolic acidosis are all poor prognostic signs. Death may result if prompt treatment is not instituted.

The heat stroke victim may present with heat-related collapse, heat exhaustion, heat cramps, or a progressive feeling of illness. Core temperature may be as high as 107°F to 108°F (41.66°C to 42.22°C). The Sports Medicine Team must not rely on oral, axillary, or tympanic temperature readings if exertional heat stroke is suspected. Although esophageal temperature is considered the most reliable measure of core temperature, it is not practical in the field. Rectal temperature gauges the magnitude of hyperthermia. Relying on tympanic temperature, which has been found to be 2.3°C (36.14°F) lower than rectal temperatures in hyperthermic runners, may delay appropriate and necessary treatment (26). Traditionally, it was felt that the sweating mechanism had failed in heat stroke, resulting in the hot, dry, and flushed patient, but often they will still be perspiring. Altered CNS responses are prominent presenting signs.

The ABCs should first be addressed, followed by calling 911 and rapid cooling. The faster the core temperature can be reduced, the greater the chance for ultimate recovery. Cold or ice water immersion (5–15°C [41–59°F]) of the entire body is critical for survival (27). If an ice tub is not available, cooling fans, ice packs to the head, axillary, and groin regions and behind are needed, and cool towels that encourage evaporation should be used. The temperature should be reduced to 38°C (100.4°F). Intravenous lines should be placed in the antecubital vein and IV hydration may be instituted. Fluid infusion should be based on the hydration status, and may contain normal saline or simple sugars to combat hypoglycemia. Laboratory values should be monitored acutely and often to determine electrolytes, blood glucose, complete blood count, and renal and liver function. A bladder catheter should be placed to monitor urine output. Proper ventilation and oxygenation should be monitored. The main physiological component of treatment is to restore normal perfusion to the organ systems. This will eliminate waste products, restore normal function, and prevent tissue failure.

Return to sport after exertional heat stroke has not been formalized. Delaying exercise for several days to a week post hospitalization is suggested. Appropriate follow-up by a physician and supervision of exercise is also recommended for several weeks. Progressive and gradual increase in the intensity and duration of exercise over several weeks followed by re-establishment of heat acclimation should occur. The athlete who had heat stroke is at risk for further heat intolerance and should be monitored closely. Proper education of the athlete, parents, coaching staff and medical staff may assist in preventing this condition.

Emergency Protocols

The Sports Medicine Team should establish written emergency protocols appropriate to the coverage of events and circumstances. Components of an emergency actions plan are as follows: (a) establishing appropriate medical coverage for the event, whether it is a practice or game; (b) developing emergency communication plans for every facility and situation; (c) utilization, availability, and maintenance of necessary emergency equipment and supplies; (d) availability of transportation; and (e) establishing written policies and procedures for common emergencies.

Medical Event Coverage

Identifying the member of the emergency team may be taken for granted, but is a necessary step in developing appropriate protocols. At some individual events, the only person present, other than the athlete, is the coach. Education of coaches in basic first aid and emergency evaluation is a necessary step. At other events, the entire Sports Medicine Team will be available. Knowing the attending medical personnel, such as the certified athletic trainer, student athletic trainers, EMS providers, team physicians and medical specialty consultants, and defining their roles and responsibilities before an emergency presents itself is paramount. Individuals with limited credentials should yield to those with the most appropriate training. In an emergency, individual egos should be checked for the care of the injured athlete.

Emergency Communication

One of the most disturbing, yet most common, failures is the unavailability of telecommunication when an event occurs. Access to a working telephone or cellular phone is crucial when athletes are participating in practice or games. Identifying the location of the nearest telecommunication device is extremely important and should be a primary focus of the attending Sports Medicine Team member. Never assume that there is access to this device. Availability and workability must be performed for each event covered. Directions on how to gain access to the athletic venue should also be written and kept near the available telephone.

Emergency Equipment and Supplies

All necessary supplies and equipment should be on-site, quickly available and in good working order. This requires checking the equipment on a regular basis. The available equipment should be appropriate for the level of training of the covering medical personnel. Advanced training on how to use the equipment is necessary. Periodic practice and mock events are indicated to keep skills and knowledge updated. An emergency is not the time to learn how to use the devices.

Transportation

Access to either on-site ambulance or appropriate transportation is crucial when high-risk sporting events occur. EMS response time is an additional factor that may determine whether on-site personnel will be required to attend events. Foreseeing traffic delays must be done in this regard. Emergency providers should refrain from transporting unstable patients in inappropriate vehicles. Establishing relationships with police, fire, and EMS providers before an emergency occurs should also be undertaken. Written directions should be available and prominently displayed so as not to delay access to the event site.

Written Policies and Procedures

Before an emergency, written protocols appropriate for the patient population should be developed. The following is a suggested list:

1. Basic airway management
2. Use of a pocket mask
3. How to insert an oropharyngeal airway
4. How to insert a nasopharyngeal airway
5. Suctioning
6. Use of bag-valve mask
7. How to administer supplemental oxygen
8. Use of epinephrine auto-injector
9. Use of oral glucose gel
10. Use of automated external defibrillator
11. Guidelines in prevention of heat-related illness
12. Use of metered dose inhalers (MDI) and small volume nebulizers (SVN)
13. Use of cervical spine boards
14. Removal of face mask
15. Removal of helmet
16. How to logroll a prone athlete

In each of these conditions, written procedures regarding indications and contraindications, technique, side effects, complications, appropriate reassessment, and how to notify others in the Sports Medicine Team should be established. Training of new members should be done on a scheduled basis.

CONCLUSION

Although emergencies are not avoidable, their management should be anticipated and well planned. Identification of potential emergency situations appropriate to individual sporting events is a part of the responsibility of the Sports Medicine Team. When emergencies occur, chaos can quickly follow. Establishing protocols and practicing them before hand will lead to sound and stable management and fewer complications.

REFERENCES

1. 2005 American Heart Association. Guidelines for cardiopulmonary resuscitation and emergency cardiovascular care. *Circulation* 2005;112 (24 Suppl):IV1–203.
2. Banerjee R. Catastrophic cervical spine injuries in the collision sport athlete, part 1: epidemiology, functional anatomy, and diagnosis. *Am J Sports Med* 2004;32(4):1077–1087.
3. Mueller F, Cantu R, Van Camp S. Football. In: Mueller F, Cantu R, Van Camp S, eds. *Catastrophic injuries in high school and college sports,* 1st ed. Champaign IL: Human Kinetics, 1996:41–56.
4. Luke A, Micheli L. Sports injuries: emergency assessment and field-side care. *Pediatr Rev* 1999;20(9):293.
5. National Spinal Cord Injury Statistical Center. *Spinal cord information network: facts and figures at a glance.* Birmingham: University of Alabama at Birmingham, Available at www.ncddr.org/rpp/hf/hfdw/mscis/nscisc/html. 2003.
6. Luke A, Micheli L. Sports injuries: emergency assessment and field-side care. *Pediatr Rev* 1999;20(9):694.
7. Kraus JF. Epidemiology of head injury. In: Cooper PR, ed. *Head injury,* 2nd ed. Baltimore: Lippincott Williams & Wilkins, 1987:1–19.
8. Nobunga AL, GO BK, Karunas RB. Recent demographic and injury trends in people served by the model spine cord injury care systems. *Arch Phys Med Rehabil* 1999;80:1372–1382.
9. Cantu RC, Mueller FO. Fatalities and catastrophic injuries in high school and college sports, 1982–1997. *Phys Sportsmed* 1999;27:705.
10. Herzog RJ, Wiens JJ, Dillingham MF, et al. Normal cervical spine morphometry and cervical spinal stenosis in asymptomatic professional football players: plain film radiography, multiplanar computed tomography, and magnetic resonance imaging. *Spine* 1991;16(Suppl 6):178–186.
11. Mussack T, Wiedeman E. Pneumoperitoneum, pneumoretroperitoneum, and pneumomediastinum caused by laryngeal fracture after multiple trauma. *Am J Emerg Med* 2001;19(6):523–524.
12. Ades PA. Preventing sudden death. *Phys Sportsmed* 1992;20:75.
13. Balley KA. Cardiac arrest in saunders *Manual of medical practice.* Rakel, RE: WB Saunders, 1996:235.
14. Atkins DL, Bossaert LL, Hazinski MF, et al. Automated external defibrillation/ public access defibrillation. *Ann Emerg Med* 2001;37(Suppl 4):S60–67.
15. Drezner JA, Rogers K, Zimmer R, et al. Use of automated external defibrillators at NCAA division I Universities. *Med Sci Sports Exerc* 2005; 37(9):1487–1492.
16. Perron AD, Brady WJ, Erling BF. Commotio cordis: an underappreciated cause of sudden cardiac death in young patients: assessment and management in the ED. *Am J Emerg Med* 2001;19(5):406–409.
17. Maron BJ, Link MS, Wang PJ, et al. Clinical profile of commotio cordis: and underappreciated cause of sudden death in the young during sports and other activities. *J Cardiovasc Electrophysiol* 1999;10:114–120.
18. Yeh GL, Williams GR. Conservative management of sternoclavicular injuries. *Orthop Clin North Am* 2000;31(2):189–203.
19. Williams CC. Posterior sternoclavicular joint dislocations. *Phys Sportsmed* 1999;27(2):105–113.
20. Mello A. Fat embolism. *Anaesthesia* 2001;56(2):145–154.
21. Matthews BD. Fatal cerebral fat embolism after open reduction and internal fixation of femur fracture. *J Trauma* 2001;50(3):585.
22. Rudman N, McIlmail D. Emergency department evaluation and treatment of hip and thigh injuries. *Emerg Med Clin North Am* 2000;18:1.
23. Brautigan B, John DL. The epidemiology of knee dislocation. *Clin Sports Med* 2000;19(3):387–398.
24. Hegyes MS, Richardson MW, Miller MD. Knee dislocation: complication of nonoperative and operative management. *Clin Sports Med* 2000; 19(3):387–398.
25. National Center for Catastrophic Sport Injury Research. *Twenty-second annual report: fall 1982—spring 2004.* Chapel Hill: University of North Carolina, 2004.
26. Knight JC, Casa DJ, McClung JM, et al. Assessing if two tympanic temperature instruments are valid indicators of core temperature in hyperthermic runners and does drying the ear canal help. *J Athl Train* 2000;35(2):S21.
27. Costrini A. Emergency treatment of exertional heatstroke and comparison of whole-body cooling techniques. *Med Sci Sports Exerc* 2000;22: 15–18.

Respiratory System

11

Jeffrey R. Kovan   *James L. Moeller*

ASTHMA

Typically characterized as intermittent narrowing of the airways due to chronic inflammation and bronchial hyperactivity, asthma often is provoked by irritants or "triggers" that come in contact with the bronchi. Airway inflammation appears to be the precipitating factor leading to increased airway reactivity. Wheezing, cough, chest tightness, and shortness of breath are the typical presenting symptoms, but frequently are not found at the time of examination. The prevalence of asthma in children is approximately 6% to 7% in the general population (1). The incidence appears to increase in heavily industrialized areas where potential allergens are the greatest. Chronic asthma is the result of cellular changes within the airway epithelium. Inflammatory cells migrate to the bronchi and chemical mediator alterations occur resulting in airway narrowing and increased permeability of the epithelium. Narrowing of the airways secondary to smooth muscle contraction, edema, and increased mucous production ensues. Many potential allergens have been described, which act as triggers for an asthmatic flare. This appears to be more commonly found in patients with a personal or family history of atopy. A few of these include typical house dusts and molds, environmental pollutants, and food allergens. Other precipitating mechanisms to create an asthmatic response include respiratory tract infections, hot and/or cold exposure, smoke, stress, and exercise (2).

Diagnosis and Management

The previously described symptoms of wheezing, cough, and shortness of breath should alert the physician to the possibility of asthma. Demonstrating reversible airway obstruction is essential in confirming clinical suspicions. Use of peak flow measurements and/or spirometry provides an objective means of confirming the diagnosis. The standard classification of asthma severity by the National Heart, Lung, and Blood Institute, known as the *National Asthma Education and Prevention Program* (NAEPP), set guidelines in 2002 for the diagnosis and management of asthma, which are listed in Table 11.1.

EXERCISE-INDUCED ASTHMA

Exercise-induced asthma (EIA) is a transient airflow obstruction triggered by physical exertion. Airway narrowing occurs in those with increased airway reactivity, and symptoms similar to those described with asthma occur, but on a transient basis. EIA effects approximately 12% to 15% of the general population and has been found in 90% of asthmatic patients (4). EIA is seen in 40% of allergy or "hay fever" sufferers (5). No apparent age or gender differences are reported. The effects of exercise are not clearly understood, although the type, intensity, and duration of exercise, along with varied environmental conditions such as tobacco smoke, molds, dust, and cold temperatures appear to play a role in triggering a flare.

Pathophysiology

The pathophysiology of EIA is commonly described by two theories (6). **"The water loss theory"** is based on water loss through the bronchial mucosa following exercise as a means to warm and saturate inspired air. Hyperosmolarity of the airways occurs with a subsequent release of mediators leading to bronchial constriction. A second theory describes **"heat exchange"** as a means to cool the airways with increased ventilation due to exercise. Once cooling is completed, the bronchial vasculature dilates and engorges to rewarm the epithelium. A rebound effect occurs, with hyperemia of the bronchial vascular beds and ultimately airway narrowing. As described earlier, hyper-reactivity with any of the environmental allergens may stimulate an exaggerated EIA response with even minimal exertion.

TABLE 11.1

LONG-TERM MANAGEMENT OF ASTHMA IN CHILDREN

Asthma Classification[a]	Symptom Frequency	Lung Function[b]	Medications Required to Maintain Long-term Control
Mild intermittent	Daytime: 2 d/wk or less Nighttime: 2 nights/mo or less	PEF or FEV_1: 80% or more of predicted function	No daily medication needed
Mild persistent	Daytime: more than 2 d/wk, but less than one time/d Nighttime: more than 2 nights/mo	PEF or FEV_1: 80% or more of predicted function	Low-dosage inhaled corticosteroid delivered by nebulizer or metered dose inhaler with holding chamber, with or without a face mask, or by dry-powder inhaler in children 5 yr and younger
Moderate persistent	Daytime: daily Nighttime: more than 1 night/wk	PEF or FEV_1: 60%–80% of predicted function	Children 5 yr and younger: low-dosage inhaled corticosteroid and long-acting $beta_2$ agonist or medium-dosage inhaled corticosteroid Children older than 5 yr: low- to medium-dosage inhaled corticosteroid and long-acting inhaled $beta_2$ agonist.
Severe persistent	Daytime: continual Nighttime: frequent	PEF or FEV_1: 60% or less of predicted function	High-dosage inhaled corticosteroid and long-acting $beta_2$ agonist

PEF = peak expiratory flow; FEV_1 = forced expiratory volume in 1 sec.
[a]-Clinical features before treatment or adequate control.
[b]-Lung function measurements are used only in patients older than 5 years.
Source: Adapted from National Asthma Education and Prevention Program. *Expert panel report: guidelines for the diagnosis and management of asthma: update on selected topics, 2002.* Bethesda, MD: U.S. Department of Health and Human Services, Public Health Service, National Institutes of Health, National Heart, Lung, and Blood Institute, 2003; NIH publication no. 02–5074:115; From the Courtney AU, McCarter DF, Pollart SM. Childhood asthma: treatment update. *Am Fam Physician* 2005;71(10):1959–1968, (3).

Signs and Symptoms

EIA is classically described as wheezing and chest tightness within the first 5 to 10 minutes of strenuous exercise. Typically, episodes will remit 30 to 60 minutes after the completion of exercise. History of the signs and symptoms described here with a strong allergy and/or family history of asthma should heighten suspicion for this condition. These symptoms and the less common complaints of cough, fatigue, the inability to keep up with peers, and recurrent "stomach aches" should also alert the care provider to the possibility of EIA. Physical examination is rarely beneficial when the athlete is at rest. Occasionally, signs of allergies, including allergic shiners, nasal polyps, and less commonly, watery and blood shot eyes will be noted. Respiratory findings are also typically absent at rest. Any suggestion of wheezing at rest should raise suspicion of underlying chronic asthma. In an acute event following activity, respiratory wheezing, cough, and poor inspiratory effort will be evident.

Diagnosis

The diagnosis of EIA begins with identification of irritants that may trigger an attack, followed by simple avoidance techniques. When history and clinical findings suggest EIA, supportive care with a trial of nonsedating antihistamines and minimizing cold exposure may relieve or at least delay symptoms. Alternative conservative measures of submaximal exercise for 15 to 30 minutes before sport participation may provide a refractory period of 1 to 3 hours and help a small percentage of sufferers. Self-reported symptoms for EIA diagnosis in the athletic population will likely yield high frequencies of both false positive and false negative results. Diagnosis should include spirometry using an exercise or environmental challenge in combination with the athlete's history of asthma symptoms (7).

Pulmonary Function Testing

Pulmonary function testing (PFT) provides an accurate assessment of baseline pulmonary function. PFT at rest provides the pre- and postexercise norms for an individual. The use of an office spirometer allows for determination of forced expiratory volumes (FEV) in 1 second (FEV_1). FEV_1 is typically normal in pre-exercise individuals and roughly 90% to 100% of the predicted norms in those with normal lung function following exertion. In chronic asthmatics, baseline FEV_1 values will often be less than 80% of predicted norms (6). In EIA, the most objective measure for diagnosis is the pulmonary function test following an appropriate exercise challenge.

Exercise Challenge Testing

Exercise challenge testing requires enough exertion to achieve the desired heart rates at 80% to 90% of the maximum for 5 to 8 minutes. This can be achieved with the use of a treadmill or ergometer, but should be a sport specific exercise challenge in the appropriate environment when possible (e.g., the ice rink for skaters, the swimming pool for swimmers). FEV_1, along with FVC (forced vital capacity) and FEF25–75 (forced expiratory flow 25%–75%) are measured postexercise and frequently thereafter for roughly 20 to 30 minutes. Typically, FEV_1 will be used to assess respiratory response following an exercise challenge. A fall in FEV_1 of greater than or equal to 15% from pre-exercise values is diagnostic (6). Healthy controls will maintain FEV_1 values above 85% to 90% of the baseline. A 15% to 20% fall in FEV_1 suggests mild EIA, whereas a 20% to 30% decline is suggestive of a moderate level. A 30% or greater reduction of FEV_1 from baseline would be classified as severe.

Peak Flow Monitoring

When spirometry is unavailable, peak flow monitoring with hand held devices can serve as a useful tool in assessing respiratory status and adjusting treatment options. It is very important that the exercise challenge is adequate to produce a response. Patients should become quite adept at assessing current respiratory status and therefore adjusting workouts and treatments by this method.

Methacholine Challenge Testing

Less commonly used, but quite advantageous when equivocal results are found on traditional testing measures, methacholine challenge testing can be performed to help facilitate a drop in FEV_1. Nebulized methacholine has been shown to have negative effects in asthmatics, thereby lowering FEV_1 and ultimately pulmonary function when administered. In nonasthmatic sufferers, a significantly higher dosage of medication will be required to see similar results. Frequently, repeat PFT at 1 to 2 months after the initiation of treatment is required to measure its effects and adjust medications, dosing frequency, and concentrations to maximize an athlete's respiratory function.

Eucapnic Voluntary Hyperventilation Test

Eucapnic voluntary hyperventilation (EVH) testing is used to verify EIA and the need for the use of bronchodilators before competition (8). According to Eliasson et al. (9) sensitivity is reported to be at 50% with specificity up to 100%. Inhalation of a dry gas consisting of carbon dioxide, oxygen, and nitrogen gases is performed at a rate of 85% maximum voluntary ventilation (MVV) for 6 minutes. FEV_1 measurements are made throughout the study and compared to baseline values before inhalation. A 20% decline in FEV_1 is diagnostic for EIA. Bronchodilator use following conclusion of the study should reverse respiratory compromise and the patient's symptoms. Reversibility of airway hyperresponsiveness and clinical improvement should be documented. Despite utilization by the International Olympic Committee, availability of this testing measure is otherwise difficult and is therefore less frequently used than previously mentioned testing measures.

Treatment

Treatment of EIA begins with conservative measures. Well-controlled chronic asthma must be achieved in athletes with a predisposition to respiratory compromise with exercise (see Table 11.1). Avoidance of any predetermined triggers and/or the use of appropriate nonsedating antihistamines to control allergic flares is essential. Peak aerobic conditioning to improve oxygen utilization and thus decrease the number of ventilations with exercise may provide relief in some athletes. The use of sub-maximal exercise before exertion may allow for a symptom-free refractory period in some and should be attempted as well. Inhaled short-acting beta-agonists (e.g., albuterol) remain the first line treatment of EIA (10). Dosing is recommended as 1 to 2 inhalations through a metered dose inhaler 15 to 30 minutes before exercise. Onset of action is expected within 5 to 15 minutes, with duration of action typically 2 to 4 hours. For prolonged events a second dose may be required. Long-acting beta-agonists (e.g., salmeterol) are available and can be used twice daily to offer extended relief, with boosting before competition from a short-acting agent.

Unsuccessful control or undesired side effects may warrant a trial of short-acting anti-inflammatory agents. Cromolyn and nedocromil are mast cell stabilizers that provide potent anti-inflammatory effects through inhibition of the mediator release from mast cells. Decreased degranulation of mast cells leads to reduction in bronchoconstriction. These agents are typically given 15 to 30 minutes before exercise, but unlike beta-agonists these are less useful for acute symptoms and generally more effective as a second line agent in prophylaxis. Occasionally, use of both beta-agonists and anti-inflammatory agents are required to maximize control. Daily maintenance dosing of one or both of these agents may be required in those not responsive to pre-exercise medication alone. Inhaled corticosteroids are first line medications for the treatment of chronic asthma, but are less frequently used in EIA.

Corticosteroids prevent airway obstruction from inflammation before exercise. Generally not effective for pre-exercise treatment alone, corticosteroids require 2 to 4 weeks of maintenance dosing to achieve desired effects. In combination with short-acting beta-agonists, corticosteroids may provide relief from EIA when other measures fail.

Less commonly used agents in EIA, inhaled anticholinergics (e.g., ipratropium) and leukotriene inhibitors, have shown promise in controlling chronic inflammation and specific allergic triggers. The leukotriene inhibitors (e.g., montelukast, zafirlukast) offer oral dosing and relatively few side effects. These agents are beneficial in children and adults with mild, stable chronic asthma. Montelukast, in two double blind, placebo-controlled trials, has been shown to be more effective than salmeterol in long-term treatment of EIA in children with asthma (11,12). Inhaled ipratropium has not been shown to be effective in the treatment of EIA (13).

A thorough knowledge of the current banned substance listings for specific organizations is essential before dosing with any of the agents mentioned here. Adjustments in medications may be necessary and should be done well in advance of competition.

Differential Diagnosis

Other clinical entities should be considered in an athlete with respiratory compromise during exercise when traditional diagnostic and treatment measures fail. Vocal cord dysfunction (VCD), anxiety disorders, and gastroesophageal reflux disease may all present with clinical signs and symptoms mimicking EIA (see Table 11.2).

OTHER RESPIRATORY DISORDERS

Pulmonary Contusion

Generally regarded as the most common chest injury in children, pulmonary contusions involve a blunt injury to the chest wall with subsequent injury to the lung parenchyma. Subsequent edema and blood collection in the alveolar spaces lead to loss of normal lung structure and function. Injury to the lung develops over the following 24 hours and commonly the extent of injury is not truly apparent for up to 48 hours.

Diagnosis

Diagnosis is typically made following reported chest wall trauma and subsequent bruising, rib fractures, and/or flail chest. Physical examination rarely assists with diagnosis in the early stages. Evidence of hypoxia with severe cases and inspiratory crackles may be heard but are

TABLE 11.2
CAUSES OF DYSPNEA IN THE ATHLETE

	Timing of Symptoms	Symptoms	Physical Findings	Diagnostic Tests	Treatment
Asthma	At rest and with exertion	Wheezing, cough, chest tightness and SOB, signs of atopy	Based on stage and severity at presentation; tachypnea, tachycardia, expiratory wheezes at rest	Spirometry, peak flow measurements	Based on severity of asthma (see Table11.1)
Exercise-induced asthma	Onset 5–10 min into exercise and then throughout exercise	Wheezing, cough, chest tightness, SOB, fatigue with exercise	Tachypnea, tachycardia, inspiratory and expiratory wheezes	Exercise, pulmonary function, methacholine challenge test, eucapnic voluntary hyperventilation	Avoidance of triggers, control of allergies, beta-agonists, cromolyn, inhaled corticosteroids, leukotriene inhibitors, and anticholinergics
Vocal cord dysfunction	Within first 5–10 min of exertion; may only be present in competition setting	SOB, stridor, dysphonia, throat tightness	Upper airway wheezing and respiratory distress	Laryngoscopy with direct visualization	Behavior modification, speech therapy, anti-inflammatory agents, surgery
Gastroesophageal reflux disease	Early to middle stages of the exercise	Heartburn, dyspepsia, bloating, belching, sour taste, cough, SOB	None	Upper endoscopy	Lifestyle modification, avoidance of alcohol and tobacco, antacids, H_2 blockers, protein pump inhibitors
Anxiety/panic attacks	Before competition	SOB, nervousness, palpitations, sweating, faintness	Tachycardia, tachypnea	When indicated: cardiac monitoring, pulmonary function tests, thyroid laboratory panel, electrolytes	Cognitive behavior therapy, benzodiazepines, SSRIs

SOB = shortness of breath; SSRI = selective serotonin reuptake inhibitor.

nonspecific. Chest x-ray can be diagnostic in significant pulmonary contusions, but often lags behind clinical findings. Computed tomography (CT) scanning is the diagnostic measure of choice and appears quite sensitive for identification of pulmonary contusions and the extent of injury.

Treatment

Management of pulmonary contusions is generally supportive as resolution generally occurs within a few days. Oxygen support is rarely required but may be needed in more extensive injury and subsequent hypoxemia. Pain control measures are vital as restricted inspiratory and expiratory efforts may predispose patients to pneumonia. Close observation is necessary with more severe injury as complications such as adult respiratory distress syndrome (ARDS) may occur and can be fatal.

Pneumothorax

Typically described as air (pneumothorax) or blood (hemothorax) that occurs in the pleural space between the lung and the chest wall, a pneumothorax develops either spontaneously or as the result of direct trauma. The most common etiology of a *spontaneous pneumothorax* is the result of a congenital bleb on the surface of the visceral pleura that ruptures (14). Typically seen in young, thin males between the ages of 20 to 40, a spontaneous pneumothorax may occur both at rest and with exertion. Clinical symptoms vary from mild to moderate shortness of breath with a small pneumothorax (<15%–20%) to acute pleuritic chest pain, cough, and severe shortness of breath for the more advanced cases (>20%).

Diagnosis

Diagnostic evaluation for suspicion of a pneumothorax begins with a thorough physical examination. Findings on chest auscultation may include absent breath sounds on the affected side, wheezing, and poor air exchange on inspiration and expiration. Radiographic evaluation should include a posterior/anterior (PA) chest x-ray and a lateral decubitus view with the suspected side uppermost (see Figure 11.1). The PA chest x-ray should be performed at forced, full expiration to intensify the radiographic appearance. An arch of lucency adjacent to the lung margin will be noted and then classified according to the degree of collapse.

Treatment

Treatment for a pneumothorax of 15% to 20% or less can often be accomplished conservatively with observation, supplemental oxygen, rest and repeat chest x-rays until clear. A 20% or greater collapse typically requires extended hospitalization and chest tube placement. Most leaks seal spontaneously within 24 hours. Continued re-expansion must be demonstrated following clamping of the chest tube before removal can be attempted. Return to play following a pneumothorax is somewhat unclear. Return to noncontact activity can be resumed within 3 to 6 weeks following hospital discharge. Progression of activity is based on tolerance level and symptom-free exertion. Flying is typically delayed for 4 to 6 weeks and underwater (scuba) diving is completely discouraged (15). Some report recurrence rates as high as 50% for pneumothoraces, increasing in frequency with additional events (16). A careful and slow progression to symptom-free exertion and a delayed return to physical activity may assist in reducing this likelihood.

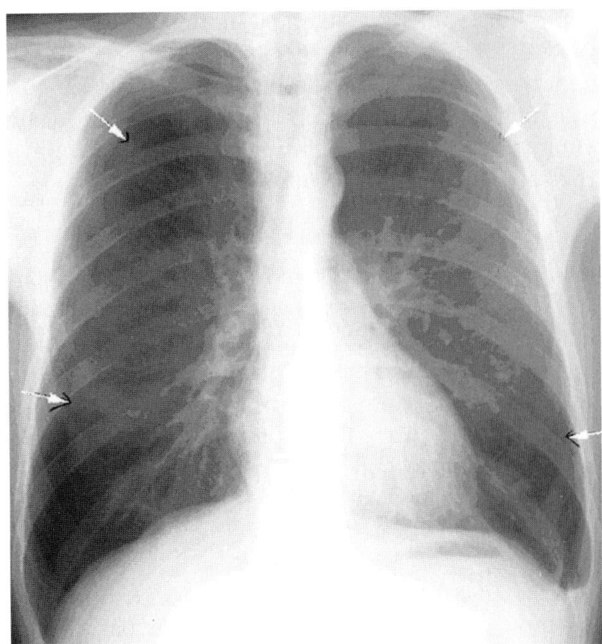

Figure 11.1 Radiographic evaluation for suspicion of a pneumothorax should include a posterior/anterior (PA) chest x-ray and a lateral decubitus view with the suspected side uppermost. (*Source:* From American College of Radiology CD ROM series, *Chest*, 2001.)

Hyperventilation Syndrome

An injured athlete or one who is experiencing severe anxiety or stress may begin breathing rapidly and develop hyperventilation syndrome. The effects of prolonged hyperventilation include decreased P_{CO_2} and increase in arterial pH (respiratory alkalosis). The patient usually becomes panic-stricken while gasping for breath, and may suffer carpopedal spasm or frank tetany. Less severe complaints include dyspnea, faintness, confusion, numbness of the extremities, and paraesthesia. Syncope without loss of consciousness may occur (17,18).

Diagnosis

On examination, there are no rales, wheezes, or other chest findings to account for the dyspnea. Carefully evaluate the patient for findings that might suggest severe underlying cardiopulmonary disease. Laboratory tests are of little assistance except to rule out more serious diseases. The electrocardiograph (ECG) is usually normal. Measurements of arterial P_{CO_2} and pH generally are unrewarding, but pulmonary function tests maybe helpful. Look for other causes of hyperventilation as this syndrome can be the first symptom of a multitude of other diseases (19). However, hyperventilation in athletes often is a response to stress.

Treatment

Reassure the athlete that there is no serious disease and advise him/her to breathe slowly or rebreathe into a paper bag for a few minutes in order to raise the alveolar air CO_2 content. Once the athlete is breathing at a more normal rate, he/she may return to sports participation. An effort should be made to see that a proper diagnosis has been made and to look more carefully into the psychological aspects of the individual.

Foreign Body Aspiration

Aspiration of a foreign body during sports participation happens to both children and adults. It can include the accidental inhalation of dental appliances, food substances, gum, or chewing tobacco. If the object is located between the larynx and carina, acute symptoms of cough, wheezing, stridor, hoarseness, and dyspnea are present. The athlete may display marked retraction of the chest with use of the accessory muscles of respiration. If the obstruction is below the carina, only one lung or a portion of one lung may be affected so that the symptoms are not as dramatic or immediately life threatening. Early symptoms include cough, malaise, fever, and wheezing and can be mistaken for infection, asthma, or other respiratory diseases.

Diagnosis

Indirect laryngoscopy should be performed where possible to look for evidence of a foreign body. Auscultation of the chest may reveal localized wheezing. A PA and lateral x-ray of the neck and chest will reveal evidence of an opaque object.

Treatment

When aspiration is suspected, a Heimlich maneuver should be performed immediately. If symptoms persist and respiratory compromise worsens, a tracheostomy should be performed unless the obstruction is located below the tracheostomy site. Tracheostomy is seldom needed for objects at or below the carina. Patients should be seen by an ENT specialist for endoscopic extraction of the foreign body when indicated.

Complications following foreign body aspiration may come from perforations of the respiratory tree by the aspirated object or from incidental trauma involved in extraction. In order to prevent accidental aspiration, athletes should be instructed to avoid placing any and all objects in their mouths (except for mouthguards) when playing sports.

Vocal Cord Dysfunction

Frequently overlooked when evaluating an athlete with exercise-associated respiratory compromise, VCD is typically described as paradoxical inspiratory closure of the vocal cords. Adduction of the cords with inspiration limits the airflow, and respiratory distress ensues. As described in EIA, patients with VCD generally complain of wheezing, stridor, and shortness of breath with exertion. Laryngoscopy with direct visualization during inspiration is the diagnostic measure of choice (20). Treatment measures vary based on the etiology of cord dysfunction. Behavioral modification and speech therapy along with medications and surgical interventions may be warranted.

Chronic Lung Diseases and Exercise

Chronic obstructive pulmonary disease (COPD) is a condition of deteriorating pulmonary function due to obstruction of expiratory airflow. The primary cause is tobacco use, but other environmental exposures along with alpha-1-antitrypsin deficiency can play a role. Severe restrictions in lung function with associated chronic hypoxemia lead to a fear of exercise in many adults and therefore further deconditioning. This deterioration in aerobic and anaerobic fitness leads to further exertional fatigue, a more sedentary lifestyle, and eventual loss of independence. Exercise has not been shown to reverse the physiological or anatomical changes seen in COPD (21). Many studies support the belief that exercise improves the dyspnea, reduces ventilation, and improves overall exercise tolerance. Moderate exercise on a daily basis has shown the most benefit in improving functional capacity. Owing to other co-morbidities frequently seen with COPD, medical clearance by a physician is recommended before beginning a new exercise program.

Cystic fibrosis (CF) is an autosomal recessive disorder affecting multiple organ systems. Of chief importance for this chapter are its affects on the lungs. Thick mucous production seen in CF often leads to infection and compromise of the respiratory system. Regular exercise has been reported to be an essential part of the physiotherapy management of children with CF. Improved cardiorespiratory fitness, enhanced strength, and improved endurance and mobility are useful to enhance self-esteem and improve daily function. Additional support for exercise in CF patients comes from studies by Thomas, Cook, and Brooks in 1995 (22). They reported significant augmentation of secretions when exercise was combined with chest physiotherapy. Mild cases of CF are essentially cleared for exercise as allowed by their pulmonary function. More severe cases may require supplemental oxygen and a formal rehabilitation program. Fluid balance is a key element in all forms of exercise and especially with CF. Avoidance of exercise in the heat, or at least an awareness of water and salt losses, followed by appropriate hydration is necessary.

REFERENCES

1. Rupp NT, Brudno S, Guill M. The value of screening for risk of exercise-induced asthma in high school students. *Ann Allergy* 1993;70:339–342.
2. Storms W. Exercise-induced asthma: diagnosis and treatment for the recreational or elite athlete. *Med Sci Sports Exerc* 1999;31(1):S33–S38.
3. Courtney AU, McCarter DF, Pollart SM. Childhood asthma: treatment update. *Am Fam Physician* 2005;71(10):1959–1968.
4. Feinstein RA, LaRussa J, Wang-Dohiman A, et al. Screening adolescent athletes for exercise exercise-induced asthma. *Clin J Sport Med* 1996;6(2):119–123.
5. Wilkerson L. Exercise-induced asthma. *J Am Osteopath Assoc* 1998;98(4): 211–215.
6. Lacroix VJ. Exercise-induced asthma. *Phys Sportsmed* 1999;27(12):75–92.
7. Rundell KW, Im J, Mayers LB, et al. Self-reported symptoms and exercise-induced asthma in the elite athlete. *Med Sci Sports Exerc* 2001;33:208–213.
8. Anderson SD, Argyros GJ, Magnussen H, et al. Provocation by eucapnic voluntary hyperpnea to identify exercise-induced bronchoconstriction. *Br J Sports Med* 2001;35:344–347.
9. Eliasson AH., Phillips YY, Rajagopal KR, Howard RS: Sensitivity and specificity of bronchial provocation testing. An evaluation of four techniques in exercise-induced bronchospasm. *Chest* 1992;102:347–355.
10. Weiler J. Exercise-induced asthma: a practical guide to definitions, diagnosis, prevalence and treatment. *Allergy Asthma Proc* 1996;7(6):315–325.
11. Villaran C, O'Neill SI, vanNoord JA, et al. Montelukast versus salmeterol in patients with asthma and exercise-induced bronchonstriction. *Eur Respir J* 1999;104:547–553.
12. Edelman JM, Turpin JA, Bronsky EA, et al. Oral montelukast compared with inhaled salmeterol to prevent exercise bronchoconstriction: a randomized, double blind trial. *Ann Intern Med* 2000;132:97–104.
13. Poppius H, Sovijarvi AR, Tammilehto L. Lack of protective effect of high-dose ipratropium on bronchoconstriction following exercise with cold air breathing in patients with mild asthma. *Eur J Respir Dis* 1986;68(5):319–325.
14. Vukich D, Markovchick V. *Emergency medicine: concepts and clinical practice textbook*. CV Mosby, 1983.
15. Bracker M. *The 5-minute sports medicine consultant textbook*. Lippincott Williams & Wilkins, 2001.
16. Johnson R. *Sports medicine in primary care textbook*. WB Saunders, 2000.
17. Karofsky PS. Hyperventilation syndrome in adolescent athletes. *Phys Sportsmed* 1987;15(2):133.
18. Lewis BL. The hyperventilation syndrome. *Ann Int Med* 1983;38:918.
19. Anderson SD. Issues in exercise-induced asthma. *J Allergy Clin Immunol* 1985;76:763–772.
20. Morris MJ, Deal LE, Grbach VX, et al. Vocal cord dysfunction in patients with exertional dyspnea. *Chest* 1999;116:(6):1676–1682.
21. American College of Sports Medicine. *Current comment. Exercise for persons with COPD*. October 2002.
22. Thomas J, Cook DJ, Brooks D. Chest physical therapy management of patients with cystic fibrosis: a meta-analysis. *Am J Respir Crit Care Med* 1995;151:846.

Gastrointestinal System

12

Scott A. Paluska

Athletes may experience a diverse array of minor to serious gastrointestinal (GI) disorders in association with physical activity. The complex interactions among the various hollow viscus and solid abdominal organs generate a number of possibilities for activity-related injuries or functional perturbations. For example, GI motility and bleeding disorders have been noted in athletes after cycling or running sessions. Other disquieting symptoms such as eructation, dyspepsia, bloating, regurgitation, and reflux may also occur during physical activity. Medications that are used by athletes, including nonsteroidal anti-inflammatory drugs (NSAIDs), may significantly increase the risk of bleeding, gastritis, or other unpleasant GI symptoms (1,2). In addition, blunt or penetrating abdominal trauma from contact sports may damage vulnerable solid abdominal organs. This chapter will address the etiology and management of several common GI conditions to assist clinicians in managing these disorders among their athletic populations.

MOTILITY DISORDERS

A significant number of recreational and competitive athletes complain of GI motility disturbances during exercise (3,4). Symptoms are reported more frequently with running than with other endurance sports that utilize a more stable body position such as cycling or rowing (5–9). As a result, GI motility disorders were first labeled as "runner's trots" in reference to the stool changes associated with running (10). Nonetheless, athletic motility symptoms are highly variable and may include nausea, vomiting, bloating, cramping, the urge to defecate, or a change in the frequency of bowel movements (4,5,11–14). Lower GI disturbances are generally more common than upper GI ones (4,8,12). Symptoms of the lower GI tract are also noted more often by female athletes, potentially due to the altered GI transit that occurs during the luteal phase of the ovulatory cycle (4,6,15). In general, inexperienced or untrained athletes are more likely to experience GI motility disorders (4,5,7,10).

Etiology

Significant controversy surrounds the etiology of exercise-related GI motility disorders. Some have speculated that compression of the colon by psoas muscle hypertrophy alters GI motility (3). Others have proposed that increased sympathetic nerve tone during exercise disrupts GI transit by preferentially shunting blood away from the gut to skin and skeletal muscles (3,6). Investigators have also postulated that running alters bowel transit time by jostling the abdomen, although the bouncing of abdominal contents during exercise has not been clearly shown to alter GI motility significantly (16,17). Hormonal fluctuations of catecholamines, secretin, glucagon, motilin, gastrin, beta-endorphin, and vasoactive intestinal peptide (VIP) have all been observed during exercise and may play an additional role in affecting GI motility (4–6,14,18–21).

The impact of physical activity on whole gut transit has not been clearly determined. Most researchers have concluded that mild to moderate physical activity does not lead to significantly altered mouth-to-cecum transit time (7,12–16,18,22,23), but some have suggested that exercise does accelerate this process (3,4,19). It is clear that each organ, from the esophagus to the colon, plays a unique role in gut transit time during exercise. Esophageal peristaltic contractions undergo altered durations, amplitudes, and frequencies as exercise intensity increases (7,20,22,24–26). However, there is no clear consensus that the functional esophageal changes that occur with physical activity significantly modify esophageal motility (9,27). Light to moderate exercise (<70% $VO_{2\ max}$) minimally impacts gastric emptying, whereas more intense exercise significantly delays emptying of the stomach (3,6,7,9,12,14,18,22,23,28). Small bowel data is conflicting, but transit time and propulsion speed typically decline as physical activity levels increase (6,12,14,15,29). Exercise negligibly alters large intestine motility, the single greatest contributing factor to whole gut transit (3,6,12,13,29). Thus, the overall impact of exercise on the speed with which food passes from the mouth to the anus during physical activity is likely clinically insignificant (21,28,29).

Although GI motility disorders that occur in association with exercise most likely have a multifactorial etiology, relative ischemia of the GI tract contributes significantly (3–6,10,18). Visceral blood has been noted to decrease by 30% during mild to moderate activity (11) and by up to 80% during maximal exertion (5,19,22,30). Hyperthermia during exercise may also exacerbate relative ischemia (10). In addition, intense physical exertion may disrupt the intestinal barrier, increase permeability, enhance the uptake of toxic substances, and augment ischemic-related GI distress (5,14,31). Hydration status is also significant, and a greater percentage of body weight lost during a marathon is a strong predictor of increased GI motility complaints (3,6). Of note, routine ingestion of sports drinks containing carbohydrates during exercise leads to more GI complaints than water consumption (8).

Management

Owing to the mild symptoms of most GI motility disorders, athletes often do not seek medical attention (10). Among those athletes who present for evaluation, consideration should be given to other causes including inflammatory bowel disease, irritable bowel syndrome, travel-related illnesses, infectious diarrhea, and colon cancer. Clinical suspicion of these conditions merits testing for fecal leukocytes, erythrocytes, ova, parasites, fat, and bacterial pathogens (5). Upper and lower endoscopy may also be necessary in certain cases. Initial therapy should focus on hydrating the athlete with cold, low-osmolarity solutions (3). Severely dehydrated athletes may need intravenous (IV) hydration or hospitalization. After symptoms subside, training intensity and duration should be reduced for 1 to 2 weeks. Cross training in temperate conditions may help minimize symptoms when resuming exercise (5).

Awareness and prevention of GI motility disorders among athletes is essential to minimize the frequency and severity of symptoms. Exacerbating substances such as high fiber or high fat foods, milk, and fruits should be avoided for several hours before exercise (5,13). Moderate consumption of caffeinated beverages is acceptable, as there do not appear to be any significant negative GI motility effects of consuming limited amounts of caffeine before exercise (8). The routine use of cathartics or laxatives should be avoided (3,12). Supplemental protein and herb extracts may induce GI upset, so their use before activity should be minimized (6). Urination or bowel movements before exercise may also help attenuate symptoms (12). If symptoms regularly occur despite the interventions mentioned in the previous text, then a trial of antiperistalsis agents such as loperamide may be considered, although their use may negatively affect performance (3,5). In general, most GI motility disorders are relatively benign and can be conservatively managed with limited medical intervention.

GASTROINTESTINAL BLEEDING

Episodes of GI bleeding have been well documented following strenuous or endurance activities (3,12,32). In some instances, GI bleeding occurs in conjunction with motility disorders or other systemic conditions (6,13). Exercise intensity is related to the incidence of GI bleeding. Notably, 7% to 30% of marathoners and 80% to 85% of ultramarathoners have event-related hemoccult-positive stools (5,12,14,32,33). The risk of bleeding peaks during the 24 to 48 hours following athletic activities (30). Several reported cases of GI bleeding have occurred in runners, but cyclists and other athletes are also at risk (3,32,34). Although occult bleeding, iron deficiency, or mild anemia frequently occurs as a result of intense exercise, significant bleeding is rare (3,11,12,28,30,33,34). Because occult bleeding is the norm, affected athletes may only note exertional dyspnea, fatigue, or decreased endurance (21). However, it may be difficult to assess the actual level of anemia, because pseudoanemia resulting from a relatively increased plasma volume may also be present (12).

Etiology

Identifying an upper GI or lower GI source of an athlete's bleeding is usually challenging. Hemorrhagic gastritis is the most commonly identified cause of exercise-related GI bleeding (3,12,14). The colon is the second most frequently implicated site, but no confirmed cases of esophageal bleeding have been reported in association with physical activity (12,14,30). Although small bowel bleeding is rare, exercise-related anemia due to ileal ulcers diagnosed by capsule endoscopy has been reported (35). Exercise-induced GI bleeding may also be related to irritated hemorrhoids or anal fissures. Nonetheless, the causes of athletic GI bleeding often remain obscure, and most cases have no identified sources (12,30,32).

Some have suggested that the use of NSAIDs may increase the risk of GI bleeding among active individuals (6,32–34), but others have found no significant associations between athletic NSAID use and GI bleeding (3,5,12,30,36). One study of 34 healthy runners who completed the Chicago marathon found that runners who ingested ibuprofen had significantly increased intestinal permeability, but the reported GI symptoms did not correlate with the observed alterations in permeability (31). Moreover, the use of NSAIDs was not associated with the frequency or severity of subjective GI symptoms. Nonetheless, NSAID-induced toxicity results in over 100,000 hospitalizations and 16,500 deaths yearly in the United States for serious GI complications, often without any prior symptoms of GI distress (2). As such, NSAID use should be limited by athletes, especially because there is no conclusive evidence supporting the routine use of NSAIDs in treating most soft tissue injuries (37).

Several etiologies have been proposed to explain exercise-related GI bleeding. Most researchers believe that relative bowel ischemia produces regional blood flow attenuation (3,11–13,30,32,36). As noted previously, intestinal blood flow may decrease by 30% to 80%, depending on the intensity and duration of activity, and this diminished bowel perfusion may subsequently increase the risk of bleeding (5,11,14,17,19,28). However, the amount or intensity of exercise has not been consistently correlated with GI bleeding, so other factors likely also play a role (12). The proximal colon appears to be particularly susceptible to ischemia and may be traumatized by high-impact mechanical jarring during exercise, the "cecal-slap syndrome"(5,30,32). Decreased lower esophageal sphincter pressures that occur during exercise increase the risk of bleeding due to irritation of the gastroesophageal junction by the stomach contents (33). Arachidonic acid is the precursor of the mucosal-protecting prostaglandins through the cyclooxygenase enzymes (COX-1, COX-2), and decreased levels of arachidonic acid in the membranes of GI mucosa have been postulated to be another risk factor for GI bleeding in active older adults (38). Finally, athletic GI bleeding may occur as a result of inflammatory bowel disease, coagulation disorders, systemic connective tissue disorders, or GI cancer (3,5,39).

Management

Small amounts of GI bleeding have not been shown to produce detrimental health effects, and most sports-related cases are self-limited and spontaneously resolve. Nonetheless, significant or life-threatening blood loss may occur among athletes (12,30). Athletes with brisk GI bleeding need prompt stabilization and treatment. The athlete should be placed supine with the legs elevated to assist blood return to the heart (Trendelenburg position). Intravenous access should be obtained with two large-bore (16-gauge) catheters. Fluid resuscitation may be accomplished with normal saline or Ringer's lactate solution. Athletes with substantial blood loss should be transferred to an appropriate facility for endoscopic evaluation and further treatment. Blood transfusions may rarely be necessary. Physical activity should be discontinued until symptoms have fully resolved and a comprehensive evaluation completed (5). Athletes who have successfully recovered from significant exercise-related GI bleeding will need to advance activities slowly under careful supervision.

Prevention of GI bleeding may be effective in some instances. Dehydration and hypovolemia should be avoided, as they both can augment intestinal ischemia (33). In addition, the routine use of an H_2-receptor antagonists (H_2RAs) before exercise may help prevent GI bleeding due to hemorrhagic gastritis (3,5,30). If NSAIDs are regularly used by athletes with a history of GI bleeding, concomitant treatment with a proton pump inhibitor (PPI) should be considered, but H_2RAs do not appear to have the same protective effect (1,2). Routine, moderate intensity exercise among older adults has been associated with a decreased risk of severe GI bleeding and may have preventive effects in certain populations (36). Appropriate training with gradual activity progression may minimize episodes of GI bleeding by enhancing GI blood flow, although the gut generally adapts poorly to the increased physiological stress of high-intensity exercise (6).

GASTROESOPHAGEAL REFLUX DISEASE

Numerous upper GI symptoms including eructation, fullness, heartburn, and regurgitation occur during athletic activities (17,21,28,40,41). Gastroesophageal reflux disease (GERD), a condition in which gastric contents shift from the stomach into the esophagus, affects more than 30% of adults, increases linearly with age, and causes symptoms that are frequently reported to physicians (42–45) (see Figure 12.1). Multiple intrinsic and extrinsic factors contribute to GERD, including age, postprandial exercise, smoking, and dietary fat intake (17,28,41). Moreover, an increased body mass index (BMI) is a significant risk factor for GERD, and the burgeoning worldwide rates of childhood and adult obesity will likely increase the incidence of symptomatic reflux (44,46–48). Gastroesophageal reflux is

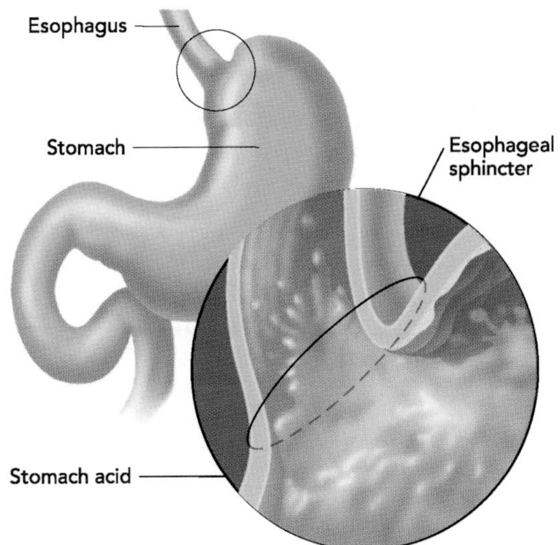

Figure 12.1 Gastroesophageal reflux disease (GERD) occurs when gastric contents shift from the stomach into the esophagus.

frequently noted by athletes, and up to 50% complain of reflux symptoms during exercise (40,49). A prior history of GERD also increases the likelihood of noticeable symptoms during exercise. The mode of physical activity is an important predisposing factor; runners and weight lifters have particularly high rates of documented gastroesophageal reflux (17,25,27,40,41,50,51).

Untreated GERD may not only produce disquieting symptoms but also pose other health risks to athletes. Gastroesophageal reflux may potentially exacerbate asthmatic symptoms, although there is no clear correlation between exercise-induced bronchoconstriction and GI reflux among individuals with asthma (52). Chronic GERD may also cause posterior laryngeal changes that predispose an athlete to paradoxical vocal cord dysfunction and interfere with physical activity (53). Some athletes with reflux may report symptoms that mimic cardiac pain and require extensive evaluation resulting in unnecessary anxiety and delayed participation. Physical activity may decrease the lower esophageal sphincter pressure and increase the risk of GI bleeding or anemia due to irritation of the gastroesophageal junction (33). Chronic gastric acid reflux may also lead to ulcerations, strictures, metaplastic esophageal changes (Barrett's esophagus), or esophagitis (see Figure 12.2). Finally, strong evidence has supported an association between chronic, symptomatic GERD and adenocarcinoma of the esophagus (42).

Etiology

Several hypotheses have been offered to explain the increased incidence of gastroesophageal reflux during physical activity. Vigorous running or jumping may jostle the abdomen, increase air swallowing, and promote acid reflux. Although physical activity may increase gastric acid production or delay gastric emptying, there is little change in gastric pH or emptying during exercise bouts at up to 70% of VO_2 max (6,9,22,23,41). Regional blood flow may decrease by 30% to 80% depending on the activity intensity and produce relative bowel ischemia (3,11–13,30,32,36). This ischemia may interfere with normal esophageal contractility, clearance, or metabolism of protective luminal factors (38). Exercise may also augment the release of plasma hormones (especially glucagon and VIP) that alter the lower esophageal sphincter pressure and delay gastric emptying (14,17,20,21,40,41). Compromised integrity of the esophagogastric junction has also been strongly associated with a susceptibility for exercise-associated reflux (27). Physical activity induces more frequent transient lower esophageal sphincter relaxations (tLESrs) than normally occur in sedentary individuals (12,20,21,51,54). However, it is unclear that these tLESrs account for significant episodes of exercise-associated reflux (40).

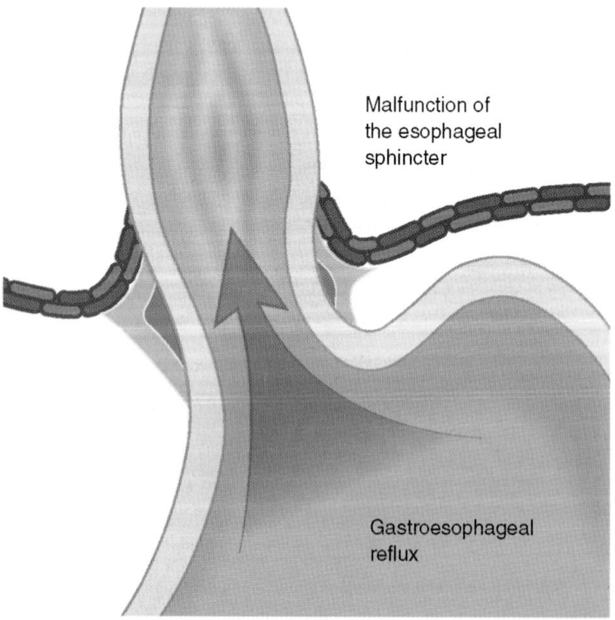

Figure 12.2 Decreased lower esophageal sphincter pressure causes gastric acid reflux and may lead to lower esophageal ulcerations, strictures, metaplastic changes (Barrett's esophagus), or esophagitis.

Body position or intense straining during exercise may both increase reflux episodes because the altered pressure gradient and positional relation between the stomach and the esophagus allow the movement of gastric acid into the lower esophagus. In support of the effect of intra-abdominal pressure changes on athletic GERD, one study of conditioned runners, cyclists, and weight lifters found that weight lifters experienced the most heartburn and reflux, especially during the fed state (40). However, weight lifters experienced the same amount of reflux regardless of whether they remained upright or reclined during activity, suggesting that increased intra-abdominal pressure present during weight lifting may be more important than the gravitational forces. Other studies have also found that running exacerbates measurable reflux, confirming the likeliness that gravity does not influence exercise-related reflux as much as other factors (49–51,54,55).

Fluid intake plays an uncertain role in exercise-related reflux. Athletes can become dehydrated during exercise and develop decreased salivary production. Saliva functions as an important esophageal defense mechanism that helps neutralize stomach acid, but reduced salivary volume also attenuates swallowing frequency and esophageal contractions (20,25,56). Many physically active individuals consume sports drinks containing 4% to 8% carbohydrate in addition to water during prolonged athletic participation to prevent dehydration and replenish energy stores. One study noted that exercise-related reflux was significantly greater after carbohydrate beverage ingestion than after water supplementation (54). In contrast, others have found no differences in reflux or gastric pH between carbohydrate-electrolyte solution sports drinks and water during vigorous exercise (23). Further research is needed to clarify the possible roles of salivary production and fluid replacement in promoting exercise-related GERD.

Exercise intensity variably affects the frequency of gastroesophageal reflux episodes. On one hand, light- to moderate-intensity activities, such as walking, have been shown to reduce esophageal acid exposure time among individuals with known reflux (56). More vigorous activities, on the other hand, disrupt esophageal motor activity and increase gastroesophageal reflux episodes among both trained athletes and untrained individuals (20,24–26,40,44,49,50).

Ambulatory pH monitoring has been used to monitor reflux episodes during physical activity, as it generally has good reproducibility, sensitivity, and specificity (57). One study using ambulatory intraesophageal pH recordings in asymptomatic, physically fit individuals during vigorous stationary bicycling and running found that reflux episodes occurred more often during running than cycling (50). Moreover, postprandial reflux was quantitatively greater than fasting reflux during both cycling and running. Other studies have confirmed the finding that postprandial running induces more measurable reflux episodes in an intensity-related manner (12,25,26,40,54).

It is important to note that upper abdominal and atypical chest pain symptoms are very common in the general population and may be unrelated to reflux (12). In addition, healthy individuals have confirmed brief gastroesophageal reflux episodes in the upright position during ambulatory esophageal pH monitoring without noting any symptoms (55,56). In general, objectively measured reflux is typically found more frequently than subjectively reported symptoms during exercise. Therefore, the clinical applicability and relevance of ambulatory intraesophageal pH-documented reflux as a correlate of exercise-related symptoms is uncertain. Dynamic position testing may be preferable to identify symptomatic GERD, because it has been shown to be more definitive, informative, and efficient (results in <1 hour) in detecting significant reflux than 24-hour pH testing (58). Moreover, it is possible that the upper GI symptoms reported during physical activity are not solely related to acid reflux, so other etiologies should also be considered (49).

Management

Overall, the impact of gastroesophageal reflux on athletic performance needs further clarification but appears to be relatively minimal (22,40). Lifestyle modifications are occasionally helpful in relieving symptoms among athletes with mild to moderate GERD (see Table 12.1) (21,44, 46,59). Refraining from vigorously exercising for at least 3 hours after eating may decrease the likelihood of symptomatic GI reflux (28,57). However, maintaining a program of light- to moderate-intensity physical activity is important, as regular exercise has been shown to have a beneficial effect on symptomatic GERD and may strengthen the lower esophageal sphincter (46,59). Chewing gum or taking oral lozenges after a meal stimulates salivary secretion, promotes swallowing and may also reduce postprandial esophageal acid exposure for a few hours (56). Weight loss is an essential step to diminish reflux, because abdominal obesity displaces the lower esophageal sphincter and gastroesophageal junction superiorly from the peritoneal cavity into the lower pressure intra-thoracic region and facilitates acid shifts from the stomach into the distal esophagus (27,47) (see Figure 12.3).

If lifestyle modifications and nonpharmacological measures are not effective, several therapeutic agents may be

TABLE 12.1
NONPHARMACOLOGICAL MEASURES USED IN THE TREATMENT OF GASTROESOPHAGEAL REFLUX DISEASE

Dietary
Avoid caffeinated products
Avoid chocolate or mint
Avoid fatty foods or large meals
Avoid eating 3–4 hr before lying down
Avoid citrus fruits, onions, tomatoes, or spicy foods
Minimize alcohol consumption
Use lozenges or gum to stimulate salivary secretion
Lifestyle
Elevate the head of the bed on blocks
Discontinue smoking
Lose weight
Avoid exercise for 3 hr after eating

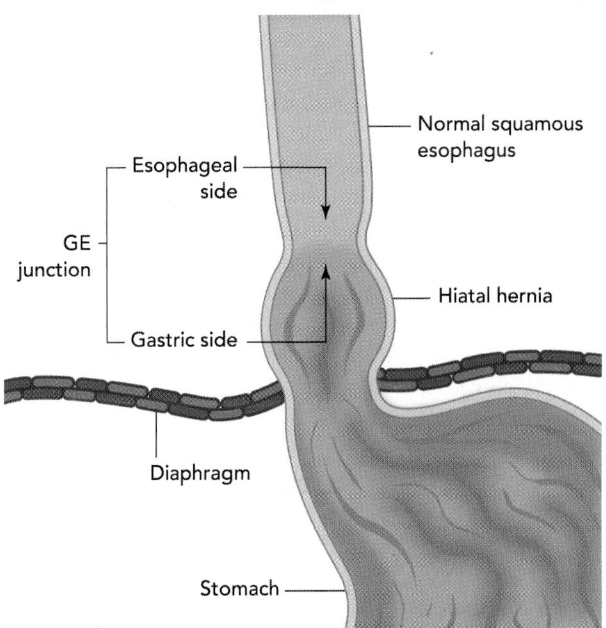

Figure 12.3 Abdominal obesity may displace the lower esophageal sphincter and gastroesophageal (GE) junction superiorly from the peritoneal cavity into the lower pressure intra-thoracic cavity, facilitating acid shifts from the stomach into the distal esophagus.

TABLE 12.2
MEDICATIONS USED IN THE TREATMENT OF GASTROESOPHAGEAL REFLUX DISEASE

Medication (Trade name)	Class	Typical dosage	Generic available
Aluminum hydroxide **(Amphojel)**	Antacid	5–10 mL or one to two tablets, maximum six tablets/d	Yes
Calcium carbonate **(Tums)**	Antacid	1–3 g, maximum 8 g/d	Yes
Aluminum hydroxide/magnesium hydroxide **(Maalox)**	Antacid	10–20 mL or one to four tablets, maximum 12 tablets/d	Yes
Cimetidine **(Tagamet)**	H_2-receptor antagonist	400 mg 2/d or 800 mg at night	Yes
Famotidine **(Pepcid)**	H_2-receptor antagonist	20 mg 2/d or 40 mg at night	Yes
Nizatidine **(Axid)**	H_2-receptor antagonist	150 mg 2/d or 300 mg at night	Yes
Ranitidine **(Zantac)**	H_2-receptor antagonist	150 mg 2/d or 300 mg at night	Yes
Esomeprazole **(Nexium)**	Proton pump inhibitor	20–40 mg/d	No
Lansoprazole **(Prevacid)**	Proton pump inhibitor	15–30 mg/d	No
Omeprazole **(Prilosec)**	Proton pump inhibitor	20–40 mg/d	Yes
Pantoprazole **(Protonix)**	Proton pump inhibitor	40 mg/d	No
Rabeprazole **(Aciphex)**	Proton pump inhibitor	40 mg/d	No

tried in the treatment of reflux (see Table 12.2). Most of the medications commonly used for GERD are safe and well tolerated by athletes (41). Potential adverse reactions include somnolence, confusion, headache, dizziness, diarrhea, nausea, vomiting, constipation, and abdominal pain. Antacids neutralize gastric acid and diminish acidic irritation of the lower esophagus during exercise. However, calcium and aluminum-based antacids may cause constipation, and magnesium-based ones may produce diarrhea. H_2RAs reversibly inhibit histamines, binding to gastric parietal cells and decrease gastric acid secretion. When taken before exercise, H_2RAs have been shown to reduce intraesophageal acid exposure significantly during running (51). Although the currently available H_2RAs differ in cost, potency, and duration, they are equally effective (57). PPIs decrease gastric acid secretion to a greater degree than either antacids or H_2RAs by irreversibly inhibiting the H+/K+ adenosine triphosphatase (ATPase) pump on parietal cells and are very effective for controlling GERD (57). The PPI omeprazole has been shown to diminish acid reflux substantially on intraesophageal pH recording during strenuous physical activity (49). In general, there are no clear efficacy differences among the currently available PPIs, but they should be taken at least 30 minutes before eating (57). An empirical trial of 4 to 8 weeks of a PPI for symptomatic reflux is reasonable for most athletes (57,60).

Many athletes respond well to lifestyle modifications and brief courses of medications. Athletes, particularly those older than 55 years, with dyspepsia and alarm symptoms such as early satiety, unintended weight loss, bleeding, persistent vomiting, a strong family history of GI cancer, odynophagia, or progressive dysphagia should undergo upper endoscopy (60). Nonetheless, the low absolute risk of esophageal cancer in most athletes with reflux symptoms combined with the lack of demonstrated efficacy of endoscopic screening usually makes routine upper endoscopy unnecessary (42,57). Antireflux surgery may rarely be necessary for those with chronic GERD who have failed conservative therapy or developed complications such as Barrett's esophagus. The goal of surgery is to improve the integrity of the lower esophageal sphincter, and laparoscopic or open surgical techniques are effective for long-term symptom relief (43,57).

SPLEEN INJURIES

The spleen is one of the most commonly injured abdominal organs due to its rigid capsule and vulnerable location (3,61). In general, solid abdominal organs such as the spleen and liver are more susceptible to injury than hollow viscera (61). A direct abdominal blow or indirect injury from overlying rib fractures is the most common cause of activity-related spleen injury or rupture (see Figure 12.4). Tenderness that is noted over the left ninth, tenth, or eleventh ribs should heighten one's suspicion of an underlying spleen injury (3,61) (see Figure 12.5). While some spleen injuries bleed slowly, most bleed briskly and pose a substantial morbidity and mortality risk (3). Splenomegaly increases the likelihood of a spleen injury, and rupture of an enlarged spleen is the most common cause of death in association with infectious mononucleosis (IM) (62). Unfortunately, it is often clinically difficult to identify splenomegaly during the abdominal examination because palpation detects splenomegaly only 17% to 50% of the time (62–67).

Etiology

Although athletic trauma is a risk factor for a spleen injury, injuries may occur spontaneously during everyday activities

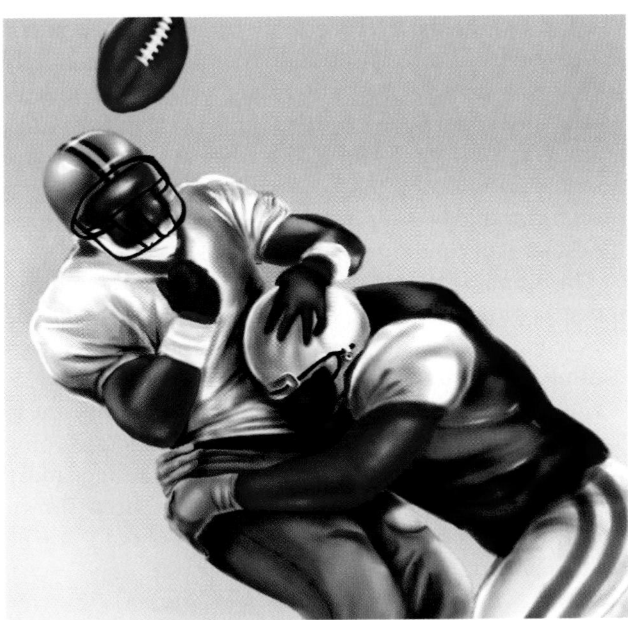

Figure 12.4 A direct abdominal blow to the left upper quadrant may cause a spleen injury or rupture.

such as coughing or lifting (63,68). As noted, spleen injuries should be considered after any rib fractures of the left lower thorax or blows to the left upper quadrant of the abdomen. The rapid acceleration–deceleration forces that occur during contact sports can also tear the spleen's rigid capsule (69).

Acute IM poses a significant risk factor for sustaining a spleen injury due to the presence of splenomegaly. IM is caused by the Epstein-Barr virus and peaks without seasonality in individuals aged 15 to 19 years in industrialized countries. It has a variable systemic presentation and infrequently presents with the classic triad of fever, pharyngitis, and lymphadenopathy (62,65,70–73). Splenomegaly is a common finding in IM and occurs in approximately 50% of acute infections (62,70,71). The risk of spleen rupture is greatest during days 4 to 21 of acute IM, and ruptures occur in 0.1% to 0.5% of infected individuals (3,62,64,74–76). Most IM-related spleen injuries occur in men as a result of contact sports, but athletic ruptures may have no correlation with traumatic episodes (66,69,73,75,76). Although the risk of spleen injury during abdominal palpation in IM is minimal, repeated palpation of an enlarged spleen should be avoided (77). A more extensive discussion of IM can be found in Chapter 18.

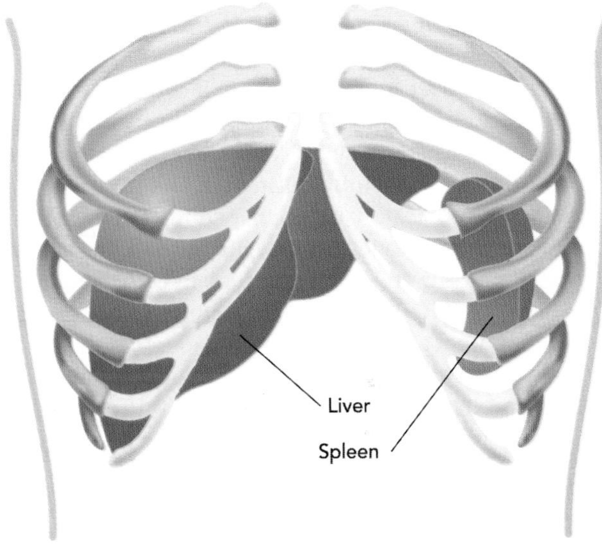

Figure 12.5 The spleen typically lies behind the left ninth, tenth, and eleventh anterior ribs.

Management

Suspected spleen injuries require a rapid, thorough assessment. Athletes with acute injuries may be hemodynamically unstable and present with pallor, tachycardia, orthostasis, or shock (75). A capsular rupture may cause a hemoperitoneum, and a positive Kehr's sign (referred pain to the left shoulder due to diaphragmatic irritation from free intraperitoneal blood) occurs in 50% of spleen injuries (75,76). The presence of persistent tachycardia or right shoulder pain may also indicate the presence of a spleen rupture (77). Initial management of suspected spleen injuries should include assessing vital signs and establishing two large-bore IV lines (3,69). Blood should be drawn and sent for type and cross-match (69). Cases of suspected spleen rupture or bleeding should be immediately transported to a hospital after initial stabilization has been performed.

Various methods have been used to identify the extent of spleen injuries. Abdominal computed tomography (CT) has been considered the study of choice to assess injury grade, but ultrasound (USN) can rapidly identify spleen injuries in many instances (74,75,78,79) (see Figure 12.6). Infrequently, spleen injuries are not detected by abdominal USN, and minimal or no intraperitoneal fluid is visible on CT scanning. Such injuries are generally of minimal clinical significance (80). Diagnostic peritoneal lavage (DPL) has historically been used to evaluate cases of suspected spleen injury, but has little modern value (61,69,79,81).

Splenectomy, which has a relatively low morbidity and mortality, may be necessary following a significant spleen injury (68,74–76). Nonetheless, selective nonoperative management is appropriate for hemodynamically stable individuals and minimizes the risk of post-splenectomy complications or sepsis due to encapsulated bacteria (61,73–76,81–83). Close monitoring is essential if a nonoperative approach is employed. Pneumococcal conjugate and/or polysaccharide vaccine and quadrivalent meningococcal vaccine are indicated for all asplenic athletes aged 2 years or more. Previously unimmunized athletes should also receive immunization against *Haemophilus influenzae* Type b infections. Daily antimicrobial prophylaxis with penicillin for protection against pneumococcal infections should be

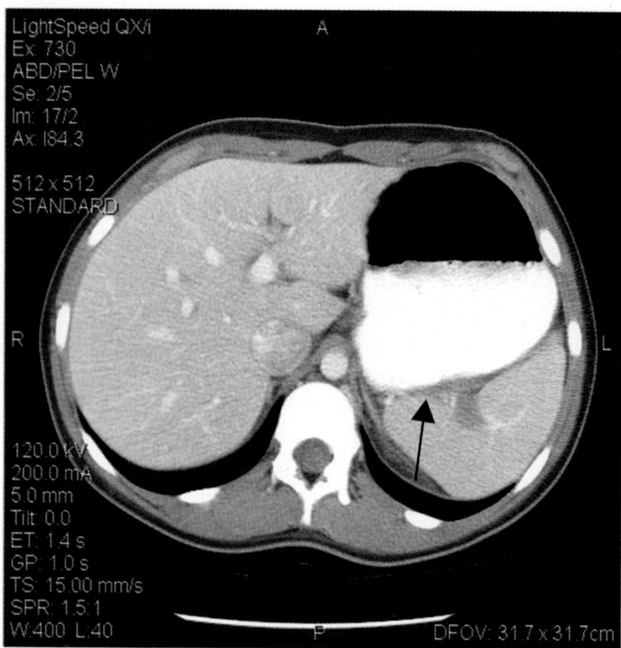

Figure 12.6 Abdominal computed tomography (CT) is an excellent way to identify and grade a spleen injury or rupture (arrow).

considered for certain asplenic athletes, especially those with sickle cell anemia, neoplasia, or thalassemia (83).

Making the decision when to allow athletes with spleen injuries to return to play is challenging, and a wide range of periods have been proposed. Athletes who have had a splenectomy or a laceration repair should wait at least 6 weeks before returning to full activity (61,75). Individuals who have had a nonoperatively treated spleen injury should wait 2 to 6 months, depending on the severity of the injury, before returning to athletic activities (75).

A variety of recommendations for return to play have also been advocated for an athlete with acute IM. Unfortunately, no clear correlation exists among the disease's clinical severity, illness duration, liver enzyme levels, spleen size, and subsequent risk of spleen rupture (66,67,73). Classically, the potential risk of a spleen rupture in IM was felt to necessitate restriction of athletics for 6 months after symptom onset (77). Because most spleen injuries associated with IM occur during the first 21 days of illness, clinicians currently recommend that athletes avoid vigorous activity, weight lifting, and contact sports for at least 3 weeks after the onset of symptoms or the date of diagnosis (62,64,66–68). Although USN is occasionally employed to evaluate the presence and degree of splenomegaly before returning an athlete to contact sports, there is little evidence to support its routine use (3,62,65,71,84). Moreover, adult spleen length nomograms may be misrepresentative of the normal spleen dimensions in tall athletes because spleen size correlates with height (67,85). As such, revised mean and upper limits of the normal range of spleen length for several increments of body height for both men and women have been developed (85).

After 3 weeks, the level of activity can be slowly advanced as tolerated, but clinicians should monitor athletes closely for existing or new abdominal symptoms. Most athletes with acute IM can safely return to limited activities 4 weeks after symptom onset and slowly increase intensity and duration as tolerated (84). However, it may take several months for highly competitive athletes to regain their pre-illness level of conditioning (73).

Uncomplicated IM typically needs only supportive therapy with fluids and analgesics. Aspirin should be avoided, as its use may contribute to the risk of spleen rupture or systemic thrombocytopenia (73). Because IM is a viral illness, antibiotics are not helpful and may cause side effects such as skin rashes. Corticosteroids are only indicated for significant pharyngeal edema causing airway compromise (65,66,73). Acyclovir has not been shown to have a consistent clinical benefit and should not be routinely used (62,63,71).

LIVER INJURIES

The liver plays an essential physiological role as the largest, most versatile solid abdominal organ (85). Although significant liver injuries are relatively rare during athletics, the liver and spleen are the most commonly injured abdominal organs due to trauma (86,87). In contrast to spleen injuries, however, liver injuries rarely result in immediate, significant bleeding (3,86). Nonetheless, substantial blood loss may occasionally accompany a liver injury, and exsanguination accounts for more than 50% of liver-injury–related deaths (69). Most of the athletic-related liver injuries result from football, rugby, wrestling, and soccer participation (61). Liver damage may also rarely occur in association with episodes of hypotension or heatstroke during endurance events (12). Acute or chronic hepatitis may predispose an athlete to systemic symptoms, but routine exercise does not appear to exacerbate hepatitis or meaningfully interfere with the recovery process once acute symptoms have subsided (28,88,89).

Diagnosing liver injuries can be difficult, as physically active individuals may have abnormal liver tests in the absence of liver pathology (12). Moreover, hepatomegaly is often difficult to identify during the abdominal physical examination. Regional muscular contusions, choledocholithiasis or gall bladder disease may also mimic hepatic injuries. Because liver injuries may present with few clinical signs and no obvious bleeding, any athlete who has persistent right upper quadrant pain or tenderness should be clinically evaluated for a possible liver injury. In suspicious cases, CT or magnetic resonance imaging (MRI) should be considered before returning the athlete to activity (3).

Etiology

Athletic liver injuries can occur as a result of blunt or penetrating trauma. A forceful impact to the mid-to-upper

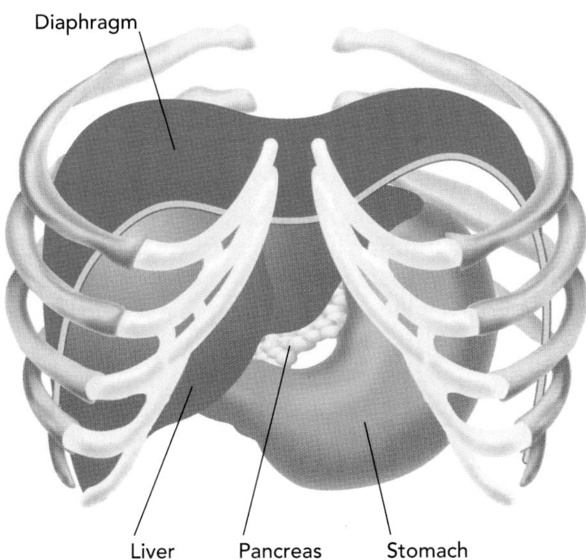

Figure 12.7 A blunt or sharp impact to the right upper quadrant or lower anterior ribs may injure or lacerate the liver.

abdomen or right lower chest may damage the liver and overlying ribs (see Figure 12.7). Resultant liver contusions can produce subcapsular or intraperitoneal hemorrhage and generate right upper quadrant pain and tenderness. Penetrating injuries are rare among athletes but may result from certain atypical mechanisms such as impalement on a sharp object (61). Hepatomegaly may occur with acute hepatitis or IM and predispose an athlete to liver injury (62,64,71,72). Several additional hepatic conditions that increase the likelihood of liver injuries during athletic activities are listed in Table 12.3.

TABLE 12.3
CONDITIONS THAT INCREASE THE RISK OF A LIVER INJURY DURING PHYSICAL ACTIVITY

Infectious
Viral hepatitis type A, B, C, or D
Schistosomiasis
Cytomegalovirus
Mononucleosis
AIDS
Neoplastic
Hepatocellular carcinoma
Lymphoma
Leukemia
Myeloproliferative disease
Metastatic disease
Congenital or Acquired
Congestive heart failure
Pulmonary hypertension
Reticuloendotheliosis
Hemochromatosis
Acute cirrhosis
Venocclusive disease (i.e., Budd-Chiari syndrome)
Alcoholic hepatitis
Valvular heart disease (i.e., tricuspid stenosis)
Steatohepatitis
Constrictive pericarditis
Amyloidosis
Lipid metabolism disorders (i.e., Gaucher's disease)
Sarcoidosis
Mastocytosis
Thalessemia
Castleman's disease (angiofollicular lymph node hyperplasia)
Primary biliary cirrhosis
Primary sclerosing cholangitis
Sickle cell disease

AIDS = acquired immune deficiency syndrome

Management

Initial stabilization of an athlete with a known or suspected liver injury should include placing two large-bore IV lines, positioning the athlete in the Trendelenburg position, giving isotonic fluids, and performing laboratory studies including blood type and cross-match (61,69). If the athlete is free of peritoneal signs (abdominal rigidity, spasm, or guarding) and hemodynamically stable, then he or she may be closely monitored in a supervised setting. However, any athlete who develops increasing pain, peritoneal signs, or hemodynamic instability needs prompt additional evaluation (61,90).

Because the physical examination and abdominal x-rays are often inaccurate for identifying liver abnormalities, ancillary studies are frequently needed to confirm the presence of a liver injury (69,79,89,91). DPL had previously been the preferred method to detect an occult liver injury due to its high sensitivity (90%–98%) and specificity (90%–100%) (61,69,79). Nonetheless, DPL is invasive, produces serious complications in 1% of patients and is infrequently utilized (79). Recently abdominal CT and USN have gained acceptance as accurate, non-invasive ways to evaluate liver injuries. CT has a higher sensitivity and specificity than USN, but requires more time to perform and exposes the athletes to radiation (79,87,91). The addition of an oral contrast solution to CT scanning following blunt abdominal trauma is needed and significantly delays the time necessary to complete the study (92). USN offers the advantages of safety, decreased expense, portability, and speed. As a result, many centers are using USN as their initial diagnostic study to evaluate athletes with suspected liver injuries (78,79,91) (see Figures 12.8 and 12.9). Some liver injuries are not detected by abdominal USN, and minimal or no intraperitoneal fluid is visible on CT scanning. Generally, such injuries are of minimal clinical significance (80).

Most blunt liver injuries (85%) are hemodynamically stable and can be managed conservatively. As such,

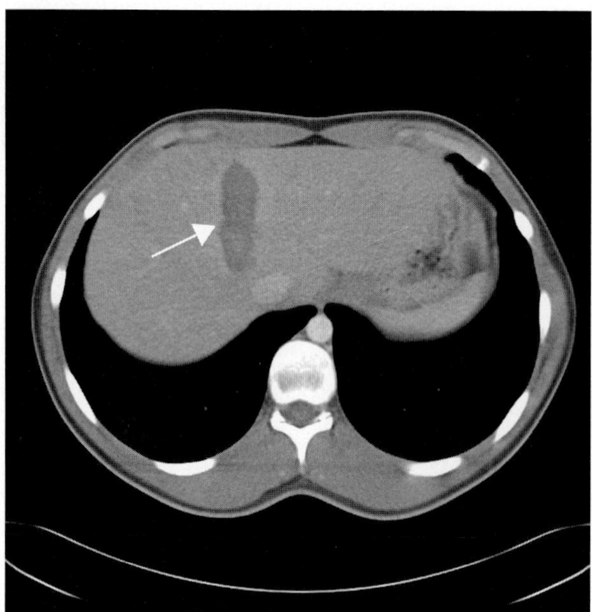

Figure 12.8 Abdominal computed tomography (CT) is a highly sensitive and specific way to identify and grade liver injuries (arrow).

nonoperative management of liver injuries in most children and certain adults has become routine (80,86,87,90,93). Potential complications of nonoperative management include hepatobiliary dysfunction, delayed hemorrhage, undetected injuries to other abdominal organs, and decreased abdominal organ blood flow due to peritoneal hypertension (abdominal compartment syndrome) (93). In general, penetrating liver injuries are associated with greater morbidity and mortality than blunt trauma, and nonoperative treatment of these injuries is not recommended (94).

Appropriate patient selection and documented bleeding cessation are important components of successful nonoperative management (86). Standardized organ injury scales have been developed and updated for liver injuries, but nonoperative treatment decisions should be based on an athlete's hemodynamic stability and not on his or her injury grade (86,87,95). The injury grade may also be helpful to predict which athletes are at increased risk of postoperative hepatobiliary complications (94). By itself, the presence of a hemoperitoneum does not necessitate a laparotomy, but the need for transfusion or ongoing parenchymal bleeding requires operative evaluation (86,87). When operative therapy is indicated following a liver injury, laceration repair or lobectomy can typically be performed without sufficiently affecting postoperative hepatic function (3).

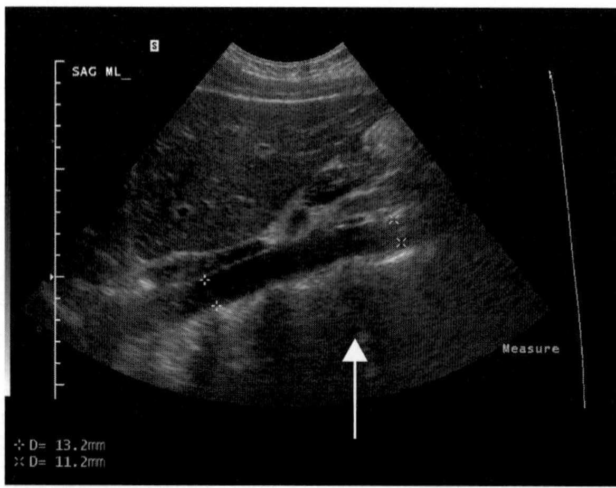

Figure 12.9 Liver injuries may also be identified quickly using ultrasound (arrow).

An athlete must be hemodynamically stable and pain-free before returning to activities after a liver injury. Heavy work or contact sports should be avoided for at least 6 to 8 weeks (61,87). Routine monitoring of liver function tests is not necessary in managing athletes following liver injuries (96). A follow-up CT scan or USN should be used to document healing for an athlete managed nonoperatively (87,90,91). Because complications or hemorrhage may occur days to weeks after a traumatic liver injury, any athlete complaining of right upper quadrant pain, lightheadedness, weakness, or hemodynamic instability warrants prompt additional investigation (87,90). Protective equipment, gradual activity progression, appropriate hydration, and proper technique modifications may minimize recurrent liver injuries. Although most athletes recover uneventfully following blunt liver injuries, the mortality rate from significant, high-grade liver injuries ranges from 17% to 80% (93,94).

SUMMARY

Clinicians who work with physically active individuals need to be mindful of several potential GI disorders or injuries. The abdomen is relatively unprotected and vulnerable to traumatic injury during contact sports. In addition, physical activity may disrupt the complex process of digestion and result in motility, bleeding, or reflux disorders. Appropriate nutrition, hydration, conditioning, and gradual activity progression usually attenuate GI motility disturbances. Most cases of activity-related GI bleeding are self-limited and spontaneously resolve. Gastroesophageal reflux is common in the general population and may become more prominent during exercise. Lifestyle modifications and the judicious use of medications usually control symptoms of exercise-related reflux. Protective equipment and technique modifications may prevent some spleen and liver injuries. In addition, athletes with acute IM or hepatitis should abstain from vigorous activities or contact sports for at least 3 weeks after symptom onset. Any hemodynamically compromised athlete with a GI disorder or injury requires immediate stabilization and a thorough evaluation. Fortunately, most GI disorders can be managed conservatively, and clinically stable athletes may progress their activity levels as symptoms allow.

REFERENCES

1. Chan FKL, Hung LCT, Suen BY, et al. Celocoxib versus diclofenac and omeprazole in reducing the risk of recurrent ulcer bleeding in patients with arthritis. *N Engl J Med* 2002;347(26):2104–2110.
2. Singh G, Triadafilopoulos G. Epidemiology of NSAID-induced gastrointestinal complications. *J Rheumatol* 1999;26(Suppl 56):18–24.
3. Green GA. Gastrointestinal disorders in the athlete. *Clin Sports Med* 1992;11(2):453–470.
4. Riddoch C, Trinick T. Gastrointestinal disturbances in marathon runners. *Br J Sports Med* 1988;22(2):71–74.
5. Butcher JD. Runner's diarrhea and other intestinal problems of athletes. *Am Fam Physician* 1993;48(4):623–627.
6. Brouns F, Beckers E. Is the gut an athletic organ? Digestion, absorption, and exercise. *Sports Med* 1993;15(4):242–257.
7. Soffer EE, Summers RW, Gisolfi C. Effect of exercise on intestinal mobility and transit in trained athletes. *Am J Physiol* 1991;260(Pt I):G698–G702.
8. Van Nieuwenhoven MA, Brouns F, Kovacs EMR. The effect of two sports drinks and water on GI complaints and performance during an 18-km run. *Int J Sports Med* 2005;26:281–285.
9. Van Nieuwenhoven MA, Brouns F, Brummer RJM. Gastrointestinal profile of symptomatic athletes at rest and during physical exercise. *Eur J Appl Physiol* 2004;91:429–434.
10. Fogoros RN. Runner's trots: gastrointestinal disturbances in runners. *JAMA* 1980;243(17):1743–1744.
11. Heer M, Repond F, Hany A, et al. Acute ischaemic colitis in a female long distance runner. *Gut* 1987;28:896–899.
12. Moses FM. The effect of exercise on the gastrointestinal tract. *Sports Med* 1990;9(3):159–172.
13. Sullivan SN, Wong C. Runner's diarrhea: different patterns and associated factors. *J Clin Gastroenterol* 1992;14(2):101–104.
14. Berg A, Müller HM, Rathmann S, et al. The gastrointestinal system: an essential target organ of the athlete's health and physical performance. *Exerc Immunol Rev* 1999;5:78–95.
15. Meshkinpour H, Kemp C, Fairshter R. Effect of aerobic exercise on mouth-to-cecum transit time. *Gastroenterology* 1989;96(3):936–941.
16. Kayaleh RA, Meshkinpour H, Avinashi A, et al. Effect of exercise on mouth-to-cecum transit on trained athletes: a case against the role of runners' abdominal bouncing. *J Sports Med Phys Fitness* 1996;36(4):271–274.
17. Simons SM, Kennedy RG. Gastrointestinal problems in runners. *Curr Sports Med Rep* 2004;3:112–116.
18. Robertson G, Meshkinpour H, Vandenberg K, et al. Effects of exercise on total and segmental colon transit. *J Clin Gastroenterol* 1993;16(4):300–303.
19. Oettlé GJ. Effect of moderate exercise on bowel habit. *Gut* 1991;32:941–944.
20. Soffer EE, Merchant RK, Duethman G, et al. Effect of graded exercise on esophageal motility and gastroesophageal reflux in trained athletes. *Dig Dis Sci* 1993;38(2):220–224.
21. Casey E, Mistry D, MacKnight JM. Training room management of medical conditions: sports gastroenterology. *Clin Sports Med* 2005;24:525–540.
22. Van Nieuwenhoven MA, Brouns F, Brummer RJM. The effect of physical exercise on parameters of gastrointestinal function. *Neurogastroenterol Motil* 1999;11:431–439.
23. Van Nieuwenhoven MA, Brummer RJM, Brouns F. Gastrointestinal function during exercise: comparison of water, sports drink, and sports drink with caffeine. *J Appl Physiol* 2000;89:1079–1085.
24. Ravi N, Stuart RC, Byrne PJ, et al. Effect of physical exercise on esophageal motility in patients with esophageal disease. *Dis Esophagus* 2005;18:374–377.
25. Choi SC, Yoo KH, Kim TH, et al. Effect of graded running on esophageal motility and gastroesophageal reflux in fed volunteers. *J Korean Med Sci* 2001;16:183–187.
26. Soffer EE, Wilson J, Duethman G, et al. Effect of graded exercise on esophageal motility and gastroesophageal reflux in nontrained subjects. *Dig Dis Sci* 1994;39(1):193–198.
27. Pandolfino JE, Bianchi LK, Lee TJ, et al. Esophagogastric junction morphology predicts susceptibility to exercise-induced reflux. *Am J Gastroenterol* 2004;99:1430–1436.
28. Bi L, Triadafilopoulos G. Evidence and gastrointestinal function and disease: an evidence-based review of risks and benefits. *Clin Gastroenterol Hepatol* 2003;1:345–355.
29. Rao KA, Yazaki E, Evans DF, et al. Objective evaluation of small bowel and colonic transit time using pH telemetry in athletes with gastrointestinal symptoms. *Br J Sports Med* 2004;38:482–487.
30. Moses FM. Gastrointestinal bleeding and the athlete. *Am J Gastroenterol* 1993;88(8):1157–1159.
31. Smetanka RD, Lambert GP, Murray R, et al. Intestinal permeability in runners in the 1996 Chicago marathon. *Int J Sport Nutr Exerc Metab* 1999;9(4):426–433.
32. Wilhite J, Mellion MB. Occult gastrointestinal bleeding in endurance cyclists. *Phys Sportsmed* 1990;18(8):75–78.
33. Mechrefe A, Wexler B, Feller E. Sports anemia and gastrointestinal bleeding in endurance athletes. *Med Health R I* 1997;80(7):216–218.
34. Stewart JG, Ahlquist DA, McGill DB, et al. Gastrointestinal blood loss and anemia in runners. *Ann Intern Med* 1984;100(6):843–845.
35. Valle J, Morillas J, Pérez-Grueso MJ, et al. Ileal ulcers in a long-distance runner diagnosed by capsule endoscopy. *Rev Esp Enferm Dig (Madrid)* 2004;11:801–802.
36. Pahor M, Guralnik JM, Salive ME, et al. Physical activity and risk of severe gastrointestinal hemorrhage in older persons. *JAMA* 1994;272(8):595–599.
37. Stanley KL, Weaver JE. Pharmacologic management of pain and inflammation in athletes. *Clin Sports Med* 1998;17(2):375–392.
38. Phinney SD. Physical activity and risk of gastrointestinal hemorrhage in the elderly (letter to the editor). *JAMA* 1994;273(7):521–522.
39. Rubin RB, Saltzman JR, Zawacki JK. Bicycle racing, Raynaud's phenomenon, and gastrointestinal bleeding. *Am J Gastroenterol* 1994;89(2):291–292.
40. Collings KL, Pratt FP, Rodriguez-Stanley S, et al. Esophageal reflux in conditioned runners, cyclists, and weightlifters. *Med Sci Sports Exerc* 2003;35(5):730–735.
41. Parmelee-Peters K, Moeller JL. Gastroesophageal reflux in runners. *Curr Sports Med Rep* 2004;3:107–111.
42. Shaheen N, Ransohoff DF. Gastroesophageal reflux, Barrett esophagus, and esophageal cancer: scientific review. *JAMA* 2002;287(15):1972–1981.
43. Scott M, Gelhot AR. Gastroesophageal reflux disease: diagnosis and management. *Am Fam Physician* 1999;59(5):1161–1169.
44. Nandurkar S, Locke GR III, Fett S, et al. Relationship between body mass index, diet, exercise and gastroesophageal reflux symptoms in a community. *Aliment Pharmacol Ther* 2004;20(5):497–505.
45. Nilsson M, Johnsen R, Ye W, et al. Prevalence of gastro-oesophageal reflux symptoms and the influence of age and sex. *Scand J Gastroenterol* 2004;11:1040–1045.
46. Nocon M, Labenz J, Willich SN. Lifestyle factors and symptoms of gastroesophageal reflux: a population-based survey. *Aliment Pharmacol Ther* 2006;23(10):169–174.
47. Jacobson BC, Somers SC, Fuchs CS, et al. Body-mass index and symptoms of gastroesophageal reflux in women. *N Engl J Med* 2006;354(22):2340–2348.
48. Ogden CL, Carroll MD, Curtin LR, et al. Prevalence of overweight and obesity in the United States, 1999–2004. *JAMA* 2006;295(13):1549–1555.
49. Peters HPF, De Kort AFCC, Van Krevelen H, et al. The effect of omeprazole on gastro-oesophageal reflux and symptoms during strenuous exercise. *Aliment Pharmacol Ther* 1999;13:1015–1022.
50. Clark CS, Kraus BB, Sinclair J, et al. Gastroesophageal reflux induced by exercise in healthy volunteers. *JAMA* 1989;261(24):3599–3601.
51. Kraus BB, Sinclair JW, Castell DO. Gastroesophageal reflux in runners. Characteristics and treatment. *Ann Intern Med* 1990;112(6):429–433.
52. Weiner P, Konson N, Sternberg A, et al. Is gastro-oesophageal reflux a factor in exercise-induced asthma? *Respir Med* 1998;92:1071–1075.
53. Powell DM, Karanfilov BI, Beechler KB, et al. Paradoxical vocal cord dysfunction in juveniles. *Arch Otolaryngol Head Neck Surg* 2000;126:29–34.
54. Peters HPF, Wiersma JWC, Koerselman J, et al. The effect of a sports drink on gastroesophageal reflux during a run-bike-run test. *Int J Sports Med* 2000;21:65–70.
55. Saraswat VA, Dhiman RK, Mishra A, et al. Correlation of 24-hr esophageal pH patterns with clinical features and endoscopy in gastroesophageal reflux disease. *Dig Dis Sci* 1994;39(1):199–205.
56. Avidan B, Sonnenberg A, Schnell TG, et al. Walking and chewing reduce postprandial acid reflux. *Aliment Pharmacol Ther* 2001;15:151–155.
57. DeVault KR, Castell DO. Updated guidelines for the diagnosis and treatment of gastroesophageal reflux disease. *Am J Gastroenterol* 2005;100:190–200.
58. Schowengerdt CG. Dynamic position testing for the detection of esophageal acid reflux disease. *Dig Dis Sci* 2005;50(10):100–102.
59. Nilsson M, Johnsen R, Ye W, et al. Lifestyle risk factors in the aetiology of gastroesophageal reflux. *Gut* 2004;53:1730–1735.
60. Talley NJ, Vakil N. The Practice Parameters Committee of the American College of Gastroenterology. Guidelines for the management of dyspepsia. *Am J Gastroenterol* 2005;100:2324–2337.
61. Diamond DL. Sports-related abdominal trauma. *Clin Sports Med* 1989;8(1):91–99.
62. Godshall SE, Kirchner JT. Infectious mononucleosis: complexities of a common syndrome. *Postgrad Med* 2000;107(7):175–186.
63. Chetham MM, Roberts KB. Infectious mononucleosis in adolescents. *Pediatr Ann* 1991;20(4):206–213.
64. Haines J. When to resume sports after infectious mononucleosis: how soon is safe? *Postgrad Med* 1987;81(1):331–333.
65. Ebell M. Epstein-Barr virus infectious mononucleosis. *Am Fam Physician* 2004;70(7):1279–1287.
66. MacKnight J. Infectious mononucleosis: ensuring a safe return to sport. *Phys Sportsmed* 2002;30(1):27–41.
67. Waninger KN, Harcke HT. Determination of safe return to play for athletes recovering from infectious mononucleosis: a review of the literature. *Clin J Sport Med* 2005;15(6):410–416.
68. Eichner ER. Infectious mononucleosis: recognizing the condition, 'reactivating' the patient. *Phys Sportsmed* 1996;24(4):49–54.
69. Burns RK, Ross SE. Emergency: blunt abdominal trauma. *Hosp Med* 1993;29(2):73–86.
70. Bisno AL. Primary care: acute pharyngitis. *N Engl J Med* 2001;344(3):205–211.
71. Straus SE, Cohen JI, Tosato G, et al. Epstein-Barr virus infectious: biology, pathogenesis, and management. *Ann Intern Med* 1993;118(1):45–58.

72. Rea TD, Russo JE, Katon W, et al. Prospective study of the natural history of infectious mononucleosis caused by Epstein-Barr virus. *J Am Board Fam Pract* 2001;14(4):234–242.
73. Auwaerter PG. Infectious mononucleosis in active patients: definitive answers to common questions. *Phys Sportsmed* 2002;30(11):43–50.
74. Schuler J, Filtzer H. Spontaneous splenic rupture: the role of nonoperative management. *Arch Surg* 1995;130:662–665.
75. Farley DR, Zietlow SP, Bannon MP, et al. Spontaneous rupture of the spleen due to infectious mononucleosis. *Mayo Clin Proc* 1992;67(9):846–853.
76. Safran D, Bloom GP. Spontaneous splenic rupture following infectious mononucleosis. *Am Surg* 1990;56(10):601–605.
77. Rutkow IM. Rupture of the spleen in infectious mononucleosis. *Arch Surg* 1978;113(6):718–720.
78. Boulanger BR, McLellan BA, Brenneman FD, et al. Prospective evidence of the superiority of a sonography-based algorithm in the assessment of blunt abdominal injury. *J Trauma* 1999;47(4):632–637.
79. Lentz KA, McKenney MG, Nuñez DB, et al. Evaluating blunt abdominal trauma: role for ultrasonography. *J Ultrasound Med* 1996;15:447–451.
80. Ochsner MG, Knudson MM, Pachter HL, et al. Significance of minimal or no intraperitoneal fluid visible on CT scan associated with blunt liver and splenic injuries: a multicenter analysis. *J Trauma* 2000;49(3):505–510.
81. Pearl RH, Wesson DE, Spence LJ, et al. Splenic injury: a 5-year update with improved results and changing criteria for conservative management. *J Pediatr Surg* 1989;24(1):121–125.
82. Guth AA, Pachter HL, Jacobowitz GR. Rupture of the pathologic spleen: is there a role for nonoperative therapy? *J Trauma* 1996;41(2):214–218.
83. American Academy of Pediatrics. Immunization in special clinical circumstances. In: Pickering LK, ed. *Red book: 2003 report of the committee on infectious diseases*, 26th ed. Elk Grove Village: American Academy of Pediatrics, 2003:80–81.
84. Beck CK. Infectious diseases in sports. *Med Sci Sports Exerc* 2000;32(7):S431–S438.
85. Spielmann AL, DeLong DM, Kliewer MA. Sonographic evaluation of spleen size in tall healthy athletes. *AJR Am J Roentgenol* 2005;184(1):45–49.
86. Knudson MM, Lim RC Jr, Oakes DD, et al. Nonoperative management of blunt liver injuries in adults: the need for continued surveillance. *J Trauma* 1990;30(12):1494–1500.
87. Carillo EH, Platz A, Miller FB, et al. Non-operative management of blunt hepatic trauma. *Br J Surg* 1998;85(4):461–468.
88. Ritland S. Exercise and liver disease. *Sports Med* 1988;6:121–126.
89. Anish EJ. Viral hepatitis: sports-related risk. *Curr Sports Med Rep* 2004;3:100–106.
90. MacGillivray DC, Valentine RJ. Nonoperative management of blunt pediatric liver injury-late complications: case report. *J Trauma* 1989;29(2):251–254.
91. Röthlin MA, Näf R, Amgwerd M, et al. Ultrasound in blunt abdominal and thoracic trauma. *J Trauma* 1993;34(4):488–495.
92. Stafford RE, McGonigal MD, Weigelt JA, et al. Oral contrast solution and computer tomography for blunt abdominal trauma: a randomized study. *Arch Surg* 1999;134(6):622–627.
93. Yang EY, Marder SR, Hastings G, et al. The abdominal compartment syndrome complicating nonoperative management of major blunt liver injuries: recognition and treatment using multimodality therapy. *J Trauma* 2002;52(5):982–986.
94. Knudson MM, Lim RC, Olcott EW. Morbidity and mortality following major penetrating liver injuries. *Arch Surg* 1994;129(3):256–261.
95. Moore EE, Cogbill TH, Jurkovich GJ, et al. Organ injury scaling: spleen and liver (1994 revision). *J Trauma* 1995;38(3):323–324.
96. Mure AJ, Josloff R, Rothberg J, et al. Serum amylase determination and blunt abdominal trauma. *Am Surg* 1991;57(4):210–213.

13 Cardiovascular System

Vivien Lim *Aravind Rao Kokkirala* *Paul D. Thompson*

Exertion-related death is most frequently caused by trauma and cardiac events, and more rarely by conditions such as heat stroke and rhabdomyolysis. The widespread publicity given to such exercise-related cardiac events as the deaths of author Jim Fixx, college basketball star Hank Gathers, and professional basketball legend Pete Maravich have increased both physician and public awareness of the cardiovascular risks of exercise. This awareness, in turn, has increased both the frequency with which primary care physicians are asked to evaluate cardiac problems in athletes and the physician's concern about the consequences of any decision. The present chapter provides an overview of cardiac problems in active individuals and a general approach to common cardiac conditions in athletes. Readers are referred elsewhere for a more detailed discussion of this topic (1).

CAUSES AND FREQUENCY OF EXERCISE-RELATED CARDIOVASCULAR EVENTS IN THE YOUNG

Genetic and congenital cardiac conditions are the primary cause of exercise-related cardiac events in young subjects (see Table 13.1) (2). Acquired conditions such as myocarditis, idiopathic dilated cardiomyopathy, infiltrative myocardial disease, and atherosclerotic disease are responsible for a small proportion of these events in young subjects (3). The causes of exertion-related deaths in young subjects may vary by geographical location. In the United States, hypertrophic cardiomyopathy (HCM) accounts for 36% to 50% of sudden death in young athletes (3) and arrhythmogenic right ventricular cardiomyopathy (ARVC) is an unusual cause accounting for only 1% of such events (3). In contrast, ARVC is the dominant cause of exercise-related deaths in young Italian athletes accounting for 20% of events in the Veneto region of that country (4). It is unclear whether these differences are due to varying prevalence of disease or differences in screening procedures and diagnostic criteria. Other common causes of exercise-related cardiac deaths in young subjects include anomalous origin and course of the coronary arteries (13%), valvular and subvalvular aortic stenosis (8%), and aortic dissection in association with inherited connective tissue disorders such as Marfan's syndrome (2%) (2,3).

The frequency of exercise-related sudden death in high school and college athletes has been estimated as one death/year for every 133,000 men and 796,000 women (2). Deaths were included if they occurred within 1 hour of practice or competition. These numbers can only be regarded as estimates, and each death is a tragedy for the individual and the family, but these estimates do provide reassurance that the absolute incidence of sudden death during athletic participation is low. These results also place the value of screening in question. The Cardiovascular Disease in Adolescents (CARDIA) Study demonstrates that the incidence of unexplained echocardiographically documented left ventricular hypertrophy (LVH), consistent with HCM, is one to two cases per 1,000 individuals in the general population (5). Because HCM is the most frequent cause of exercise-related cardiac deaths in American athletes, it is surprising that the death rate is not higher. Indeed, if all cases of unexplained LVH and HCM resulted in exercise-related events, the incidence of death could be as high as 200 cases per 100,000 male athletes. Such observations suggest that most athletes with unexplained LVH and possible HCM tolerate the condition and athletic activity without being affected by sudden death (6). Such observations also question the wisdom of routinely screening all athletes and disqualifying all with possible HCM.

TABLE 13.1
CARDIAC CAUSES OF DEATH IN HIGH SCHOOL AND COLLEGE ATHLETES (N = 100)

	Men	Women
Hypertrophic cardiomyopathy[a]	50	1
Probable hypertrophic cardiomyopathy	5	0
Coronary artery anomalies[b]	11	2
Myocarditis	7	—
Aortic stenosis	6	—
Cardiomyopathy	6	—
Atherosclerotic coronary disease	2	1
Aortic rupture	2	—
Subaortic stenosis	2	—
Coronary aneurysm	—	1
Mitral prolapse	1	—
Right ventricular dysplasia	—	1
Cerebral arteriovenous malformation	—	1
Subarachnoid hemorrhage	—	1

[a]Three also had coronary anomalies, one had Wolff-Parkinson-White syndrome.
[b]Includes anomalous left coronary artery (LCA) from right sinus of Valsalva (n = 4); intramural left anterior descending (LAD) (n = 4); anomalous LCA from pulmonary artery (n = 2); anomalous right coronary artery (RCA) from left sinus (n = 2); hypoplastic RCA (n = 2); and ostial ridge of the LCA (n = 2). Three subjects with coronary anomalies also had hypertrophic cardiomyopathy and are tabulated with that group.
Source: Adapted from Van Camp SP, Bloor CM, Mueller FO, et al. Nontraumatic sports death in high school and college athletes. *Med Sci Sports Exerc* 1995;27:641–647.

CAUSES AND FREQUENCY OF EXERCISE-RELATED CARDIOVASCULAR EVENTS IN ADULTS

Atherosclerotic vascular disease is the primary cause of almost all exercise-related deaths in adults. Ragosta examined the cause of death in 75 men and 1 woman older than 29 years who died during or immediately after recreational exercise (7). All deaths were related to atherosclerotic vascular disease including atherosclerotic coronary artery disease (CAD) in 71, hypertensive heart disease in 2, dissecting aortic aneurysm in 1, and cerebrovascular accident in 1 victim. In addition to being the primary cause of exercise-related death, atherosclerotic CAD causes virtually all exercise-related myocardial infarctions (MIs). Sudden cardiac death and acute MI in *previously healthy adults* in the general population are generally produced by atherosclerotic plaque rupture with acute coronary thrombosis (8,9) although erosion, rather than rupture, of the atherosclerotic plaque has been noted by some observers in up to 32% of exertion-related deaths (10).

The absolute incidence of cardiac events during exertion is low, but increased relative to the incidence during nonvigorous activities. From a collection of deaths during exertion, we estimated the annual incidence of death during jogging as only one death per 15,640 previously healthy adults, but the hourly frequency of death during exercise was seven times that at rest (11). Others determined an absolute annual incidence of exercise-related cardiac arrest as only 1 per 18,000 previously healthy men, but again the incidence during exercise was greater than at rest (12). Interestingly, for the habitually least active men, the risk of a cardiac arrest was 56-fold greater during exercise than at rest whereas the relative risk of exercise was only 5-fold greater in the habitually most active men. We observed a similar pattern for exercise-related MI (9). Physically inactive men were 30 times more likely to suffer an MI during vigorous exertion whereas the relative risk was only 20% higher (relative risk of 1.2) and not significantly increased in the most active subjects. These results demonstrate that exercise increases the risk of exercise events, but such events in adults are largely restricted to physically inactive individuals, primarily men, performing unaccustomed physical activity.

All of these studies on the incidence of exercise-related cardiac events suffer from small sample sizes because the absolute incidence of events is low. Results have been reported but only in abstract form for almost 3 million members of a national chain of fitness facilities who engaged in 182 million exercise sessions (13). There were only 71 fatal events occurring in 61 men and 10 women. Almost 55% of those suffering cardiac events exercised on average less than once weekly and 10 had participated in less than three sessions. The incidence of events was one death per 25,000 subjects per year. These results are important because they confirm with more events in a larger population the figures reported in smaller studies (12,13) and also support the conclusion that exercise-related cardiac events are more frequent in infrequent exercisers (9,13,14).

This study also has the potential to provide important data on the incidence of cardiac events in adult women who have not been studied previously because of the rarity of exercise events in this group.

The mechanism by which exercise increases acute plaque rupture is not clear. Thompson in 2000 postulated that the increased "twisting and bending" of coronary arteries during vigorous exertion increased the frequency of plaque rupture (1). This motion is exacerbated by the increases in heart rate and contractility produced by exercise. Other possibilities also exist and probably contribute. Exercise dilates normal coronary arteries, but can produce vasoconstriction in atherosclerotic segments (15). Such spasm over a thickened, noncompliant atherosclerotic plaque could itself induce plaque rupture. Exercise also acutely increases platelet aggregability, which would increase thrombosis; platelet to leukocyte aggregation, which could increase leukocyte adherence to an injured arterial wall; and elastase levels, which can attack elastic fibers in the extracellular matrix and facilitate plaque disruption (16).

It should be emphasized that plaque rupture and thrombosis as a cause of exercise-related cardiac death applies primarily to previously *asymptomatic* subjects. Patients with known coronary heart disease who die during exertion may, but often do not, demonstrate evidence of an acute coronary lesion or recent myocardial injury, but often show evidence of a previous infarction (17). This suggests that these patients died of ventricular fibrillation (VF), which originated from the infarction site.

THE ATHLETIC HEART SYNDROME

Physicians performing cardiac evaluations of highly trained competitive athletes should be aware that the clinical findings characteristic of the athletic heart syndrome can mimic disease and increase the complexity of the evaluation. Clinical distinctions between physiologic athlete's heart and pathological conditions have critical implications for athletes, because cardiovascular abnormalities can trigger disqualification from competitive sports and a misdiagnosis can result in unnecessary restrictions, depriving athletes of the psychological, social, and economic benefits of sports (18–24). The athletic heart syndrome was first described by Henschen in 1889 (25) and is characterized by electrocardiographic (ECG) changes and by changes in cardiac conduction and architecture. There are three salient points regarding the athletic heart syndrome. First, cardiovascular findings in the athletic heart syndrome rarely exceed the normal range. Second, cardiac abnormalities are generally found only in endurance-trained athletes. Third, findings that do exceed the normal range are generally restricted to well-trained athletes engaged in endurance sports requiring the use of a large muscle mass, such as rowing and Nordic skiing. The corollary of these principles is that findings exceeding normal parameters in nonendurance or noncompetitive athletes should prompt a search for other etiologies.

The ECG findings of the athletic heart syndrome include ST segment changes of early repolarization, abnormal T waves, and evidence of chamber enlargement. The ST-T segment elevations of early repolarization and T inversions are attributed to the augmented parasympathetic tone characteristic of exercise training.

Habitual endurance exercise produces a global cardiac enlargement, which may affect both the right and left atria and ventricles in the presence of normal systolic and diastolic function (20). The most consistent enlargement is seen in the left ventricular chamber. Mild enlargement of both atria and the right ventricle can occur, but marked enlargement of these structures is suggestive of a disease process, and is not observed in the athletic heart syndrome. The magnitude of physiologic hypertrophy may also vary according to the particular type of sports training (26).

The ECG in well-trained athletes may show mildly increased P wave amplitude suggesting right atrial enlargement, P wave notching suggesting left atrial enlargement, incomplete right bundle branch block (RBBB), and voltage criteria for right and LVH (27). Among endurance athletes, voltage criteria for right ventricular hypertrophy are noted in 18% to 69% of subjects (28). Incomplete RBBB is also common. ECG voltage evidence for LVH is common in endurance athletes and the voltage may be quite large in some athletes. Frequent/complex ventricular tachyarrhythmias, increased R or S wave voltages, Q waves and repolarization abnormalities may also be seen in the ECG, mimicking certain cardiac diseases (21,22).

The resting bradycardia, sinus arrhythmia, and atrioventricular conduction delay of the athletic heart syndrome are due to enhanced parasympathetic and reduced sympathetic tone. These abnormalities in sinus rate, A-V conduction, and early repolarization should disappear with exertion because exercise decreases vagal tone and increases sympathetic activity. A heart rate less than 60 beats/minute is found in up to 91% of endurance athletes (28) and rates as low as 25 beats/minute have been reported (29). Sinus bradycardia and sinus pauses of more than 2 seconds have been documented during sleep in endurance athletes (28). First degree A-V block, defined as a PR interval greater than 0.20 seconds is reported in 10% to 33% of endurance athletes (29). Second degree A-V block of the Mobitz I or Wenchebach pattern or progressive prolongation of the PR interval before a nonconducted P wave is also seen more commonly in the athletic heart syndrome (29) (see Table 13.2). Second degree A-V block with Mobitz II appearance, which appears as a nonconducted P wave without preceding PR prolongation, is not typical

TABLE 13.2
COMMON FINDINGS IN ENDURANCE-TRAINED ATHLETES

Auscultation
S_3 (third heart sound)
S_4 (fourth heart sound)
Systolic murmurs (grade I or II)
Chest x-ray
"Cardiomegaly"
Electrocardiogram
"Left ventricular hypertrophy" (prominent voltage, usually not meeting Estes criterion)
T-wave inversion (inferiorly)
ST-T-wave evaluation (juvenile repolarization pattern)
Incomplete (or complete) right bundle branch block
Rhythm
Bradycardia (sinus)
Sinus arrhythmia
First-degree heart block (Wenckebach)
Functional bradycardia
Premature atrial contractions
Premature ventricular contractions

Source: From Kuland, D.N. *The Injured Athlete*. Philadelphia, PA I.P. Lippincott Co., 1982:120.

of the athletic heart syndrome. A-V block with Mobitz II appearance may occur in well-trained athletes, but is rare (28) and should be attributed to the athletic training only if the athlete is asymptomatic and no other abnormalities are detected. The prolongation of the A-V interval and decrease in A-V conduction velocity described earlier may also unmask ventricular pre-excitation seen in the Wolff-Parkinson-White (WPW) syndrome (28).

ST elevation of the "early repolarization pattern" is common in endurance-trained athletes whereas ST depression is extremely unusual. Peaked, biphasic, and inverted T waves in the precordial leads may also be seen in endurance athletes. Deeply inverted T waves can also be normal in athletes, but are rare and should be evaluated by echocardiography because they may be a sign of HCM.

Echocardiographic studies have documented global chamber enlargement in the athletes. At least 59 studies have consistently documented increased left ventricular dimensions. Thirteen studies noted that right ventricular dimensions averaged 24% greater in athletes than controls (30). Fourteen studies examined left atrial dimensions and demonstrated that the transverse dimension was 16% larger in the athletes. At least one study has documented a larger right atrial size in the athletes (18).

Pelliccia et al. examined left ventricular wall thickness in 783 nationally ranked Italian male athletes and 209 women (18). Only 16 athletes or 1.7% had a left ventricular wall thickness of more than 12 mm, the upper limit of normal. Fifteen of these athletes were rowers or canoeists, sports that require both isotonic and isometric effort and involve a large muscle mass. All athletes with increased wall dimensions were internationally ranked. The largest wall thickness in any athlete was 16 mm. All of the female athletes had wall thickness values below 11 mm.

These same investigators examined left ventricular cavity dimensions in 1,300 elite athletes participating in 38 different sports (19). left ventricular end diastolic dimension (LVEDD) was greater in male (55 mm) than in female (48 mm) athletes. LVEDD was greater than 55 mm, the upper limits of normal, in 45% of the athletes and exceeded 60 mm in 14%. The largest LVEDD was 66 mm in a woman and 70 mm in a man. The sports that were most associated with an LVEDD equal or greater than 60 mm were those that required a large endurance component or a combination of moderate endurance training and increased body size such as cycling (49% of cycling athletes), ice hockey (42%), basketball (40%), rugby (39%), canoeing (39%), and rowing (34%). Despite enlarged intrachamber dimensions only 14 of the athletes or 1.1% had a septal thickness of more than 12 mm and only 4 athletes (0.3%) exceed this posterior wall thickness.

These results are useful in differentiating the athletic heart syndrome from pathological conditions. Left ventricular wall thickness more than 12 mm affected less than 2% of elite athletes and should not be seen in healthy recreational athletes. No athlete had a left ventricular wall thickness more than 16 mm so that values above this range should raise the possibility of HCM. The largest cardiac dimensions occurred in elite athletes performing sports that require a large amount of endurance training and increased body size. Also, despite enlarged end diastolic ventricular volumes in the athletes, systolic and diastolic function was normal. However, there are occasional ambiguous situations. The two most common are (a) diagnosing HCM in an athlete with mildly increased left ventricular wall thickness, normal ventricular function, and no systolic anterior motion of the mitral valve and (b) differentiating an early dilated cardiomyopathy from athletic heart syndrome in an athlete with normal left ventricular cavity dimensions and a low-normal left ventricular ejection fraction (50% to 55%). Such cases may be clarified by observing the response of cardiac mass to deconditioning, assessment of diastolic filling parameters (23), genotyping and serial observation and echocardiographic studies of the athlete over time (26).

FUNCTIONAL CARDIAC MURMURS IN ATHLETES

Functional murmurs are also part of the athletic heart syndrome and are produced by the cardiac adaptations to exercise training. Endurance exercise training reduces resting heart rate, increases resting stroke volume, and enhances cardiac performance. These adaptations produce a larger stroke volume. Much of the larger stroke volume is delivered more vigorously in early systole increasing blood velocity and producing systolic "flow murmurs." Flow murmurs in young athletes are due to flow across the pulmonic valve and often vary with respiration. Athletes aged 50 years and above may have mild sclerosis of the aortic valve leaflets and their flow murmurs are often due to both aortic valve sclerosis and the increased blood velocity. These murmurs may be less "innocent" because they can progress over time to become important aortic stenosis of adults or what has been called *"aortic stenosis of the elderly."* This sclerotic process resembles atherosclerosis and shares many of the same risk factors (31,32).

PREPARTICIPATION CARDIOVASCULAR SCREENING IN THE YOUNG

There is considerable debate about the value of screening individuals before athletic participation and what components are required for adequate screening. Fortunately, the rarity of cardiac events among young athletes limits the utility and increases the effective cost of any screening procedure (24). Some authors recommend routine ECG in screening high school athletes (33) and others advocate routine echocardiography to detect HCM (34). The American Heart Association has developed (35) and updated (26) (see Table 13.3) recommendations based on the opinions of an expert writing group to evaluate this issue. This document does not recommend routine echocardiography

TABLE 13.3

AHA CONSENSUS PANEL RECOMMENDATIONS FOR PREPARTICIPATION ATHLETIC SCREENING

Family History
- Premature sudden cardiac death
- Heart disease in surviving relatives younger than 50 years

Personal History
- Heart murmur
- Systemic hypertension
- Fatigue
- Syncope/near-syncope
- Excessive/unexplained exertional dyspnea
- Exertional chest pain
- Heart murmur—supine and standing
- Femoral pulses to exclude coarctation of the aorta
- Stigmata of Marfan's syndrome
- Brachial artery pressure—sitting

Source: Adapted from Maron BJ, Douglas PS, Graham TP, et al. Task Force 1: preparticipation screening and diagnosis of cardiovascular disease in athletes. *J Am Coll Cardiol* 2005;45(8):1322–1326.

or ECG, but does recommend an evaluation before participation and reexamination at least every 4 years.

Perhaps the most important part of this examination is that it should be performed by someone who is knowledgeable about the athletic heart syndrome as well as about those conditions likely to cause exercise-related events, and who is qualified to perform the cardiac examination. We advocate that such examinations should be performed by the athlete's personal physicians because this person will often know the athlete and family and thereby be more likely to be aware of important medical issues and a family history of cardiac disease.

The evaluation should include a personal and family history and a physical examination. The history should include questions about exertional symptoms including chest discomfort, syncope, dyspnea, and fatigue; known cardiac disease; and a family history of sudden death or of any of the conditions known to be associated with sudden death. The physical examination performed in screening situations is often somewhat cursory, but should be *carefully* cursory to exclude the potentially fatal conditions noted earlier. The athlete's general appearance should be assessed for Marfan features such as pectus deformity, high arched palate, kyphoscolioses, and arm span greater than height. Blood pressure should be measured. The patient should be examined for radial—femoral pulse delay and other signs of aortic coarctation if hypertension is present. The carotid upstrokes should be checked for delayed upstroke suggestive of aortic stenosis. Auscultation should be performed with the patient standing or sitting because this position maximizes the chance of hearing abnormal

TABLE 13.4

DIFFERENTIATING THE HYPERTROPHIC CARDIOMYOPATHY (HCM) MURMUR FROM "PHYSIOLOGIC" MURMURS

	Intensity of HCM Murmur	Intensity of Innocent Murmur
Valsalva maneuver	Increased	Decreased
Standing	Increased	Decreased
Squatting	Decreased	Increased
Sustained hand grip	Decreased	No change

splitting of the second sound found in atrial septal defects and the murmur of obstructive HCM. Auscultation in the sitting position is also useful if possible. We also ask the athlete to do a Valsalva maneuver during the standing examination because this can provoke a murmur in HCM. Unfortunately, murmurs in HCM are heard in less than 25% of patients because the disease is often not obstructive and so does not provoke a murmur (see Table 13.4).

There is currently increased emphasis on diagnosing genetic causes of exercise-related sudden cardiac death because sudden cardiac death can be prevented in such patients with implanted defibrillators. These conditions include HCM, ARVC, long-QT (LQT) syndrome, Brugada syndrome, and other inherited arrhythmogenic channelopathies. Unfortunately, a genetic diagnosis does not necessarily indicate a bad prognosis because of differences in genetic expression. Consequently, how to deal with genetic diagnoses in asymptomatic athletes is not currently clear (36,37).

PREPARTICIPATION CARDIOVASCULAR SCREENING IN ADULTS

Older athletes constitute a large percentage of the participants in individual athletic events such as road running races (38). Preparticipation screening in this population should include screening for atherosclerotic CAD (26).

The preparticipation screening of adults before exercise should consist of a history and physical examination designed to detect symptoms such as chest discomfort, dyspnea, and syncope that may be manifestations of unappreciated cardiac disease. The physical examination should focus on detecting hypertension requiring treatment or murmurs suggesting occult valvular disease.

The use of exercise stress testing to screen adults before initiating an exercise program is controversial because of its high cost and its poor predictive value for cardiac complications during exercise. Exercise testing fails to identify most individuals who will have exercise-related cardiac events (39), probably because it requires a hemodynamically significant coronary obstruction to become truly positive, whereas acute coronary events often involve plaque rupture and thrombosis at the site of previously non-obstructive atherosclerotic plaque (40). Indeed, a positive exercise test in asymptomatic adults is a better predictor of angina than of acute MI or sudden death (41). In one study, less than 20% of patients with an exercise-related MI or sudden cardiac death had a prior positive stress test (42).

The American College of Cardiology and American Heart Association have developed Guideline for Exercise Testing (41). This group considered the use of exercise testing in men older than 40 and women older than 50 years to be an area with conflicting evidence and divergent opinion, but where the evidence for its usefulness was not well established. Nevertheless, opinion is divided. Our approach is not to recommend routine exercise stress testing, but to advise the individual to begin exercise gradually and to progress slowly. We describe the nature of cardiac discomfort to active individuals and inform them of the importance of having such symptoms evaluated promptly. When the individual has symptoms, exercise testing can be extremely useful to evaluate the importance of the complaint.

EVALUATING CARDIAC ABNORMALITIES AND SYMPTOMS IN ATHLETES

It is evaluating cardiovascular abnormalities in athletes, it is extremely important to distinguish between abnormalities found during screening examinations and those found during the evaluation of possible cardiac symptoms. Cardiac abnormalities detected during screening examinations are often variants of the athletic heart syndrome and therefore really variants of normal. They should be evaluated by someone knowledgeable about this syndrome and treated appropriately. It is important to emphasize that the cardiac variants of the athletic heart syndrome rarely exceed the upper limits of normal cardiac dimensions. Abnormalities detected during the evaluation of real cardiac symptoms cause much greater concern and should be attributed to the athletic heart syndrome only when pathological conditions can be excluded.

We use the term *"real cardiac symptoms"* because symptomatic complaints from athletes are common and can be magnified by family and physician concerns generated in part by the widespread publicity given to exercise-related cardiac deaths. Rather than being fun, athletics are stressful for some adolescents who may worry about their health or subconsciously prefer a medical explanation for poor performance to the loss of self or peer esteem. This does not mean that any symptoms in an athlete should be dismissed out of hand, but simply that when symptoms are equivocal for serious disease, the evaluating physician should attempt to understand the athlete and their social situation so that the diagnosis and evaluation is consistent with the ultimate problem, be it social or otherwise.

In this context, a common syndrome in our experience in young athletes is what we have named the *"the athletic swoon syndrome."* These athletes often present with "syncope," but rarely have lost total consciousness. They usually have experienced a period of more than 5 minutes during which they were poorly responsiveness, but vaguely aware of their surroundings. This often happens near the finish line of competitions when they athlete was not performing up to expectations. The athletic swoon syndrome must be differentiated from true exercise-induced syncope and from the prolonged QT Syndrome. True exercise-induced syncope is a threatening symptom associated with important cardiac disease such as aortic stenosis, HCM, and anomalous coronary arteries. We are repeatedly impressed with the number of athletes who die during exercise after presenting with symptoms that were ignored or inadequately evaluated. It must be remembered that significant disease can be misdiagnosed as hysteria. Patients with LQT syndrome, for example, are occasionally misdiagnosed as having hysterical syncope before the correct diagnosis is made (43). Consequently, the physician must be cautious in reaching a psychological diagnosis, but such psychological issues in athletes are considerably more frequent than life-threatening cardiac diseases and making a correct psychological diagnosis can often spare an expensive evaluation.

MANAGING COMMON CARDIAC PROBLEMS IN ATHLETES

Hypertension

Hypertension is the most common cardiovascular condition observed in competitive athletes. The diagnosis of hypertension depends on three blood pressure readings on three separate occasions (44). Blood pressure readings of greater than 140 mm Hg systolic or greater than 90 mm Hg diastolic are labeled as hypertension in individuals older than 18 years (45). Hypertension is by itself not a cause of exercise-related sudden cardiac death, but increases the risk of exercise-related cerebrovascular accidents and aortic dissections (see Table 13.5).

Secondary causes of hypertension must be excluded in the young athlete. A wide pulse pressure (systolic minus diastolic pressure) greater than 60 mm Hg suggests aortic valvular insufficiency. A higher blood pressure in the arms than in legs and a radial to femoral delay in the pulse is consistent with coarctation of the aorta.

Athletes with stages I and II hypertension with no concomitant heart disease or target end organ damage can compete in all sports. Athletes with stages III and IV hypertension should be restricted from sports requiring a high isometric or static effort during training or competition until the pressure is controlled (class IIA to IIIC)

TABLE 13.5
CLASSIFICATION OF HYPERTENSION

Age >18 yr	Mild (stage I) (mm Hg)	Moderate (stage II) (mm Hg)	Severe (stage III) (mm Hg)	Very Severe (stage IV) (mm Hg)
Systolic BP	140–159	160–179	180–209	≥210
Diastolic BP	90–99	100–109	110–119	≥120

BP = blood pressure.
Source: Adapted from Kaplan NM, Deveraux RB, Miller HS. Tak force 4: systemic hypertension. *J Am Coll Cardiol* 1994;24(4):885–889.

(Table 13.5) (46). Alcohol, sympathomimetics including ephedrine containing compounds and cocaine, anabolic steroids, and nonsteroidal anti-inflammatory medications can all increase blood pressure and should be considered before starting antihypertensive medications (47). Treatment of hypertension in athletes should be initiated with low doses of a diuretic such as hydrochlorthiazide 25 mg daily plus either an angiotensin converting enzyme inhibitor or a calcium channel blocker as needed. Beta-blockers can interfere with athletic and sexual performance, which limits compliance. In some sports such as shooting and diving beta-adrenergic receptor blockers may be contraindicated (48). The diuretic should be held for before training or competition likely to reduce plasma volume (see Table 13.6).

Chest Discomfort in the Young Athlete

The causes of chest discomfort are multiple even in young athletes. In contrast with adults, however, chest discomfort in young athletes is due to cardiac problems in less than 5% of cases (49).

Most times no etiology is found in adolescents and the pain is termed *idiopathic.* When a specific diagnosis can be made, musculoskeletal etiologies are the most frequent (50). Pain on direct palpation of the area and deep inspiration worsens the pain of both traumatic injuries and costochondritis. Fractured ribs and sternum should be ruled out in athletes involved with direct chest trauma. Athletes participating in sports involving upper trunk rotation (i.e., tennis and baseball) are at risk for muscular sprain, which is exacerbated by normal breathing. The precordial catch syndrome is a nontraumatic and benign condition which is characterized as anterior chest pain that is sudden, sharp, brief, nonradiating, associated with deep inspiration, unrelated to exertion, and relieved by stretching the painful area (51).

Gastrointestinal causes of chest pain include gastroesophageal reflux, esophageal spasm, and peptic ulcer

TABLE 13.6
CLASSIFICATION OF SPORTS

	A. Low Dynamic	B. Moderate Dynamic	C. High Dynamic
I. Low Static	Billiards, bowling, cricket, curling, golf, riflery	Baseball, softball, table tennis, tennis (doubles), volleyball	Badminton, cross-country skiing (classic technique), field hockey, race walking, raquetball, running (long distance), soccer, squash, tennis (singles)
II. Mod. Static	Archery, auto racing, diving, equestrian, motorcycling	Fencing, figure skating, football, rodeoing, rugby, running (sprint), surfing, synchronized swimming	Basketball, ice hockey, cross-country skiing (skating technique), lacrosse, running (middle distance), swimming, team handball
III. High Static	Bobsledding, gymnastics, karate/judo, sailing, rock climbing, waterskiing, weight lifting, windsurfing	Body building, downhill skiing, wrestling	Boxing, canoeing/kayaking, cycling, decathlon, rowing, speed skating

Source: Adapted from Mitchell JH, Haskell WL, Raven PB. Classification of sports. *J Am Coll Cardiol* 1994;24(4):864–866.

disease. Patients tend to complain of symptoms at rest following eating. Exercise-related gastrointestinal symptoms do occur, but often when exercise is after consuming coffee or spicy foods, and rest symptoms are also usually present (52).

One of the most common causes of chest discomfort in athletes is exercise-induced asthma (EIA). In one study, up to 73% of otherwise healthy children with chest pain tested positive for EIA (53). Coughing or inspiration often worsens chest pain, and forceful expiration may initiate wheezing on the clinical examination.

Psychological causes may be operative in approximately 9% of chest pain cases in adolescent athletes with an equal distribution between male and females (49). The chest pain is often related to a recent psychological stress. Panic attacks often include chest pain associated with intense fear, hyperventilation, and a feeling of impending doom.

Cardiac causes of chest pain are similar to the causes listed under the following section on "Syncope". Aortic dissection typically presents with chest pain, and may occur in individuals with disorders of connective tissue including Marfan's syndrome. HCM and aberrant coronary arteries can present with chest discomfort, but often present with syncope.

The approach to athletes with chest discomfort is to obtain a careful history, ECG, and chest x-ray when indicated. Additional testing including exercise stress testing and echocardiography should be considered when the diagnosis is uncertain and possibly cardiac. Difficult cases with the possibility of such unusual conditions as aberrant coronary arteries should be referred to a cardiologist for evaluation.

Syncope

Syncope is a sudden, transient loss of consciousness with loss of postural tone and spontaneous recovery (54). Ostensibly healthy athletes who experience exercise-related syncope are much more likely to have an organic cause than are athletes with nonexertional syncope (54–57). Athletes who are described as being "unconscious" but who are able to assist in their own care are unlikely to have a life-threatening arrhythmia, but could still have metabolic conditions such as hyponatremia or hypoglycemia.

Syncope can be classified as neurocardiogenic syncope or a simple faint, metabolic, neurological, allergic, and/or cardiac related. Neurocardiogenic syncope is the most common cause of syncope in young adults. Neurocardiogenic syncope occurs as a result of sudden reflex vasodilatation or bradycardia or both usually in response to a sudden increase in catecholamine levels, and increased stimulation of left ventricular wall vagal efferent receptors. It is most frequently provoked in athletes by venous pooling when they remain upright and stationary following exercise. Athletes are particularly susceptible to neurocardiogenic syncope because of their high levels of resting vagal tone, relative hypovolemia resulting from insensible fluid losses (perspiration, and rapid breathing), and the sudden withdrawal of sympathetic tone as exercise ceases. The sudden cessation of activity may also predispose athletes to neurocardiogenic syncope because the lack of muscular activity to increase venous return may reduce cardiac output. The physical examination and ECG should be normal. Upright tilt-table testing should not be performed in well-trained athletes because of an increased incidence of false positives (58,59). Neurocardiogenic syncope in athletes is generally benign and has a favorable long-term prognosis (60).

Metabolic causes of syncope include hypoglycemia, hypernatremia, and hyponatremia. Neurological manifestations of hypoglycemia are usually preceded by autonomic symptoms of palpitations, sweating, anxiety, tremor, and hunger. Early cognitive dysfunction is noted in healthy subjects when the blood glucose level is less than 50 mg/dL (61). Diabetic patients taking insulin and athletes with eating disorders are at risk for developing hypoglycemia. Athletes may be susceptible to hyponatremia when ingesting large amounts of water during an athletic event (i.e., marathon), whereas hypernatremia may be caused by dehydration. Both conditions can impair mentation. Hypernatremia can even cause focal intracerebral and subarachnoid hemorrhage (62,63).

Neurological causes of syncope include seizure, hypocapnia, hypoxia, and hyperthermia or heat stroke. Athletes in prolonged endurance events occurring during high-temperature conditions are susceptible to heat stroke. Black athletes with exercise-associated collapse associated with high altitude training, dehydration, or hyperthermia should be screened for sickle cell trait. Exercise-induced anaphylaxis is a rare condition that is preceded by erythema, pruritic urticaria, and angioedema before vascular collapse.

Exercise-related syncope that is cardiovascular related is of most concern because of its life-threatening nature. The causes of exercise-related syncope or sudden death differ greatly between young (age $\leq$35 years) athletes and older (age $\geq$35 years) athletes. The most common cause of exercise-related syncope in older athletes is CAD, in contrast to congenital structural abnormalities in young athletes. Evaluation of patients with exercise-related syncope should include assessment of any cardiac prodromal symptoms, such as chest pain, shortness of breath, palpitations, and presyncope. The incidence of prodromal symptoms preceding exercise-related syncope ranges from 8% to 46% (64,65). Athletes should avoid exertion if such symptoms appear.

An ECG in patients with exercise-related syncope may be helpful in diagnosing LQT syndrome. LQT syndrome is associated with a high risk of torsade de pointes, syncope, and sudden death. LQT syndrome is a heterogeneous disorder caused by defective myocardial ion channels. It is characterized by a corrected QT (QTc) of more than 460 milliseconds. Currently, there are many recognized LQT phenotypes, each associated with different genetic variations (66). LQT1 accounts for 55% of the LQT syndrome subtypes. Arrhythmia in LQT1 is exacerbated by increased catecholamines, and cardiac events in LQT1 patients are associated with exercise 62% of the time versus only 3% of the time with rest. Swimming is independently associated with cardiac events 33% of the time. Most individuals with LQT1 destined for cardiac-related events have them before the age of 20 (67).

The diagnosis of LQT1 is based on detecting a prolonged QTc on the resting ECG. Genotyping for LQT1 is also available, but its use is primarily employed as a research technique and for confirming the diagnosis. Although patients with LQT1 more frequently experience cardiac events during exercise than do LQT2 and LQT3 patients, all patients with LQT syndrome should be restricted from vigorous sports and exertion. Patients with LQT1 should avoid swimming without supervision. The clinical management of LQT1 involves lowering sympathetic tone. Treatment with beta-blockers has been shown to decrease cardiac-related events by 80% and 3 year mortality from 26% to 6% (67). The beta-blocker dose should be high enough to ensure that the patient's heart rate does not exceed 130 beats/minute on exercise stress testing. Patients at high risk for sudden cardiac death or with a QTc of more than 520 milliseconds should be considered for implanted defibrillator therapy.

GENERAL APPROACH TO EVALUATING CARDIAC ARRHYTHMIAS IN ACTIVE PEOPLE

Palpitations and skipped heartbeats are a frequent complaint among active people. Benign conditions such as premature atrial and ventricular contractions (PACs and PVCs) are often first detected by the patient when palpating the pulse during exercise training. Arrhythmias are judged both by the arrhythmia itself, and the structural integrity of the heart. Consequently, the first step in evaluating an arrhythmia is to diagnose the arrhythmia. Often tapping out the rhythm can make a tentative diagnosis for the patient. A regular rate with an early beat can be used to mimic PACs and PVCs. The pattern of atrial fibrillation (A-fib) can be mimicked by an irregularly irregular cadence. A regular rapid rhythm at approximately 150 beats/minute represents atrial flutter whereas regular rapid rhythms faster than this suggest paroxysmal atrial tachycardia (PAT). Arrhythmias that occur daily or almost daily can usually be recorded on a 24-hour ECG whereas use of a long-term event monitor is usually required for less frequent arrhythmias. An arrhythmia routinely occurring with exercise may be provoked with a standard exercise test, but such tests are usually of insufficient duration to reproduce the arrhythmia. Patients can be exercised for a more prolonged time in a setting such as a cardiac rehabilitation program where monitoring can be performed. They can also exercise near the hospital so that they can come in for recording if the arrhythmia appears. Long-term loop ECG recorders and implantable rhythm detectors are also available.

The second step is to determine if the arrhythmia is an isolated phenomenon or associated with important symptoms or structural cardiac disease. Arrhythmias that produce no or few symptoms and are infrequent can be evaluated less aggressively if the heart is normal. Alternatively, frequent arrhythmias or those associated with symptoms such as dyspnea or presyncope and those associated with occult heart disease require more extensive evaluation or referral to a cardiologist. Ultimate treatment of the arrhythmia depends on both the diagnosis and associated symptoms or associated disease.

Premature Atrial Contractions

PACs are common and benign. When they require treatment because they are annoying to the patient, they can usually be suppressed with beta-blockers or a calcium channel blocker with effects on the sinus node, such as diltiazem. Athletes with PACs can participate in all competitive sports.

Atrial Fibrillation

A-fib is a common arrhythmia in general and may be more frequent in active subjects (68). The explanation for this possible increased frequency in athletes is not clear. A-fib occurring at rest in athletes may be related to their increased vagal tone and concurrent atrial electrophysiologic changes. A-fib induced by exercise is usually provoked by exercise-related catecholamine discharge. The situations associated with the onset of A-fib help guide initial treatment. For example, A-fib occurring at rest in totally healthy athletes may be treated with an agent such as flecanide, which is effective in preventing A-fib associated with increased vagal tone. The use of flecanide has risks, however, and should be directed by a cardiologist. A-fib provoked by exertion is often best managed with beta-blockers. All patients with A-fib require an evaluation which includes a thyroid stimulating hormone (TSH) level to exclude hyperthyroidism as a cause. A 12-lead and a long-term 24-hour ECG is necessary, along with an echocardiogram (69).

A-fib can occur without structural heart disease. Medications such as theophylline, adenosine, and digitalis (70–72); alcohol; and drugs such as cocaine should be excluded as causes, although A-fib is often associated with hypertension or CAD in elderly athletes. In an athlete with no structural heart disease and with idiopathic A-fib, which is frequent or symptomatically bothersome, 24 hour or longer ECG recording should be performed to determine if atrial tachycardia precedes the A-fib. Because A-fib in patients younger than 40 years is unusual, further investigation for associated rhythms, and cardiac conditions, such as atrial septal defect, paroxysmal supraventricular tachycardia (PSVT), and accessory conduction pathways, should be considered in these patients. Further, A-fib may be initiated by a focus located in a pulmonary vein near its insertion into the left atrium. These focal arrhythmias in some cases can be obliterated by radiofrequency ablation and the athlete may be cured (73).

The management of A-fib is divided into the management of the arrhythmia as an acute or as a chronic condition. Asymptomatic athletes who have episodes of A-fib of 5 to 15 seconds that do not increase in duration during exercise can be active in all sports (69). The goal in managing acute A-fib is to restore normal sinus rhythm. Thromboembolus is the primary concern in converting A-fib to normal sinus rhythm. A-fib produces blood stasis in the left atrium with the possibility of thrombus formation. Restoration of normal sinus rhythm can reestablish effective atrial contraction and dislodge atrial thrombi. Classic teaching maintains that acute A-fib of less than 48 hours duration can be acutely cardioverted without fear of arterial embolization. Currently, concern about thromboembolism and the devastation it can produce as well as the availability of such techniques as transesophageal echocardiography to image left atrial thrombi have prompted a more cautious approach.

Most athletes experience sudden, new onset A-fib often at a rapid rate, and so they are aware of the arrhythmia onset. If the patient is certain that the A-fib has been present for less than 10 hours and the patient has no history for heart disease and has an otherwise normal ECG, we initiate heparin and electrically cardiovert the patient immediately. The patient can then be discharged from immediate medical care. For patients with A-fib of more than 10, but less than 24 hours duration, we initiate heparin immediately, perform a transesophageal echocardiogram, and cardiovert such patients only if there is no evidence of left atrial thrombus on transesophageal echocardiography. For patients with fibrillation lasting more than 24 hours or who have thrombus on echocardiography, we initiate heparin and warfarin therapy promptly. After at least 4 weeks of full anticoagulation, we repeat the transesophageal echocardiography and cardiovert the patient if there is no evidence of thrombus. We maintain anticoagulation with warfarin for an additional month after successful cardioversion.

Physicians managing chronic A-fib of unknown duration face several difficult decisions, and most patients should be managed in combination with a cardiologist. First, should the patient be cardioverted? We attempt cardioversion with or without adjunctive medical therapy to maintain sinus rhythm in virtually all of our A-fib patients, although the success decreases with A-fib of more than 6 months duration. Such patients must be anticoagulated for atleast 4 weeks with INR between (2 and 3), before, and after cardioversion and we perform transesophageal echocardiography to exclude residual thrombi before proceeding. Second, what agents should be used, if any, to maintain normal sinus rhythm after cardioversion? Third, should the patient with A-fib be chronically anticoagulated? Anticoagulation is recommended in patients with A-fib with structural heart disease, heart failure, diabetes, hypertension, history of transient ischemic attack (TIA), or stroke, or age more than 65 years. There is no consensus regarding anticoagulation in patients and without these risk factors. Aspirin should be prescribed to patients with no thromboembolic risk factors and short bursts of paroxysmal atrial fibrillation (PAF). Patients with recurrent PAF of durations approaching 10 hours should probably be considered for chronic warfarin therapy. Current guidelines permit athletes with asymptomatic A-fib without structural heart disease and a normal ventricular response to activity while on no A-V nodal blockers to participate in all competitive sports. Athletes who have been treated with ablation techniques may return to all competitive sports after 4 to 6 weeks if they have no recurrence or after an electrophysiological study has confirmed noninducibility of A-fib. Athletes with structural heart disease, A–fib, and an appropriate ventricular rate response to exertion can participate in sports as appropriate for their primary cardiac condition. Patients on anticoagulation with warfarin should be prohibited from sports with collision risk (69). We are not as restrictive as these guidelines and permit athletes with acute A-fib to return to sports within 2 weeks, and athletes with recently converted chronic A-fib to return to sports after 3 months of normal sinus rhythm. We permit athletes with persistent A-fib to participate in all sports as long as they are asymptomatic.

Paroxysmal Supraventricular Tachycardia

PSVT is frequent in athletes and frequently produced by exercise. It can often be terminated acutely with vagal maneuvers such as Valsalva, carotid sinus pressure, or initiating the diving reflex by facial immersion or even by applying a wet towel to the face. PSVT can often be easily managed by beta-blockers and calcium channel blockers such as diltiazem or verapamil. Patients with frequent episodes, medication intolerance, or disabling infrequent episodes should be referred for radiofrequency ablation of the offending electrical circuit.

Ventricular Pre-Excitation

An ECG showing the WPW pattern of a short PR interval, a widened QRS complex, and a delta wave on R wave, is more common in athletes probably because increased resting vagal tone blocks normal A-V conduction to reveal the accessory conduction pathway (17). The concern with accessory A-V conduction pathways is that in the presence of A-fib, the accessory pathway may be capable of conducting very rapidly, producing a rapid ventricular response that may degenerate into VF. WPW syndrome is a rare cause of exercise-related cardiac events (17), but athletes with this ECG pattern should be referred to a cardiologist for evaluation. In general, if the athlete is asymptomatic and if the WPW pattern disappears suddenly (from one beat to the next) during exercise testing, the accessory pathway is most likely benign and the athlete can participate in all competitive sports. The accessory pathway can often be obliterated by radiofrequency ablation in symptomatic athletes or in those with potentially dangerous pathways.

Atrial Flutter

The untreated normal atrial flutter is close to 300 beats/minute with the ventricular response rate usually at 150, but occasionally at 100 beats/minute or half to one third the flutter atrial rate. Structural heart disease must be excluded because atrial flutter is unusual in normal hearts and may indicate underlying cardiomyopathy (68). Radiofrequency ablation of the ectopic focus can approach a cure rate of 80% in athletes (74), and may be a preferred to long-term antiarrhythmics.

Premature Ventricular Contractions

PVCs, if not bothersome to the patient, can usually be managed by benign neglect once structural heart disease is excluded by echocardiography. Patients can be managed with beta-blockers if treatment is required for symptoms. Frequent PVCs, more than 10/minute, should be evaluated more extensively with cardiologic guidance to exclude myocarditis or some other cardiac cause.

Ventricular Tachycardia

Ventricular tachycardia (VT) at rates greater than 110 beats/minute should be referred to a cardiologist for evaluation. VT less than 110 beats/minute is benign and can be treated with beta-blockers if treatment is required. Recommendations for cardiologists managing athletes with VT have been presented (69).

Ventricular Fibrillation

Athletes who have experienced a cardiac arrest or who are at great risk for cardiac arrest should be treated with an implanted cardiac defibrillator (ICD) and are restricted from moderate to high intensity competitive sports. However, athletes with ICDs may participate in low-intensity sports provided they have had not required device therapy for 6 months (69).

Heart Block

As discussed in the section on athletic heart syndrome, A-V conduction disturbances including first and second degree A-V blocks are common in athletes. Asymptomatic athletes with a structurally normal heart and no worsening of the heart block with exercise can participate in all competitive sport. Transient third degree or complete heart block may occasionally be seen in well-trained endurance athletes during sleep, but is rare and should be carefully evaluated before permitting full athletic competition. In symptomatic athletes with complete heart block, pacing is required and competitive sports with a risk of bodily collision should be avoided to prevent injury to the pacemaking system (69).

Commotio Cordis (Cardiac Contusion)

Blunt cardiac trauma can cause ST segment elevation and life-threatening arrhythmias. The incidence of commotio cordis is rare and occurs usually in athletes younger than 16 years and in males. The typical presentation is an athlete who receives a direct blow to the left chest and then instantly collapses, or has a brief period of consciousness preceding collapse. The most common rhythm is VF. After resuscitation, marked ST elevation can occur without evolution to Q waves or elevation of cardiac enzymes. Survival in commotio cordis approaches 10%.

Exercise in the Prevention and Treatment of Coronary Artery Disease

Physical activity and exercise training have important roles in the prevention and treatment of CAD. These topics have recently been discussed in detail elsewhere (75,76) and are beyond the scope of this chapter.

Acknowledgements

Supported by grants from Hartford Hospital Research Fund and gifts from William Jakober, the McNulty Family, and the Haire Family.

REFERENCES

1. Thompson PD, ed. *Exercise and sports cardiology*. New York, NY: McGraw-Hill, 2000.
2. Van Camp SP, Bloor CM, Mueller FO, et al. Nontraumatic sports death in high school and college athletes. *Med Sci Sports Exerc* 1995;27:641–647.
3. Maron BJ, Shirani J, Poliac L, et al. Sudden death in young competitive athletes: clinical, demographic and pathologic profiles. *JAMA* 1996;276:199–204.
4. Thiene G, Nava A, Corrado D, et al. Right ventricular cardiomyopathy and sudden death in young people. *N Engl J Med* 1988;318:129–133.
5. Maron BJ, Gardin JM, Gidding SS, et al. Prevalence of hypertrophic cardiomyopathy in a general population of young adults: echocardiographic analysis of 4111 subjects in the CARDIA study. *Circulation* 1995;92:785–789.
6. Maron BJ, Klues HG. Surviving competitive athletics with hypertrophic cardiomyopathy. *Am J Cardiol* 1994;73:1098–1104.
7. Ragosta M, Crabtree J, Sturner WQ, et al. Death during recreational exercise in the state of Rhode Island. *Med Sci Sports Exerc* 1984;16:339–342.
8. Hammoudeh AJ, Haft JI. Coronary-plaque rupture in acute coronary syndromes triggered by snow shoveling. *N Engl J Med* 1996;335:2001.
9. Giri S, Thompson PD, Kiernan FJ, et al. Clinical and angiographic characteristics of exertion-related acute myocardial infarction. *JAMA* 1999;282:1731–1736.
10. Burke AP, Farb A, Malcom GT, et al. Plaque rupture and sudden death related to exertion in men with coronary artery disease. *JAMA* 1999;281:921–926.
11. Thompson PD, Funk EJ, Carleton RA, et al. Incidence of death during jogging in Rhode Island from 1975 through 1980. *JAMA* 1982;247:2535–2538.
12. Siscovick DS, Weiss NS, Fletcher RH, et al. The incidence of primary cardiac arrest during vigorous exercise. *N Engl J Med* 1984;311:874–877.
13. Franklin BA, Conviser JM, Stewart B, et al. Sporadic exercise:a trigger for acute cardiovascular events. *Circulation* 2000;102(Suppl II):612.
14. Mittleman MA, Maclure M, Tofler GH, et al. Triggering of acute myocardial infarction by heavy exertion: protection against triggering by regular exercise. *N Engl J Med* 1993;329:1677–1683.
15. Gordon JB, Ganz J, Nabel EG, et al. Atherosclerosis influences the vasomotor response of epicardial coronary arteries to exercise. *J Clin Invest* 1989;83:1946–1952.
16. Li N, Wallen H, Hjemdahl P. Evidence of prothrombotic effects of exercise and limited protection by aspirin. *Circulation* 1999;100:1374–1379.
17. Cobb LA, Weaver WD. Exercise: a risk for sudden death in patients with coronary heart disease. *J Am Coll Cardiol* 1986;7:215–219.

18. Pelliccia A, Maron BJ, Spataro A, et al. The upper limit of physiologic cardiac hypertrophy in highly trained elite athletes. *N Engl J Med* 1991;324:295–301.
19. Pelliccia A, Culasso F, Di Paolo FM, et al. Physiologic left ventricular cavity dilatation in elite athletes. *Ann Intern Med* 1999;130:23–31.
20. Pluim BM, Zwinderman AH, van der Laarse A, et al. The athlete's heart a meta-analysis of cardiac structure and function. *Circulation* 2000;101: 336–344.
21. Pelliccia A, Maron BJ, Culasso F, et al. Clinical significance of abnormal electrocardiographic patterns in trained athletes. *Circulation* 2000;102:278–284.
22. Biffi A, Pelliccia A, Verdile L, et al. Long-term clinical significance of frequent and complex ventricular tachyarrhythmias in trained athletes. *J Am Coll Cardiol* 2002;40:446–452.
23. Maron BJ, Pelliccia A, Spirito P, et al. Cardiac disease in young trained athletes insights into methods for distinguishing athlete's heart from structural heart disease, with particular emphasis on hypertrophic cardiomyopathy. *Circulation* 1995;91:1596–1601.
24. Maron BJ. Sudden death in young athletes. *N Engl J Med* 2003;349:1064–1075.
25. Rost R. The athlete's heart. Historical perspectives-solved and unsolved problems. *Cardiol Clin* 1997;15:493–512.
26. Maron BJ, Douglas PS, Graham TP, et al. Task Force 1: preparticipation screening and diagnosis of cardiovascular disease in athletes. *J Am Coll Cardiol* 2005;45(8):1322–1326.
27. Estes NAM, Link MS, Homoud M, et al. Electrocardiographic variants and cardiac rhythm and conduction disturbances in the athlete. In: Thompson PD III, ed. *Exercise and sports cardiology*. New York, NY: McGraw-Hill, 2000:211–232.
28. Huston TP, Puffer JC, Rodney WM. The athletic heart syndrome. *N Engl J Med* 1985;313:24–32.
29. Chapman J. Profound sinus bradycardia in the athletic heart syndrome. *J Sports Med Phys Fitness* 1981;22:294–298.
30. Thomas LR, Douglas PS. Echocardiographic findings in athletes. In: Thompson PD, ed. *Exercise and sports cardiology*. New York, NY: McGraw-Hill, 2000:43–70l.
31. Stewart BF, Siscovick D, Lind BK, et al. Clinical factors associated with calcific aortic valve disease. Cardiovascular health study. *J Am Coll Cardiol* 1997;29:630–634.
32. Wilmshurst PT, Stevenson RN, Griffiths H, et al. A case-control investigation of the relation between hyperlipidaemia and calcific aortic valve stenosis. *Heart* 1997;78:475–479.
33. Fuller CM, McNulty CM, Spring DA, et al. Prospective screening of 5,615 high school athletes for risk of sudden cardiac death. *Med Sci Sports Exerc* 1997;29:1131–1138.
34. Corrado D, Basso C, Schiavon M, et al. Screening for hypertrophic cardiomyopathy in young athletes. *N Engl J Med* 1998;339:364–369.
35. Maron BJ, Thompson PD, Puffer JC, et al. Cardiovascular preparticipation screening of competitive athletes. A statement for health professionals from the Sudden Death Committee (clinical cardiology) and Congenital Cardiac Defects Committee (cardiovascular disease in the young), American Heart Association. *Circulation* 1996;94:850–856.
36. Maron BJ, Shen WK, Link MS, et al. Efficacy of implantable cardioverter-defibrillators for the prevention of sudden death in patients with hypertrophic cardiomyopathy. *N Engl J Med* 2000;342:365–373.
37. Corrado D, Leoni L, Link MS, et al. Implantable cardioverter-defibrillator therapy for prevention of sudden death in patients with arrhythmogenic right ventricular cardiomyopathy/dysplasia. *Circulation* 2003;108:3084–3091.
38. Maron BJ, Araújo CG, Thompson PD, et al. Recommendations for preparticipation screening and the assessment of cardiovascular disease in Master's athletes an advisory for healthcare professionals from the working groups of the World Heart Federation, the International Federation of Sports Medicine, and the American Heart Association Committee on Exercise, Cardiac Rehabilitation, and Prevention. *Circulation* 2001;103:327–334.
39. Thompson PD. Sudden death in the athlete: athlerosclerotic coronary artery disease. In: Estes M III, Salem DN, Wang PJ, eds. *Sudden cardiac death in the athlete*. Armonk, New York: Futura Publishing, 1998:393–402.
40. Little WC, Constantinescu M, Applegate RJ, et al. Can coronary angiography predict the site of a subsequent myocardial infarction in patients with mild-to-moderate coronary artery disease? *Circulation* 1988;78:1157–1166.
41. Gibbons RJ, Balady GJ, Beasley JW, et al. ACC/AHA guidelines for exercise testing. *J Am Coll Cardiol* 1997;30(1):260–315.
42. Siscovick DS, Ekelund LG, Johnson JL, et al. Sensitivity of exercise electrocardiography for acute events during moderate and strenuous physical activity. The lipid research clinics coronary primary prevention trial. *Arch Intern Med* 1991;151:325–330.
43. Viskin S, Fish R, Roth A, et al. Clinical problem-solving. QT or not QT? *N Engl J Med* 2000;343:352–356.
44. Kaplan NM, Deveraux RB, Miller HS. Tak force 4: systemic hypertension. *J Am Coll Cardiol* 1994;24(4):885–889.
45. Chobanian AV, Bakris GL, Black HR, et al. The seventh report of the Joint National Committee on Prevention, Detection, Evaluation, and Treatment of High Blood Pressure: JNC 7 Report. *JAMA* 2003;289:2560–2572.
46. Mitchell JH, Haskell WL, Raven PB. Classification of sports. *J Am Coll Cardiol* 1994;24(4):864–866.
47. Kaplan NM, Gidding SS, Pickering TG, et al. Task Force 5: systemic hypertension. *J Am Coll Cardiol* 2005;45:1346–1348.
48. Niedfeldt MW. Managing hypertension in athletes and physically active patients. *Am Fam Physician* 2002;66(3):445–452.
49. Selbst SM, Ruddy RM, Clark BJ, et al. Pediatric chest pain: a prospective study. *Pediatrics* 1988;82:319–323.
50. Selbst SM. Chest pain in children. *Am Fam Physician* 1990;41:179–186.
51. Billups D, Martin D, Swain RA. Training room evaluation of chest pain in the adolescent athlete. *South Med J* 1995;88(6):667–672.
52. Peters HP, Bos M, Seebregts L, et al. Gastrointestinal symptoms in long-distance runners, cyclists, and triathletes: prevalence, medication, and etiology. *Am J Gastroenterol* 1999;94(6):1570–1581.
53. Weins L, Sabath R, Ewing L, et al. Chest pain in otherwise healthy children and adolescents is frequently caused by exercise-induced asthma. *Pediatrics* 1992;90:350–353.
54. Kapoor WN. Approach to the patient with syncope I. In: Goldman L, Braunwald E, eds. *Primary cardiology*. Philadelphia: WB Saunders, 1998:144–153.
55. Driscoll DJ, Jacobsen SJ, Porter CJ, et al. Syncope in children and adolescents. *J Am Coll Cardiol* 1997;29:1039–1045.
56. Maron BJ, Shirani J, Polliac LC, et al. Sudden death in young competitive athletes. Clinical, demographic, and pathological profiles. *JAMA* 1996;276:199–204.
57. Sakaguchi S, Schultz JJ, Remole SC, et al. Syncope associated with exercise, amanifestation of neurally mediated syncope. *Am J Cardiol* 1995;75:476–481.
58. Puffer JC, Bergfeld JA, et al. When does fainting represent a deadly condition? Exertional syncope: benign hypotension or life-threatening abnormality? Part 1. *Sports Med Dig* 1997;19:118–120.
59. Grubb BP, Temmsey-Armos PN, Samoil D, et al. Tilt table testing in the evaluation and management of athletes with recurrent exercise-induced syncope. *Med Sci Sports Exerc* 1993;25:24–28.
60. Calkins H, Seifert M, Morady F, et al. Clinical presentation and long-term follow-up of athletes with exercise-induced vasodepressor syncope. *Am Heart J* 1995;129:1159–1164.
61. Mitokou A, Ryan C, Veneman T, et al. Hierarchy of glycemic thresholds for counterregulatory hormone secretion, symptoms and cerebral dysfunction. *Am J Physiology* 1991;260:E67.
62. Rose BD, Post TW. *Clinical physiology of acid-base and electrolyte disorders*, 5th ed, New York: McGraw-Hill, 2001:716–720, 761–764.
63. McManus ML, Churchwell KB, Strange K, et al. Genotype-phenotype correlation in the long-QT syndrome- gene specific triggers for life-threatening arrhythmias. *Circulation* 2001;103:89–95; Disease. *N Engl J Med* 1995;333:1260.
64. Ciampricotti R, Deckers JW, Taverne R, et al. Characteristics of conditioned and sedentary men with acute coronary syndromes. *Am J Cardiol* 1994;73:219–222.
65. Thompson PD, Stern MP, Williams P, et al. Death during jogging or running: a study of 18 cases. *JAMA* 1979;242:1265–1267.
66. Vincent GM, Jaisawal D, Timothy KW. Effects of exercise in heart rate, QT, QTc, QT/AS2 in the romano-ward inherited long QT syndrome. *Am J Cardiol* 1991;68:498–503.
67. Schwartz PJ, Priori SG, Spazzolini C, et al. Genotype-phenotype correlation in the long-QT syndrome- gene specific triggers for life-threatening arrhythmias. *Circulation* 2001;103:89–95.
68. Furlanello F, Bertoldi A, Dallago M, et al. Atrial fibrillation in elite athletes. *J Cardiovasc Electrophysiol* 1998;9:S63–S68.
69. Zipes DP, Ackerman MJ, Estes NAM III, et al. Task Force 7: arrhythmias. *J Am Coll Cardiol* 2005;45:1354–1363.
70. Van der HCS, Heeringa J, van Herpen G, et al. Drug-induced atrial fibrillation. *J Am Coll Cardiol* 2004;44:2117.
71. Varriale P, Ramaprased S. Aminophylline induced atrial fibrillation. *Pacing Clin Electrophysiol* 1993;16:1953.
72. Strickberger SA, Man KC, Daoud EG, et al. Adenosine-induced atrial arrhythmia: a prospective analysis. *Ann Intern Med* 1997;127:417.
73. Link NMS, Homoud MK, Wang PJ, et al. Cardiac arrhythmias in the athlete. *Cardiol Rev* 2001;9(1):21–30.
74. Fischer B, Haissaguerre M, Garrigues S, et al. Radiofrequency catheter ablation of common atrial flutter in 80 patients. *J Am Coll Cardiol* 1995;25:1365–1372.
75. Thompson PD, Buchner D, Williams MA, et al. American Heart Association Council on Clinical Cardiology Subcommittee on Exercise, Rehabilitation, and Prevention; American Heart Association Council on Nutrition, Physical Activity, and Metabolism Subcommittee on Physical Activity. Exercise and physical activity in the prevention and treatment of atherosclerotic cardiovascular disease: a statement from the Council on Clinical Cardiology (Subcommittee on exercise, rehabilitation and prevention) and the Council on Nutrition, Physical Activity, and Metabolism (Subcommittee on physical activity). *Circulation* 2003;107:9053–9054.
76. Thompson PD. Exercise prescription and proscription for patients with coronary artery disease. *Circulation* 2005;112:2354–2363.

Head Injuries

14

Margot Putukian

Head injuries occur commonly during sports participation, and can have serious consequences if not treated properly. Detecting injury, assessing severity, and making appropriate return to play (RTP) decisions are important responsibilities of the physician caring for athletes of all ages. An organized comprehensive evaluation, with special attention to exclude cervical spine injury, vascular or other focal injuries are essential for the physician caring for athletes on the sideline. Understanding the complications and long-term sequelae of head injuries and how these impact RTP decisions is important. This chapter will discuss these issues and review current literature regarding head injuries in athletes.

In general, the head injuries that occur in the athletic setting are mild in comparison to those that occur in motor vehicle accidents or other high velocity impact injuries. Despite this, the physician taking care of the athlete must always consider the possibility of a catastrophic injury. Of the catastrophic injuries that occur on the athletic field, head and spine injuries, along with cardiac fatalities, are the most common. Recognizing serious head and spine injuries and understanding their progression is therefore essential. For the head injured athlete, the most common serious injuries include vascular intracranial injuries and cervical spine injuries. Vascular catastrophes can present immediately or be delayed by several hours. Other complications of brain injury include "second impact syndrome" (SIS) (1,2), repetitive and/or cumulative injury, and post-concussion syndrome. The morbidity and mortality of these complications are significant for the athlete. Cervical spine injuries often occur in association with head injuries, and can be missed because of the attention paid to the brain injury. A comprehensive method of evaluating and following up the injuries of these athletes remains paramount in order to minimize the potential for missing these other related injuries. Whether there are age- or gender-related risks for head injury is a question that remains unanswered. What are the risks present with RTP before complete cognitive recovery or with recurrent head injury and are there prognostic factors that help determine which athletes are at greater risk for long-term complications of injury? These are issues that have begun to be addressed.

The assessment of head injury includes recognizing that an injury has occurred, managing the acute injury, determining referral status, and eventually making RTP decisions. Many head injuries go undetected, and are not reported to the medical or coaching staff. This may be in part due to the lack of availability of medical staff for certain sports or levels of participation, but in many cases it is due to the nature of the sport, where sustaining a "ding" or "bell-ringer" is felt to be part of the game. Some athletes will try to minimize their injury, knowing that if they report their symptoms, they will be kept out of play. This can obviously have significant consequences. Athletes and coaches must be educated on the importance of these injuries in terms of the athlete's long-term health and function (3). In one study of rugby athletes, 56% of 544 athletes sustained at least one head injury associated with memory loss (amnesia) after the event. In those athletes who had amnesia lasting more than 1 hour, only 38 of 58 athletes were admitted to the hospital for treatment (4). Fortunately, over the last several years, the impact of these injuries has become more apparent, and an increased awareness by both the athletic training staff and medical personnel has allowed for a higher index of suspicion and earlier detection of these injuries.

Post-traumatic encephalopathy, or the "punch drunk syndrome"(5), has been described in boxers and is felt to be due to repetitive injuries that result in cumulative injury to the brain. This repetitive, cumulative head trauma may increase the risk for the development of Alzheimer's disease (5–7). The long-term risks of repetitive head trauma is an area of sports medicine research that is gaining significant attention, and with the advent of neuropsychological and balance testing, more sensitive tools for assessing cognitive function after mild traumatic brain injury (MTBI) are available.

EPIDEMIOLOGY

According to the National Head Injury Foundation, sports causes 18% of all head injuries, compared to motor vehicle accidents (46%), falls (23%), and assaults (10%). In 1984, traumatic brain injuries accounted for approximately 500,000 hospital admissions, with 3% to 10% of these related to sport activities (8). One million head injuries are seen in North American emergency departments annually. Head injury causes 19% of all nonfatal injuries in football, and 4.5% of all high school sports injuries (9,10). At the elementary, junior, and high school levels, football accounts for the highest incidence of head injury among any sport (11).

Amongst young children in Australia, closed head injury was six times more likely to be a result of organized sports activities versus leisure activities (12). In the United States it is estimated that 1 million children sustain head injuries annually, 85% of them being mild, with 250,000 admissions, accounting for 10% of all emergency room visits (13).

As mentioned previously, the incidence of concussion is likely greater than what is reported, especially in younger athletes for whom medical care is less available. A recent retrospective study of 1,532 high school football players from 20 schools found that 29.9% of players reported a history of concussion, with 15.3% reporting a concussion in the current season. Of these recent injuries, only 47.3% were reported, predominantly to a certified athletic trainer. Of the unreported injuries, 66.4% of the respondents felt that their injuries were medically insignificant, 41% did not report their injuries because they did not want to be kept out of play, and the remainder did not realize their injury was a concussion (14).Concussions account for roughly 1.6% to 6.4% of all injuries at the college level, with an incidence of 0.06 to 0.55 injuries/1,000 athlete exposures (15). Over the recent years, ice hockey and football tend to account for the highest percentage of head injuries. However, men's and women's soccer also have relatively high incidence rates of concussion. In addition, sports that utilize head protection (ice hockey, football, men's lacrosse) have a similar incidence to those sports without head protection (men's and women's soccer, field hockey). Player to player contact is the most common mechanism of injury reported in most sports tracked by the National Collegiate Athletic Association (NCAA), with the exceptions being field hockey (contact with the stick), women's lacrosse, women's softball, and baseball (contact with the ball). Understanding the mechanism of injury is very important in the attempts to decrease injuries by considering changes to rules or equipment.

Helmets

In several sports, wearing of helmets has been proposed as a means to decrease head injury. It is important to use injury surveillance data to make decisions with evidence-based data to support these changes. Although appealing at first glance, one must be aware of the potential that wearing a protective equipment may have. In other words, by wearing a helmet, some athletes may feel invulnerable, play more aggressively, and this may potentially change the nature of the sport. Wearing a weighted, hard plastic helmet may inadvertently increase the risk of either head injury or cervical spine injury. Therefore, it is important that one considers the true incidence of injury as well as the potential, even untoward, effects that the proposed changes may have on sports.

The use of helmets has decreased the frequency of head injury in ice hockey and football (16,17). The 50% decrease in injuries in football since 1976 (18) has been attributed to both changes in helmet fit and design, as well as rule changes that forbid spear tackling. The data has been more controversial for ice hockey because, although there has been a decrease in head injury, there has been an increase in cervical spine injuries. The use of helmets with face guards has significantly reduced the number of orofacial injuries. Pforringer (19) found that 75% of 246 injuries in ice hockey were a result of violence outside game play (high sticking, deliberate pushing, fist fighting). Therefore, enforcement of existing rules may be as important in protecting athletes from head injury as proper equipment.

In baseball and softball, helmets are used effectively to decrease the incidence of head injury. Athletes in these sports use helmets while batting and running bases. Ample evidence exists to demonstrate that head injury, involving a batted or thrown ball, has decreased (15,20). Possibly the most compelling evidence for the use of helmets in decreasing head injury is bicycling. When a fall occurs while bicycling, there is a 50% chance that a head injury will occur, and if the cyclist is traveling 20 mi/hour, there is a higher risk of fatality (20). Every year, 1,300 deaths occur as a result of cycling accidents, with most occurring due to head injury. When an appropriate helmet is used, the risk of traumatic brain injury is decreased by 88% (21). Given this data, the use of helmets by the cycling athlete is imperative.

DEFINITIONS

Head injuries occur on a spectrum, with or without focal abnormalities. Focal injuries include subdural hematoma, epidural hematoma, cerebral contusion, and intracranial hemorrhages, both subarachnoid and intracerebral. Diffuse brain injuries do not have focal lesions associated with them, but can be associated with significant deficits in cognitive function. Focal injuries often occur as a result of blunt trauma and are associated with focal neurological deficits and loss of consciousness (LOC). If LOC is brief or does not occur, these injuries can go undetected, making it more important that injury assessment is complete and thorough. Early recognition and treatment of these focal injuries is essential in optimizing successful recovery.

Subdural Hematoma

Subdural hematomas occur as a result of disruption of the venous blood vessels, causing a low-pressure accumulation of blood in an enclosed space. These "subdurals" are the most common focal injuries in the sport setting, and are often associated with LOC and slow deterioration of mental status and focal neurological deficits. If there is no associated underlying cerebral contusion or edema, the subdural is considered simple, yet the mortality rate approximates 20%. If there is underlying cerebral contusion or edema, then it is considered a complex subdural, and the mortality rate increases to 50% (see Figures 14.1 and 14.2). Depending on the age of the athlete, subdural hematomas may be more or less symptomatic. Cerebral atrophy correlates with age, and therefore there is more room for accumulation of blood in the older athlete. For a younger athlete, the same amount of bleeding will result in more and earlier onset of symptoms. Early recognition is therefore more important in the younger athlete in whom deterioration can occur quickly and become life threatening. In the older athlete the symptoms are due to a mass effect, whereas in the younger athlete the symptoms are often a result of compression of the normal brain substance (22).

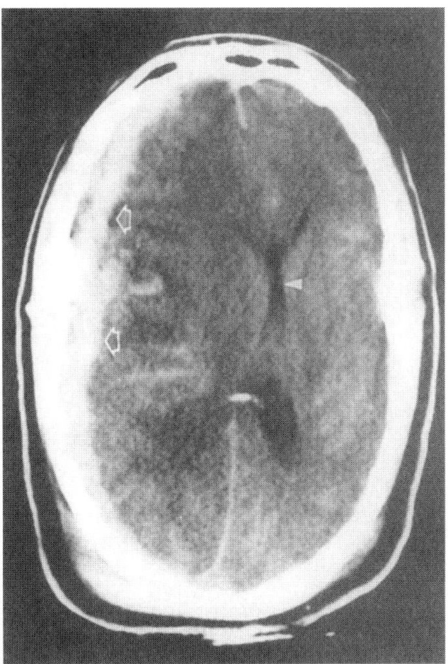

Figure 14.2 Typical appearance of an acute subdural hematoma (*open arrows*) on an axial computed tomography image. The degree of shift of the midline structures (*arrowhead*) is greater than the thickness of the subdural hematoma, suggesting significant parenchymal injury to the hemisphere, in addition to the hematoma. (*Source*: Reprinted with permission from Fu FH, Stone DA, eds. *Sports injuries: Mechanisms, prevention, treatment*. Baltimore: Williams & Wilkins, 1994.)

Epidural Hematoma

Epidural hematomas are not as common as subdural hematomas, and are high-pressure vascular injuries. They are due to disruption of a meningeal artery, most often the middle meningeal artery. The classic presentation of an epidural hematoma is an initial LOC followed by a lucid interval and apparent recovery. Then, after minutes to hours, headache, rapid deterioration of mental status, LOC with pupillary abnormalities (ipsilateral pupil dilates), and decerebrate posturing with weakness on the opposite side of the bleed will occur (23). Only one third of the patients will demonstrate this "classic" presentation (see Figure 14.3), underscoring the need to maintain a high index of suspicion for these emergencies.

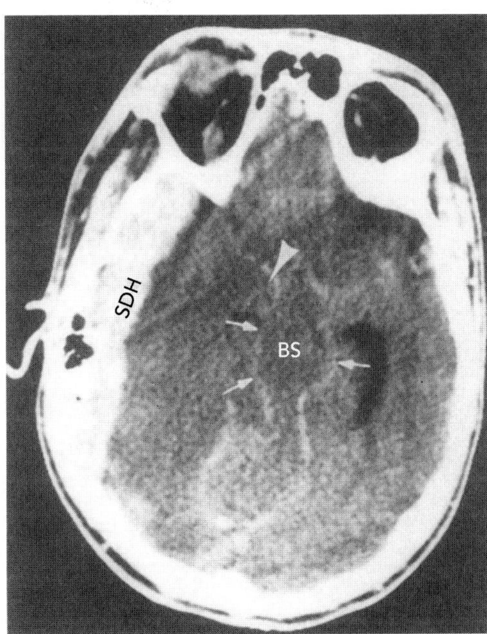

Figure 14.1 Axial computed tomography image demonstrating an acute subdural hematoma (SDH) on the right side, with herniation of the medial temporal lobe into the tentorial notch (*arrowhead*). The midbrain is outlined by subarachnoid hemorrhage in the perimesencephalic cistern (*arrows*). BS = brain stem. (*Source*: Reprinted with permission from Fu FH, Stone DA, eds. *Sports injuries: Mechanisms, prevention, treatment*. Baltimore: Williams & Wilkins, 1994.)

Other Focal Injuries

Other focal injuries include cerebral contusions, intracerebral hemorrhages, and subarachnoid hemorrhages. Common symptoms of these injuries include headache, post-traumatic amnesia (PTA), and confusion, but not LOC. Intracerebral hemorrhages occur within the substance of the brain, whereas subarachnoid hemorrhages occur on the surface of the brain. Cerebral contusions and hemorrhages can both occur in association with mass changes and hydrocephalus (see Figures 14.4 and 14.5).

Computed tomography (CT) as well as magnetic resonance imaging (MRI) and electroencephalography (EEG) are useful tools for detecting focal injuries (22, 24–28). MRI is a sensitive tool, and MRI findings in those individuals with persistent LOC admitted to the

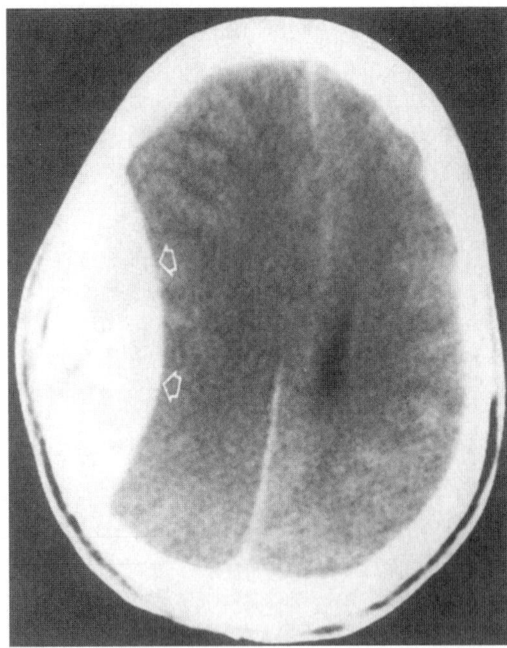

Figure 14.3 Typical appearance of an epidural hematoma on an axial computed tomography image. (*Source*: Reprinted with permission from Fu FH, Stone DA, eds. *Sports injuries: Mechanisms, prevention, treatment.* Baltimore: Williams & Wilkins, 1994.)

intensive care unit correlate with the depth and severity of injury. Lesions were present in 88% of these patients with severe clinical compromise (29). The diagnostic test of choice in the first 48 hours for evaluation of the head injured athlete is CT, given the sensitivity of this test to detect blood and fracture better than MRI. After 48 hours, MRI is favored for detecting subtle injuries (30–32). Both CT and MRI are equally sensitive in detecting focal injuries requiring surgical treatment (33). For those lesions requiring neurosurgical treatment, the time from detection to treatment is critical in terms of reducing morbidity and mortality.

Diffuse Axonal Injury

Diffuse brain injuries are nonfocal injuries with no identifiable lesion. The spectrum of these injuries correlates with the amount of anatomical disruption. Diffuse axonal injury represents the most severe injury along the spectrum and is often associated with prolonged LOC. It is commonly associated with residual psychological personality and neurological deficits. Cerebral concussion is often considered at the other end of the spectrum and represents a nonfocal injury, although it can be associated with structural abnormalities.

Cerebral Concussion

Cerebral concussion has been defined as "a clinical syndrome characterized by immediate and transient impairment of neurological function secondary to mechanical forces" (34). The hallmarks of concussion are confusion and amnesia. LOC does not necessarily occur during concussion, and varying amounts of memory dysfunction can occur. Headache is the most common symptom of concussion, and this symptom can occur by itself without concussion, making it difficult to discern and evaluate athletes with more severe injury from those with only mild trauma and headache. Additional symptoms that are typical in cerebral concussion are given in Table 14.1. Typically, concussions involve the rapid onset of short-lived neurological impairment that resolves spontaneously. Though neuropathological changes may occur, the acute symptoms seen are generally due to a functional disturbance, not

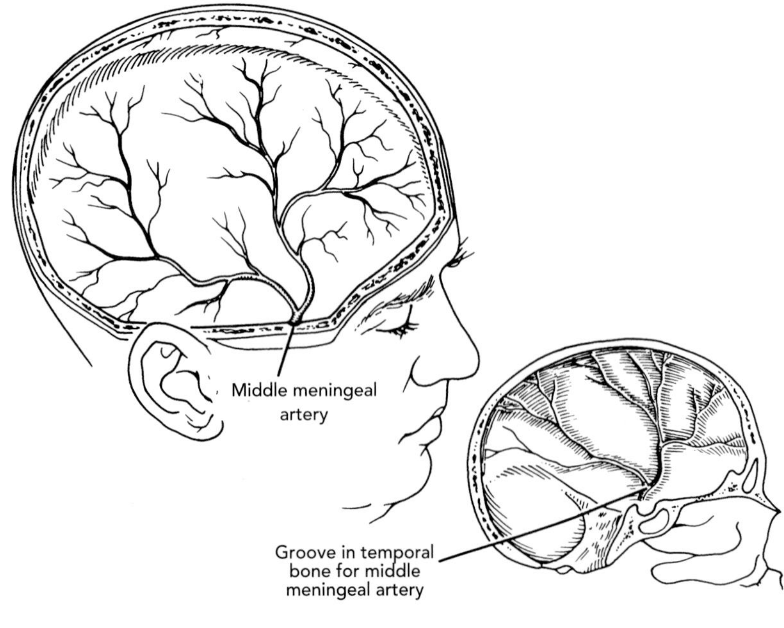

Figure 14.4 The middle meningeal artery is tethered in a groove in the temporal bone and is easily lacerated by fractures through this bone. Hemorrhage from the middle meningeal artery causes an epidural hematoma. (*Source*: Reprinted with permission from Fu FH, Stone DA, eds. *Sports injuries: Mechanisms, prevention, treatment.* Baltimore: Williams & Wilkins, 1994.)

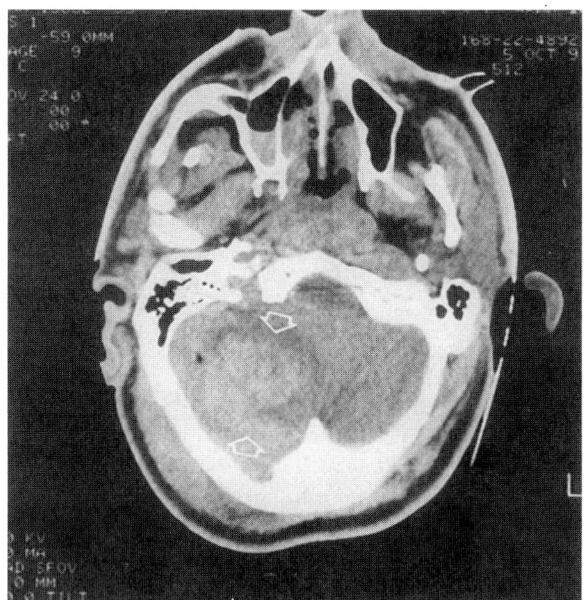

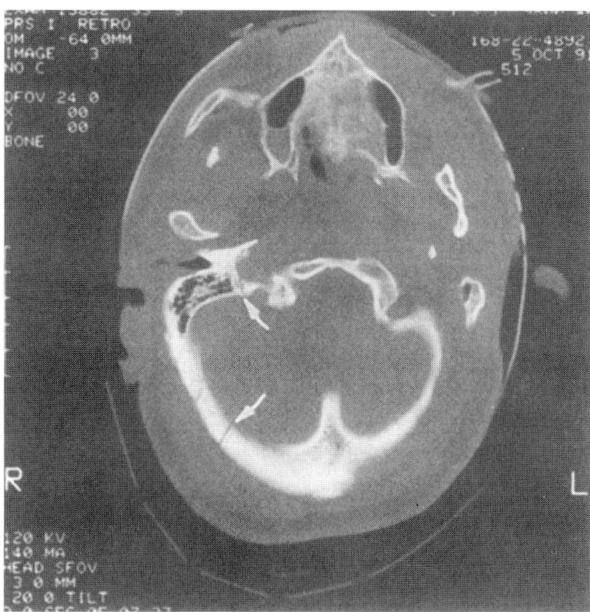

Figure 14.5 Axial computed tomography images demonstrate a hemorrhagic contusion of the right cerebellar hemisphere **(A)** associated with a fracture through the floor of the posterior fossa on the right side **(B)**. (*Source*: Reprinted with permission from Fu FH, Stone DA, eds. *Sports injuries: Mechanisms, prevention, treatment.* Baltimore: Williams & Wilkins, 1994.)

structural injury. Resolution of injury generally occurs in a sequential course, and neuroimaging studies are generally grossly normal. Cerebral concussion, commonly referred to as MTBI, is the most common head injury seen in athletic practice or competition. MTBI can occur independently or in association with the focal injuries described earlier. MTBI can be associated with significant morbidity and mortality, especially if not treated appropriately.

MECHANISMS AND PATHOPHYSIOLOGY

Understanding injury mechanisms can be useful in predicting the severity and recovery from head injury (35,36), as well as potentially avoiding injuries from occurring. Diffuse brain injuries are associated with anatomical changes, including disruption of axonal and myelin sheath structures throughout the white matter of the hemispheres and brain stem, petechial hemorrhages in periventricular regions, and chromatolysis and cell loss throughout the cortical gray matter and brain stem nuclei (37–40). With repetitive injury, atrophy of the cerebral hemispheres can occur (39). Research models of head injury demonstrate acceleration and impact forces similar to that seen in sports, and both of these are important in the pathophysiology of injury.

Recent reviews have discussed the correlation of specific traumatic forces with different types and severities of head injuries (41). Rotational forces and their subsequent shearing stresses are felt to be the most important factors in causing severe structural injuries (37,39,42,43). An example of a rotational force in sports is the boxer being struck by a left hook. Acceleration forces can occur when an athlete's moving head strikes a nonmoving object, such as the ground. Impact or compressive forces occur when a stationary head is struck with a forceful blow, such as when a football player is struck in the head. These forces often occur in various combinations, with the combination of both acceleration and rotational forces associated with the most significant deleterious effects (43).

Injuries are considered "coup" injuries when the area maximally injured is the area just beneath where the head was struck, which is often the case in impact injuries. "Contra-coup" injuries occur when the maximal area of injury is on the opposite side of the skull where the impact occurred, as is often the case with acceleration injuries. These are easy to understand if one considers that the brain is floating in a fluid within the rigid confines of the skull. When an acceleration or rotational injury occurs, the brain lags slightly behind the skull at impact, and then strikes the opposite side of the skull. The attachments of the dura mater to the bony ridges of the skull create potential forces where this tethering occurs, such that when the skull is impacted, these attachments are pulled on (44).

The strength of the neck musculature is important in providing stability to the head when struck. When a force strikes the skull, the force imparted depends in part on whether the musculature is rigid. Using Newton's second law (mass × acceleration = force), if the neck musculature is rigid, then more acceleration is necessary to impart the same force to the skull. This explains why a football player prepared for a hit is less likely to sustain an injury, and why a soccer player who forcibly strikes a ball may not be at the same risk as the player who is struck while not expecting

TABLE 14.1
SIGNS AND SYMPTOMS OF CEREBRAL CONCUSSION

Loss of consciousness
Confusion
Post-traumatic amnesia
Retrograde amnesia
Disorientation
Delayed verbal and motor responses
Inability to focus
Headache
Nausea/vomiting
Visual disturbances (photophobia, blurry vision, double vision)
Disequilibrium
Feeling "in a fog," "zoned out"
Vacant stare
Emotional lability
Dizziness
Slurred/incoherent speech
Excessive drowsiness
Symptoms Consistent with Postconcussive Syndrome
Loss of intellectual capacity
Poor recent memory
Personality changes
Headaches
Dizziness
Lack of concentration
Poor attention
Fatigue
Irritability
Phono/photophobia
Sleep disturbances
Depressed mood
Anxiety

a blow. Therefore, neck muscle strengthening and teaching athletes the proper techniques in certain sport-specific skills may be useful in decreasing injuries.

Mild traumatic injury is associated with neurochemical and neurometabolic changes, which can put cells at risk for insult. In animal research models, the release of excitatory amino acids, such as glutamate, can cause ionic fluxes that disrupt the way cell's utilize oxygen (45–48). When a head injury occurs, there is an increased need for glycolysis (45,46,49). At the same time, there is a decrease in cerebral blood flow (46,50), resulting in an imbalance between glucose supply and demand. It has been theorized that this imbalance creates cell dysfunction, which then puts the cell at an increased risk for a second insult (41,51).

In the limited human research that has been performed, the data appears consistent with what is seen in animal research. Cerebral glucose metabolism is increased as a result of ionic shifts (38,52), and reductions in cerebral blood flow and oxidative metabolism occur is association with changes in glutamate, potassium, and calcium. [18F]Fluorodeoxyglucose-positron emission tomography (FDG-PET) scanning studies have shown that these changes occur in severely brain injured patients (53,54). The basic and clinical science of concussion has been reviewed and is discussed in detail elsewhere (55,56).

EVALUATION OF THE HEAD INJURED ATHLETE

It is essential that the initial evaluation and management of the head injured athlete be thorough, orderly, and performed by appropriate medical personnel in an appropriate setting. The first step in evaluation is recognition that an injury has occurred. On-field evaluation must first assess the need for basic emergency services such as airway, breathing, and circulation (ABC) and assure that a cervical spine injury has not occurred. Observing the mechanism of injury can help the medical staff determine the severity of injury. Observing and recording any LOC that occurs is helpful, as well as noting the time the injury occurred. For the conscious athlete, evaluation should include assessment for any symptoms of concussion, and most importantly, any retrograde or PTA that is present. In the unconscious athlete, the medical personnel should assume that a cervical spine injury is present, and emergency care procedures should be initiated. The Glasgow Coma Scale (GCS) is a useful tool in predicting long-term prognosis, although in most sport-related head injuries, the GCS is often normal (see Table 14.2). Eighty percent of patients with a GCS less than 5 will die or remain in a vegetative state, whereas if the GCS is greater than 11, more than 90% will have complete recovery (44). An increase in GCS is associated with improved prognosis, underscoring the importance for serial assessments.

Cervical spine injuries occur in 5% to 10% of severe head injuries (57). The Inter-Association Task Force for Appropriate Care of the Spine-Injured Athlete published a manuscript that reviews the prehospital care of the injured athlete with cervical spine injuries. This manuscript also reviews the importance of the Emergency Action Plan (58). These guidelines, along with those from the American College of Sports Medicine, recommend that for the football player with a helmet, the helmet should be left in place unless an airway must be secured or the facemask cannot be cut away (59).

During the initial assessment, in addition to confirming that the cervical spine is stable, it is also important to exclude associated skull fracture. Findings seen in association with skull fracture are given in Table 14.3. If skull fracture is suspected, there may be an increased risk for intracranial infection, due to the compromise of the skin and skull into the surface of the brain. There is also a 20-fold increase in the risk of intracranial bleed when skull fracture occurs in association with head injury compared

TABLE 14.2
GLASGOW COMA SCALE

	Score
Eye opening	
Eyes open spontaneously	4
Eyes open to verbal command	3
Eyes open only with painful stimuli	2
No eye opening	1
Verbal response	
Oriented and converses	5
Disoriented and converses	4
Inappropriate words	3
Incomprehensible sounds	2
No verbal response	1
Motor response	
Obeys verbal commands	6
Response to painful stimuli (upper extremities)	
Localizes pain	5
Withdraws from pain	4
Flexor posturing	3
Extensor posturing	2
No motor response	1
Total score = eye opening + verbal response + motor response	

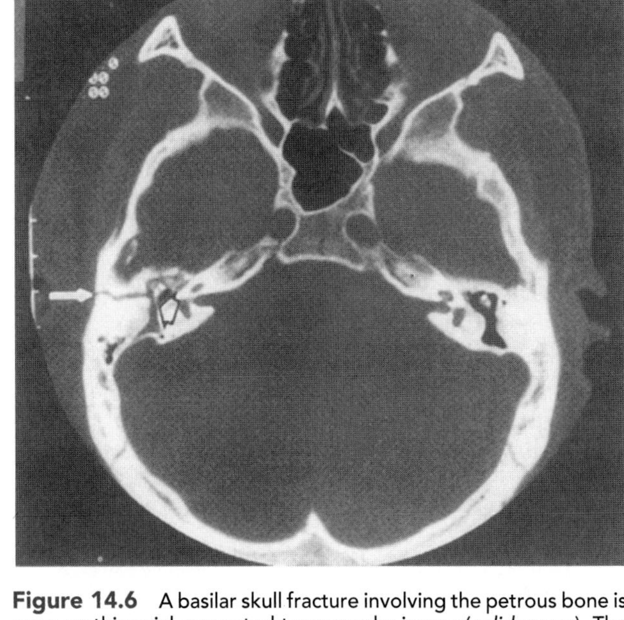

Figure 14.6 A basilar skull fracture involving the petrous bone is seen on this axial computed tomography image (*solid arrow*). The fracture extends into the middle ear (*open arrow*) and can cause a conducive hearing loss by disrupting the tympanic membrane or the ossicles of the middle ear. The fracture also can cause hemorrhage into the middle ear cavity, which will result in hearing loss. (*Source*: Reprinted with permission from Fu FH, Stone DA, eds. *Sports injuries: Mechanisms, prevention, treatment.* Baltimore: Williams & Wilkins, 1994.)

with head injury without skull fracture (60). If any concern for potential skull fracture is present, the athlete should be transported emergently to a medical facility where imaging studies can be obtained (see Figures 14.6 and 14.7) and a neurosurgical consultation can be secured if indicated.

On the field, the athlete should be asked questions that assess their orientation, memory status, and overall cognitive function. Once the athlete's cervical spine is deemed to be stable, further assessment can occur on the sideline. Additional questions, such as what the score of the game is, what color jersey the opponent is wearing, the site of the game, and previous game results, as well as questions on events that occurred before the injury are helpful. Asking about specific plays or defensive/offensive strategies with confirmation by a teammate or coach is also a useful way to determine if the athlete's memory is intact. If the injured athlete is seen in the office setting, or several days after the injury occurred, it may be important that an athletic trainer, teammate, coach, or family member accompanies the athlete, especially if memory dysfunction or altered levels of consciousness has occurred. Determining if LOC occurred, and for how long, is best reported by an individual who has witnessed the injury. Athletes often mistake the period in which they were confused or disoriented as "unconscious."

TABLE 14.3
SIGNS OF SKULL FRACTURE

Battle's sign	Postauricular hematoma
Rhinorrhea	CSF leaking from the nose
Otorrhea	CSF leaking from the ear canal
Raccoon eyes	Periorbital ecchymosis due to leakage of blood from anterior fossa into periorbital tissues
Hemotympanum	Blood behind the eardrum
Cranial nerve injuries	Especially involving the facial nerve
Palpable malalignment of calvarium	

CSF = cerebrospinal fluid.

Determination of the extent of memory loss for events before the injury (retrograde amnesia [RGA]) or after the injury (PTA) is also essential when evaluating the head injured athlete and, as will be discussed later, may be the most sensitive markers for the severity of injury. In addition, if it is clear that the athlete is struggling in answering these questions, it is often more obvious to the athlete, coach, or parent that the athlete should not be allowed to return to participation. Aspects of the examination that are difficult to measure, yet remain important, include the athletes' ability to follow commands and how quickly and smoothly they perform aspects of the examination. For example, a useful sideline evaluation of memory and information processing

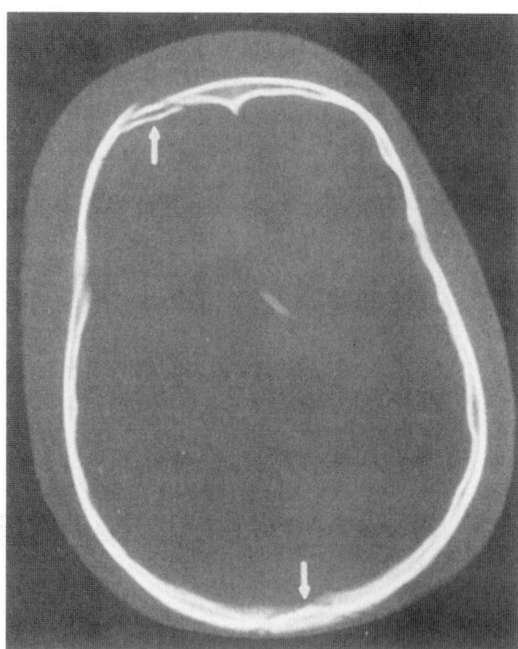

Figure 14.7 Axial computed tomography image of right frontal and occipital comminuted skull fractures. The occipital fracture is particularly ominous because it lies over the superior sagittal sinus and may have lacerated it, causing an intracranial hematoma. (*Source*: Reprinted with permission from Fu FH, Stone DA, eds. *Sports injuries: Mechanisms, prevention, treatment.* Baltimore: Williams & Wilkins, 1994.)

speed is to ask an athlete to give the months of the year backwards from a selected month. Although the athlete may be 100% accurate with the information they provide, observing the difficulty and speed with which they are able to perform this is useful in the overall evaluation process. Unfortunately, unless these same tests have been performed by the athlete earlier, it is often difficult to know the exact extent of their deficits.

Other symptoms of head injury, other than RGA, PTA, and LOC, include headache, nausea, dizziness, tinnitus, balance problems, and "feeling in a fog." Difficulties associated with gait, vision, speech, or cranial nerve deficits may also occur. Common signs and symptoms of cerebral concussion are given Table 14.1. A complete neurological examination should be performed as soon as the athlete is cleared of cervical spine injury and/or skull fracture. This should include pupillary response, cranial nerve testing, upper and lower extremity strength and sensory function, reflexes, cerebellar examination, and evaluation of complex tasks, such as gait. Deficits should be noted, and serial examinations performed along with the assessment of symptoms. The athlete should be assessed immediately and serially after head injury to ensure that deterioration does not occur.

If symptoms worsen on examination, or mental status deteriorates, the athlete should be referred for further emergent evaluation. Guidelines regarding when further evaluation in an emergency facility is warranted are presented by the NATA (National Athletic Trainers' Association) Consensus Statement on Concussion (61), as well as the Team Physician Consensus Statement on MTBI (62). In addition, the American Academy of Pediatrics has made recommendations in 1999 for the management of minor closed head injury in children (63).

Determining when diagnostic imaging is indicated is often difficult. If there is sustained LOC, concern for skull fracture, or any evidence of focal deficits, imaging should be considered. If an athlete has an initial lucid interval, then demonstrates a decline in mental status or worsening symptoms, imaging is indicated. The American Academy of Pediatrics found no indication for routine skull radiographs for minor head injury, and also stated that CT scanning was no different in individuals with or without LOC, and was no better than observation alone, thereby questioning the routine use of CT scanning in head injured children (63). Close observation is very important for the athlete who sustains MTBI, and it is essential to ensure that the athlete is not left alone. Determining which athletes require inpatient observation is often a challenge to the team physician. CT scanning is felt to be the best initial neuroimaging test acutely, given its ability to detect fracture and blood. These imaging studies are generally normal in concussion injuries, and are obtained to exclude skull or cervical spine fracture and/or other focal abnormalities discussed previously, such as intracranial bleeding and subdural or epidural hematomas.

MANAGEMENT OF THE CONCUSSED ATHLETE

Once an athlete has been diagnosed with concussion, it is important to watch him/her closely, perform serial evaluations, and determine whether he/she requires inpatient observation, observation at home, or RTP. Though there is controversy regarding several aspects of concussion treatment and management, all agree that athletes with symptoms should not be allowed to continue play. Ensuring that no athlete is symptomatic requires diligent questioning of the athlete and calls for more than merely asking him/her "are you alright?" It is often beneficial to use a symptom checklist to ensure that no additional symptoms have developed. For those athletes who are symptomatic, placing them in a quiet and dark environment, away from severe environmental conditions, is helpful. Decisions regarding whether the athlete stays on the sideline or goes into the locker room can be made based on individual cases, but the injured athlete should remain supervised by qualified medical personnel at all times to watch for decompensation. Athletes who are not kept under observation should be given written instructions; these are often also given to a teammate, roommate, and/or parent/guardian. The take-home instructions should include avoiding alcohol or other drugs, avoiding aspirin or nonsteroidal anti-inflammatory medications, and signs and symptoms to watch for that warrant emergency referral. Athletes should also be told to avoid any significant physical or mental exertion, which may exacerbate their symptoms. Finally, athletes should be given a time for follow-up evaluation, and should not perform any weight lifting or other exertional activities (gym class, bicycling, etc.) until re-evaluation has occurred.

Athletes who are symptomatic should not participate and should be instructed to follow-up with athletic medicine personnel, the timing of which is individualized, depending on the situation. The use of neuropsychological (NP) testing is often used early in the evaluation of the concussed athlete as a more sensitive measure of cognitive function. These tests are especially useful when compared with preinjury tests obtained as a baseline measure.

RETURN TO PLAY

After the acute treatment of MTBI is complete and symptoms have resolved, the challenge of making RTP decisions remains. Several factors should be considered, including previous head or neck injury, extent of neurological involvement and the clinical course of previous injuries, the temporal relation of previous injuries, and the extent and severity of the present injury. In addition, the age of the athlete, the sport and position the athlete participates in, and emotional readiness of the athlete should also be considered.

Before 2000, several classification systems were published that provided guidelines for determining the severity of concussion and when to allow RTP (44,64–68). Although well intentioned, many of these classification systems were based on personal experience and poorly controlled research. In addition, depending on the classification system used, different "grades" existed. For example, an injury without LOC but with RGA and PTA (69) could be considered a Torg grade IV, Nelson III, Cantu II, or Colorado Medical Society III. Although these guidelines were useful in certain settings, new research has changed the evaluation and treatment of the athlete with MTBI.

Recent data using NP testing has raised significant questions regarding the accuracy and reliability of previous classification systems in determining the severity of injury and therefore RTP. For example, almost all of the earlier classification systems associate LOC with the most severe classification of MTBI. Recent research using NP testing has demonstrated that LOC is not necessarily associated with more severe injury (70). NP testing is an established method of measuring cognitive function, and has been used in the assessment of, and recovery from, head injury (71,72). NP testing has been used specifically in the athletic setting with documented success (33,44,69,71, 73–75) and is becoming an increasingly important part of the preparticipation evaluation of athletes engaged in sports with a risk for head injury. NP testing provides a reliable assessment and quantification of brain function by examining brain-behavior relationships. NP tests can measure a broad range of cognitive functions, including speed of information processing, attention, concentration, reaction time, visual scanning and visual tracking ability, memory recall, and problem solving abilities (33,71,72, 76–78). Acute and chronic injuries can be assessed, and NP testing is more sensitive in assessing cognitive function than classic medical testing (69,73–75,79).

In one study, individuals who sustained minor or moderate closed head injury were evaluated by MRI, CT scanning, and NP testing. MRI demonstrated intracranial lesions more often than CT, although both imaging studies detected the lesions requiring surgical treatment. Memory and cognitive function by NP testing correlated to the location and size of deficits seen on MRI scans, as well as their improvement at 1 and 3 months follow-up (29,33).

The Penn State Concussion Program was initiated in 1995 as a research protocol to prospectively assess athletes at risk for head injury using a battery of NP tests. Sports that were assessed included football, men's and women's soccer, men's and women's basketball, and ice hockey. If an athlete sustained a MTBI, he/she was retested, along with a yoked control, within 2 hours, 48 hours, 1 week, and 1 month. The results of this program indicate that, at the college level, NP testing is a useful tool in assessing MTBI and can be useful in making RTP decisions (74). This study also demonstrated that the severity of head injury correlates with a higher frequency of abnormalities in a number of tests, that the length of time an abnormality persists increases as the severity of injury increases, that there are significant individual differences between athletes, and that symptoms do not always correlate with NP findings. Most tests return to baseline within 5 days after injury.

Recently, computerized versions of various NP test batteries have been utilized in the athletic realm, and show promise for making it easier to test large numbers of athletes with minimal inconvenience (80). Paper and pencil tests have limitations in that they were designed to assess severe brain injury, and were not designed for serial assessment. Paper and pencil tests often lack alternate forms, and require a "tester," which introduces another variable in test outcome. In addition, many of these tests have a "practice effect," whereby the results improve with repeated testing, especially if the test–retest time interval is short (81–88). A detailed review of testing is performed elsewhere (89).

Computerized batteries of NP tests have been developed to assess MTBI in sports (Automated Neuropsychological Assessment Metrics [ANAM], CogSport, Concussion Resolution Index, and Immediate Postconcussion Assessment and Cognitive Testing [ImPACT]) (75,90,91). Unlike paper and pencil tests, these computerized batteries were designed for sport-related concussion, and also for serial assessments. In addition, they require less time, are associated with lower costs, and can often be administered to a large number of athletes simultaneously. In addition, reaction time is measured by the computer, in milliseconds, allowing for the measurement of thousands of levels of performance. The test–retest reliability measures and sensitivity of these computerized batteries are also favorable (90,92–94). Computerized batteries have the disadvantage of relying heavily on reaction time tests, which is only one facet of cognitive function. These batteries may not assess subtle deficits in cognitive function that occur with concussion (95). In addition, many of these batteries are brief, with only a small number of tests and therefore a less extensive evaluation of overall cognitive function assessed. Finally, because these tests are often administered to a large group of athletes, the possibility of confounding variables, such as distraction, exists.

Attention and concentration (74,82,96,97) reaction time, measures of psychomotor function and information processing and decision making, working memory and learning memory (98–100) have all been found to be sensitive to sport-related head injury. There is minimal data regarding the specificity and sensitivity of NP testing. One study reported a sensitivity of 80% and a specificity of 77% for a battery when individual postinjury tests were compared with preinjury baseline tests. If preinjury baselines were unavailable, the sensitivity dropped to 75% (83). Another study of a computerized battery has reported a sensitivity of 81.9% and a specificity of 89.4% (101).

Several factors that may effect NP testing but have not been adequately evaluated include age, psychiatric or medical problems, test anxiety, previous MTBI, attention deficit disorder or other learning disorders, disability, cultural or educational background, sleep deprivation, medications, and drugs.

Another area that remains unclear is the correlation of NP testing with symptoms. Symptoms are the subjective report provided by athletes, and therefore may be inaccurate and/or may not provide prognostic information (55,102). Athletes often minimize their symptoms in an attempt to be allowed back into activity (103). In addition, many symptoms, such as headache and dizziness, are common in the general population, and not specific to concussion (104). Several researchers report deficits in cognitive function as assessed by NP testing, which persist after symptoms have resolved (74,98,99,105,106).

SIDELINE TOOLS

Sideline tools have been developed in an attempt to standardize the evaluation that occurs acutely. The Standardized Assessment of Concussion (SAC) was initially developed as a sideline tool (107), and although attractive, because it is short and easy to administer, it has limitations clinically. In one study, the SAC was used to evaluate high school and college athletes who sustained concussion (108). The SAC was administered as a baseline, and then again at the time of injury (time 0), and again administered 1, 3, and 10 days after injury. Although the SAC was able to differentiate between the concussed and nonconcussed athletes at time 0, it did not do so at any point of time thereafter. One third of the individuals were able to improve their score to within normal limits, despite remaining symptomatic, raising the concern that the SAC may not be sensitive to the subtle effects of concussion. Although no practice effect is evident with repeated SAC testing (109), this may be due to a "ceiling" effect, in which there is so little room for improvement that no practice effect is evident. Most importantly, the SAC should not be used to make the diagnosis of concussion; clinical judgment is paramount. More recently, the Prague Guidelines have been published and developed another sideline tool called the *Sideline Concussion Assessment Tool* (102). This tool is more extensive than the SAC and remains promising as a standardized sideline tool, although further research validating this tool is needed.

SEVERITY

As discussed previously, older classification systems of concussion used LOC to denote the most severe injuries. Lovell demonstrated that this was not the case in emergency room patients seen for head injury (70). This finding was subsequently confirmed in the athletes participating at the high school and college levels (105). These researchers assessed on-field markers of concussion severity and postinjury NP scores and symptoms, including disorientation, PTA, RGA, and LOC. ImPACT scores and symptom composite scores performed at baseline and postinjury were their outcome measures. They found that athletes who had a "poor" presentation 2 days after injury were 10 times more likely to have RGA (<0.001), over four times more likely to have PTA, and at least 5 minutes of mental status change ($p < 0.013$) than those athletes considered "good" at presentation. LOC did not differentiate between "poor" or "good" outcomes.

One study of 101 concussions in athletes participating in various sports found that several signs and symptoms were significantly associated with delayed RTP. These included headache for more than 3 hours duration, any RGA, or any LOC. These authors concluded that athletes with these symptoms or signs should be followed-up and treated more cautiously (110). Though this study would at first glance support the idea that LOC may be associated with more severe injury, the study design was such that clinicians did not follow any particular protocol, and therefore may have kept the athletes with LOC out longer because of their own reluctance, thereby affecting the outcome.

Other studies have demonstrated that severity appears to be associated with memory dysfunction that persists for more than 1 day (99). More recently, guidelines have suggested that determining the severity can only occur after all the symptoms have cleared, and both the neurological and cognitive examination of the athlete has returned normal results (62,102,111). Although this approach is somewhat frustrating for the athlete, parent, or coach, who would want to know right away when the injured athlete can be expected to return to full play, it likely represents the best approach currently.

THE RETURN TO PLAY PROGRESSION

The decision to allow an athlete to RTP must be made only after determining that the athlete is asymptomatic and he/she has both a normal neurological examination and normal cognitive examination. The latter can be difficult to discern without NP testing, and if not available, the physician should err on the side of caution. The RTP progression is an incremental increase in demands, specific to the sport and athlete, and one which gradually reintroduces the athlete to activity. The progression often starts with a cardiovascular challenge, then sport-specific skills, where no risk of contact or collision occurs, then eventually back into full practice activities, and finally game activities. Although there is agreement that the head injured athlete should progress incrementally from no activity, to light cardiovascular activity, to noncontact sport-specific activity, to practice activities, and finally to full activity, there is no agreement as to how quickly this progression can occur. Some physicians will permit this progression quite quickly and allow RTP the same day of injury, whereas others recommend that a minimum of 24 hours should pass between stages, and that no athlete should return to full activity the same day of any injury (102). Each situation must be treated individually, taking into account all of the factors discussed. Further research regarding the importance of repetitive injury in making the RTP decision is needed, and has been reviewed elsewhere (112).

In young athletes, the progression should occur at a much slower rate than in adults. There is significant controversy surrounding the concept of RTP during the same contest, with some advocating that once a concussion is identified, the athlete is "done for the day." Others, most notably at the professional and college level, will allow RTP during the same contest if the athlete quickly clears, does not have symptoms for more than 20 minutes, and does not experience significant memory dysfunction. RTP is an individualized decision that must be made by the clinician after taking into account several factors.

The RTP decision should be more conservative in the athlete who has had a previous history of concussion, especially if the injury was recent. In addition, clinical considerations, such as the nature, burden, and duration of symptoms, should be considered when making the RTP decision (62,113). If injury occurs because of a disproportionate force, then delaying the RTP decision should be considered. Other factors that should be considered include the sport played, the psychological readiness of the athlete (114), and the feelings and concerns of others, such as parents, guardians, and/or coaches.

NP tests, if available, help in making the RTP decision, especially if they can be compared to preinjury results. In the absence of NP tests, the clinician has the athlete's subjective report of symptoms, which may not be reliable, and it is more difficult to have confidence that the cognitive function of the athlete is where it should be. Considering this, without NP data, a more conservative approach to RTP should be considered. It is important to understand the limitations of NP testing; it is "one tool in the toolbox" for physicians to use in their assessment of an injured athlete, and does not take the place of clinical judgment.

CUMULATIVE INJURY

In making the RTP decision, the athletes' previous history of concussion along with the temporal relation of the current injury to previous injuries should be considered. In addition, the nature of the previous injury and the burden and duration of symptoms are all important, especially if symptoms were persistent or memory dysfunction occurred. There is controversial data regarding the cumulative nature of concussion. Some studies have failed to show an effect of cumulative injury (84,97). In a study of collegiate and high school football players, however, the relative risk for MTBI was 5.8 times greater for those individuals who gave a history of concussion compared to those with no previous history of concussion (115). In another study of college athletes, a threefold greater risk of concussion was present in those athletes who gave a history of three or more concussions in the past 7 years (116). Athletes who had a previous history of two or more concussions took more time to become asymptomatic after a subsequent concussion. In this study, they also found that athletes who had a concussion were three times more likely to sustain another concussion than those who did not, and that 92% of these occurred within the first 10 days after their first injury.

Recent research has raised concern for cumulative concussive injury. Athletes with a history of three or more concussions were 8 times more likely to experience LOC, 5.5 times more likely to have anterograde amnesia, and 5.1 times more likely to have confusion than those without such a history (117). In another study, Iverson found that amateur athletes with a history of multiple concussions were more likely to have memory deficits measured 2 days after injury when compared to athletes without a history of concussion (118). These studies certainly raise concern for the athlete with repetitive injury, and therefore more caution should be taken when making the RTP decision regarding these athletes. In addition, the temporal relation between injuries is important, such that there should be more concern for the athlete with several injuries within the past few months when compared to his/her history of injuries 4 years previously.

AGE OF THE ATHLETE

The RTP decision must take into account the age of the athlete, because the effects of concussion are different for the young athlete and the older adult. There is little well-controlled prospective data to evaluate the reasons for the differences seen, and this is further confounded by the number of research studies that have grouped college and high school athletes together. However, the professional athlete is able to RTP more quickly and apparently without significant complications (119).

Although the deficits seen and the duration of symptoms that occur as a result of MTBI are similar in both children and young adults, it appears that the cognitive deficits seen in children aged 14 to 18 persist longer than in athletes aged 18 to 25 (120). Problems with behavior have been seen after concussion, despite normal NP test results (121). Very little is known about the effects of concussion on the ability of the developing brain to learn new information, interact socially, and on growth and maturation.

NEUROPSYCHOLOGICAL TESTING

The use of NP Testing has evolved over the past decade and is now utilized by many professional, college, and high school team physicians as part of their concussion management program. There are, however, many limitations and questions that remain unanswered about the use of NP testing. Several of the most recent guidelines and position statements have endorsed the use of NP testing (61,62,122), with the Vienna guidelines stating that NP testing is the "cornerstone" of the evaluation process. This same group, in its subsequent Prague Guidelines (102), backed down on their recommendations, instead stating that NP testing need not be used for "simple" concussion, but remains a tool for evaluating "complex" injuries. They also stated that if NP testing is used, having the baseline, preinjury test results to compare it with is preferable. These recommendations are difficult to follow because it is impossible to know which injuries will be simple and which will be complex, in advance. The Team Physician Consensus Conference (TPCC), the most recent of the guidelines published, states that the use of NP tests is desirable, but not essential for the team physician taking care of the head injured athlete (62). If NP testing is available, it can provide objective and sensitive measures of cognitive function, and perhaps allow for an earlier RTP.

An area that has not been researched adequately is the time course for formal NP testing as well as options for NP batteries. Certainly, aspects of the sideline evaluation, such as word recall, months backward, and other measures of memory, are considered NP tests. Because some deficits in cognitive function are not evident until 24 to 48 hours after injury, some have recommended that this should be the time that a formal postinjury assessment is made (74). Once an athlete becomes asymptomatic, a clinical progression would allow them to advance to a cardiovascular challenge. If their NP tests are markedly abnormal, one might extend the time frame for rest or noncontact activities. Some advocate waiting for the athlete to become completely asymptomatic before performing formal NP testing, in order to minimize the number of times the athlete is exposed to the battery and thereby minimizing the practice effect that occurs with repetitive testing (102,106).

The use of NP testing in children and young adults has also raised some controversy. It has been suggested that if NP testing is used before the age of 16, repeat testing should be performed every 6 months to account for the natural change in cognitive function that occurs with growth and development (123).

The combination of a computerized battery along with select paper and pencil tests is also an effective method of incorporating NP testing into the concussion management program. This allows several athletes to be baseline tested, and yet allows for a more comprehensive battery to be used if concussion occurs and also for using baseline data for those individuals who give a prior history of multiple and/or severe concussions. This program is currently being used with great success (Princeton Concussion Program, unpublished).

In 2004, the NATA published guidelines for the evaluation and treatment of concussion (61). This is a very useful document for athletic trainers and physicians who take care of concussed athletes. It provides a comprehensive review of many of the salient issues regarding concussion assessment, has recommendations regarding when an athlete should be evaluated by a physician, and home care instructions. Most recently, the team physician consensus statement was published in late 2005 (62). This document addresses several issues, including on-field, sideline, and office settings of evaluation, as well as other RTP controversies.

There is little data to guide RTP decisions in the case of athletes who sustain focal lesions. Cantu (44) has developed guidelines that are based on his clinical judgment and vast experience. If an athlete sustains an intracranial hemorrhage (epidural, subdural or intracerebral hematoma, or subarachnoid hemorrhage), a SIS, or diffuse axonal injury, then a focal injury has occurred. The athlete with a focal injury should not return to participate if they have (a) persistent postconcussive symptoms, (b) permanent central neurological sequelae (organic dementia, hemiplegia, homonymous hemianopsia), (c) hydrocephalus, (d) spontaneous subarachnoid hemorrhage from any cause, or (e) symptomatic neurological or pain-producing abnormalities about the foramen magnum (44). If surgery is performed, athletes should be seriously discouraged from continued participation in contact and collision sports. For other focal lesions with no underlying brain injury not requiring surgical treatment, many authors suggest remaining out of contact or collision sports for at least one full year after recovery from injury (44).

NEW TOOLS IN ASSESSING HEAD INJURY

Postural sway has been studied and found to be sensitive in assessing head injury. Guskewicz measured postural sway along with limited NP testing (Trail Making Test, Digit Span Test, Stroop Test, and Hopkins Verbal Learning Test) and found that at 1 day after mild head injury, postural sway was more sensitive in detecting deficits than NP tests (124). Further research is necessary to assess whether an athlete with normal cognitive function but minimal disturbances in postural sway is at risk for a second impact injury. In other words, sports medicine physicians often allow an athlete with a mild ankle sprain to RTP even when he/she is not back to 100% fitness, and whether there is an acceptable margin of deficit in the case of MTBI is unclear. The risks of sustaining a second impact are obviously more severe than a second ankle sprain, but these limitations have not yet been elucidated.

Near infrared spectroscopy (125,126), single photon emission computed tomography (SPECT) (127,128) magnetic resonance angiography (129), and diffusion weighted MRI (130) are other new studies that show promise in the assessment of MTBI. There appears to be a correlation with these noninvasive studies and the neurochemical and neurometabolic changes that occur when the head is injured, and are more sensitive than traditional MRI and CT scans. These latter studies remain important in assessing focal lesions and skull fractures, but as new technologies advance, so too may our understanding of the natural history of MTBI and how to manage it.

COMPLICATIONS AND SEQUELAE OF HEAD INJURY

The complications and sequelae of head injury include cervical spine injuries, intracranial bleeds, skull fractures, post-traumatic seizures, SIS, and postconcussive syndrome. Though MTBI by definition is mild, it is important to keep these complications in mind when assessing the athlete, making RTP decisions, and counseling coaches, athletes, and their family. It is also important that the athlete, family, coach, and administrators understand that after an athlete has sustained a concussion, he/she is four to six times more likely to sustain another injury when compared to an individual who has not sustained a concussion (10,131). Seizures occur in approximately 5% of traumatic brain injuries and, if they are to occur, often occur within the first week (132). When skull fracture occurs, seizures can occur, and are often related to the undersurface brain injuries that often occur with fractures. Children younger than 16 years are less likely to experience seizures than adults. Risk factors for the development of persistent seizures after head injury include (a) seizures within 1 week of trauma, (b) PTA for greater than 12 hours, (c) intracranial bleed, or (d) neurological deficit after injury. Even if an EEG is normal, post-traumatic epilepsy can occur (133).

POSTCONCUSSION SYNDROME

Postconcussion syndrome (PCS) can occur after head injury, with symptoms that include persistent headache, inability to concentrate, irritability, fatigue, vertigo, disturbance in gait, sleep, and vision, and emotional lability. There is significant variability in the onset of symptoms as well as their persistence. Whether the presence or duration of LOC or PTA correlates with the development of PCS is unknown (134). It is difficult to differentiate PCS from either persistent symptoms, unrelated symptoms, or trauma-induced migraine. Headaches are ubiquitous, and determining their etiology is often difficult.

The criteria for PCS are presented in Table 14.4, although many of these do not use the strict definition of PCS given in the 1994 Diagnostic Statistical Manual (DSM-IV) of the American Psychiatry Association (135). Criteria include PTA for more than 12 hours, head injury with LOC, and seizure activity within the first 6 months following head injury. Two of the three must be present to meet the strict criterion. Despite these criteria, many physicians use the term PCS for any athlete who has persistent symptomatology after head injury, even if the strict criteria are not met (see Table 14.1).

Psychotherapy, behavior modifications, medications, biofeedback, and physical therapy have all been used as part of a multidisciplinary approach to the treatment of PCS. There may be biochemical changes that occur in PCS which are also present in acute MTBI and post-traumatic headache. All these may have the common findings of changes in electrolytes, excitatory amino acids, serotonin, catecholamines, and endogenous opiodes, neuropeptides, and impaired glucose utilization (136). Both tricyclic antidepressants and beta-blockers have been used in PCS and post-traumatic headaches, and additional management options are reviewed in detail elsewhere (137–139).

SECOND IMPACT SYNDROME

SIS is a potential complication of MTBI and is of significant concern in the athlete. Saunders (1) initially described SIS as the occurrence of a second head injury before an individual has fully recovered from a first insult. The "second impact" can cause brain swelling, persistent deficits, and death. The symptoms of the initial insult may be mild or severe, as may be that of the second impact (2). Once the second impact occurs, the individual deteriorates quickly within seconds to minutes, with deterioration of mental status, dilated and fixed pupils, and

TABLE 14.4

PROPOSED CRITERIA FOR POSTCONCUSSIVE SYNDROME

A. History of head injury that includes at least two of the following:
 1. Loss of consciousness for 5 min or more
 2. Post-traumatic amnesia of 12 hr or more
 3. Onset of seizures (post-traumatic epilepsy) within 6 mo of head injury

B. Current symptoms (either new symptoms or substantially worsening pre-existing symptoms) to include the following:
 1. At least the following two cognitive difficulties
  a. Learning or memory (recall)
  b. Concentration
 2. At least three of the following affective or vegetative symptoms:
  a. Easy fatiguability
  b. Insomnia or sleep/wake cycle disturbances
  c. Headache (substantially worse than before injury)
  d. Vertigo/dizziness
  e. Irritability and/or aggression on little/no provocation
  f. Anxiety, depression, or lability of affect
  g. Personality change (e.g., social or sexual inappropriateness, child-like behavior)
  h. Aspontaneity/apathy

C. Symptoms associated with a significant difficulty in maintaining premorbid occupational or academic performance or with a decline in social, occupational, or academic performance

Source: From Brown SJ, Fann JR, Grant I. Postconcussional disorder: time to acknowledge a common source of neurobehavioral morbidity. *J Neuropsychiatry Clin Neurosci* 1994;6:15–22, with permission.

subsequent respiratory failure and death. Although some have suggested that SIS does not exist (140), it remains a concern, and underscores the need for full recovery from the initial injury before return to participation.

Changes in cerebral blood flow with recurrent trauma is felt to be the etiology of SIS. With a first impact, the sensitivity of the cerebral vasculature is increased. With the second impact, dysfunction in the autoregulation in cerebral blood flow results in increased vascular congestion and resultant increased intracranial pressure. This can lead to herniation of the brain, brainstem compromise, coma, and respiratory failure (2).

CHRONIC TRAUMATIC ENCEPHALOPATHY

Chronic traumatic encephalopathy (CTE) is another complication of recurrent head injury (141). CTE is the premature loss of normal central nervous system function, and was first described in athletics as "the punch drunk syndrome" in boxers in 1928 (142). Other terms such as *dementia pugilistica* (143) have been used. Alzheimer's disease is similar clinically to pathologically confirmed dementia pugilistica (144). Apolipoprotein E4 (ApoE4) is well established as a risk factor for the development of Alzheimer's disease (145). Jordan (146) found that ApoE4 was associated with an increased severity of chronic traumatic brain injury in high exposure boxers (more than 12 professional bouts), which suggests that genetics may place an individual at increased risk for developing CTE. More research is needed. Changes include abnormalities in the cerebellar, pyramidal, and extra-pyramidal systems, as well as cognitive and personality deficits. CTE can occur without LOC, and remains difficult to predict (67). In professional boxers, CTE occurs in 9% to 25% of the participants and correlates with the length of their career and the number of fights they had (5). The chronic effects of boxing on neurological function have been reviewed (147), and imaging studies have also documented the pathological changes (148–150). One study demonstrated that in 338 professional boxers 7% had abnormal CT scans and another 22% had borderline scans (150).

The boxing community has made significant improvements in the sport to minimize these risks. Many states mandate a suspension in participation after head injury to prevent the athletes from returning prematurely. One of the states issues a 45-day suspension after a mild concussion, a 60-day suspension for moderate concussions, and a 90-day suspension and normal CT and EEG for severe concussions (151). These changes, as well as an increased awareness by the medical staff in watching for and detecting these injuries, should reduce the complications and sequelae seen in the sport of boxing.

In soccer, there has been recent concern that the repetitive sport-specific skill of heading, where the head is purposely used to strike the ball, may also be associated with

CTE. There have been cross-sectional, retrospective studies in European soccer players demonstrating cervical spine changes (152), cerebral atrophy (105), EEG changes (153), and cognitive dysfunction (154,155). However, many of these studies have significant flaws in methodology, and are poorly controlled for other problems such as alcohol use and previous motor vehicle accidents. In addition, an assumption has been made in these studies that heading is the culprit. The effect of concussion has not been separated. In fact, in Matser's study (155), he demonstrated that a history of previous concussion was inversely related to performance on NP testing. In cross-sectional studies in which soccer players have been compared to boxers or track athletes, no differences were seen on MRI, CT, EEG, and NP testing (147). In a well-controlled study, Jordan assessed U.S. National Team soccer players and compared them with track and field athletes using MRI scans, and found no difference between the two groups of athletes (156).

In prospective data using NP testing, no differences have been seen in both a pilot study addressing the effect of heading on college soccer players' cognitive function during a single practice, as well as over the course of a single season (157,158). Research addressing this over the course of a 4 to 5 year college career is underway. Recent research with elite Norwegian soccer players has demonstrated no effect of heading exposures and previous concussion history with neuropsychological differences (159). A workshop in 2002 reviewing the data regarding the effect of heading on cognitive function sponsored by the Institute of Medicine concluded that there is no significant data suggesting that heading leads to cognitive dysfunction (160).

Concussions occur commonly in soccer, with high incidence rates at both the college and high school levels (15,161). Most of these injuries are mild, and the mechanism of injury is most often contact with another player, the ground, or the goal posts, with none due to purposeful heading (162). It may be that repetitive or severe concussions may explain the dysfunction noted in the older European studies. In addition, many of these players were evaluated when they were in their fifties, suggesting that the length of a career may play a role in the development of these deficits. The forces in soccer during heading are linear (163), compared to boxing, where the forces are more rotational, the latter is associated with more risk for injury. More prospective research is needed to determine the separate effects of heading and concussion on cognitive function over a longer period in soccer players.

CONCLUSIONS

MTBI occurs in the realm of sports, and may be associated with significant sequelae and complication, especially if recognition and/or treatment is delayed. A spectrum of injury occurs in sports, with the mildest representing an injury with minimal, if any, long-term effects, to the most severe injury, which precludes return to collision or contact sports. Early recognition of injury is important, and assessment for associated cervical spine, cerebrovascular, and intracranial injuries is essential. Thorough evaluation including mental status examination and neurological examination are important. NP testing can help assess cognitive function. Determining the initial management of the athlete and subsequent RTP decisions remain a challenge to the sports physician, with several factors to consider.

RTP decision after repetitive MTBI is often difficult, and must be individualized. Athletes who are symptomatic should not be allowed to RTP (61,62,102,122,164,165). Severity of injury should be determined once the athlete is asymptomatic, and should be based on the nature, burden, and duration of symptoms. Whenever possible, NP testing should be included in the baseline preseason evaluation of athletes with a history of prior concussion as well as for sports with an inherent risk of concussion. Subsequent NP testing can be performed within 48 hours of injury, and then again once the athlete is asymptomatic both at rest and exertion. Once the athlete has a normal neurological and cognitive examination, a progressive advancement from sport-specific skills to noncontact drills to full contact play can be initiated. This progression must be tailored to the age of the athlete, with extreme caution in the young athlete. It is imperative to account for prior history of concussion as well as the severity of concussion when individualizing the RTP decision.

Several newer guidelines exist, which together provide good information for the team physician taking care of the head injured athlete (61,62,122,164–166). More research is needed to help determine the extent of recovery necessary to allow the athletes to protect themselves and avoid subsequent injury. In addition, more long-term prospective studies are necessary to delineate the natural history of MTBI, and define the utility of assessment tools such as NP, EEG, and neuroimaging studies.

REFERENCES

1. Saunders RL, Harbaugh RE. The second impact in catastrophic contact-sports head trauma. *JAMA* 1984;252:538–539.
2. Cantu RC. Second-impact syndrome. *Clin Sports Med* 1998;17(1):37–44.
3. Wojtys EM, Hovda D, Landry G, et al. Concussion in sports. *Am J Sports Med* 1999;27:676–688.
4. McLatchie G, Jennett B. ABC of sports medicine. Head injury in sport. *Brit Med J* 1994;308:1620–1624.
5. Mortimer JA. Epidemiology of post-traumatic encephalopathy in boxers. *Minn Med* 1985;68:299–300.
6. Spear J. Are footballers at risk for developing dementia? *Int J Geriatr Psychiatry* 1995;10:1011–1014.
7. Mayeux R, Ottman R, Ming-Xin T, et al. Genetic susceptibility and head injury as risk factors for Alzheimer's disease among community-dwelling elderly persons and their first degree relatives. *Ann Neurol* 1993;33:494–501.
8. Kraus JF. Epidemiology of head injury. In: Cooper PR, ed. *Head injury*, 2nd ed. Baltimore: Williams & Wilkins, 1987:1–19.
9. Garrick JG, Requa RK. Medical care and injury surveillance in the high school setting. *Phys Sportsmed* 1981;9:115.
10. Zemper E. Analysis of cerebral concussion frequency with the most commonly used models of football helmets. *J Athl Train* 1994;29(1):44–50.
11. Bruce DA, Schut L, Sutton LN. Brain and cervical spine injuries in children and adolescents. *Prim Care* 1984;11(1):175–194.
12. Browne GJ, Lam LT. Concussive head injury in children and adolescents related to sports and other leisure physical activities. *Br J Sports Med* 2006;40:163–1688.

13. Yeates K, Luria J, Bartkowski H, et al. Post concussive symptoms in children with mild closed head injuries. *J Head Trauma Rehabil* 1999;14:337–350.
14. McCrea M, Hammeke T, Olsen G, et al. Unreported concussion in high school football players: implications for prevention. *Clin J Sport Med* 2004; 14(1):13–17.
15. National Collegiate Athletics Association (NCAA). *Injury surveillance system, 2000–2002*. Overland Park, Kansas and Indianapolis IN.
16. Bishop PJ. Impact performance of ice hockey helmets. *Safety Res* 1978;10: 123–129.
17. Hodgson VR. National operating committee on standards for athletic equipment. Football helmet certification program. *Med Sci Sports* 1975;7: 225–232.
18. Cantu RC, Mueller F. Catastrophic spine injury in football 1977–1989. *J Spinal Disord* 1990;3:227.
19. Pforringer W, Smasal V. Aspects of traumatology in ice hockey. *J Sports Sci* 1987;5:327–336.
20. Greensher J. Non-automotive vehicle injuries in adolescents. *Pediatr Ann* 1988;17:114–121.
21. Thompson RS, Rivara FP, Thompson DC. A case-control study of the effectiveness of bicycle safety helmets. *N Engl J Med* 1989;320:1361–1367.
22. Borczuk P. Predictors of intracranial injury in patients with mild head injury. *Ann Emerg Med* 1995;25:731–736.
23. Warren WL, Bailes JE. On the field evaluation of athletic head injuries. *Clin Sports Med* 1998;17(1):13–26.
24. Davis RL, Mullen N, Makela M, et al. Cranial computed tomography scans in children after minimal head injury with loss of consciousness. *Ann Emerg Med* 1994;24:640–645.
25. Hoffman JR. CT for head trauma in children. *Ann Emerg Med* 1995; 24:713–715.
26. Jordan B, Zimmerman R. Computed tomography and magnetic resonance imaging comparisons in boxers. *JAMA* 1990;263:1670–1674.
27. Lampert PW, Hardman JM. Morphological changes in brains of boxers. *JAMA* 1984;251(20):2676–2679.
28. Tysvaer AT, Storli OV, Bachen NI. Soccer injuries to the brain: a neurologic and electroencephalographic study of former players. *Acta Neurol Scand* 1989;80:151–156.
29. Levin HS, Williams D, Crofford MJ, et al. Relationship of depth of brain lesions to consciousness and outcome after closed head injury. *J Neurosurgery* 1988;69(6):861–866.
30. Mittl RL, Grossman RI, Heihle JF, et al. Prevalence of MR evidence of diffuse axonal injury in patients with mild head injury and normal CT findings. *Am J Neuroradiol* 1994;15:1583–1589.
31. Gentry LR, Godersky JC, Thompson B, et al. Prospective comparative study of intermediate field MR and CT in the evaluation of closed head trauma. *Am J Neuroradiol* 1988;150:673.
32. Jenkins A, Teasdale G, Hadley DM, et al. Brain lesions detected by magnetic resonance imaging in mild and severe head injuries. *Lancet* 1986;iii:445.
33. Levin HS, Amparo E, Eisenberg JM, et al. Magnetic resonance imaging and computerized tomography in relation to the neurobehavioral sequelae of mild and moderate head injuries. *J Neurosurg* 1987;66:706–713.
34. Report of the Ad Hoc Committee to Study Head Injury Nomenclature. Proceedings of the congress of neurological surgeons in 1964. *Clin Neurosurg* 1966;12:386–394.
35. Ryan AJ. Protecting the sportsman's brain. *Br J Sports Med* 1991;25(2): 81–86.
36. Macciocchi SN, Barth JT, Littlefield LM. Outcome after mild head injury. *Clin Sports Med* 1998;17(1):27–36.
37. Elson LM, Ward CC. Mechanisms and pathophysiology of mild head injury. *Semin Neurol* 1994;14:8–18.
38. Adams H, Mitchell DE, Graham DI, et al. Diffuse brain damage of immediate impact type. Its relationship to "primary" brain stem damage. *Brain* 1977;100(3):489–502.
39. Peerless SJ, Rencastle NB. Shear injuries of the brain. *Can Med Assoc J* 1967;96:577–582.
40. Chason JL, Hardy WG, Webster JE, et al. Alterations in cell structure of the brain associated with experimental concussion. *J Neurosurg* 1958;15: 135–139.
41. Graham DI. Neuropathology of head injury. In: Narayan RK, WIlberger JE Jr, Povlishock JT, eds. *Neurotrauma*. New York: McGraw-Hill, 1996: 46–47.
42. Ommaya AK, Gennarelli TA. Cerebral concussion and traumatic unconsciousness. Correlation of experimental and clinical observations in blunt head injuries. *Brain* 1974;97:633–654.
43. Ommaya AK. Head injury mechanisms and the concept of preventative management: a review and critical synthesis. *J Neurotrauma* 1996;12:527–546.
44. Cantu RC. Return to play guidelines after a head injury. *Clin Sports Med* 1998;17(1):45–60.
45. Yoshino A, Hovda DA, Kawamata T, et al. Dynamic changes in local cerebral glucose utilization following cerebral concussion in rats: evidence of a hyper- and subsequent hypometabolic state. *Brain Res* 1991;561: 106–119.
46. Yoshino A, Hovda DA, Katayama Y, et al. Hippocampal CA3 lesion prevents the post-concussive metabolic derangement in CA1. *J Cereb Blood Flow Metab* 1991;11(Suppl 2):S343.
47. Katayama Y, Becker DP, Tamura T, et al. Massive increases in extracellular potassium and the indiscriminate release of glutamate following concussive brain injury. *J Neurosurg* 1990;73:889–900.
48. Katayama Y, Cheung MK, Alves A, et al. Ion fluxes and cell swelling in experimental traumatic brain injury: the role of excitatory amino acids. In: Hoff JT, Betz AL, eds. *Intracranial pressure VII*. Berlin: Springer-Verlag, 1989: 584–588.
49. Kawamata T, Katayama Y, Hovda DA, et al. Administration of excitatory amino acid antagonists via microdialysis attenuates the increase in glucose utilization seen following concussive brain injury. *J Cereb Blood Flow Metab* 1992;12(1):12–24.
50. Yamakami I, McIntosh TK. Alterations in regional cerebral blood flow following brain injury in the rat. *J Cereb Blood Flow Metab* 1991;11:655–660.
51. Jenkins LW, Moszynski K, Lyeth BG, et al. Increased vulnerability of the mildly traumatized rat brain to cerebral ischemia: the use of controlled secondary ischemia as a research tool to identify common or different mechanisms contributing to mechanical and ischemic brain injury. *Brain Res* 1989;477:211–224.
52. Hovda DA, Lee SM, Smith ML, et al. The neurochemical and metabolic cascade following brain injury: moving from animal models to man. *J Neurotrauma* 1995;12(5):143–146.
53. Nevin NC. Neuropathological changes in the white matter following head injury. *J Neuropathol Exp Neurol* 1967;26:787–784.
54. Bergsneider M, Hovda DA, Shalmon E, et al. Cerebral hyperglycolysis following severe traumatic brain injury in humans: a positron emission tomography study. *J Neurosurg* 1997;86:241–251.
55. McCrory P, Johnston KM, Mohtadi NG, et al. Evidence-based review of sport-related concussion: basic science. *Clin J Sport Med* 2001;11(3): 160–165.
56. Johnston KM, McCrory P, Mohtadi NG, et al. Evidence-based review of sport-related concussion: clinical Science. *Clin J Sport Med* 2001;11(3): 150–159.
57. Maron DW. Head injuries. In: Fu FH, Stone DA, eds. *Sports injuries; mechanisms, prevention, treatment*. Baltimore: Williams & Wilkins, 1994:813–831.
58. Kleiner DM, Almquist JL, Bailes J, et al. *Prehospital care of the spine-injured athlete: a document from the Inter-Association Task Force for appropriate care of the spine-injured athlete*. Dallas, Texas: National Athletic Trainers' Association, 2001.
59. Kleiner DM, Cantu RC. *Football helmet removal*. Indianapolis, IN: American College of Sports Medicine, Current Comment, 1996.
60. Edna TH. Acute traumatic intracranial hematoma and skull fracture. *Acta Chir Scand* 1983;149:449–451.
61. Guskiewicz KM, Bruce SL, Cantu R, et al. National Athletic Trainers' Association position statement: management of sport-related concussion. *J Athl Train* 2004;39(3):280–297.
62. Herring S, Bergfeld J, Indelicato P, et al. Concussion (Mild traumatic brain injury) and the team physician: a consensus statement. *Med Sci Sports Exerc* 2005;37(11):2012–2016.
63. American Academy of Pediatrics. The management of minor closed head injury in children. *Pediatrics* 1999;104:1407–1415.
64. Colorado Medical Society, Sports Medicine Committee. *Guidelines for the management of concussion in sports*. (revised May 1991). Denver: Colorado Medical Society, Sports Medicine Committee, 1990.
65. Kelly JP, Rosenburg JH. Diagnosis and management of concussion in sport. *Neurology* 1997;48:575–580.
66. Nelson WE, Jane JA, Gieck JH. Minor head injury in sports: a new classification and management. *Phys Sportsmed* 1984;12(3):103–107.
67. Quality Standards Subcommittee, American Academy of Neurology. Practice parameter; the management of concussion in sports (summary statement). *Neurology* 1997;48:581–585.
68. Torg JS. *Athletic injuries to the head, neck, and face*. St. Louis: Mosby-Year Book, 1991.
69. Putukian M, Echemendia RJ. Managing successive minor head injuries; which tests guide return to play? *Phys Sportsmed* 1996;24(11):25–38.
70. Lovell MR, Iverson GL, Collins MW, et al. Does loss of consciousness predict neuropsychological decrements after concussion? *Clin J Sport Med* 1999;9:193–198.
71. Abreau F, Templer DI, Schuyler BA, et al. Neuropsychological assessment of soccer players. *Neuropsychology* 1990;4:175–181.
72. Rimel RW, Giordani B, Barth JT, et al. Moderate head injury: completing the clinical spectrum of brain trauma. *Neurosurgery* 1982;11(3):344–351.
73. Alves WM, Rimel RW, Nelson WE. University of Virginia prospective study of football-induced minor head injury: status report. *Clin Sports Med* 1987;6(1):211–218.
74. Echemendia RJ, Putukian M, Mackin RS, et al. Neuropsychological test performance prior to and following sports-related mild traumatic brain injury. *Clin J Sports Med* 2001;11:23–31.
75. Lovell MR, Collins MW. Neuropsychological assessment of the college football player. *J Head Trauma Rehabil* 1998;13:9–26.
76. McLatchie G, Brooks N, Galbraith S, et al. Clinical neurological examination, neuropsychology, electroencephalography and computed tomographic head scanning in active amateur boxers. *J Neurol Neurosurg Psychiatry* 1987;50:96–99.
77. Porter MD, Fricker PA. Controlled prospective neuropsychological assessment of active experienced amateur boxers. *Clin J Sports Med* 1996;6:90–96.

78. Rimel RW, Giordani B, Barth JT, et al. Disability caused by minor head injury. *Neurosurgery* 1981;9(3):221–228.
79. Collins MW, Grindel SH, Lovell MR, et al. Relationship between concussion and neuropsychological performance in college football players. *JAMA* 1999;282:964–970.
80. Maroon JC, Lovell MR, norwig J, et al. Cerebral concussion in athletes: evaluation and neuropsychological testing. *Neurosurgery* 2000;47(3):659–669. discussion 669–672.
81. Hinton-Bayre AD, Geffen G, McFarland K. Mild head injury and speed of information processing: a prospective study of professional rugby league players. *J Clin Exp Neuropsychol* 1997;19:275–289.
82. Guskiewicz KM, Ross SE, Marshall SW. Postural stability and neuropsychological deficits after concussion in collegiate athletes. *J Athl Train* 2001; 36:263–273.
83. Hinton-Bayre AD, Geffen GM, Geffen LB, et al. Concussion in contact sports: reliable change indices of impairment and recovery. *J Cin Exp Neuropsychol* 1999;21:70–86.
84. Guskiewicz KM, Marshall SW, Broglio SP, et al. No evidence of impaired neurocognitive performance in collegiate soccer players. *Am J Sports Med* 2002;30:157–162.
85. Macciocchi SN. Practice makes perfect: the retest effects in college athletes. *J Clin Psychol* 1990;46:628–631.
86. Oliaro SM, Guskiewicz KM, Prentice WE. Establishment of normative data on cognitive tests for comparison with athletes sustaining mild head injury. *J Athl Train* 1998;33:36–40.
87. Heaton RK, Timken N, Daiken S, et al. Detecting change: a comparison of three neuropsychological methods, using normal and clinical samples. *Arch Clin Neuropsychol* 2001;16:75–91.
88. Putukian M, Echemendia RJ, Mackin RS. The acute neuropsychological effects of heading in soccer: a pilot study. *Clin J Sports Med* 2000;10: 104–109.
89. McCaffrey RJ, Duff K, Westervelt JH. *Practitioner's guide to evaluating change with neuropsychological assessment instruments*. New York: Kluwer Academic, 2000.
90. Erlanger D, Saleba E, Barth J, et al. Monitoring resolution of concussions symptoms in athletes. Preliminary results of a web based neuropsychological test protocol. *J Athl Train* 2001;36:280–287.
91. Collie A, Darby D, Maruff P. Computerized cognitive assessment of athletes with sports related head injury. *Br J Sports Med* 2001;35: 297–302.
92. Stuss DT, Pogue J, Buckle L, et al. Characterization of stability of performance in patients with traumatic brain injury: variability and consistency on reaction time tests. *Neuropsychology* 1994;8:316–324.
93. Bleiberg J, Garmoe WS, Halpern EL, et al. Consistency of within-day and across-day performance after mild brain injury. *Neuropsychiatry Neuropsychol Behav Neurol* 1997;10:247–253.
94. Iverson G, Lovell M. Validity of impact for measuring the effects of sports related concussion. *Presented at the National Academy of Neuropsychology Annual Conference*. Miami, FL: February 25–March 3, 2002.
95. McKeever CK, Schatz P. Current issues in the identification, assessment, and management of concussions in sports-related injuries. *Appl Neuropsychol* 2003;10:4–11.
96. Macciocchi SN, Barth JT, Alves W, et al. Neuropsychological functioning and recovery after mild head injury in collegiate athletes. *Neurosurgery* 1996; 39:510–514.
97. Macciocchi SN, Barth J, Littlefield L, et al. Multiple concussions and neuropsychological functioning in collegiate football players. *J Athl Train* 2001;36:303–306.
98. Collins MW, Field F, Lovell MR, et al. Relationship between postconcussion headache and neuropsychological test performance in high school athletes. *Am J Sports Med* 2003;31:168–173.
99. Lovell MR, Collins M, Iverson G, et al. Recovery from concussion in high school athletes. *J Neurosurg* 2003;98:293–301.
100. Collie A, Maruff P. Computerised neuropsychological testing. *Br J Sports Med* 2003;37:2–3.
101. Schatz P, Pardini JE, Lovell MR, et al. Sensitivity and specificity of the ImPACT Test Battery for concussion in athletes. *Arch Clin Neuropsychol* 2006;21(1):91–9.
102. McCrory P, Johnston K, Meeuwisse W, et al. Summary and agreement statement of the 2nd International Conference on Concussion in Sport, Prague 2004. *Br J Sports Med* 2005;39:196–204.
103. Echemendia R, Julian L. Mild traumatic brain injury in sports: neuropsychology's contribution to a developing field. *Neuropsychol Rev* 2001;11:69–99.
104. Mittenberg W, Strauman S. Diagnosis of mild head injury and the postconcussion syndrome. *J Head Trauma Rehabil* 2000;15:783–791.
105. Collins MW, Iverson GL, Lovell MR, et al. On-field predictors of neuropsychological and symptom deficit following sports-related concussion. *Clin J Sport Med* 2003;13:222–229.
106. McCrory P, Makdissi M, Davis G, et al. Value of neuropsychological testing after head injuries in football. *Br J Sports Med* 2005;39:58–63.
107. McCrea M. Standardized mental status assessment of sports concussion. *Clin J Sport Med* 2001;11:176–181.
108. Hecht S, Puffer JC, Clinton C, et al. Concussion assessment in football and soccer players. *Clin J Sports Med* 2004;14:310.
109. McLeod TCV, Perrin DH, Guskiewicz K, et al. Serial administration of clinical concussion assessments and learning effects in healthy young athletes. *Clin J Sport Med* 2004;14:287–295.
110. Asplund C, McKeag DB, Olsen C. Sport-related concussion: factors associated with prolonged return to play. *Clin J Sport Med* 2004;14(6): 339–343.
111. Cantu RC. Concussion severity should not be determined until all postconcussion symptoms have abated. *Lancet* 2004;3:437–484.
112. Putukian M. Repeat mild traumatic brain injury: how to adjust return to play guidelines. *Curr Sports Med Rep* 2006;5:15–22.
113. Cantu RC. Recurrent athletic head injury: risks and when to retire. *Clin Sports Med* 2003;22:593–603.
114. Herring S, Boyajian LA, Coppel DC, et al. Psychological issues related to injury in the athlete and the team physician: a consensus statement. *Med Sci Sports Exerc* 2006;38(11):2030–2034.
115. Zemper ED. Two year prospective study of relative risk of a second cerebral concussion. *Am J Phys Med Rehabil* 2003;82:653–659.
116. Guskiewicz KM, McCrea M, Marshall SW, et al. Cumulative effects of recurrent concussion in collegiate football players: the NCAA concussion study. *JAMA* 2003;290:2549–2555.
117. Collins MW, Lovell M, Iverson G, et al. Cumulative effects of concussion in high school athletes. *Neurosurgery* 2002;51:1175–1179.
118. Iverson GL, Gaetz M, Lovell MR, et al. Cumulative effects of concussion in amateur athletes. *Brain Inj* 2004;18:433–443.
119. Pellman EJ, Powell JW, Viano DC, et al. Concussion in professional football: epidemiological features of game injuries and review of the literature—part 3. *Neurosurgery* 2004;54:81–96.
120. Field M. Does age play a role in recovery from sports-related concussion? A comparison of high school and collegiate athletes. *J Pediatr* 2003;142: 546–553.
121. Ponsford J, Wilmott C, Rothwell A, et al. Cognitive and behavioral outcome following mild traumatic head injury in children. *J Head Trauma Rehabil* 1999;14:360–372.
122. Johnston K, Aubry M, Cantu R, et al. Summary and agreement statement of the first International Conference on Concussion in Sport, Vienna 2001. *Phys Sportsmed* 2002;30(2):57–63.
123. McCrory P, Collie A, Anderson V, et al. Can we manage sport related concussion in children the same as in adults? *Br J Sports Med* 2004;38: 516–519.
124. Guskiewicz KM, Riemann BL, Perrin DH, et al. Alternative approaches to the assessment of mild head injury in athletes. *Med Sci Sports Exerc* 1997; 27(7):213–221.
125. Kirkpatrick PJ. Use of near-infrared spectroscopy in the adult. *Philos Trans R Soc Lond B Biol Sci* 1997;352(1354):701–705.
126. Robertson CS, Gopinath SP, Chance B. A new application for near-infrared spectroscopy: detection of delayed intracranial hematomas after head injury. *J Neurotrauma* 1995;12(4):591–600.
127. Lewis DH. Functional brain imaging with cerebral perfusion SPECT in cerebrovascular disease, epilepsy, and trauma. *Neurosurg Clin N Am* 1997; 8(3):337–344.
128. Masdeu JC, Abdel-Dayem H, Van Heertum RL. Head trauma: use of SPECT. *J Neuroimaging* 1995;5(Suppl 1):S53–S57.
129. James CA. Magnetic resonance angiography in trauma. *Clin Neurosci* 1997; 4(3):137–145.
130. Ono J, Harada K, Takahashi J, et al. Differentiation between dysmyelination and demyelination using magnetic resonance diffusional anisotropy. *Brain Res* 1995;671(1):141–148.
131. Gerberich SG, Priest JD, Boen JR, et al. Concussion incidence and severity in secondary school varsity football players. *Am J Public Health* 1983; 73:1370–1375.
132. Cantu RC. Epilepsy and athletics. *Clin Sports Med* 1998;17(1):61–69.
133. Henderson JM, Browning DG. Head trauma in young athletes. *Med Clin North Am* 1994;78(2):289–303.
134. Bornstein RA, Miller HB, van Schoor JT. Neuropsychological deficit and emotional disturbance in head-injured patients. *J Neurosurg* 1989;70: 509–513.
135. Brown SJ, Fann JR, Grant I. Postconcussional disorder: time to acknowledge a common source of neurobehavioral morbidity. *J Neuropsychiatry Clin Neurosci* 1994;6:15–22.
136. Packard RC, Ham LP. Pathogenesis of post traumatic headache and migraine: a common headache pathway? *Headache* 1997;37(3):142–152.
137. Rizzo M, Tranel D. Overview of head injury and postconcussive syndrome. In: Rizzo M, Tranel D, eds. *Head injury and postconcussive syndrome*. New York: Churchill Livingstone, 1996:1–18.
138. Troncoso JC, Gordon B. Neuropathology of closed head injury. In: Rizzo M, Tranel E, eds. *Head injury and postconcussive syndrome*. New York: Churchill Livingstone, 1996:47–56.
139. Barcellos S, Rizzo M. Post traumatic headaches. In: Rizzo M, Tranel D, eds. *Head injury and postconcussive syndrome*. New York: Churchill Livingstone, 1996:1–18.
140. McCrory PR. Second impact syndrome. *Neurology* 1998;50:677–683.
141. Critchley M. Medical aspects of boxing, particularly from a neurological standpoint. *Br Med J* 1957;1:357–362.
142. Martland HS. Punch drunk. *JAMA* 1928;91:1103–1107.
143. Millspaugh JA. Dementia pugilistica. *U.S. Naval Med Bull* 1937;35:297.

144. Tsuang D, Kukull W, Shepard L, et al. Impact of sample selection on APOEe4 frequency: a comparison of two Alzheimer's disease samples. *J Am Geriatr Soc* 1996;44:704–707.
145. Jordan BD, Kanick AB, Horwich MS, et al. Apolipoprotein e4 and fatal cerebral amyloid angiopathy associated with dementia pugilistica. *Ann Neurol* 1995;38:698–699.
146. Jordan BD, Relkin NR, Ravdin LD, et al. Apolipoprotein Ee4 associated with chronic traumatic brain injury in boxing. *JAMA* 1997;278:136–140.
147. Haglund Y, Eriksson E. Does amateur boxing lead to chronic brain damage? A review of some recent investigations. *Am J Sports Med* 1993;21: 97–109.
148. Bogdanoff B, Natter H. Incidence of cavum septum pellucidum in athletes: a sign of boxer's encephalopathy. *Neurology* 1989;39:991–992.
149. Jordan BD. Head injury in sports. In: Jordan BD, Tsairis P, Warren R, eds. *Sports neurology*. Maryland: Aspen Publishers, 1990.
150. Jordan B, Jahre C, Hauser A, et al. CT of 338 active professional boxers. *Radiology* 1992;185:509–512.
151. Wilberger JE, Maroon JC Jr. Head injuries in athletes. *Clin Sports Med* 1989;8:1.
152. Sortland O, Tysvaer AT, Storli OV. Changes in the cervical spine in association football players. *Br J Sports Med* 1982;16:80–84.
153. Sortland O, Tysvaer AT. Brain damage in former association football players. *Neuroradiology* 1989;31:44–48.
154. Matser JT, Kessels AG, Jordan BD, et al. Chronic traumatic brain injury in professional soccer players. *Neurology* 1998 51(3):791–796.
155. Matser JT, Kessels AG, Lezak MD, et al. Neuropsychological impairment in amateur soccer players. *JAMA* 1999;282:971–973.
156. Jordan SH, Green GA, Galanty HL, et al. Acute and chronic brain injury in United States National Team Soccer Players. *Am J Sports Med* 1996; 24(2):205–210.
157. Putukian M, Echemendia RJ, Mackin RS. The acute neuropsychological effects of heading in soccer: a pilot study. *Clin J Sports Med* 2000;10:104–109.
158. Putukian M, Echemendia RJ, Evans TA, et al. Effects of heading contacts in collegiate soccer players on cognitive function; prospective neuropsychological assessment over a season. In review. *Presented at American Medical Society for Sports Medicine Annual Meeting*, San Antonio, Texas, April 9, 2001.
159. Straume-Naesheim TM, Anderson TE, Dvorak J, et al. Effects of heading exposure and previous concussion on neuropsychological performance among Norwegian elite footballers. *Br J Sports Med* 2005;39:70–77.
160. Institute of Medicine (IOM) Report. *Is soccer bad for children's heads? Summary of the IOM workshop on neuropsychological consequences of head impact in youth soccer*. Washington, DC: National Academy Press, 2002: 1–26. www.nap.edu.
161. Powell JW, Parber-Foss KD. Traumatic brain injury in high school athletes. *JAMA* 1999;282:958–963.
162. Boden BP, Kirkendall DT, Garrett WE. Concussion incidence in elite college soccer players. *Am J Sports Med* 1998;26(2):238–241.
163. Burslem I, Lees A. Quantification of impact accelerations of the head during the heading of a football. In: Reilly T, Lees A, Davids K, et al. eds. *Science and football: proceedings of the First World Congress of Science and Football*. London; E&FN Spon Ltd., 1987:243–248.
164. Cantu RC. Posttraumatic retrograde and anterograde amnesia: pathophysiology and implications in grading and safe return to play. *J Athl Train* 2001; 36:244–248.
165. Kissick J, Johnston KM. Return to play after concussion: principles and practice. *Clin J Sport Med* 2005;15(6):426–431.
166. Echemendia RJ, Cantu RC. Return to play following sports-related mild traumatic brain injury: the role for neuropsychology. *Appl Neuropsychol* 2003;10:48–55.

Peripheral Neuropathy 15

Philip D. Zaneteas

Injuries to the peripheral nervous system remain an important area of pathology for the sports medicine physician. It may be difficult to diagnose these lesions and even more difficult to fully delineate their severity and type. Electromyography (EMG) remains the singular procedure for diagnosing neurological injuries. The following discussion, involving brachial plexus injury as well as trauma to its peripheral nerve branches, will proceed with this notion in mind.

BRACHIAL PLEXUS INJURIES

The brachial plexus is vulnerable to injury from a number of etiologies. The clinical manifestations additionally can be protean. Delineating the correct diagnosis, the degree of severity and the optimal treatment are dependant upon detailed knowledge of the neuroanatomy of the region as well as a comprehensive electrodiagnostic examination (EMG). Care must be taken to distinguish between a brachial plexus lesion (which may affect more than one portion of the plexus), a cervical radiculopathy, or a peripheral nerve injury. Often, this is difficult in that the clinical presentation may be similar or identical. The task, although difficult, is crucial as the treatment and ultimate prognosis remain dependant on this distinction.

Brachial Plexus—Anatomy (C5-8, T1)

The brachial plexus is initially formed by the ventral or anterior primary rami of C5-T1. The anterior rami of the C5-6 roots join to form the upper trunk. The anterior ramus from C7 becomes the middle trunk. The anterior rami from C8 and T1 join to form the lower trunk. Anatomical variants may occur with contributions from C2-4 and T2 (i.e., prefixed and postfixed plexuses correspondingly). At the clavicle, the trunks bifurcate into their anterior and posterior divisions. The anterior divisions of the upper and middle trunk coalesce to form the lateral cord. The medial cord is formed by the anterior component of the lower trunk. The posterior divisions of all three trunks form the posterior cord. The cords themselves extend from the midpoint of the clavicle to the inferomedial portion of the coracoid process of the scapula. At this point, the cords give rise to their respective peripheral nerve branches (see Figure 15.1).

From the standpoint of clinical conceptualization of brachial plexus injuries, one approach is to separate injuries as occurring either proximal or distal to the clavicle. Supraclavicular and infraclavicular injuries often have different biomechanical mechanisms of injury with different prognoses. Within this paradigm, the electromyographer-sports medicine physician can expect characteristic electrodiagnostic findings, specific and typical of the site of injury.

Mechanisms of Injury

Mechanisms of injury to the brachial plexus include blunt and penetrating trauma, traction injuries, compression, and inflammatory/autoimmune (e.g., Parsonage-Turner syndrome/brachial plexitis) conditions. Nerve injury classification systems continue to be delineated in the electrodiagnostic literature. For our purposes, three general categories of nerve injury can be cited. Neuropraxic injuries are consistent with demyelination of the axon sheath. The axon itself remains intact. Conduction block may occur at the site of injury. Nerve repair occurs with remyelination. Axonotmesis is characterized by trauma to the axon itself along with the myelin sheath. Wallerian degeneration occurs in variable degrees depending on the severity of the injury. An intact epineurium implies the capacity for nerve regeneration. Electrodiagnostic findings on needle examination are notable for the presence of spontaneous axonal loss findings in the form of fibrillation potentials and positive sharp waves. Moreover, motor unit dropout may occur with decreased motor unit recruitment characterized by large amplitude, increased duration motor units. Neurotmesis occurs with more serious nerve injuries

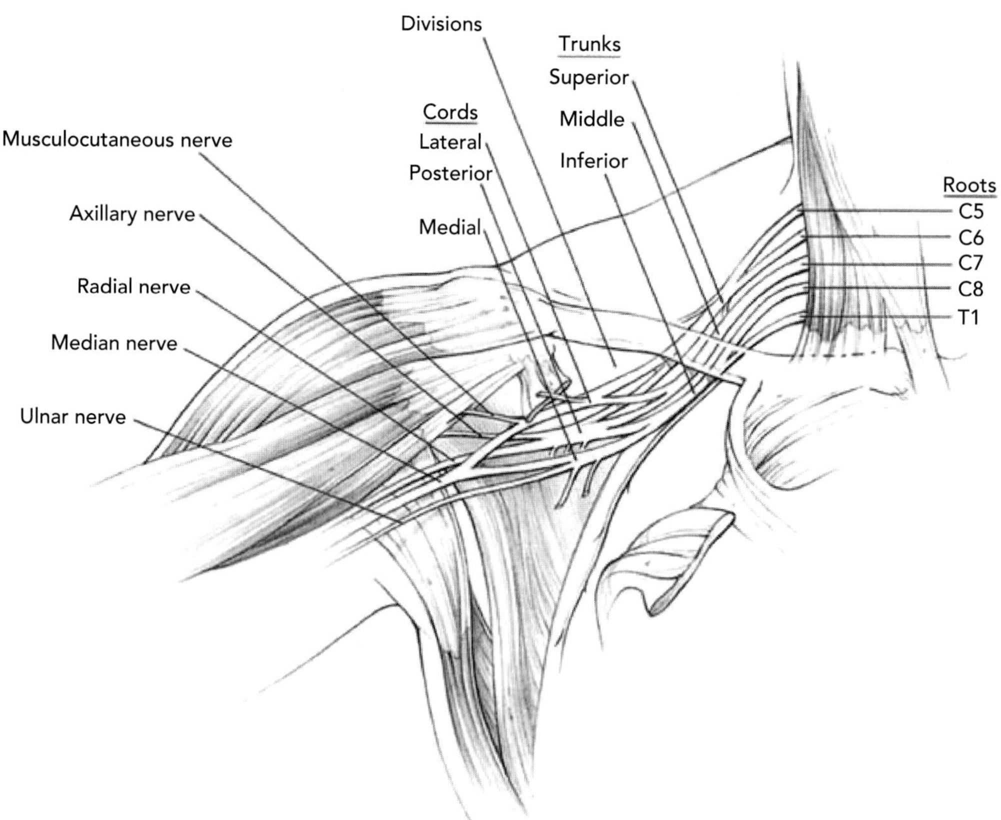

Figure 15.1 The brachial plexus and its branches in a dissection of the axilla and neck.

where the endoneurium is disrupted. The nerve and its fibrous sheath are transected, rendering axonal regeneration unlikely. Denervation patterns on electrodiagnostic examination predominate.

Physical Examination

Observation of the patient's anatomy at rest should focus on the shoulder girdle musculature as well as the distal upper extremities to discern the presence or absence of atrophy, skeletal deformity, scapular winging, and posture (see Table 15.1). Palpation of the patient should include regions of discomfort to assess for fracture, masses, swelling, and possible signs of inflammation. Range of motion, both actively and passively in all of the upper extremity joints including the cervical spine, may reveal evidence of contractures (both fixed and variable), spasticity, and instability. The motor-sensory examination may also help differentiate between root, trunk, cord, and peripheral nerve lesions. Finally, the examination of reflexes and upper motor neuron testing should be included.

Specific Brachial Plexus Injuries

The "Burner/Stinger" Syndrome

The burner/stinger syndrome represents a trauma-induced symptom complex involving the shoulder girdle region. It is generally characterized by a sharp, burning pain radiating from the supraclavicular region extending distally down the arm. It is associated with generalized paresthesias and/or anesthesia (nondermatomal) that tend to resolve within minutes. Shoulder girdle motor weakness may subsequently develop either immediately or within a few days. Associated signs and symptoms include muscle spasm and neck pain. In severe brachial plexus injuries of this type, the athlete (commonly a linebacker or defensive back in football) will come off the field holding his involved upper extremity in an internally rotated, adducted position.

The physical examination of the patient should include a detailed neuromuscular examination not only of the shoulder girdle region (i.e., all three heads of the deltoid, supraspinatus, infraspinatus, rhomboids, teres major/minor) but also of the cervical spine, the serratus anterior (scapular "winging" must be ruled out), and the more distal musculature of the upper extremity (e.g., those muscles innervated by the radial, median and ulnar nerves). It is important to note that motor testing immediately after the injury may be normal or minimally compromised. For this reason, given the potential of evolving neurological pathology, the athlete should be followed up closely over the following 2 to 3 weeks to determine if there are any residual motor or sensory deficits. Within this context, the delineation of the baseline motor-sensory status is

TABLE 15.1
UPPER EXTREMITY MOTOR INNERVATION: ROOT, TRUNK, AND CORD LOCALIZATION

Upper Trunk (C5-6)	Middle Trunk (C7)	Lower Trunk (C8-TI)
Supraspinatus	Triceps	Extensor carpi ulnaris
Infraspinatus	Pronator teres	Flexor carpi ulnaris
Deltoid	Flexor carpi radialis	Flexor digitorum profundus (digits four, five)
Biceps extensor digitorum communis		Flexor pollicis longus
Pectoralis major		Abductor pollicis brevis
Extensor carpi radialis		First dorsal interosseous
Pronator teres		Abductor digiti quinti
Flexor carpi radialis		
Brachioradialis		
Triceps		
Lateral Cord	**Posterior Cord**	**Medial Cord**
Biceps	Deltoid	Flexor carpi ulnaris
Pronator teres	Triceps	Flexor digitorum profundus (digits four, five)
Flexor carpi radialis	Brachioradialis	Abductor digiti quinti
	Extensor carpi radialis	First dorsal interosseous
	Extensor carpi ulnaris	Abductor pollicis brevis

fundamental as a reference point to the later neuromuscular examinations.

Localization of the site of injury may be related to the mechanism of injury. Supraclavicular injuries tend to be secondary to traction mechanisms with involvement at both root and trunk levels. The upper and middle trunks tend to be more commonly involved. Infraclavicular injuries tend to be secondary to shoulder abduction/extension biomechanics, which involve cords and terminal nerves generally, and the posterior cord and axillary nerve more specifically. In both types of injury, the suprascapular nerve is commonly involved. In such instances, the athletes develop weakness in shoulder abduction initiation (supraspinatus involvement) as well as shoulder external rotation (infraspinatus involvement). Distal peripheral nerves may also be involved at their origins including the musculocutaneous, radial, median, and ulnar nerves. With musculocutaneous nerve involvement, weakness of the biceps occurs with elbow flexion with the forearm fully supinated. Weakness of the brachialis may be tested with the forearm fully pronated. Both the biceps and the brachialis are innervated by the musculocutaneous nerve and testing of elbow flexion should be performed not only with the forearm fully supinated and pronated as described earlier but also in "neutral" in order to test the brachioradialis, which is innervated by the radial nerve. The physical examination, therefore, is an important precursor to the electrodiagnostic examination in performing a preliminary delineation of areas of weakness and involvement in the injured upper extremity.

From the standpoint of further evaluation of brachial plexus "stinger/burner" injuries, the sports medicine physician should always be cognizant of the differential diagnoses in such a clinical milieu.

Simultaneous injuries to adjacent or contiguous neuromuscular structures should be entertained when clinically indicated. The more common differential diagnostic concerns in the "burner/stinger" syndrome include cervical spine injury as well as potential shoulder, clavicular, and scapular bony trauma. For this reason, radiographic studies of all of these regions may be clinically indicated. From a neurological standpoint, it is important to remember in cases where there is any question of cervical spine instability or spinal cord trauma, continued radiographic workup is clearly indicated. Initially, a standard cervical radiographic series including anteroposterior (AP, including open mouth view), lateral, and oblique views may be obtained. If the findings are normal and the athlete is neurologically intact, flexion–extension lateral views may be obtained if there is a question of instability.

In the presence of symptoms and physical examination findings suggesting a cervical radiculopathy, magnetic resonance imaging (MRI) of the cervical spine may be considered. Bony lesions such as fractures are better demonstrated by cervical computed tomography (CT). Although uncommon, one must also be alert to any symptoms or findings that may suggest bony trauma to the shoulder girdle region (including the clavicle, glenohumeral joint, and scapula). Radiographic evaluation is generally sufficient to rule out any bony abnormalities. Finally, in severe shoulder girdle injuries of which the "singer/burner" presentation may be just one component, the possibility of a rotator cuff tear (full or partial thickness) may be ruled out by means of an MRI study.

In considering the neurophysiological status of the patient, an electrodiagnostic examination may be necessary to further delineate the extent and severity of the athlete's neurological injury. The electrodiagnostic and sports medicine literature historically has debated the relative distinctions concerning potential trauma at the cervical root, trunk, cord, and peripheral nerve levels. At this time, the only means to evaluate the neurophysiology of the brachial plexus and its cervical root origins is EMG. Acute, traumatic brachial plexus injuries (burners/stingers) may have several potential biomechanical causes involving different levels of the neuroaxis in the neck and upper extremity. To delineate this pathology physiologically, the patient must be studied with an EMG examination. The term "burner/stinger" has probably caused more confusion and uncertainty in both diagnosis and treatment in that it remains nonspecific. Clinically, what exists rather is a varied spectrum of potential pathology that has been classified as the "stinger syndrome." An alternative approach would be to incorporate the use of a paradigm utilizing the following differential diagnoses: spinal cord contusion, cervical radiculopathy, trunk/cord (brachial plexus) injury, peripheral nerve injury, or any combination of the above. Any of the above lesions may exist either singly or in some combination. The clinical imperative does not exist that would require that they exist in a mutually exclusive presentation.

An important point for the clinician to remember is to distinguish between a spinal cord injury and root injury as well as between an intraspinal and extraspinal injury. Chronic root scarring (especially at C5, C6) along with compression by musculature (e.g., scalene muscle compression) can result in repetitive numbness/weakness. Distinguishing between preganglionic and postganglionic lesions at the root level is also important in that the prognosis can be significantly different. What exists then is an "extraspinal nerve injury syndrome" that may occur anywhere from the cervical roots (either pre or postganglionic) to the trunk or possibly at the cord level of the brachial plexus. In attempting to simplify the "stinger phenomenon," the diagnostic waters have been muddied by attributing the "stinger" to a single etiology.

Return to Play

There remains the issue of return to activity. First, a clear diagnosis must be made electrodiagnostically distinguishing the presumed from the actual site of the lesion(s). Second, EMG findings may remain abnormal for years with findings consistent with residual, chronic axonal loss and demyelinative pathology. This should not remain the determining criterion for return to play or activity as some have argued. Rather, the electrodiagnostic findings should be utilized in the overall evaluation of the patient once a comprehensive rehabilitation program has been utilized. Recommendations in the sports medicine literature urge the development of relative symmetry in both strength and flexibility parameters with symptom-free status before returning to play or activity. Finally, variables that would seem to predispose the athlete to injuries of this type should be targeted and addressed, such as improper biomechanics specific to the sport, relative muscle and flexibility imbalances, and return to play before sufficient healing occurs. Athletes who complain of repeated episodes of "burning" or paresthesias appear to be at particular risk and probably should be withheld temporarily from active participation in contact sports. In this capacity, the sports medicine physician performs a preventative role in avoiding further nerve injury while rehabilitation continues.

SUPRASCAPULAR NERVE INJURY

The suprascapular nerve originates from the upper trunk with C5-6 (C4) root innervation. It is relatively susceptible to injury during its course (see Figure 15.2). It crosses the posterior triangle of the neck to the superior border of the scapula where it passes through the suprascapular notch and supplies the supraspinatus. It then passes around the spinoglenoid notch and terminates in the infraspinatus. Sensory branches innervate the posterior capsule of the glenohumeral joint and the acromioclavicular joint.

Suprascapular neuropathies may have a variable presentation depending on the location of injury along the course of the nerve as well as the inciting type of pathology. Traumatic injuries secondary to fractures of the scapula or blunt trauma rarely result in significant nerve damage. In contrast, compression injuries either at the suprascapular notch or the spinoglenoid notch have been well documented in the literature. Compression may occur secondary to ligamentous structures, callus formation, ganglions, or ossified bone. Traction injuries either secondary to athletic biomechanics or traumatic mechanisms are also possible etiologies. Additionally, the suprascapular nerve is commonly involved in patients experiencing acute brachial plexitis (Parsonage-Turner syndrome), but this exists as a generalized neuropathic condition with an autoimmune etiology, which can simultaneously involve multiple peripheral nerve branches as well as the supplying roots of the brachial plexus.

The clinical presentation of suprascapular neuropathy includes poorly localized pain in the shoulder girdle region, weakness in shoulder abduction initiation, as well as external rotation with intact sensation. Physical examination can reveal atrophy in both the supraspinatus and infraspinatus. If deltoid function is found to be abnormal, a more generalized process is likely. Electrodiagnostic evaluation is necessary to delineate the level, degree, and type of suprascapular nerve injury. The EMG needle examination is utilized to determine whether spontaneous axonal loss pathology is present. Motor unit recruitment should be assessed to rule out the possibility of a "neurogenic" (decreased) motor unit recruitment pattern secondary to motor unit dropout. Side-to-side suprascapular

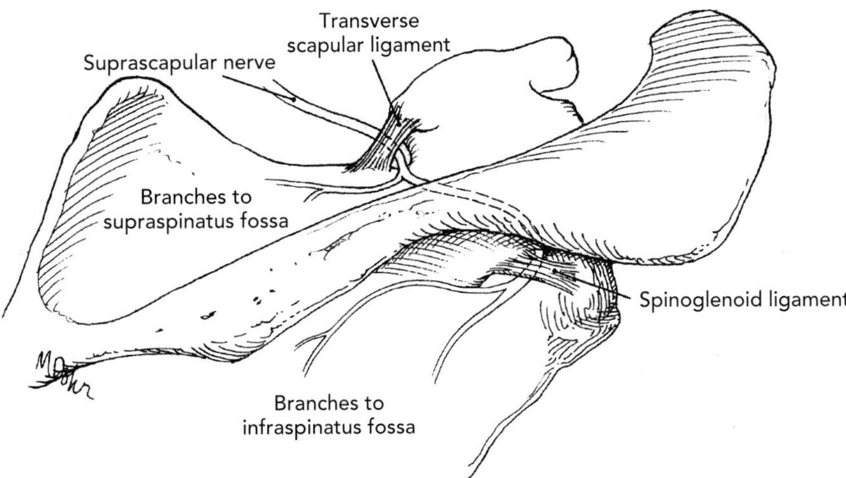

Figure 15.2 Suprascapular nerve injury.

motor nerve conduction studies with pickups on both the supraspinatus and infraspinatus can be of benefit in determining the presence of demyelination in the form of conduction block. When present, this would result in relatively lower motor amplitudes on the affected side. This in turn gives the clinician an approximate value of the percentage of elicitable motor units innervated by the involved suprascapular nerve. Within this electrodiagnostic and clinical context, it is important to remember that traction injuries involving the suprascapular nerve tend to occur at the nerve's origin (Erb's point), whereas kinking and compression of the nerve can occur both at the suprascapular notch as well as the spinoglenoid notch (an MRI of the spinoglenoid notch may reveal a surgically amenable ganglion cyst).

Treatment options include conservative management, analgesics (both oral NSAIDs as well as a short course of a steroid taper), a comprehensive shoulder girdle rehabilitation program that focuses on strengthening and biomechanics, as well as correction of any sport/activity-specific biomechanical errors in technique utilizing the upper extremity. Surgical exploration and decompression of any compressive lesions may be required in more severe injuries.

THORACIC OUTLET SYNDROME

"Thoracic outlet syndrome" (TOS) (see Figure 15.3) refers to a symptom complex that occurs secondary to compression of the subclavian blood vessels ("vascular" TOS) as well as the brachial plexus ("neurogenic" TOS), although involvement of the former is exponentially much greater than the latter. TOS has been characterized as a neurovascular phenomenon in the surgical literature although its neurogenic form is rarely confirmed electrodiagnostically. Symptom presentation can be quite variable depending upon the neurological structures traumatized. Involvement of the lower trunk (C8-T1) of the brachial plexus can mimic carpal tunnel syndrome (CTS) with regard to weakness in the abductor pollicis brevis (APB). The patient may complain of pain or paresthesias along the medial aspect of the arm and ulnar aspect of the forearm. Symptoms can extend into the fourth and fifth digits with a decrease in intrinsic muscle strength. Upper trunk (C5-6) involvement is less frequent (unlike "acute brachial plexitis"—Parsonage-Turner syndrome). In this instance, shoulder girdle complaints may occur circumferentially (the differential diagnosis should also include C5 and/or C6 radiculopathies). Vascular compression may include venous obstruction (characterized by upper extremity edema, cyanosis with potential collateralization to the shoulder and thorax) as well as arterial obstruction (typified by numbness diffusely, coolness to touch, decreased pulses, and exertional fatigue).

Etiologies of TOS include congenital and structural anomalies (e.g., cervical ribs, fibrous bands, anomalous fibrous bands in the scalene musculature), trauma, dysfunctional upper extremity, and shoulder biomechanics that may all cause narrowing of the costoclavicular outlet. Potential sites of compression include the interscalene triangle (where the brachial plexus and subclavian artery

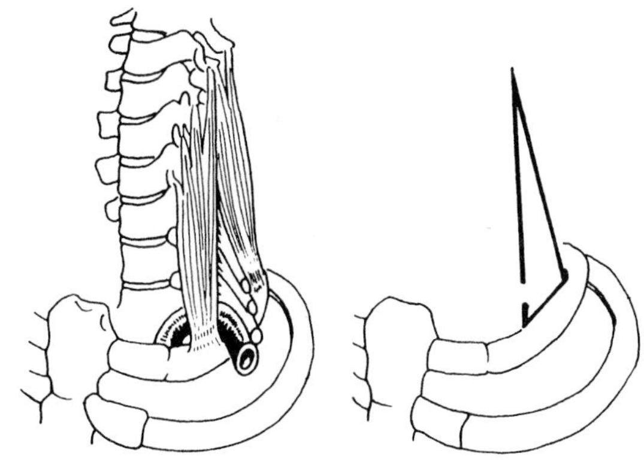

Figure 15.3 Thoracic outlet syndrome.

pass between the anterior and middle scalene muscles and over the first rib), the costoclavicular outlet, and proximal to the axilla (compression under the pectoralis minor insertion on the coracoid process, which may occur in hyperabduction activities, e.g., swimming, throwing, and the tennis serve).

From a diagnostic standpoint, classic tests on physical examination have been shown to be equivocal at best with a high rate of false positives (e.g., Adson's test, Wright's maneuver, overhead exercise test). Radiographs of the cervical spine and medial clavicle may rule out a cervical rib as a potential etiology. Electrodiagnostic evaluation remains the centerpiece to evaluation of the "neurogenic" form of TOS. The amplitude of the compound motor action potential (CMAP) of the median nerve is the parameter most commonly affected. The ulnar sensory nerve action potential (SNAP) is less than 10 uV in 50% of patients. Needle examination most often reveals findings localized to the lower trunk musculature (especially the APB and first dorsal interosseous). A detailed needle study is required to rule out other pathologies such as distal entrapment neuropathies and cervical radiculopathy. Most patients referred for evaluation of possible TOS that manifest abnormal findings on EMG turn out to have CTS. With regard to "vascular" TOS, a venogram and/or arteriogram are generally required to determine the presence of venous obstruction, aneurysms, or regions of arterial insufficiency.

Treatment of TOS is often problematic, but can include correction of posture malalignments, strengthening of the shoulder girdle and scapular musculature, as well as symptom-directed physical medicine techniques and modalities including trigger point injections, ultrasound, electrical stimulation, and a desensitization program. Surgical options are to be considered only as a last resort in patients with documented vascular or neurogenic pathology.

AXILLARY NERVE INJURY

The axillary nerve receives its innervation from the C5-6 roots through the posterior cord. It enters the "quadrilateral space" and gives off articular branches to the inferior medial aspect of the glenohumeral joint capsule and subsequently divides into anterior/posterior branches supplying the anterior/posterior components of the deltoid. A small branch supplies the teres minor and the overlying skin of the deltoid.

The greatest incidence of axillary nerve trauma occurs with blunt trauma, for example, shoulder dislocation. Contact sports including football and wrestling possess a high incidence of injury (see Figure 15.4). Secondary complications from trauma such as glenohumeral joint instability, humeral fractures, hematoma, chronic fibrous adhesions, and vascular compromise ("quadrilateral space syndrome"—compression of the posterior humeral circumflex artery and axillary nerve in the quadrilateral space) may all contribute to creating a potentially fertile environment for nerve damage, either acutely or chronically.

Clinically, patients present with muscle weakness/atrophy in the deltoid musculature. Care should be taken to examine all three components of the deltoid (anterior/middle/posterior heads) in that the nerve injury may not be uniform in all three branches. From a prognostic and rehabilitation standpoint, this is an important consideration in that the greater the specificity in terms of the physical examination and diagnosis, the greater likelihood of an optimal course of treatment and rehabilitation. EMG supplements the physical examination and can assist in following up the more severe injuries to monitor potential ongoing nerve reinnervation and clinical recovery. A needle examination of all three heads of the deltoid will allow for the determination of the distribution and extent of the axillary nerve injury. Evaluation of motor unit recruitment as well as investigation for the presence of axonal loss findings can provide objective information with regard to the type and degree of nerve trauma and its relevant prognosis for recovery. As with the electrodiagnostic workup of suprascapular nerve injuries (see previous text), side-to-side axillary motor nerve conduction studies can provide valuable information with regard to motor amplitude asymmetry and by inference the relative percentage of elicitable and therefore potentially viable motor units in the involved extremity.

LONG THORACIC NERVE INJURY

The long thoracic nerve receives innervation from the anterior rami of C5-7. It is a purely motor nerve that innervates the serratus anterior. Branches from the C5-7 roots join to form the long thoracic nerve before they unite to create the upper and middle trunks of the brachial plexus. Anatomically, the long thoracic nerve passes beneath the clavicle and runs along the anterolateral chest wall supplying the interdigitations of the serratus anterior. The functional anatomical role of the serratus anterior is to provide stabilization of the scapula against the chest wall to create a foundation for the scapular musculature to contribute and modify glenohumeral joint motion. Injuries to the long thoracic nerve (see Figure 15.5) can occur in a variety of athletic endeavors and is commonly seen with blunt and recurrent trauma, surgical and operative positioning injuries, as well as traction injuries and acute brachial plexitis.

The clinical presentation is typified by scapular "winging" and compromised glenohumeral biomechanics. Forward flexion and abduction of the shoulder is impaired and the patient often complains of a dull ache with dysesthesias about the shoulder. The physical examination may also reveal "variants" of scapula winging findings caused by injuries to the dorsal scapular nerve (supplying the rhomboids) and the spinal accessory nerve (supplying the trapezius). A C7 radiculopathy may also present in this

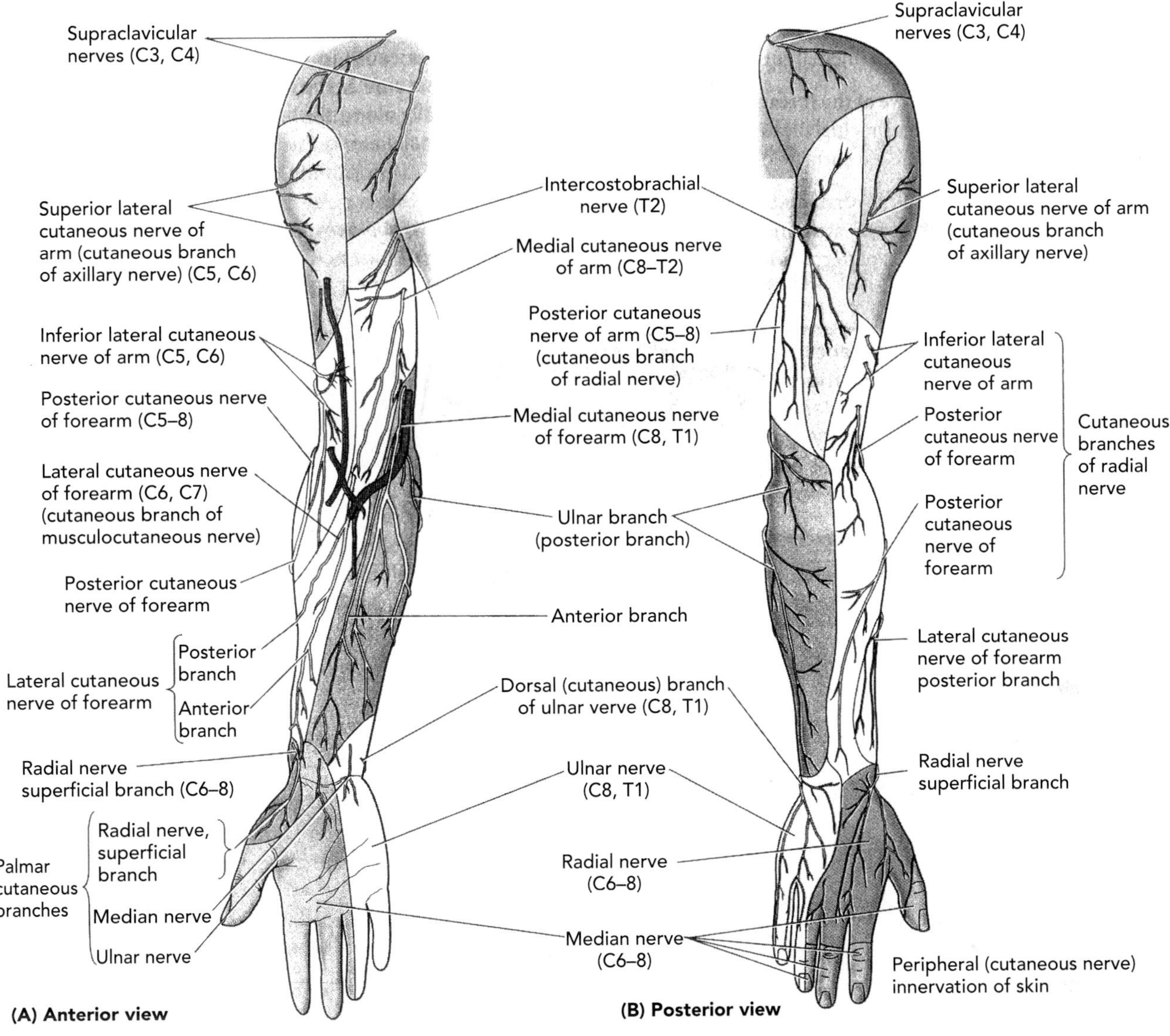

Figure 15.4 Axillary nerve.

manner. For this reason, an electrodiagnostic examination should consider all of these potential etiologies of scapula "winging." A "positive" EMG needle examination generally reveals spontaneous axonal loss findings at rest (e.g., fibrillation potentials, positive sharp waves) with polyphasic motor units in instances where regenerative "collateral sprouting" from the remaining viable motor units has occurred. Motor unit recruitment may be decreased in more severe cases. Side-to-side long thoracic motor nerve conduction studies may also be performed to determine any evidence of demyelinative conduction block leading to motor amplitude decrement in the affected extremity when compared with the uninvolved side.

Treatment options include conservative management with cessation of overhead activities. This avoids further traction of the nerve and facilitates healing. Shoulder girdle strengthening (focusing on the rhomboids, trapezius, and pectoralis musculature) and passive/active range of motion below 90 degrees of abduction/flexion is recommended, because this positioning restriction limits ongoing/exacerbating traction/torque mechanisms. In more severe cases, bracing of the scapula can be utilized to further prevent serratus anterior strain although this is generally poorly tolerated. In more severe cases, surgical options such as a scapulothoracic fusion or muscle transfer procedures may be considered.

SPINAL ACCESSORY NERVE INJURY

The spinal accessory nerve (cranial nerve XI) is a pure motor nerve. It communicates with the nerve roots C2-4 and innervates the sternocleidomastoid and trapezius muscles. (see Figure 15.6 here). Mechanisms of injury include stretch injuries, blunt trauma, surgical trauma (especially with lymph node dissection and exploration

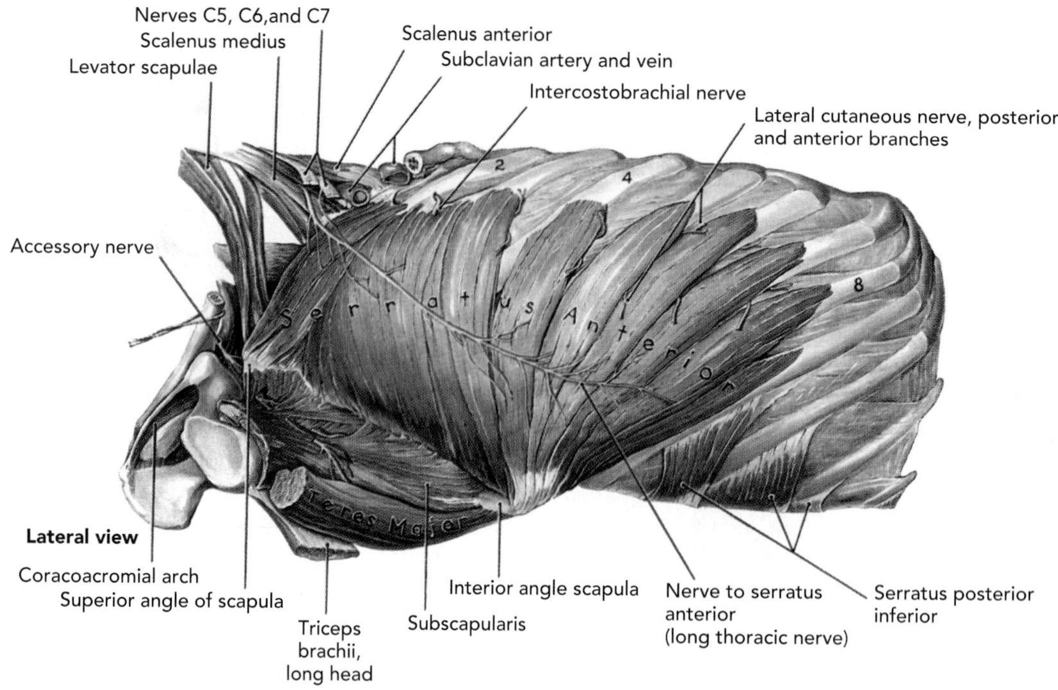

Figure 15.5 Long thoracic nerve injury.

of the posterior triangle), and irradiation. The clinical presentation may include nonspecific shoulder girdle and paracervical pain, weakness and limited shoulder abduction, "lateral" winging of the scapula, and decreased or absent shoulder shrug. Potential complications include adhesive capsulitis, increased traction on the brachial plexus along with an increased risk for subacromial impingement.

Electrodiagnostic findings on needle examination are notable for axonal loss findings in the sternocleidomastoid and the trapezius musculature. An incomplete lesion will manifest incomplete motor unit recruitment with "nascent" motor unit potentials. All three portions of the trapezius should be examined in that the middle and lower components tend to receive a greater proportion of their innervation from the cervical plexus.

Treatment is generally conservative from a pain management standpoint. A comprehensive shoulder girdle/scapular rehabilitation program should be initiated in a graduated manner. Shoulder stabilization may be required

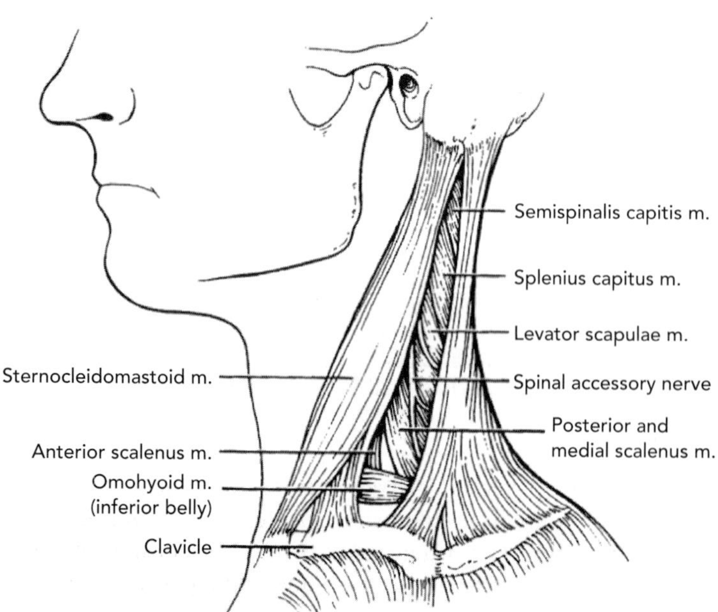

Figure 15.6 Spinal accessory nerve.

initially utilizing shoulder slings when the patient is upright. Proximal stabilization of the shoulder and its relationship to the scapula should be addressed to avoid traction on the brachial plexus itself as well as avoiding incipient shoulder subluxation. Electrical stimulation should be avoided acutely to prevent overloading of regenerating motor units. In patients without neurological recovery, orthopedic consultation should be obtained to assess suitability for scapula stabilization procedures.

MUSCULOCUTANEOUS NERVE INJURY

The musculocutaneous nerve derives its root innervation from C5-6 (with C7 contribution inconsistently). It arises from the lateral cord of the brachial plexus innervating the biceps, coracobrachialis, and brachialis muscles. Its terminal sensory branch, the lateral cutaneous nerve, bifurcates into anterior and posterior branches innervating the lateral forearm.

Musculocutaneous nerve injuries (Figure 15.1) are uncommon but can occur secondary to acute shoulder dislocations. Clinically, the patient presents with biceps and brachialis weakness with sensory deficits or dysesthesias in the lateral forearm. Electrodiagnostic examination should include both sensory (lateral cutaneous nerve) and motor (active pickups on the biceps) nerve conduction studies, as well as a needle examination of the C5, C6, and C7 innervated muscles, including the cervical paraspinal muscles.

Treatment of an isolated musculocutaneous nerve injury should be predicated on a number of factors including the etiology or mechanism of injury (blunt trauma, traction, or part of a more widespread entity, e.g., acute brachial plexitis, burner/singer syndrome), the physical examination findings, and the extent of neurological damage as defined by the electrodiagnostic study. This discussion also assumes that the patient has been ruled out for a biceps tendon rupture, a C5 and/or C6 radiculopathy, as well as a more proximal brachial plexus injury.

As a general rule, in the initial treatment stages, the athlete should avoid excessive traction or torque to the musculocutaneous innervated muscles as well as high resistance exercises. Active and active-assisted range of motion exercises are to be performed to maintain optimal flexibility and to avoid flexion contractures which would make the later stages of rehabilitation more problematic. Once the athlete is felt to be electrodiagnostically stable (this may require a follow-up EMG study in the more serious injuries), a strengthening program may commence characterized by low-resistance exercises. Simultaneous strengthening of the shoulder girdle muscles and the radial innervated brachioradialis (the only nonmusculocutaneous innervated elbow flexor) should also be addressed. It is the aim of the final stage of rehabilitation to attain bilateral symmetry with regard to the musculocutaneous innervated elbow flexors (i.e., biceps and brahialis) in terms of motor strength and range of motion.

Isolated injuries of the musculocutaneous nerve are rare. More commonly, a musculocutaneous neuropathy is part of a more generalized brachial plexopathy. The differential diagnosis includes C5 and/or C6 radiculopathies and a biceps tendon rupture. Neuropraxic injuries can also occur secondary to positioning, such as prolonged abduction and external rotation of the shoulder.

ULNAR NERVE INJURY

The ulnar nerve originates as the terminal branch of the medial cord of the brachial plexus with its innervation supplied by the anterior primary rami of C8 and T1. Its innervation includes the following muscles: flexor carpi ulnaris (two heads), flexor digitorum profundus (fourth and fifth digits), abductor digiti minimi, ulnar intrinsic hand muscles (e.g., first digit), adductor pollicis, third and fourth lumbricals. The dorsal cutaneous ulnar branch provides sensory innervation along the dorsal, medial surface of the hand and leaves the main branch proximal to the ulnar styloid before the main branch enters the Guyon's canal. It is, therefore, an important branch to study in distinguishing between ulnar nerve lesions at the wrist and elbow.

The most common site of ulnar nerve trauma is the elbow. Most lesions (see Figure 15.4) occur either within the ulnar groove (e.g., bone spurs/osteoarthritis), or below the medial epicondyle (cubital tunnel). Rarely, lesions may occur above the medial epicondyle (e.g., "arcade of Struthers"). Etiological factors include repetitive trauma with episodic elbow flexion (the ulnar nerve elongates 4.7 mm and is displaced medially 7 mm when compressed by the medial head of the triceps), traction injuries secondary to valgus and overhand biomechanics (baseball pitching), recurrent subluxation of the nerve anterior to the medial epicondyle, higher incidence of peripheral neuropathies generally with diabetic patients with superimposed polyneuropathies, space occupying lesions (e.g., ganglions, neoplastic lesions, rheumatoid nodules), and blunt trauma/fracture about the elbow.

The clinical presentation with ulnar neuropathies at the elbow is not unlike that of a wrist/hand ulnar nerve lesion. One cannot assume the location of the injury solely by history and physical examination. An electrodiagnostic examination is required to delineate the nature of the pathology and the degree of its severity. Having said this, patients generally present with either continuous or intermittent paresthesias in the fifth and, to a lesser degree, in fourth digits. Pain may radiate distally from the medial epicondylar region of the elbow. The patient may note hand weakness with fine motor deficits. Symptoms may be exacerbated with overhand activities. The physical examination may reveal a positive "elbow flexion test" with exacerbation of complaints with continuous elbow flexion (this test is akin to the Phalen's test for CTS testing), intrinsic muscle atrophy (first dorsal interosseous fascicle location along the periphery of the main ulnar nerve trunk makes it more vulnerable to repetitive trauma early in the clinical course of the neuropathy), flexor carpi ulnaris atrophy (although less common than first digit atrophy), positive Tinel's sign (although unreliable generally), structural bony/ligamentous deformities at the level of the medial epicondyle (especially in patients with rheumatological disease), and hyperesthesias in an ulnar distribution with sensory testing.

The differential diagnosis includes C8 and/or T1 radiculopathies, a brachial plexopathy involving either the lower trunk or the medial cord, a peripheral polyneuropathy, and "overuse syndrome" in a workman's compensation situation. The electrodiagnostic examination of patients being evaluated for a potential ulnar neuropathy must take into account not only the specific etiology of the ulnar nerve trauma (if it in fact exists) but also the neuropathological type (demyelinating versus axonal loss pathology) and degree of injury severity, because surgical decision making is often dependent on these results.

The electrodiagnostic study should include a detailed nerve conduction examination focusing on the ulnar motor nerve at the elbow. Slowed ulnar motor conduction velocities across the elbow (<50 m/second) along with an amplitude drop with proximal stimulation above the elbow (suggestive of conduction block), both suggest demyelinative pathology. Across the elbow, conduction velocities can be compared to both below and above elbow conduction velocities to determine any "relative" difference (multiple studies have delineated suitable diagnostic "cutoffs" for satisfying the diagnosis of ulnar nerve pathology based on the conduction velocity "delta" value). More detailed studies with stimulation at 2-cm intervals across the elbow region can be performed ("short segment stimulation study") to further localize the lesion site. This is followed by a detailed needle examination of the ulnar innervated musculature not only to determine the presence or absence of axonal loss but also to help rule in or out more proximal lesions (e.g., brachial plexopathy, C8 and/or T1 radiculopathy). Axonal loss findings generally present in the form of spontaneous fibrillation potentials and/or positive sharp waves along with decreased motor unit recruitment should a significant degree of motor unit dropout exist. Nerve reinnervation is suggested by the presence of large amplitude, polyphasic motor units.

The physical examination of patients with possible ulnar nerve trauma in the hand/wrist may reveal tenderness in the region of Guyon's canal with a positive Tinel's sign, a positive Froment's sign on motor testing (flexor pollicis longus substitution for the adductor pollicis with resistive testing of strength in key pinch), or a positive Wartenberg's sign (abducted fifth digit at rest with ulnar nerve pathology). Allen's test should also be performed to differentiate between vascular disease/spasm and nerve compression.

Ulnar neuropathy at the wrist/hand (Guyon's canal) remains a more difficult entity to examine electrodiagnostically from the standpoint of determining the ultimate clinical management. This is because the clinical presentation may be variable with both sensory and motor complaints depending on the site of trauma. Additionally, the presence of a proximal ulnar nerve injury at the elbow does not preclude the presence of a concurrent ulnar nerve lesion at the wrist/hand. The electrodiagnostic study should include both motor and sensory nerve conduction studies along with a detailed needle examination of the ulnar innervated musculature both above and below the wrist. Given that the ulnar nerve divides into a deep motor branch, multiple sensory branches, and a branch to the hypothenar muscles, a cursory needle study will not suffice in patients with "ulnar nerve" complaints. Finally, the dorsal cutaneous nerve should be examined, because it arises proximal to the main trunk's entrance to Guyon's canal. Evidence of trauma to this nerve implies a lesion proximal to the wrist/hand. Commonly, with lesions of the ulnar nerve at Guyon's canal, the ulnar deep motor branch is involved but assumptions of relative involvement are to be avoided. Indeed, only upon the completion of the EMG can one retrospectively evaluate the data and reach a conclusion as to the distribution and severity of the pathology present.

The differential diagnosis includes "hypothenar hammer syndrome" characterized by vascular insufficiency, fracture of the hook of the hamate, ganglion cyst, as well as those entities cited in the discussion of ulnar neuropathy at the elbow. Treatment options of ulnar nerve lesions at both the elbow and wrist include surgical intervention, if clinically warranted, as well as assessing biomechanics, repetitive trauma variables, and an integrated upper extremity rehabilitation program focusing on the relationship between the cervical spine, shoulder, elbow, and wrist regions.

RADIAL NERVE INJURY

The radial nerve represents the terminal branch of the posterior cord. Its cervical root contribution is from C5-8. Its musculature innervation includes the following: the triceps, anconeous, supinator, brachioradialis, extensor carpi radialis, extensor digitorum, extensor carpi ulnaris, extensor pollicis longus, abductor pollicis longus, and extensor indicis proprius. Its initial axillary branch supplies the long head of the triceps with a cutaneous sensory branch to this region. Distally, at the "spiral groove," fractures of the humerus commonly result in a "proximal" radial neuropathy. The innervation to the brachioradialis and the extensor carpi radialis longus (ECRL) occurs just proximal to the forearm. Within the forearm, the radial nerve divides into a pure motor branch (posterior interosseous nerve) and a superficial sensory branch. The terminal superficial sensory branch becomes subcutaneous in the distal lateral forearm supplying the sensory innervation to the dorsum of the lateral hand, the first web space, and the proximal phalanges of digits one to three.

Proximal radial nerve lesions (see Figure 15.4) in the arm may be caused by the following: humeral shaft fractures, improper use of axillary crutches, tourniquet compression, deep intramuscular injections into the posterior/lateral region of the arm, and "Saturday night compression/palsy." Nontraumatic causes of compression are rare but can occur with weight lifting (repetitive and resisted elbow extension). A common site of compression is the "spiral groove" of the humerus where the radial nerve passes inferior to the lateral head of the triceps. Clinical findings may include decreased motor return/paralysis in wrist/digital extension with decreased sensation over the dorsal lateral aspect of the hand.

Radial neuropathies in the forearm are somewhat more difficult to delineate in that their presentation can be quite variable. The "pure motor syndrome" ("posterior interosseous nerve syndrome) is characterized classically by weakness in wrist dorsiflexion in a radial direction (ECRL is intact) given the involvement of the extensor carpi ulnaris. Additionally, the digital extensors including the thumb are weakened. Interphalangeal joint extension remains intact secondary to the viable intrinsic musculature. "Complete" patterns of injury are rare. An "incomplete" pattern is more common.

Potential sites of compression or entrapment of the radial nerve distal at the spiral groove include the following: (a) the posterior interosseous nerve may become entrapped in the supinator muscle (supinator channel syndrome) and is especially vulnerable at the "arcade of Froshe," which may act as a restraining entity to the radial nerve when swollen or actively contracted with repetitive rotatory movements; (b) compression of the radial nerve may occur at the extensor carpi radialis brevis; (c) compression may occur in the "radial tunnel" (a region demarcated by the lateral epicondyle and the supinator muscle) which exists as a "potential space" with numerous sites and mechanisms of potential compression and trauma to the radial nerve including fibrous bands, blood vessels, and the arcade of Froshe itself.

Two important points should be emphasized at this juncture. First, the clinical presentation of patients with lateral epicondylitis is quite similar to that of patients with radial nerve entrapment syndromes either at the elbow or in the forearm. The patient may note pain and/or dysesthesias in the lateral epicondylar region with exacerbation of symptoms with resisted wrist extension. Decreased sensation in a radial distribution can occur but it is generally not the overriding presenting symptom. Moreover, the biomechanical causes of lateral epicondylitis (i.e., repetitive wrist extension with rotatory forearm supination/pronation) also tend to predispose the patient to radial nerve trauma at the elbow and forearm. Distinguishing between these two entities can be difficult because the pre-eminent symptom is generally pain and not numbness or tingling. Therefore, in this instance, radial neuropathy remains a difficult diagnosis clinically without the aid of an electrodiagnostic evaluation.

This brings us to our second point. To make the diagnosis of a radial neuropathy at the elbow or forearm (e.g., radial tunnel syndrome, supinator channel syndrome, or posterior interosseous nerve syndrome) a detailed needle examination must be performed in the radial innervated musculature distal to the triceps. All too often, the patient is given the diagnosis of lateral epicondylitis initially. Patients are then seen at a later date when their conservative management of this presumed entity fails. Even then, an incomplete or limited needle examination on the EMG study may fail to make the diagnosis of a distal radial neuropathy. Additionally, the incidence of concurrent lateral epicondylitis along with a radial neuropathy is common and the existence of one does not preclude the existence of the other. Finally, nerve conduction studies should also be performed but are generally of limited usefulness due to their relative inexactitude when compared to the needle examination, which can more clearly delineate axonal loss pathology.

The final radial neuropathy to consider is traumatic involvement of its terminal sensory branch. This generally occurs at the distal forearm and may be secondary to repetitive pronation/supination of the forearm (with increased compression of the ext. carpi radialis longus and brachioradialis tendons), compression or blunt trauma in the form of contusions or lacerations, as well as the presence of neuromas or ganglion cysts. The presentation is characterized by impaired sensation in the dorsolateral hand with absent motor deficits. Symptoms may be reproduced with forearm pronation with ulnar wrist flexion. A nerve conduction examination of the superficial radial nerve with comparison to the contralateral side should be sufficient to make the diagnosis.

With regard to the electrodiagnostic examination, it has already been emphasized that the needle examination in the forearm remains the sin qua non from the standpoint of diagnosing a radial neuropathy in this region. Additionally, motor conduction studies in the forearm, although technically difficult, should also be performed. Comparison of below (i.e., forearm) and across elbow conduction velocities and amplitudes should be made to determine absolute and relative differences. The conduction velocity in the forearm can be normal or borderline in confirmed cases of "radial tunnel syndrome" (i.e., fastest conducting fibers may still be relatively intact and myelinated). Finally, as with all electrodiagnostic evaluations of upper extremity peripheral nerves and the brachial plexus, a generous needle sampling of multiroot innervated musculature and the cervical paraspinal muscles should be performed to help rule out a cervical radiculopathy or a brachial plexopathy. As one can see, the diagnosis of a radial neuropathy in the forearm remains a challenging but attainable task for the electromyographer-sports medicine physician.

MEDIAN NEUROPATHY

The median nerve is supplied by the C6, C7, C8, and T1 cervical roots and is formed by branches emanating from the medial and lateral cords of the brachial plexus. Its motor innervation includes the pronator teres, flexor carpi radialis, palmaris longus (when present), flexor digitorum superficialis, flexor digitorum profundus (digits land II), pronator quadratus, flexor pollicis longus, first and second lumbricals, APB, and the opponens pollicis. Its anatomical course in the forearm is clinically notable for potential sites of compression at the pronator teres (pronator teres syndrome), more distally in the forearm involving the anterior interosseous nerve (anterior interosseous nerve syndrome—a pure motor syndrome), as well as the carpal tunnel (CTS). Interestingly, a rare compression may occur before the median nerve enters the forearm at the distal humerus. The nerve may be entrapped by a ligament (ligament of Struthers) fixed to a bony spur.

The sensory innervation of the median nerve includes the lateral palmer surface as well as the dorsal region of the distal phalanges. Additionally, the lateral three digits as well as the lateral half of the fourth digit are supplied.

Compression neuropathies of the median nerve (see Figure 15.4) in the forearm may occur at a number of potential sites: (a) The "ligament of Struthers"—here, compression occurs secondary to a supracondylar spur and its ligamentous attachment. A palpable bony mass may often be localized proximal to the elbow along the medial border of the distal brachialis muscle. All of the median innervated musculature would be vulnerable to demyelinative and axonal loss pathology. The median motor conduction velocity could also be slowed. (b) The lacertus fibrosis or bicipital aponeurosis, which is a fibrous membrane overlying the flexor musculature, may be a source of compression. Symptoms are exacerbated with recurrent elbow flexion and forearm supination. (c) The pronator teres muscle, with its two heads (along with the flexor superficialis), may cause compression of the median nerve as it passes between these two structures as well as by fibrous bands, local tenosynovitis, bleeding, and repetitive trauma. Symptoms may be exacerbated by repetitive pronation of the forearm or elbow flexion.

In the proximal forearm median nerve lesions, the clinical presentation may be similar to CTS with numbness and tingling in a median distribution. Unlike CTS, however, nocturnal symptomatology is rare and a positive Phalen's sign is generally absent. Important to note with regard to "pronator teres syndrome" is the absence of axonal loss findings on EMG needle examination in the pronator teres muscle itself, because its innervation resides proximal to the muscle, thereby sparing it. The presence of axonal loss findings in the median innervated musculature of the forearm serves to distinguish this syndrome from CTS. It is for this reason that a screening needle examination of the proximal median innervated musculature remains a necessary component of the overall EMG workup of CTS. The possibility of dual sites of compression of the median nerve (both at the carpal tunnel distally and proximally in the forearm) must always be entertained. Failing to do so will result in partial and, therefore, incomplete treatment of these patients with dual lesions. (d) Compression of the anterior interosseous nerve (which is a pure motor nerve) may occur secondary to a number of etiologies including fibrous bands, muscular anomalies, fractures, hematomas, muscular hypertrophy, and neuromas. The classic sensory complaints of CTS as well as more proximal median nerve entrapments are absent given the pure motor nature of this branch. For this reason, a high degree of suspicion is necessary for its diagnosis along with a detailed needle examination of its innervated musculature, namely the flexor pollicis longus, flexor digitorum (digits two and three), and the pronator quadratus.

Compression of the median nerve at the carpal tunnel has been studied extensively in the electromyographic as well as the sports medicine literature. Electrodiagnostic nerve conduction techniques have developed significantly over the last 20 years with regard to increased sensitivity and specificity allowing early detection of this entity. Compression of the median nerve occurs deep to the transverse retinacula ligament in the volar wrist. Sensory and motor branches may be affected in a variable manner. The clinical presentation generally includes pain or dysesthesias in the hand and wrist with numbness in a median distribution. Symptoms may radiate proximally into the volar forearm and tend to be worse nocturnally. Decreased grip strength along with a positive Phalen's sign may be present. Late findings include thenar muscle wasting.

From an electrodiagnostic standpoint, it is important to note that sensory nerve conduction studies have been developed that allow the early detection of CTS. A number of these studies utilize the relative sensory latency differences between the median nerve (with the median sensory latency having the greatest value) and the radial as well as ulnar nerves. Comparative sensory studies at digit one (median/radial D1 sensory study) and digit four (median/ulnar D4 sensory study) enable the electromyographer to compare the respective latencies and thereby determine a latency "delta" value. Generally, latency delta values greater than or equal to 0.4 millisecond are considered diagnostic of CTS.

In cases of severe CTS, a number of studies comparing the median and ulnar motor nerve latencies have also been compared while obtaining a median/ulnar motor delta value resulting in heightened sensitivity in making the CTS diagnosis. It is important to reiterate that a detailed needle examination, not only of the APB in the hand but also of the proximal median musculature, should also be performed to help rule out a median nerve lesion in the forearm or at the elbow. The differential diagnosis should include a cervical radiculopathy or a brachial plexopathy, if clinically indicated.

Management of CTS includes conservative measures (e.g., wrist splinting, local corticosteroid injections, diuretics, avoidance of precipitating activities, NSAIDs). Surgical decompression of the median nerve may be necessary for symptom resolution.

SUGGESTED READINGS

Andary M, Williams F. *Carpal Tunnel syndrome: sensitive techniques for diagnosis. An AAEM Workshop*. October 1993.

Bartosh R, Dugdale TW, Nielsen R, et al. Isolated musculocutaneous nerve injury complicating closed fracture of the clavicle. *Am J Sports Med* 1992;20(3):356–359.

Braddom R. Musculocutaneous nerve injury after heavy exercise. *Arch Phys Med Rehabil* 1978;59:290–293.

Bradshaw D, Shefner J. Ulnar neuropathy at the elbow. Entrapment and other focal neuropathies. *Neurol Clin* 1999;17(3):447–461.

Brown W, Bolton C. *Clinical electromyography*, 2nd ed. Butterworth-Heinemann, 1993.

Burke D. Conservative management of carpal tunnel syndrome in physical medicine and rehabilitation clinics of North America. *Carpal Tunnel Syndr* 1997;8(3):513–528.

Campbell W. AAEE case report # 18: ulnar neuropathy in the distal forearm. *Muscle Nerve* 1989;12:347–352.

Carlson N, Logigian E. : Radial neuropathy. Entrapments and other focal europathies. *Neurol Clin* 1999;17(3):499–523.

Cassvan A, Ralescu S, Shapiro E, et al. Median and radial sensory latencies to digit I as compared with other screening tests in carpal tunnel syndrome. *Am J Phys Med Rehabil* 1988;67:221–224.

Cifu D, Saleem S. Median-radial latency difference: its use in screening for carpal tunnel syndrome in twenty patients with demyelinating peripheral neuropathy. *Arch Phys Med Rehabil* 1983;74:44–47.

Clancy W, Brand R, Bergfield J. Upper trunk brachial plexus injuries in contact sports. *Am J Sports Med* 1977;5(5):209–216.

Clinchot D. Motor conduction studies and needle electromyography in carpal tunnel syndrome in physical medicine and rehabilitation clinics of North America. *Carpal Tunnel Syndr* 1997;8(3):459–475.

DeLisa J, Lee H, Baran E, et al. *Manual of nerve conduction velocity and clinical neurophysiology*, 3rd ed. New York: Raven Press, 1994.

Dillin L, Hoaglund FT, Scheck M, et al. Brachial neuritis. *J Bone Joint Surg* 1985;67-A(6):878–880.

Dumitru D, Amato AA, Zwarts MJ, et al. *Electrodiagnostic medicine*, 2nd ed. Philadelphia: Hanley & Belfus, Inc, 2002.

Eisen A. The electrodiagnosis of plexopathies. In: Brown W, Bolton C. *Clinical electromyography*, 2nd ed. Boston: Butterworth-Heinemann, 1993:211–225.

Feinberg J. Burners and stingers in physical medicine and rehabilitation clinics of North America. 2000;11(4):771–784.

Felsenthal G, Freed M, Kalafut R, et al. Across-elbow ulnar nerve sensory conduction technique. *Arch Phys Med Rehabil* 1989;70:668–672.

Giuliani M. *Electrodiagnostic approach to brachial plexus trauma in 1998 AAEM course C: electrodiagnosis in traumatic conditions*. Orlando, FL, 1998:13–20.

Glousman RE. Ulnar nerve problems in the athlete's elbow in clinics in sports medicine. *Neurovasc Inj* 1990;9(2):365–377.

Goodman C, Kenrick M, Blum M. Long thoracic nerve palsy: a follow up story. *Arch Phys Med Rehabil* 1975;56:352–355.

Goslin K, Krivickas L. Proximal neuropathies of the upper extremity. Entrapments and other focal neuropathies. *Neurol Clin* 1999;17(3):525–548.

Green R, Brian M. Accessory nerve latency to the middle and lower trapezius. *Arch Phys Med Rehabil* 1985;66:23–24.

Gregg J, Labosky D, Harty M, et al. Serratus anterior paralysis in the young athlete. *J Bone Joint Surg* 1979;61-A(6):825–832.

Gross P, Tolomeo E. Proximal median neuropathies. Entrapment and other focal neuropathies. *Neurol Clin* 1999;17(3):425–445.

Hadley M, Sonntag VKH, Pittman HW, et al. Suprascapular nerve entrapment. *J Neurosurg* 1986;64:843–848.

Hennessey W, Kuhlman K. The anatomy, symptoms, and signs of carpal tunnel syndrome in physical medicine and rehabilitation clinics of North America. *Carpal Tunnel Syndr* 1997;8(3):439–457.

Hershman E, Asa JW, Bergfeld JA, et al. Acute brachial neuropathy in athletes. *Am J Sports Med* 1989;17(5):655–659.

Hershman EB. Brachial plexus injuries in clinics in sports medicine. *Neurovasc Inj* 1990;9(2):311–329.

Hill N, Howard F, Huffer B. The incomplete anterior interosseous nerve syndrome. *J Hand Surg* 1985;1(1):4–16.

Howard F, Hill N. Entrapment of the anterior interosseous nerve. *Contemp Orthop* 1986;12(6):43–47.

Johnson E, Terebuh B. Sensory and mixed nerve conduction studies in carpal tunnel syndrome in physical medicine and rehabilitation clinics of North America. *Carpal Tunnel Syndr* 1997;8(3):477–501.

Kanakamedala R, Simons D, Porter R, et al. Ulnar nerve entrapment at the elbow localized y short segment stimulation. *Arch Phys Med Rehabil* 1988;69:959–963.

Karas SE. Thoracic outlet syndrome in clinics in sports medicine. *Neurovasc Inj* 1990;9(2):297–310.

Kincaid J. AAEE minimonograph #31: the electrodiagnosis of ulnar neuropathy at the elbow. *Muscle Nerve* 1988;11:1005–1015.

Kothari M. Ulnar neuropathy at the wrist. Entrapment and other focal neuropathies. *Neurol Clin* 1999;17(3):463–476.

Lee H, DeLisa J. *Surface anatomy for clinical needle electromyography*. New York: Demos, 2000.

Levine B, Jones J, Burton R. Nerve entrapments of the upper extremity: a surgical perspective. Entrapments and other focal neuropathies. *Neurol Clin* 1999;17(3):540–565.

Liveson J. *Peripheral neurology: case studies in electrodiagnosis*, 2nd ed. Philadelphia: FA Davis Co, 1991.

Matz S, Welliver P, Welliver D. Brachial plexus neuropraxia complicating clavicle fracture in a college football player. *Am J Sports Med* 1989;17(4):581–583.

McCarroll HR. Nerve injuries associated with wrist trauma. *Orthop Clin North Am* 1984;15(2):279–287.

Mendoza F, Main K. Peripheral nerve injuries of the shoulder in the athlete in clinics in sports medicine. *Neurovasc Inj* 1990;9(2):331–342.

Miller R. AAEM case report #1: ulnar neuropathy at the elbow. *Muscle Nerve* 1991;14(2):97–101.

Morris H, Peters B. Pronator syndrome: clinical and electrophysiological features in seven cases. *J Neurol* 1976;39:461–464.

Moss S, Switzer H. Radial tunnel syndrome: a spectrum of clinical presentations. *J Hand Surg* 1983;8(4):414–420.

Neviaser T, Ain B, Neviaser R. Suprascapular nerve denervation secondary to attenuation by glionic cyst. *J Bone Joint Surg* 1986;68-A(4):627–628.

Olney R, Hanson M. AAEE case report # 15: ulnar neuropathy at or distal to the wrist. *Muscle Nerve* 1988;11:828–832.

Pianka George, Hershman E. *Neurovascular injuries—the upper extremity in sports medicine*. Chapter 31, Nicholas JA, Hershman EB, eds. 1990:702–704.

Poindexter D, Johnson E. Football shoulder and neck injury: a study of the "stinger". *Arch Phys Med Rehabil* 1984;65:601–602.

Posner MA. Compressive neuropathies of the median and radial nerves at the elbow in clinics in sports medicine. *Neurovasc Inj* 1990;9(2):343–363.

Post M, Jayer J. Suprascapular nerve entrapment. *Clin Orthop Relat Res* 1987;223:126–136.

Rayan G. Lower trunk brachial plexus compression neuropathy due to cervical rib in young athletes. *Am J Sports Med* 1988;16(1):77–79.

Rehak DA. Pronator syndrome in clinics in sports medicine. *Overuse Inj Upper Extremity* 2001;29(3):531–540.

Ringel S, Treihaft M, Carry M, et al. Suprascapular neuropathy in pitchers. *Am J Sports Med* 1990;18:80–86.

Robertson W, Eichman P, Clancy W. Upper trunk brachial plexopathy in football players. *JAMA* 1979;241(14):1480–1482.

Rockett F. Observations of the "burner": traumatic cervical radiculopathy. *Clin Orthop Relat Res* 1982;164:18–19.

Rorabeck C, Harris W. Factors affecting the prognosis of brachial plexus injuries. *J Bone Joint Surg* 1981;63-B(3):404–407.

Ross M, Kimura J. AAEM case report #2: the carpal tunnel syndrome. *Muscle Nerve* 1995;18(6):567–573.

Sable A. Median and ulnar nerves in the hand in physical medicine and rehabilitation clinics of North America. *Electromyography* 1998;9(4):737–753.

Stanish W, Lamb H. Isolated paralysis of the serratus anterior muscle: a weight training injury. *Am J Sports Med* 1978;6(6):385–386.

Steveens J. AAEE minimonograph #26: the electrodiagnosis of carpal tunnel syndrome. *Muscle Nerve* 1987;10:99–113.

Subramony SH. AAEE case report #14: neuralgic amyotrophy (acute brachial neuropathy). *Muscle Nerve* 1988;11:39–44.

Weinstein S, Herring S. Nerve problems and compartment syndromes in the hand, wrist, forearm in clinics in sports medicine. *Inj Hand Wrist* 1992;11(1):161–188.

Weinstein S. Assessment and rehabilitation of the athlete with a "Stinger" in clinics in ports medicine. *Neurol Athl Head Neck Inj* 1998;17(1):127–135.

Wilbourn A, Aminoff M. AAEE minimonograph # 32: the electrophysiologic examination patients with radiculopathies. *Muscle Nerve* 1988;11(11):1099–1114.

Wilbourn A. *AAEM case report #7: true neurogenic thoracic outlet syndrome*. October 1982.

Wilbourn A. Electrodiagnosis of plexopathies. *Neurol Clin* 1985;3(3):511–529.

Wilbourn A. Thoracic outlet syndromes. Entrapment and other focal neuropathies. *Neurol Clin* 1999;17(3):477–497.

Wilbourn A. Electrodiagnostic testing of neurologic injuries in athletes in neurovascular injuries. *Clin Sports Med* 1990;9(2):229–245.

Woodhead A. Paralysis of the serratus anterior in a world class marksman. *Am J Sports Med* 1985;13(5):359–362.

Wright T. Accessory spinal nerve injury. *Clin Orthop Relat Res* 1975;108: 15–18.

Wu J, Morris J, Hogan G. Ulnar neuropathy at the wrist: case report and review of literature. *Arch Phys Med Rehabil* 1985;66:785–788.

Zaneteas PD. Brachial plexus injuries and the electrodiagnostic examination. *Curr Sports Med Rep* 2003;2(1):7–14.

Genitourinary System

16

Kevin B. Gebke

PERSPECTIVE

The genitourinary (GU) system comprises of the internal and external organs that make up the urinary system (kidney, ureter, urinary bladder, and urethra) and the genital organs. Both systems are located in the lower abdomen and pelvic area. Injuries to the kidney, ureter, and bladder are common in athletics. The most common symptom reported in GU system injuries is hematuria.

ANATOMY

For the most part, the organs of both the genital and urinary systems are well protected. The kidneys are located in the retroperitoneal upper lumbar area of the abdomen, with the upper third of the right kidney and the upper half of the left kidney located underneath the 12th rib. The psoas, paravertebral, and latissimus dorsi muscles protect the remaining parts of the kidneys. The kidneys themselves rest in a bed of pericapsular fat.

The ureters run their course along the posterior peritoneal wall and are primarily protected by the vertebrae and muscles of the posterior abdominal wall. The ureters are vulnerable only where they course over the pelvic rim and into the bladder. The bladder lies within the pelvis except when it is full and rises above the pelvic rim. The bladder is thinnest and most vulnerable when full. The entire female reproductive system is situated within the pelvis, as are the prostate and internal portion of the male urethra. The external male genitalia (penis, scrotum, and testes) are obviously the most vulnerable portions of the male GU system. During sports, these organs are protected and held close to the body by an athletic supporter.

KIDNEY INJURIES

Injury to the kidney can result from direct trauma, repetitive jarring, decreased renal blood flow, and medication side effects.

Traumatic Injuries

The kidney can be injured by a direct blow to the exposed flank area or abdomen, such as when a football player reaches up to catch a pass and is tackled. The kidney also is subject to a contrecoup type of injury after a high-speed collision. The following kidney injuries are common in sports: contusion, intra- and extracapsular injury, capsular tear or rupture, renal parenchymal tear or rupture, and tear of the renal pedicle.

Injury to the kidney is typically accompanied by pain, tenderness, ecchymosis and/or hematuria. In rare instances, renal colic can occur from blockage of the renal pelvis by blood clots. Hypovolemic shock may be a result of extensive bleeding. There is a weak correlation between the degree of hematuria and the degree of kidney injury. Occasionally, there will be no blood in the urine if the renal collecting system is spared. An indication of significant bleeding is the loss of renal outline and psoas muscle shadow on plain kidney, ureter, and bladder (KUB) films of the abdomen (Figure 16.1). Associated rib fractures, renal capsular and renal cortex tears, or bleeding may be detected on plain x-rays or intravenous pyelogram (IVP).

If an athlete has flank pain following an injury but the urinalysis is normal, successive urine studies should be done to ensure that the urine remains clear. If the team physician doubts the presence of a kidney injury and the urinalysis and plain films of the abdomen are negative, further diagnostic tests are unnecessary and observation is all that is required to manage this situation. If an injury

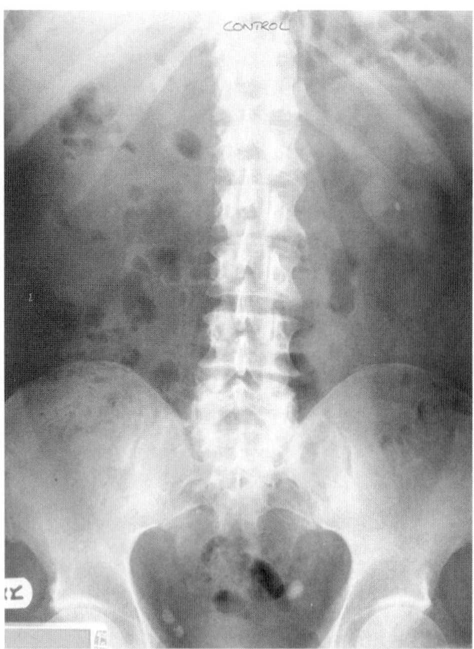

Figure 16.1 Kidney, ureter, and bladder (KUB) demonstrating normal psoas muscle shadow and renal outline.

to a kidney is strongly suspected, an IVP or computed tomography (CT) with intravenous contrast should be obtained. CT has emerged as the preferred diagnostic test; Definitive diagnosis can be established and associated abdominal and retroperitoneal injuries are easily identified.

The incidence of renal trauma in sports is unknown. Kidneys that are large, malformed, or have tumors are more prone to injury. There are five classes of injury as follows:

- *Class I—contusion.* These represent most (>85%) sports-related injuries to the kidney (1). There is usually a history of trauma but signs of trauma may or may not be present. Hematuria is usually present and the IVP is negative. CT (Figure 16.2) will identify the renal contusion (1), but most class I injuries do not require such extensive evaluation. Treatment of most contusions initially involves observation, hydration, bed rest, and repeat urinalysis. Most athletes return to sports after approximately 2 to 3 weeks of rest.
- *Class II—cortical laceration.* Cortical laceration is usually related to trauma and has findings similar to a contusion. On a plain radiograph, the psoas shadow may be lost and an IVP will show extravasations of dye. CT may be useful to identify the degree of injury. Again, observation, hydration, bed rest, and a repeat urinalysis are indicated. As with class I injuries, most athletes return to play within 2 to 3 weeks.
- *Class III—caliceal laceration.* Caliceal laceration involves intrarenal hemorrhage and disruption of the caliceal collecting system. CT establishes diagnosis, and repeat scanning is recommended to establish stabilization of the injury and healing (Figure 16.3). IVP, if utilized, will show an intact capsule with intrarenal extravasation of dye and loss of definition of the calices. Treatment involves observation and surgery for more serious cases.
- *Class IV—complete renal fracture.* This is a rare sports injury and the patient usually presents in shock. CT or IVP can establish diagnosis if the athlete is stable. Immediate surgery is indicated.
- *Class V—vascular pedicle injury.* This injury is also rare in sports and the patient presents in hypovolemic shock. Hematuria may or may not be present and the kidneys are usually not visualized on IVP. Visualization of the renal pedicle is possible with CT. A selective renal arteriogram shows renal vascular damage. Treatment always involves surgery, usually emergently.

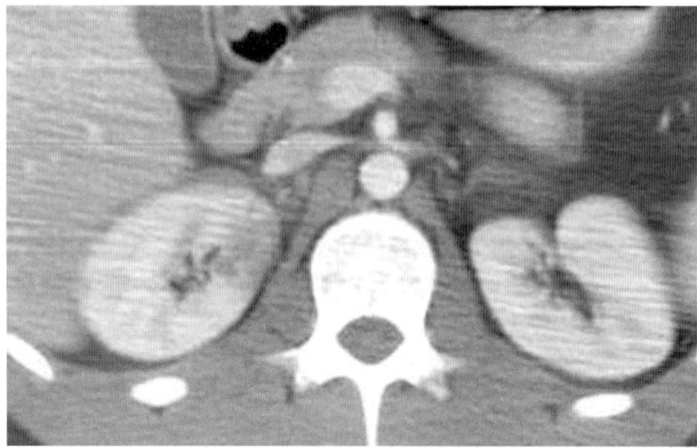

Figure 16.2 Computed tomography (CT) of the abdomen demonstrating a right renal contusion (without laceration).

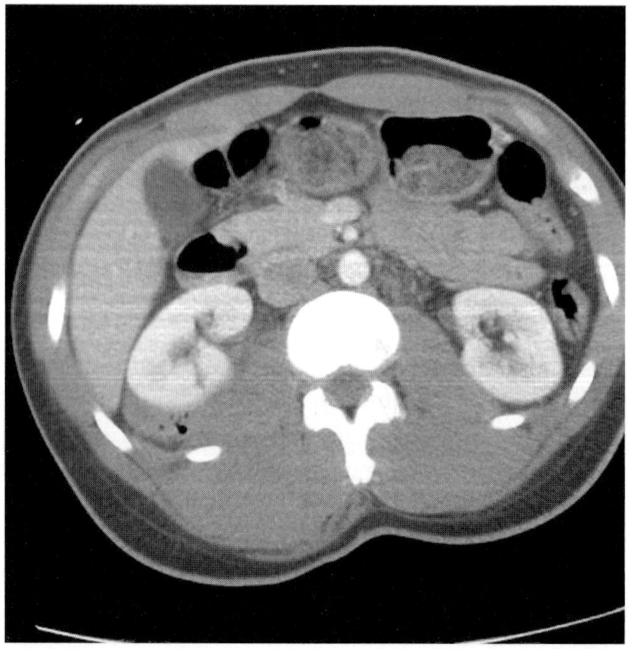

Figure 16.3 CT of the abdomen demonstrating a right renal laceration.

Most kidney trauma results in intracapsular or contusion injuries and heals without sequelae or complications. The athlete should be at complete bed rest until the urine is completely free of hematuria. Any athlete who develops hematuria after a blow to the flank or abdomen should be monitored closely. Extracapsular kidney injuries respond well to bed rest and close follow-up by the team physician in 50% of cases. The other 50% of cases may have continued bleeding (2). If diagnostic testing shows a nonfunctioning kidney or major injury with extracapsular extravasation, prompt referral is indicated. Referral to a urologist and appropriate treatment, including bed rest and/or surgery, is preferable in managing this situation.

The examining physician should check for injury to other intra-abdominal organs whenever a serious kidney injury is suspected. The athlete should not exercise further and hospital transport should be expedited. Surgery is usually indicated for pedicle tears, kidney lacerations, and massive hemorrhage of the kidney. It should be noted that there is a risk for rebleed following major renal vascular surgery. The occurrence rate is approximately 15% and is typically seen 15 to 20 days postoperatively, corresponding with clot resolution. Also, postinjury hypertension has been described at various rates of occurrence.

Prevention of severe kidney injuries should be considered in collision sports. Hip pads do not generally extend high enough to protect the kidneys, but kidney pads can be hung by straps from the shoulders. The use of a flak jacket also provides excellent kidney protection in most cases. Proper coaching techniques and adherence to regulations about protective equipment can reduce the incidence of severe kidney injuries.

Kidney Injuries from Prolonged Heavy Exercise

Renal function is affected by prolonged exercise. Renal blood flow decreases in response to exercise as blood is shunted to exercising muscles (3,4). Renal blood flow decreases more in exercising dehydrated or hypovolemic patients, but will generally return to pre-exercise levels within approximately 60 minutes. The mechanism for decreased renal blood flow is related to sympathetic nervous system–induced constriction of afferent and efferent arteries and increased levels of epinephrine and norepinephrine. Dramatic decreases in renal blood flow up to 50% may result in ischemia of the kidney and hematuria.

The following changes in renal physiology have been observed during exercise: (1) a drop in renal blood flow is proportionate to the severity of the exercise performed; (2) glomerular filtration rate (GFR) is usually well maintained but may decrease; (3) free water clearance decreases during even short exercise periods in well-hydrated subjects; (4) transient proteinuria may develop; (5) significant reduction in sodium excretion is observed because of increased tubular reabsorption; (6) antidiuretic hormone (ADH) may increase threefold with heavy exercise, and urinary water excretion is usually decreased as there is a decrease in urine flow during exercise, and (7) an increased excretion of white blood cells (WBCs) and red blood cells (RBCs) in addition to increased urinary excretion of casts (hyaline and granular) occurs.

These renal changes are transient and disappear after exercise. For the most part, renal function typically normalizes within 10 to 36 hours. Damage to renal parenchyma does not occur during heavy exercise. All renal changes noted in the preceding text are attributed to constriction of the renal vasculature. It has been postulated that an increase in core body temperature will increase permeability and also lead to some of the renal changes noted during exercise.

Acute renal failure (ARF) may be seen with renal ischemia during heat injury or severe dehydration. Severe muscle damage will produce myoglobinemia. The physician should be aware that nephrotoxins are usually excreted in this situation. Treatment of ARF should follow normal guidelines for this diagnosis. Prevention of this problem is related to proper hydration of the athlete before and during competition and exercise activities.

INJURY TO THE URETER AND BLADDER

Ureters

Injury to the ureter is commonly associated with severe renal damage. Fractures of the pelvis and lower lumbar vertebrae should be considered when assessing this type of injury. IVP is useful in diagnosis. Traumatic injuries to the ureter are rare and should be referred to a urologist.

Bladder

An empty bladder is rarely damaged by trauma. Traumatic bladder injuries do occur in the martial arts. The most common type of bladder injury is a contusion. Complete rupture of the bladder is rare. Most bladder injuries are related to blunt trauma on a distended bladder. Bladder trauma is present in 10% to 15% of patients with a fractured pelvis (5). Repetitive jarring of the bladder in long-distance racing may cause transient bladder contusions. The patient presents with a history of trauma, suprapubic pain, and guarding. Diagnostic evaluation should include a cystogram with a postdrainage film. Athletes with bladder trauma can pass small blood clots and often report dysuria and hematuria.

Two types of bladder injury are common. The first is a contusion where the degree of hematuria does not correlate well with the severity of the injury. Patients with a contusion are treated with bed rest and observation. Severe contusions require the use of an indwelling catheter for 7 to 10 days and antibiotic treatment. The second type of injury involves a bladder rupture, which can be intra- or extraperitoneal, or a combination of both. These injuries are usually associated with a pelvic fracture and require immediate surgery.

The urologist should dictate treatment. Follow-up with frequent urinalysis examinations will be necessary. The athlete may return to competition when symptom free and all evidence of hematuria has cleared. Prevention of most bladder injuries is accomplished by having the athlete completely empty the bladder before competition.

Biker's Bladder

A possible complication of aggressive bicycling is the development of "biker's bladder" (detrusor muscle irritability). The athlete usually has an abrupt onset of urinary frequency, diminished urinary stream, nocturia, and terminal dribbling. This symptom complex is similar to that described secondary to prostate irritation from prolonged cycling. These problems may be avoided by frequently and properly emptying the bladder during long bicycle rides. Once symptomatic, athletes will usually respond favorably to rest from the offending activity. Some cases will require urologic referral.

URETHRAL INJURIES

Injuries to the anterior urethra can be seen in athletes. The injury is typically sustained when an athlete falls into a straddle position on a hard object or suffers a direct blow to the perineum. This injury can predispose to future urethral stricture secondary to scarring. Diagnosis is established by history and physical examination findings (blood at the urethral meatus, perineal or penile hematoma). The diagnosis should be confirmed by retrograde urethrogram. Partial injuries can be treated conservatively with urethral cauterization and/or stenting. More severe injuries require surgical repair. Posterior urethral injuries are rarely seen and are usually associated with severe trauma and pelvic fracture. Urologic evaluation is recommended for most urethral injuries.

URINARY INCONTINENCE

Stress incontinence has an unknown relation to exercise. Athletes may notice symptoms sooner than their nonathletic peers (6). Treatment is the same in athletes as it is in nonathletes. Referral to a urologist or gynecologist may be required for female athletes to treat severe cases of urinary incontinence that interfere with daily activities and exercise.

HEMATURIA

Hematuria is the most common urinary symptom seen after vigorous athletic activity (6). Distance swimmers and runners usually have the greatest incidence of exercise-induced hematuria, although it has been commonly reported in lacrosse, running, football, and rowing athletes. Most studies in the literature report clearing of hematuria within 48 hours after vigorous exercise (7–14). Direct kidney injury, renal vein kinking, bladder contusion, or preexisting renal pathology may also cause hematuria. The problem for the team physician is to distinguish significant organic disease from transient, benign conditions that cause hematuria.

Gardner (15) was the first to use the term *athletic pseudonephritis* when he described hematuria and proteinuria in 45% of football players examined. Microscopic hematuria is very common in the general population. In a population-based study at the Mayo clinic, 13% of men and postmenopausal women had asymptomatic microscopic hematuria (16). A study at Kaiser Medical Center, Honolulu, on patients undergoing multiphasic screening revealed a 15% incidence of microhematuria (11). Microscopic hematuria is also common in younger patients. In a survey of 8,954 Finnish school children, microscopic hematuria was found in one or more specimens in 4% of the children (14). The lower urinary tract is regarded as the most common source of hematuria after prolonged and exhaustive exertion. The existence of renal stones, urinary tract infection, or exercise-induced irritation of the urethral meatus from contusion or cold exposure should be eliminated in the differential diagnosis of hematuria.

No consensus exists on the upper limit of normal for urinary RBC. Urinary RBC count may rise after events such as mild trauma, exercise, or sex (17). A 1990 review says the most commonly accepted upper limit of normal is 3 RBCs/HPF or 1,000 RBCs/mL of urine (13). False negatives may occur from contamination of the urine by menses in the female or by masturbation in the male. Any African-American athlete with hematuria should be evaluated for sickle cell disease/trait. A history of drug and medication use should be obtained. The timing of hematuria is important to note: (1) initial hematuria is most likely urethral in origin; (2) terminal hematuria is most likely bladder or posterior urethral in origin; and (3) continuous hematuria most likely originates from the upper urinary tract (kidney, ureter, or bladder). Urinalysis can provide some understanding of the location of the bleeding site. Dark brown urine usually signifies upper tract bleeding, whereas salmon pink or pink/red coloration most often results from lower tract bleeding.

The presence of casts in a postexercise urinalysis has also been described. The incidence and significance of casts in this setting is unclear. Casts generally signify renal disease, and athletes with this finding should receive a meticulous evaluation of additional urine samples.

Proof of reversion to normal urine after exercise-related hematuria is important in order to exclude such diseases as nephritis, nephrolithiasis, or tumors occurring in the urinary tract (10). Papillary necrosis, infection, and vascular diseases should be considered if hematuria persists. In younger athletes (<40 years old) with asymptomatic hematuria following exercise, a repeat urinalysis should be performed at 24 and 48 hours. Clean-catch urine should be cultured if cystitis or infection is suspected. No further testing is indicated if repeated urinalyses are negative. If hematuria persists, is recurrent, or is associated with continued symptoms such as pain, dysuria, or fever, further investigation is indicated.

The identification of hematuria should always prompt further evaluation. A repeat urinalysis at 24 to 48 hours after the initial observation of microscopic hematuria should always be performed. The follow-up urinalysis is a critical branching point and indicates the need for medical evaluation if gross or microscopic hematuria persists. If the repeat urinalysis is abnormal, a urine culture should be obtained and any urinary infection treated appropriately. Abnormal levels of serum creatinine and blood urea nitrogen (BUN), sickle cell prep, and/or IVP will require further evaluation and possibly referral to a nephrologists (see Figure 16.4). Therapy for athletes and nonathletes with hematuria is mostly dependent on making an accurate diagnosis. If these tests are negative, cystoscopy should be arranged to exclude bladder lesions, especially if the patient is older than 40 years.

Further work-up at this point should not be repeated after subsequent episodes of exercise-related hematuria that clears with rest. Abnormalities on IVP or cystoscopy are pursued in a conventional manner as shown in the figure. Athletes with negative tests but persistent hematuria should undergo additional investigation for causes of intrinsic renal disease. The IVP confers a risk of osmotic injury to the kidney and some experts argue that a renal ultrasound could replace IVP with a minimal decrease in diagnostic yield and a substantial decrease in risk (13). CT scan can best detect small or peripheral renal lesions and may outperform magnetic resonance imaging (MRI). Retrograde pyelography is done if the IVP completely illuminates the lower urinary tract (12,13). Cystoscopy is the next step, and it may provide the best initial results in an actively bleeding patient. Cystoscopy is the best method for studying the bladder and entire male urethra and can provide cytological materials (9). The indications for renal angiography and renal biopsy are controversial. Discussions of the pros and cons are available as are diagnostic algorithms (9,12,13,18). Therapy should be based on a specific diagnosis and be performed by a nephrologist. Athletes with benign hematuria secondary to exercise may continue to be active but they should be encouraged to drink appropriate quantities of fluids before exercise and to avoid dehydration. A general rule-of-thumb recommendation is for such athletes to ingest 16 to 24 ounces of fluids before exercise, and 5 to 8 ounces for every 15 minutes of exercise thereafter.

In summary, pseudonephritis is more common than nephritis. Asymptomatic microscopic hematuria, especially if it occurs only once or twice and is transient, is probably best followed up without an invasive work-up. On the other hand, persistent or recurrent microhematuria can

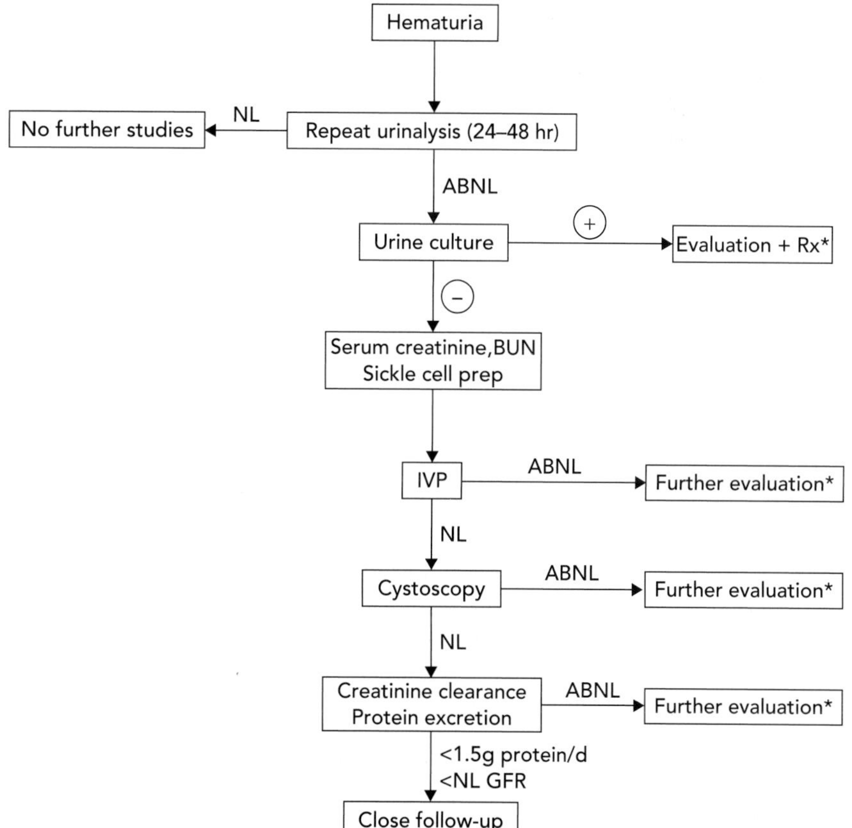

Figure 16.4 Evaluation of the patient with hematuria. NL = Normal; ABNL = Abnormal; BUN = blood urea nitrogen; IVP = intravenous pyelogram; GFR = glomerular filtration rate; Rx = treatment. *Retrograde ureterogram, angiography, ultrasound, and renal biopsy as indicated. (*Source*: Adapted from Goldszer RC, Siegel AJ. Renal abnormalities during exercise. In: Strauss RH, ed. *Sports medicine*. Philadelphia: WB Saunders, 1984:133.)

signal disease and requires further evaluation. Hematuria should always rouse suspicion in patients with risk factors for bladder cancer such as tobacco use, phenacetin abuse, or exposure to aniline dyes (13,19).

Physicians can help prevent hematuria through education. Hematuria from bladder contusions can be prevented through proper hydration and avoidance of complete bladder emptying just before running. Urethritis associated with cycling can be prevented by lowering the nose of the saddle, using a special seat or seat cover, and rising off the saddle for bumps. Athletes with sickle cell trait and infrequent episodes of gross hematuria can continue to participate in sports and exercise.

PROTEINURIA

Proteinuria occurs in many types of exercise such as rowing, football, boxing, track, long-distance running, swimming, and calisthenics. It happens more often with severe, strenuous, or prolonged exertion. Normal protein excretion is 30 to 45 mg/day. The degree of exertional proteinuria is usually no more than 2+ (>0.062 mg/dilution) by dipstick determination, and is always transient if due to exercise alone. Common associated findings on urinalysis include hemoglobinuria, hematuria, and myoglobinuria (20). Quantitative measurements of proteinuria range from 100 to 300 mg or less in a 24-hour period.

Alterations in renal hemodynamics associated with vigorous exercise are responsible for the proteinuria. A decrease in intravascular volume from acute dehydration may be responsible for proteinuria in athletes undertaking severe exercise. The most commonly observed pattern of renal function in exercising athletes includes an acute decrease in renal blood flow with maintenance of normal GFR. Elevations in the levels of renin, angiotensin II, and ADH following sustained, vigorous exercise cause alterations in renal hemodynamics. Most exercise-induced proteinuria occurs within 30 minutes of exercise and clears within 24 to 48 hours. When proteinuria is due to exercise alone, most athletes have no long-term sequelae (21,22).

Proteinuria initially observed after exertion may be independent of exercise or be secondary to underlying renal disease (6). There is a direct relation between the intensity of exercise and the amount of proteinuria (6). If the proteinuria does not clear within 24 to 48 hours after exercise, further investigation is indicated. A personal or family history of renal disease or the presence of hypertension, edema, or anemia suggests a need for further diagnostic testing. Proteinuria that persists for 24-hours after resting should be evaluated by collecting an overnight or supine and upright urine samples to exclude benign orthostatic proteinuria. If proteinuria persists in the sample collected while in the supine position, serum tests for renal function and a 24-hour urine collection for creatinine and total protein are useful. The physician also should determine the serum creatinine and BUN levels and obtain a fasting blood glucose and complete blood count.

Urinary protein electrophoresis, creatinine clearance levels, and IVP testing should be performed on patients with proteinuria while the patient is in a supine, resting position. Athletes with more than 1 g of protein in a 24-hour urine collection should be referred to a nephrologist for consultation and possible renal biopsy to exclude renal tubular interstitial disease (Figure 16.5). In general, exercise-induced proteinuria is likely to be recurrent in athletes after physical exertion. There is no evidence to support an increased risk for chronic renal disease or reason to limit physical activity in such individuals. All athletes with proteinuria should have a medical checkup and urinalysis for protein on a yearly basis. No further evaluation is necessary unless other abnormalities are present.

HEMOGLOBINURIA

Runners may pass dark red urine that contains hemoglobin pigment. This is commonly due to mechanical damage of RBCs in the soles of the runner's feet causing hemolysis. This condition can also be seen in individuals who participate in the martial arts secondary to repetitive hand and sole trauma. When hemolysis occurs, free hemoglobin is bound to haptoglobin for transport. If the haptoglobin stores are exhausted, hemoglobin is spilled into the urine. The presence of dark red urine 1 to 3 hours after these activities should indicate the possibility of hemoglobinuria (7). Running on softer surfaces or padding the areas of repetitive trauma can eliminate the condition. This condition usually clears spontaneously, but may require referral to a nephrologist in more complex cases.

MYOGLOBINURIA

Myoglobinuria may mimic the presence of hematuria. Myoglobin may appear in the urine of athletes secondary to the breakdown of muscle fibers. It is typically seen within 24 to 48 hours of exertion. Urine dipstick test does not distinguish myoglobin from hemoglobin. Urinalysis should be performed. Common findings include dark brown urine with the presence of myoglobin, hemoglobin, albumin, erythrocytes, and erythrocyte casts.

Acute tubular necrosis (ATN) may follow rhabdomyolysis, the breakdown of muscle. ARF associated with myoglobinuria is often associated with dehydration. The incident myoglobinuria can be very mild. However, with more severe ATN/ARF, a nephrologist should evaluate this condition. Myoglobinuria can be prevented by proper conditioning techniques and by avoiding dehydration. Exercise programs that gradually increase intensity levels will help prevent this syndrome.

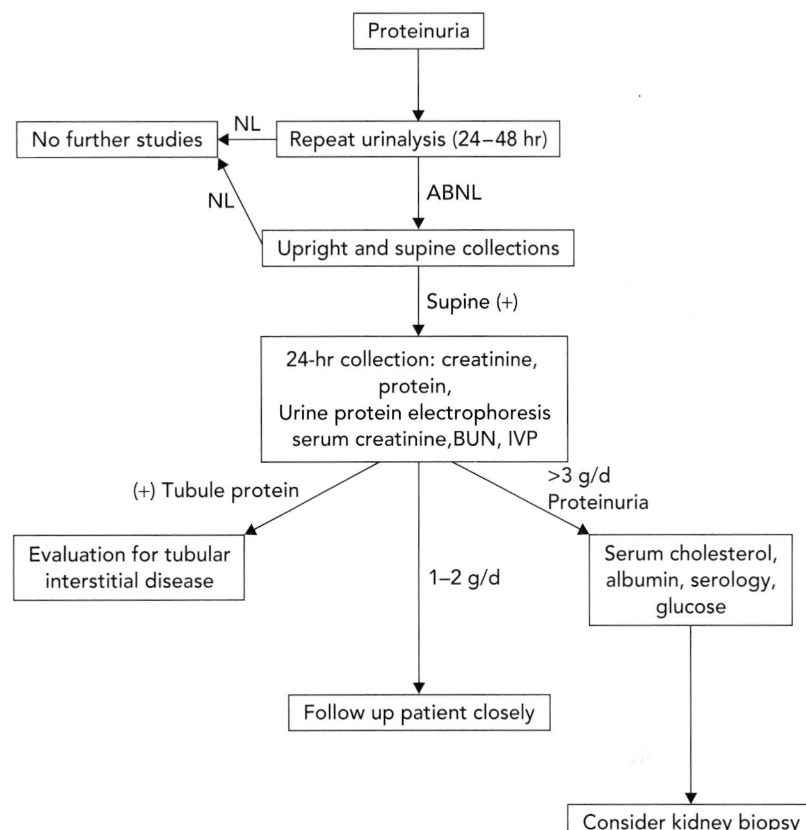

Figure 16.5 Evaluation of the Patient with Proteinuria. NL=Normal; ABNL=Abnormal; BUN = blood urea nitrogen; IVP = intravenous pyelogram. (*Source*: Adapted from Goldszer RC, Siegel AJ. Renal abnormalities during exercise. In: Strauss RH, ed. *Sports medicine*. Philadelphia: WB Saunders, 1984:134.)

NONSTEROIDAL ANTI-INFLAMMATORY DRUG–ASSOCIATED NEPHROTOXICITY

The widespread use and availability of nonsteroidal anti-inflammatory drugs (NSAIDs), and their use by athletes for prophylaxis of minor soft tissue injuries, presents a potentially serious cause of glomerular damage that manifests as proteinuria. Extensive review of the literature supports the view that combinations of antipyretic analgesics taken in large doses over long periods of time may cause kidney disease and chronic renal failure (23,24). No evidence has been presented to indicate that the use of single NSAIDs taken in small dosages will cause chronic renal disease. NSAID-associated nephrotoxicity accounts for approximately 2% of end-stage renal disease. The prophylactic use of multiple NSAIDs by some athletes to prevent soft tissue inflammation may lead to long-term renal disease and its complications. The team physician should actively educate athletes on the potential risk of NSAID abuse.

GENITAL INJURIES

A variety of genital injuries may occur in sports, especially in gymnastics, cycling, and martial arts. Trauma to the unprotected perineal area of either sex can result in hematoma formation. In women, the vulva is highly vascular and hematoma formation may result from a water skiing accident or a fall onto the balance beam in gymnastics. The male scrotum is highly vascular and prone to hematoma or hematocele formation. This can be a result of a kick to the groin or from trauma that traps the testicle and scrotum against the thigh or bony pubis (long-distance cycling). Ice application and rest are the treatments of choice. More difficult cases should be referred to the urologist.

Injury to the Testicles

The testicles are commonly injured if they are not well protected. These paired structures develop in the retroperitoneum adjacent to the fetal kidney and descend into the scrotum during the eighth fetal month. Many male athletes should use an athletic supporter to elevate the testicles and decrease the discomfort caused by freely hanging organs.

The testes are prone to the development of contusion, epididymitis, or torsion. Direct trauma to the scrotum may cause testicular contusion. The athlete presents with severe pain, nausea, palor, and anxiety. Place the athlete on his back and flex the thighs to his chest to release the spasm of the cremasteric muscle. The use of ice to control bleeding and swelling as well as elevation for 12 to 24 hours is indicated. If pain and nausea persist, torsion of the testicle must be ruled out and the athlete should be referred to a urologist. The team physician should see all significant testicular injuries as soon as possible. If there is an expanding mass that cannot be transilluminated, or if the epididymis cannot be separated from the testicle, a diagnosis of fracture of the testicle or epididymis should be considered.

Scrotal ultrasound may show disruption of the tunica albuginea or epididymis, but may be falsely negative. Radionuclide testicular scan is not very helpful except in delayed evaluation when the viability of the testicle is being considered. Testicular ultrasound with color Doppler should be done quickly to decide whether surgery is needed. If it is needed, it should be accomplished rapidly with a generous scrotal incision. An orchiectomy is performed in most cases (1).

Preexisting scrotal abnormalities may predispose the testicle to increased injury. Consequently, the preparticipation physical examination should carefully evaluate for the presence of undescended testicles, which may be due to anorchia, retractile testes, or undescended testes. Unilateral anorchia is found in 5% of the boys presenting for surgical exploration. This is most often due to torsion of the testicle and infarction before birth and not due to hormonal or fertility abnormalities (1). Most commonly, the undescended testicles reside permanently within the inguinal canal or just inside the internal inguinal ring and cannot be pulled into the scrotum. These testicles require surgical intervention. Patients with undescended testicles are at increased risk for developing testicular cancer and they have decreased fertility.

Torsion of the Spermatic Cord

A single ligament normally prevents mobility of the testis by attaching the lower end of the spermatic cord and epididymis to the scrotum. If the tunica vaginalis is loosely attached to the scrotal lining, extravaginal torsion may occur as the spermatic cord rotates above the testis. Intravaginal torsion occurs when the tunica vaginalis is attached unusually high on the spermatic cord and allows motion of the testis below the deformity. Contraction of the athlete's cremasteric muscle draws the testis up over the pubis and twists it clear of the cord. Torsion of the spermatic cord is less likely to occur if the athlete wears an athletic supporter. Torsion of the appendix testes can also be seen. This clinical presentation can be indistinguishable from torsion of the testis and occurs in a similar age-group (25).

Diagnosis of torsion of the spermatic cord should be kept in mind whenever an athlete has scrotal pain or swelling. It usually occurs in young athletes (10–20 year age-group) who develop increasing abdominal or groin pain. The athlete often experiences abrupt, excruciating testicular pain, vomiting, and eventual collapse. A history of a mobile testis should be ascertained. The patient may also present with an abnormal position of the epididymis, induration of the overlying scrotal skin, a high-riding testicle, or possible obliteration of the space between the epididymis and the cord. All of these conditions should alert the physician to the possibility of testicular cord torsion. Testicular cord torsion is a true emergency and warrants prompt urological evaluation. The torsion is commonly related to vigorous activity, but it is unlikely that activity is responsible for the torsion (26).

The physician normally will find localized tenderness, edema, and hyperemia of the scrotal skin, with the scrotal contents adherent to the skin. The vas deferens is inseparable from the swollen, twisted cord. Epididymitis is a common problem to be differentiated from torsion of the spermatic cord. Elevation of the scrotum usually relieves the pain caused by epididymitis. By contrast, a twisted spermatic cord will cause an increase in testicular and abdominal pain when the scrotum is manually elevated. Other distinguishing features between epididymitis and testicular torsion include (1) loss of cremasteric reflex in testicular torsion, and (2) insidious onset of pain in epididymitis. Torsion of the appendix testis may present with the clinical finding of a small blue dot in the region of the torsion when the scrotal skin is pulled tight over it (25).

If the patient presents within 4 to 6 hours after cord torsion occurs, cooling of the scrotal skin, xylocaine cord block, and manual derotation may be accomplished but should not delay surgical exploration and repair. Color Doppler ultrasonography can be employed to distinguish torsion from epididymitis; Clinical suspicion, however, should override a negative scan. Also, surgical intervention should not be delayed in order to obtain a scan. Testicular torsion usually can be reduced by external manipulation with orchiopexy performed by a urologist at a later date. An irreducible torsion of the spermatic cord should undergo operative exploration to prevent infarction of the testis, which can occur within hours after the onset of torsion. At surgery, the testis is fixed to the scrotum, a procedure that usually prevents further difficulty. It has been described that an ischemic testicle, if left in place, may cause future infertility secondary to a testicular defect on the contralateral side (27).

Scrotal Masses

Testicular cancer is the most common malignancy in 16- to 35-year-old men. When a scrotal mass is discovered, early urologic consultation should be obtained. The presence of a mass in the testicle that is separate from the cord and epididymis is probably due to a malignancy and demands prompt exploration. A mass separate from the testicle should be evaluated by transillumination with a bright light. Masses that cannot be transilluminated should be evaluated by ultrasound and possibly surgical exploration.

Varicocoeles are present in 9% to 19% of all men (25). Such varicosities of the internal spermatic veins may be described as *"a bag of worms"* adjacent to the testicle. Seventy percent of varicocoeles are found on the left side, 20% are bilateral, and 10% are on the right side. Surgical correction of these lesions may be indicated for pain control, diminished ipsilateral testicular size, or infertility.

Cystic masses within the epididymis or adjacent to the testicle are probably spermatoceles, caused by extravasation of sperm from the epididymis following trauma or infection. They require no treatment unless they are extremely large or painful (1). A cystic mass that surrounds the testicle and epididymis is usually a hydrocele, which is caused by decreased absorption of the normal tunica vaginalis secretions due to trauma, infection, or tumors. An acute hydrocele may contain an underlying malignancy and should be investigated by ultrasound or possibly surgical exploration. Traumatic or infectious hydrocele may become large enough to cause significant pain, and surgical correction may be required.

Epididymitis

Testicular pain in male athletes commonly involves a differential diagnosis of spermatic cord torsion or epididymitis. A tender, indurated epididymis may be felt in early epididymitis. Later, the area will become hard and fixed to the skin and the spermatic cord will be swollen and indurated. The patient may develop a fever and an elevated WBC count. Urinalysis is usually positive for leukocytes. Treatment consists of bed rest, Sitz baths, and scrotal support on towels. The most common etiologic agent in men younger than 35 years is chlamydia, and *Escherichia coli* in men older than 35 years. Cultures should be obtained to evaluate for gonococcal infection. If gonococcal organisms are not found on culture, treatment with doxycycline 100 mg PO b.i.d. or tetracycline 500 mg PO q.i.d. is required for 10 to 14 days (15). Gonococcal infection can be effectively treated with ceftriaxone 250 mg IM (15). Athletes with a suspected sexually transmitted disease should be treated empirically for gonorrhea and chlamydia without waiting for culture confirmation.

Penile and Urethral Injuries

The penis is seldom injured in sports. Traumatic irritation of the pudendal nerve in cyclists may cause priapism or ischemic neuropathy of the penis. These symptoms usually resolve when the bicycle race is over. Cyclists should be advised to use a furrowed saddle and avoid squeezing the saddle on uphill climbs.

The erect penis is susceptible to acute trauma and acute fractures of the tunica albuginea. The area of fracture is swollen and ecchymotic and the penis is bent to the affected side. This injury is a true urologic emergency necessitating evacuation of the hematoma and repair of the tunica tear. The patient usually neglects to mention his sexual activity that caused the fracture and ascribes the injury to work or sport-related trauma. Direct blows to the flaccid penis or perineum may lead to vascular injuries and potential impotency. Straddle-type injuries or direct blows to the pubis such as spearing with football helmets cause these injuries. Similar mechanisms could lead to total disruption of the male urethra although this has not been described during sports activities. In the presence of these injuries, a retrograde urethrogram should be performed. Primary repair may be an option, but recent reports indicate that insertion of a transcutaneous suprapubic catheter leads to resolution of the urethral tear in approximately 20% of cases (28). Penile frostbite has been described in runners who wear inadequate clothing in very cold weather. Obviously, adequate protection of the penis and perineum in extremely cold weather is mandatory.

Injuries to the Female Genitalia

Blunt trauma can damage the distal urethra of the female but this is rare as the urethra is well protected. Forced water douche resulting from a fall during waterskiing may cause an incomplete, spontaneous abortion as well as salpingitis. Such a douche can inject water past the vulva into the vagina and oviducts. To avoid this type of injury, female water skiers should wear rubber pants while skiing. Application of ice packs is useful in treating most vulvar hematomas and other common injuries to external female genitalia.

GENITOURINARY INFECTIONS

Urethritis

Sexually transmitted diseases are the most common urologic problem of the athlete. Non-gonococcal urethritis (NGU) is the most common disorder found in the athletic population. Patients will present with dysuria and a urethral discharge. The work-up should include serologic testing for syphilis as well as evaluation for gonococcus and chlamydia. Chlamydia infections respond to a 14-day course of doxycycline 100 mg PO b.i.d. Alternative regimens for chlamydia include azithromycin 1 g PO as a single dose and erythromycin 500 mg PO q.i.d. for 7 days (15,29). A complete sexual history should be obtained, as these infections may be reportable, depending on state law. Sexual partners should be appropriately treated and the patient should be cautioned either to abstain from sexual activity or to use a condom during treatment until the infection has been cleared.

Gonococcal urethritis involves a history of dysuria, penile discharge 2 to 8 days postexposure, and the presence of a positive gonococcal culture. Concomitant chlamydial infection is found in 25% to 45% of cases (1). Owing to the prevalence of penicillinase producing Neisseria and tetracycline-resistant strains, the patient should be treated with intramuscular ceftriaxone 250 mg followed by doxycycline orally 100 mg b.i.d. for 14 days. All sexual contacts should be appropriately cultured and treated. Testing for syphilis and human immunodeficiency virus (HIV) should be offered to the patient.

Prostatitis

Prostatitis involves a history of lower abdominal pain, urethral discharge, and dysuria. The prostate is usually swollen on physical examination, but not always. A urinalysis will typically show increased numbers of leukocytes in the urine. Preferred treatment for acute prostatitis involves ofloxacin 400 mg PO once, then 300 mg PO b.i.d. for 7 days. Chronic prostatitis is best treated with a 14-day course of ciprofloxacin 500 mg PO b.i.d.

Venereal Warts

Condyloma acuminatum is a commonly seen sexually transmitted disease. An increased finding of abnormal cervical pap smears due to the papilloma virus has made it important that venereal warts are appropriately diagnosed and treated. These warts appear as papillary growths on the shelf of the penis, perineum, scrotum, and anal areas. If no lesions are visible, the affected areas are wrapped with a 2% acetic acid–soaked gauze pad for 10 minutes and then examined under magnification. Areas of papilloma virus will appear in a bright light.

Treatment of venereal warts involves freezing, electrical cautery, laser ablation, or local application of one of the various topical agents currently available. The recurrence rate for venereal warts is up to 80% regardless of the treatment. The use of carbon dioxide laser at 1 to 2 watts seems to lead to fewer recurrences with minimal ulceration and scar formation. The use of condoms for 3 months with frequent examinations during that time is indicated. Intraurethral lesions should be treated with urethroscopy and laser ablation or daily intraurethral installation of 5-fluorouracil (5%) for a month.

Herpes Simplex

Herpes progenitalis is a chronic disease with no known cure and presents as an edematous wheal with small vesicles that resolve in 7 to 10 days. These lesions are painful and can become secondarily infected. Topical application of acyclovir ointment or cream decreases pain and works best when the first prodromal symptoms occur. Oral acyclovir, 200 mg 5 times daily for 7 to 10 days may decrease pain or shorten the active period of these lesions during an initial manifestation. Alternative therapies for a first clinical episode include (1) acyclovir 400 mg PO t.i.d. for 7 to 10 days, (2) famciclovir 250 mg PO t.i.d. for 7 to 10 days, or (3) valacyclovir 1 g PO b.i.d. for 7 to 10 days (15,29). The virus will reside continually within the nerve ganglia so that no form of therapy completely resolves the problem. Recommended therapies for recurrent genital herpes include (1) acyclovir 400 mg PO t.i.d. for 5 days, (2) acyclovir 200 mg PO 5 times daily for 5 days, 3) Acyclovir 800 mg PO b.i.d. for 5 days, 4) Famciclovir 125 mg PO b.i.d. for 5 days, or (5) valacyclovir 1 g PO q.d. for 5 days (15,29). Patients with frequent recurrences (>6/year) will benefit from viral suppression therapy (70–80% reduction in frequency) (29). Daily suppression therapy for recurrent genital herpes can be achieved with (1) acyclovir 400 mg PO b.i.d., (2) famciclovir 250 mg POb.i.d., (3) valacyclovir 500 mg PO q.d., or (4) valacyclovir 1 g PO q.d. (29). Owing to the extreme contagiousness of herpes simplex, patients should abstain from sexual activity during the infection stage.

REFERENCES

1. York JP. Sports and the male genital-urinary system. *Phys Sportsmed* 1990;18(10):92–100.
2. Mandell J, Cromie WJ, Caldamone AA, et al. Sports-related genitourinary injuries in children. *Clin Sports Med* 1982;1:483–492.
3. Castenfors J. Renal clearance of urinary sodium and potassium excretion and supine exercise in normal subjects. *Acta Physiol Scand* 1967;70:204–214.
4. Castenfors J. Renal function during prolonged exercise. *Ann N Y Acad Sci* 1978;301:151.
5. Morelli V, Smith V. Groin injuries in athletes. *Am Fam Physician* 2001;64:1405–1414.
6. Goldszer RC, Siegel AJ. Renal abnormalities during exercise. *Your Patient Fitness* 1987;1(3):6–9.
7. Arbarbanel J, Benet A, Lask D, et al. Sports hematuria. *J Urol* 1990;143:887–890.
8. Blacklock MJ. Bladder trauma in the long-distance runner (10,000 meters hematuria). *Br J Urol* 1977;49(2):129–132.
9. Finney J, Baum N. Evaluation of hematuria. *Postgrad Med* 1989;85(8):44–47, 51–53.
10. Hoover DL, Cromie WJ. Theory and management of exercise-related hematuria. *Phys Sportsmed* 1981;9:91.
11. Mariani AJ, Mariani MC, Macchioni C, et al. The significance of adult hematuria: 1000 hematuria dilations including a risk/benefit and cost/effective analysis. *J Urol* 1989;414(2):350–355.
12. Restepo MC, Carey PO. Evaluating hematuria in adults. *Am Fam Physician* 1989;40:149–156.
13. Sutton JM. Evaluation of hematuria in adults. *JAMA* 1990;263(18):2475–2480.
14. Vehaskari VM, Rapola J, Koskimiwa O, et al. Microscopic hematuria in school of children: epidemiology and clinicalpathologic evaluation. *J Pediatr* 1979;95(5 Part I):676–684.
15. Gilbert DN, Moellering RC, Sande MA. *The sanford guide to antimicrobial therapy*. Hyde Park, VT: Antimicrobial Therapy, 2005.
16. Mohr DN, Offord KT, Owen RA, et al. Asymptomatic microhematuria and neurologic disease. A population-based study. *JAMA* 1986;256(2):224–229.
17. Eichner ER. Hematuria—a diagnostic challenge. *Phys Sportsmed* 1990;18(11): 53–63.
18. Siegel AJ. Urinary abnormalities in athletes. *Your Patient Fitness* 1987;1(3): 6–9.
19. Raghavan D, Shipley WU, Garnick MB, et al. Biology and management of bladder cancer. *N Engl J Med* 1990;322(16):1129–1138.
20. Allen TJ. Urology. In: *The merck manual*. Rahway, NJ: 1992:1554, 1557, 1595.
21. Peggs JF, Reinhardt RW, O'Brien JM, et al. Proteinuria in adolescent sports physical examinations. *J Fam Pract* 1986;22:80–81.
22. West CD, Shapiro FL, Swartz CD. Proteinuria in the athlete. *Phys Sportsmed* 1981;9:45.
23. Johnson PJ. Nephrotoxicity associated with the use of nonsteroidal anti-inflammatory drugs. *JAMA* 1984;251(23):3123.
24. Kraus SE, Siroky MB, Babayan RK, et al. Hematuria and the use of non-steroidal anti-inflammatory drugs. *Urologia* 1984;132(2):288–290.
25. Presti JC. Urology. In: *Current medical diagnosis and treatment*. New York, NY: Lange/McGraw-Hill, 2000:920–921.
26. Skoglund RW, McRoberts JW, Ragde H. Torsion of the spermatic cord: a review of the literature and an analysis of 17 cases. *J Urol* 1970;104(4):604–607.
27. York JP, Drago JR. Torsion and the contralateral testicle. *J Urol* 1985;133(2):294–297.
28. Morehouse DD. Delayed management of external urethral injuries. In: Cass A, ed. *Genital urethral trauma oxford*. England: Blackwell Science, 1988:209–222.
29. Centers for Disease Control and Prevention. Sexually transmitted diseases treatment guidelines 2002. *MMWR Recomm Rep* 2002;51(RR-6):1–78.
30. Gardner KD Jr. Athletic pseudonephritis—alteration of urine sediment by athletic competition. *JAMA* 1956;161:1613–1617.
31. O'Brien K. Biker's bladder. *N Engl J Med* 1981;304(22):1367.
32. Galejs LE, Kass EJ. Diagnosis and treatment of the acute scrotum. *Am Fam Physician* 1999.
33. Strauss, RH, ed. *Sports medicine*. Philadelphia: WB Saunders, 1984:130–139.

Dermatologic Conditions in Athletes

17

Delmas J. Bolin

During the course of training and competition, athletes develop numerous skin conditions that are directly related to sports participation. The team physician must appropriately recognize and treat these conditions both in the training room and on the field. Skin problems in athletes generally arise from mechanical, environmental, and infectious causes. The age, skin type, and sex of the athlete influence susceptibility. The physician must consider the physical demands, required equipment, training environment, and the intensity and amount of training when making management decisions. Some skin injuries are directly attributable to technical faults or equipment.

Skin infections are of much higher concern in high contact sports, such as wrestling, where there is significant risk of epidemic spread. The recent increase in methicillin-resistant *Staphylococcus aureus* (MRSA) requires prompt recognition and treatment. Athletes with MRSA, impetigo, molluscum contagiosum, and herpes can spread the disease to opponents, coaches, and teammates, necessitating precompetition skin checks and specific guidelines for return to play.

The management of skin conditions is made easier when identified early by athletic trainers, athletes, and coaches. In many cases, prompt recognition and intervention can prevent many skin problems associated with athletic activity. Developing a treatment plan and preparing a well-stocked coverage bag and training room are essential to return athletes with skin conditions quickly and safely to optimal performance.

TRAUMATIC INJURIES

Lacerations

Skin lacerations during athletic contests must be handled efficiently. Athletes are barred from competition if they are actively bleeding or if they have blood-soiled uniforms. Strict universal precautions should be observed. Often, these wounds can be quickly closed and the athlete returned to competition. Informed consent from the athletes' parent's, particularly in the high school setting, is essential.

After adequate anesthesia is established, the wound should be thoroughly cleaned and irrigated with sterile saline to remove loose debris. Lavage should be accomplished with no smaller bore than an 18-gauge needle to avoid "jet injury" to the tissue. Iodine-containing solutions will sterilize the surrounding tissue, but care should be taken not to introduce them directly into the wound as they can hinder tissue healing. Following sterile preparation, the wound can be closed and protectively bandaged. If stitches are required during competition, it may be most efficient to close the wound temporarily with Steri-strips, then definitively close the wound with stitches at halftime or after the competition.

Planning before the event can assist in efficient return to play for the injured athlete (see Table 17.1). The coverage bag should include a variety of syringes and needles as well as small-unit sterile lidocaine or other anesthetic. Closure material including Steri-strips and tincture of benzoin,

TABLE 17.1
SUGGESTED WOUND MANAGEMENT SUPPLIES FOR THE MEDICAL COVERAGE BAG

Wound cleansing
Sterile saline
Syringe
18-Gauge needle
Antiseptic cleanser
Betadine
Alcohol swabs
Sterile gauze
Antibiotic cream
Anesthetic
Lidocaine
Lidocaine without epinephrine
Ethyl chloride spray
Lidocaine applicator ampules (bee stings)
Wound closure
Bandages and tape
Acrocyanate skin glue (e.g., Dermabond)
Steri-strips
Tincture of benzoin
Suture material
Sterile suture kit
Cold pack
Hemostasis
Aluminum chloride (Drysol) or Lugol's solution
Protection
Second skin
Padding/moleskin

suture material, and sterile kits should be available. Acrocyanate "skin glue" is now commonly used and very effective at closing wounds with good cosmetic result (1). The injury must be clean, dry, and free from active bleeding. Thorough cleaning of the wound is essential before closure to prevent infection. After closure, the athlete can return to play. In settings where there is limited time to address injuries during the competition, such as wrestling or tennis, "skin glue" may provide more efficient closure than stitches.

MECHANICAL INJURIES

Familiarity with the demands of sport and its associated equipment is often overlooked in the prevention of skin injuries. For example, Lacrosse players frequently develop bruising from blocking impact by opponent's crosses. If a player has an injured thigh or shoulder muscle, these areas can be padded to protect them during competition. Familiarity with the required equipment and inspection for improper padding is essential. Unpadded sharp corners may predispose to injury (see Figure 17.1).

Sports participation places the skin at risk primarily through friction and impact, either with the athlete's own equipment or the playing surface. Shear forces or repetitive impacts can lead to subcutaneous hemorrhages. There are numerous conditions that are sports specific, with similar underlying mechanisms.

Talon noir (literally, black heel) is commonly seen in young adults. It consists of horizontal petechiae usually on the posterior or lateral heel (see Figure 17.2). It is most commonly seen in sports that require frequent stops and starts, such as tennis, racquetball, or basketball. The condition is benign, painless, and resolves spontaneously after the season. Similar lesions can appear on the palms (Tache noir) of gymnasts, golfers, and weight lifters. It can be mistaken for melanoma, leading some to biopsy the site. If definitive diagnosis is necessary, the skin can be scraped, mixed with saline and tested for occult blood (2).

Although not involving the skin *per se*, shear forces can separate the skin from underlying tissues, resulting in hematoma formation. In wrestling, shear forces secondary to contact of the ear with the mat can separate skin from underlying cartilage and lead to auricular hematoma (see Figure 17.3). Auricular hematomas must be rapidly recognized, drained, and splinted with a compression dressing to prevent the development of a chronic deformity, cauliflower ear.

Jogger's Nipples are raw, painful, and eroded skin that develops more commonly in male long-distance runners. Friction between the nipple/areolar complex and the shirt fabric during the run results in raw, irritated nipples. Women are usually protected by sports bras. Men can avoid the condition by running without a shirt or by covering the nipples with adhesive bandages or petroleum jelly immediately before running.

There are several other common sports specific conditions that are similar. **Golfer's nails** are small subungual splinter hemorrhages that develop from gripping the club too tightly. Proper grip technique prevents the problem (3). **Mogul skier's palms** are ecchymoses that are seen over the hypothenar eminence secondary to repetitive trauma. Like tache noir, they clear at the end of the season (4).

Piezogenic papules are small, often painful collections of extruded fat on the lateral aspect of the heels (see Figure 17.4). They are usually flesh colored and may only be noticeable when standing. They are commonly seen in long-distance runners. A heel cup may reduce symptoms (5).

Long-distance runners may develop a small area of ecchymosis in the gluteal cleft, known as "**runner's rump**." It is thought to be secondary to prolonged friction at the site, and reassurance is indicated. Rowers develop gluteal lichen simplex chronicus ("**rower's rump**") from prolonged rowing on unpadded seats. Seat padding lessens friction and resolution is speeded with topical fluorinated steroids (2). A thorough understanding of the demands

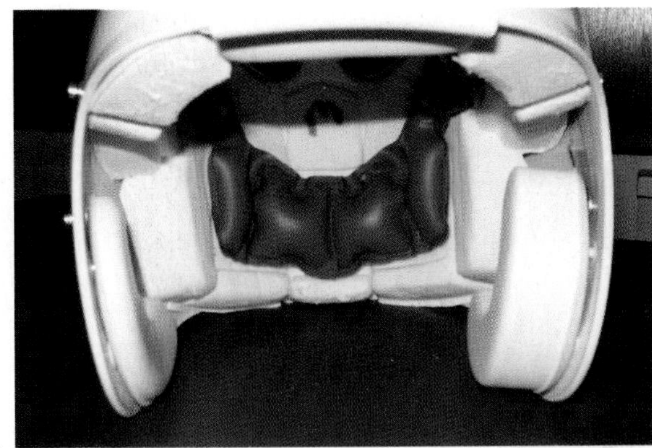

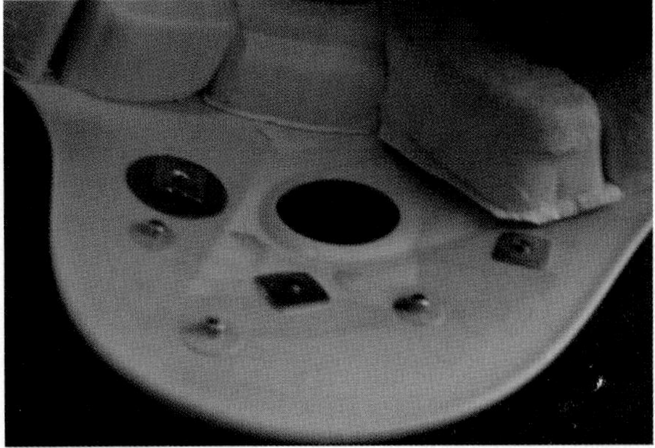

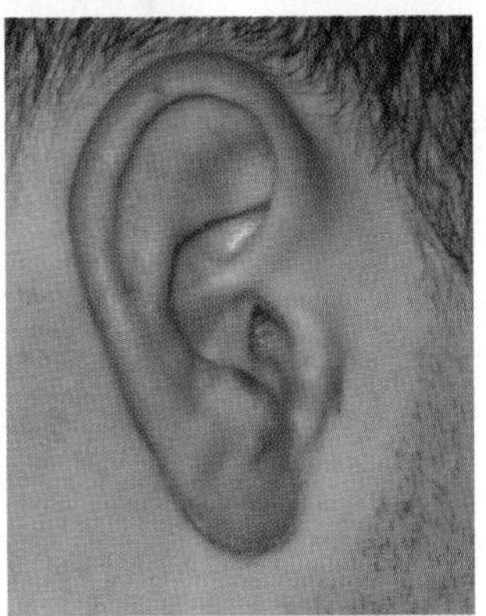

Figure 17.1 **A:** Football helmet ear pads. The 0.5-in. pads on the left side were mistakenly used instead of the unusual 1.5-in. pads on the right. **B:** Three athletes had ear lacerations against the in-beveled ear holes. With the change to 1.5-in. ear pads and smoothing of the ear hole edge, no further lacerations were reported. **C:** An "ear hole" laceration 3 weeks after closure with acrocyanate "skin glue."

of the sport may provide insight into the etiology of the resulting skin lesions.

Abrasions may occur secondary to impact with natural or artificial turf or wrestling mats or by rubbing against improperly fit equipment. During the course of the season, chronic exposure to friction can lead to skin changes, hair loss, or callous formation. For example, soccer goalkeepers often lose the hair of their lateral leg in season due to repetitive diving and sliding (friction alopecia).

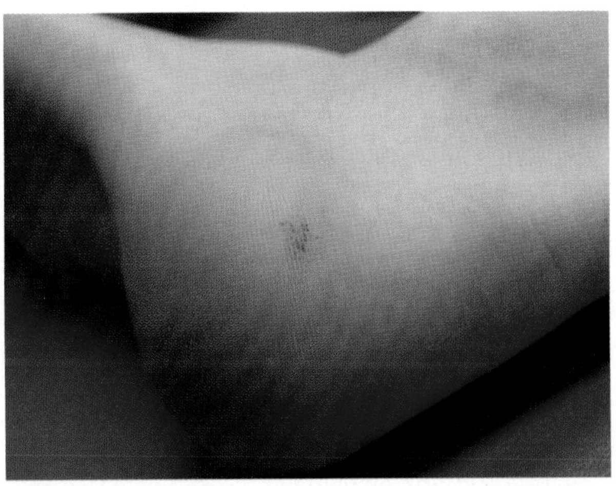

Figure 17.2 Talon noir on the heel of a lacrosse player. The condition results from shear forces on the heel that lead to subcutaneous pinpoint hemorrhage. The lesion resolved spontaneously after the season.

The goals of treatment are symptom relief, protection to prevent further injury, and prevention of infection. The skin is erythematous and there may be clear serous crusting and weeping. The area should be thoroughly cleansed with soap and water. Protective and antifriction lubricants can protect the skin and provide symptomatic relief. Telfa padding with petroleum jelly or antibiotic ointment to reduce friction is often effective.

Blisters from repetitive friction may develop (see Figure 17.5). Common sites are sport-dependent, but are usually on the feet or behind the heels. These usually develop because the athlete has poorly fitting shoes or new shoes at the start of the season. Blisters are typically managed closed, but can be opened and drained if large. Drainage up to three times in the first 24 hours speeds up healing (6). The goal of drainage is to reestablish connection between separated tissue layers. The overlying skin should be left intact to offer protection to the affected area. The practice of injecting blisters with a variety of creams is not supported by the literature as promoting healing and prevents reapproximation of the

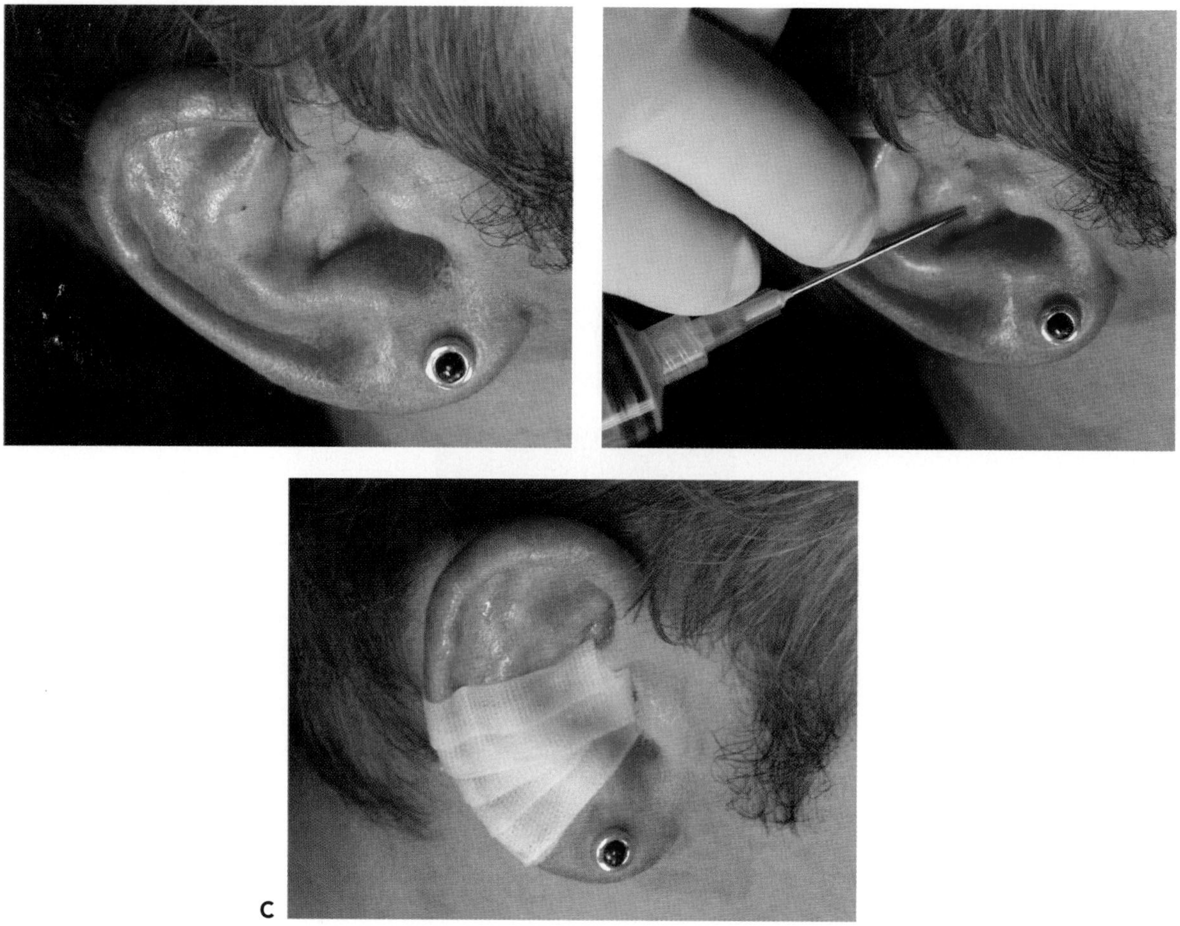

Figure 17.3 **A:** Acute on chronic auricular hematoma in a collegiate wrestler. **B and C:** After drainage, a colloid splint was applied to prevent reaccumulation.

injured tissues. Doughnut bandages made from moleskin can protect and relieve pressure. Moleskin doughnuts can lead to localized fluid collection and should be used with caution in dependent locations.

Athletes should be cautioned about breaking-in new shoes gradually before the start of the season to help prevent calcaneal blisters. Wearing two pairs of socks may prevent blisters, especially if a synthetic fiber is worn against the skin. Synthetic socks wick sweat away from the foot and protect the skin from maceration. Hydrocolloidal antifriction products can be used underneath ankle taping to decrease risk. If infection is a concern, silver sulfadiazine cream can be applied and offers both antifriction and antibiotic protection.

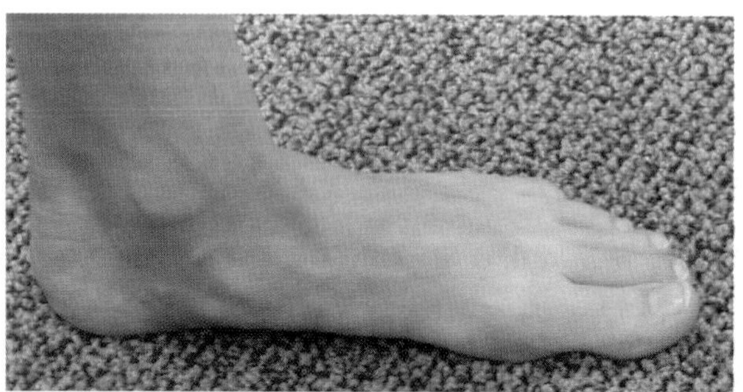

Figure 17.4 Benign piezogenic papules on the instep of a collegiate volleyball player. Papules represent extruded subcutaneous fat and are rarely symptomatic.

Calluses are secondary to hyperplasia of the epidermis and are the most common dermatosis associated with sports. Callus formation is protective and may actually offer a competitive advantage, as they can permit endurance to repetitive trauma that might otherwise cause blisters or pain (7). In weight lifters, palmar calluses (from gripping the bar) or lichenification on the neck (from resting the bar on the neck during "clean and jerk" technique) are signs of dedication and hours of practice (8). Plantar calluses can be difficult to manage in season for most weight-bearing athletes. If symptomatic, the callus can be gently pared or debrided with a pumice stone. Topical salicylic acid plasters or keratolytic emollients (with lactic acid, urea, or salicylic acid) can be used (7). As with management of warts, discussed later, aggressive paring in season should be avoided as it can induce inflammation and make the athlete more uncomfortable. For plantar keratosis, a pad made

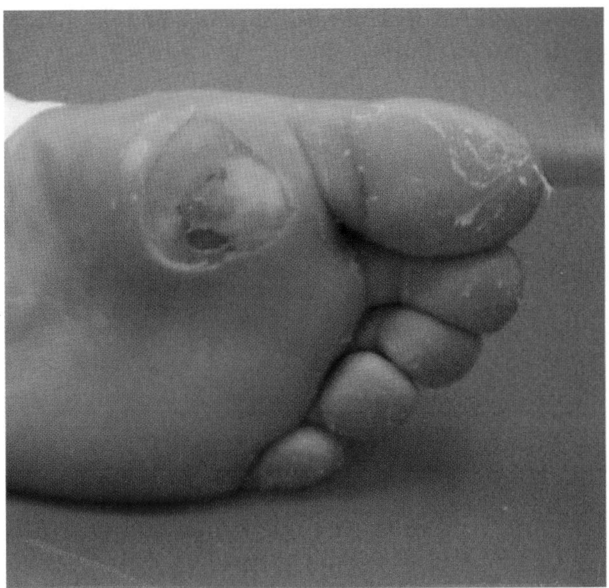

Figure 17.5 Blister on the plantar surface of the first metatarsal head. This athlete drained and removed the skin overlying the blister on the first day of injury. There is peripheral callous formation and a second blister has formed and drained in the base of the first. The overlying skin should be left in place for protection after drainage.

from moleskin or wool can be designed to decrease pressure over the callus and spread the forces to less symptomatic areas of the foot.

Corns are focal accumulations of keratin that develop over pressure points and bony prominences. They are most commonly seen on the toes. Thorough evaluation of shoe fit and appropriate padding may prevent recurrence. Large or symptomatic corns may be treated with debridement or keratolytic emollients, as described earlier (7).

Subungual hematomas are described in many sports (jogger's toe, skier's toe, hiker's toe, climber's toe) and may develop acutely or after prolonged repetitive trauma (see Figure 17.6). Acute traumatic subungual hematoma, resulting from being stepped on by the opponent's cleat, can be quite painful and limit participation. These can be easily released with a portable cautery unit. A small drain hole is made with cautery through the nail. Once the pressure is released, padding can be applied and the athlete returned to play. Long-standing subungual hematomas require no treatment. The discoloration will grow out with the nail. If multiple shades of pigment are noticed under the nail, or if the discoloration leaches to the proximal nail fold, the lesion should be biopsied to rule out melanoma.

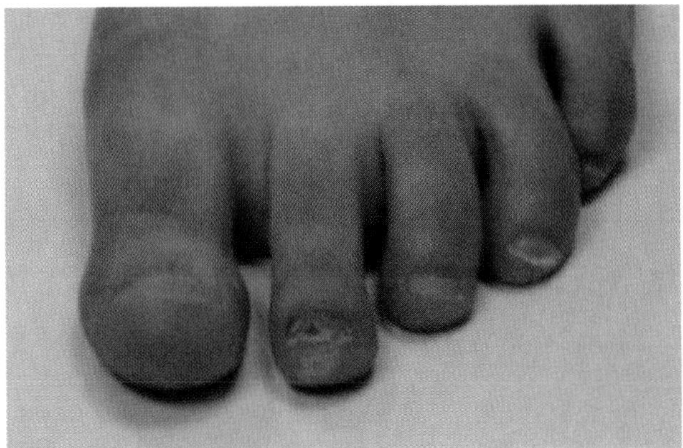

Figure 17.6 Jogger's nails. Subungual hematoma in the second toe of a runner from repetitive trauma.

Connective tissue nodules (collagenomas) may develop at sites of repetitive pressure or trauma. These have been described as "**surfers nodules**" but may be seen in football players or boxers. If the athlete has severe pain, the nodules can be injected with corticosteroid or excised. Often, no treatment is required (9).

Swimmer's shoulder is usually seen in unshaven male freestyle swimmers. It is an erythematous plaque on the shoulder that occurs secondary to beard friction against the skin. Shaving prevents the problem (10).

ENVIRONMENTAL INJURIES

Sun Exposure

Because many sports are played outside, chronic exposure to sun may increase the athlete's risk for long-term complications of sun exposure, including thinning of the skin and skin cancer. Sunburn is the most common sun-related skin disorder. Care should be taken to avoid high intensity sunlight without protection, especially during the period of 10 a.m. to 3 p.m. Complications of sunblock use include risk of contact dermatitis from sunscreen additives and slightly increased incidence of folliculitis with oily preparations (11). Some athletes do not like the residue from oily sunblocks; however, the benefits far outweigh the risks. The sports physician should counsel athletes to limit sun exposure as much as possible, especially those with fair complexions who burn easily. As year-round tanning has become trendy, athletes should be counseled to limit exposure in tanning beds as well.

Sunscreens are available that protect against ultraviolet (both UVA and UVB) rays. These should be applied copiously 30 minutes before exercise and repeated after periods of intense sweating or water immersion. Use of water-resistant formula enhances protection. A shirt may be used for protection; however, the effectiveness is decreased as the material becomes wet. Darker materials absorb more photo-energy and are more protective. Sunblock should be used under the clothing (12).

Treatment consists of symptomatic treatment for minor burns. Cool compresses and low-dose topical steroids may be used. Second-degree burns may require systemic corticosteroids as well as topical treatments. The burn can be covered with a nonadherent dressing for protection. The burn should be re-evaluated in 2 to 3 days, as the full extent of injury is often not apparent until 48 to 72 hours after exposure.

There has recently been controversy suggesting that swimmers are at increased risk of skin cancer because of exposure to sun. Epidemiological studies suggest that the greater risk is to swimmers who swim in polluted water, where the skin is exposed to potential carcinogens. The sports physician should counsel young athletes to use appropriate sunblock and avoid swimming in open waters where contamination may be present (12).

Photosensitivity may develop in athletes who are taking one of the several general classes of medications. There are more than 50 medicines that are associated with photodermatitis; the likelihood of a reaction with any one of these drugs is highly variable (13). Photosensitivity may develop with certain soap, deodorant, and perfume additives. The symptoms may be similar to sunburn, but can also include blisters, swelling, and rash. The athlete should be counseled to avoid direct sunlight while taking these medications. If a reaction occurs, the medication should be discontinued. In severe cases, corticosteroids or immunosuppressant therapy may be used. If sun exposure cannot be avoided, alternative appropriate medication, if available, should be considered. Table 17.2 lists several commonly prescribed medicines and additives that are associated with photosensitivity.

TABLE 17.2

MEDICATIONS, SUPPLEMENTS, AND ADDITIVES THAT ARE ASSOCIATED WITH PHOTODERMATITIS

Prescription medication
Antibiotics
- Tetracyline
- Doxycycline
- Minocycline
- Ciprofloxacin (Cipro)
- Cotrimoxazole (Batrim, Septra)

Anti-inflammatory
- Indomethacin (Indocin)
- Nambutone (Relafen)
- Naproxyn sodium (Aleve)
- Ibuprophen (Motrin, Advil)

Diuretic
- Thiazides (hydrochlorothiazide)

Antiallergy
- Diphenhydramine

Over-the-counter and herbal medicines
- Benzoyl peroxide (Clearasil, Oxy-10)
- St John's wart
- Anise
- Dong Quoi
- Tribulus terrestris (Tribestan)

Additives
- Bergamot oil (mint or citrus scented soaps, shampoo)
- Citrus fruit (psoralens)
- Coal tar (eczema creams)

There are more than 50 medicines that can cause photosensitivities, the most common are presented here.

Heat

Hot and humid conditions may lead to miliaria. Two forms are commonly encountered. Miliaria crystalline consists of "dew drop" vesicles on a warm erythematous base. Treatment includes cold compresses that lead to a rapid resolution of this self-limiting condition. Miliaria rubra consists of deeper, erythematous papules. These can be longer lasting, and exercise should be limited to times when the ambient temperature is lower (7).

Cold Exposure

Extremities exposed to prolonged periods of cold may be injured. There is a continuum between early superficial injury (frostnip) and deeper tissue injury (frostbite). Frostnip is the most common form of cold injury, representing freezing of the skin and superficial subcutaneous tissues. It commonly occurs on exposed areas such as the nose and ears. It presents as numb white areas of skin. Symptoms can persist for up to 72 hours. Vesicles may form. Treatment involves gentle rewarming using warm damp compresses or running warm water. Rubbing should be avoided as it can denude the vesicles. Prevention can be achieved by covering the skin. Creams offer some protection against the sun and cold, but thin insulated ski-masks are available and should be used for outdoor sports requiring prolonged exposure to low temperatures (14). Multiple layers are protective.

Frostbite is a deeper tissue injury that progresses from numbness to blisters and necrosis. Rapid rewarming in water at 39°C to 44°C (102.2°F to 111.2°F) for 20 minutes is the treatment of choice. Rewarming should only be completed once the athlete has been rescued and there is minimal risk of refreezing. This avoids further tissue damage caused by freeze–thaw cycles. Once cold injury has occurred, the effected area is often cold sensitive for prolonged periods thereafter (15).

Pernio is a localized area of vasoconstriction resulting in painful nodules. Women are more commonly affected. Exposed extremities are most at risk, including the dorsal aspect of the toes and distal toes, hands, ears, and nose. It may be associated with a paresthesia and pruritus. Skiers, mountain climbers, and other cold weather sport athletes are at risk. Warm woolen socks are helpful for its prevention.

Allergic Dermatitis

The most common contact dermatitis is "poison ivy" (see Figure 17.7). The allergic reaction is to ursinol, a chemical in the sap of Toxicodendron plants, which leads to vesicle formation on an erythematous base. The lesions are typically in a linear distribution and can last 10 days to several weeks. Golfers, hunters, and cross-country runners

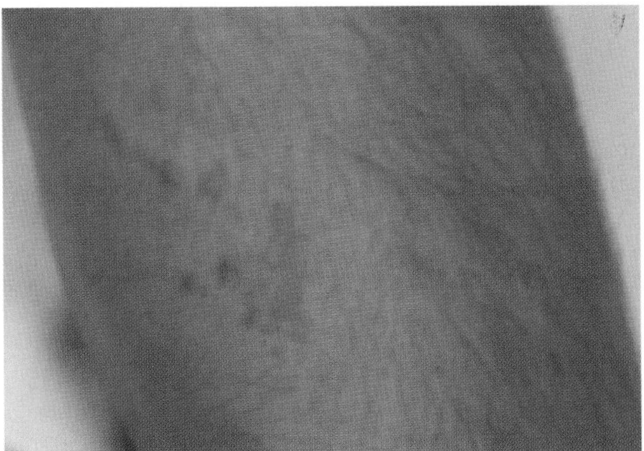

Figure 17.7 "Poison ivy" resulting from contact with the resin of toxicodendron plants. Note the linear pattern of reaction, typically caused by leaves brushing against skin.

are at greatest risk. Athletes who are exposed should quickly clean any contaminated skin, clothing, and shoes. Resin can remain on the clothes and later provoke an allergic reaction. Immediate skin cleansing with plain soap, emulsifiers, or with chemical modifiers is between 50% and 70% effective in preventing the rash (16). Traces of resin can remain under the fingernails. Exposed persons should clean under the nails with soap or a lipid emulsifier, water, and a nailbrush to avoid further spread. The sites themselves are not contagious once cleaned. They should be covered to prevent secondary infection. Treatment is often with topical or systemic steroids, usually for 10 to 21 days to prevent reflare, which can occur if treatment is withdrawn too early (17). Newer topical agents, such as pimecrolimus (Elidel), have not been demonstrated to be effective (18). Nonsedating antihistamines or topical aluminum acetate can be helpful in controlling the itch.

Irritant contact dermatitis can also be seen with common field line markings, such as calcium oxide. Mixed with water or sweat, it becomes a potent base and can induce rash (19).

Contact dermatitis can also arise from synthetic components of sports equipment, including swim masks (ethyl butyl thiourea) and hockey sticks (fiberglass). The diagnosis is usually made by the history and characteristic distribution of the erythematous and pruritic eruption. Equipment made with alternative materials should be acquired. Topical steroids are helpful to control the reaction (20).

Urticaria (hives) occur in response to many triggers, including activity. Exercise-induced urticaria is commonly seen in runners. Cholinergic urticaria occurs in response to increased body temperatures. Swimmers can have aquagenic urticaria. Cold urticaria may be precipitated by exposure to ice or cold temperatures (see Figure 17.8). Hives are usually pruritic, well-defined edematous erythematous plaques of varying sizes. Treatment involves antihistamines with variable response. Systemic steroids are not usually effective. Lesions usually remit spontaneous within 24 hours. Signs of difficulty breathing, swallowing, or talking should be sought to rule out anaphylaxis.

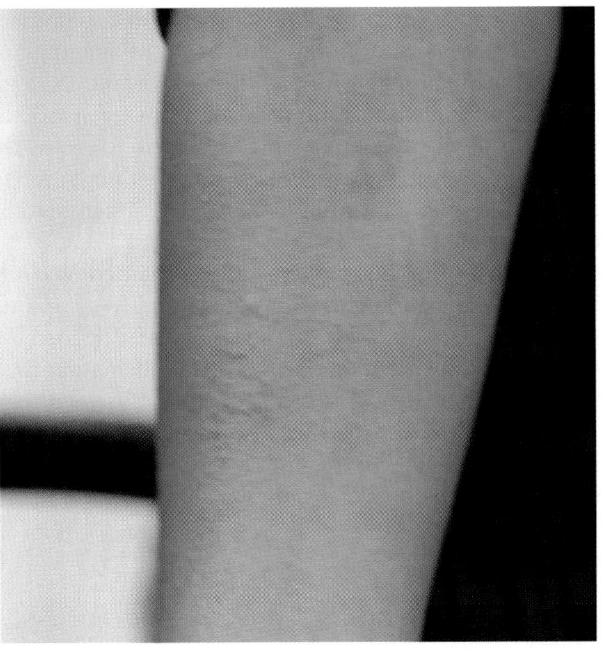

Figure 17.8 Cold urticaria. The papules developed on this cross-country runner's forearm after 5 to 7 minutes of cold pack exposure. The athlete complained of generalized hive formation during outdoor running in the winter months. The symptoms resolved with administration of a systemic antihistamine.

Sting of insects should be anticipated during outdoor sports. Although usually experienced as an irritation, systemic symptoms can and do occur. For the patient who experiences anaphylaxis, rapid administration of epinephrine (EpiPen) should be available. For those who merely have pain and little local reaction, topical anesthesia in a small ampule can be rapidly applied to the skin, and results in several minutes to 2 hours of pain relief. If the stinger is still in place on the wound site, care should be taken to remove it without squeezing more of the venom into the wound and increasing the severity of the response. If a player experiences systemic symptoms, both the player and the traveling medical staff should have an EpiPen each available at the field.

INFECTIOUS DISEASE

Sea-bather's and Swimmer's Itch

A common condition seen in recreational swimmers and scuba divers with prolonged contact with seawater. The eruption is an irritating pruritic dermatitis that is usually confined to the areas covered by bathing suits. The causative organism is the larva of *Edwardsiella lineata* and *Linuche unguiculata*. Each larva has a multiple stinging mechanism and injects toxin to the skin, which results in the pruritus (21). Swimmer's itch is caused by actual invasion of the skin by the parasites (22).

In sea-bather's itch, the first symptoms are usually seen within 24 hours of exposure and consist of stinging and a maculopapular rash with or without urticaria. The rash can persist for a week and severe cases, usually associated with skin allergy to the toxin, may last up to 6 weeks. The distribution is usually in the region of the bathing suit. The condition responds to antihistamines, topical steroids, and antipruritics (21).

Swimmer's itch tends to spare areas protected by clothing and appears only on water-exposed skin. The symptoms start on evaporation, with organisms penetrating the skin, accompanied by a prickling sensation. Erythematous macules appear and may be associated with diffuse erythema and urticaria. Vesicles or pustules suggest secondary infection. Treatment is symptomatic and the condition is self-limited, usually resolving over 10 days to 2 weeks (22).

Viral Infections

Herpes: epidemics of herpes have been reported in wrestling (Herpes gladiatorum) and rugby (Herpes rubeiorum). Skin lesions are caused by Herpes Simplex virus type 1 and are mainly seen on the head and upper torso of athletes in sports in which direct skin-to-skin contact and trauma occur. Infection may have a short prodrome of tingling or itching at the site. The typical lesion is a cluster of small vesicles on an erythematous base. Late infections may demonstrate only erosions (see Figure 17.9). The lesions are painful and may be accompanied by fever or regional lymphadenopathy. Diagnosis is confirmed with Tzanck smear, culture, or immunofluorescence (20). Treatment includes careful unroofing of the vesicles and treatment with a desiccant, such as benzoin or aluminum chloride, to facilitate drying. Treatment of initial infections with oral valacyclovir 1,000 mg twice daily for 10 days decreases symptoms and speeds up healing compared to other antiviral agents. Three- to 5-day courses are prescribed for recurrent outbreaks (23). Topical preparations are less effective than oral preparations and continue to be controversial (24). The trainer and physician should protect their skin from direct contact with the lesions to prevent herpetic whitlow, a painful herpes infection of the hand or finger.

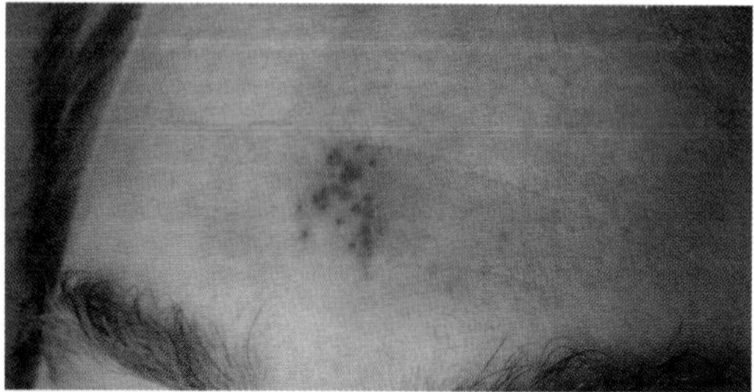

Figure 17.9 Herpes gladiatorum on the forehead of a collegiate wrestler. The lesions are several days old and demonstrate erosions. Early symptoms may include paresthesia, followed by the appearance of small vesicles on an erythematous base.

Return to play guidelines for wrestling are frequently revised. The current requirements are that the lesions be dry, crusted, and covered, and the athlete be treated with antiviral medication 5 days before competition (25).

Prophylaxis is an important issue as herpes gladiatorum can be an epidemic. With the National Collegiate Athletic Association (NCAA) treatment requirements, there is a significant risk of missing competitions with new or recurrent infection. For those known to have had herpes gladiatorum, but no outbreaks in the past 2 years, valacyclovir 500 mg is effective in preventing outbreaks in the season. Others with herpes gladiatorum should use valacyclovir 500 mg twice daily as prophylaxis (26).

Warts

Human papilloma virus causes warts on the hands and feet. Warts are usually well defined, verrucous plaques and papules on the hands and soles. They can be differentiated from callous and corns by paring. Pinpoint hemorrhages are seen in pared warts, but not with callous. A central core is seen with corns. Destructive treatments, such as excision, cryosurgery, bleomycin injection or salicylic acid, induce inflammation and the resulting pain can cause an athlete to lose practice and competition time. Topical acid treatment can be inconvenient for the athlete, as it requires soaking the wart in warm water for several minutes before application. The dead skin must be pared away daily. Several weeks or months may be necessary to achieve results.

Immunotherapy has recently been promoted to help clear viral warts. Intralesional candida injections may stimulate an immune response. A recent small trial found that 74% of participants who were injected with either candida or mumps antigen had resolution of the injected lesion; 78% had complete resolution of all noninjected warts (27). Cimetidine has been used in doses of 30 to 40 mg/kg/day to treat warts. The mechanism is thought to be its ability to stimulate T cell activity. A study in children demonstrated that cimetidine is as effective as topical treatments or cryotherapy (28).

Topical imiquimod has recently been used to treat lesions and is gaining in popularity because of its convenience and relatively few side-effects (23). In general, if lesions are large, paring can be used in season to control the symptoms; more definitive treatments can wait until the off-season, when inflammation interferes less with competition. Athletes should wear shower-sandals in the locker room and shower to prevent spread of infection.

Molluscum contagiosum are small (2–3 mm) papules with a central dimple (umbilication). These are frequently found on the abdomen or thighs of wrestlers and swimmers. This infection is more frequently associated with nonathletic activities. Treatment is usually by sharp curettage and cauterization of the base. Alternative treatments such as topical imiquimod (1%) for 1 month (29) or systemic griseofulvin for 3 to 4 months can also be effective (14).

Bacterial Infections

Impetigo is a bacterial infection caused by Streptococci or Staphylococci species. It is found most commonly in sports with traumatic skin-to-skin contact such as football, wrestling, and rugby. The lesions are erythematous plaques with "honey-crusted" lesions usually on the upper extremity, torso, head, and neck. Antibiotics are indicated. Oral regimens include cephalexin 500 mg t.i.d. to q.i.d. or dicloxacillin 500 mg t.i.d. Erythromycin can be used if the athlete is penicillin allergic. Topical mupirocin has been demonstrated to be equally efficacious in treatment when used twice daily for 10 days. Return to play is suggested after treatment for 5 days, but there are no evidence-based studies to demonstrate that this prevents transmission. Athletes can reduce transmission by not sharing equipment or towels. There is no evidence to suggest that equipment serves as a reservoir for infection.

Furunculosis (a "boil") is a Staphylococcus or Streptococcus infection of the hair follicles. Up to 20% of basketball players and 25% of football players will develop furunculosis (30). In this population, the athlete is more likely to develop a furuncle if they have skin trauma and direct skin-to-skin contact with a furuncle. The lesions are erythematous painful nodules on the upper extremity and torso. Treatment is similar to that for impetigo, with oral or topical antibiotics and warm soaks. If fluctuance is present, the lesion can be opened for drainage. The lesions should be covered with occlusive dressings to prevent contact during activity. There is no evidence to guide return to play decisions; if no systemic signs are present and the lesion can be reliably covered, then the athlete may be allowed to participate while under treatment. Multiple cases should alert the sports medicine team to the possibility of Staphylococcus colonization of the nares. Colonization can be eradicated with intra-nares mupirocin twice daily for 1 week. Complications are rare, but cases of poststreptococcal glomerulonephritis ("scrum kidney") have been reported after furunculosis (31).

Furunculosis caused by MRSA has become much more prevalent in training rooms since 2000 (see Figure 17.10). MRSA has now been reported in epidemic outbreaks on football and wrestling teams. Spread is associated with close contact, colonization with the MRSA bacteria, skin trauma from synthetic turf, and cosmetic shaving (32).

The impact of MRSA in athletic populations has recently been reviewed (33,34). The USA-300 MRSA strain is the most common community acquired type (CA-MRSA) seen in athletic populations and has a different virulence than the hospital-acquired variety. Hospital strains of MRSA have a larger Staphylococcus cassette chromosome (SCC) coding for *Panton-Valentine leukocidin*, a gene that increases tissue penetration. CA-MRSA SCC lacks this complete virulence factor.

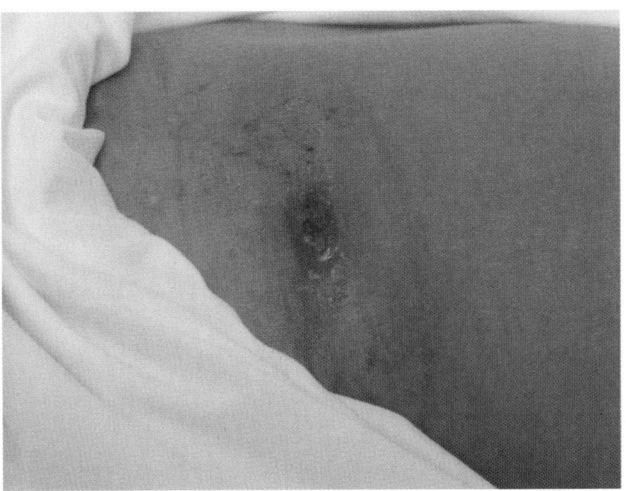

Figure 17.10 Methicillin-resistant *Staphylococcus aureus* (MRSA) infection in the left thigh of a high school volleyball player. Despite the patient's effort to drain the lesion, pockets of purulence remained. With drainage, cleaning, and a course of trimethoprim/sulfamethoxazole at 10 mg trimethoprim/kg/day, the lesion resolved uneventfully.

In managing MRSA infections of skin and soft tissues, some general principles should be followed. High index of suspicion should be maintained. Areas that are exposed and subject to minor skin trauma are frequent sites of MRSA infection. The wound should be cleaned and any purulence should be incised, drained, and well irrigated. It is important to culture the wound and determine antibiotic sensitivities. CA-MRSA is often sensitive to more commonly used antibiotics. A retrospective study found that most infections did not require hospitalization or surgical debridement but could be managed as outpatients when treated in this way (35). Antibiotic treatments are required and the treating physicians should consult the latest recommendations. Trimethoprim/sulfamethoxazole combinations should be administered twice daily in the dosage 10 mg Trimethoprim/kg/day and is currently considered effective for treating CA-MRSA. This is equivalent to two double strength tablets twice daily (33). There are many new antibiotics available. These should be reserved for more aggressive infections.

Pseudomonas or "hot-tub" folliculitis is frequently seen in athletes who use whirlpool and hot tubs for recreation or as part of rehabilitation. The lesions are small erythematous follicular and occasionally green papulo-pustules (20). They are seen on submerged skin surfaces around the axilla and groin and are sometimes associated with areas covered by bathing suits. Abraded skin appears to be most commonly affected. In about half the cases, associated systemic symptoms of fatigue, lymphadenopathy, and fever may be present (36). *Pseudomonas aeruginosa* type O:11 is most commonly isolated from cultures (37,38). Treatment has been suggested to increase the risk of recurrence and is thought necessary only when systemic signs and symptoms are present (37). When treatment is indicated, ciprofloxacin

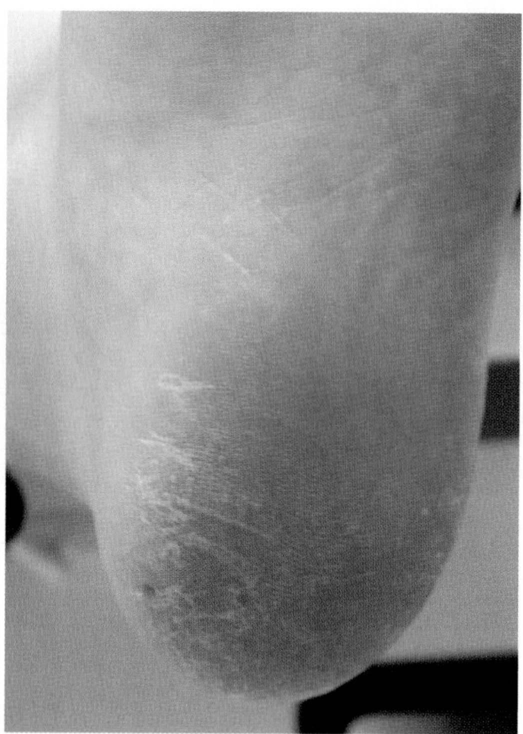

Figure 17.11 Pitted keratolysis on the heel of a cross-country runner. This condition had been present off and on for many years, but resolved with topical clindamycin treatment for 2 weeks.

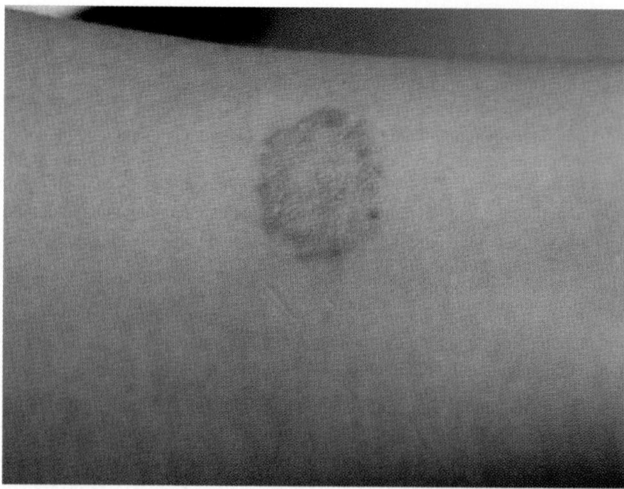

Figure 17.12 Tinea Corporis. Ringworm present on the arm of a collegiate athlete. The central clearing is typical, but may be absent if the athlete presents very early for care.

250 mg twice daily for 10 days is effective (37). Pool conditions, including proper cleaning and adequate pH and chlorine levels, can help prevent infections (12). Athletes with lesions or abrasions should use occlusive dressings before using the pool (37).

Pitted keratolysis (see Figure 17.11) is an infection found on the soles of athletes whose feet are macerated after long exposure to moist, warm, occlusive conditions. Tennis and basketball players are commonly affected. The infection is caused by Corynebacterium and micrococcus species and is characterized by discrete pits and foul odor in the heel of the foot (12). Treatment includes topical clindamycin or erythromycin (20). It is prevented by the use of synthetic socks and avoidance of prolonged occlusion in athletic shoes.

Acne mechanica occurs due to heat, friction, and tight occlusive equipment, such as knee or shoulder pads. The typical appearance is small pustules and papules on an erythematous base, usually on the back, shoulders, and chin. Lesions can be difficult to treat, requiring topical antibiotics or keratolytic agents. Good hygiene and sweat-wicking underclothing can be helpful in clearing the outbreak (20).

Fungal Infection

In wrestling, where epidemic spread has been reported, fungal infections can result in temporary disqualification from competition. Tinea corporis gladiatorum is the fungal infection found on the torso, upper extremities, head, and neck of wrestlers (see Figure 17.12). Epidemiological studies show that 24% to 77% of team members have positive fungal cultures (39–41). The causative organism is commonly *Trichophyton tonsurans*. Direct skin-to-skin contact and sharing of towels and equipment are considered significant sources of spread (42). Mats are not thought to be a significant reservoir for fungal infection, although fungus was cultured from a mat in one study (43). Infection occurs in sports such as wrestling, football, and rugby, in which sweating, maceration, and skin trauma increase the chance of transmission.

The typical lesion is a well-demarcated erythematous scaling plaque with central clearing. Unfortunately, hypervigilant wrestlers often present early for evaluation, before the typical central clearing is present. Diagnosis is often clinical, but can be confirmed by examining the lesion scraping treated with potassium hydroxide under a microscope. Potassium hydroxide reveals branching hyphal elements with a sensitivity of 88% and specificity of 95% (44).

Treatment with either topical or systemic antifungal medication is effective. Topical treatments may take several weeks, but are well tolerated and available in relatively inexpensive generic forms. Systemic treatments are more expensive, have more side-effects, and require greater monitoring. Systemic treatments show promise for rapid treatment and perhaps prophylaxis of tinea corporis. In a recent study, 100% of athletes taking weekly fluconazole (100 mg) had negative cultures at 3 weeks (45). Precompetition skin checks are required for NCAA matches, and athletes may not compete unless the lesions can be covered and treatment has been ongoing for 120 hours before competition (25). A recent survey of Pennsylvania scholastic wrestlers indicated that 85% of schools had at least one wrestler diagnosed with ringworm and 33%

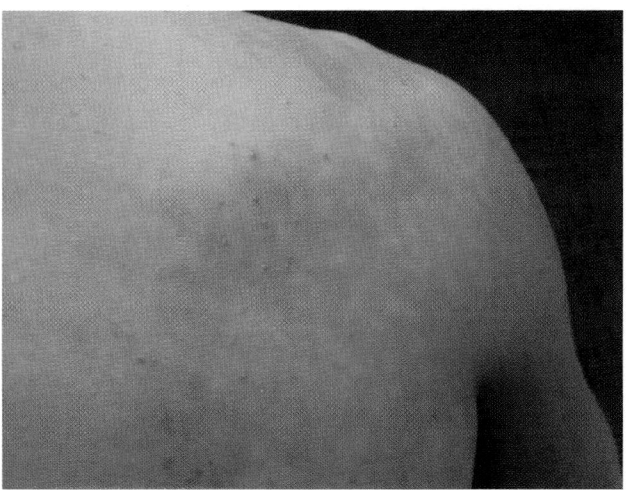

Figure 17.13 Tinea Versicolor. Caused by *Malassezia furfur*, the infection leads to hypopigmentation and is marked by a high rate of recurrence in susceptible individuals.

had a wrestler held from competition (46). Consequently, systemic antifungals are frequently used during periods of frequent competition when a wrestler has a history of fungal infection.

Tinea versicolor is a common benign infection caused by *Malassezia furfur*. As the name implies, its presentation is varied, but is most commonly marked by hypopigmentation (see Figure 17.13). Hypopigmentation can persist for some time after the infection is treated. The lesions are often more pronounced on darkly pigmented skin. Treatment includes topical antifungal preparations and selenium sulfide. Systemic antifungal medications can also be used, but do not prevent the high rate of recurrence in susceptible individuals.

Athlete's foot, tinea pedis, is commonly seen on the soles, insteps, and interdigital areas (see Figure 17.14). Risk factors include occlusive footwear, skin maceration, and trauma. Topical medications are effective for limited disease, whereas systemic medications can be used for extensive or recalcitrant cases. Topical treatments have cure rates of 47% to 70% whereas systemic treatments have cure rates of 72% to 94% (see Table 17.3) (47). Prevention includes keeping the feet dry by using synthetic socks, and limiting exposure in the locker room and shower by using sandals (20).

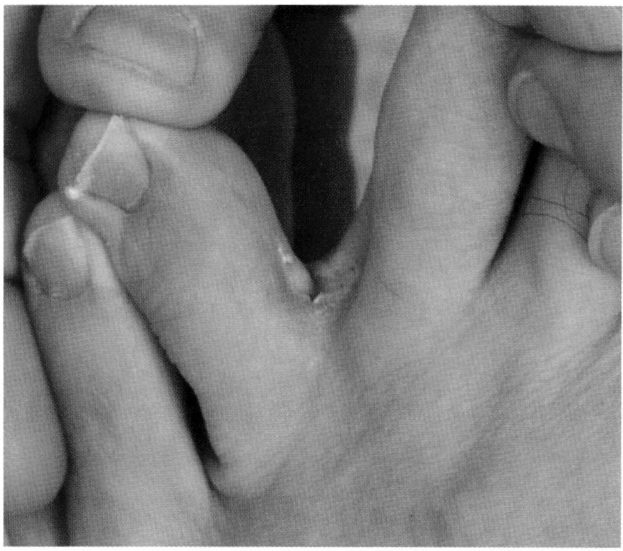

Figure 17.14 Tinea Pedis. Maceration and yeast superinfection in the fourth interdigital space in a collegiate soccer player. Interdigital spaces should be inspected to rule out occult sources of infection. The condition is easily treated with good foot hygiene and topical antifungal medications.

SUMMARY

Numerous skin conditions can affect athletic performance. Coaches, athletic trainers, and players should be allies in identifying problems early and seeking care. A well-stocked training room and event bag are essential for returning athletes to play as quickly and safely as possible after injury. Infections pose a significant risk for epidemic spread among certain athletic populations and should be

TABLE 17.3
SELECTED MEDICATIONS FOR TREATMENT OF FUNGAL SKIN INFECTIONS

Drug	Cure Rate	Form	Frequency and Duration	Price, Availability
Miconazole	47%	2% Lotion, cream	b.i.d. 2–4 wk	Inexpensive, OTC
Ketoconazole	—	2% Cream	b.i.d. 2–4 wk	Inexpensive, prescription
Terbinafine	70%	1% Cream	b.i.d. 1–2 wk	Shorter, Rx, OTC
Fluconazole	90%–100%	100-mg tablet	qwk, length Rx Prophylactic, q1–2wk	Expensive, Rx only
Itraconazole	90%–100%	400 mg	q2wk, prophylactic (41)	Expensive, Rx only

OTC = over the counter; Rx = by prescription; b.i.d. = twice daily; qwk = once weekly.

rapidly identified and treated. The sports medicine team can anticipate and prevent numerous skin conditions by understanding the demands of the sport, the environmental conditions, and the equipment used.

REFERENCES

1. Mattick A. Use of tissue adhesives in the management of paediatric lacerations. *Emerg Med J* 2002;19:382–285.
2. Pharis DB, Teller C, Wolf JE. Cutaneous manifestations of sports participation. *J Am Acad Dermatol* 1997;36:448–459.
3. Ryan AM, Goldsmith LA. Golfer's nails. *Arch Dermatol* 1995;131:857–858.
4. Swinehart JM. Mogul skier's palm. *Cutis* 1992;24:318.
5. Basler RSW. Skin lesions related to sports activity. *Prim Care* 1983;10:479–494.
6. Cortese TA, Fukuyama J, Epstein WL, et al. Treatment of friction blisters. *Arch Dermatol* 1968;97:717–721.
7. Helm TN, Bergfeld WF. Sports dermatology. *Br J Sports Med* 1998;16:159–165.
8. Scott MJ, Scott NI, Scott LM. Dermatologic stigmata in sports: weightlifting. *Cutis* 1992;50:141–145.
9. Cohen PR, Eliezri YD, Silvers DN. Athlete's nodules: sports related connective tissue nevi of the collagen type (collagenomas). *Cutis* 1992;50:131–135.
10. Koehn GC. Skin injuries in sports medicine [letter]. *J Am Acad Dermatol* 1991;24:152.
11. Conklin RJ. Common cutaneous disorders in athletes. *Sports Med* 1990;9:110–119.
12. Adams BB. Sports dermatology. *Adolesc Med* 2001;2:305–322.
13. Gonzalez E, Gonzalez S. Drug photosensitivity, idiopathic photodermatoses and sunscreens. *J Am Acad Dermatol* 1996;35:871–885.
14. Basler RSW. Managing skin problems in athletes. In: Mellion MB, Walsh WB, Madded C, et al. eds. *The team physician's handbook*, 3rd ed. Philadelphia: Hanley and Belfus, Inc, 2002:311–325.
15. Fisher AA. Sports-related cutaneous reaction. Part I: dermatoses due to physical agents. *Cutis* 1999;63:134–136.
16. Stibich AS, Yagan M, Sharma V, et al. Cost effective post-exposure prevention of poison ivy dermatitis. *Inj J Dermatol* 2000;39(7):515–518.
17. Craig K, Meadows SE. What is the best duration of steroid therapy for contact dermatitis (rhus)? *J Fam Pract* 2006;55(2):166–167.
18. Amrol D, Keitel D, Hagaman D, et al. Topical pimecrolimus in the treatment of human allergic contact dermatitis. *Ann Allergy Asthma Immunol* 2003;91(6):563–566.
19. Fisher AA. Sports-related cutaneous reactions. Part III: sports identification marks. *Cutis* 1999;63:256–258.
20. Adams BB. Dermatologic disorders of the athlete. *Sports Med* 2002;32(5):309–321.
21. Basler RSW, Basler GC, Palmer AH, et al. Special skin symptoms seen in swimmers. *J Am Acad Dermatol* 2000;43:299–305.
22. Mulvihill CA, Burnett JW. Swimmer's itch: a cercarial dermatitis. *Cutis* 1990;46:211–213.
23. Brown TJ, McCrary M, Tyring SK. Antiviral agents: non-antiviral drugs. *J Am Acad Dermatol* 2002;47:581–599.
24. Nikkels AF, Pierard GE. Treatment of mucocutaneous presentations of herpes simplex virus infections. *Am J Clin Dermatol* 2002;3(7):475–487.
25. Bubb R, ed. *2002–2003 NCAA wresting rules and interpretations.* Indianapolis: NCAA, 2002.
26. Anderson BJ. The effectiveness of valacyclovir in preventing reactivation of herpes gladiatorum in wrestlers. *Clin J Sports Med* 1999;9:86–90.
27. Johnson SM, Robertson PK, Horn TD. Intralesional injection of mumps or candida skin test antigens, a novel immunotherapy for warts. *Arch Dermatol* 2001;137:451–455.
28. Rogers CJ, Gibney MD, Sigfried EC, et al. Cimetidine therapy for recalcitrant warts in adults: is it any better than placebo? *J Am Acad Dermatol* 1999;41:123–127.
29. Syed TA, Goswami J, Ahmadpour OA, et al. Treatment of Molluscum contagiosum in males with analog of imiquimod 1% in cream: a placebo-controlled double blind study. *J Dermatol* 1998;25:309–313.
30. Conclin RJ. Common cutaneous disorders in athletes. *Sports Med* 1990;9:100–119.
31. Mast EE, Goodman RA. Prevention of infectious disease transmission in sports. *Sports Med* 1997;1:1–7.
32. Begier EM, Frenette K, Barrett NL, et al. A high-morbidity outbreak of methicillin-resistant Staphylococcus aureus among players on a college football team, facilitated by cosmetic body shaving and turf burns. *Clin Infect Dis* 2004;39(10):1446–1453.
33. Ellis MW, Lewis JS. Treatment approaches for community-acquired methicillin-resistant Staphylococcus aureus infections. *Curr Opin Infect Dis* 2005;18(6):496–501.
34. Rihn JA, Michaels MG, Harner CD. Community acquired methicillin resistant Staphylococcus aureus—an emerging problem in the athletic population. *Am J Sports Med* 2005;33(12):1924–1929.
35. Romano R, Lu D, Holtom P. Outbreak of community-acquired methicillin resistant staphylococcus aureus skin infection among a collegiate football team. *J Athl Train* 2006;41(2):141–145.
36. Centers for Disease Control and Prevention (CDC). Pseudomonas dermatitis/folliculitis associated with pools and hot tubs—Colorado and Maine, 1999—2000. *MMWR* 2000;49:1087–1091.
37. Green JJ. Localized whirlpool folliculitis in a football player. *Cutis* 2000;65:359–362.
38. Silverman AR, Nieland ML. Hot tub folliculitis: a familial outbreak of Pseudomonas folliculitis. *Arch Dematol* 1983;8:153–156.
39. Adams BB. Tinea corporis gladiatorum: a cross-sectional study. *J Am Acad Dermatol* 2000;43:1039–1041.
40. Beller M, Gessner BD. An outbreak of tinea corporis gladiatorum on a high school wrestling team. *J Am Acad Dermatol* 1994;31:197–201.
41. Hazen PG, Weil ML. Itraconazole in the prevention and management of dermatophytosis in competitive wrestlers. *J Am Acad Dermatol* 1997;36:481–482.
42. Kohl TD, Lisney M. Tinea gladiatorum: wrestling's emerging foe. *Sports Med* 2000;29:439–447.
43. El Fari M, Gräser Y, Presber W, et al. An epidemic of tinea corporis caused by Trichophyton tonsurans among children (wrestlers) in Germany. *Mycoses* 2000;43:191–196.
44. Haldane DJ, Robart E. A comparison of calcofluor white, potassium hydroxide, and culture in the laboratory diagnosis of superficial fungal infections. *Diagn Microbiol Infect Dis* 1990;13:337–339.
45. Kohl TD, Martin DC, Nemeth R. Fluconazole for the prevention and treatment of tinea gladiatorum. *Pediatr Infect Dis J* 2000;19:717–722.
46. Kohl TD, Giesen DP, Moyer J, et al. Tinea gladiatorum: Pennsylvania's experience. *Clin J Sports Med* 2002;12:165–171.
47. Markova T. What is the most effective treatment for tinea pedis? *J Fam Pract* 2002;51:21.

Acute Infections

18

Christopher A. McGrew

Acute infections are a common source of morbidity and time loss from sports-related activity for all types of athletes. Within college and professional athletic training rooms, acute infections can be the cause of up to 50% of the visits to the trainer or physician (1). Most of these infections will be evaluated and treated in athletes in a similar way to those patients not involved in sports and athletic activity, but there are a variety of special circumstances that the health care provider who works with these populations should be aware of. Additionally, health care providers involved in the care of athletes need to be cognizant of the effects of acute infection on exercise as well as special considerations for treatment of specific illnesses and return-to-play decisions. (Skin infections such as tinea, herpes gladiatorum and methicillin-resistant Staphylococcus aureus (MRSA) are covered in Chapter 17 on Dermatology)

GENERAL EFFECTS OF EXERCISE ON THE IMMUNE SYSTEM

The innate immune system includes anatomic and physiologic barriers (e.g., skin, mucous membranes, temperature, pH), specialized cells (natural killer (NK) cells and phagocytes including neutrophils, monocytes, and macrophages) and inflammatory barriers. When the innate immune system fails to effectively combat an invading pathogen, the body mounts an acquired immune response. The acquired immune system includes special cells called B and T lymphocytes that are capable of secreting specialized chemicals such as antibodies and cytokines to regulate the immune response. T lymphocytes can also engage in direct cell-on-cell warfare. Acute episodes of vigorous activity have the following effects on the immune system (lasting 3 to 72 hours): stress hormone induced neutrophilia and lymphopenia, decrease in NK cell cytotoxic activity, decrease in the delayed type hypersensitivity response, increase in plasma cytokines, decrease in nasal and salivary Immunoglobulin A (IgA) concentrations and nasal neutrophil function and blunted major histocompatibility complex (MHC) II expression and antigen presentation in macrophages. Chronic exercise effects have been more difficult to document. Attempts thus far to compare resting immune function in athletes and nonathletes have failed to provide evidence that athletic endeavor is linked to many specific changes in the immune system, although epidemiologic studies have shown decreased upper respiratory infections in some groups of regular exercisers when compared to nonexercisers ("the J-curve theory"). Of all immune measures only NK cell activity has emerged as a somewhat consistent indicator differentiating the immune systems of athletes and nonathletes. NK cell activity has been reported to be higher in athletes when compared to nonathletes in several studies (2,3).

EFFECTS OF ACUTE INFECTIONS ON EXERCISE CAPACITY—GENERAL CONSIDERATIONS

Acute infectious disease is often associated with a fever and it is difficult to differentiate some of the effects of fever on exercise from the effects of the acute illness. In general it is recognized that fever impairs muscle strength, aerobic power, endurance, coordination, fluid/temperature regulation and concentration (4–6). All of these effects are obviously detrimental to optimal performance. Additionally, acute infections are associated with a variety of immune system responses that are triggered by cytokines and are correlated to fever, malaise and anorexia along with other signs and symptoms (7). Acute viral illnesses can potentially hinder exercise capacity not only by the direct fever effects noted earlier, but also with such influences as muscle protein catabolism, tissue wasting and negative nitrogen balance. These effects result in decreased muscle performance, the full recovery of which may require weeks to months after a week long febrile illness (8). Although the relation is not completely understood, exercise during or just after an acute viral illness may be a risk factor for rhabdomyolysis (9). Respiratory infections, probably the leading cause of acute illness in athletes, have been shown to have negative effects on respiratory function (10).

PHARMACOTHERAPY CONSIDERATIONS

Most of the acute infections in athletes are viral in nature such as upper respiratory tract infections and gastroenteritis. Athletes often present requesting that everything possible be done to ensure that they train and compete. The temptation to presumptively treat these infections with antibiotics is great but should be resisted. Antibiotic treatment side effects such as diarrhea, rashes, nausea, yeast infection, and allergic reactions can negatively influence training and competition and are hard to justify when the antibiotics are not really treating a viral illness. (On the other hand, there does not appear to be a direct ergolytic effect on either muscle strength or endurance from the use of antibiotics.) The increasing problems of resistant strains of bacteria along with unnecessary costs of treatment are other issues to be considered as well. Photosensitivity is a potential problem with some antibiotics such as doxycycline. Quinolones are contraindicated in young athletes with open growth plates and there are case reports about fluoroquinolones and Achilles tendon problems (11). Additionally, potential performance decreasing effects need to be considered when prescribing to the athlete (e.g., sedating antihistamines would not be a good choice for many athletes). Even some antibiotics have been linked to decreased performances.

The use of agents to treat the symptoms of these acute infections must also be evaluated in the context of drug testing that athletes might be subjected to in various sports. Decongestants, antihistamines, cough suppressants, antidiarrheals, and bronchodilators are all commonly used. The health care professional treating athletes must be aware of various banned drug lists for the different sports and organizations that oversee these sports. Toll free telephone hot lines and internet websites are available for most of these groups such as the United States Olympic Committee and the National Collegiate Athletic Association (NCAA), which give details of the medications that are prohibited (http://www.usantidoping.org/).

RESPIRATORY TRACT ILLNESSES

Colds and Upper Respiratory Tract Infections

The upper respiratory tract is the most common site of infection in humans accounting for more than half of all acute illnesses. Upper respiratory tract infections (URTIs) involved affect the respiratory mucosa from the nose to the lower respiratory tree, not including the alveoli. Over 200 viruses are implicated as the cause of common colds/URTIs of which rhinoviruses, coronaviruses, respiratory syncytial virus, influenza virus and adenoviruses are the leading agents of infection. (Several bacteria are responsible for a small percentage of URTIs.) Viral URTIs occur throughout the year although there are seasonal peaks in the autumn and spring. Transmission occurs by aerosol and droplet spread, direct saliva contact and indirect saliva contact. These modes of transmission raise the obvious need for good hygiene in order to limit outbreaks among athletic teams. Frequent washing of hands by athletes and their coaches and attendants is the most vital step. Other important measures include avoidance of sharing of implements such as water bottles and towels, along with proper hydration and carbohydrate replacement before, during, and after exercise (12).

Symptoms and signs of URTIs are manifold and can include both local and systemic findings. The latter suggest a more serious infection and a greater need for restriction of activities (see "neck check" described later).

Some of the specific concerns for athletes include the following:

1. Intense exercise during the incubation phase of an infection may result in a more severe illness (13).
2. Intense exercise while infected with enteroviruses (such a coxsackievirus) may increase the risk for contracting myocarditis that has been reported as a cause of sudden death during exercise (8).
3. The aforementioned risk of rhabdomyolysis (9) has been reported in athletes performing intense exercise during, or just after the acute phase of a viral illness.

   Unfortunately, there are no clinically proven methods of determining in advance which athletes are likely to be susceptible. Fortunately, myocarditis and rhabdomyolysis are rare sequelae.

In general the treatment of URTIs is aimed at symptom relief and support of the athlete's fluid and energy needs. There are thousands of brand names and generic cold remedies on the market and most them include mixtures of antihistamines and decongestants. Oral and topical decongestants may help relieve upper respiratory symptoms. Topical nasal decongestants work better and faster than oral agents, but, because of rebound congestion or tolerance, the topical products can be used for only 3 to 5 days. If they are used continuously for 1 to 2 weeks or more, rhinitis medicamentosus—chronic nasal stuffiness—can occur as a result of drug dependency. First-generation antihistamines appear to reduce sneezing and nasal discharge but have no effect on nasal stuffiness. Though their benefits are thought to be due to anticholinergic effects rather than to their effect on histamine, anticholinergic side effects such as orthostasis and disruption of thermoregulation can impair athletic performance. There is no evidence that decongestants or antihistamines change the natural history of the illness.

Herbal and "natural" remedies have become increasingly popular but support for them is sparse. Fluids and easily digestible carbohydrate sources should be made readily available to the athlete and saltwater gargles and saline nasal irrigation are useful adjuncts to symptom relief without unwanted side effects. Warm fluids such as soups and teas may have temporary effects on relieving congestion symptoms along with cultural psychological benefits. Aspirin should not be used in athletes under the age of 21 for fever and myalgia relief because of the association with Reye's Syndrome (13); instead acetaminophen and ibuprofen should be utilized. A few studies have supported the use of zinc gluconate lozenges in the first 24 to 48 hours of the onset of URTI for reduction of the duration and intensity of symptoms (13).

Athletes are responsible for everything that goes into their bodies. Some over the counter (OTC) preps contain banned substances. Athletes also need to be reminded that supplements are not Food and drug Administration (FDA) regulated and may also contain banned substances.

It is unlikely that heavy training during acute febrile illness would be very beneficial. When advising an athlete with acute illness on when to exercise, an intuitive "neck check" approach (14) has been suggested:

> If the athlete only has symptoms "above the neck" such as sore throat, nasal congestion, and rhinorhea, then he/she can probably continue to exercise to the level of tolerance if symptoms improve during the first few minutes of the exercise session.
>
> If the athlete has symptoms below the neck, such as chest congestion that causes respiratory compromise, fever (temperature greater than 38°C), chills, or mylagias, then abstinence from all but the mildest exercise is recommended.

It is useful to evaluate the type of activity that is planned when advising the athlete who is acutely ill. Distinctions can be made between sports as well as between training versus competition within a single sport. For example golf and diving obviously have different demands than soccer and basketball and the effects of an acute infection might be better tolerated in the former two examples as opposed to the latter. Training for football (e.g., a 2 to 3-hour continuous practice) is much more demanding metabolically than the 10 to 15 minutes of actual playing time for a given player with all of the "down time" that is involved in the football contest. In contrast, soccer with its continuous activity would present a much more continuous demand on the athlete that is similar to his/her practice. Another issue to consider is that an athlete may tolerate skills training in a particular area of their sport (e.g., batting practice or free throw shooting), but wouldn't be able to tolerate intense conditioning drills for their sport. These are just a few examples of the variability for each athlete that should be considered when evaluating what activities are appropriate to partake in when an acute infection is present.

Influenza A and B deserve special consideration, due to their potential severity and potential for specific prevention. Pulmonary function is frequently abnormal for weeks and constitutional symptoms can be quite severe. This may have a tremendous impact on athletes and an outbreak in a team can be devastating. It seems to be of pragmatic value to recommend vaccination of athletes, especially those whose seasons are primarily during the winter months.

(Classic Influenza Vaccination Recommendations for inactivated influenza vaccination have targeted specific groups for annual immunization, including persons older than 6 months who are at high risk for complications from influenza because of age or presence of certain medical conditions, persons who are in close contact with those at high risk, persons aged 50 to 64 years, and close contacts of infants aged 0 to 6 months (1). Vaccination is also encouraged, when feasible, for children aged 6 to 23 months and their close contacts and caregivers. In addition, physicians should administer the flu vaccine to any person who wishes to reduce the likelihood of becoming ill with influenza. http://www.cdc.gov/mmwr.)

Influenza A and B have been shown to respond to oseltamivir orally and zanmivir by inhalation. These therapies are only effective if started within 24 to 36 hours of the onset of symptoms. Outbreaks in nonvaccinated teams may be curtailed with daily prophylaxis with one of these agents for 2 weeks after administration of vaccine (14).

The diagnosis of a URTI is usually straightforward; however, in some cases there may be some confusing issues. Chronic, recurrent and seasonal occurrence may indicate the possible contribution of allergic and/or vasomotor rhinitis that can mimic a URTI, especially if there is a strong cough component. These entities can often be very effectively treated with a well-planned treatment of nasal saline irrigation, oral antihistamines and/or nasally applied corticosteroids or cromolyn sodium. URTIs are often associated with concurrent wheezing and subclinical bronchospasm during the time of acute illness and frequently there are postinfection problems with training such as unaccustomed dyspnea and/or exercise related coughing. The measurement of expiratory peak flow rates may be helpful in evaluation of such patients and a trial of albuterol for preexercise inhalation may be useful in alleviating symptoms. Another problem is the overuse of antibiotics for URTIs that are overwhelmingly caused by viral agents. Antibiotics should be reserved for use in the very small percentage of patients with a URTI who develop purulent sinusitis, or whose URTI symptoms are due to Group A beta-hemolytic streptococcal pharyngitis, or whose severe, prolonged (>10 days) course might indicate infection with an antibiotic susceptible entity such as *Mycoplasma pneumoniae, Chlamydia pneumoniae* or *Bordetella pertussis* (14).

Pharyngitis

Most cases of pharyngitis are viral in nature, and require only symptomatic treatment such as warm saline gargles, antipyretics, analgesics, fluids, and appropriate rest. In athletes with large hydration and caloric demands, aggressive treatment of pain of the sore throat is very important so that the athlete will not forego appropriate intake of food and liquids. As mentioned previously, the use of zinc gluconate lozenges may be useful for reducing the duration and severity of symptoms if started early after their onset (13). Sore throat associated with fever, swollen tonsils, exudates and tender anterior cervical adenopathy with the absence of coryza, cough, sinus congestion and other peripheral symptoms is suggestive of Group A beta-hemolytic streptococcus (GABHS) and/or infectious mononucleosis (IM); these entities call for more specific attention in diagnosis and treatment.

Group A Beta-hemolytic Streptococcus

Rapid strep tests are available for the diagnosis of GABHS, but throat culture is still the gold standard for diagnosis. Treatment for GABHS is primarily for prevention of rheumatic heart disease and can be started up to 10 days after the onset of illness. There is limited evidence that early treatment within 24 hours of onset of symptoms is effective in reducing the duration and severity of symptoms of streptococcal pharyngitis by a short period (less than a day) (15). Some athletes who have experienced GABHS previously may express a sentiment that they "get better quicker" with treatment and this will often prompt them to request antibiotic treatment at the first sign of any sore throat, so careful evaluation and education of these patients is necessary to avoid overtreatment. Penicillin is the first choice for treatment, but many options are available for the penicillin allergic such as erythromycin, clarithromycin, azithromycin and clindamycin. Return-to-activity criteria are the same as for any acute febrile illness.

Infectious Mononucleosis

IM is an acute, generally self-limiting, viral lymphoproliferative disease caused by the Epstein-Barr Virus (EBV). EBV is secreted in saliva and has an incubation period of 30 to 50 days so there is ample opportunity for the disease to be spread unknowingly. The attack rate is highest from ages 15 to 25 with 25% to 50% of those infected developing the classic syndrome which includes a 3 to 5 day prodrome with headache, fatigue, loss of appetite, malaise and myalgias, followed by the classic signs and symptoms over days 5 to 15 of sore throat with tonsillar enlargement, moderate fever, tender anterior and posterior cervical lymph nodes, petechiae of the palate, and swollen eyelids. A palpable enlarged spleen is present in 50% to 75% of cases; jaundice can occur in 10% to 15%. Serologic diagnosis (IgM) can be made with a rapid slide test based on heterophil antibody absorption (Monospot), but it may be negative in the first week to 10 days after onset of symptoms, so it should be repeated weekly if initially negative. Up to 10% to 15% of patients with clinical IM will repeatedly test negative for heterophil antibody (16). Other techniques such as immunoflourescence or enzyme linked immunosorbent assay may be necessary to make the diagnosis. Aggressiveness in "nailing down" the diagnosis is justified in some cases because of the return-to-play implications for the athlete (17).

Other laboratory tests are useful in IM. A complete blood count (CBC) may show moderately elevated concentration of WBCs with a marked lymphocytosis (>50%) and atypical lymphocytes (10% to 20% of white blood corpuscles (WBCs)). Liver function tests will show increased results in most cases reflecting mild hepatitis. GABHS is concurrent in 5% to 30% of cases and appropriate testing should be done. (Although the GABHS may not always be pathogenic, it seems prudent to treat with appropriate antibiotics—not ampicillin—when GABHS is cultured.)

Although IM affects most organ systems, complications occur in less than 5% of cases (17). Complications associated with IM can include splenic rupture, airway obstruction, peritonsillar abscess, autoimmune hemolytic anemia, thrombocytopenia, aplastic anemia, Guillan-Barre syndrome, encephalitis, aseptic meningitis, transverse myelitis, optic neuritis, severe hepatitis, hepatic necrosis, myocarditis, pericarditis, pneumonia, orchitis, and glomerulonephritis. There is no evidence to suggest that, with the possible exception of splenic rupture, significant complications are either triggered by exercise or more common in those who exercise as tolerated during and after the acute phase of the disease (18).

The spectrum of patient responses to IM ranges widely: many patients have significant acute symptoms along with significant weakness and extreme fatigue; on the other hand, some patients will only have mild symptoms that do not prompt a visit to a health care provider. After resolution of the acute clinical symptoms, fatigue and malaise may persist for longer periods—usually not longer than 6 weeks. Up to 10% of patients experience the fatigue and malaise for much longer. Some elite athletes may take up to 3 to 6 months to regain full performance capacity (18).

The treatment for IM is primarily symptomatic and supportive. This will include relative rest, acetaminophen or non-aspirin nonsteroid anti-inflammatory drugs (NSAIDs) for fever, aches, and throat pain. (NSAIDs should be avoided when there is thrombocytopenia or hemolysis.) Sore throat may also be aided by lozenges, salt water gargles, and in some cases viscous lidocaine. Codeine may be useful in those with refractory pain, but may cause constipation. Stool softeners can be used to avoid straining during bowel movements. Fluids and adequate nutrition that is palatable is important for minimizing weight loss and/or muscle wasting. Corticosteroids are only indicated for complications such as impending upper-airway obstruction (19,20).

Return to some amount of activity can be relatively soon for most patients with IM. Welch et al. studied the aerobic capacity of military cadets who were recovering from IM and concluded that they could begin a non-contact exercise program as soon as they became afebrile and did not have any significant complications (21). If the athlete feels well, is afebrile, and has normal liver functions, return to noncontact activity can progress as tolerated. The time for such developments may range from a few days after diagnosis to weeks or in some cases, months. Most patients will be well in 4 to 6 weeks (18,19).

Probably the most common question about return to contact activity for the athlete with IM concerns splenomegaly and the risk for splenic rupture. Although splenomegaly is present in most IM cases, splenic rupture is rare, occurring in 0.1% to 0.5% of all IM cases. Some of these ruptures may occur in spleens that are not significantly enlarged. Almost all cases of splenic rupture occur within the first 3 weeks from the onset of illness. Most splenic ruptures are associated with routine daily activities such as lifting, bending, and straining at defecation, not with direct trauma and/or sports activity. Although for many it seems intuitive that splenomegaly and splenic rupture are closely related, it really is not clear what the connection is. What might be more important than the actual spleen enlargement are structural and cellular changes that occur in the spleen during the first few weeks of the illness in relation to the profuse lymphocyte infiltration. This process may stretch and weaken the splenic capsule and supporting internal architecture of the spleen resulting in a "fragile state," regardless of its size (20,22).

It is important to note that physical examination techniques for evaluation of spleen size have poor sensitivity and specificity (23). Although the use of sonography or computerized tomography (CT) is very accurate in determining spleen size, recent data describing normative spleen size in a population of 631 collegiate athletes demonstrated considerable variability of normal spleen size. Because of this wide variability, a single diagnostic imaging measurement is considered unreliable as conclusive proof of splenic enlargement (24). At this time there is no specific evidence to either definitively support or refute the use of ultrasound or CT assessment of spleen size in the routine management of mononucleosis in athletes. Diagnostic imaging such as ultrasound or CT is indicated in cases of suspected splenic injury (24).

A pragmatic approach to management of the athlete with mononucleosis and return-to-play is as follows: educate the athlete about the need for "listening to one's body" during recovery and appropriate supportive care for symptoms. Inform the athlete (and his/her family if a minor) that splenic rupture is a rare but real complication that has the potential for significant morbidity and potential mortality. Additionally, information should be given about the signs of splenic rupture and an emergency plan of action, should they occur. Finally, advise the patient that splenic rupture is statistically more likely to occur in an everyday, nonsport activity. With this background information, the athlete should be allowed to progress in activity as they feel fit to do so, except with restrictions on heavy Valsalva activities and contact until 3 weeks from the first day of the illness (the period for most splenic ruptures). Obviously, any complicating factors (e.g., hepatitis, encephalitis, etc.) will extend this return to play according to the individual athlete's recovery pattern.

Acute Sinusitis

Acute sinusitis is defined as an inflammatory condition, often associated with infection, that involves the paranasal sinuses and air spaces. Although any athlete can be affected, those involved in water sports such as swimming, diving, surfing, and water polo appear to have a higher risk of developing sinusitis (25). The primary pathology in sinusitis is the obstruction of the ostial openings. This obstruction is commonly due to swelling/inflammation of mucosa in and around the ostia caused by allergies and URTIs. This leads to decreased oxygen tension, decreased clearance of foreign material, accumulation of fluid, mucosal edema, and secondary infection. Approximately 30% of cases of sinusitis are allergic or viral. The most common bacterial causes are *S. pneumoniae*, *H. influenzae*, and *B. cartarrhalis*; up to 10% of cases may be caused by anaerobes (26).

Recent trends in medical treatment have questioned the appropriateness and timing of antibiotic use in uncomplicated acute sinusitis (27). Three-day treatment courses have been shown to be as effective as 10-day courses in acute, noncomplicated maxillary sinusitis. First-line antibiotics (amoxicillin, trimethoprim/sulfamethoxazole [TMP/SFX], erythromycin) are as effective as, and much less expensive than, newer agents. Topical decongestants along with saline nasal irrigation are useful in attempts to open ostia that are obstructed. Control of allergy effects on ostia with appropriate antihistamines or topical agents may also be indicated.

Return-to-play considerations with acute sinusitis are similar to those of the common URTIs (see "neck check" described earlier). Scuba diving should not be allowed until the sinusitis is resolved, as the atmospheric-sinus pressure disequilibrium from an obstructed ostia can cause sinus wall mucosal damage and bleeding (barosinusitis) (28).

Acute Bronchitis

Acute bronchitis is defined as a respiratory infection characterized by inflammatory change in the bronchial tree, leading to recurrent cough. Viral infections cause most cases of bronchitis; a much lesser number have bacterial etiologies. As with acute sinusitis, there are many controversies and uncertainties in the general medical literature concerning bronchitis, and thus it is not surprising that little information has arisen to help direct the treatment of athletes with acute bronchitis (29). One extensive review article showed no significant difference between drug and placebo, and the two studies that did showed only small clinical differences. In terms of helping symptoms, albuterol had an impressive advantage over erythromycin in the studies reviewed. The authors concluded that antibiotics should not be used in the treatment of acute bronchitis in healthy persons unless convincing evidence of a bacterial infection is present (30). In one large meta-analysis the findings suggested a small benefit from the use of the antibiotics erythromycin, doxycycline, or trimethoprim/sulfamethoxazole in the treatment of acute bronchitis in otherwise healthy patients (less than half day in reducing the duration of illness symptoms). As this small benefit must be weighed against the risk of side effects and the societal cost of increasing antibiotic resistance, the authors believed that the use of antibiotics was not justified in these patients (31). However, many athletes might consider even a small change in the duration of symptoms worthwhile, if in the middle of their competitive season.

Once the diagnosis is made and a general management plan is initiated, there are some special considerations for athletes: (a) impairment in respiratory flow dynamics—the use of peak flow measurements may be useful as an objective measure for making decisions on return to play as well as the use of bronchodilators, (b) intense exercise may cause impairment of mucociliary clearance as well as brief periods of immune suppression—the athletes who attempts to train vigorously through bouts of acute bronchitis may place themselves at risk by lowering their resistance to secondary bacterial infections, pneumonia, and a prolonged course of illness (29).

Pneumonia

Pneumonia is a lower respiratory infection characterized on the chest radiograph by interstitial or alveolar infiltrates. In studies of healthy young adults, common respiratory viruses cause 30% to 50% of pneumonias with some variation based on the time of the year. *S. pneumoniae, H. influenzae, M. pneumoniae* and *Chlamydia pneunomiae* are the primary nonviral pathogens. Diagnosis and treatment are well described in standard medical textbooks and journals (32,33).

Pneumonia causes a much greater insult to pulmonary function than does bronchitis. Rapid return to training and competition should not be the primary goal of any therapeutic program, rather the healthcare provider should focus on the complete resolution of the infection. Without taking appropriate recovery time, the athlete may face a greater risk of complications such as persistent infection, abscess, or empyema (29).

Mycoplasma pneumonia is common in college students; fortunately this has the shortest duration of any common pneumonia. Often all pulmonary changes resolve in 2 to 4 weeks and relatively little pulmonary scarring occurs, so training may proceed relatively rapidly after the acute phase resolves. On the other hand, pneumococcal pneumonia resolves more gradually and may require 4 weeks to several months to return to normal pulmonary status. The other common entities fall somewhere within this spectrum. Before return to extensive activity for any athlete, an objective measure of normal or near-normal pulmonary function is desirable. As the athlete returns to activity, monitoring of heart rate and perceived exertion levels can be helpful in guiding the intensity of workouts (29,34).

ACUTE OTITIS MEDIA AND EXTERNA

Acute otitis media (AOM) refers to inflammation (often associated with infection) of the middle ear and the mucosal-lined air spaces of the temporal bone. Eustachian tube dysfunction following a URTI, or as a response to an environmental allergen, can result in fluid collection in the middle ear. This fluid acts as a growth medium for various microbes (25). Of the 22 million visits annually to United States physicians for AOM, almost 4 million are by patients 15 years or older. In a prospective study involving 500 patients 15 years or older, neither type nor duration of antibiotic treatment affected outcome. Recovery was more related to individual patient characteristics (multiple previous episodes of AOM and increasing age) (35). Additionally, a significant body of evidence suggests that antimicrobials offer only a marginal advantage in the treatment of uncomplicated AOM in healthy patients older than 2 years and there is no contemporary evidence that management through the use of symptomatic therapy (e.g., analgesics, decongestants) heightens the risk for complications (e.g., mastoiditis) (36).

There are no published studies specific to athletes, AOM and the use of antibiotics for therapy. In general, symptomatic therapy with decongestants and analgesics should suffice for most situations; however, in selected cases, antibiotic therapy may be seen as appropriate. Diving should be avoided until there is normal tympanic membrane mobility by Valsalva or tympanogram, because of the risk of tympanic rupture at depths greater than 4.3 feet when there is eustachian tube dysfunction (25). Additionally the tympanic membrane should be intact before returning to water activity. For those athletes involved in surface swimming with chronic otitis media, the use of grommets (tympanostomy tubes) may be useful if they avoid diving (37,38).

Otitis externa ("swimmer's ear") is defined as inflammation (often associated with infection) of the external ear canal. It is a common problem among athletes participating in sports or training which involve repetitive water exposure and/or mechanical trauma to the external ear. It is caused primarily by bacteria, most commonly *Pseudomonas aeruginosa*. Occasionally there are fungal contributors (aspergillus) as well. It is important to carefully evaluate the tympanic membrane, which may require cleansing of the ear canal with hydrogen peroxide and/or saline washes. Clearance of debris also facilitates topical treatment with antibiotic/anti-inflammatory drops such as polymyxin b/hydrocortisone drops (applied liberally over a cotton wick for improved retention) twice a day for 7 days followed by prophylactic use of acetic acid in isopropyl alcohol after each swimming session. Swimmers should be advised to tilt the head and shake the water from the ear canals after swimming and dry the area with a hair dryer. The use of earplugs is controversial as some authors have suggested that trauma from their use may predispose to infection. Return to water activity is based on resolution of symptoms and patient tolerance (25,39). If earplugs are deemed necessary the most effective form appears to be cotton wool coated in paraffin jelly, which out performed custom made synthetic plugs at a considerable cost savings (40).

CONJUNCTIVITIS

Conjunctivitis is conjunctival inflammation which may be caused by allergen, toxic insult, or infection. The most common infectious causes are viral. The most common bacterial causes include *Staphyloccus aureus, Staphylococcus epidermis* and various Streptococcus and Haemophilus species. Treatment of allergic and viral causes is primarily symptomatic; bacterial causes are commonly treated with appropriate topical broad spectrum antibiotic preparations (41).

Other less common, but potentially more serious, causes are *Neisseria gonorrheoeae* and herpes simplex virus (HSV). Neisseria infection should be considered in any sexually active adolescent or young adult presenting with a prominent purulent discharge. Culture and Gram's stain should be used to confirm the diagnosis and parenteral antibiotic treatment is required (25). HSV may be transmitted during participation in contact sports (notably wrestling and rugby), and has potential for severe complications including dendritic keratitis and corneal scarring. In the athlete with copious clear watery discharge, vesicular lesions on the lids and preauricular nodes, this diagnosis must be considered and appropriate ophthalmologic consultation obtained. (The patient with HSV eye involvement often has a history of active skin lesions) (42).

Prevention of transmission of conjunctivitis is the primary return-to-play consideration. Infectious athletes should be excluded from competition in high contact sports such as wrestling and rugby until they have been adequately treated and the symptoms have cleared. Because of the potential for transmission of viral agents such as adenovirus 3 in chlorinated pools, swimmers should also be isolated for an appropriate time (43).

MYOCARDITIS

Myocarditis is an inflammatory condition of the myocardial wall. Most acute infectious myocarditis is caused by viruses, with coxsackievirus B being the most common agent, although numerous other viruses have been implicated. Myocarditis is a rare cause of reported sudden death in athletes where a diagnosis is made (44). Coxsackie infections usually occur in epidemics, most often in summer and early fall. Animal data suggest that exercise during experimentally induced septicemic viral infections may increase the risk for the development of acute myocarditis (45,46). No such studies have been performed in humans and, as usual, the degree to which animal data can be transferred to humans is unclear.

Systemic signs and symptoms at the time of a typical viral infection can include fever, headache, myalgia, respiratory/gastrointestinal distress, exanthem and lymphadenopathy. Less frequent, but still possible are splenomegaly, meningitis, and hepatitis. Typically, symptoms are mild and nonspecific. There are no clinical predictors for which patients with these symptoms are likely to develop myocarditis. Additionally no clear historical or physical findings can confirm the early diagnosis of myocardial involvement, although retrospectively, myalgia may be a significant clue.

A typical clinical picture of myocarditis consists of fatigue, chest pain, dyspnea, and palpitations, yet except for palpitations one might have these same symptoms with the acute phase of a general, systemic viral illness. In myocarditis, however, these manifestations rarely occur at the height of the infectious illness, but instead become evident during the convalescent phase as the acute systemic viral illness subsides. Not all patients who are diagnosed with viral myocarditis recall having a viral illness. Additionally, most myocarditis episodes are subclinical (i.e., the patient is asymptomatic). In the face of all these nonspecific scenarios, one can certainly appreciate the incredible difficulty in management decisions for the clinician, especially one dealing with teams/institutions where numerous athletes present in a short period with nonspecific acute infections. There is no research that can offer clear evidence-based guidelines about exercise during viral infections. For the time being the clinician's advice to athletes with an acute, nonspecific infection will be dependent on common sense and collaboration with the athlete.

Return to activity with myocarditis: currently, there are no clinically accurate predictors of sudden death risk in patients with myocarditis (47). The 36th Bethesda Conference (48) made the following recommendations for the athlete in regard to return to activity:

1. Athletes with probable or definite evidence of myocarditis should be withdrawn from all competitive sports and undergo a prudent convalescent period of approximately 6 months following the onset of clinical manifestations.
2. Athletes may return to training and competition after this period if
   (a) LV function, wall motion, and cardiac dimensions return to normal (based on echocardiographic and/or radionuclide studies at rest and with exercise)
   (b) clinically relevant arrhythmias such as frequent and/or complex repetitive forms of ventricular or supraventricular ectopic activity are absent on ambulatory Holter monitoring and graded exercise testing
   (c) serum markers of inflammation and heart failure have normalized
   (d) the 12-lead electrocardiograph (ECG) has normalized. Persistence of relatively minor ECG alterations such as some ST-T changes are not, per se, the basis for restriction from competition.

MENINGITIS

Meningitis is a potentially life-threatening medical emergency associated with multiple neurological complications and sequelae. Fortunately, the most reported meningitis cases in the literature concerning athletes are described as aseptic. The primary etiology of aseptic meningitis is the enterovirus (echovirus, Coxsackie A and B viruses, polioviruses, and the numbered enteroviruses). Enteroviruses are responsible for most of the aseptic meningitic cases. Other viral causes include arboviruses, herpesviruses, zoster, adenovirus, human immunodeficiency virus (HIV), lymphocytic choriomeningitis virus (LCM), measles, mumps, rubella, rabies, influenza A and B, parainfluenza virus, parvovirus, and rotavirus. Aseptic meningitis is most prevalent during the summer and early fall months (ranging from July to December). Enteroviruses are spread through the fecal-oral route (ie, shared infected water sources, in the form of containers, bottles, or ice cubes). Seasonal predilection and fecal-oral route of spread may explain why aseptic meningitis is more prevalent in football and soccer athletes.

Aseptic meningitis is a commonly encountered disease process with a clinical presentation similar to that of bacterial meningitis. These similarities can present a diagnostic dilemma. The presentation of meningitis can be acute (less than 24 hours) or subacute (occurring over 1 to 7 days). Obvious signs in the clinical presentation of meningitis include the classic triad of fever, headache, and neck stiffness (meningismus). This triad is often accompanied by other nonspecific symptoms, including nausea, vomiting, pharyngitis, diarrhea, photophobia, and focal neurologic signs. Symptoms can be accompanied by mental status changes ranging from lethargy to coma. (It is important to note only about half of patients over the age of 16 present with the classic triad.) Bacterial meningitis can have both a rapidly progressive and fulminant course, or an indolent course consisting of vague symptoms. An indolent course is common when an individual has been pretreated with oral antibiotics.

Prevention revolves around good hand washing and decreasing use of shared water sources. Meningococcal vaccine immunization, with the quadrivalent vaccine, (meningococcal polysaccharide vaccine - 4) MPSV-4 (Menomume; serogroups A, C, Y, W-135), has been recommended by the United States Advisory Committee on Immunization practices (ACIP) for individuals older than 2 years who have functional or surgical asplenia or who have terminal complement deficiencies, for those traveling or living in areas of the world where meningococcal infection is endemic, and for college age students (18- to 23-year-olds) living in dormitories (threefold risk compared with age-matched controls) (12).

HUMAN IMMUNODEFICIENCY VIRUS

HIV is a blood borne pathogen that is transmitted through sexual contact, direct contact with infected blood or blood products such as blood transfusions and IV drug use with contaminated needles/syringes and from mother to baby in the antepartum/perinatal periods along with breast-feeding. The clinical manifestations of HIV disease are widespread and varied. Acute infection is often asymptomatic, but may be associated with symptoms similar to many common benign viral syndromes such as infectious mononucleosis (IM). Individuals who experience the "acute HIV syndrome," which occurs to varying degrees in approximately 50% of individuals with primary infection, have high levels of viremia that last for several weeks (described later). The acute mononucleosis-like symptoms are well correlated with the presence of viremia. Virtually all patients appear to develop some degree of viremia during primary infection, which contributes to virus dissemination, although they remain asymptomatic or do not recall experiencing symptoms. Careful examination of lymph nodes from more than one site in patients with established HIV infection that did not report symptoms of a primary infection strongly indicate that wide dissemination to lymphoid tissue occurs in most patients (49).

There is no evidence that exercise of a mild to moderate intensity is detrimental to the health of HIV infected athletes. The decision to participate in sports should be based on the individual's current health status (obviously, many athletes with acute infection will not be suspected initially of being infected with HIV). If the athlete is asymptomatic and without evidence of deficiencies in immune function, then no restrictions are necessary.

Transmission of HIV by sports participation has not been documented in a valid manner (50). The estimated risk of transmission has been evaluated for professional (American) football setting and is infinitesimal (51).

Routine mandatory testing of athletes for HIV (or hepatitis B virus [HBV], for that matter) is not recommended by any sportsmedicine group. Individuals who desire voluntary testing based on personal reasons and risk factors should be assisted in obtaining such testing through appropriate public health resources.

HEPATITIS

Infections with viral hepatitis are predominantly caused by one of five viruses (A, B, C, D and E). HAV and HEV occur by the fecal-oral route or from contaminated water or food. HBV, HCV and HDV are blood borne pathogens. Viral hepatitis can present as a broad spectrum of clinical syndromes ranging from asymptomatic disease to fulminant and fatal acute infections (chronic infections are not discussed in this chapter). Common presenting symptoms of acute hepatitis include anorexia, nausea, myalgia and fatigue. These symptoms typically develop seven to fourteen days before the onset of jaundice. Other common symptoms include headache, arthralgias and, in children, diarrhea. These symptoms are virtually the same in all forms of acute hepatitis no matter what the cause. Symptoms will persist for a few weeks. Hepatitis A is usually self-limited and does not result in a chronic carrier state or cirrhosis. Progression to chronic hepatitis is primarily a feature of HBV, HCV and HDV. One of the most feared complications of acute hepatitis is fulminant hepatitis, which has a very high mortality rate. It is primarily seen in adults infected with hepatitis B, D, and E and only rarely occurs in A and C.

Acute liver insult with viral hepatitis predisposes to hypoglycemia and altered lipid metabolism compromising energy availability during exercise. Additionally, liver dysfunction results in altered protein synthesis and metabolism that cause a variety of physiologic disturbances including coagulopathy and hormonal imbalances. It has been shown that exercise can significantly alter the hemodynamics of the liver in healthy subjects. This included decreases in portal vein cross sectional area, portal venous velocity, and flow. The decreases were transient and completely reversible. No problems were noted in healthy subjects, but theoretically could lead to complications in subjects with liver dysfunction associated with acute hepatitis (52). Considering these parameters including fatigue symptoms, altered physiology, and the potential for fulminant complications, the traditional recommendation for the athlete with acute hepatitis, to comply with a regimen of rest and refrain from exertion, seems intuitively reasonable (53,54). However, experience from several studies challenges this conservative approach (55–58). Available data suggest that mild to moderate exercise can be safely permitted as tolerated in the previously healthy individual with an episode of acute viral hepatitis. This training should be guided by the clinical condition of the patient. This approach is consistent with position statements/guidelines from the American Medical Society for Sports Medicine, the American Orthopedic Society for Sports Medicine and the American Academy of Pediatrics (59,60). There is no data that address exercise training at an extreme exertion or competitive levels. It seems prudent to avoid extreme exercise and competition until liver tests are normal and hepatomegaly (if present) resolves.

The concerns for transmission of "blood borne pathogens" such as Hepatitis B, C and D during sporting events has been addressed by various sports medicine authorities (59–61). The athlete with either acute or chronic HBV infection presents very limited risk of disease transmission in most sports. Two situations in which the transmission of Hepatitis B related to sports participation have been reported in Japan (62,63). These situations did not include the attendance of an athletic trainer or other health care provider at training sessions and there is no evidence that appropriate blood and body fluid precautions were taken. No cases have been reported in other countries. The NCAA has suggested the following for those athletes with Hepatitis B: "*if the student-athlete develops acute HBV illness, it is prudent to consider removal of the individual from combative, close contact sports (e.g., wrestling) until loss of infectivity is known. (The best marker for infectivity is the HBV antigen, which may persist up to 20 weeks in the acute stage) Student-athletes in such sports who develop chronic HBV infections (especially those who are e-antigen positive) should be removed from competition indefinitely, due to the small but realistic risk of transmitting HBV to other student-athletes*"(61).

Practically speaking, health care providers working with athletes should be much more concerned with the likely transmission of blood borne pathogens such as Hepatitis B through the common routes of needle use and sexual intercourse. In particular, the increasing popularity of tattoos and piercings in athletes at all levels is alarming. There are no reported cases of transmission of Hepatitis C or D from sports participation. Transmission of Hepatitis A or E seems more likely because of the oral route, but cases have not been reported that link transmission from athlete to athlete during sports participation, although environmental causes have been implicated such as a polluted body of water that the sport is taking place in (64).

REFERENCES

1. McGrew C, Lillegard W. Profile of patients seen in a primary care sports medicine fellowship. *Clin J Sports Med* 1992;2(2):126–131.
2. Shepard R, Shek P. Exercise, immunity and susceptibility to infection. *Phys Sportsmed* 1999;27(6):47–71.
3. Niemen D. Does exercise alter immune function and respiratory infections? *President's Counc Phys Fit Sports Res Dig* 2001;3(13):10.
4. Alluisi E, Beisel W, Morgan B, et al. Effects of Sandfly fever on isometric muscular strength, endurance and recovery. *J Mot Behav* 1980;12:1–11.
5. Mellion M. Infections in athletes. In: Mellion, et al. ed. *The team physician's handbook*. 1996:255–267.
6. Friman G, Wright J. Ilback: does fever or myalgia indicate reduced physical performance capacity in viral infections? *Acta Med Scand* 1985;217(4): 353–361.
7. Brenner I, Shek P, Shephard R. Infection in athletes. *Sports Med* 1994; 17:86–107.
8. Friman G, Ilback N. Acute infection: metabolic responses, effects on performance, interaction with exercise, and myocarditis. *Int J Sports Med* 1998;19:S172–SS18.
9. Line R, Rust G. Acute exertional rhabdomylosis. *Am Fam Physician* 1995; 52(2):502–506.
10. Cate T, Roberts J, Russ M, et al. Effects of common colds on pulmonary function. *Am Rev Respir Dis* 1973;108(4):858–865.
11. van der Linden P, van Puijenbroek E, Feenstra J, et al. Tendon disorders attributed to fluoroquinolones: a study on 42 spontaneous reports in the period 1988 to 1998. *Arthritis Rheum* 2001;45(3):235–239.
12. Hosey RG, Rodenberg RE. Training room management of medical conditions: infectious diseases. *Clin Sports Med* 2005;24:477–506.
13. Quam D. Recognizing a case of reye's syndrome. *Am Fam Physician* 1994;59:1491–1496.
14. Primos W. Sports and exercise during acute illness: recommending the right course for patients. *Phys Sportsmed* 1996;24(1):44–53.
15. Glasziou P, Del Mar C. Upper respiratory tract infection. In: Godlee F, ed. *Clinical evidence*, Vol. 3. BMJ Publishing Group, 2000:737–742.
16. Beck C. Infectious diseases in sports. *Med Sci Sports Exerc* 2000;32(7):S431–S438.
17. Maki DG, Reich RM. Infectious mononucleosis in the athlete. *Am J Sports Med* 1982;10(3):162.
18. Doolittle R. Pharyngitis and infectious mononucleosis. In: Fields K, Fricker P, eds. *Medical problems in athletes*. Cambridge: Blackwell Science, 1997:11–20.
19. Howe W. Infectious mononucleosis in athletes. In: Garett W, Kirkendall D, Squire D, eds. *Principles and practice of primary care sports medicine*. Philadelphia: Lippincott Williams & Wilkins, 2001:239–246.
20. Eichner ER. Infectious mononucleosis: recognizing the condition, 'reactivating' the patient. *Phys Sportsmed* 1996;24(4):49–54.
21. Welch MJ, Wheeler L. Aerobic capacity after contracting infectious mononucleosis. *J Othop Sports Phys Ther* 1986;8:199–202.
22. Ali J. Spontaneous rupture of the spleen in patients with infectious mononucleosis. *Can J Surg* 1993;153:283–290.
23. Tamayo SG, Rickman LS, Mathews WC, et al. Examiner dependence on physical diagnostic test for the detection of splenomegaly: a prospective study with multiple observers. *J Gen Intern Med* 1993;8(2):69–75.

24. Hosey RG, Quarles JD, Kriss VM, et al. Spleen size in athletes—a comparison of BMI, gender, race, and past history of mononucleosis. *Med Sci Sports Exerc* 2004;36(5):S-312.
25. Butcher J, Lillegard W. *Sinusitis, otitis media, otitis externa and conjunctivitis pages 21–25 IN Medical problems in athletes.* Fields K, Fricker P, ed. Blackwell Science Publishers, 1997.
26. Josephon J, Rosenberg S. Sinusitis. *CIBA Clin Symp* 1994;46:1–32.
27. Stalman W, van Essen G, van Der Graaf Y. Determinants for the course of acute sinusitis in adult general practice patients. *Postgrad Med J* 2001; 77(914):778–782.
28. Kizer K. Scuba diving and dysbarism. In: Auerbach P, ed. *Wilderness medicine: management of wilderness and environmental emergencies,* 3rd ed. St. Louis: Mosby, 1995:1176–1208.
29. Field K. Infectious bronchitis and pneumonia in athletes. In: *Medical problems in athletes.* Blackwell Science, 1997:26–33.
30. MacKay D. Treatment of actue bronchitis without underlying lung disease. *J Gen Intern Med* 1996;11(9):557–562.
31. Bent S, Saint S, Vittinghoff E, et al. Antibiotics in acute bronchitis:a meta-analysis. *Am J Med* 1999;107(1):62–67.
32. Levison M. *Chapter 255: pneumonia, including necrotizing pulmonary infections (Lung Abscess) part 9: disorders of the respiratory system.* http://www.harrisonsonline.com/server-java/Arknoid/amed/harrisons/co_chapters/ch255/ch255_p09.html, 2006.
33. Kim MK, Nightingale C, Quintiliani R. Guidelines for treatment of community acquired pneumonia. *Conn Med* 2001;65(8):473–475.
34. Melham T. Atypical pneumonia in active patients: clues, causes, and return to play. *Phys Sportsmed* 1997;25(10):43–59.
35. Culpepper L, Froom J, Bartelds A, et al. Acute otitis media in adults: a report from the International Primary Care Network. *J Am Board Fam Pract* 1993;6(4):333–339.
36. Marcy M. Treatment of otitis media. *Pediatr Infect Dis J* 2000;19(10):1023.
37. Pringle M. Grommets, swimming, and otorhea- a review. *J Laryngol Otol* 1993;107:190–194.
38. Cohen H, Kauschansky A, Ashkenasi A, et al. Swimming and grommets. *J Fam Pract* 1994;38:30–32.
39. Brukner P, Khan K. *Clinical sports medicine chapter 10 facial injuries.* McGraw-Hill, 1993:170–180. pages in
40. Robinson A. Evaluation of waterproof ear protectors for swimmers. *J Laryngol Otol* 1989;103(12):1154–1157.
41. Sheikh A, Hurwitz B. Treatment of conjunctivitis. *Br J Gen Pract* 2001; 51(467):473–477.
42. Holland E, Mahanti R, Belongia E. Ocular involvement in an outbreak of herpes gladiatorum. *Am J Opthalmol* 1992;114:680–684.
43. Weinberg S. Medical aspects of synchronized swimming. *Clin Sports Med* 1986;5:159–167.
44. Maron B, Shirani J, Poliac L, et al. Sudden death in young competitive athletes. *JAMA* 1996;276:199–204.
45. Illback N, Fohlman J, Friman G. Exercise in coxsackie B3 myocarditis: effects on heart lymphocyte subpopulations and the inflammatory reaction. *Am Heart J* 1989;117:1298–1302.
46. Gatmaitan B, Chason J, Lerner A. Augmentation of the virulence of murine coxsackie virus B-3 myocardiopathy by exercise. *J Exp Med* 1970; 131:1121–1136.
47. Portugal D, Smith J. Myocarditis and the athlete. In: Estes N, Dame D, Wong P, eds. *Sudden cardiac death in the athlete.* Armonk, NY: Futura Publishing, 1998:349–371.
48. Maron B, Ackerman M, Nishimura R, et al. Task Force 4: HCM and other cariodmyopathies, mitral valve prolapse, myocarditis and Marfan syndrome. *Am Coll Cardiol* 2005;45:1340–1345.
49. Fauci A, Lane H. *Human immunodeficiency disease (HIV) disease: AIDs and related disorders: in Harrison's principles of internal medicine.* On-line edition chapter 309 pages http://www.harrisonsonline.com/server-java/Arknoid/amed/harrisons/co_chapters/ch309/ch309_p01.html. 1–44.
50. Calabrese L. HIV infections, exercise and athletes. *Sports Med* 1993;15(1): 1–7.
51. Brown L. Bleeding injuries in professional football:estimating the risk for HIV transmission. *Ann Intern Med* 1995;111(4):271–274.
52. Ohnishi K. Portal venous hemodynamics in chronic liver disease: effects of posture change and exercise. *Radiology* 1985;155:757–761.
53. Krickler DM, Zilberg B. Activity and hepatitis. *Lancet* 1966;2(7472):1046–1047.
54. De Celis G. Hepatitis A and vigorous physical activity. *Lancet* 1998; 352(9124):325.
55. Chalmers TC, Eschkardt RD, Reynolds WE, et al. The treatment of acute infectious hepatitis: controlled studies of the effects of diet, rest and physical reconditioning on the acute course of the disease and on the incidence of relapses and residual abnormalities. *J Clin Invest* 1955;34:1163–1194.
56. Chalmers TC. Rest and exercise in hepatitis. *N Engl J Med* 1969;281:1393–1396.
57. Edlund A. The effect of defined physical exercise in the early convalescence of viral hepatitis. *Scand J Infect Dis* 1971;3:189–196.
58. Repsher LH, Freeborn RK. Effects of early and vigorous exercise on recovery from infectious hepatitis. *N Engl J Med* 1969;281:1393–1396.
59. American Medical Society for Sports Medicine and American Orthopedic Society for Sports Medicine. Joint position statement: human immunodeciency virus and other blood borne pathogens in sports. *Clin J Sport Med* 1995;5:199–204.
60. American Academy of Pediatrics, Committee on Sports Medicine and Fitness. Medical conditions affecting sports participation. *Pediatrics* 2001; 107(5):1205–1209.
61. Guideline 2-H blood-borne pathogens and intercollegiate athletics. In: *NCAA sports medicine, handbook.* 2004–2005:35–39.
62. Kashiwagi S. Outbreak of hepatitis B in members of a high school sumo wrestling club. *JAMA* 1982;1248:213–214.
63. Tobe K, Matsuura K, Ogura T, et al. Horizontal transmission of hepatitis B virus among players of an American football team. *Arch Intern Med* 2000;160(16):2541–2545.
64. Philipp R, Waitkins S, Caul O, et al. Leptospiral and hepatitis A antibodies amongst windsurfers and waterskiers in Bristol City docks. *Public Health* 1989;103(2):123–129.

Hematology

19

Thomas H. Trojian   Diana L. Heiman

Blood has a central focus in athletics. Its oxygen and nutrient carrying properties make it a matter of concern for many coaches and athletes. Athletes with anemia may present with signs and symptoms only during strenuous exercise (1). Athletes will present with subtle findings, such as fatigue while sprinting. It is important to identify anemia because improvements can be seen in the athletic performance after its correction.

Anemia is a common finding in athletes, as well as in the general population. The signs and symptoms are multiple. Most often, the cause of the anemia is benign, but thorough evaluation is needed to rule out other more serious causes. Evaluations for poor dietary intake, as well as blood or nutrient loss through various sources, such as the gastrointestinal (GI) and genitourinary (GU) systems, and sweat, will provide the cause of anemia in most cases. When the anemia does not follow as per standard evaluation, then abnormal hemoglobin and hemoglobin electrophoresis should be considered.

Variations of the normal alpha and beta unit are not uncommon and can be found in at least 8% of African-American athletes (2). Controversy exists about the true risks of variations, such as sickle cell trait, and exercise. Some concerns are minor but others are very serious, including sudden death. This chapter will review all of these concerns.

On the other end of the continuum is erythrocythemia. This is most often caused by some form of manipulation of blood levels through altered living conditions or some form of blood doping. Athletes are often on the forefront of medical experimentation in the area of hemoglobin (Hgb) boosting. This was emphasized by the alleged use of darbepoetin (a drug not yet available for general use, similar to erythropoietin [EPO]) during the 2002 Winter Olympics in the hope that it would be undetectable in testing.

PSEUDOANEMIA (SPORTS ANEMIA)

In 1970, Yoshimura coined the phrase "sports anemia" (3). This is actually a false anemia secondary to plasma expansion from exercise. The red blood cell (RBC) mass is actually normal to slightly increased, but there is a plasma expansion, such as in pregnancy, which causes a lower hematocrit level (4). Therefore, this is actually a dilutional pseudoanemia.

The decreased hematocrit values found are explained by the repeated relative hemoconcentration that occurs from dehydration, loss of plasma in sweat, and increased osmotic pressure in the muscles from lactic acid and other byproducts. After exercise, a plasma expansion occurs. Even a single bout of exercise can cause a 10% change in plasma volume and a hematocrit drop of 3.8% (5). This subsequent overshoot from the post-workout plasma volume expansion will cause a dilutional pseudoanemia. This type of anemia is found in endurance athletes. Therefore, its occurrence should not be high on the differential diagnosis in nonendurance sports such as American Football. The hemoglobin levels can be 1.0 to 1.5 g/dL below normal levels. It is important to evaluate for iron-deficiency anemia, as both can be present. Sports anemia should be considered a diagnosis of exclusion.

Pseudoanemia is not pathological but an adaptive response to endurance training (6). Therefore, supplementation with iron or other vitamins is not necessary. Normalization of the Hgb can be seen after 5 days from cessation of exercise. There is no need for an alteration in training. Dilutional pseudoanemia is functionally beneficial to the endurance athlete. It should not be corrected.

MICROCYTIC ANEMIA

Iron Deficiency

Iron-deficiency anemia is the most common form of true anemia seen in athletes. It can be seen in any athlete but is most often seen in menstruating female athletes. In menstruating female athletes, the rate is as high as 20%, and it is approximately 6% in postmenopausal women. The rate is 4% in male athletes (7). The incidence of anemia in the athletic population is no different than in the general population (8). Many studies have examined the incidence of iron deficiency in athletes as compared to controls and have given varying results. There are some studies that show significant differences (9) and others that show no difference when compared to appropriately matched controls (10). Studies looking at endurance athletes showed this population to be at increased risk for iron deficiency (11). These studies used serum ferritin, which looks at body iron stores and overestimates anemia. A recent study does not show any difference in the prevalence of the disease in athletes compared to nonathletes (12). The rate of anemia may not be different in athletes, but the effects can be detrimental. Therefore, it is important to identify and correct this problem.

An increased rate of iron deficiency in athletes may be controversial. However, when compared to the general population, there is an increase in nonanemic iron deficiency. The ferritin level is predictive of iron stores. Increased rates of low ferritin levels have been seen in endurance athletes. The significance of a low ferritin on performance is uncertain, as iron replacement has not been shown to change performance outcomes (13). In endurance athletes, pseudoanemia (dilutional anemia) can coexist with a low ferritin level, and an iron-deficiency anemia with a dilutional pseudoanemia must be considered. A trial of iron levels with a follow-up reticulocyte count and hemoglobin level would be appropriate to rule out iron-deficiency anemia (see Table 19.1).

TABLE 19.1
SIGNS AND SYMPTOMS OF IRON-DEFICIENCY ANEMIA

Signs	Pallor Glossitis Angular cheilitis Koilonychia
Symptoms	Weakness Lassitude Palpitations Shortness of breath Pica (craving for ice, starch, etc.)

In athletes, as in nonathletes, the cause of iron deficiency is either from iron loss or insufficient intake. Iron losses are either from GI or GU sources or, questionably, sweat. GI is the most significant cause, and GI bleed can be a sign of a more serious illness. Appropriate tests should be done for any athlete with frank hematochezia.

Many athletes will develop microscopic GI bleeding while performing endurance sports. The exact mechanism is unknown, but many causes have been touted (14). The ones of note are non-steroidal anti-inflammatory agents (NSAIDs) and prednisone. Both can cause GI bleeding and their use is common among athletes (see Chapter 12 for further discussions on GI bleeding in athletes).

Other areas of iron loss have been described in athletes (15). Their significance is most often minimal. Loss of iron from sweat is negligible and unlikely to be the cause of iron deficiency. Losses from hematuria and foot-strike destruction are seen in the same group of athletes that have blood loss from the GI tract. Therefore, evaluation of possible GI losses of blood should be thoroughly investigated first.

In female athletes, obtaining a menstrual history is important in the evaluation. Heavy or prolonged menses is a common source of blood and iron loss. Menstrual history may lead to the diagnosis of amenorrhea, and if so, further questions need to address the possibility of disordered eating. In the amenorrheic athlete, evaluation of GI blood loss is important, once again, as this is still the most common source of iron-deficiency anemia.

Nutritional deficiencies are common in the general population as well as in athletes. Iron intake is as important as iron loss as the causes of iron-deficiency anemia. There are many athletes who adhere to restrictive and fad diets trying to get a real or perceived competitive advantage. In addition, anemia may be a sign of an eating disorder. A thorough dietary history is needed to identify low iron intake. A 2-week diet record is helpful in identifying iron nutritional deficiencies.

Evaluating anemia is best done in a stepwise approach. A complete blood count (CBC) with manual differential (diff) to identify and evaluate the anemia is very useful. The manual differential is an evaluation of all the cell types (white blood cells (WBC), RBC, Platelets). The CBC with differential will guide you to decide on the other needed studies. Additional blood can be drawn and held for further studies. The presence of target cells, Howell-Jolly bodies, schistocytes, elliptocytes, and other abnormal cell types can be found in the differential and will help in determining the cause of anemia. Also, the differential will identify if the anemia is microcytic or macrocytic.

If a microcytic anemia is diagnosed, then the reticulocyte count and ferritin level should be performed. A low ferritin (less than 20) and a reticulocyte index less than 1 almost confirm an iron-deficiency anemia. The athlete should be started on iron replacement. Follow-up hemoglobin and reticulocyte count is performed in 14 days. The reticulocyte index should be greater than two.

When the ferritin level is low normal, other tests can help identify an iron-deficiency anemia. Iron studies including serum iron and total iron binding capacity are useful tests. At times, differentiating the anemia is complex. A helpful test in separating iron-deficiency anemia from the anemia of chronic disease is the serum transferrin receptor ferritin ratio. It is elevated in iron-deficiency anemia, whereas normal in the anemia of chronic disease.

When the reticulocyte index does not increase after the start of iron replacement or a microcytic anemia is concurrent with normal iron studies, then performing hemoglobin electrophoresis is appropriate. Many forms of abnormal hemoglobin will produce low hematocrit levels with microcytosis but have normal or elevated reticulocyte counts. In addition, full compliance with iron replacement may not be tolerated, and questioning the athlete regarding barriers to compliance can identify why there is no bone marrow response to treatment.

Oral iron replacement is the treatment of choice. There is rarely, if ever, a reason for the use of parental iron therapy. Replacement should be 20 to 60 mg of elemental iron divided into three doses and given between meals. Ferrous sulfate tablets of 30 mg will supply 60 mg of elemental iron. There is a large reduction (50%) in absorption if given at mealtime. Some evidence supports the use of vitamin C with iron to increase absorption. The length of treatment to fully replenish iron stores is generally 3 to 6 months.

When the athlete expresses difficulty with iron replacement, you should investigate the reason. If it is an upset stomach, then taking the dose with food will help. Constipation can be corrected with a stool softener. Diarrhea is seldom a problem, but taking the iron with food can help. If needed, pediatric liquid formulation can be used. Altering oral iron therapy is far better than using parental iron. Because of the many serious local and systemic reactions, parental iron should be avoided.

Thalassemia

Thalassemia is the result of deletion or mutation of the genes responsible for the alpha and beta globin chains. Hemoglobin consists of two alpha and two beta globin units. The alpha globin is located on chromosome 16 along with the alpha-like globin zeta. The beta globin is on chromosome 11 in a linked cluster in the order epsilon, gamma, delta, and beta. There are many variations and degrees of deletion of the globin units. The presentation can range from asymptomatic to fetal death in-utero.

Mediterranean, African, and Middle Eastern patients commonly have alpha-thalassemia. African-Americans have alpha-thalassemia trait at a rate of approximately 2%. Beta-thalassemia presents in people from the Middle East, Indian Subcontinent, Northern Africa, and the Mediterranean at a rate of 1%. It is often seen with other hemoglobinopathies, such as sickle cell.

Beta-thalassemia

Beta-thalassemia minor or thalassemia trait describes the asymptomatic forms of the disease. The athlete's CBC with differential usually presents as profound microcytosis and hypochromia with target cells and elliptocytes, but the anemia is only mild. The reticulocyte count is elevated. Hemoglobin electrophoresis classically reveals an elevated hemoglobin A_2 (Hgb A_2) (3.5% to 7.5%). Normal Hgb A_2 with elevated fetal hemoglobin (HgbF) can be seen in some forms. Genetic counseling and patient education are essential.

In athletes with beta-thalassemia trait, their CBC with differential will often resemble iron deficiency and can be misdiagnosed as such. Ferritin and reticulocyte counts are useful in differentiating beta-thalassemia and iron-deficiency anemia. Athletes should avoid the unnecessary use of iron but must be aware that iron-deficiencies may develop with heavy menses, pregnancy, and GI bleeds.

Alpha-thalassemia

Alpha-thalassemia is characterized by the number of deletions in the four alpha gene loci. A single locus deletion, most common in Southeast Asians, produces the common alpha-thalassemia-2 trait. This form is asymptomatic. Two loci deletions produce alpha-thalassemia-1 trait, which resembles beta-thalassemia minor.

Presentation

Normally, the athlete presents with the signs or symptoms of anemia. Tests reveal a microcytic anemia that does not respond to iron therapy or, if iron studies are done, normal levels are found. Ferritin may be low in athletes without anemia. That is why follow-up laboratory studies are needed to determine the response to iron therapy. The reticulocyte count in thalassemia is elevated, not low as in iron-deficiency anemia, on initial presentation.

Hgb electrophoresis in alpha-thalassemia group shows a decrease in Hgb A_2, and beta group shows increases in Hgb F and Hgb A_2. The other tests are summarized by normal iron studies, low mean cell volume (MCV) (often 60 or less) and occasionally basophilic stippling seen on manual differential. Care must be taken not to cause iron overload in these athletes.

MACROCYTIC ANEMIA

Macrocytic anemias are not nearly as common as microcytic anemias in athletes. The main causes of macrocytic anemia are vitamin B12 deficiency, folate deficiency, drugs that effect folate metabolism (see Table 19.2), and hypothyroidism (16). Ethanol can cause a macrocytosis with a MCV greater than 100, without signs of liver damage.

Vitamin B12 Deficiency

Macrocytic anemia from vitamin B12 deficiency is uncommon. The cause is frequently from an absorption problem

TABLE 19.2
DRUGS THAT CAUSE MACROCYTIC ANEMIA

- Methotrexate
- Sulfamethoxazole-trimethoprim
- Sulfasalazine
- Triamterene
- Oral contraceptives
- Anticonvulsants

due to the lack of an intrinsic factor. Deficiency in the intake of vitamin B12 is possible in vegans (people who eat no animal products, including dairy and eggs). Most vegans are well aware of the need for vitamin B12 and will use supplements. It is rare to find of a person with vitamin B12 deficiency who does not have pernicious anemia or a chronic GI disorder.

Folate Deficiency

Folate is available now in most foods in the United States and Canada. Folate deficiency is most often due to severe restriction diets, inflammatory diseases, and pregnancy. Folate stores last 4 months compared to the 2-year stores of B12. Vitamin B12 levels need to be evaluated if folate deficiency is detected.

Diagnosis

The athlete will present with symptoms of anemia. Macrocytic anemias are insidious in nature; the first presentation can be as severe as congestive heart failure. The CBC with differential will show a low hematocrit with an MCV greater than 100. The microscopic examination will show macrocytic cells with elliptocytes or **Howell-Jolly bodies.** Multilobed neutrophils can also be seen in the peripheral smear. A pancytopenia can occur.

The follow-up tests should include vitamin B12 and red cell folate levels. The red cell folate (RBC folate) test is a superior test than the folate level test, which is quickly elevated with feedings. The RBC folate is a measure of the folate stores in the body. A person who has recently received blood transfusion will have an altered RBC folate level. Liver function, thyroid function, reticulocyte count, and serum protein electrophoresis should be considered in the evaluation of macrocytic anemia.

Therapy

Therapy is replacement of the missing vitamin or cessation of the offending medicine. Folate replacement is 5 mg/day for 4 months. Vitamin B12 should be tried orally, even in pernicious anemia. Vitamin B12 injections can be painful and difficult for patients. 1,000 to 2, 000μg of oral vitamin B12 has been shown to treat pernicious anemia (17). Most, but not all, absorption of B12 is intrinsic factor dependent, so oral supplementation is successful and should be the route of first choice.

Folate is an important vitamin in the development of the fetus and prevention of neural tube defects (NTD). In 1998, the Food and Drug Administration (FDA) in the United States and the Canadian government ordered that folate be added to all cereal grain products. The rate of spina bifida has since dropped by 20%. Dietary folic acid is likely to be inadequate for maximal protection against NTD (18). Approximately half of all pregnancies in the US are unplanned, therefore birth defect prevention is recommended for all women of childbearing age. The recommended daily dose is 400μg of synthetic folic acid. This could reduce the overall incidence of NTD from 2 to 0.6/1,000 pregnancies and prevent disease in approximately 2,000 babies per year in the US.

HEMOLYTIC ANEMIA

Sickle Cell Anemia

Sickle cell anemia is an autosomal recessive trait that occurs due to the change of a single glutamic acid for a valine at position 6 on the Hgb beta chain. The RBCs with sickle hemoglobin have a protective effect against malaria. Sickle cell anemia is common in areas where malaria is prevalent. On the other hand, at low oxygen tensions the cells can form a sickle shape and occlude the capillaries, causing ischemia. Sickle cell disease is associated with chronic anemia, with Hgb in the 6 to 7 range.

Sickle Cell Trait

Sickle cell trait is the heterozygous form, Hgb AS. Most people with Hgb AS will have 60% A and 40% S; for the most part they are asymptomatic. In the general population, the incidence of sickle cell trait in African-Americans is approximately 8%, and 1 in 10,000 in Caucasians. Under extreme environmental conditions, the athletes with sickle cell trait may have sickling events. These include conditions such as travel to altitudes 6,000 feet above sea level, scuba diving, or dehydration.

Athletes with Hgb AS participate in sports regularly. Surveys among professional athletes reveal similar rates of Hgb AS to that in the general population (19). Studies analyzing $\dot{V}O_{2max}$, exercise capacity, and other measures do not show differences with normal controls. Therefore, sickle cell trait does not appear to inhibit athletic performance.

There are three main complications seen in athletes with sickle cell trait. The first is hematuria, second is splenic infarction at altitudes, and the third is sudden death. These complications vary in severity and probability.

Athletes with sickle cell trait may present with hematuria. It is usually benign and is often recurrent. It occurs mostly in male athletes and most often in the left kidney. The etiology is unknown but thought to be due to vaso-occlusive phenomena. Treatment is hydration, and urine alkalization. Urine alkalization can be done using $NaCO_2$ at 10 mg/kg before training. Recurrent episodes are treated with epsilon-aminocaproic acid (ACA), or desmopressin.

Splenic infarcts at high altitudes (as low as 6,000 feet but mostly higher than 10,000 feet) can be seen due to the hypoxic environment and subsequent sickling. Splenic infarct is a significant consequence for skiers or athletes training at altitudes. The warning signs of acute abdominal pain and left-sided stitch when at heights should be treated as potential splenic infarct. The person should descend to a lower height, oxygen should be given, and bed rest and hydration initiated if possible.

Concern has been raised because increased rates of sudden death with Hgb AS have been reported among Army recruits (20). The rate of sudden death in military recruits with sickle cell trait is higher than in the general military recruit population. The absolute risk seems to be 1 in 3200. Cases are usually associated with heat exhaustion and dehydration (21). Certain situations may trigger sickling episodes in athletes with Hgb AS. The increased death rate has been postulated to be due to an increased susceptibility to exertional rhabdomyolysis with Hgb AS from exertion heat illness in untrained recruits (2). This is definitely controversial, but most clinicians believe that athletes with sickle cell trait are at increased risk. Caution against the risks of sickle cell trait is warranted at difficult altitudes, and with severe dehydration (hot environments, and post illness). The importance of proper training techniques and hydration cannot be overemphasized for this group of athletes.

There is no consensus on the appropriateness of testing for sickle cell trait in athletes. Currently, the Air Force and the Navy carry out this test on all their recruits. The disease is more common in African-Americans, but is seen in most racial groups. Therefore, carrying out selective screening for sickle cell will miss athletes with sickle cell trait.

Foot-strike Hemolysis

Evidence for foot-strike hemolysis comes from studies that show an association between foot impact and excess hemolysis as a cause of hematuria (22), and from other studies showing that less of heel-strike causes less hematuria (23). Hemolysis occurs because of the rupture of RBCs in the heel due to heavy impact. It has been reported that soft-soled running shoes decrease hematuria.

Foot-strike hematuria is the best-known exertional hemolysis, but it is also seen in sports like swimming, a non-foot-strike sport. Intense exercise causes the production of factors that destroy RBCs. Measurement of haptoglobin levels pre- and postexercise will help in the evaluation of foot-strike hemolysis. A reduction in haptoglobin levels and a frank anhaptoglobinemia can be found (24). The exact mechanism for the RBC destruction is not known as yet.

TABLE 19.3

DRUGS THAT CAUSE HEMOLYSIS IN G6PD DEFICIENCY

- Dapsone
- Doxorubicin
- Methylene blue
- Nitrofurantoin
- Phenacetin
- Phenazopyridine
- Primaquine
- Sulfacetamide
- Sulfamethoxazole
- Sulfapyridine

G6PD = Glucose-6-phosphate dehydrogenase deficiency

Glucose-6-phosphate Dehydrogenase Deficiency

Glucose-6-phosphate dehydrogenase deficiency (G6PD) is the loss of the enzyme involved in the oxidative protective pathway. Millions of people are affected in the same racial groups that are affected by the thalassemias. There is no specific evidence that individuals with heredity hemolytic disorders are adversely affected by exercise. The deficiency is sex linked and affects males predominantly. It can cause sensitivity to *fava beans* (broad beans), and hemolytic responses to oxidant drugs. It is certainly appropriate to be aware of drugs that can elicit hemolysis in G6PD deficient athletes. Table 19.3 shows a list of drugs that can cause hemolysis.

BLEEDING DISORDERS

Bleeding disorders are commonly discovered in childhood and adolescence. Therefore, bleeding disorders may present in young athletes. The three most common problems are hemophilia, von Willebrand's disease (vWD), and immune thrombocytopenia. vWD is the most common of the three disorders.

Work-up of bleeding disorders may be complicated and a hematologist referral may be needed. Work-up of all bleeding disorders should include CBC with differential, prothrombin time, partial thromboplastin time (PTT), and bleeding time tests. More tests for specific factors can be obtained afterward. A prolonged PTT can be the first clue of hemophilia and vWD (see Table 19.4).

von Willebrand's Disease

vWD is an inherited platelet disorder along with a partial defect of factor VIII. These defects cause an increase in bleeding time. It is estimated to occur in 1 in 100 to

TABLE 19.4
BLEEDING DISORDERS

Disease	Cause	Genetics	Gender Affected
Hemophilia A	Decreased factor VIII	Sex linked recessive trait	Males
Hemophilia B	Decreased factor IX	Sex linked recessive trait	Males
Hemophilia C	Decreased factor XI	Autosomal trait	Males and females
vWD	Dysfunction in platelet adhesiveness and defect in factor VIII	Autosomal trait	Males and females
Immune thrombocytopenia	Platelet adhesion problem usually secondary to immunoglobulins	None	Males and Female

vWD = von Willebrand's disease

1,000 people. Aspirin and NSAIDs make vWD worse by inhibiting platelet aggregation. Recurrent nose-bleeds are a common sign of vWD. This disorder is often undetected until a female athlete presents with menorrhagia. Menstrual history before surgery is useful in order to screen for vWD.

Immune Thrombocytopenia

Immune thrombocytopenia is either autoimmune or drug-induced. Petechiae and purpura are signs of thrombocytopenia and the athlete should be tested for these. Any offending drugs need to be stopped. In adolescents, this condition is usually autoimmune, and steroids need to be given. Contact sports should be avoided when platelet counts are less than 100,000/mm^3.

Hemophilia

Hemophilia is an inherited deficiency in factor VIII or IX (see Table 19.4). It is often diagnosed before the start of athletics. During earlier times, exercise was discouraged due to potential of hemarthrosis. Recently, there has been a change in attitude toward exercise. Increased activity is now being promoted because of the positive physical and psychological effects. Once detected in an athlete, replacement therapy is often recommended for those engaging in contact sports. Some trial and error is necessary.

The type of exercise needs to be selected on an individual basis and centered on what the athlete considers enjoyable. Swimming, bicycling, skating, and walking are considered safe. Contact sports should be avoided, but the severity of the disease needs to be considered.

Weight training has been shown to be safe (25). Factor VIII seems to increase with strength training. There are improvements in coagulation parameters in mild and moderately affected patients carrying out weight lifting (26).

Risks are present for athletes with hemophilia. No running should be done when joint swelling is present, as hemarthrosis is a frequent problem. Athletes with hemophilia are susceptible to the same injuries as other athletes. There is documented data regarding delayed recovery from injury and this should be kept in mind for planning return to play. Protective equipment is emphasized to prevent bruising. This disease should not prevent people from participating in athletics (see Table 19.5) (27).

TABLE 19.5
SPORTS PARTICIPATION IN HEMOPHILIA

Highly Recommended Sports	■ Swimming ■ Golf ■ Table Tennis ■ Walking ■ Fishing
Strongly Discouraged Sports (contact sports)	■ Football ■ Karate ■ Wrestling ■ Skateboarding
Questionable	■ Field sports

BLOOD BOOSTING/BLOOD DOPING

Introduction

The manipulation of the amount of erythrocytes in blood has become a common practice in endurance athletics. Blood boosting is said to happen when blood, either autologous stored packed RBC or packed RBCs from a blood bank, is given intravenously to an athlete before an event. From the first report of the usefulness of supplementing erythrocytes for improved performance in 1947 (28), this has now become a regular practice. The use of blood boosting and blood doping techniques was highlighted (or lowlighted) in the 2002 Winter Olympics.

There are other techniques employed by athletes with a design to manipulate the production of erythrocytes in order to produce an erythrocythemia. The three main techniques are as follows: live at a higher altitude and train at a lower elevation (live high, train low); produce a pseudo-elevated sleeping environment (altitude house); and the use of recombinant hormones that stimulate RBC production. The first two are legitimate techniques and the third is a banned practice.

Blood Boosting

Intravenous blood boosting has been rumored to be a practice in sports for many years now. The advantages of such transfusions were shown in a study in 1972, in which Vo_{2Max} was increased by 9% with transfusions (29). The benefit of transfusions is probably the result of overcoming the aerobic endurance's rate-limiting step, the oxygenation of the muscles. It is estimated that a pint of whole blood can add a significant amount (about 100 dL) of oxygen to the total oxygen carrying capacity (30). The increase in RBCs is one way to increase the delivery of oxygen.

Along with the apparent success in the manipulation of the oxygen carrying capacity of blood, there are real dangers in this practice, including the deaths of healthy, young cyclists from overtransfusions. The transfusions cause an increased viscosity, which can reduce cardiac stroke volume, and the increased viscosity is exacerbated by hemoconcentration during endurance exercise. Transfusions of heterologous RBCs are also a risk, as transfusion reactions are not uncommon in the normal hospital setting, and will potentially be even more of a problem in a hotel setting. This is a dangerous practice that should be stopped.

The cycling community has been under scrutiny for many years for the practice of blood boosting and doping. During the Tour de France, riders' hotels and vans have been raided to prevent blood doping. Cycling is not the only sport in which this practice occurs. Since the 1984 Olympics, the International Olympic Committee has banned transfusions, but detection is difficult. From reports at the 2002 Winter Olympic Games, the practice is still going on.

Live High Train Low

The idea of living high and training low is to reap the benefits of both environments. Studies have shown an increased exercise performance with this technique. At elevations, there is a compensatory erythropoiesis due to the relative hypoxia. Living at high altitudes increases 2,3-Diphosphoglycerate. This molecule binds to hemoglobin and aids in the delivery of oxygen. Over time, the hematocrit increases to compensate for the low oxygen environment. Training at low altitudes circumvents the problems of decreased Vo_{2Max} seen at higher altitudes. The athlete gains oxygen carrying capacity and maintains optimal training.

Altitude Houses

Altitude houses are a way of living high and training low without needing to move from the sea level. The athlete will spend 12 hours a day in a house or sleeping-chamber in which the environment is adjusted with nitrogen to decrease the oxygen content to 15% from the normal 21%. This is not inexpensive. The "thin air" leads to an increase in endogenous EPO levels and an increased hematocrit without the need for travel.

Recombinant Human Erythropoietin

The use of recombinant human erythropoietin (rhEPO) started in 1987 in Europe. It is used mostly in patients with renal failure and patients undergoing chemotherapy, in order to stimulate RBC production. Uncontrolled studies have shown that it is beneficial in athletics (31). Like blood boosting, use of rhEPO can lead to excessive erythrocythemia and viscosity. This leads to increased thrombogenicity and clotting. Currently no reliable test is available to detect blood doping by this technique. It is difficult to test for rhEPO in urine. Monitoring of hematocrit concentrations is used in cross-country skiing, cycling, and long track speed skating, with a cutoff of 50% for participation. Drug companies continue to invent newer forms of recombinant EPO (darbepoetin), but fortunately they are also developing detection methods in conjunction with these drugs. Further research in the detection of rhEPO from endogenous EPO will benefit sports by curbing rhEPO use.

THROMBOSIS

Deep Vein Thrombosis

The yearly incidence of Deep Vein Thrombosis (DVT) in the general population is 1 in 1,000. The risk of developing a DVT increases with estrogen use, smoking, obesity, prolonged sedentary situations (long plane ride, being bedridden), and surgery. People with certain genetic defects in protein C, protein S, factor V Leiden, Antithrombin III, and Prothrombin G20210 mutation are at a higher risk of thrombosis. The increased risk from each defect varies from threefold to 80-fold. A report on elite athletes showed no increased rate of defects compared to the normal population (32). Pretreatment of athletes with genetic defects is not warranted.

A DVT can often be missed in athletes. The athlete will present with calf pain, unilateral leg swelling, edema, tenderness, or erythema. DVTs have been reported in many sports, from football to skiing. The rate of DVT in postarthroscopic surgery is reported to be 0.7% to 12% (33,34).

Diagnosis is difficult clinically and a high index of suspicion is needed. The most notable clinical test, Homan's sign, is not reliable, with a positive likelihood ratio of 1.0 (35). Homan's sign does not change the pretest probability of DVT. The use of d-dimer test to rule out significant DVTs has been suggested (36). A low value can rule out a DVT. The standard test for detection is duplex sonography. Venogram is the gold standard for diagnosing DVTs. A venogram has high morbidity related to it and is limited in its usefulness clinically for the detection of DVT.

The exact treatment of distal leg DVTs (below the knee) is controversial. Some people believe that the treatment should be with heparin than with warfarin. Others feel that aspirin and repeat duplex sonography are acceptable, as most distal DVTs do not progress. Proximal DVTs are different and can be dangerous. They run a significant risk of causing pulmonary embolism. Treatment is necessary to reduce complications.

Treatment is IV heparin or low molecular weight heparin (LMWH) with oral warfarin started concurrently. Warfarin is continued for 3 to 6 months. The recommendation of duration varies, depending on risk factors and underlying thrombophilia. LMWH is being used more now for treatment of DVTs because of the safety profile, absence of the need to monitor PT/INR (prothrombin time/International Normalization Ratio) levels, and lower cost associated with outpatient treatment.

The formation of a DVT in an athlete is a rare occurrence. This group of people should not normally have thrombotic disease. DVT formation in an athlete should prompt further work-up for thrombophilias, such as prothrombin gene mutation, hyperhomocystinemia, antithrombin III deficiency, or antiphospholipid syndrome. The problem may be in a mutation in the Factor V gene called *Factor V Leiden* or *activated protein C resistance* (37). Factor V gene mutations are the most common cause of recurrent DVTs. Investigative testing to determine prothrombin G20210 mutation or inherited deficiencies of antithrombin, protein C, or protein S should be undertaken (38). These are less common causes but pose significant risk for reoccurrence. Current recommendations are unclear regarding lifelong anticoagulation for patients with thrombophilias (39).

When to return the athlete to play is not well defined. Little research is available in this area. Graded 6 week return has been suggested in noncontact athletic events after clearance of thrombus. An athlete on warfarin should not participate in contact sports. No athlete with an active thrombus should participate in sports.

Effort Thrombosis

Effort thrombosis occurs in the upper extremity. It is most often seen in wrestlers, swimmers, baseball players, and tennis players. It is a rare occurrence, with two cases per year reported in a major urban hospital.

Paget-Schroetter's syndrome is a thrombus in the axillary-subclavian vein, most commonly on the left side. The cause of Paget-Schroetter's syndrome is injury to the subclavian and axillary veins by retroversion or hyperabduction of the arm. This can cause trauma to the venous intimae, producing a successive local activation of coagulation and development of a thrombosis within the vessel (40). It is related to thoracic outlet syndrome or excessive overhead activity. It presents as arm swelling and acute or subacute pain.

Treatment is needed emergently, especially in the case of athletes who make strong use of their dominant arm, as outcomes are grossly different with delayed treatment. The disorder seldom causes pulmonary embolism, but can cause destruction of venous valves and chronic venous insufficiency. Appropriate treatment is important to prevent long-term sequelae.

REFERENCES

1. Eichner ER, Scott WA. Exercise as disease detector. *Phys Sportsmed* 1998;26(3):41–52.
2. Kark JA, Ward FT. Exercise and hemoglobin S. *Semin Hematol* 1994;31:181–225.
3. Yoshimura H. Anemia during physical training (sports anemia). *Nutr Rev* 1970;28:251.
4. Balaban EP. Sports anemia. *Clin Sports Med* 1992;11:313–325.
5. Gillen CM, Lee R, Mack GW, et al. Plasma volume expansion in humans after a single intense exercise protocol. *J Appl Physiol* 1991;71(5):1914–1920.
6. Eichner ER. Sports anemia, iron supplements, and blood doping. *Med Sci Sports Exerc* 1992;24:s315–s318.
7. Chatard JC, Mujika I, Guy C, Lacour JR. Anaemia and iron deficiency in athletes. Practical recommendations for treatment. *Sports Med* 1999;27:229–40.
8. Shakey DJ, Green GA. Sports haematology. *Sports Med* 2000;29:27–38.
9. Clement DB, Asmundson RC. Nutritional intake and hematological parameters in endurance runners. *Phys Sportsmed* 1982;10(3):37–43.
10. Balaban EP, Cox JV, Snell P, et al. The frequency of anemia and iron deficiency in the runner. *Med Sci Sports Exerc* 1989;21:643–648.
11. Garza D, Shrier I, Kohl HW III, et al. The clinical value of serum ferritin tests in endurance athletes. *Clin J Sport Med* 1997;7:46–53.
12. Ashenden MJ, Martin DL, Dobson GP, et al. Serum ferritin and anemia in trained female athletes. *Int J Sports Med* 1998;19:474–478.
13. Garza D, Shrier I, Kohl HW III, et al. The clinical value of serum ferritin tests in endurance athletes. *Clin J Sport Med* 1997;7(1):46–53.
14. Moses FM. Gastrointestinal bleeding and the athlete. *Am J Gastroenterol* 1993;88:1156–1159.
15. Trojian TH. Medical problems. Chapter 7 In: Fu F, Stone D, eds. *Sports injuries- mechanisms, prevention, treatment*, 2nd ed. Philadelphia: Lippincott Williams & Wilkins, 2001.
16. Hoffbrand V, Provan D. ABC of clinical haematology: macrocytic anaemias. *Br Med J* 1997;314:430.
17. Lederle FA. Oral cobalamin for pernicious anemia. Medicine's best kept secret? *JAMA* 1991;265(1):94–95.
18. Green NS. Folic acid supplementation and the prevention of birth defects. *J Nutr* 2002;132(8 Suppl):2356S–2360S.
19. Murphy JR. Sickle cell hemoglobin (Hb AS) in black football players. *JAMA* 1973;225:981–982.
20. Kark JA, Posey DM, Schumacher HR, et al. Sickle-cell trait as a risk factor for sudden death in physical training. *N Engl J Med* 1987;317:781–787.
21. Murray J, Evans P. Sudden exertional death in a soldier with sickle cell trait. *Mil Med* 1996;161(5):303–305.
22. Falsetti HL, Burke ER, Feld RD, et al. Hematological variations after endurance running with hard and soft-soled running shoes. *Phys Sportsmed* 1983;11:118–120, 122–124.
23. Miller BJ, Pate RR, Burgess W. Foot impact force and intravascular hemolysis during distance running. *Int J Sports Med* 1988;9:56–60.
24. Robinson Y, Cristancho E, Boning D. Intravascular hemolysis and mean red blood cell age in athletes. *Med Sci Sports Exerc* 2006;38(3):480–483.
25. Greene WB, Strickler EM. A modified isokinetic strengthening program for patients with severe hemophilia. *Develop Med Child Neurol* 1983;25:189–196.
26. Koch B, Luban NL, Galioto FM, et al. Changes in coagulation parameters with classic hemophilia. *Am J Hematol* 1984;16:227–233.
27. Buzzard BM. Sports hemophilia: antagonist or protagonist. *Clin Orthoped Relat Res* 1996;328:25–30.
28. Pace N. The increase in hypoxia tolerance of normal men accompanying the polycythemia induced by transfusion of erythrocytes. *Am J Physiol* 1947;148:152–163.
29. Ekblom B, Goldbarg AN, Gullbring B. Response to exercise after blood loss and reinfusion. *J Appl Physiol* 1972;33:175–180.
30. Shaskey DJ, Green GA. Sports haematology. *Sports Med* 2000;29(1):27–38.
31. Ekblom B, Berglund B. Effect of erythropoietin administration on maximal aerobic power. *Scand J Med Sci Sports* 1991;1:88–93.
32. Hilberg T, Jerschke D, Gabriel HH. Hereditary thrombophilia in elite athletes. *Med Sci Sports Exerc* 2002;34:218–221.

33. Poulsen KA, Borris LC, Lassen MR. Thromboembolic complications after arthroscopy of the knee. *Arthroscopy* 1993;9(5):570–573.
34. Obernosterer A, Schippinger G, Lipp RW, et al. Thromboembolic events following arthroscopic knee surgery. *JAMA* 1999;282(5):431.
35. Anand SS, Wells PS, Hunt D, et al. Does this patient have deep vein thrombosis? *JAMA* 1998;279:1094–1099.
36. Lippi G, Mengoni A, Manzato F. Plasma D-dimer in the diagnosis of deep vein thrombosis. *JAMA* 1998;280(21):1828–1829.
37. Sheppard DR. Activated protein C resistance: the most common risk factor for venous thromboembolism. *J Am Board Fam Pract* 2000;13(2):111–115.
38. Meinardi JR, Middeldorp S, de Kam PJ, et al. Risk of venous thromboembolism in carriers of factor V Leiden with a concomitant inherited thrombophilic defect: a retrospective analysis. *Blood Coagul Fibrinolysis* 2001;12(8):713–720.
39. Buller HR, Agnelli G, Hull RD, et al. Antithrombotic therapy for venous thromboembolic disease: the seventh ACCP conference on antithrombotic and thrombolytic therapy. *Chest* 2004;126(3):410S–428S.
40. Zell L, Kindermann W, Marschall F, et al. Paget-schroetter syndrome in sports activities–case study and literature review. *Angiology* 2001;52(5):337–342.

Endocrine

20

Thomas H. Trojian

SECTION A
DIABETES MELLITUS

Diabetes mellitus (DM) is a group of metabolic diseases characterized by hyperglycemia secondary to defects in insulin secretion, insulin receptors, or both (1). The vast majority of cases of DM fall into two broad categories. In type 1 DM, the cause is an absolute deficiency of insulin secretion, often related to pancreatic beta-cell destruction. In the absence of exogenous insulin, individuals with type 1 DM are prone to develop ketoacidosis. Much more common is type 2 DM, a combination of resistance to insulin action and an inadequate compensatory insulin secretory response (1). Other major causes of DM are listed in Table 20A.1.

The diagnosis of DM can be made based on one or more of the following criteria: (a) fasting plasma glucose of 126 mg/dL or more on two separate occasions; (b) symptoms of diabetes plus a random plasma glucose concentration of 200 mg/dL or more; (c) 2-hour postprandial glucose of 200 or more following a 75-g glucose load during an oral glucose tolerance test (1).

In the United States alone, it is estimated that more than 20 million people currently have been diagnosed with DM (2). By the year 2025, this number will increase to approximately 22 million. The increasing prevalence of DM is occurring not only in the United States, but it is being witnessed around the world. By 2025, approximately 300 million people worldwide will be diagnosed with DM. The chronic hyperglycemia of diabetes is associated with the development of several adverse medical conditions including retinopathy, nephropathy, and neuropathy. Individuals with DM are also at an increased risk for developing cardiovascular disease, which remains a major cause of morbidity and mortality in this population. As a result, diabetes and its complications will result in an increasing burden on health care costs in the United States and abroad (3).

Refer to Chapter 7 for a discussion on the benefits of exercise in patients with DM.

MANAGING THE ATHLETE WITH DIABETES

Exercise of short duration (<10 minutes) is managed very differently than sports of longer duration. Many athletes in short sprints do not worry about elevated glucose levels before events because there is little concern about the onset of hyperglycemia. Athletes participating in longer duration events, such as 10 km runs, marathons, basketball, or soccer do not want to start an event in a hypoinsulinemic state with elevated glucose because their glucose levels can climb to dangerous levels during the event. Athletes participating in both short and long duration events do not want to start an event in a low glucose or hyperinsulinemic state because it will produce very low glucose levels and dangerous consequences. For sprint events, elevated serum glucose without ketones is acceptable. For longer duration events, serum glucose more than 250 mg/dL with ketones or any serum glucose measurement more than 300 mg/dL pre-exercise should not be initiated until glucose is under better control.

The intensity and duration of exercise will determine specific modifications in the insulin regimen. These include: eating a low glycemic index meal 3 hours before exercise; having a small snack 1 hour before exercise; exercising after the peak action of subcutaneous insulin injection; and, delaying exercise until glucose and ketones are under control (4). Before exercise, depending on the predicted intensity, athletes should modify insulin dosage accordingly. Typically, this reduction ranges from 20% to 50% (5). Taking into account the peak action of each insulin type (see Table 20A.2), it is advised to decrease the dose of the specific insulin that would peak during an upcoming sporting event. For example, for a morning workout, the morning

TABLE 20A.1
OTHER FORMS OF DIABETES

Gestational diabetes	■ Placenta produces estrogen, cortisol, and human placental lactogen which block insulin effects ■ Worsens as pregnancy progresses and placenta enlarges ■ 25% of gestational diabetic patients go on to have type 2 DM
Insulinopathies	■ Rare cases of DM ■ Clinical characteristics of type 1 DM ■ Secretion of insulin that does not bind normally to the insulin receptor ■ Greatly elevated plasma immunoreactive insulin levels ■ Normal plasma glucose responses to exogenous insulin
Diabetes secondary to pancreatic disease	■ Chronic pancreatitis, particularly in alcoholics ■ Mildly hyperglycemic and sensitive to low doses of insulin ■ Destruction of insulin and glucagon cells ■ Frequently suffer from rapid onset of hypoglycemia
Diabetes secondary to other endocrine diseases	■ Clinical characteristics of type 2 DM ■ Secondary to Cushing's syndrome, acromegaly, pheochromocytoma, glucagonoma, primary aldosteronism, or somatostatinoma ■ Peripheral or hepatic insulin resistance ■ Type 1 DM is increased in patients with certain autoimmune endocrine diseases, e.g., Graves' disease, Hashimoto's thyroiditis, and idiopathic Addison's disease
Diabetes induced by beta-cell toxins	■ Clinical characteristic of type 1 DM ■ Vacor, a rodenticide, is cytotoxic for human islets ■ Streptozocin can induce experimental diabetes in animals but rarely causes diabetes in humans

DM = diabetes mellitus.

dose of short-acting insulin (regular insulin—onset: 1–2 hours, peak: 2–4 hours) should be reduced whereas an afternoon activity requires reduction of the morning dose of intermediate-acting insulin (NPH or Lente insulin—onset: 1–3 hours, peak: 4–10 hours). The physician must understand that some trial and error occurs to meet each athlete's insulin and carbohydrate requirements (4).

When administering exogenous insulin, the insulin level may remain elevated during exercise leading to inhibition of both glycogenolysis and gluconeogenesis. To avoid the resultant hypoglycemia, adequate calorie intake and blood glucose monitoring is critical. The athlete needs to replace fluid losses adequately. The athlete with diabetes, if appropriately managed, will initially experience a drop

TABLE 20A.2
INSULIN DURATION

Type	Name (brand name)	Onset of Action	Peak of Action	Duration of Action
Rapid-acting	Insulin lispro (Humalog) Insulin aspart (NovoLog)	10–30 min	1/2–3 hr	3–5 hr
Short-acting	Insulin regular (Humulin R, Novolin R, others) Insulin regular buffered (Velosulin)	30–60 min	2–5 hr	5–8 hr
Intermediate-acting	Isophane insulin (Humulin N, Novolin N) Insulin zinc (Humulin L)	1–2 hr	2–12 hr	14–24 hr
Long-acting	Insulin zinc extended (Humulin U)	1/2–3 hr	4–20 hr	20–36 hr
	Insulin glargine (Lantus)	1/2–3 hr	No peak	Up to 24 hr

in glucose levels. As insulin levels begin to decrease after cessation of the insulin pump or from properly timed subcutaneous injection, frequent monitoring is necessary to assess subsequent glucose elevation. Because it is important for the athlete to replenish glycogen stores during and immediately after exercise, they should ingest 40 g of carbohydrate for every half hour of intensive exercise.

Following exercise, the athlete with diabetes should anticipate late-onset hypoglycemia. If the exercise intensity was unusually high, blood glucose monitoring should occur frequently in the hours following activity, even throughout the night. Any sense of exhaustion, or weakness, or increase in appetite hours after exercise may warn the athlete of possible hypoglycemia. Prevention requires frequent blood glucose checks, upward adjustments of caloric intake, and lowering of longer acting insulin dosage that typically would peak overnight.

For the athlete with DM using multiple injections, the site of injection and rate of absorption is important. Insulin absorption is more rapid and less predictable when injected into the leg before exercise (4). Care should be taken to avoid accidental intramuscular injection. The most common site used by athletes for injection is the abdomen, given its ease of access during meals and more predictable insulin absorption time (6).

INSULIN PUMP

The insulin pump or continuous subcutaneous insulin injection (CSII) system allows more flexibility for skipped meals, sleeping late, and spontaneous exercise. The subcutaneous insulin delivery with the pump allows for precise dosing of insulin. The CSII delivers a continuous basal rate and then boluses can be given by the user for meals. In order to reduce hypoglycemia, the basal rate of the pump is reduced by 50% approximately 1 hour before activity (7). For exercise of lower intensity or shorter duration, the standard basal rate can be maintained and a simple reduction in the premeal bolus is sufficient.

Insulin pumps can malfunction during exercise. The athlete must be mindful of displacement of the infusion set which can lead to a hypoinsulinemic state and diabetic ketoacidosis (DKA) in a short period. Continuing to exercise, unaware of a displaced catheter results in lower insulin levels than expected and can easily quicken the progression to DKA.

Sweating can displace the pump; liquid skin preparations can be used to prevent displacement. The use of antiperspirants around the infusion site has helped reduce sweating around the infusion set. Insulin is heat sensitive and overheating can occur when exercising in the heat with the pump next to the body. The environment (cold and heat) can affect the overall effectiveness of an insulin pump. If unexplainable hyperglycemia occurs, the infusion catheter and insulin cartridge should be replaced. Proper care and monitoring of the equipment is essential for successful use of the pump during exercise.

If removal of the pump is needed during contact and collision sports, it should be stopped 30 minutes before short duration exercise (<1 hour) due to the persistent action of insulin after pump removal. Care should be taken in order to ensure protection of the catheter that will remain in the athlete. Small boluses during exercise may be needed for longer activities (>1 hour) to prevent hypoinsulinemic states during prolonged activities such as marathons and soccer. These boluses should be given hourly and the amount of insulin given should represent approximately 50% of the usual hourly basal rate (8).

HYPOGLYCEMIA

The athlete with DM should be aware of the warning signs of hypoglycemia, which tend to be reproducible for each individual. Symptoms typically involve headache, hunger, and dizziness, which indicate mild hypoglycemia (blood glucose levels between 50 and 70 mg/dL). Both the practitioner and athlete should be prepared to treat acute hypoglycemia with glucose containing liquids, hard candy, or oral glucose tablets. More severe hypoglycemia occurs when glucose levels drop below 40 mg/dL and athletes may be unconscious, combative, or severely obtunded. If the level of consciousness does not allow for protection of the airway, glucose by the oral route should be avoided. In these cases, intravenous glucose administration is indicated. It is always preferable to have confirmation of hypoglycemia by finger stick testing; however, initiating glucose therapy should not be delayed. In those experiencing severe hypoglycemia, glucagon (1 mg SC or IM) should be administered to produce a rapid release of liver glycogen. This is ineffective if all liver glycogen stores have been depleted after prolonged, intense exercise. Given that glucagon is relatively short-acting, once mental status has improved, oral carbohydrate supplements should be given to avoid rebound hypoglycemia. A glucagon emergency kit is a required addition to every field-side coverage bag for events in which athletes with diabetes participate.

SECTION B
THYROID

Thyroid disease is common, affecting approximately 5% of the population during their lifetime. Women have a five to seven times higher incidence of thyroid disease than men. The peak incidence of the disease is over the age of 40 but is common in the college-age population.

Screening for thyroid disease in the general population is controversial, even more so in the athletic population. The recommendation for screening in the general population is every 5 years in women over 35 years of age (2).

Thyroid problems will affect performance and should be considered in athletes with reduced performance. Thyroid screening has been proposed for the Elite Athlete during the preparticipation physical examination (9). This is hardly justifiable and should not be recommended in the general asymptomatic athletic population. Screening of symptomatic individuals should start with the thyroid-stimulating hormone (TSH) because it is a very sensitive screening test for thyroid disease. Once an abnormal value is obtained, further testing should be done based on symptoms and clinical suspicion.

FUNCTION

Thyroxine (T_4) is a tyrosine-based hormone, which is iodinated in the thyroid gland. T_4 is released from the thyroid upon stimulation from TSH. The TSH is released from the anterior pituitary gland by a thyroid releasing factor made in the hypothalamus. T_4 is then converted to tri-iodothyronine (T_3) in the peripheral tissues by a selenium-dependent enzyme (see Figure 20B.1). Thyroid hormone functions by increasing oxidative metabolism in mitochondria and by increasing tissue responsiveness to catecholamines. Problems in the thyroid system stem from interference of proper stimulation of the gland, production of thyroxine, or peripheral conversion. Most frequently, it is a primary thyroid problem. Problems at the hypothalamus or peripheral tissues are uncommon. Medications can effect thyroid function and thyroid hormone binding (see Table 20B.1).

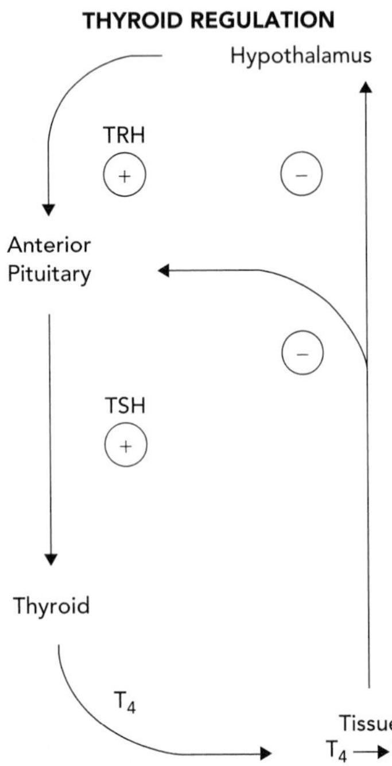

Figure 20B.1 Thyroid function. TRH = thyrotropin releasing hormone; TSH = thyroid-stimulating hormone; T_4 = thyroxine; T_3 = tri-iodothyronine.

TABLE 20B.1
DRUGS THAT EFFECT THE THYROID

Drug(s)	Effect(s)
Amiodarone	↑ TSH secretion
Androgens, carbamazepine	↓ Levels of binding proteins
Dopamine and dopamine agonists	↓ TSH secretion
Estrogen, clofibrate, heroin	↑ Levels of binding proteins
Iodide	↓↑ T_4 synthesis and release from thyroid
Lithium	↓ T4 synthesis and release from thyroid
Phenytoin	↓ TSH secretion, ↓ T_4 metabolism, ↓ levels of binding proteins
Rifampicin, anticonvulsants	↑ T_4 metabolism
Salicylates, frusemide, mefenamic acid, amiodarone, beta-blockers	↓ T_4/T_3 binding to protein
Steroids	↓TSH secretion, ↓ T_4/T_3 binding to protein, ↓ levels of binding proteins

T_4 = thyroxine; T_3 = tri-iodothyronine.

HYPOTHYROID

Hypothyroidism is not conducive to athletics. A large reduction in VO_{2max} and endurance is seen. There is a decrease in cardiac output (CO) and increase in total peripheral resistance (TPR) in patients with hypothyroidism, resulting in a decrease in exercise tolerance.

In hypothyroidism, there is decreased oxidative capacity in the muscle. A decrease in perfusion to the muscle has also been noted. This decreased perfusion is seen in type 2a and type 1 muscle fibers but not in type 2b fibers (10). There is a change in muscle types from fast twitch to slow twitch fibers. The normal energy supply is altered and there is a decrease of lipid (free fatty acids [FFA]) substrate and an increase dependence on muscle glycogen. This results in early fatigability.

There are many different causes of hypothyroidism. The prevalence of overt hypothyroid disease is 1.0% to 1.5% (11). The athlete with thyroid disease will often present complaining of fatigue (91% of patients with hypothyroidism have fatigue) among other complaints. However, fatigue is a common complaint in athletes and is most often not due to thyroid disease. Besides fatigue, the female athlete with thyroid dysfunction will frequently present with menstrual dysfunction, either menorrhagia with hypothyroid or amenorrhea with hyperthyroidism. It

TABLE 20B.2
SIGNS AND SYMPTOMS OF HYPOTHYROIDISM

Symptoms and Signs	Positive Likelihood Ratio	Sensitivity (%)
Slow movement	27.7	36
Puffiness	16.2	60
Ankle reflex	11.8	77
Hearing	8.8	22
Sweating	3.9	54
Constipation	3.2	48
Coarse skin	3.2	60
Paraethesia	3.0	52
Hoarseness	2.7	34
Cold skin	2.5	50
Weight increase	2.4	54
Dry skin	2.1	76

Source: Adapted from Zulewski H. Estimation of tissue hypothyroidism by a new clinical score: evaluation of patients with various grades of hypothyroidism and controls. *J Clin Endocrinol Metab* 1997;82:771–776. (Ref. 12)

is important to consider thyroid disease in female athletes with menstrual irregularities.

The main signs and symptoms of hypothyroidism are slow movement, puffiness, slowed ankle reflex, and dry skin (see Table 20B.2). In this chapter, the two most common forms of hypothyroidism, Hashimoto's thyroiditis and subclinical hypothyroidism, will be discussed.

Hashimoto's Thyroiditis

Hashimoto's thyroiditis is the most common cause of primary hypothyroidism with peak occurrence in middle age, but it is seen frequently in the college athlete. It is an autoimmune disorder with a genetic predisposition. The two most important autoimmune antibodies are the antithyroglobulin antibodies and antithyroid peroxidase antibodies (13).

The usual presentation of Hashimoto's thyroiditis is a goiter. The gland is rubbery and both lobes are enlarged, but not necessarily symmetrically. The patient is usually euthyroid with an elevated TSH. The presence of autoantibodies is found. Levels of free T_4 are often normal initially, but will eventually decrease so monitoring is needed on a bimonthly basis. Occasionally, the patient will present with hyperthyroidism either from concurrent Graves' disease or anti-TSH receptor antibody and then progress from euthyroid to hypothyroid over time.

Treatment is recommended when patients have increased TSH and antibodies are present. Pregnant women with elevated antibody levels have increased miscarriage rates, despite treatment. The use of exogenous thyroxine can reduce the goiter size and relieve symptoms.

Subclinical Hypothyroidism

Screening for subclinical hypothyroidism in women over 35, or during the first prenatal visit is recommended by some authors (14). Subclinical hypothyroidism is disproportionately seen in women. There is an increase in the incidence of the disorder with age. Reports vary from 1% to 10% of patients depending on age-group and location. People with subclinical hypothyroidism describe slightly more thyroid-related symptoms than controls.

Treatment leads to symptom reduction in 25% of patients treated for subclinical hypothyroidism (15). Long-term benefits of treatment are postulated because of the changes in cholesterol with treatment and the noted increase in atherosclerosis in patients with untreated subclinical hypothyroidism. Prevention of overt hypothyroidism by treatment of subclinical hypothyroidism is postulated as elevated TSH or presence of thyroperoxidase antibodies in population studies correlate with an increased rate of 2.1% and 2.6% per year of developing overt hypothyroidism.

Treatment is recommended in patients with TSH greater than 10 mU/L along with either antithyroid antibodies or elevated lipid panel. Treatment with thyroxine should start at 0.05 to 0.075 mg/day. Caution in treatment is needed in patients with coronary artery disease because over treatment with thyroxine can precipitate angina. Patients should be retested in 4 to 6 weeks to check that thyroid function has normalized.

HYPERTHYROID

Hyperthyroidism causes an increase in cardiac output and reduction in TPR. Despite these changes, VO_{2max} is decreased by 10% and endurance is reduced (16). An increase in blood flow to muscles occurs, which might predict an advantage during exercise but decrease in total endurance is seen. Glycogen is depleted at a much faster rate along with elevated lactate levels (17). These metabolic changes and the hyperthermia seen with hyperthyroidism both account for the decreased endurance associated with this disorder.

Hyperthyroid is associated with many overt symptoms. The elevation in circulating thyroid hormone affects cardiac and skeletal systems. Patients with thyroid toxicosis are at a higher risk for atrial fibrillation (AF) and osteoporosis. The incidence of hyperthyroidism has been reported as more than 0.1/1000 in men and 0.8/1000 in women per year (18). Graves' disease is the most common cause of hyperthyroidism. Subacute thyroiditis and subclinical hyperthyroidism are also addressed in this chapter.

Graves' Disease

Graves' disease is the most common cause of hyperthyroidism. It is seen seven times more frequently in females than males. Graves' disease is most common in adults 20 to 50 years old with peak incidence in the third and fourth decade of life (19). The exact cause is unknown but it is characterized by the presence of thyrotropin receptor antibodies (TRAb) and familial predisposition. TRAb are IgG autoantibodies (20).

Patients who have hyperthyroidism commonly have nervousness, fatigue, a rapid heartbeat or palpitations, heat intolerance, and weight loss. These symptoms are seen in more than 50% of all patients who have the disease. Ophthalmological changes, such as proptosis, are probably the most well-known physical characteristics with Graves' disease and can be noted in 50% to 75% of patients. The most common eye findings are eyelid retraction or lag and periorbital edema. Although exophthalmos (proptosis) is commonly described with Graves' disease, it occurs in only a third of patients. The ophthalmological changes seem to be a cross reactivity with receptor antibodies seen in Graves' disease affecting a preadipose subpopulation of the orbital fibroblast.

Some patients who have Graves' disease (1%–2%) may develop dermopathy over the shin area. This pretibial myxedema is typified by hyperpigmented patches and plaques that indurate with touch. The dermopathy is seen almost exclusively with severe ophthalmopathy. As with ophthalmopathy, dermopathy may develop the year before or into the course of the disease.

Diagnosis of Graves' disease is improved with new second generation assays with reported sensitivity and specificity of 99.6% and 98.8% (21). The RAIU (Radioactive Iodine Uptake) scan can help differentiate Graves' disease (diffusely increased uptake) from toxic nodules (with focal uptake) and subacute, chronic, or postpartum thyroiditis (with low uptake).

Treating Graves' disease should include reducing symptoms and controlling the overactive thyroid. Beta-blockers are useful at reducing the symptoms of tremor and tachycardia until the patient is euthyroid. Controlling the overactive thyroid can be accomplished in three ways: antithyroid medications, radioactive iodine ablation, and thyroidectomy.

The medications propylthiouracil and methimazole inhibit thyroid hormone synthesis by inhibition of the thyroid peroxidase enzyme. Remission rates 40% to 65% have been reported with 2 years of antithyroid medication use and thyroid replacement (22). Addition of thyroxine prevents TSH production and theoretically reduces antireceptor antibody production. Side effects of antithyroid medications include leukopenia, rash, pruritus, arthralgias, and, rarely (0.3%), agranulocytosis. Complete blood count should be monitored appropriately while on this medication. Total T_3 and free T_4 should be monitored every 6 weeks until euthyroid then every 3 to 4 months for 2 years. Once medication is stopped, TSH, total T_3 and free T_4 should be monitored every 6 weeks for 18 weeks (22).

Radioactive iodine is the treatment of choice in North America. It is a safe and common treatment (23). The treatment should not be used in patients who are pregnant or might become pregnant in the next 4 months. The main side effect of radioactive iodine treatment is post-treatment hypothyroidism. It can initiate or exacerbate the ophthalmological symptoms of Graves' disease, which can be treated with prednisone. Antithyroid medications should not be used immediately before or after radioactive iodine. Medications such as propylthiouracil can be radioprotective for up to 55 days. Patient thyroid states usually stabilize 6 to 12 months after treatment, and can be followed up every 3 to 4 months, or as needed, with a T_4 index and TSH tests. Once euthyroid, these patients should be followed up yearly with a serum TSH test.

Subtotal thyroidectomy is the preferred treatment for certain subgroups of patients with Graves' disease including those who are pregnant and those allergic to antithyroid medications. After surgery, patients may be hypothyroid and will need supplemental thyroid hormone. It is important to follow up patients for 6 months following surgery as hypothyroidism may develop over that period. Yearly thyroid testing is recommended, whether the patient needs thyroid replacement or is euthyroid postoperatively.

Graves' ophthalmopathy may not improve with thyroid treatment, because the antibodies attack the eye as well as the thyroid. Mild to moderate ophthalmopathy may improve without a thyroid treatment and supportive care is all that is needed. Proptosis can produce symptomatic corneal exposure, which can be treated by taping the eyelids closed overnight. Other eye symptoms can be usually treated with sunglasses and artificial tears. Ophthalmology should be consulted for any severe symptoms (such as for severe proptosis, orbital inflammation, or optic neuropathy). Approximately two thirds of patients with severe ophthalmopathy improve with high dose glucocorticoid and/or orbital radiation (24).

Subacute (de Quervain's) Thyroiditis

de Quervain's thyroiditis is viral in origin. It presents after an upper respiratory infection with prolonged malaise, asthenia, and pain over the thyroid due to stretching of the capsule from the expanding thyroid. The thyroid is most often tender to palpation. The symptoms may smolder and be vague in nature.

The diagnosis is made with an elevated erythrocyte sedimentation rate (ESR) and a depressed RAIU. Other tests (free T_4, total T_3, and TSH) can vary depending on the stage of the illness. If the symptoms smolder, the thyroid may be painless and can mirror Graves' disease. Differentiating the two clinical entities will be difficult in these cases.

Treatment of subacute thyroiditis is mostly supportive because the problem will resolve spontaneously. Propranolol is used to control the symptoms of thyrotoxicosis. To decrease the inflammatory response, aspirin is used if the case is mild or prednisone if more severe. When the RAIU and free T_4 return to normal, therapy can be stopped.

Subclinical Hyperthyroidism

Subclinical hyperthyroidism is defined by low TSH but normal thyroxine and T_3. The incidence varies by location, associated thyroid abnormalities, and increasing age. Reported amounts vary from 2% to 16%. The disease may be transient or persistent in nature (25). There is a very small likelihood of subclinical hyperthyroidism developing into overt hyperthyroidism. The main concerns and controversies in treatment are the associated increased risk in cardiac and musculoskeletal diseases.

Population studies have shown an increased chance of AF over 10 years; incidences of 8%, 12%, and 21% for TSH concentrations of normal, 0.1 to 0.4 (μ)U/mL, and less than 0.1 (μ)U/mL respectively (26). These increases in AF are correctable with treatment. This is not a reason for immediate therapy as the natural course of the disease is often transient. Monitoring is appropriate.

An increase in bone demineralization is noted in subclinical hyperthyroidism (27). In premenopausal women the rate was not significant, but increased. In postmenopausal women the rate was higher and significant. The athlete with subclinical hyperthyroidism and stress fractures should be considered for earlier treatment.

REFERENCES

1. Report of the expert committee on the diagnosis and classification of diabetes mellitus. *Diabetes Care* 1997;20:1183–1197.
2. Danese MD, Powe NR, Sawin CT, et al. Screening for mild thyroid failure at the periodic health examination. A decision and cost-effectiveness analysis. *JAMA* 1996;276:285–292.
3. Peirce NS. Diabetes and exercise. *Br J Sports Med* 1999;33:161–173.
4. Lisle DK, Trojian TH. Managing the athlete with type 1 diabetes. *Curr Sports Med Rep* 2006;5(2):93–98.
5. American Diabetes Association. Diabetes mellitus and exercise. *Diabetes Care* 2001;24:S51–S55.
6. Frid A, Ostman J, Linde B. Hypoglycemia risk during exercise after intramuscular injection of insulin in the thigh of IDDM. *Diabetes Care* 1990;8:337–343.
7. Sonnenberg GE, Kemmer FW, Berger M. Exercise in type 1 diabetic patients treated with continuous subcutaneous insulin infusion. Prevention of exercise induced hypoglycemia. *Diabetologia* 1990;33:696–703.
8. Schiffrin A, Parikh S. Accommodating planned exercise in type 1 diabetic patients on intensive treatment. *Diabetes Care* 1985;8:337–342.
9. Mellman MF, Podesta L. Common medical problems in sports. *Clin Sports Med* 1997;16:635–662.
10. McAllister RM, Delp MD, Laughlin MH. Thyroid status and exercise tolerance- cardiovascular and metabolic considerations. *Sports Med* 1995;20:189–198.
11. Tunbridge W, Evered DC, Hall R, et al. The spectrum of thyroid disease in a community: the Whickham survey. *Clin Endocrinol (Oxf)* 1977;7:481–493.
12. Zulewski H. Estimation of tissue hypothyroidism by a new clinical score: evaluation of patients with various grades of hypothyroidism and controls. *J Clin Endocrinol Metab* 1997;82:771–776.
13. Barbesino G, Chiovato L. Autoimmune thyroid disease: the genetics of Hashimoto's disease. *Endocrinol Metab Clin* 2000;29:357–374.
14. Cooper DS. Subclinical hypothyroidism. *N Engl J Med* 2001;345:260–265.
15. Cooper DS, Halpern R, Wood LC, et al. L-thyroxine therapy in subclinical hypothyroidism: a double-blind, placebo-controlled trial. *Ann Intern Med* 1984;101:18–24.
16. Martin Wh, Spina RJ, Korte E, et al. Mechanism of impaired exercise capacity in short duration experimental hyperthyroidism. *J Clin Invest* 1991;88:2047–2053.
17. Sestoft L, Saltin B. Working capacity and mitochondrial enzyme activities in muscle of hyperthyroid patients before and after 3 months of treatment. *Biochem Soc Trans* 1985;13:733–734.
18. Boelaert K, Franklyn JA. Thyroid hormone in health and disease. *J Endocrinol* 2005;187:1–15.
19. McIvers B, Morris JC. The pathogenesis of graves' disease. *Endocrinol Metab Clin North Am* 1998;27:73–89.
20. Gough SC. The genetics of Graves' disease. *Endocrinol Metab Clin North Am* 2000;29:255–266.
21. Costagliola S, Morgenthaler NG, Hoermann R, et al. Second generation assay for thyrotropin receptor antibodies has superior diagnostic sensitivity for Graves' disease. *J Clin Endocrinol Metab* 1999;84:90–97.
22. Hashizume K, Ichikawa K, Sakurai A, et al. Administration of thyroxine in treated Graves' disease: effects on the level of antibodies to thyroid stimulating hormone receptors and on the risk of recurrence of hyperthyroidism. *N Engl J Med* 1991;324:947–953.
23. Singer PA, Cooper DS, Levy EG, et al. Treatment guidelines for patients with hyperthyroidism and hypothyroidism: standards of care committee, American Thyroid Association. *JAMA* 1995;273:808–812.
24. Bartalena L, Marcocci C, Pinchera A. Treating severe Graves' ophthalmopathy. *Baillieres Clin Endocrinol Metab* 1997;11:521–536.
25. Shrier DK, Burman KD. Subclinical hyperthyroidism: controversies in management. *Am Fam Physician* 2002;65:431–438.
26. Sawin CT, Geller A, Wolf PA, et al. Low serum thyrotropin: a risk factor for atrial fibrillation in older persons. *N Engl J Med* 1994;331:1249.
27. Faber J, Galloe M. Changes in bone mass during prolonged subclinical hyperthyroidism due to L-thyroxine treatment: a meta-analysis. *Eur J Endocrinol* 1994;130:350–356.

Environment

21

Thomas H. Trojian

Environment changes the outcome of athletic events on a regular basis. The effects of fog, rain, cold, heat, and altitude alter the performance of athletes, interfering with the body's ability to maintain homeostasis. In this chapter, the effects of the environment on the human body are discussed. Ways of preventing environmental related illness are detailed. Treatments for these environmental illnesses are also addressed.

HEAT STRESS

Introduction

As heat stress increases, there is a reduction in physical performance (see Figure 21.1). Heat is a limiting factor during exercise, irrespective of dehydration or fuel availability status. The body must divert blood flow from muscles to the skin to regulate core temperature (1). This shunting causes a reduction in physical performance. Compounding the problem is the loss of fluid volume due to sweating causing a hypohydrated state. The diversion of blood flow from the muscles and loss of volume due to sweating leads to a decrease in cardiac function. A reduction in stroke volume and cardiac output occurs. This causes the muscles to use more carbohydrates, burning up stored glycogen and producing lactic acid (2). There is an increased perceived exertion and earlier onset of fatigue (3). All these factors bring about a decrement in physical performance.

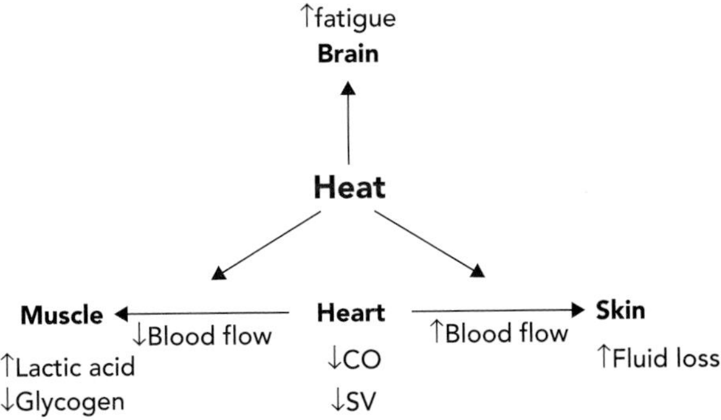

Figure 21.1 Effects of heat on exercise tolerance.

The body's ability to thermoregulate during exercise depends upon a myriad of factors (ambient temperature, humidity, and wind velocity, radiant heat from the sun, and the intensity and duration of exercise). To protect against the development of heat stress, exercise intensity and duration can be altered. Factors such as the weather cannot be altered, but they can be monitored. This is an important means of assessing environmental heat stress, an important factor in planning any outdoor sporting event.

Wet bulb globe temperature (WBGT) is the most efficient method (4) for determining environmental heat stress. The WBGT is determined by using several instruments: (a) a dry bulb thermometer, which measures ambient temperature (T_{db}), (b) a wet bulb thermometer that measures humidity, (T_{wb}) and (c) a black globe thermometer (T_g) that measures radiant heat. If the WBGT Index and wind speed are both measured, an effective temperature can be calculated. Table 21.1 correlates WBGT measurements and exercise safety. A useful website is http://www.smasa.asn.au/resources/hotweather.htm (September 2006.)

Thermoregulation

The main forms of heat loss in humans are evaporation, conduction, convection, and radiation. Evaporation is the loss of heat by evaporation of sweat from the skin. Conduction is the loss of heat passively through tissue to the periphery from the core. Convective heat loss occurs when heat is transferred from the core by the blood to the skin, warm air next to the body is displaced by cool air. The biggest factor contributing to convective heat loss is wind. Radiation is the loss of heat from the warmer body

TABLE 21.1
GUIDELINE FOR EXERCISE IN HEAT

WBGT	Exercise Safety
<27.8°C (82°F)	Safer
27.8°C–29.4°C (82°F–85°F)	Caution ("Danger")
29.4°C–32.2°C (85°F–90°F)	Extreme Caution ("Severe Danger")
>32.2°C (90°F)	No Exercise ("STOP")

WBGT = wet bulb globe thermometer. Amount of clothing, duration of event and the physical health of participants should be considered. You should error on the side of caution.

to the colder environment. Exercising muscles produce a large amount of heat. Roughly, 75% of the energy produced by the utilization of carbohydrates and free fatty acids is converted into heat. The human body acts as a literal furnace. At rest, humans utilize different methods of regulating core temperature compared to times of activity. At rest, the body relies on radiation over evaporative heat loss. The normal percentages are 50% and 20% for radiation and evaporation, respectively, at rest compared to 5% and 80% to 90% when exercising. The change to heat loss by way of evaporation is necessary to maintain core temperature in a narrow physiologic range.

The human body maintains a core temperature in the range of 35°C to 40°C (95°F to 104°F). The core temperature increases with exercise reaching a plateau level of homeostasis tolerated by the athlete. This level can be as high as 41°C (105.8°F) in elite athletes. The maintenance of core temperature is accomplished by the use of thermodetectors in the hypothalamus, spinal cord and limb muscles to maintain and regulate core temperature during exercise. Well-conditioned athletes can produce and dissipate over 1,000 kcals/hour safely. Radiation and convection dissipate most heat when the ambient temperature is greater than 20°C (68°F) and less than 35°C (95°F). Radiation is very important when the ambient temperature is below the body temperature. The body uses conduction and convection to transfer heat less effectively.

Evaporation is the main defense against heat stress. The body sweats to remove heat. This is accomplished by the evaporation of the sweat from the skin. Evaporative heat lost can remove a large amount of energy with 1 L of sweat removing approximately 600 Kcal of energy. An athlete will sweat varying amounts with the normal range being 0.5 to 1.5 L/hour but enormous rates of 4 L/hour have been noted. Sweat is only useful when it is in contact with the skin. If it is wiped off or rolls off the body, then the heat cannot be transferred away from the skin by this method.

The body is able to compensate for the energy produced in exercise to a certain point after which the compensatory factors fail (5). This occurs when the amount of heat generated by the human furnace is greater than the amount possible to dissipate. This varies by the intensity of the activity and the surrounding environment. The core temperature increases as the body is unable to further remove heat by evaporation. The two main reasons for the inability to shed further heat by evaporation are (a) a high WBGT in which the humidity is such that evaporation is diminished, and (b) hypohydration or dehydration in which the production of sweat is decreased. As the loss of body fluid increases, the core temperature increases faster. Compounding the problem, with dehydration the core temperature during exercise that an athlete is able to tolerate is lower. This is due to the reduction in stroke volume as well as the reduction of the volume of blood to the skin and decrease in sweating with dehydration. Hypohydration, as low as 1%, can produce an elevation in core temperature during exercise (6). The amount of increase in core temperature ranges is significant with 0.1°C to 0.25°C (32.18°F to 32.45°F)/percent body weight lost. As the amount of hypohydration increases so does the core temperature.

Predisposition

Several factors increase the susceptibility of an athlete to heat stress (7). Dehydration is the prime factor as discussed in the previous section. Preventing dehydration is important in preventing heat stress. A few facts are important to understand. Regular replacement of fluids is needed because thirst is a poor predictor of fluid status. Most athletes do not develop thirst until they have loss more than 2% body weight. One should note that sweat is hypotonic. There is very little salt in sweat, as well as the amount of salt in sweat decreases with training and acclimatization. Therefore, cold water is the best replacement fluid during exercise. When prolonged activity of greater than 1 hour is performed, a hypotonic salt solution with a 6% to 7% glucose polymer will aid in absorption of fluids.

Acclimatization is important in dealing with heat stress during exercise. This develops with 7 to 10 days of exposure. The benefits of heat acclimatization come from improved skin blood flow rates, earlier onset of sweating, an increased plasma volume, and a lower metabolic rate. Exercising in the heat for 100 minutes is the most effective method of adapting. It is important to increase the core temperature during exercise to develop the adaptive effects quickly. Even sedentary people will adapt to heat but not as quickly as exercising people. The effect is transient and is retained for 2 weeks after last exposure, which proceeds to rapid lost of acclimatization over the next 2 weeks. The more fit an athlete is, the slower the loss of the adaptive benefits.

Clothing and equipment can be significant inhibitors of heat dissipation. Dry clothes soak up sweat and prevent evaporative heat loss. Dark clothes will cause radiant heat gains instead of loss. Football equipment prevents heat loss, thereby at a lower WBGT heat related problems can occur. Adjustments in practices are needed to protect against heat stress (8). These include using less equipment (such as helmet and shorts) during high WBGT and switching practices to early morning or after sundown when the WBGT is lower.

There is a greater potential for heat stress during a febrile illness. These conditions can produce dehydration. Fever will cause an increase in the core temperature and decrease the body's ability to compensate to the heat. Exercising with fever is a dangerous practice especially in the heat.

There are many prescription and over-the-counter medications that can augment the heat stress. Medications such as diuretics cause dehydration. Amphetamines and stimulants can increase metabolic rate and therefore heat production. Anticholinergic agents can decrease sweat production and therefore the evaporation of sweat and removal of heat. These medications should be avoided during exercise.

Women seem to have better thermoregulation than males. Variation in heat dissipation is noted over the menstrual cycle with a slight decrease in the luteal phase. This decrease does not appear to be clinically significant. Estrogen replacement therapy is falling out of favor for numerous reasons but it appears to give a minimal benefit in thermoregulation in postmenopausal women.

Heat Cramps

Heat cramps occur from involuntary contractions of exercising muscles. Calf muscles are by far the most common but any muscle in the body can be affected. The cause is presumed to be an electrolyte imbalance during exercise. However, there is evidence that a spinal neural mechanism may induce cramping that is unrelated to biochemical changes either in the blood or in the affected skeletal muscle (9). The best treatment is prevention with proper hydration, sodium, and calcium supplementation. The standard treatment of heat cramps involves rest, massage, passive stretch, and rehydration. Some people swear by the use of pickle juice or yellow mustard to relieve cramps. The reason for the anecdotal success of these two treatments is unknown but both are high in sodium.

Heat Syncope

The syncopal episode occurs in the elderly and the poorly acclimatized individual due to volume depletion, peripheral vasodilatation, and decreased vasomotor tone. The athlete is vasodilated with large pooling of blood in the leg muscles, the heart rate and cardiac output decreases, resulting in insufficient blood supply to the brain. This is made worse by dehydration or a poor cool down after running. Treatment involves elevating the legs (to increase preload and stroke volume), rehydration, and transfer to a cool shaded location. Cardiac and neurological causes need to be considered in the evaluation

Heat Exhaustion

Athletes with heat exhaustion present with fatigue, weakness, piloerection, lightheadedness, headache, and neuromuscular incoordination. They typically have elevated rectal temperatures below 104°F (40°C). The problem is due to inadequate cardiac response to heat stress. Blood is shunted to the muscles and the skin and there is a lack of cardiac preload to maintain cardiac output. Athletes may develop neurological symptoms of headache, irritability, and mild confusion. Treatment is the same as heat stroke.

Heat Stroke

Heat stroke is an emergency that needs to be recognized early (10). The athlete will present with an elevated rectal temperature more than 40°C (104°F) and altered mental status. The classic heatstroke patient will present with dry hot skin without sweating. The heat stroke athlete may still be sweating. Obtaining the rectal temperature of anyone with neurological symptoms is essential. The success of treatment is in early recognition. Difference in symptoms between heat cramps, heat exhaustion, and heat stroke is listed in Table 21.2.

Exertional heat stroke can cause major organ system problems. Acute renal failure, rhabdomyolysis, and disseminated intravascular coagulation are more common in victims of exertional heat stroke than in victims of classic heat stroke (elderly during heat waves). Laboratory abnormalities can include elevated white blood cell count, elevated liver function tests, and hypokalemia in the initial stages with hyperkalemia manifesting later. Sodium levels can be normal or slightly elevated, depending on the hydration status of the patient. Patients can also have

TABLE 21.2
COMPARISON BETWEEN HEAT CRAMPS, HEAT EXHAUSTION, AND HEATSTROKE

Heat Cramps	Heat Exhaustion	Heatstroke
Elevated body temperature	Heat cramps, plus	Heat exhaustion, plus
Thirst	Nausea/vomiting	Anhydrosis
Sweating	Headache	Hyperventilation
Tachycardia	Malaise	Renal failure
Muscle cramps	Myalgias	Hepatocellular necrosis
	Blood Pressure	Pulmonary edema
	Lightheadedness	Arrhythmia
	Oliguria	Rhabdomyolysis
	Uncoordination	Seizure
	Irritability	Disseminated Intravascular Coagulation
	Confusion	Shock/coma

Source: adapted from Wexler RK. Evaluation and treatment of heat-related illnesses. *Am Fam Physician* 2002;65(11):2307–2314, (11).

elevated creatinine phosphokinase (CPK) secondary to rhabdomyolysis. Patients who have peak CPK levels above 10,000 IU/L are at significant risk for the development of acute renal failure.

Acute reduction of the body temperature is the key to recovery and prevention of organ damage. This can be accomplished with ice water immersion or ice packs to the groin and axillary regions. Cool mist fans or alcohol rubs can aid in cooling. Unlike fever from infection in which toxins reset the hypothalamic set point, the elevation in temperature in this case, is due to excessive energy produced. Nonsteroidal anti-inflammatory medicines are not useful in these patients and should be avoided.

In a study of exertional heat stroke cases, ice water immersion lowered core temperature to less than 39°C (102.2°F) in 10 to 40 minutes (12). There were no fatalities in this group. In another study, ice water immersion cooled twice as fast as evaporative cooling (13). The author recommends rapid cooling using ice water immersion whenever possible.

The athlete with altered mental status may have a condition other than heat stroke such as infection, midbrain cerebral vascular accident, drug use, hyponatremia, and hypoglycemia. These other diagnoses need to be remembered when considering treatment. For example, the use of intravenous hydration (half normal saline) would be inappropriate for a runner with altered mental status caused by hyponatremia so obtaining a serum sodium level is important before rehydration is started.

In endurance athletes, hyponatremia can be found secondary to over rehydration with excessive free water. There are seldom mental status changes until the serum sodium level is less than 120 mEq/L. The athlete with a history of large fluid intake in a race or with a later finishing times (usually the less fit runners) is most susceptible. The athlete will have headaches, confusion, and seizures (rare). The same is seen in heatstroke and the rectal temperature is essential in differentiating. Normal temperatures and distal swelling (rings too tight) are reasons for further evaluation of hyponatremia.

Return to activity should be restricted for anyone with syncope, core temperature of greater than 39°C, and neurological symptoms. The person should acclimatize to the heat more and avoid high-intensity activities for 48 hours. Athletes with lesser heat illnesses need to be cooled and closely monitored. There is a higher risk for reinjury in athletes with prior heat illnesses.

Precooling

Prolonged exercise causes body temperature to rise; the increase in core temperature occurs rapidly and reaches steady state values when heat production matches heat loss. A critical limiting temperature exists; so to reduce the risk of cellular injury or heat related illness, athletes must reduce their exercise intensity so that exercise can continue. In hot conditions, the temperature gap between the start and the critical temperature is narrowed and the situation is exacerbated, often resulting in the termination of exercise. When exercising in high temperature environments, it would therefore be sensible to start exercise with a lower body temperature. Precooling (core body temperature cooling) before exercise would be expected to widen the temperature gap and delay the time before the critical limiting temperature is reached (14).

Studies confirm that increasing body heat is a limiting factor during exercise. Precooling is probably only beneficial for endurance exercise of up to 30 to 40 minutes rather than for intermittent or short-duration exercise (15–17). Studies show precooling before an endurance event may be worthwhile if the facilities are available. Precooling takes approximately 30 minutes to complete and can be done in either a swimming pool or a cold shower (18). Ice vests have been used and are more portable than immersion techniques. Precooling could be advantageous for endurance exercise in warm conditions (18).

COLD STRESS

Physiology

During cold weather, the body tries to maintain core body temperature while heat loss continues to occur due to conduction and convection mechanisms. The wind chill index is a measurement used to evaluate the effects of increased wind speed on heat loss. Wind increases conductive heat loss, therefore increasing cooling. A difference in ambient temperature and body temperature increases conduction heat loss. The loss of body heat by conduction is 25-fold greater in water than in air (19). A person in 20°C (68°F) water will become hypothermic depending on clothes and size of person in 2 to 40 hours whereas a dry person in 20°C (68°F) temperature on dry land would not become hypothermic.

In an attempt to maintain core body temperature, basal heat production increases slightly in the cold. Yet, it is not sufficient to maintain body temperature. A layer of subcutaneous fat is helpful to act as an insulator against the cold, but again the benefit is small. Intake of calories and exercise is important to generate sufficient calories to stay warm.

Voluntary and involuntary methods of heat generation are used to maintain core temperature in humans. The body will produce 3 to 6 times the basal amount of heat by involuntary shivering. Shunting of blood from the skin to the core also occurs to prevent heat loss. Thermoreceptors in the skin signal the hypothalamus to increase heat generation both voluntarily and involuntarily and to constrict peripheral circulation.

Voluntary exercise can generate significant heat. The body acts as a furnace keeping the core temperature in the narrow physiologic range. Approximately 75% of muscle contraction energy is released as heat. The amount of energy the body can generate diminishes as energy stores are used up. Mild to moderate intensity exercise produces sufficient heat and helps to keep the temperature in the physiologic range. It generates less heat than severe intensity exercise but longer duration exercise is possible. Mild intensity exercise often does not produce enough heat to prevent shivering.

As the body's core temperature starts to drop, a cold-induced diuresis occurs. This occurs because the cardiac output increases and the systemic vascular resistance is higher. The kidneys receive an increase in blood flow and an increased of amount of fluid is filtered. As the body's core temperature drops lower, the renal perfusion decreases as cardiac output becomes less and less.

Hypothermia

Hypothermia is a seen in prolonged athletic events where the temperature is below 10°C (50°F), precipitation is occurring and wind speed is elevated. Most cases, in sports, will be mild but in extreme sports during winter, the severity of hypothermia can increase. Care needs to be implemented to maintain reheating of the individual.

Mild Hypothermia

Mild hypothermia is when the body core temperature is between 32.2°C and 35°C (89.96°F and 95°F) (20). The person will have confusion, slurred speech, impaired judgment, and amnesia. Cardiac output increases with tachycardia and increases preload secondary to the peripheral constriction. Shivering still occurs at these temperatures to stimulate heat. An athlete with confusion, dysarthria and ataxia with prolonged exposure to the cold should be considered to have hypothermia. A rectal temperature is needed to evaluate core temperature. It is useful to assess consciousness and shivering. A shivering conscious athlete probably has a core temperature above 31°C (87.8°F); whereas a severely disoriented or unconscious athlete not shivering is likely to have a core temperature below 31°C (87.8°F).

Moderate/severe Hypothermia

Moderate hypothermia presents with lethargy, disorientation, and unconsciousness. As the core body temperature lowers, cardiac output decreases and respiration is decreased and shallow. Before loss of consciousness, people have been known, paradoxically, to undress. This phenomenon is secondary to the loss of peripheral vasoconstriction and sudden warming of the extremity and sense of over heating. This severe impairment in judgment does not allow them to realize that this is a poor choice. Paradoxical undressing is a poor prognostic sign.

Severe hypothermia is often confused with death. The person has fixed dilated pupils, poor pulse that could be missed on palpation, severe muscular stiffness, and areflexia, even to noxious stimuli. Electrocardiography (EKG) may show asystole, ventricular fibrillation and other findings. The person without an EKG abnormality can have an arrhythmia triggered with sudden jarring. Careful assessment of the person with hypothermia is needed to guarantee no pulse before starting cardiopulmonary resuscitation (CPR). If possible, cardiac monitoring should be done.

Treatment

Treatment for hypothermia has common components for mild, moderate and severe forms. Further heat loss should be prevented (21). The person should have any wet clothes removed. Rectal temperature should be measured and monitored if possible. Prevention of worsening orthostatic hypotension is done by placing them supine. A barrier to the cold ground such as a sleep pad, blanket, or sleeping bag is needed to prevent conductive heat loss. All of these things should be done for every hypothermic patient.

The person with mild hypothermia needs to be kept warm, supplied with warm beverages and allowed to shiver. The shivering will effectively reheat the body. Exogenous rewarming is not needed. Actually, it may slow reheating. Heated humidified air is not going to add a significant temperature increase. It is important to prevent further heat loss.

Moderate to severe hypothermia needs close observation and cardiac monitoring. Careful transport to a hospital is the best option/action. Active external rewarming is needed in these patients once recooling can be prevented. The use of heat packs to the groin, axilla and neck, as well as feet in hot water or force heated air device (e.g., Bair Huggers, Arizant Healthcare Inc., Eden Prairie, MN) can be useful. Care is needed to avoid thermal burns.

For severe hypothermia, active internal rewarming is recommended. Warmed intravenous solution (normal saline) at 43°C (109°F), peritoneal lavage with warmed fluids and, if possible, warmed (42°C to 46°C [108°F to 115°F]) humidified oxygen during bag-mask ventilation is to be administered. If the victim is pulseless with no detectable signs of circulation, start chest compressions immediately. Follow advance cardiac life support principals (22).

Frostnip

Frostnip is what most people get when they go out in the cold and their nose, ears, toes, fingers, cheeks, or chin get white and cold. Often ice crystals will be seen on the surface of the skin. It occurs slowly and painlessly. Reheating occurs quickly and redness, pain, and hypersensitivity will develop over the affected area. There is no permanent damage after reheating. It is important to warm the affected area and keep the area warm to prevent further freezing and damage.

Frostbite

Frostbite is a problem in athletes exposed to freezing or near freezing weather such as those participating in orienteering, cross-country skiing, hiking, kayaking, skiing, ice climbing, and skating. Any sport performed outdoors can increase the risk for frostbite if the athlete is outdoors for prolonged periods. Length of exposure is the most important risk factor in the severity of injury.

Injury occurs by three different and simultaneous pathways: tissue freezing, inflammatory mediator release and tissue hypoxia. The tissue forms ice crystals, and then intracellular dehydration and death occur. At first, something called the "hunting response" (21) occurs with constriction and then dilation of the peripheral vessels to keep the tissue oxygenated. Once the core temperature drops with prolonged cold exposure, the body closes off the peripheral blood supply to maintain core temperature. Tissue hypoxia followed by cell death occurs. The local tissue damage causes the release of inflammatory mediators such as prostaglandin F2 (PGF_2), thromboxane A2 (TA_2), and oxygen radicals. The release of these mediators reaches their peak with rewarming and increases with refreezing and thawing again. The inflammatory mediators are the prime cause of further tissue damage after rewarming. A "secondary" zone of injury can cause worsening injury. Table 21.3 reviews the four stages of frostbite.

Clinically it can be divided into two stages.

1. Superficial Injury (first and second degree) is when there is only damage to the skin, no deep structures are involved and with no permanent damage.
2. Deep Injury (third and fourth degree) is when the structures below the skin are frozen. They are usually permanent injuries. The muscle or bones of the extremity are involved. It is not possible to identify the extent of injury initially. It takes 22 to 45 days before the definite extent of permanently injured tissue is identified.

The extent of damage is not identifiable definitively in the first 3 to 5 days. The use of magnetic resonance imaging (MRI) or bone scintigraphy to assess the extent of tissue damage should be delayed for at least 14 days. Vascular studies (i.e., Doppler ultrasound) may be useful at 1 week. Care should be the same for each stage of frostbite at the initial stage.

It is important in the care of the athlete with frostbite not to warm the affected area and then allow it to freeze. As mentioned previously this allows excessive release of mediators and subsequent further tissue damage. It would be better to leave the tissue frozen if prompt care cannot be instituted.

Care of the athlete in the hospital setting initially involves prevention of further damage by the three pathways. The affected area is rewarmed, usually in a warm water bath of 40°C to 42°C (104°F to 107.6°F). The mediators are blocked by the administration of a nonsteroidal anti-inflammatory agent. Blisters are drained and a potent topical anti-inflammatory agent, aloe vera, is applied every 6 hours. The person is prohibited from smoking to prevent further hypoxia and if possible, hyperbaric oxygen is used to decrease hypoxia. Prevention of tetanus and bacterial infection by the administration of tetanus toxoid and immunization, I.V. penicillin, and daily hydrotherapy with hexachlorophene is done. The patient is made comfortable with narcotic pain medication, as rewarming will cause severe pain. Elevation and splinting is used to prevent swelling.

In deep injuries, amputation may be needed even with the best care. These decisions should be delayed until 22 to 45 days, when the extent of necrotic tissue is clearer (23). Debridement should be limited unless infection spread cannot be stopped. It will not be initially obvious which tissue is viable and nonviable, so patience is needed to prevent excessive amputations. Swelling and edema may cause compartment syndromes and earlier fasciotomies are done when needed.

TABLE 21.3
STAGES OF FROSTBITE

Four Stages of Frostbite	
First degree	Numbness, white plague, and surrounding erythema
Second degree	Blistering, erythema, and edema
Third degree	Hemorrhagic blisters
Fourth degree	Complete necrosis and loss of tissue

Prevention of Cold Injury

Clothing Units (CLO) is a measure of the insulator ability of clothing (19). Clothes help prevent conduction heat loss. One CLO is equal to the insulator effects of normal business attire at room temperature (see Table 21.4). An athlete performing intense exercise can maintain body temperature in cold weather. As the activity level decreases, more and more insulation is needed. The dry athlete in calm winds needs different clothes than the athlete in wind and rain. As clothes get wet, the water pulls the heat from the body. It is important to have a waterproof layer in wet weather to stay warm. There are many synthetic clothes that act to keep warmth close to the body. Layering is important so that overheating does not occur and subsequent excessive sweating, causing clothes to become wet and decrease insulation ability, should be avoided. Wind protection is necessary to maintain heat retention because wind helps increase conductive heat loss. The body will spare peripheral tissue to maintain the core temperature. Therefore, it is important to ensure proper protection for ears, fingers, and toes.

LIGHTNING INJURIES

Lightning is responsible for more deaths in the United States than any other natural phenomena. The overall

TABLE 21.4

THE NUMBER OF CLOTHING UNITS NEEDED FOR THE RESPECTIVE APPARENT TEMPERATURE

Activity Levels ↓	20°C (68°F)	0°C (32°F)	−20°C (−4°F)	−40°C (−40°F)	−60°C (−76°F)	−80°C (−112°F)
Rest	1	4	7.5	10.5	13.75	17
Walking 5 Km/hr	1	2	3	4	5	6
Running 10 Km/hr	1	1.5	2.25	2.75	3.4	4
Running 16 Km/hr	1	1	1	1	1	1

Note how the amount of clothing units greatly increases at rest but not when running, because of the heat generated during activity.

mortality rate in lightning strike injuries from Colorado data is 1 in 10 (24). The morbidity rate in survivors approaches 70% (25). Two paramount rules to reduce the morbidity and mortality rates from lightning strikes during sport activities are as follows: (a) have a proactive plan that has been considered before undertaking the sports activity, and (b) seek and stay in a safe shelter until the lightning risk is gone. A safe shelter has been defined as any sturdy building that has been electrically ground by metal plumbing and/or wiring (26).

Mountain Sports

There is a high-risk time for lightning strikes in the mountains. An analysis of lightning related injuries showed that the injuries occur in July and August, in late morning to early evening. Therefore, the recommendation is that hikers should be off the mountain by 11 a.m. in high lightning risk periods (27).

Cold weather does not eliminate danger from lightning. Skiers are not immune from lightning strikes. Thunder snowstorms may occur from October to May but most are in the spring. In addition to the normal signs of lightning, during winter the skier should watch for the appearance of convective clouds, and Graupel (a type of precipitation referred to as soft hail or snow pellets). This precipitation is associated with lightning strikes and can be seen before the visualization of any lightning (28).

Skiing and hiking are not the only sports in which lightning can cause injury. Bicyclists should be aware that rubber tires do not provide protection from lightning. Many injuries occur from being thrown from the cycle due to the force of the lightning strike. Safe structures should be found during a lightning storm while cycling.

Golf

At times, lightning causes more mortality in golf in 1 year than any other cause in any sport. Some problems specific to golf are the paucity of safe shelters on many courses, and the habit of golfers to stand under single tall trees for protection. Open golf carts do not provide protection from lightning. Finding safe shelter is important to live to play another round. If suitable shelter cannot be found, individuals should squat with both feet together and cover their ears with their hands ("lightning position") to minimize risk of strike and acoustic trauma.

Ball Field

Lightning strikes on ball fields are more common in younger athletes. Dugouts are not considered safe protective structures from lightning strikes (28). Automobiles or homes should be sought or other closed structures such as those described previously.

Water Sports

As unbelievable as it may sound, many people do not realize that they need to leave the water during a thunderstorm. The cause of death from lightning strikes in water is not well defined. The proposed mechanisms include the normal electrical effects seen on dry land without an entrance or exit wound due to tissue cooling from the water. Death may also be caused by temporary paralysis and subsequent drowning. Kayaks and sculls are not safe structures for prevention of lightning injuries. A safe shelter needs to be found out of the water.

Lightning Injuries

There are three types of injuries:

Minor injury—Patients are conscious but confused. Most common symptoms are muscle pain and paresthesia, but no burns or paralysis. Complete recovery can be expected.

Moderate Injury—Signs of disorientation are present. Mottled extremities and an absence of peripheral pulses along with first and second-degree burns that appear over several hours are common. The tympanic membrane of the ear is often ruptured. These patients may have an incomplete recovery accompanied by chronic sleep problems and coordination difficulties due to neurological problems.

Severe Injury—Patients may present with ventricular fibrillation or systole. Prognosis in this group is uniformly poor unless CPR is immediate. Treatment of these patients should follow the basic advanced life support guidelines. Cervical spine injuries, secondary to the initial lightning strike, are possible and should be suspected in the unconscious person so that excessive movement of the cervical spine is avoided.

Prevention

Prevention of lightning strike injuries is the best treatment. It is important that available safe cover is readily accessible. Monitoring of lightning is important and can be accomplished by two methods: a lightning monitor, which measures static electricity in the air and gauges distance of lightning strikes, second is the count method in which the time from visual lightning strikes to thunder sound is recorded. The time in seconds is multiplied by 0.2 mi. A safe distance is greater than 6 miles. Therefore, there will be a gap of 30 seconds between flash and sound. For a flash to bang of 30 seconds all sporting activity should be suspended and safe cover should be found. Waiting 30 minutes or longer after the last flash of lightning or sound of thunder is recommended before athletic or recreational activities are resumed (29).

Treatment

If you are present at a lightning strike, it is important to first assess the airway, breathing, and circulation (ABCs) and initiate CPR if appropriate. The person who is unconscious should be considered to have a cervical spine injury. Once stabilized, the person should be safely moved to a medical center for observation. A complete blood cell count and urinalysis, including a test for myoglobinuria should be performed. An electrocardiogram is essential in all patients with lightning strike due to the common presence of QT prolongation after injury. The patient with severe injury warrants further diagnostic testing including electrolyte screen, blood urea nitrogen, and serum creatinine. Serial cardiac enzymes are indicated in the patient with moderate to severe injury. Other tests should be performed as warranted.

WATER EXPOSURE INJURY

Near-drowning

Near-drowning is the ingestion of water into the lungs from submersion/immersion. Near-drowning in lakes and unchlorinated waters is associated with inhalation of bacteria and pneumonia. Prophylactic antibiotics are not recommended (30). Cervical spine injuries should be considered in divers with near-drowning. Assessment of the basic ABCs is needed. Keep the person warm and comfortable. The near-drowning victim often suffers psychological trauma from the event.

Drowning

Drowning is often preventable; it is estimated that 80% of all cases are preventable (31). The new uniform definition of drowning—"the process of experiencing respiratory impairment from submersion/immersion in liquid," as was agreed upon during the World Congress on Drowning in Amsterdam, Netherlands, in 2002 (32) implies that respiratory insufficiency or respiratory failure may follow soon after the incident of immersion or submersion. The brain is the most vulnerable organ for asphyxia, and cerebral impairment occurs before cardiac problems in submersion. CPR should be attempted on drowning victims. Things to consider are cervical spine injury, brain damage, cardiac arrest, respiratory arrest, and hypothermia. The exact cause of brain damage is unknown but asphyxia is the most postulated cause.

Barotraumas

Barotrauma is injury to tissue when there is failure of a gas-filled space to equalize the internal pressure with the pressure in the surrounding environment. Barotrauma to the ears is the most common disorder in divers during decent. Barotrauma to the sinuses causing severe headaches is another. All organs can be affected by barotrauma with the lung being one of the most dangerous due to pneumothorax. Pulmonary barotrauma can produce an air-embolism, which needs immediate attention to reduce damage to the brain. The treatment of air-embolism is hyperbaric oxygen. The increased oxygen pressure forces nitrogen out of the body and equilibrates the gaseous environment. The nearest hyperbaric oxygen chamber should be located before diving.

Decompression Sickness

Decompression sickness (DCS) is defined as the release of inert gas bubbles (most often nitrogen) into the bloodstream and tissues after ambient pressure is reduced (33). This can generally be divided into two broad categories: (a) those due to physical injury as a result of an expansion of gas, and (b) those due to liberation of a gas phase in tissues. The gas in a space is reduced as a diver descends (at a 10 m descent the volume is half of that at the surface). The diver breathes compressed air mixture and the volume expands. As the diver ascends to the surface the gas in the lungs expands and needs to be released or physical injury will occur. Gas in tissues will be released and gas bubbles will develop in the blood if ascent is too rapid (34). Divers with a patent foramen ovale may have these bubble transported to the brain from the venous system (34). There are two main types of DCS. Type I is a mild form that is characterized by joint pains, urticarial rash, and pruritus. The incidence of DCS among recreational scuba divers is estimated to be one case per 5,000 to 10,000 dives. The problem usually resolves in a short period without treatment but observation is warranted (35). Type II is severe and needs immediate transfer to a recompression chamber. Symptoms of type II DCS are mental status changes, weakness, headaches, gait abnormalities, and breathing problems. The recompression chamber redissolves the nitrogen bubbles in the blood. The addition of 100% oxygen and IV hydration is helpful in the treatment of the patient with decompress sickness (36). The use of nonsteroidal anti-inflammatory medication is controversial (35). The best treatment is prevention. The rate of ascent should be controlled by stopping regularly to allow equilibralization. The U.S. Navy has developed diving tables to guide ascent. These can be found at http://www.ndc.noaa.gov/gi.html (September 2006).

ALTITUDE

Altitude changes affect the human body because of the relative hypoxic environment and decreased atmospheric pressure. These changes can be pathological or used for enhancing training (see Table 21.5).

Altitude Training

The 1990s were the beginning of the popularization of the "live high–train low" strategy (35). This has led to the use of a number of new altitude training devices by athletes. These include the following: (a) normobaric hypoxia through nitrogen dilution (hypoxic apartment), (b) supplemental oxygen, (c) hypoxic sleeping devices, and (d) intermittent hypoxic exposure (IHE). Each method uses alterations in the F_IO2 to stimulate changes in the body that could be advantages to competition.

A normobaric hypoxic apartment simulates elevations equivalent to 2,000 to 3,000 m. The barometric pressure within the apartment is equivalent to sea level. The Finnish "nitrogen-houses" are actually well-furnished hotel rooms, with nitrogen gas pumped into the rooms to decrease the F_IO2 to approximately 15%. This simulates the living at high altitude and then training at "sea level," when the athlete goes outside to the normal "higher" F_IO2. Long term use of a normobaric hypoxic apartment (12 to 18 hours/day for 10 to 25 days) stimulates the release of serum erythropoietin (EPO) (37) and significantly increases reticulocyte count. Not all studies demonstrate this effect (38). These differences between studies may be the result of assessment methods, simulated altitudes, and the training status of the athletes.

TABLE 21.5
EFFECTS OF ALTITUDE ON THE BODY

Heart	↑Heart rate, ↔Cardiac output
Pulmonary	↑Respiratory rate ↑Volume
Sleep	↓Restful sleep ↑Periodic breathing/apnea

There is evidence that peak cardiovascular function is reduced during maximal exercise in both acute and chronic hypoxia with no evidence for any primary alterations in myocardial function. Peak skeletal muscle electromyographic activity is also reduced during hypoxia. Both support a model in which a central, neural governor constrains the cardiac output by regulating the mass of skeletal muscle that can be activated during maximal exercise in both acute and chronic hypoxia.

Published data on the use of supplemental O2 training suggest that high-intensity workouts at moderate altitude and endurance performance at sea level may be enhanced through hyperoxic training utilized at an altitude over a period of several weeks (39). Training with supplemental oxygen is a modification of the "live high–train low" philosophy. The athlete is increasing their F_IO2 while training compared to their living conditions. A study showed the efficacy of hyperoxic training suggesting that high-intensity workouts at moderate altitude (1,860 m) and endurance performance at sea level may be enhanced when supplemental oxygen training is used (40). The full benefit from hyperoxic training is not yet known. Much more research is needed.

IHE and Intermittent Hypoxic Training (IHT) allow athletes to "live low–train high". IHE is based on the assumption that brief exposures to hypoxia (1.5 to 2.0 hours) are sufficient to stimulate the release of EPO, bring about an increase in red blood corpuscles (RBC) concentration. Athletes typically use IHE while at rest, or in conjunction with a training session. It is unclear whether passive IHE or IHT leads to improvements in hematological measures. In addition, there are minimal data to support the claim that IHE or IHT enhance Vo_{2max} and endurance performance. Anaerobic power and anaerobic capacity may be improved as a result of IHT (41).

Hypoxic sleeping devices include the Colorado Altitude Training (CAT) Hatch (Boulder CO) (hypobaric chamber) and Hypoxico Tent System (Hypoxico Inc. New York, NY) (normobaric hypoxic system), both of which are designed to allow athletes to sleep high and train low. These devices simulate altitudes up to approximately 4,575 m and 4,270 m, respectively. They are similar to the hypoxic apartments but on a smaller scale. The chambers are cheaper than the hypoxic apartments but not equivalent. RBC production, maximal oxygen uptake, and/or performance in elite athletes do not appear to be affected by the use of these systems despite theoretical advantages (42).

Acute Mountain Sickness

Pathophysiology

The Lake Louise Consensus Group (43) defined Acute Mountain Sickness (AMS) as the presence of headache and one or more of the following symptoms: gastrointestinal (anorexia, nausea, or vomiting), insomnia, dizziness, and lassitude or fatigue, in an unacclimatized person who has recently arrived at an altitude above 2,500 m. Symptoms seem to correlate with decreased urine output. Altitude related illness is rare at altitudes below 2,500 m but is common in travelers above 3,500 m. The occurrence is increased by a rapid gain in altitude and reduced by a slow ascent, allowing time for acclimatization. Most (approximately 65%) people who develop AMS become symptomatic within the first 6 to 12 hours of arrival to that altitude. Acclimatization schedules of 600 m ascent above 2,000 m/day and preexposure of 5 or more days above 3,000 m in the last 2 months help reduce AMS.

The exact mechanism of AMS is unknown. Either hypoxia-induced cerebral vasodilatation or mild cerebral edema most likely produces the headache. The headache itself can cause nausea and malaise and thereby account for mild AMS. Impaired cerebral autoregulation, the release of vasogenic mediators, and alteration of the blood-brain barrier by hypoxia may also be important (44). Similar mechanisms are thought to cause cerebral edema at high altitude, which may represent a more severe form of AMS. Differences in individual susceptibility to AMS are striking and are not fully understood.

AMS may be confused with many other ailments but it responds to restful acclimatization within 1 to 3 days. Influenza-like illness, intracerebral hemorrhage, exhaustion, migraine-vascular headaches, dehydration, alcohol hangover, substance abuse, carbon monoxide toxicity, hypothermia, and even mild stroke are in the differential diagnosis especially if symptoms develop more than 1 day after ascent. Alcohol and sedative drugs should be avoided as they alter sleep patterns, decrease ventilation, and intensify hypoxemia. The most important reason to recognize AMS is that it may represent the first stage in the progression to severe HAPE (High Altitude Pulmonary Edema) or High-altitude cerebral edema (HACE) or both. HAPE and HACE are serious conditions (discussed later below); high-altitude illness is associated with rapid ascent above 2,500 m. Alaska climbers sleep at altitude from 3,000 to 5,300 m, a high incidence of HAPE and HACE (2% to 3%) is seen on Denali. Very high altitude, 3,500 to 5,500 m, is associated with extreme hypoxemia during exercise and sleep and is the most common range for severe altitude illness. At above 5,500 m altitudes, above the highest permanent human habitation, deterioration of physiologic function eventually exceeds acclimatization ability.

The three major determinants of developing AMS are 1) a prior history of AMS (increased odds ratio (OR) of 3.0), 2) preexposure (decreased OR 3.2), and 3) slow ascent (decreased OR of 3.0). There has been no significant association of AMS prevalence with gender or smoking. Most studies find no association between training status and likelihood of developing AMS. Most studies reported determinants of risk factors for AMS such as age and obesity; which were factors with an increased risk of AMS (38).

Prevention

For the prevention of high-altitude illness, the best strategy is a gradual ascend to promote acclimatization. The suggested guidelines are an increase of 600 m/day once above 2,000 m with an extra day added for acclimatization for every increase of 1,200 m. Some people need a slower ascent of 400 m/day. Some people would choose not to climb if they had to ascend that slowly (45).

Medications that aid in reducing AMS symptoms with rapid ascent are dexamethasone, acetazolamide, and ginkgo biloba (46). Above 4,000 m, dexamethasone (8 and 16 mg) and acetazolamide (250 mg t.i.d.) are equally efficacious in preventing AMS when ascent rates are higher than 500 m/day. With low rates of ascent, prophylaxis is shown to be worthwhile. The usefulness of acetazolamide is demonstrated by the fact that fewer than three people need to use acetazolamide for one subject not to experience AMS as compared to placebo (46). Severe rebound illness can occur when dexamethasone is discontinued at high altitude and its use is controversial. For these reasons, dexamethasone should not be used immediately before or while ascending to a higher altitude. It should be reserved for treatment with descent or treatment at an altitude when there is an inevitable delay in descent. Meta-analysis showed lower doses of dexamethasone (0.5 mg or 2 mg) and lower doses of acetazolamide (500 mg) were not effective in preventing AMS (46). Others feel that acetazolamide (500 mg) is helpful and there needs to be a randomized control trial to find the optimal dose of acetazolamide (47,48). Ginkgo biloba has been used to prevent AMS. The prophylactic ginkgo dosage of 60 mg t.i.d. for 5 days decreases the incidence of AMS during gradual ascent (49). Ginkgo biloba is a supplement and in the United States caution needs to be used because quantity and quality are not guaranteed. None of the medications will prevent AMS in all people.

Treatment

AMS usually resolves in 2 to 3 days. The person should not increase their altitude and should be monitored for signs of HAPE or HACE. Aspirin (325 mg q4 hours) has been studied and it reduces the headache associated with AMS (50). If rest and symptomatic headache treatment are not effective, descent to lower altitude is indicated. Possibly, giving the patient acetazolamide (500 mg b.i.d.) as treatment can be helpful. Dexamethasone may be used if there is delay in descent or a worsening condition. Treatment with dexamethasone in an oral dose of 8 mg initially followed by 4 mg every 6 hours results in clinical improvement. Continuous use is necessary. Nausea symptoms can be treated with antiemetics. Descent and supplementary oxygen are the treatments of choice, and for severe illness, the combination provides optimal therapy. Astonishingly, only 500 to 1,000 m descent leads to resolution of symptoms in most cases of AMS. Simulated descent with portable hyperbaric chambers is also effective. With the use of these chambers at a pressure of 2 psi

(13.8 kPa), the equivalent altitude is roughly 2,000 m lower. For example, at altitude of 5,000 m being inside the bag is like being at 3,000 m (51). If descent is not possible, combination of hyperbaric chamber and dexamethasone is very useful. AMS treatment can start as watchful waiting but close monitoring is needed and descent of 500 m for 1 day may be helpful.

High-altitude Pulmonary Edema

Patients with HAPE typically presents with dyspnea, cough, weakness, and chest tightness within 1 to 3 days of arrival at altitude (52). Resting tachypnea, tachycardia, and rales are often present. Patients frequently describe a "gurgling" in their lungs. Physical findings include tachypnea, tachycardia, rales, and cyanosis. HAPE can occur rapidly, presenting with exertional fatigue, mild dyspnea, and cough, progressing to severe hypoxic coma overnight. Fatalities related to HAPE have been reported at altitudes as low as 2,440 m (43). HAPE is the most common cause of fatality at high altitude. It is caused by high pulmonary artery pressures that lead to a protein-rich and mildly hemorrhagic edema. HAPE is a form of hydrostatic pulmonary edema with altered alveolar-capillary permeability (53).

For many years, it was misdiagnosed as pneumonia occurring within several days of ascent in healthy young men. HAPE has become increasingly recognized. Many factors have been associated with HAPE including amount of exertion, individual susceptibility, rate of ascent, maximum altitude, and sedative drug use. However, a person's physical conditioning before the climb does not seem to decrease occurrence. Gradual acclimatization as well as avoidance of sedatives and alcohol may lower the risk of HAPE. Salmuterol 125μg inhaled b.i.d. reduced episodes of HAPE in susceptible individuals (54).

To treat HAPE, immediate descent is essential; this may require medical evacuation. Oxygen saturation of 90% or more is important, which may require 4 to 6 liters/minute or more of supplementation. Nifedipine (10 mg) is used for reduction of the pulmonary vascular resistance and pulmonary artery pressure. Acetazolamide at 250 mg orally every 6 hours has also been used in acute disease. Dexamethasone, 8 mg orally for the first dose, then 4 mg every 6 hours can be used. The use of a portable hyperbaric chamber is recommended while awaiting descent.

High-altitude Retinal Hemorrhages

High-altitude retinal hemorrhages (HARH) occur at altitudes above 4,250 m and are common 5,500 m. They are usually asymptomatic. Nonsteroidal anti-inflammatory use, previous elevated intraocular pressure, rapid ascent, and exertion with hypoxemia are thought to be precipitating stresses (55). They are probably related to increased blood flow and retinal vessel dilatation. The hemorrhages usually resolve over 7 to 10 days. They go unnoticed unless they involve the macular area (56). Fundoscopic examination is recommended if other signs of altitude illness are seen (57). If vision is impaired or hemorrhages are severe, descent is advised.

High-altitude Cerebral Edema

HACE is a potentially fatal metabolic encephalopathy associated with exposure to the hypobaric hypoxia of altitude (58). Common symptoms include headache, ataxia, and confusion progressing to stupor and coma. Often AMS worsens to HACE or even HACE and HAPE. Focal signs may be seen in severe HACE. HACE can progress within hours but can also take days. Isolated HACE without HAPE occurs at higher altitudes. The mean altitude of HACE is 4,730 m versus 3,920 m when it is coupled with HAPE (59).

Hypertension is not believed to be a major factor in HACE, although minor blood pressure elevation is seen with rapid ascent. It has been postulated that there is a predominantly vasogenic edema mechanism related to a subacute hypobaric hypoxia component in severe HACE (60). This is secondary to a beneficial response to steroids in patients with HACE. One hypothesis that could account for many of the pathophysiologic features of HACE and provide a common link with HAPE is related to capillary leakage from hypoxia-induced endothelial damage.

The treatment of HACE is similar to HAPE except one main feature. Nifedipine is known to reduce pulmonary vascular resistance and pulmonary artery pressure in suspected HAPE. The difficulty is that it can lower systemic arterial pressure, which would impair the cerebral perfusion pressure in HACE; nifedipine should be avoided. Main treatment is immediate descent or evacuation. HACE is completely reversible with expeditious treatment. The use of 100% oxygen, if possible, should be administered until oxygen saturation can be monitored. Dexamethasone, 8 mg orally then 4 mg every 6 hours should be used and a hyperbaric bag can be helpful if immediate evacuation or descent is not possible. Recovery from HACE is not as rapid as from AMS or HAPE and may be prolonged or incomplete if descent or medical therapy is delayed.

JET LAG

The internal clock (circadian rhythm) of your body gets out of step when you cross several time zones over a short period. Jet lag can cause athletes to have trouble falling asleep, early rising, fatigue, irritability, difficulty concentrating, clumsiness, memory problems, weakness, headache, loss of appetite, and an upset stomach. These symptoms may last up to several days.

There are a number of aggravating factors. These include travel across three or more time zones, age or impaired health, lack of previous travel, sleep deprivation, dehydration, stress, alcohol use, and large meals. It is best to maintain good sleep habits, eat light, avoid alcohol and maintain hydration when traveling. Traveling west to east is more difficult than east to west because the actual "biological clock" is slightly longer than 24 hours.

It is best to maintain a positive and relaxed attitude. Pretravel changes may help prevent jet lag. Starting 3 days before departure, begin adjusting your schedule (1 hour a day) of eating, sleeping, and training to that of your destination time. Set your watch to destination time at start the start of the trip. Remain as active as allowed during travel. Sleep on the plane at the appropriate time that is in accordance with the time at the arrival destination. Use pillows, blankets, eyeshades, earplugs, and recline during sleep. Get your preferred seat (aisle, window, etc.) at the onset of the flight. Avoid boredom and stress during travel with relaxing books, music, and so on. You should avoid overeating. Drink plenty of water to stay hydrated. Avoid alcohol because it will affect your circadian rhythm. Upon arrival, you should adopt local time and eating habits, get sun exposure, and stay awake during the day.

Athletes have unique issues to consider. Training intensity should be lighter in the first days after arrival. Fine coordination may be transiently diminished. There is often decreased confidence and increased accidents. Exercise is recommended to help adjust to the new time zone. Although research shows mixed results, studies have shown reduced performance in both the eastward and westward direction with worse performance found in the westward direction (61,62)

Medications can be helpful in adjusting to travel. Slow release caffeine taken in the morning (300 mg) has been shown to help with daytime symptoms (63). Though there are no studies specifically in athletes, zolpidem (Ambien), a nonbenzodiazepine hypnotic medication, appears to be helpful in decreasing jet lag symptoms in travelers. Two studies looking at reducing effects of jet lag with eastward travel have shown the medication to be helpful (64,65)

Melatonin is effective in preventing and reducing jet lag symptoms. Five mg of melatonin from a reliable source should be recommended to adult travelers flying across five or more time zones. Melatonin has not been shown to be as effective as zolpidem. Timing is important with melatonin dosing. It should be taken at bedtime corresponding to the arrival time zone. Better results are found when traveling in the easterly direction, and if they have experienced jet lag on previous journeys. Travelers crossing <5 time zones may find benefit. The use of melatonin in people with epilepsy has had negative results, and there exists a possible interaction with warfarin (66).

Jet lag can cause detrimental effects in athletic performance. These effects can be limited or eliminated with proper planning and medication. The team physician can play a significant role in the success of athletes traveling long distances.

REFERENCES

1. Charkoudian N. Skin blood flow in adult human thermoregulation: how it works, when it does not, and why. *Mayo Clin Proc* 2003;78:603–612.
2. Febbraio MA. Alterations in energy metabolism during exercise and heat stress. *Sports Med* 2001;31(1):47–59.
3. Nielsen B, Nybo L. Cerebral changes during exercise in the heat. *Sports Med* 2003;33(1):1–11.
4. Cheuvront SN, Haymes EM. Thermoregulation and marathon running: biological and environmental influences. *Sports Med* 2001;31:743–762.
5. Moran DS. Potential applications of heat and cold stress indices to sporting events. *Sports Med* 2001;31:909–917.
6. Cheuvront SN, Haymes EM. Thermoregulation and marathon running: biological and environmental influences. *Sports Med* 2001;31(10):743–762.
7. Cheung SS, McLellan TM, Tenaglia S. The thermophysiology of uncompensable heat stress. Physiological manipulations and individual characteristics. *Sports Med* 2000;29(5):329–359.
8. Kulka TJ, Kenney WL. Heat balance limits in football uniforms. How different uniforms ensembles alter the equation. *Phys Sportsmed* 2002;30:29–22, 37–39.
9. Wexler RK. Evaluation and treatment of heat-related illnesses. *Am Fam Physician* 2002;65:2307–2314.
10. Noakes TD. Fluid and electrolyte disturbances in heat illness. *Int J Sports Med* 1998;19(Suppl 2):S146–S149.
11. Wexler RK. Evaluation and treatment of heat-related illnesses. *Am Fam Physician* 2002;65(11):2307–2314.
12. Costrini A. Emergency treatment of exertional heatstroke and comparison of whole body cooling techniques. *Med Sci Sports Exerc* 1990;22(1):15–18.
13. Armstrong LE, Crago AE, Adams R, et al. Whole-body cooling of hyperthermic runners: comparison of two field therapies. *Am J Emerg Med* 1996;14(4):355–358.
14. Marino FE. Methods, advantages, and limitations of body cooling for exercise performance. *Br J Sports Med* 2002;36(2):89–94.
15. Cheung S, Robinson A. The influence of upper-body pre-cooling on repeated sprint performance in moderate ambient temperatures. *J Sports Sci* 2004;22(7):605–612.
16. Duffield R, Dawson B, Bishop D, et al. Effect of wearing an ice cooling jacket on repeat sprint performance in warm/humid conditions. *Br J Sports Med* 2003;37(2):164–169.
17. Marino FE. Methods, advantages, and limitations of body cooling for exercise performance. *Br J Sports Med* 2002;36(2):89–94.
18. Quod MJ, Martin DT, Laursen PB. Cooling athletes before competition in the heat : comparison of techniques and practical considerations. *Sports Med* 2006;36(8):671–682.
19. Noakes TD. Exercise and the cold. *Ergonomics* 2000;43:1461–1479.
20. Shephard RJ. Metabolic adaptations to exercise in the cold. An update. *Sports Med* 1993;16(4):266–289.
21. Fritz RL, Perrin DH. Cold exposure injuries: prevention and treatment. *Clin Sports Med* 1989;8:111–128.
22. American Heart Association. Part 10.4 hypothermia. *Circulation* 2005;112; 136–138.
23. Ulrich AS, Rathlev NK. Hypothermia and localized cold injuries. *Emerg Med Clin North Am* 2004;22(2):281–298.
24. Cherington M, Walker J, Boyson M, et al. Closing the gap on the actual numbers of lightning casualties and deaths. *Eleventh Conference of Applied Climatology*; 1999 Jan 10–15; Dallas, Boston: American Meteorological Society, 1999:379–380.
25. Ghezzi KT. Lightning injuries. A unique treatment challenge. *Postgrad Med* 1989;85:197–198, 201–203, 207–208.
26. Bennett BL. A model lightning safety policy for athletics. *J Athl Train* 1997;32:251–253.
27. O'Keefe Gatewood M, Zane RD. Lightning injuries. *Emerg Med Clin North Am* 2004;22(2):369–403.
28. Cherington M, Breed DW, Yarnell PR, et al. Lightning injuries during snowy conditions. *Br J Sports Med* 1998;32(4):333–335.
29. Walsh KM, Bennett B, Cooper MA, et al. National Athletic Trainers' Association position statement: lightning safety for athletics and recreation. *J Athl Train* 2000;35(4):471–477; errata *J Athl Train* 2003;38(1):83.
30. Ender PT, Dolan MJ, Dolan D, et al. Near-drowning–associated Aeromonas pneumonia. *J Emerg Med* 1996;14:737–741.
31. Bierens JJ, Knape JT, Gelissen HP. Drowning. *Curr Opin Crit Care* 2002;8(6):578–586.
32. Papa L, Hoelle R, Idris A. Systematic review of definitions for drowning incidents. *Resuscitation* 2005;65(3):255–264.
33. Newton HB. Neurologic complications of scuba diving. *Am Fam Physician* 2001;63(11):2211–2218.
34. Schwerzmann M, Seiler C. Recreational scuba diving, patent foramen ovale and their associated risks. *Swiss Med Wkly* 2001;131(25–26):365–374.
35. Levin BD, Engfred K, Friedman DB, et al. High altitude endurance training: effect in aerobics capacity and work performance. *Med Sci Sports Exerc* 1990;22:S35.
36. Neuman TS. Arterial gas embolism and decompression sickness. *News Physiol Sci* 2002;17:77–81.
37. Rodriguez FA, Casas H, Casas M, et al. Intermittent hypobaric hypoxia stimulates erythropoiesis and improves aerobic capacity. *Med Sci Sports Exerc* 1999;31:264–268.
38. Vallier JM, Chateau P, Guezennec CY. Effects of physical training in a hypobaric chamber on the physical performance of competitive triathletes. *Eur J Appl Physiol* 1996;73:471–478.

39. Perry CG, Reid J, Perry W, et al. Effects of hyperoxic training on performance and cardiorespiratory response to exercise. *Med Sci Sports Exerc* 2005;37(7):1175–1179.
40. Morris DM, Kearney JT, Burke ER. The effects of breathing supplemental oxygen during altitude training on cycling performance. *J Sci Med Sport* 2000;3:165–175.
41. Wilber RL. Current trends in altitude training. *Sports Med* 2001;31(4):249–265.
42. Kinsman TA, Hahn AG, Gore CJ, et al. Respiratory events and periodic breathing in cyclists sleeping at 2,650-m simulated altitude. *J Appl Physiol* 2002;92(5):2114–2118.
43. Hackett PH, Oelz O. The Lake Louise consensus on the definition and quantification of altitude illness. In: Sutton JR, Coates G, Houston. CS, eds. *Hypoxia and mountain medicine*. Burlington, Vermont: Queen City Printers, 1992:327–330.
44. Hackett PH. High altitude cerebral oedema and acute mountain sickness: a pathophysiology update. *Adv Exp Med Biol* 1999;474:23–45.
45. Barry PW, Pollard AJ. Altitude illness. *BMJ* 2003;26; 326(7395):915–919.
46. Dumont L, Mardirosoff C, Tramèr M. Efficacy and harm of pharmacological prevention of acute mountain sickness: quantitative systematic review. *BMJ* 2000;321:267–272.
47. Hackett P. Pharmacological prevention of acute mountain sickness: many climbers and trekkers find acetazolamide 500 mg/day to be useful. *BMJ* 2001;322:48.
48. Bartsch P, Schneider M. Pharmacological prevention of acute mountain sickness: same ascent rates must be used to assess effectiveness of different doses of acetazolamide. *BMJ* 2001;322:48.
49. Roncin JP, Schwartz F, D'Arbigny P. EGb 761 in control of acute mountain sickness and vascular reactivity to cold exposure. *Aviat Space Environ Med* 1996;67:445–452.
50. Burtscher M, Likar R, Nachbauer W, et al. Effects of aspirin during exercise on the incidence of high-altitude headache: a randomized, double-blind, placebo-controlled trial. *Headache* 2001;41(6):542–545.
51. Hackett PH, Roach RC. High-altitude illness. *N Engl J Med* 2001;345:107–114.
52. Bartsch P. High altitude pulmonary edema. *Respiration* 1997;64:435–443.
53. Swenson ER, Magiorini M, Mongovin S, et al. Pathogenesis of high latitude edema: inflammation is not an etiologic factor. *JAMA* 2002;287:2228–2235.
54. Sartori C, Allemann Y, Duplain H, et al. et al Salmeterol for the prevention of high-altitude pulmonary edema. *N Engl J Med* 2002;346:1631–1636.
55. Butler FK, Harris DJ Jr, Reynolds RD. Altitude retinopathy on Mount Everest, 1989. *Ophthalmology* 1992;99(5):739–746.
56. Honigman B, Noordewier E, Kleinman D, et al. High altitude retinal hemorrhages in a Colorado skier. *High Alt Med Biol* 2001;2(4):539–544.
57. MacLaren RE. Asymptomatic retinal haemorrhage is common at altitude. *BMJ* 1995;311(7008):812–813.
58. Hackett PH. High altitude cerebral edema and acute mountain sickness. A pathophysiology update. *Adv Exp Med Biol* 1999;474:23–45.
59. Hultgren HN. *High altitude medicine*. Stanford, CA: Hultgren Publications, 1997.
60. Yarnell PR, Heit J, Hackett PH. High-altitude cerebral edema (HACE): the Denver/Front range experience. *Semin Neurol* 2000;20(2):209–217.
61. Waterhouse J, Edwards B, Nevill A, et al. Identifying some determinants of "jet lag" and its symptoms: a study of athletes and other travellers. *Br J Sports Med* 2002;36(1):54–60.
62. Reilly T, Atkinson G, Waterhouse J. Travel fatigue and jet-lag. *J Sports Sci* 1997;15(3):365–369.
63. Beaumont M, Batejat D, Pierard C, et al. Caffeine or melatonin effects on sleep and sleepiness after rapid eastward transmeridian travel. *J Appl Physiol* 2004;96(1):50–58.
64. Jamieson AO, Zammit GK, Rosenberg RS, et al. Zolpidem reduces the sleep disturbance of jet lag. *Sleep Med* 2001;2(5):423–430.
65. Suhner A, Schlagenhauf P, Hofer I, et al. Effectiveness and tolerability of melatonin and zolpidem for the alleviation of jet lag. *Aviat Space Environ Med* 2001;72(7):638–646.
66. Herxheimer A, Petrie KJ. Melatonin for the prevention and treatment of jet lag. *Cochrane Database Syst Rev* 2002;(2):CD001520.

Challenged Athletes

22

Katherine L. Dec

Special populations in athletics have been mentioned throughout this text. One area of sports medicine, for the physically challenged and mentally challenged, is sometimes overlooked in general sports medicine texts. It is suggested that there are over four million recreational and competitive athletes with disabilities in the United States. The different physiological and neuromusculoskeletal components of those disabilities present additional areas of medical management for the sports medicine physician. These include unique issues in medical management, aerobic and anaerobic conditioning, and equipment used in the performance of sport. This chapter will address issues of importance in each of these areas. Please refer to the suggested readings at the end of the chapter for some of the textbooks devoted to these different athletic populations.

The nomenclature used to define this population has been varied and confusing. These are athletes with impairment that restricts or decreases their ability to participate in athletic arenas within the manner considered "normal" for the sport. "Impairment" refers to any loss or abnormality of psychological, physical, or anatomic structure or function. "Disabled" refers to any restriction imposed by an impairment that limits the individual's ability to perform an activity within the manner considered normal for a person. Therefore, "disabled," "impaired," or "challenged" are descriptive of the functional issues present in this area of sports.

Sports for athletes with physical impairment have been present since 1888, when the Sport Club for the Deaf in Berlin, Germany opened its doors. The first international competition for disabled athletes is thought to be the International Silent Games in 1924. The Stoke Mandeville Games for the Paralyzed, held in 1948, was the first noted international sports competition for athletes with various physical disabilities. It has only been since the 1980s that junior divisions have developed in some of these athletic arenas. Most areas of sports for children have been through adaptive physical education, hippotherapy, horseback riding therapy, and aquatic therapy.

MENTALLY CHALLENGED ATHLETES

Eunice Shriver organized a program of physical fitness for individuals with mental impairment in 1968. This program, Special Olympics, has grown tremendously in size: it is international and involves over 2.2 million athletes, pediatric through older adult ages. Eligibility for participation requires the individual to be at least 8 years of age (for competitions) and have intellectual ability significantly below average for biological age and social culture, as measured by formal assessment, or significant learning or vocational problems owing to cognitive delay that require or have required specially designed instruction. More information can be obtained from Special Olympics' website: www.specialolympics.org. Special Olympics is typically considered to be the competition, that is, the Summer Special Olympic Games, held by the organization. There is also a Skills Program that is available and detailed in a written format for several summer and winter sports. This is an 8-week training program, 3 days per week with goals and assessment tools. These guides/skill programs are available from Special Olympics International and assist those who wish to be active but do not actually wish to compete in the Games.

Special Olympics uses a system called "divisioning" versus a medical or functional classification system, in order to match the skills of similar competitors in a sport. Age, sex, and ability are used to create a score. Each division has three to no more than eight competitors or teams. Within a division, the top and bottom scores may not exceed each other by more than 10%. In team sports, 4 to 5 sport-specific skills are evaluated in every team member. These scores are summated to create the team score for divisioning.

Special Olympic athletes have a higher rate of abnormalities on screening evaluation (1) than able-bodied athletes;

such as gastrointestinal disorders, visual impairment and congenital heart conditions. A high incidence of visual problems has been sited in these athletes (2). Of 905 participants at the 1995 Special Olympics World Summer Games, refractive errors, poor distance acuity, and strabismus were among the vision anomalies (2).

Congenital heart conditions are present in up to 50% of athletes with Down syndrome (3). The most common congenital heart disease in western medicine literature is atrioventricular septal defect. A recent retrospective study in Saudi Arabia (4) found a similar frequency (61.3%); however, ventricular septal defect was the most common congenital heart anomaly they reported. There has also been an increased association of obesity and high cholesterol in athletes with Down syndrome (5). Some of these conditions can limit participation in sports (6), depending on the type of activity. Sports injuries in mentally challenged athletes are similar to those that occur in nonimpaired athletes and are sport specific (7).

Clinical issues potentially uncovered on preparticipation examination can include decreased neck range of motion (ROM), abnormal gait, ligamentous laxity, neurological symptoms, seizure history, and sensory symptoms. There is a reported 8.7% incidence of scoliosis in these athletes (8). The athlete may also report being easily fatigued during activity. Atlantoaxial instability is of higher incidence in Down syndrome than in nonchallenged athletes. Most athletes with atlantoaxial instability are asymptomatic (9). Lateral cervical x-rays with flexion and extension views are required in the Special Olympics screening program in all athletes with Down syndrome. There is controversy regarding using the "atlanto-dens interval" as criteria for competition in sports (10,11). The American Academy of Pediatrics suggests that presence of atlantoaxial instability be considered a contraindication for contact sports (6).

PHYSICALLY CHALLENGED

There are several groups of athletes with physical impairment as their athletic classification. Examples of the different groups of physically challenged athletes include wheelchair athletes, athletes with cerebral palsy (CP), *les autres* (meaning "the others", which includes those with various disabilities such as muscular dystrophies, multiple sclerosis [MS], etc.) and athletes with limb difference or deficiency. Hearing impaired and visually impaired are not exclusive to physically challenged competitions as many compete in athletic competitions without physical impairment as a qualification, for example, hearing impairment in wrestling. They are eligible, according to the National Collegiate Athletic Association (NCAA), "...if they qualify for a team without any lowering of standards for achievement...and do not put others at risk." Those hearing impaired athletes that compete in the physically challenged arena demonstrate a hearing impairment of greater than 55 db loss in the better ear as their qualification.

CLASSIFICATION SYSTEMS

Among the physically challenged athletes, there are classification systems developed to remove bias based on innate level of function. These systems have considered classification based on medical diagnosis alone, functional ability, and a hybrid model considering issues of function and the medical diagnosis. These systems attempt to place persons with a particular impairment on equal functional terms with other competitors. An example is noted in comparing medical and functional classification systems of *les Autres* athletes:

- L1 level in medical class is severe involvement of the four limbs—for example, MS, muscular dystrophy (MD), juvenile rheumatoid arthritis (JRA) with contractures;
- L1 level in functional class is use of wheelchair with reduced function of muscle strength and/or spasticity in throwing arm, and, poor sitting balance.

Some sports have sport-specific classification, such as alpine skiing (Table 22.1).

Figure 22.1 shows an athlete with limb deficiency using outriggers for assistance. Some of the classification systems, for Athletics (Track and Field) in Limb deficiency or difference, and, for physical condition of movement impairment/CP, are given in Tables 22.2 and 22.3. The presence of physically challenged competitions does not limit the involvement of some physically challenged athletes in able-bodied arenas. A few examples including physically challenged athletes in able-bodied arenas are archery and wrestling (athletes with hearing loss). Jim Abbott, a well-known athlete, competed as a professional major league baseball pitcher with a congenital limb deficiency of his right hand.

These classification systems are frequently revised and it is important to know the system in place for the particular

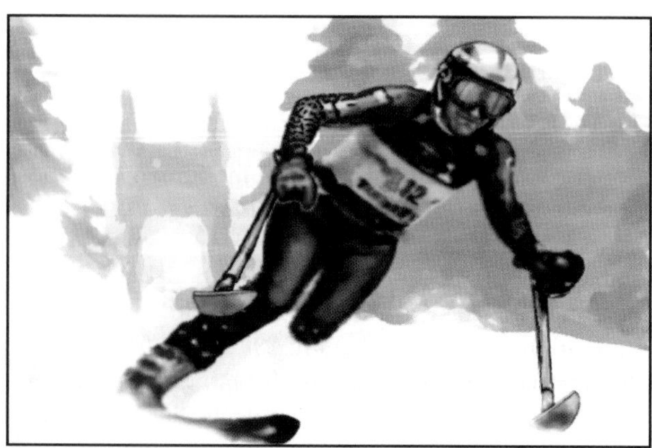

Figure 22.1 Alpine skiing; skiing with outriggers.

TABLE 22.1
ALPINE SKIING CLASSIFICATION: ATHLETES WITH MOBILITY IMPAIRMENT

LW1	Severe disability both legs (LE). Outriggers and two skis, or one ski with prosthesis
LW2	Severe disability one LE. Skiing with outriggers or poles and on one ski
LW3	Disability of both LE, skiing on two skis with two poles or stabilizers
LW3/1	Double BKA, or disabilities of both LE with maximum of 60 muscle points*
LW3/2	CP with moderate to slight diplegic involvement, or moderate athetoid or ataxic impairment
LW4	Disability one LE, skiing on two skis with poles
LW5/7	Disability both upper extremity (UE), skiing on two skis without poles
LW6/8	Disability one UE, skiing on two skis with one pole
LW9	Disability of one UE and LE, using equipment of choice
LW9/1	Disability one UE and LE (such as AKA); CP classification 7 with severe hemiplegia
LW9/2	Disability one UE and one LE (such as BKA); CP classification 7 with moderate to slight hemiplegia
Sitting Classes	
LW10	All disability in mobility and no functional sitting balance. CP limitations of all four limbs
LW11	All disability in mobility and fair sitting balance. CP with disabilities of LE
LW12	Disability in LE and good sitting balance.
LW12/1	SCI or other disabilities
LW12/2	Limb differences of deficiencies in LE

LE = lower extremity; UE = upper extremity; CP = cerebral palsy; SCI = spinal cord injury; AKA = above knee amputation; BKA = below knee amputation;
*"muscle points" considers function and strength of muscle groups tested during classifying.

TABLE 22.2
CLASSIFICATION: ATHLETICS (TRACK AND FIELD) FOR LIMB DEFICIENCY/*LES AUTRES*

Class	
T42	Single AKA; combined LE and UE amputations/ limb differences; minimum disability
T43	Double BKA; combined LE and UE amputations/ limb differences; normal function in throwing arm
T44	Single BKA; combined LE and UE amputations; moderate reduced function in one or two limbs
T45	Double AEA; double BEA
T46	Single AEA; single BEA, UE function present in throwing arm
F40	Double AKA; combined LE and UE amputations; severe problems walking
F41	Standing athletes with maximum of 70 muscle points

T = Track; F = Field; AKA = above knee amputation; BKA = below knee amputation; AEA = above elbow amputation; BEA = below elbow amputation.

competition of your athletic patient. The corresponding governing sports body can assist in clarifying any classification changes. They are typically used in sanctioned competitions but not as strictly followed for local events. International competition involves the following disabilities: paraplegia, amputation, locomotor disorders, CP, mental impairment, visual impairment, and hearing impairment. In the Atlanta Paralympics there were 3,500 athletes from 120 nations; most of these were athletes with limb deficiencies (12).

There are several sports organizations associated with physically challenged athletes. Some examples are: National Disability Sports Alliance (NDSA) formerly known as the United States Cerebral Palsy Athletic Association, United States Les Autres Sports Association (USLASA), and Dwarf Athletic Association of America (DAAA). There are also single sport organizations, such as the National Foundation of Wheelchair Tennis (NFWT), that are open to people with all types of physical impairments who use wheelchairs for sports. This organization works with United States Tennis Association (USTA) wheelchair tennis committee to achieve opportunities for competition in tennis. Internationally, there are the International Paralympic Committee (IPC), the International Stoke Mandeville Wheelchair Sports Federation (ISMWSF), and the International Sports Organization for the Disabled (ISOD), among others. The rules and regulations can vary between local, national and international competitions. In treating athletes training for competitions, be aware of what regulations may be in place for competition and classification.

PREPARTICIPATION EXAMINATIONS

Through the course of development (in congenital acquired impairments), or rehabilitation after a change in physical function (such as traumatic spinal cord injury (SCI)), the team of medical professionals are supportive and encourage the patient to pursue an active lifestyle. There are pre-participation examinations readily available in the able-bodied sports arena. Some of these also address questions to consider in physically- and mentally challenged athletes (13). These can also be used as guides for the physically challenged, however there are additional considerations

TABLE 22.3
CLASSIFICATION: CEREBRAL PALSY

Class 1	Unable to propel a manual wheelchair(w/c), involvement in all four limbs.
Class 2	Able to propel a manual wheelchair, slowly with upper or lower extremities.
Class 3	Able to propel a w/c, near normal function in one extremity. Moderate control issues in UE and torso
Class 4	Propel chair with no limitations, good functional strength, primarily LE moderate to severe involvement
Class 5	Ambulates with assistive devices; good functional strength and minimal control issues in UE
Class 6	Ambulates without assistive devices; decreased coordination. Balance problems with run/throw. Greater UE involvement.
Class 7	Involvement hemiplegic; walk/run with limp. Good function unaffected side.
Class 8	Very minimal involvement; minimal coordination issues.

LE = lower extremity; UE = upper extremity.

during the pre-participation evaluation. These medical issues are covered in more detail in other texts (14). The medical team during acute rehabilitation phases is attuned to these issues. However, some physically challenged athletes do not turn to competitive sports until after several years following their injury. It is important to gather additional information in the history and determine the presence of co-morbidities in these athletes. In a study reviewing medical comorbidities in long-term SCI individuals, the most prominent included urinary tract infection (UTI), spasticity, and hypertension—regardless of the severity of the SCI (15). Typical historical questions to review the pre-participation assessment are noted in Table 22.4. Laboratory studies must be considered in the context of concurrent medical conditions. For example, an athlete with SCI may have elevated C-reactive protein and interleukin-6 due to the bladder management program or skin breakdown; these can also be elevated in metabolic syndrome of able-bodied athletes (16,17). Potential participation limitations in physically-challenged athletes are listed in Table 22.5.

In this population, there are many medications that are used to treat problems related to various physical impairments. For example, anti-convulsants may be used for treatment of central pain, phantom limb pain, spasticity, and mood disturbances in athletes with a brain injury. Antidepressants and neuromodulation medications such as bromocriptine, baclofen, and methylphenidate are also commonly utilized. The intrathecal baclofen pump (a gamma aminobutyric acid-B [GABA-B] agonist) may be used to manage spasticity. Modafinil has been used in individuals with MS to address fatigue. The World Anti-Doping Code (WADC) applies to the physically challenged athlete in competitive arenas (18). Some of the medications used in treatment of the athlete's physical impairment may be on the prohibited list, such as modafinil, selegiline, or methylphenidate. It is important to understand the principles of the WADC and to stay updated on the list of prohibited substances as these are reviewed and updated. Therapeutic use exemption process, on a sport- and case-specific basis, is in place for those athletes, who may need a prohibited substance to manage their medical condition and which does not offer a competitive advantage.

EQUIPMENT

Medical clearance of the athlete for sport is one step; however, this athletic population may also have adaptive equipment requirements. Equipment can be sport specific, such as a quad rugby wheelchair or field event chair. It can involve modification of an everyday prosthesis, as in different terminal devices for athletes with limb deficiencies. In the general recreational, non-competitive arena, there are other types of adaptive equipment such as a swim fin for a person with lower extremity deficiency. When evaluating equipment needs, it is important to utilize a team approach as prosthetic advances for limb deficient athletes and wheelchair modifications for sports require an understanding of the sport and benefits of a particular modification or component.

Wheelchair seating and customizing is individualized. There are different seating systems, depending on the needs of the athlete and sport. Figure 22.2 shows one type of racing wheelchair. In distance racing, some options are the kneeling cage, upright cage, or kneeling bucket. Selection depends on the comfort of the athlete, the amount of torso control and the presence of joint contractures. Optimal positioning for efficient racing stroke is very important. Efficient upper extremity motion in stroke mechanics may decrease overuse injury incidence in the shoulder. There are specialized chairs for basketball, tennis and quad rugby; the latter a hybrid of the other court sport wheelchairs.

In field events there are chairs utilized to provide a level base of support. Wheels are no longer required on the chair during field events. There is a rigid base with quick release support straps. Padding and rails are provided to support and protect the body during the throwing motion.

SPECIFIC POPULATIONS OF PHYSICALLY CHALLENGED ATHLETES

Medical issues are briefly discussed in the subsequent text in the different populations of physically challenged athletes. As an overview, autonomic dysreflexia (AD), pressure

TABLE 22.4
HISTORY QUESTIONS IN THE PHYSICALLY CHALLENGED ATHLETE

History Issues	Examples
Prior secondary medical issues related to the impairment	SCI: recurring pressure sores
	Muscular dystrophy: restrictive lung disease
Concurrent systemic illnesses	TBI: uncontrollable seizures
	All athletes: diabetes, arthritis, heart disease, hypertension, and so on.
Presence of multiple impairments	Amputation and SCI visual impairment and amputation
Current medications	Antiepileptics, antispasmodics, tricyclic antidepressants, anticholinergics, baclofen pumps, pain medicines effecting cognition
History of previous surgeries	SCI: past spinal fusion—may limit the truncal movement and strength necessary for seating or activity. Past surgical muscle transfers for improved upper extremity function in high level SCI.
Gastrointestinal/Genitourinary	SCI, Neuromuscular diseases: type and success of bowel/bladder program; recurring urinary tract infections.
	SCI, Neuromuscular diseases, TBI: gastrostomy tubes
Level of functional independence	Independence in transfers from wheelchair
	Independence donning adaptive equipment
Level of independence in mobility	Wheelchair athletes, *les autres*
Adaptive equipment needs	Prosthesis, orthosis, sports equipment
Prior training	Weather conditions, familiarity with adaptive equipment used
Prior exercise program	Level of aerobic and anaerobic conditioning flexibility

SCI = spinal cord injury; TBI = traumatic brain injury;
Further questions specific to the individual's impairment should be asked as needed to clarify the athlete's ability to compete; however, space is limited to fully explore these potential questions in the context of this chapter. One of several physical medicine and rehabilitation textbooks can further address these impairment specific issues. *Source*: Dec K, Sparrow K, McKeag D. The physically-challenged athlete: medical issues and assessment. *Sports Med* 2000;29(4):245–258.

sores, thermoregulatory issues, spasticity, heterotopic ossification, exercise capacity, and the unique limitations musculoskeletal injury can impose on the athlete are mentioned. When considering an athlete new to sports, it is important to consider cardiopulmonary fitness as the demands are different in ambulating with prosthesis, propelling a wheelchair, and so on. Research delineating optimal training regimes for physically challenged athletes on the basis of biomechanics is limited. The research is most prominent in the athletes with physical impairments (due to SCI), wheelchair propulsion, and limb deficiency/difference. Studies in adult wheelchair propulsion and upper extremity exercise have demonstrated improved cardiopulmonary function (19,20). Karagoz et al. (21) note the benefit of wheelchair propulsion, upper extremity exercise, in increasing left ventricular ejection fraction in adolescents. Also, training in wheelchair sports is receiving more clarification in the scientific literature (22–24). Validating exercise tests that can be used in designing the training prescription of wheelchair athletes is an additional area of interest (22). Biomechanics of propulsion in the racing wheelchair athlete has received a great deal of attention. Optimal arm stroke pattern has been discussed and this, in turn, assists in designing weight training protocols and wheelchair design (25,26).

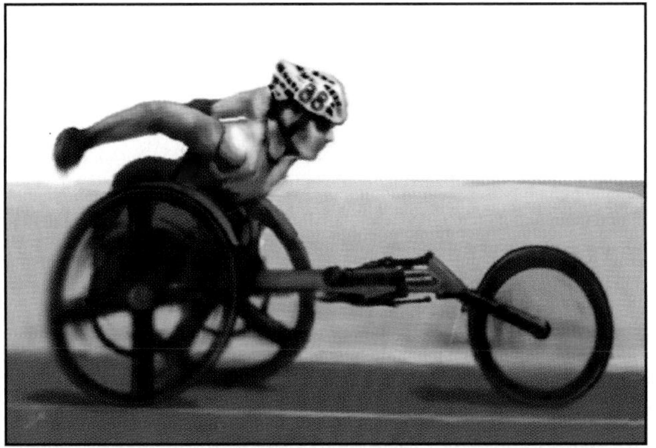

Figure 22.2 Track and field (athletics); wheelchair racing.

Energy expenditure in a person with limb deficiency or difference is greater than in an able-bodied person. Adults with below knee amputation (BKA) require16% to 25% more energy in ambulation; those with above knee amputation (AKA) require 56% to 65% more energy, and

TABLE 22.5

POTENTIAL PARTICIPATION LIMITATIONS UNIQUE TO THE PHYSICALLY CHALLENGED

Potential Athlete Subgroup	Potential Limiting Factors to Sports Participation[a]
Muscular dystrophy	Poor pulmonary function, restrictive lung disease PFT values (nocturnal study important)
Wheelchair athletes (i.e., SCI, neuromuscular impairment) or amputee athletes	Infected pressure sores effecting seating or prosthesis use. Complete rotator cuff tear (wheelchair athletes).
Down's syndrome	Significant atlanto-axial instability
All athletes	Congenital cardiac problems
Traumatic brain injury	Poorly controlled seizures

PFT = pulmonary function test; SCI = spinal cord injury
[a]Certain sports may be contraindicated, such as archery or swimming in the presence of poorly controllable seizures; other sports may be possible and need to be individually assessed for the risk to self and others.
Source: Dec K, Sparrow K, McKeag D. The physically-challenged athlete: medical issues and assessment. *Sports Med* 2000;29(4):245–258.

adults with bilateral AKA require 280% more energy in ambulation (27–29). Although research parameters vary in studies looking at energy expenditure, the increasing number of studies and interest in exercise tolerance in these individuals will assist the physician in determining training parameters for novice athletes and fine-tuning the training of Elite Athletes.

Short Stature Syndromes

There are two general types of short stature syndromes (also known as dwarf classification): 1. disproportionate—average-size torsos, unusually short limbs, and 2. proportionate—overall unusually small size for age. Causes are skeletal dysplasia or chondrodystrophy due to inherited or spontaneous gene mutations in disproportionate dwarfism, and probable endocrine or growth hormone deficiency etiologies in proportionate dwarfism. The skeletal dysplasias that typically have progressive kyphosis and/or scoliosis are spondyloepiphyseal dysplasia (SED) and diastrophic dysplasia. Eye complications can be present in SED. Many individuals with short stature syndromes are able to compete in sports. Dystrophic dysplasia and conditions underlying disproportionate dwarfism can involve joint defects, limited ROM, and have a high incidence of joint dislocation.

Les Autres

"Les Autres" meaning "the others" is used to denote athletes with medical conditions involving physical disabilities that are not eligible to compete athletes with SCI or those in the group of athletes with CP. It includes neuromuscular conditions such as Friedreich's ataxia and MS; muscular dystrophies, such as Duchenne's; and other conditions that affect bones and joints, that is, Ehlers Danlos Syndrome, arthrogryposis, osteogenesis imperfecta, and JRA.

Owing to the diversity of conditions included in this group of athletes, it is difficult to discuss the medical issues involved in each subgroup thoroughly in this chapter. Restrictive lung disease can be an issue in aerobic conditioning and competition for athletes with Duchenne's MD. Pulmonary function tests (PFTs) during the day may not reflect the degree of impairment in vital capacity; PFTs during sleep are recommended. In athletes with Friedreich's ataxia additional issues in balance, speech, coordination, and vision can affect function in a competition. Limiting joint contractures and maintenance of extensor muscle strength is important in athletes with JRA. High impact sports are contraindicated in JRA. In arthrogryposis the goal is to maintain ROM; the degree of involvement in the appendicular joints varies individually.

Athletes with Limb Deficiency

There are competitions for athletes with limb deficiency and an example of classification for Athletics is noted in Table 22.2. Athletes with limb deficiencies can compete in able-bodied sports. There are certain criteria, such as the risk of contact with other players and potential injury to other athletes that govern their involvement in able-bodied sports. The same requirements for padding an accessory brace or appliance will apply to the prosthesis used in the able-bodied arena.

Equipment issues are highly technological in prosthesis options. Involving a certified prosthetist in the treatment team is recommended. Many athletes with limb deficiency do not have the financial freedom to select multiple prosthetics for their sports of choice. Therefore, when choosing the prosthesis one needs to consider cosmesis, durability, and function as they may use their everyday prosthesis for their sport. Occasionally an athlete will compete without the prosthesis. Examples include cycling, where the athlete might utilize clip system for one limb, and swimming, where no prosthesis is allowed in officially sanctioned events.

Medical issues include phantom limb pain, skin breakdown at prosthesis interface, and energy expenditure in training. Good truncal balance and strength of the quadriceps (BKA), hip abductors and adductors, are important for adapting to the prosthetic limb or any component mismatch. The biomechanical differences in gait during lower extremity limb deficiencies, especially AKA, can increase the risk of low back pain (30). In proximal upper extremity deficiency a higher frequency of overuse injury in the nonamputated upper extremity than in the able-bodied population is seen (31).

Phantom limb sensations or pain can occur in the first few weeks after amputation in approximately 70% of individuals. It is theorized that the sudden lack of afferent input and cortical reorganization after amputation is related to the onset of these symptoms (32). Medications used in phantom limb pain or sensation can include pharmaceutical classes of antidepressants and anti-convulsants. The tricyclic antidepressants continue to demonstrate success in management of phantom limb pain (33). As noted in the preceding text, be aware of the WADC. Early reports of acupuncture for treatment of phantom limb symptoms suggest this may be a potential treatment option, but larger population studies are needed (34).

Athletes with Cerebral Palsy

Within CP, there are three types of conditions: spastic CP, athetosis CP and ataxic CP. Athletes with a cerebrovascular accident (CVA) and traumatic brain injury (TBI) are also typically included in this grouping due to the governance by the NDSA (formerly known as the United States Cerebral Palsy Athletic Association [USCPAA]) for organized competition in these movement impaired conditions. Involvement can be diplegia (lower extremities more involved than upper), quadriplegia (all four extremities involved, a.k.a. tetraplegia), hemiplegia (one side, upper and lower limbs involved), and triplegia (3 limbs involved, usually both lowers and one upper). Classification and competition based on mobility function, as in wheelchair functional classification, is controversial as other neuromotor impairments can be present that further limit the athlete's functional level in competition.

Spasticity is an issue in this group of athletes as it is in SCI. Medication options are similar. The additional issue in Cp is that retained primitive reflexes and immature postural reactions can cause postural changes and effect balance and positions used in some sports. Sports, dance and other activities have been used to enhance the postural control and, when done in correct form, can help normalize muscle tone. Sometimes primitive reflexes are used to enhance performance, that is, asymmetric tonic neck reflex (turning head towards active arm) to improve power of upper extremity.

Medical issues that can be present in athletes with these conditions include learning impairment, speech difficulty, strabismus, hearing impairment and seizures. These are all less common than perceptual deficits and reflex/balance issues. It is a misconception that intelligence is impaired in most athletes with CP; while mental impairment may be present in the general population of patients with CP, those that compete under the NDSA typically have average or better intelligence. Seizures are typically controlled by anticonvulsants and rarely impede an athlete from competition. Hip dislocation can occur, most often in a nonambulatory subset of CP athletes. Scoliosis and foot deformities are also present. Pressure sores can occur due to positioning in wheelchairs and because of orthoses used to assist function. Athletes with TBI can develop heterotopic ossification.

Training includes a daily flexibility program. This is very important when strength training is undertaken. Holland and Steadward (35) noted that athletes with CP can complete a 10-week circuit training resistance program with flexibility training and no loss of ROM (except wrist and ankles).

Spinal Cord Injured Athletes

Athletes with SCI can be classified as "complete" (loss of sensation and strength below spinal cord lesion), or "incomplete" (preservation of some sensation or muscle control below spinal cord lesion). Some of the key areas to be aware of in treating athletes with SCI are given in the subsequent text. These are unique to SCI; however, other common prevention strategies in able-athletes, such as sunscreen, are equally important; with the impairment in sensation, discomfort from sun on skin may not be noticed.

Autonomic Dysreflexia

This is a potential problem most often seen in athletes that sustain a SCI at T-6 and above. "T-6" refers to the motor and sensory nerve level impairment of the SCI. At this level, no supraspinal neurological inhibition is present and the sympathetic nervous system is left unchecked. Symptoms can include headache, piloerection, sweating, paroxysmal hypertension, and/or bradyarrhythmia. The inciting factor for AD is some form of noxious stimulus to the spinal cord below the level of the SCI, such as pressure sores, UTI, fracture, tight clothes, distended bowel or bladder, heterotopic ossification, and so on. Therefore, the first step in treatment is to remove the offending stimulus. If hypertension persists, 10 mg of sublingual Nifedipine (the current preference is for "bite and swallow" capsule) or other calcium channel blocker can be given. In a review of the current treatment in AD, Braddom and Rocco (36) have outlined a comprehensive treatment approach in AD. AD is a medical emergency and should be treated quickly.

As SCI competitors attempt to enhance their advantage over an opponent or to gain the proposed improvement in race times, the potential for self-induced AD ("boosting") may become a more prevalent problem (37). Boosting also causes an increased cardiovascular demand. A small study (38) demonstrated that an increased release of catecholamines does occur during exercise; higher peak performances, heart rate, O2 consumption and blood pressure was noted.

Bladder Management

In SCI, as in other neurological lesions involving the spinal cord and urinary reflex function, the protocol for bladder management is important. As noted in the preceding text with boosting, increased bladder distension can lead to AD. What is difficult to diagnose early in some SCI athletes is the presence of a UTI. The typical symptoms of flank pain are not present in high SCI. These UTIs can lead to significant problems if left untreated (39). Symptoms vary from increased spasticity, feeling sick, sweating and AD may be the first sign.

Bladder management typically involves intermittent catheterization, suprapubic catheter, or indwelling catheter. Intermittent catheterization involves inserting a catheter into the urethra for a few seconds to drain the urine into a disposable bag, and is typically performed on a strict schedule. Long-standing indwelling catheters can contribute to recurrent UTIs; condom catheters have also been used. The effectiveness of sacral anterior root stimulation in SCI athletes is unclear. Sacral anterior root stimulation in patients with SCI has been effective and safe in a population of complete patients with SCI (40). Urinalysis results in addition to symptoms are to be considered. An abnormal bacterial count without symptoms is usually managed without antibiotics.

Pressure Sores

Pressure sores can present in amputees with improperly fitting prosthetics or in wheelchair athletes (SCI, CP, spina bifida, neuromuscular disease). Treatment involves assuring proper positioning in the wheelchair, attaining correct fit of adaptive equipment and prosthetics, performing regular pressure reliefs (wheelchair—lifting self off seat for brief periods of 10–20 seconds throughout the day), providing appropriate cushioning, reducing skin moisture (wearing absorbent fabric) and minimizing the potential for skin shear. Prolonged sitting and positioning of the knees higher than the hips in racing wheelchairs, athletes can increase the risk of pressure sores over the sacrum and ischium.

Proper wound management should be implemented immediately at the first signs of a pressure sore. Many topical skin products are available for management of early pressure sores before the dermis is breached. Combination of topical products and assisted wound care by a physician or physical therapist may be needed for the deeper pressure sores. Also recall that these can be a cause for AD in the high SCI athlete.

Thermoregulation

Hypothermia is of special concern in the athletes with SCI. Contributing factors are the decreased muscle mass below the level of lesion, loss of vasomotor and sudomotor neural control, and possible decreased input to the hypothalamic thermoregulatory centers (41). Impaired or absent sensation intensifies the risk, because such athletes may be unaware of clothing dampness which augments the loss of body heat. It is, therefore, important to educate athletes, especially swimmers, endurance racers and cold weather sport participants about hypothermia. It is crucial to monitor them both during and immediately after competition.

Sweating is often impaired below the level of the spinal cord lesion requiring the body to rely upon less surface area (e.g., arms and upper trunk) for evaporative cooling. Feeling the skin under the arms of a distressed athlete during competition has been suggested as a useful tactic: if it is hot, the athlete is likely not dissipating heat adequately—lighter clothing, more fluids, or dousing the skin with water are necessary (42,43). Alternative mechanisms of local cooling are being studied but are currently found to be ineffective (44).

Aging can affect hydration status in these athletes, as in non-challenged athletes. Fluid intake is very important during exercise. In the elderly, the decreased thirst response may limit early recognition of dehydration during exercise. Increased risk of heat-related illness could also occur in those exercising in at-risk environmental conditions. A general recommendation for sedentary elderly would be 1.5 to 2.0 L/day; this would increase with exercise. A regular water break every 15 to 30 minutes may be a general rule; once thirst is present, low fluid stores are already present.

Venous Blood Pooling and Exercise Capacity

In addition to the impairment of autonomic neural control and its effect on thermoregulation, its effect on blood flow can impair achievement of maximal exercise capacity in the athlete with SCI, who may already be hypovolemic while training/competing. The impairment of the sympathetic nervous system decreases the reflexive regulation of blood flow (45). The vasoconstrictor function is impaired; vessels do not constrict and force blood through the venous system or return it to the heart. Cardiac output is diminished and exercise capacity is limited in those athletes with paraplegia as venous pooling can occur without activity from the lower extremity musculature. Venous pooling can result in lower stroke volume; the decrease in oxygenated blood to active limbs may lead to limited aerobic endurance and fatigue. The increased pooling can also result in edema.

In athletes with quadriplegia, peak heart rate rarely exceeds 130 beats per minute during exercise and there is the potential additional risk with medications used in this population (oxybutynin chloride, phenoxybenzamine hydrochloride) of inducing hypotension (46). There is also the risk of deep venous thrombosis (DVT); especially if excessively tight garments are used around the thighs, or abdomen. One of the more common strategies for minimizing venous blood pooling during exercise includes the use of an abdominal binder (47). Fit should be checked to assure the positive effects of compression are obtained over the excessively tight fit (i.e., DVT). Wearing positive pressure garments (stockings) (45) or lower extremity functional electrical stimulation, although often impractical, is considered an option.

Heterotopic Ossification

Athletes with SCI or TBI are at an increased risk for ectopic bone formation. This will usually occur in the area of major joints. The specific cause of heterotopic ossification remains unclear. Pain, increased warmth, swelling, decreased joint motion or contracture may be present in areas of heterotopic ossification. Sport participation does not increase the risk of ectopic bone formation. In a physically challenged athlete presenting with a warm, swollen joint following a sports injury, this is also considered in the differential diagnosis.

Initial treatment after SCI will include nonsteriodal anti-inflammatory medication as this practice can decrease the risk of heterotopic ossification 2 to 3X the non-treated SCI population (48). Etidronate and other bisphosphonates are also used in treatment of heterotopic ossification and their effects effect on bone physiology in this population is of additional interest (49). Later appearance can occur in previously etidronate-treated populations; the physiological characteristics of these ossifications can assist further in determining better management of heterotopic ossification (50). Imaging preference for heterotopic ossification is usually three-phase bone scan. X-rays are often negative in the initial symptom presentation and may take 4 to 5 weeks to reveal findings. Laboratory findings will include a significant elevation in fractionated alkaline phosphatase during bone ossification (51). As always, the laboratory results need to be considered in the presence of the physical findings to be suggestive of heterotopic ossification.

Spasticity

This is a potential problem in any athlete with central nervous system injury: spina bifida, SCI, CP or some of the neuromuscular disorders. Increased spasticity is usually secondary to nociceptive stimulus, such as UTI, distended viscera, bowel obstruction, and so on, as noted (in the preceding text) in AD. Treatment involves removal of the stimulus, changing postural position if a particular posture incites the increased tone, and incorporating a stretching program if not already commenced. It is important for the athlete to have an appropriate, successful bowel and bladder program in place. The medications that may be needed to minimize spasticity interference with sports or function can have a negative effect on alertness and muscle strength. These, as with other medications selected to treat the unique medical conditions in the athlete, should be well-established in the athlete's daily training regime.

Musculoskeletal Injuries and Physical Conditioning

Wheelchair athletes are at particular risk for overuse injuries of the shoulder complex due to repetitive use of the upper extremities for propulsion. Also, compensatory muscle imbalances may develop at the shoulder from long-term wheelchair propulsion, or from a training program deficient in strengthening of the rotator cuff (52) and scapular stabilizer muscles (especially the rhomboids and lower trapezius). Scapular stabilizer muscles are used as primary muscles for upper extremity activity. Decreased flexibility in the anterior muscles, such as pectoralis, and decreased strength in the posterior rotator cuff muscles can occur due to the pushing/propulsion mechanics used by the athlete. This can lead to musculoskeletal injury in those athletes participating in sports requiring different movement patterns such as in swimming, throwing, or racquet sports.

The rehabilitation treatment approach is similar to that for non-impaired athletes; however, modification of strengthening programs (e.g., wheelchair accessible weight machines or modifications of free weights for limb deficient or function impaired), proprioceptive techniques and flexibility exercises will be needed. The limitation of the athlete to follow "relative rest" in the treatment protocol should be considered as there may be limited muscular function available to compensate for the injured area when performing activities of daily living. Therefore, prevention is paramount.

Being well-educated in the established and complementary treatment options available for these athletes will help them avoid potentially harmful medical treatments of questionable results. A questionnaire-based study with an 82% response rate suggested that massage and heat were reported by patients with SCI and pain to provide the best pain alleviation among the non-pharmacological options (53).

Strengthening and conditioning are beneficial in all physically challenged athletes. As the research improves our understanding of the physiological adaptation to exercise, we can give better parameters for training. There are a few contraindications for strength training in the physically challenged athlete. Use of weight lifting equipment is considered limited for athletes with active inflammatory myopathy, severely dystrophic muscular disease, and in free weight equipment, for those with severe coordination deficits. Isotonic or isokinetic machines may be considered in the latter population. Attention is given to using efficient movement/recruitment patterns with the lift movement. Lastly, positioning (with use of straps to secure the trunk during some lifting exercises), and spotting during lifts are important.

In strength conditioning of athletes with SCI, adaptive isotonic equipment is available, in addition to rickshaw and arm crank ergometry. Electrical stimulation research in resistance training has demonstrated increased oxidative capacity and endurance in paralyzed muscles, but no effect on muscle fiber size or strength. Increased cardiac output has been noted in different training protocols for athletes with SCI (54,55). Athletes with paraplegia can increase VO2 max from exercise with attention to intensity, frequency and duration. The recommended guidelines: 20 to 30 minute duration; 3 to 5 days/week, at an intensity of 70% to 80% maximum heart rate (56). In selecting muscle groups to emphasize in resistance training, athletes with SCI should incorporate deltoids, pectoralis, triceps and biceps for greater force in propulsion stroke. Table 22.6 lists key shoulder muscles in the propulsion of the wheelchair.

TABLE 22.6
IMPORTANT MUSCLES AT THE SHOULDER USED FOR WHEELCHAIR PROPULSION

Muscle	Origin	Insertion	Action
Pectoralis major	Med. 2/3 clavicle, sternum, costal cartilage 1–6	Lateral lip of intertubercular groove (humerus)	Adduction and medial rotation of arm; flexion and extension of arm
Pectoralis minor	Ribs 3–5	Coracoid p. scapula	Depress shoulder; downward rotation scapula
Rhomboid major	Spinous p 2–5 thoracic vertebrae	Medial scapula border	Elevation and retraction scapula; downward rotation glenoid cavity
Rhomboid minor	Lower ligamentum nuchae; spinous p. C7-T1	Medial scapula border	Elevation and retraction scapula; downward rotation glenoid cavity
Serratus anterior	Ribs 1–8 anteriolateral thorax	Medial scapula border; inferior angle	Protraction scapula; upward rotation glenoid cavity; holds medial scapula to thorax
Infraspinatus	Infraspinatus fossa scapula	Greater tubercle humerus below supraspinatus	External rotation arm
Supraspinatus	Supraspinatus fossa scapula	Greater tubercle humerus	Abduction arm
Subscapularis	Subscapular fossa scapula	Lesser tubercle and crest humerus	Internal rotation arm
Teres minor	Upper 2/3 lateral scapula	Greater tubercle humerus below infraspinatus	External rotation of scapula
Lower trapezius	Spinous p. thoracic vertebrae	Triangular space at base of scapular spine	Depression scapula; rotation glenoid cavity upward

Additional trunk stabilization muscles not included.

Rotator cuff muscles and scapular stabilizing muscles are very important in throwing athletes, overhead sports and in prevention of glenohumeral and acromioclavicular joint problems.

MD and myotonic dystrophy athletes have been studied to evaluate the effectiveness of resistance training (57,58). With careful monitoring and emphasis on submaximal isokinetic training, increased strength has been demonstrated in boys 5 to 11 years old with MD (59). Resistance training only in the muscles with "good" (at least antigravity) strength has been recommended. Training protocols and physiological effects in neuromuscular conditions is limited in the scientific research; the improvement in strength is suggested to be the result of neural factors (60).

Limited research in use of chronic electrical simulation has revealed some increase in maximal voluntary contraction (61); no conclusive recommendations exist regarding its use in myopathies. Overworked weakness has not been reported. Respiratory muscle conditioning has risks of muscle fatigue; however, in early stage MD a study has noted inspiratory muscle strength can improve (62).

For aerobic conditioning of the athlete with SCI, it is important to remember in lesions higher than T_6 the sympathetic drive is lacking and the heart rate increase, typical in able-bodied athletes with exercise, will be reduced (63). There is less information available considering endurance training. General recommendations are to follow a submaximal training program in the early clinical stages of the myopathy and to have short training sessions that do not fatigue the athlete.

Accommodating the physically challenged athlete in your sports medicine practice will have additional challenges that can be easily overcome. Realize that there are age differences in coping with the newly acquired physical impairment of the athlete: adults have potential concurrent medical issues more often, and youth have socioeconomic issues with peer interaction, prior sports teammate relationship, and so on. Time needs to be spent to redesign athletic goals, secure financial coverage (i.e., physician is involved in appeals and referrals for necessary adaptive equipment), and adjust scheduling to allow for additional history review, possible wound care, transfer to examination table (if needed), removal and evaluation of equipment.

REFERENCES

1. McCormick DP, Ivey FM, Gold DM, et al. The preparticipation sports examination in special Olympic athletes. *Tex Med* 1988;84:39–43.
2. Block SS, Beckerman SA, Berman PE. Vision profile of the athletes of the 1995 Special Olympics World Summer Games. *J Am Optom Assoc* 1997;68(11):699–708.
3. Freeman SB, Taft LF, Dooley KJ, et al. Population-based study of congenital heart defects in Down syndrome. *Am J Med Genet* 1998;80:213–217.
4. Abbag FI. Congenital heart diseases and other major anomalies in patients with Down syndrome. *Saudi Med J* 2006;27(2):219–222.
5. Rimmer J, Braddock D, Fujiura G. Blood lipid and percent body fat levels in Down syndrome versus non-DS persons with mental retardation. *Adapt Phys Act Q* 1992;9:123–129.
6. American Academy of Pediatrics Committee on Sports Medicine and Fitness. Medical conditions affecting sports participation. *Pediatrics* 2001;107(5):1205–1209.

7. Batts KB, Glorioso JE Jr, Williams MS. The medical demands of the special athlete. *Clin J Sport Med* 1998;8(1):22–25.
8. Milbrandt TA, Johnston CE. Down syndrome and scoliosis: a review of a 50-year experience at one institution. *Spine* 2005;30(18):2051–2055.
9. American Academy of Pediatrics Committee on Sports Medicine and Fitness. Atlantoaxial instability in Down syndrome: subject review. *Pediatrics* 1995;96:151–154.
10. Peuschel SM, Scola FH, Pezzullo JC. A longitudinal study of atlanto-dens relationships in asymptomatic individuals with Down syndrome. *Pediatrics* 1992;89:1194–1198.
11. Goldberg JF. Spine instability and the special Olympics. *Clin Sports Med* 1993;12(3):507–515.
12. Tiessen JA, ed. *The triumph of the human spirit. The Atlanta paralympics experience*. Oakville, Ontario, Canada: Disability Today Publishing, 1997.
13. American Academy Family Practice. *Preparticipation physical evaluation*, 3rd ed. McGraw-Hill, 2005.
14. Dec K, Sparrow K, McKeag D. The physically-challenged athlete: medical issues and assessment. *Sports Med* 2000;29(4):245–258.
15. Noreau L, Proulx P, Gagnon L, et al. Secondary impairments after spinal cord injury: a population-based study. *Am J Phys Med Rehabil* 2000;79(6):526–535.
16. Yekutiel M, Brooks ME, Ohry A, et al. The prevalence of hypertension, ischaemic heart disease and diabetes in traumatic spinal cord injured patients and amputees. *Paraplegia* 1989;27:58–62.
17. Manns PJ, McCubbin JA, Williams DP. Fitness, inflammation, and the metabolic syndrome in men with paraplegia. *Arch Phys Med Rehabil* 2005;86:1176–1181.
18. World Anti-Doping Agency. *The world anti-doping code: the 2006 prohibited list*. International Standard, Effective January 1, 2006.
19. Price DT, Davidoff R, Barady GJ. Comparison of cardiovascular adaptations to long term arm and leg exercise in wheelchair athletes versus long distance runners. *Am J Cardiol* 2000;85:996–1001.
20. Huonker M, Schmid A, Sorichter S, et al. Cardiovascular differences between sedentary and wheelchair-trained subjects with paraplegia. *Med Sci Sports Exerc* 1988;30:609–613.
21. Karagoz T, Ozer S, Bayrakci V, et al. Echocardiographic evaluation of wheelchair-bound basketball players. *Pediatr Int* 2003;45:414–420.
22. Muller G, Odermatt P, Perret C. A new test to improve the training quality of wheelchair racing athletes. *Spinal Cord* 2004;42:585–590.
23. Knechtle B, Muller G, Willmann F, et al. Fat oxidation at different intensities in wheelchair racing. *Spinal Cord* 2004;42:24–28.
24. Umezu Y, Shiba N, Tajima F, et al. Muscle endurance and power spectrum of the triceps brachii in wheelchair marathon racers with paraplegia. *Spinal Cord* 2003;41:511–515.
25. Davis R, Ferrara M. The competitive wheelchair stroke. *National Strength Cond Assoc J* 1988;10:4–10.
26. Van der Woude LH, Veeger HE, Rozendal RH, et al. Wheelchair racing: effects of rim diameter and speed on physiology and technique. *Med Sci Sports Exerc* 1988;20:492–500.
27. Gailey RS, Wenger MA, Raya M, et al. Energy expenditure of trans-tibial amputees during ambulation at self-selected pace. *Prosthet Orthot Int* 1994;18:84–91.
28. Gonzalez EG, Cocoran PJ, Reyes RL. Energy expenditure in below-knee amputees: correlation with stump length. *Arch Phys Med Rehabil* 1974;55:111–119.
29. Ward KH, Meyers MC. Exercise performance of lower-extremity amputees. *Sports Med* 1995;20(4):207–214.
30. Kulkarni J, Gaine WJ, Buckley JF, et al. Chronic low back pain in traumatic lower limb amputees. *Clin Rehabil* 2005;19:81–86.
31. Datta D, Selvarajah K, Davey N. Functional outcome of patients with proximal upper limb deficiency—acquired and congenital. *Clin Rehabil* 2004;18:172–177.
32. Melzack R. Phantom limbs and the concept of a neuromatrix. *Trends Neurosci* 1990;13(3):88–92.
33. Wilder-Smith CH, Hill LT, Laurent S. Postamputation pain and sensory changes in treatment-naive patients: characteristics and responses to treatment with tramadol, amitriptyline, and placebo. *Anesthesiology* 2005;103:619–628.
34. Bradbrook D. Acupuncture treatment of phantom limb pain and phantom limb sensation in amputees. *Acupunct Med* 2004;22(2):93–97.
35. Holland LJ, Steadward RD. Effects of resistance and flexibility training on strength, spasticity/muscle tone, and range of motion of elite athletes with cerebral palsy. *Palaestra* 1990;6(4):27–31.
36. Braddom RL, Rocco JF. Autonomic dysreflexia: a survey of current treatment. *Am J Phys Med Rehabil* 1991;70:234–241.
37. Burnham R, Wheeler G, Bhambhani Y, et al. Intentional induction of autonomic dysreflexia among quadriplegic athletes for performance enhancement: efficacy, safety, and mechanism of action. *Clin J Sport Med* 1994;4(1):1–10.
38. Schmid A, Schmidt-Trucksass A, Huonker M, et al. Catecholamines response of high performance wheelchair athletes at rest and during exercise with autonomic dysreflexia. *Int J Sports Med* 2001;22(1):2–7.
39. Vaidyanathan S, Singh G, Soni BM, et al. Silent hydronephrosis/pylonephrosis due to upper urinary tract calculi in spinal cord injury patients. *Spinal Cord* 2000;38(11):661–668.
40. Vastenholt JM, Snoek GJ, Buschman HP, et al. A 7-year follow-up of sacral anterior root stimulation for bladder control in patients with a spinal cord injury: quality of life and users' experiences. *Spinal Cord* 2003;41(7):397–402.
41. Sawka MN, Latzka WA, Pandolf KB. Temperature regulation during upper body exercise: able-bodied and spinal cord injured. *Med Sci Sports Exerc* 1989;21:S132–S140.
42. Bloomquist LE. Injuries to athletes with physical disabilities: prevention implications. *Phys Sportsmed* 1986;14(9):97–105.
43. Corcoran PJ, Goldman RF, Hoerner EF, et al. Sports medicine and the physiology of wheelchair marathon racing. *Orthop Clin North Am* 1980;11(4):697–716.
44. Armstrong LE, Maresh CM, Riebe D, et al. Local cooling in wheelchair athletes during exercise-heat stress. *Med Sci Sports Exerc* 1995;27(2):211–216.
45. Pitetti KH, Barrett PJ, Campbell KD, et al. The effect of lower body positive pressure on the exercise capacity of individuals with spinal cord injury. *Med Sci Sports Exerc* 1994;26(4):463–468.
46. Figoni SF. Spinal cord injury. In: American College of Sports Medicine. *ACSM's exercise management for persons with chronic diseases and disabilities*. Champaign: Human Kinetics, 1997:175–179.
47. Kerk JK, Clifford PS, Snyder AC, et al. Effect of an abdominal binder during wheelchair exercise. *Med Sci Sports Exerc* 1995;27(6):913–919.
48. Schuetz P, Mueller B, Christ-Crain M, et al. Amino-bisphosphonates in heterotopic ossification: first experience in five consecutive cases. *Spinal Cord* 2005;43(10):604–610.
49. Banovac K, Sherman AL, Estores IM, et al. Prevention and treatment of heterotopic ossification after spinal cord injury. *J Spinal Cord Med* 2004;27(4):376–382.
50. Banovac K. The effect of etidronate on late development of heterotopic ossification in after spinal cord injury. *J Spinal Cord Med* 2000;23(1):40–44.
51. Orzel JA, Rudd TG. Heterotopic bone formation: clinical, laboratory and imaging correlation. *J Nucl Med* 1985;26(2):125–132.
52. Burnham RS, May L, Nelson E, et al. Shoulder pain in wheelchair athletes. The role of muscle imbalance. *Am J Sports Med* 1993;21(2):238–242.
53. Nobrink Budh C, Lundeberg T. Non-pharmacological pain-relieving therapies in individuals with spinal cord injury: a patient perspective. *Complement Ther Med* 2004;12(4):189–197.
54. Figoni SF. Exercise responses and quadriplegia. *Med Sci Sports Exerc* 1993;25:433–441.
55. Faghri PD, Glaser RM, Figoni SF. FES leg cycle ergometer exercise: training effects on cardiorespiratory responses of SCI subjects at rest and during submaximal exercise. *Arch Phys Med Rehabil* 1992;73:1085–1093.
56. Bizzarini E, Saccavini M, Lipanje F, et al. Exercise prescription in subjects with spinal cord injuries. *Arch Phys Med Rehabil* 2005;86(6):1170–1175.
57. Olsen DB, Orngreen MC, Vissing J. Aerobic training improves exercise performance in fascioscapulohumeral muscular dystrophy. *Neurology* 2005;64(6):1064–1066.
58. van der Kooi EL, Lindeman E, Riphagen I. Strength training and aerobic exercise training for muscle disease. *Cochrane Database Syst Rev* 2005;25(1):CD003907.
59. De Lateur BJ, Giaconi RM. Effect on maximal strength of submaximal exercise in Duchenne muscular dystrophy. *Am J Phys Med* 1976;58:26–36.
60. McCartney N, Moroz D, Garner SH, et al. The effects of strength training in patients with selected neuromuscular disorders. *Med Sci Sports Exerc* 1988;20:362–368.
61. Scott OM, Vrbova G, Hyde SA, et al. Responses of muscles with Duchenne muscular dystrophia to chronic electrical stimulation. *J Neurol Neurosurg Psychiatry* 1986;49:1427–1434.
62. Vilozni D, Bar-Yishay E, Gur I, et al. Computerized respiratory muscle training in children with Duchenne muscular dystrophy. *Neuromuscul Disord* 1994;4:249–255.
63. Hjeltnes N. Cardiorespiratory capacity in tetra- and paraplegia shortly after injury. *Scand J Rehabil Med* 1986;18:65–70.

SUGGESTED READING

Dec K, Sparrow K, McKeag D. The physically-challenged athlete: medical issues and assessment. *Sports Med* 2000;29(4):245–258.

DeLisa JA, Gans BM, Walsh NE, et al. *Physical medicine and rehabilitation: principles and practice*, 4th ed. Lippincott Williams & Wilkins, 2006.

Paciorek MJ, Jones JA, eds. *Sports and recreation for the disabled*, 2nd ed. Indianapolis: Cooper Masters Press, 1994.

Sweden N, ed. *Women's sports medicine and rehabilitation*. Aspen, 2000.

23 Common Sports-Related Injuries and Illnesses: Generic Conditions

Douglas B. McKeag

The philosophies of care given here are meant to serve as "ground rules." We will refer to these protocols in discussing specific injuries. The general conditions covered are as follows:

- Acute injury
- Chronic injury (with emphasis on overuse syndromes)
- Allergy

ACUTE INJURY

Acute injury is the most common sports medicine condition; unfortunately, it is also the one most likely to be ignored. Injuries that require attention on the playing field are rare in comparison to the number of acute injuries incurred in less formal contests. Beyond the initial involuntary rest (usually temporary, whether symptoms have disappeared or not), the only other attention that might be given to an acute injury is the application of a pressure dressing (elastic bandage) and/or hot/cold therapy. Little else is done, and rarely is medical attention sought. Most athletic injuries do not occur in competition but in practice or unobserved, unsupervised surroundings. Granted that most acute injuries are not true medical emergencies, but they can be treated easily if proper diagnosis is made. The untoward effects of any athletic injury can be minimized by proper care, especially in the first 24-hour postinjury period.

Coverage of athletic competition and/or practice is discussed in Chapter 9; however, the following guidelines apply to the care of any acute injury.

Become familiar with the frequency level of common injuries in the sport you are covering and in the community you live in. Of the multiple factors that determine injury frequency, the two with the greatest effect are the local community environment and the specific position played by an athlete. Sports and exercise produce more than a fair share of "zebras," but for the most part we still see and care mostly for the "horses": expect them, and learn to take care of them.

There is no single true philosophy in primary care sports medicine, only guidelines. Those guidelines should reflect individual community situations. The following mind-set for covering a sports event works well in any community regardless of the situation, geography, or personnel involved:

before competition: prevention;
during competition: triage;
after competition: rehabilitation.

Someone who understands and accepts this philosophy is the best person to be responsible for the care of competitors in a sports event in your community. Contrary to what some may think, this does not require compromising any principles of medicine. Athletes are no different from nonathletes where health care is concerned. Where the groups diverge is with respect to exercise-induced injury. Athletes are in an environment that exposes them to acute macrotrauma as well as chronic *microtrauma*. In that environment the athletes will suffer more injury than the nonathletes.

Before Competition

Active intervention in the precompetitive aspects of any community sports system offers the greatest opportunity for significant injury prevention. The preparticipation screening and assessment of the sports environment are two major areas of preventive impact.

During Competition

One of the most uncomfortable and disquieting moments a team physician can have is when he must make sideline decisions while under the close scrutiny of many spectators. However, 67% of all injuries occur during practices or training, a time when the physician is unlikely to be present. The situations are different, but these are the norms in covering athletic teams and it underlines the need to have established protocols for triage in place. Coaches, trainers, and other responsible parties need to learn appropriate triage techniques for the more common injuries. Even when the physician is present, his/her major responsibility is the triage of the acutely injured athlete.

A decision on whether to allow the participant to resume play should be made only when (a) a definite diagnosis has been made, (b) the injury will not worsen with continued play so that the athlete is at *no greater risk* of further injury, and (c) the athlete can still compete fairly and is not incapable of protecting him/her because of the injury. See Table 23.1 for a list of injuries that preclude further participation. This table may seem conservative at first; please *reread* it. It is less conservative than most lists and can be helpful in assessing the most common athletic injuries in youngsters. With college-aged or professional athletes, this apparent conservatism can be addressed on an individual basis if the physician finds it necessary to move outside these vaguely defined boundaries. The best philosophy for evaluating acute athletic injuries on-site should be neither excessively conservative nor dangerously liberal. The final decision on return to competition should always be that of the physician.

Generally speaking, the evaluation of all acute injuries that occur in competition should follow the same steps (see Figure 23.1). Immediate initial assessment is mandatory and will help elicit signs and symptoms before the inevitable secondary reactions (pain, swelling, inflammation, spasm, decreased range of motion, and guarding). First, observe the position of the athlete and the injured part in relation to the rest of the body. Begin the history with the patient's account of how the injury occurred and amplify it with the physician's assessment of the biomechanics of the situation, as well as that of others who may have witnessed the injury occur (trainer, coach, teammate, or official). Determine any positive past medical history from available records if they exist. Next should be a focused clinical appraisal of the injury; that is, an examination emphasizing function, range of motion, and the neurological and vascular integrity of the injured area.

TABLE 23.1
SITUATIONS PRECLUDING RETURN TO PARTICIPATION IN COMPETITIVE SPORTS FOLLOWING AN INJURY

1. Unconsciousness (however brief). See subsection on head injuries.
2. Dazed or inappropriate responses for longer than 10 sec as a result of a blow to the head.
3. Any complaint of neurological abnormalities such as numbness or tingling.
4. Obvious swelling, with the possible exception of the digits.
5. Limited range of motion.
6. Decreased strength through normal range of motion.
7. Obvious bleeding.
8. An injury that the examiner is unsure of or does not know how to handle.
9. Obvious loss of some normal function.
10. An injury that requires the athlete needing assistance getting on or off the field, mat, or court.
11. Whenever an athlete says he/she cannot continue to participate (regardless of what the examiner thinks of the injury).

Source: Garrick JG. Sports medicine. *Pediatr Clin North Am* 1977;24:737–747, (1).

With serious injuries, a protocol is implemented that addresses whether to treat the injured player at the site or take him/her to a medical facility. If he/she is unable to walk safely, then a decision must be made on how to transport the athlete.

With less serious injuries, the first decision is whether to allow the athlete to continue to participate. Even if the decision is affirmative, he/she should be *periodically* rechecked. The interval between checks will depend on the severity and rapidity of evolving symptoms. **Any athlete with an evolving injury in which signs and symptoms are changing must be watched and not left alone.** If an athlete leaves the sideline, he/she should be accompanied by someone who is aware of the significance of the changing symptoms of the injury. Subsequent assessment on the sidelines or in the locker room should include the same components: observation, history, and re-examination. Clothing and equipment should be removed whenever possible. A later examination should focus not only on the injured area, but also above and below the area surrounding the injury. An

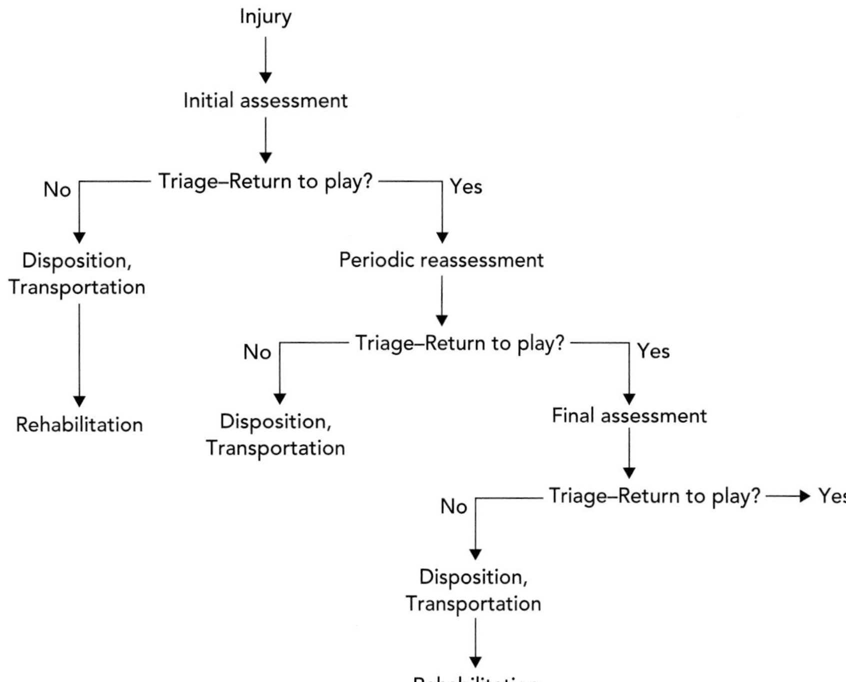

Figure 23.1 Steps used to evaluate all acute injuries that occur in competition.

appraisal of how the signs and symptoms have progressed since the first examination should also be made.

If an athlete is allowed to return to play and sustains a recurrence or exacerbation of the injury, he/she must be withdrawn from play for the remainder of the contest. If the athlete is not allowed to return, periodic assessments should continue and initial treatment and/or transportation begun.

After Competition

After a diagnosis is established and appropriate treatment given, rehabilitation can be considered and a multidisciplinary team approach involving the team physician, athlete's personal physician, other consultants (if necessary), trainer, and coach should be initiated. In reality, such a coordinated effort rarely happens. Statistics in West Virginia (2) revealed that a physician saw only 13.5% of acute injuries from a system at the high school level within 24 hours, which is the period when evaluation and treatment are the most productive. Although this low figure has hopefully increased over the past 30 years, the problems of physician accessibility remain significant. Even so, proper rehabilitation is the most important factor in the rapid return of an injured athlete to participation sports (see Chapter 35).

Common Acute Injuries by Type

One of the best and most useful surveys on sports injuries was conducted by Garrick and Requa (3). Although it dealt only with the high school level, it broke down sports injuries by type and provided a guideline on what to expect for the common acute sports injury. The numbers in parenthesis in the following text are from this study.

1. *Sprains and strains* (60.5%)—There are two ways that most sprains and strains develop. The common etiology is a sudden, abrupt, violent extension or contraction on an overloaded, unprepared, or undeveloped ligament or musculotendinous unit. There can be varying degrees of severity, from the overstretching of a few myofibrils to complete unit rupture. A second, less common, mechanism involves chronic stress placed upon the unit over time, in association with poor technique, overuse, or deformity. Strains are stretch injuries to the *musculotendinous unit;* sprains involve similar injury to *ligamentous structures.* A grading system is used to assess these injuries.

First degree/grade 1. There is little tissue injury and no increase in laxity. There usually is little immediate swelling because the tissues have not been stretched enough to produce instantaneous hemorrhage. With strains, there is usually no significant damage to the muscle or tendon and only a brief period of pain and disability if it is properly treated. Secondary tissue edema and inflammation develop within hours, restricting range of motion and resulting in minimal loss of function. Pathologically, less than 25% of the tendinous or ligamentous fibers are involved in a first-degree sprain or strain.

Second degree/grade 2. These injuries are the result of tears and disruptions of ligament or tendons. The partial tearing ranges from 25% to 75% of the fibers and there is demonstrable laxity and loss of function. There is immediate swelling and function is significantly reduced. Signs and symptoms increase until bleeding is controlled and the injury immobilized.

Third degree/grade 3. Complete disruption of the ligament or tendon usually exists with immediate pain, disability, and loss of function. However, some third-degree sprains may actually be less painful than second-degree sprains. Once a ligament is torn, there is no further stretch to cause pain sensation. Third-degree strains usually have diffuse bleeding and continuous pain.

The treatment of a third-degree injury (ligament or tendon rupture) continues to undergo change. With proper immediate care, including immobilization, these injuries can be treated conservatively without surgical intervention. Common examples of this type of injury include the medial collateral ligament in the knee, the lateral supporting structures of the ankle, and clavicular ligaments of the shoulder. Ligaments or tendons that normally are under a high amount of natural stress (Achilles tendon, biceps tendon, and the patellar ligament), as well as tendons that have retracted or ruptured, require prompt surgical intervention. Occasionally, when the tear is at the musculotendinous junction (such as an Achilles ligament rupture), the preferred treatment is immobilization. Bear in mind that severe strains and sprains may cause fewer symptoms and signs than the more moderate ones. Many young athletes have natural ligamentous laxity. Always examine and compare the injured and uninjured sides to help resolve those cases in which the findings appear equivocal.

Frequent sites of sprain are ankles (anterior talofibular ligament), knee (medial collateral ligament), and fingers (intrinsic collateral and interphalangeal ligaments). Frequent sites of strains are upper leg (hamstring muscles and adductors), back (paraspinal muscles), and the shoulder (rotator cuff tendons).

The following modalities (RICE regimen) are useful in treating strains and sprains:

R—rest the injured part to allow healing to begin and prevent further injury.

I—apply ice to the injured part to reduce swelling and extravasation of blood into the tissue (the ice should be applied directly to the skin as a massage unit at frequent intervals, but not to exceed 10 to 15 minutes per session).

C—compression with an elastic bandage, air splint, and so on, to prevent movement and further swelling.

E—elevate the injured area whenever possible to prevent pooling of blood and to control swelling.

When you know that an athlete cannot return to practice or competition, it is often beneficial to start nonsteroidal anti-inflammatory drugs (NSAIDs) to combat the inevitable soft tissue inflammatory response. Do not use these medications if the injury is minor. Some physicians now caution against early initial use of aspirin and related compounds (including NSAIDs) because they may possibly promote bleeding secondary to the inhibition of platelet function. Cyclooxygenase-2 (COX-2) NSAIDs have not been found to alter bleeding patterns. Additionally, there is evidence to suggest that NSAIDs, as a medication group, slow the healing of bone and soft tissue. Therefore, the sports medicine physician will have to balance the need for pain control and patient comfort with the need to speedup healing in the athlete.

2. *Contusions (13.7%)*—A contusion is the bruising of the skin and/or the underlying dermal tissues caused by direct trauma. Capillaries and other small vessels rupture causing extravasation of blood and effusion, followed by swelling and inflammation of the soft tissues of the surrounding areas. The secondary swelling is usually superficial and local, but occasionally may be deep if something like a hockey puck strikes an unprotected thigh. Because extravasation of blood into the soft tissue can cause extreme inflammation, a marked decrease in function may occur. Use the RICE regimen for treatment. It is important to immobilize a contusion because more bleeding may occur if the injured area is moved. An individual should not return to play until there is painless full range of motion. Complications of contusions include deep vein thrombosis and thrombophlebitis within the injured muscle mass. A more common long-term sequela of repeated contusions in the same area is *myositis ossificans,* a condition in which there is deposition of bone substance into the soft tissue areas. Thorough treatment and rehabilitation should be initiated promptly and full rehabilitation accomplished before the athlete returns to activity. The injured area should be protected from repeated trauma. The most common etiology of contusions is blunt trauma caused by an object hitting a muscle group in an extremity (a helmet against the anterior thigh of a player, or a field hockey stick hitting an opponent's forearm). The most frequent sites of contusions are the lateral upper arm and anterior thigh.

3. *Inflammation (5.9%)*—Inflammation is almost a universal sequela of acute injury and can be controlled with the RICE regimen and appropriate use of NSAIDs. Inflammation (in this situation) usually is *not* the result of *infection,* but a sign of minor injury.

4. *Fractures (5.5%)*—A fracture is a break in the continuity of bone. The major mechanism for sports injuries is a direct blow, and it is reasonable to expect a significant number of fractures in any epidemiological survey of sports injuries. The on-site care of all suspected fractures is the same. Immobilize the injured area, including the proximal and distal joint, and then transport the person to a hospital or office to obtain x-rays and definitive care. Fractures can happen at any site, and range from relatively insignificant breaks of the distal phalanx of the toe to life-threatening skull or neck fractures. Because of the possibility of further injury to the neurovascular bundle, manipulation of a fracture before radiographic examination is contraindicated. However, if the blood supply appears to be compromised, manipulation to re-establish vascularity may be necessary

in this rare orthopedic emergency. Under ordinary circumstances, immobilize the fracture, place ice and slight compression around it, and transport the patient immediately.

5. *Lacerations (1.8%)*—Lacerations are no different in sports than in any other area of medicine. Most are superficial, caused by trauma to an unprotected portion of skin. Occasionally, equipment used in the game, such as basketball hoops or high jump standards, or those worn by the athletes (braces) have been responsible. Rapid disinfection and debridement, followed by primary closure (where appropriate), produces an uneventful recovery. Neuromuscular function and vascular status of the underlying tissues should be tested before anesthesia is given. If there is any possibility of a foreign body in the wound, an x-ray should be taken to identify its location before extraction. X-rays may help when there is a non–radio-opaque foreign body by showing the pockets of subcutaneous air caused by the path of the object. Most athletes will want to play with repaired lacerations, so the wound must be protected and thoroughly disinfected before and after each participation. It is wise to cover and protect a wound longer than would be done for a nonathlete because the skin of an athlete is continually exposed to trauma and there is a significant possibility of wound dehiscence. A check of medical records from the preparticipation screening will indicate whether the athlete needs a tetanus toxoid injection.

6. *Other injuries (12.7%)*—Although the musculoskeletal and skin systems account for most of the acute injuries to athletes, other systems (internal organ trauma, thermal injury) also are involved. This highlights the need for the physician to have a primary care perspective.

CHRONIC INJURY

Less dramatic but only slightly less prevalent are chronic injuries, most of them are overuse syndromes. Significant medical intervention is often lacking with these injuries, perhaps because of the lack of intensity of the symptoms or signs. Many athletes self-treat these injuries and take the advice of fellow athletes, partly because of the inconsistencies of the medical treatment regimens that maybe given. The frequency and prevalence of chronic and overuse injuries should not be understated; they parallel the increase of exercise participation more than acute injuries do. About 71% of the patients seen in our primary care oriented sports medicine clinic present with complaints of overuse, overtraining, or overconditioning (4). In a survey of over 16,000 recreational runners, more than 1,800 overuse injuries were identified in a 2-year span (5). From the primary care perspective, the overuse syndrome, regardless of how it is defined, will account for many of the problems seen by the physician in the *recreational*, nonorganized athletic population.

The individual most likely to suffer from overuse is the regular daily exerciser. The sporadic "weekend" athlete is prone to acute injuries as described earlier. Overuse is a process, not an event. It is directly related to the amount, intensity, and frequency of exercise. The biomechanics of the sport or activity involved dictate the geographic body area affected. The overuse process causes breakdown and fatigue of body structures, usually resulting in inflammation followed by swelling. Tenosynovitis, tendonitis, fasciitis, compartment syndromes, and stress fractures are common examples of overuse syndromes. Most of these terms imply inflammation of specific types of structures, with most of them classified as soft tissues. These structures are the first to show the impact of exertional overindulgence. If exercise continues and warning signals (in the form of perceived pain) are ignored, the process continues and begins to involve the hard tissues, such as bones. In these cases, *abnormal stress* will result in damage to the *normal tissue.*

The concept of normal tissue being injured by abnormal stress is entirely consistent with the opinion held by most pathophysiologists that mechanical stress is the most important cause of overuse syndromes. We occasionally see an athlete suffering the result of another phenomenon, *normal stress* on *abnormal tissue.* Congenital defects and abnormalities, postinjury weakness or imbalance, and other types of structural malalignment may cause a predisposition to overuse problems.

Because overtraining and overconditioning happen so often and are becoming so prevalent in primary care practices, the entire concept of overuse has caused a great deal of frustration for physicians who are attempting to learn all the various treatment regimens advocated for specific areas and parts of the body. It has been contended (6) that most overuse injuries could, and should, be treated in one common "generic" way. The practical guidelines (see Table 23.2) of overuse as a spectrum of injury is a concept that assures the athlete of receiving consistent treatment regardless of the specific physician seen or the malady suffered. This protocol is based on clinical experience, taking into consideration the history, physical examination, an understanding of the pathophysiology behind a specific overuse syndrome, and the appropriateness of various diagnostic aids. Others (7,8) have advocated using similar guidelines to treat more specific injuries. These clinical guidelines cover all the musculoskeletal injuries caused by overuse, with the understanding that incorrect biomechanics and the athlete's lack of knowledge must be corrected at the same time if the condition is to be treated successfully. The protocol is designed to cover most overuse injuries encountered in the primary care settings. Overuse injuries are divided into four grades across an injury continuum. A word of caution: the clinical protocol is not intended to be used in a dogmatic way. Individual injuries may overlap grades and inconsistencies will exist. However, *most* injuries will approximate one of the clinical pictures outlined here.

Continuum of Injuries

The following is a general description of the four grades of chronic injuries used in Table 23.2:

TABLE 23.2
MUSCULOSKELETAL OVERUSE INJURIES: A CLINICAL GUIDE

Grade	History	Physical Exam	Pathophysiology	Diagnostic Aids	Treatment	Comments
1	Transient pain *after* activity, usually after hours; "Soreness" (Hx <2 wk)	Generalized tenderness	+ Lactic acid Muscle breakdown Minor inflammation	None	± Ice	Look at the training regimen Nonathlete Getting in shape
2	Longer standing pain *late* in activity or immediately after activity	Localized pain, but not discrete point tenderness	Mid musculotendinous (soft tissue) inflammation	None	Ice? Regimen reduced 10–25%	True overuse Wrong environment Wrong equipment Poor technique
3	Pain in *early* or *middle* of activity (getting closer to beginning of activity)	Point tenderness, percussion tenderness Pressure elsewhere produces pain at point Other evidence of inflammation (heat, erythema, swelling, crepitation)	Major musculotendinous inflammation Periostitis Bone microtrauma	X-ray ± bone scan +40%	Ice? Regimen reduced 25–75% Initial 5–7 day rest period with concurrent NSAID course	Prestress fracture syndrome
4	Pain before or early in exercise, preventing or affecting performance (HX >4 wk)	All of the Grade 3 signs plus disturbance in function? ROM muscle atrophy	Breakdown in soft tissue Stress fracture Compartment syndrome (especially if swelling is a major finding)	X-ray ± bone scan +95%	Ice Rest from exercise NSAID	Immobilization? Usually not required

ROM = range of motion; NSAID = nonsteroidal anti-inflammatory drug;
Source: McKeag DB. The concept of overuse: the primary care aspects of overuse syndromes in sports. *Primary Care* 1984;11(1):43–69.

Grade 1 injuries. Patients presenting with Grade 1 injuries give a vague history of transient pain, usually occurring many hours after injury. It may be perceived as soreness, is commonly present in beginner athletes attempting to "get into shape," and is accompanied by generalized tenderness. The cause of postexercise muscle soreness has been studied by various researchers (9,10). Increased levels of lactic acid, muscle breakdown, or minor inflammation have been advanced as possible explanations. There are no diagnostic aids for the physician and the only treatment is reassurance and occasional use of ice. However, the physician has an excellent opportunity to intercede in the prevention of further injury at this point by appropriate athlete education and advocacy of established exercise guidelines.

Grade 2 injuries. Grade 2 injuries describe pain of approximately 2 to 3 weeks duration that typically occurs late in activity or immediately following it. Physical examination reveals more localized pain but no true point tenderness. The signs and symptoms may suggest mild musculoskeletal inflammation, but useful diagnostic aids are absent. Treatment consists of repeated applications of ice directly to the affected area for 10 to 15 minutes at a time. In addition, relative rest is achieved by decreasing the training regimen by 10% to 25%. The physician should look at such environmental factors as use of improper or worn-out equipment, or at poor techniques or intrinsic biomechanical abnormalities. A Grade 2 injury is the most common presenting clinical picture of overuse.

Grade 3 injuries. Pain usually occurs in the middle of an activity and, over time, moves nearer to the commencement of the activity. Physical examination demonstrates point tenderness and other signs. A bone scan at this point may be positive, but the finding adds little to the clinical diagnosis or treatment plan. Treatment includes using ice and decreasing the exercise regimen by 25% to 75%. In addition, we have found that a 5 to 7 day period of complete rest with concurrent NSAIDs medication is helpful in arresting the initial inflammation and allow the individual to return to higher levels of activity quicker.

Grade 4 injuries. Grade 4 is the most serious type of injury in the continuum and has a pain pattern similar to Grade 3. Pain prevents further activity and affects performance. If swelling is a major finding, especially in the lower extremity, compartment syndrome should be considered. A positive bone scan indicating the extent of a stress fracture(s) may be helpful in obtaining better patient compliance. Treatment of Grade 4 injury consists of ice, *complete rest,* and treatment with NSAIDs. Some physicians believe that stress fractures in certain areas of the body, such as the proximal tibia, require immobilization with a cast or brace. However, this is not generally recognized as the current standard of care.

The following points about Table 23.2 should be kept in mind:

- The onset of pain as a symptom will occur closer to the start of exercise as the severity of the grade increases. Figure 23.2 illustrates the interrelation between the injury (pain) continuum and the physiological continuum.
- Tenderness changes from vague to specific as the process increases in severity.
- The duration and intensity of signs and symptoms increases with each grade.
- The findings on physical examination involves increasingly more functions as one moves through the continuum.
- The underlying pathophysiology can be subdivided: Grades 1 and 2 affect only soft tissue, and Grades 3 and 4 affect both soft and hard tissues.
- By using this table a costly test, such as a bone scan, can sometimes be avoided. A bone scan should be ordered to confirm an already suspected stress fracture, rule out multiple sites, and improve treatment compliance.

Consistency in the treatment of overuse injuries is a desired result of the widespread use of a clinical protocol such as this. A major factor contributing to patient compliance is faith in the regimen. If the regimen is consistent and the patient can be assured that the physician has not unduly restricted exercise, compliance usually will follow.

Important points to be emphasized in treating overuse syndromes are as follows:

- Decreasing the training regimen (relative rest) should be based not only on the grade of injury but also on factors known to the physician about the individual (lifestyle, motivation, and ability to comply).
- Long-term complete rest is not well accepted by most athletes as a legitimate treatment, but they will comply with 5 to 7 days of complete rest and treatment with NSAIDs. In Grade 3 injuries, this is very effective in initially controlling the inflammation and allowing a better pharmacological effect. The rest period should be followed by light intensity training (LIT).
- The application of ice should come after exercise in Grade 2 to Grade 4 injuries. Ice should be applied frequently, directly on the skin whenever possible, for 10 to 15 minutes at a time. An ice allergy may develop, but this is rare and can be controlled by stopping the ice therapy. An easy way to prepare ice for therapy is to fill small paper cups with water and freeze it for use in ice massage.
- NSAIDs should not be used if the history reveals any previous allergies or hypersensitivity reactions to these drugs.

Return to Activity

After rest, ice, and medications have been used, return to activity is the next consideration. Using the following protocol for LIT allows the patient to dictate his/her own pace of return to activity, and thus maintain some control over the process. LIT involves the following principles:

- Training should restart only when the individual is able to carry out functions of daily activity without pain. Once this is achieved, exercise can begin at a very low level of intensity and duration (half mile jog, 100 yd swim, 1 mi low gear biking).
- At the conclusion of this daily activity, the athlete then has the following three options:
  (a) If the athlete experiences pain and/or swelling during the exercise, stop the exercise immediately and decrease duration by 25% the next day.

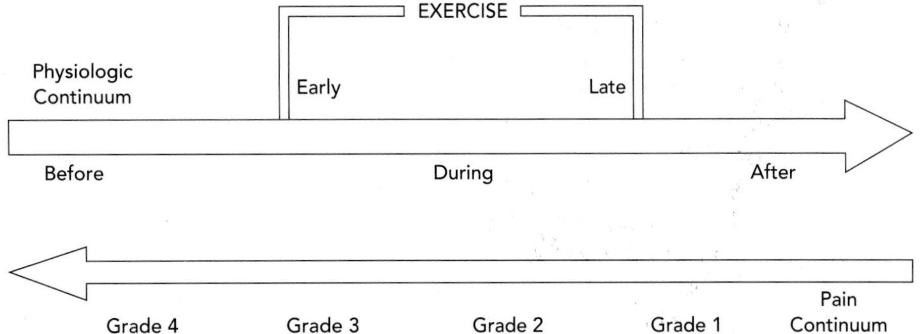

Figure 23.2 Relation of pain Continuum to physiological continuum.

(b) If the athlete experiences pain after exercise, ice the area and continue at this level of exercise the next day.

(c) If the individual experiences neither pain nor swelling during or after exercise, the program may be increased by up to 25%.

Five major points that need to be examined during the treatment of overuse injuries to try and prevent recurrence include the following:

- The athlete's philosophy about exercise should be considered.
- A brief but knowledgeable look at the training regimen may show the possibility of beneficial alterations.
- A systematic appraisal of the exercise environment of the athlete should be made, with an idea of making the needed changes.
- Congenital or injury-induced biomechanical problems, including muscle imbalance (inherent or the result of previous injury), leg length discrepancy, or self-treatment with orthotics, should be addressed.
- The athlete should be educated in the concept of pain so that he/she knows when to stop exercising and when to resume.

Treatment Modalities

Five basic modalities are used to treat most chronic injuries. Three are used in combination, occasionally with some form of electrical impulse therapy (the fourth modality), before resorting to surgery, which is the fifth modality.

Ice. Ice is the foundation treatment for all overuse injuries. It is the most effective intervention currently available.

Rest. Absolute rest from exercise has advantages and disadvantages. The ability to allow healing to progress unimpeded is one advantage. Minor reinjury, caused by using an injured part, will slow the healing process. Rest combined with medication enhances the effect of the medication. The disadvantages include noncompliance and dissatisfaction on the part of the athlete. Also, rest can cause muscle atrophy, deconditioning, and loss of fine motor skills, which may then predispose an individual to further injury once activity is resumed. Relative rest is a reasonable compromise.

Anti-inflammatory medications. Anti-inflammatory medications that are applied topically, taken orally, or injected can be used to treat overuse injuries. Topical medications have yet to come into widespread use. Dimethyl sulfoxide (DMSO), although not a federally approved medication, may be used in the self-treatment of some overuse injuries.

Oral NSAIDs are used frequently to treat overuse syndromes, and there are many different NSAIDs. All have a dual action: anti-inflammation and analgesia. They do tend to mask pain, an important consideration in caring for an athlete with a serious overuse injury. Do not prescribe any NSAIDs initially unless the patient is willing to rest completely and allow the medication to work.

The use of corticosteroid medication, either alone or in combination with an anesthetic, should be reserved for such conditions as bursitis or tenosynovitis. Injections into the tendons or ligamentous structures can significantly weaken these structures for up to 14 days following the procedure (11,12). Repeated injections can cause biomechanical disruption of soft tissue and lead directly to collagen necrosis. The possibility of tendon or ligamentous rupture is a significant side effect of such therapy and should be avoided.

Electrical impulse therapy. The use of low-grade electrical circuits set up over an injured muscle or ligamentous unit have successfully aided healing. Transcutaneous nerve stimulation not only eliminates pain feedback to the brain through the "gate theory" (13), but also stimulates the healing process peripherally and allows the soft tissue unit to relax. Similar types of therapy include galvanic stimulation, electromyostimulation, and the use of surface electrodes for serious injuries such as slow-healing stress fractures. The latter treatment usually is reserved for the most serious of overuse injuries.

Surgery. The use of surgery to treat overuse injuries, including supraspinatus tendonitis, plantar fasciitis, Achilles tendonitis, and compartment syndromes is appropriate, but only after medical measures have proven ineffective. Most clinicians argue that surgery, especially where an athlete is attempting to function at high performance levels, should be avoided at all costs.

ALLERGIES

Allergies can cause everything from chronic symptoms of the upper respiratory tract to decreased performance secondary to respiratory inefficiency. Following is a list of allergies that can be factors in athletic performance:

1. *Ice*: Ice allergies are relatively rare, affecting no more than 1% to 2%. This allergy is generally seen after ice treatment for soft tissue injury. Symptoms include the development of wheals and urticaria in the area surrounding the skin where ice was applied. Treatment is removal of the ice. Rarely, an antihistamine such as Benadryl may be necessary.
2. *Equipment*: Equipment that has been washed and cleaned in certain types of detergent can result in allergic dermatitis. Consider this in an individual with an unexplained skin rash.
3. *Medications*: Always a possible problem. This can be avoided by obtaining a history of allergies before placing an athlete on any medication.
4. *Airborne dust and molds*: Competing indoors in large arenas, athletes may be susceptible to problems caused

by dust and molds that collect in the rafters or are circulated by ventilation systems.

5. *Chlorine*: Some swimmers have an unfortunate allergy to the chlorine or bromide used to disinfect pools. This results in a contact dermatitis and should be treated as such.
6. *Personal contact*: On occasion, participants will spray or apply substances on their skin, which may be allergic to them or their opponents. During contact, an allergic reaction to the substance develops. Examples of such substances include tape, rubber, and Vaseline.

IMMUNOLOGY

The issue of immunology of exercise has been addressed by Simon (1984) (14). Habitual exercise may protect the athletes against infection. A transient increase in various host-defense factors is thought to be caused by exercise hyperthermia. Other evidence regarding immune function suggests exactly the opposite. The rigorous training programs of some aerobic sports (swimming, long distance running, bicycling) can result in anorexia and poor nutrition. While not proven, many team physicians believe that such training regimens actually decrease an athlete's resistance to endemic infections. Practices like losing a large amount of weight (wrestling, gymnastics) may put the body in a state of vulnerability. Also, many athletes, especially at the collegiate level, live in close proximity, a setting that lends itself to the spread of minor illness among team members.

It seems unlikely that exercise produces substantial functional changes in immunoglobins or complement. A number of studies have found that an increased level of habitual physical activity in a young, normal population does not result in fewer upper respiratory symptoms or shorter duration. In addition, maximal aerobic power as a measure of cardiovascular fitness is not related to the incidence or duration of upper respiratory symptoms. We can conclude that there is no clinical evidence that exercise alters the frequency or severity of human infections.

As primary care team physicians, the authors bias is that high intensity training done in the winter months or in close proximity to large groups does constitute at least a minor risk factor for developing acute contagious infections. Whenever possible, the team physician should try to aid athletes by pre-outbreak immunization or emphasizing good eating and sleeping habits.

REFERENCES

1. Garrick JG. Sports medicine. *Pediatr Clin North Am* 1977;24(4):737–747.
2. Bowers KD. Disposition of high school athletic injuries. *W V Med J* 1974;73:88–89.
3. Garrick JG, Requa R. Medical care and injury surveillance in a high school setting. *Phys Sportsmed* 1981;9(2):116–120.
4. McKeag DB. Overuse injuries: the concept in 1992. *Prim Care* 1991; 18(4):851–865.
5. Clement DB, Taunton JE, Smart GW, et al. A survey of overuse running injuries. *Phys Sportsmed* 1981;9(5):47–58.
6. McKeag DB. The concept of overuse: the primary care aspects of overuse syndromes in sports. *Prim Care* 1984;11(1):43–59.
7. Blazina DE, Fox JS, Caron SJ. Basketball injuries. *Med Aspects of Sports* 1974; 15:15–19.
8. Jackson DW. Shinsplints: an update. *Phys Sportsmed* 1978;6(10):51–62.
9. Schwane JA, Williams JS, Sloan JH. Effects of training on delayed muscle soreness and serum creatine kinase activity after running. *Med Sci Sports Exerc* 1987;19:584–690.
10. Tiidus PM, Ianuzzo CD. Effects of intensity and duration of muscular exercise on delayed soreness and serum enzyme activities. *Med Sci Sports Exerc* 1983;15:461–465.
11. Gottlieb NL, Riskin WG. Complications of local corticosteroid injections. *JAMA* 1980;243(15):1547–1548.
12. Kennedy JC, Willis RB. The effects of local steroid injections on tendons: a biomechanical and microscopic correlative study. *Am J Sports Med* 1976; 4(1):11–21.
13. Ersek RA. Transcutaneous electrical neurostimulation: a new therapeutic modality for controlling pain. *Clin Orthop* 1978;128:314–324.
14. Simon HB. The immunology of exercise. *JAMA* 1984;252(19):2735–2738.

Head and Neck

24

Scott H. Grindel

Injuries to the head, face and neck in athletics are relatively common and the leading cause of morbidity and mortality in athletes. Approximately 12% of all craniomaxillofacial injuries seen in trauma centers are attributable to sports participation (1). Since 1945, a total of 497 deaths have been attributed to football in the United States, 69% of which were due to brain injury and 19% due to spinal cord injuries (2). Significant declines in the severity and incidence of head injuries were seen from 1983 to 1999 (19% and 4%, respectively) thought to be due to improved helmet design and rule changes (3). These statistics are testimony of our constant vigilance of these injuries, use of current treatment recommendations, and continued epidemiological monitoring concerning the need for improved equipment, and changes in or increased enforcement of the rules of play.

Head injury includes trauma to the scalp, soft tissue, bone, or brain. These injuries are typically classified to reflect their acute and long-term clinical significance. Severe head injuries are those with obvious potential for chronic neurological damage or death. Mild head injuries are those that involve the soft tissue and bone of the head (excluding cranial vault fractures) and clinically reversible brain damage. On the basis of the potential for infection and injury severity, injuries may also be classified as open or closed head injuries. See Table 24A.2 for an outline. This chapter will deal primarily with injuries to the head, face, and neck; brain injuries are covered more thoroughly in other chapters in this book.

SECTION A
HEAD INJURIES

Head injuries, and the fear of them, remain one of the most powerful motivating forces for policy changes in sports. Advances in the technology of protective equipment improved the safety of sports, but may have instilled a degree of invincibility in some athletes. For instance, as shown in Table 24A.1, a significant increase in severe head and neck injuries seen in football in the 1970s sharply declined after the institution of rules outlawing "spearing" (5). Present studies estimate that 17,008 head injuries present to the emergency room per year due to hockey (rates 7–13:10,000 participants), 86,697 due to soccer (rates 6–10:10,000 participants), and 204,802 due to football (rates 9–14:10,000 participants). Concussion, skull fracture, and intracranial injuries due to hockey account for 9,883 of these visits (rates 4–9:10,000 participants), 50,035 due to soccer (rates 3–7:10,000 participants), and 128,968 due to football (rates 5–10:10,000 participants) (6).

TABLE 24A.1
MORTALITY RATES DUE TO FOOTBALL HEAD AND NECK INJURIES FOR 1977–1986 PRESENTED IN INCIDENCE PER 100,000 PARTICIPANTS

Year	High School	College
1977	0.77	2.67
1978	0.92	0.00
1979	0.62	4.00
1980	0.84	2.67
1981	0.46	2.67
1982	0.54	2.67
1983	0.84	1.33
1984	0.38	0.00
1985	0.38	2.67
1986	0.23	0.00

Source: Adapted from Mueller FO, Blyth CS. Fatalities from head and cervical spine injuries occurring in tackle football: 40 years' experience. *Clin Sports Med* 1987;6:185–196, (4).

TABLE 24A.2
ORGANIZATIONAL OUTLINE FOR HEAD INJURIES

Traumatic head injury
- I. Obvious neurological structural damage[a] (severe head injury)
  - A. Focal injuries
    1. Epidural hematoma
    2. Subdural hematoma
    3. Subarachnoid hemorrhage
    4. Cerebral contusion/hematoma
    5. Skull fractures
    6. Penetrating injuries
  - B. Diffuse injuries
    1. Diffused axonal injury
    2. Second impact syndrome
- II. No obvious neurological structural damage (mild head injury)
  - A. Mild traumatic brain injury
    1. Concussion
    2. Postconcussion syndrome
  - B. Bone and soft tissue damage
    1. Scalp and facial lacerations
    2. Ear, nose, and mouth injury
    3. Facial bone fractures
    4. Scalp and facial bone contusions/abrasions

[a]May additionally be classified as open or closed.
Source: Adapted from Grindel SH, Lovell MR, Collins MW. The assessment of sport-related concussion: the evidence behind neuropsychological testing and management. *Clin J Sport Med* 2001;11:134–143, (7).

ANATOMY

There are five distinct layers of the scalp (see Figure 24A.1):

- Epidermis and dermis. They are the most superficial layers of the scalp. The scalp is a common area for lacerations in sports not requiring a helmet and are often seen in some helmeted sports (i.e., ice hockey).
- Superficial fascia. It contains an extracranial blood supply from the external carotid artery. There is no arterial supply from the bone to nourish the scalp. The venous system of the scalp, however, communicates with the cavernous, superior, sagittal, and lateral sinuses of the brain. As a result, scalp infections can potentially spread intracranially by means of the venous system.
- Galea aponeurotica. It is a tough, dense layer of fibrous tissue separating the superficial layers of the scalp from the skull.
- Subaponeurotic layer.
- Pericranium. It acts as the periosteum or glia of the skull.

The skull consists of a bony vault made up of eight bones tightly joined at the suture lines. There are two parietal and temporal segments, and a single occipital, frontal, ethmoid, and sphenoid segment. The four distinct tissue layers between the skull and the brain are as follows (see Figure 24A.1):

- *Epidural space.* In actuality a potential space between the skull and the dura mater. Epidural hematomas develop in this tissue plane.
- *Dura mater.* It contains the venous sinuses and three meningeal arteries and veins. This is the location of the middle meningeal artery, a terminal branch of the external carotid. Injury to this artery is the most frequent mechanism of epidural hematomas (see Figure 24A.2).
- *Arachnoid.* It is a narrow space between the dura and the pia mater containing the spinal fluid of the brain. Subdural hematomas can develop here following intracranial venous lacerations.
- *Pia mater.* It is a layer closely adherent to the cerebral cortex and the site of potential subarachnoid hematomas.

The brain itself is unique because it is a fixed volume enclosed in a nonexpandable vault (the skull and dura mater). A significant increase in its mass (edema, hematomas, etc.) leads to an increase in intracranial pressure. This often leads to injury or death due to compression of brain tissue against bony prominences and herniation through the foramen magnum, neither of which is a welcome occurrence in the sports arena.

The brain is supplied by two arterial sources, the internal carotids anteriorly, and the vertebral arteries posteriorly. These two arterial sources reconnect within the cranial vault at the circle of Willis thereby providing some redundancy to protect from ischemia due to stroke or injury. The face and scalp are supplied by the external carotids, an important branch of which is the middle meningeal artery. Injury to the middle meningeal artery can result in significant intracranial bleeds. See Figure 24A.2 for details of the blood supply to the head and neck.

MECHANISMS OF HEAD INJURY

Any blow to the head can cause brain injury. Concussion and minor brain contusion have also been associated with blows to the body. In either case, injury is often due to the resultant sudden head movement and shifting of the brain within the skull. This is particularly true with rotational movements of the brain, which cause shearing forces and rotation of the brain over irregularities on the inner skull. This explains why many injuries involve brain tissue overlying the frontal lobe, temporal lobe, and the base of the brain. Even minor impacts can cause tearing of small vessels and the formation of petecchiae (8). Following a concussion, there may be a reduction in the brain's ability to process information, which typically resolves within 5 to 7 days (9–11). As the number of past concussions grows, the more severe the concussions can become, often taking

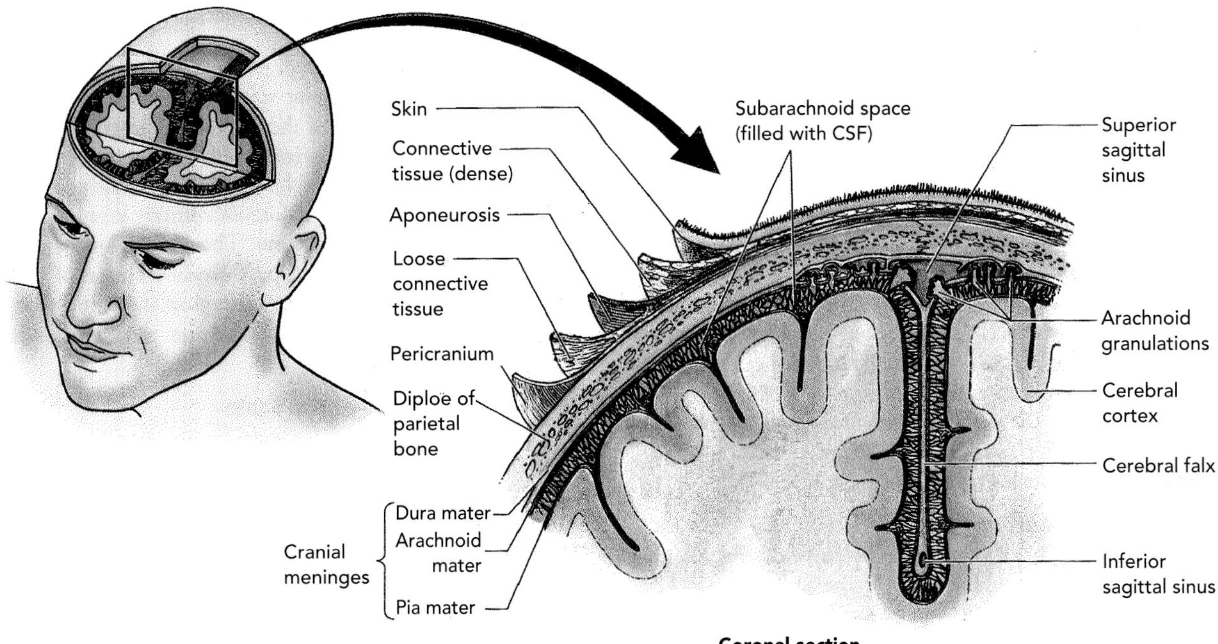

Figure 24A.1 Anatomy of the tissues overlying the brain. Important structures shown here include the dermis, epidermis, fascia, galea aponeurotica, subaponeurotic layer, pericranium, epidural space, dura mater, arachnoid CSF, cerebrospinal fluid, and pia mater. (*Source*: From Moore KL. *Clinically oriented anatomy*, 4th ed. Philadelphia: Lippincott Williams & Wilkins, 2000.)

only minor impacts to cause severe concussions. Repeated concussions may also lead to permanent damage and long-term symptoms. If a second concussion occurs before the first has resolved, massive swelling of the brain can occur resulting in death. This is the so-called "second impact syndrome" or "diffuse brain edema" (12).

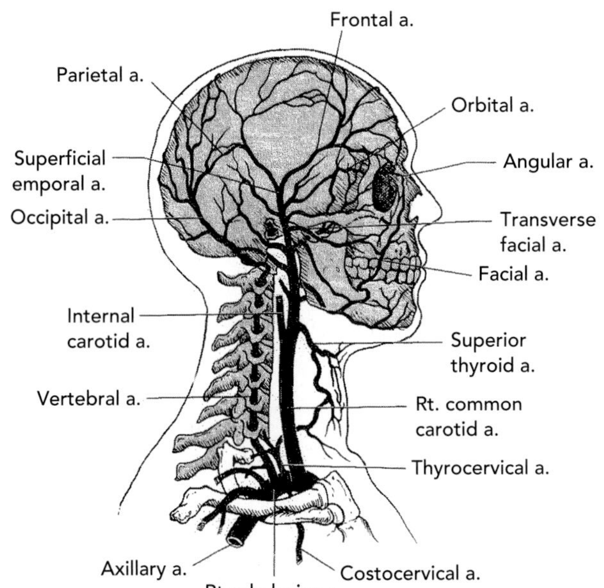

Figure 24A.2 Blood supply of the head and neck. (*Source*: From Anderson MK, Hall SJ. *Fundamentals of sports injury management*. Philadelphia: Lippincott Williams & Wilkins, 1997.)

DIRECT INJURIES

Brain injury occurs most often by direct trauma to the head. This can occur with a moving object striking the head such as seen in boxing, baseball, field hockey, or ice hockey. These injuries typically cause damage at the site of impact or a "coup injury". More often, injury occurs when a moving head impacts a fixed or slow moving object such as the turf, an opposing player, or a goal post as with football or hockey. This mechanism often results in injury on the opposite side of the brain as the impact referred to as a *countercoup injury*.

INDIRECT INJURIES

Traumatic impact to another body part can be transferred to the cranium. For example, a fall on the coccyx while ice-skating can lead to an injury at the base of the brain. Impacts to the periphery that lead to a rotational force to the brain, such as a head-on check to the lateral shoulder as seen in ice hockey, can lead to concussions, contusions and hematomas of the brain, as well as neck injuries.

BIOMECHANICS

The location and degree of head injury depends on the position of the head at the moment of impact, the magnitude and direction of impact, and the structural

Primary injury

Contusions, lacerations, shearing injuries, hemorrhage, and swelling can occur at the time of impact and cannot be reversed by treatment.

Contusions typically occur over the frontal and temporal poles of the brain regardless of the cranial impact site.

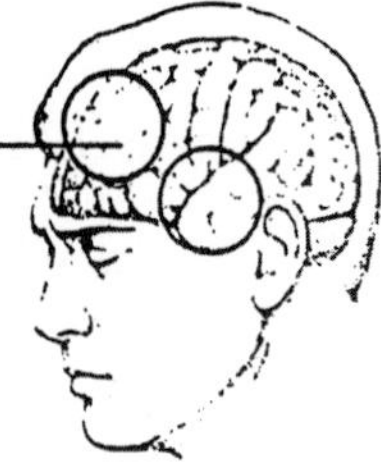

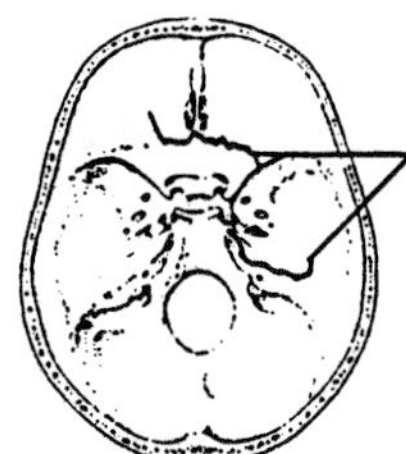

Lacerations, with or without associated fractures, are usually located near the midline, adjacent to the floor of the anterior or middle cranial fossa, and often involve the corpus callosum or pontomedullary junction.

Shearing injuries occur when the impact is accompanied by sudden angular rotation of the skull.

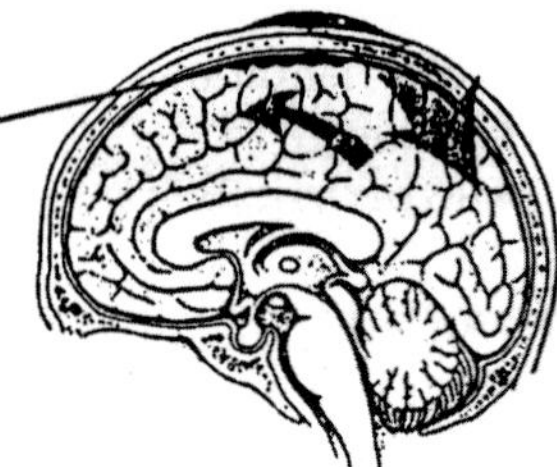

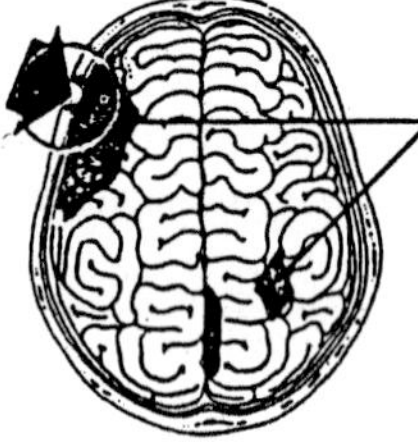

Hemorrhage can range from small intracerebral collections to large intra- or extracerebral clots that cause deterioration by their "mass" effect on brain tissue.

Figure 24A.3 Types of primary head injuries.

features and integrity of the skull. It is the response to the force rather than the force alone, which causes these injuries (13). See Figure 24A.3 for a delineation of the types of primary head injuries.

SCALP INJURIES

Lacerations

Lacerations should be treated as outlined elsewhere in this book; however, the increased vascularity of the superficial layer of the scalp make these lacerations prone to continued bleeding, in many cases hampering appropriate wound closure. Venous connections to intracranial structures heighten the concern for infections. Repair should be done under sterile conditions, after copious irrigation and shaving where necessary to clear the field (except the eye brow). Staples can be a quick repair in the heat of an event, but do not neglect to irrigate the wound and evaluate the athlete for brain or neck injury. Use prophylactic antibiotics in all human bite wounds. Double coverage is recommended such as amoxicillin/clavulanate 825/125 mg PO b.i.d. (pediatric patients use 22.5 mg/kg PO b.i.d.), or ciprofloxacin 500 mg PO b.i.d. (pediatric patients use TMP/SMX 5 mL suspension/10 kg PO b.i.d.), *and* clindamycin 125 mg PO q.i.d. (pediatric patients use 5 mg/kg PO q.i.d.) for 5 days. Testing protocols for hepatitis and HIV should be strongly considered in both individuals involved.

Subglial Hematoma

Blunt injury commonly causes blood to collect between the glia and the skull, sometimes called a *goose egg*. Initial treatment involves the application of ice as well as a skull x-ray to rule out fracture. If there is no skull fracture, pressure and ice over the area may minimize the size of the hematoma. Careful follow-up should take place to monitor for infection or neurological changes. Again, evaluating the patient for brain or neck injury should not be neglected.

SKULL FRACTURES

Skull fractures may be open or closed. Because the force of the blow may actually be absorbed during the fracturing process, the resultant intracranial damage may actually be lessened. Fracture lines crossing the grooves of meningeal arteries, particularly the middle meningeal arteries, should arouse suspicion for epidural hematoma. Battle's sign (ecchymosis behind the ear) and "raccoon eyes" (ecchymosis under the eye[s]) may be the result of a basilar skull fracture (see Figure 24A.4). Hemotympanum (see Figure 24A.5) or cerebrospinal fluid (CSF) leaking

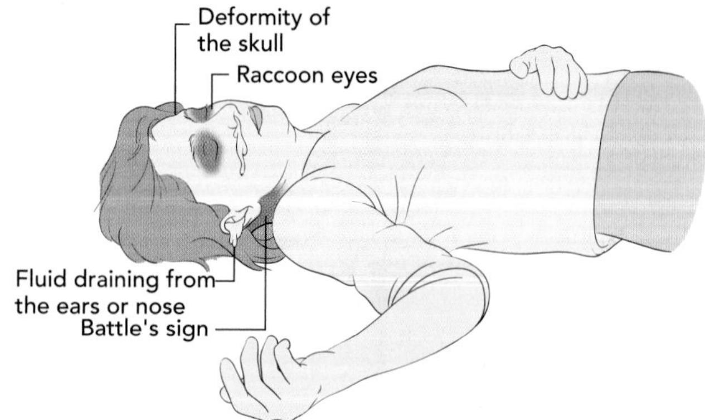

Figure 24A.4 Signs of head injury, head trauma include; **Battle's sign**, a bluish discoloration in the postauricular region signifying a basilar skull fracture; **raccoon eyes** signified by periorbital hematomas are suggestive of basilar skull, nasal, or facial bone fracture; and **CSF otorrhea** CSF leaking from the external auditory canal is due to a basilar skull fracture and resultant disruption of the middle ear and tympanic membrane. (*Source*: From LifeART.© 2007 Lippincott Williams & Wilkins, All right reserved.)

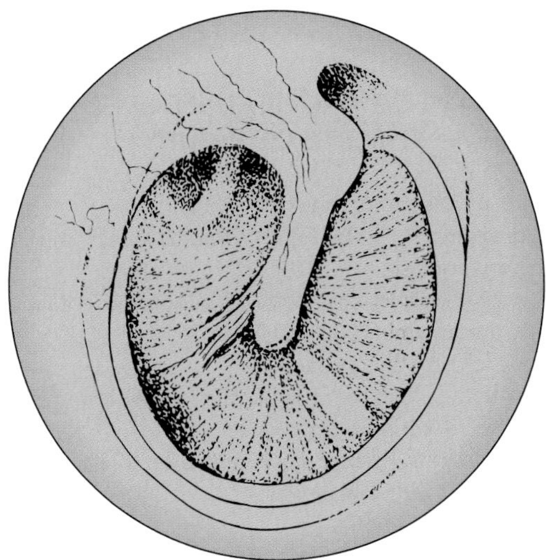

Figure 24A.5 Hemotympanum. A bluish discoloration of the tympanic membrane is due to a basilar skull fracture and resultant blood in the middle ear. (*Source*: From Weber J, Kelley J. *Health assessment in nursing*, 2nd ed. Philadelphia: Lippincott Williams & Wilkins, 2003.)

from the nose or ears (CSF rhinorrhea/otorrhea) may also be a clue to this type of fracture. In a mixture of CSF and blood, CSF separates when placed on filter paper and forms a characteristic "double ring sign" or "halo sign." Although this test is sensitive, false positives are possible.

Skull Fracture Classification

- **Linear-hairline separation fractures** may cause loss of the curvature of the skull. These are typically produced by blunt impact and represent 70% of all skull fractures.
- **Comminuted fractures** typically entail a small impact area causing indentation and fragmentation of the underlying bone.
- **Depressed-skull fractures** are displaced inwardly, the depression increasing with the pointedness of the object (baseball vs. javelin). Complications may arise if the fracture has entrapped brain or meninges or if an intracranial hematoma develops.
- **Blowout fractures of the orbit** are caused by direct blunt impact to the floor or roof of the orbit or the eye itself. This may entrap the inferior or superior oblique muscle causing loss of extraoccular movements. See section on Eye Injuries in this chapter.

See Table 24A.3 for observations supporting radiological workup for skull fracture.

BRAIN INJURY

The best way to prevent the sequelae of serious head injury is to be prepared for it and diagnose it rapidly. The team physician should carry the necessary supplies or have them at the event site. See Appendix 24.1 for a checklist. In determining the seriousness of the injury, a brief neurological examination and a tentative diagnosis should be made. The neurological examination should include an assessment as outlined in Table 24A.4 and in Appendix 24.2. With the information from this examination, a score on the Glasgow Coma Scale (GCS) can be reached. Consult Table 24A.5 for determining the proper score.

The use of the GCS at the time of evaluation correlates well with the degree of injury severity. Athletes scoring 13 to 15 on this scale are defined as having minor head injury, 9 to 12 a moderate head injury and those who score 3 to 8

TABLE 24A.3
OBSERVATIONS ON EXAMINATION THAT WOULD SUGGEST THAT FURTHER WORKUP WITH PLAIN FILM, COMPUTED TOMOGRAPHY, OR MAGNETIC RESONANCE IMAGING MAY BE NECESSARY

Unconsciousness at the time of examination
History of focal trauma capable of producing a depressed skull fracture
Penetrating injury to the head
Compromised athlete unable to give a good history
Prolonged post-traumatic symptoms such as headache, dizziness, vomiting, etc.
CSF rhinorrhea or otorrhea
Neurologic findings such as anisocoria, hemiparesis, unilateral Babinski's sign, asymmetric findings
Raccoon eyes
Battle's sign

TABLE 24A.4
PHYSICAL EXAMINATION EVALUATING ALL AREAS OF THE NERVOUS SYSTEM

Mental Status	Motor/Strength Examination
Alertness	All myotomes
Concentration	**Deep tendon reflexes**
Memory	Patellar tendons
Affect	Achilles tendons
Cranial nerves I-XII	Biceps tendons
See Appendix 24.2	Triceps tendons
Sensory examination	Brachioradialis tendons
All dermatomes	Babinski's reflex
Proprioception	**Tests of coordination and reaction time**
Finger-to-nose	Heel-to-toe walking
Heel-to-shin	Slap hands test
Romberg's sign	Rapid alternating hand movements
Pronator drift	

TABLE 24A.5
GLASGOW COMA SCALE

		Score
Eye opening	Spontaneous	E4
	To speech	3
	To pain	2
	Nil	1
Best motor responses[a]	Obeys	M6
	Localizes painful stimuli	5
	Withdraws	4
	Abnormal flexion[b]	3
	Abnormal extensions[c]	2
	No response	1
Verbal response[d]	Oriented	V5
	Confused conversation	4
	Inappropriate words	3
	Incomprehensible sounds	2
	No response	1
Total possible		15

Athletes scoring 13–15 on this scale are defined as having minor head injury, 9–12 a moderate head injury and those who score from 3–8 are in the severe category.
[a]Rub knuckles against sternum and observe arms if necessary.
[b]Indicating decorticate rigidity.
[c]Indicating decerebrate rigidity.
[d]Arouse with painful stimulus if necessary.

TABLE 24A.6
ACUTE CARE OF THE HEAD INJURED PATIENT AT THE SITE OF INJURY

1. Check for responsiveness
   - Conscious: R_x-100% O_2 (10 breaths/min) through reservoir mask
   - Unconscious: R_x-oral airway—bag mask ventilation (24 breaths/min, 100% O_2)
2. Check for breathing difficulty
   - Conscious: R_x-bag mask ventilation (24 breaths/min, 100% O_2) without oral airway
   - Unconscious: R_x-bag mask ventilation (24 breaths/min, 100% O_2) with oral airway
3. Establish Circulation
   - Absent Carotid Pulses: R_x-advanced life support under medical control
   - Hypotension: R_x—elevate foot of backboard —establish i.v. line with no. 18 percutaneous plastic catheter using 5% dextrose in Ringer's lactate
4. Get history and do physical examination
   - Establish level of consciousness (Glasgow Coma Scale)
   - Check for change in level of consciousness since injury
   - Check for pupil size, position, equality and reaction to light
   - Evaluate length of unconsciousness
5. Prevent aspiration pneumonia in unconscious patients
   - Minimal oral secretion: R_x-periodic nasopharyngeal suctioning
   - Excessive oral secretions: R_x-esophageal airway
6. Reduce intracerebral edema
   R_x-methylprednisolone (Solumedrol)
   15 years and older—2 g i.v.
   5–15 yr—1 g i.v.
   <5 yr—0.5 g i.v.
7. Transport patient to hospital base station with advanced life support capability
   - Monitor vital signs every 15 min
   - Contact hospital base station
   Communicate:

Patient's age	Neurological examination
Patient's sex	Glasgow Coma Scale score
Mechanism of injury	Pupillary response
Vital signs	Other injuries
Brief history	Treatment

- Continue communication with hospital base station

Source: Adapted from: Rimel RW, Edlich RF, Winn HR, et al. *Acute care of the head and spinal cord injured patient at the site of injury.* Charlottesville, Virginia: University of Virginia, 1978.

are in the severe category (14). Evidence suggests that brain damage increases linearly in the descending GCS scale from 12 to 6. The most severe head injuries fall into the 3 to 5 GCS category and there is little hope for these patients because most have suffered irreversible brain injury before admission to the hospital.

Depending upon the situation, the physician may need to initiate treatment for increased intracranial pressure. The initial head injury management and treatment protocol is listed in Table 24A.6.

Any head injury in sports should be treated with immediate and periodic follow-up. If treated as an outpatient, patient education and instructional materials should be given to families or roommates (see Appendix 24.3).

Concussion/Mild Traumatic Brain Injury

Concussion is defined as a temporary disturbance of the brain function, which occurs without a permanent structural change in the brain following a blow to the head or body. Clinically, it is characterized by immediate and transient impairment of neural function, such as alteration of consciousness or disturbance of vision or equilibrium. A concussion involves a change in mental behavior with or without loss of consciousness. It is the most common head injury in contact sports accounting for 250,000 concussions annually in football alone, 90% of which were "grade 1" concussions (15). Statistics from other studies showed that 20% of high school football players, 34% of college football players, and 54% of elite soccer players reported a history of at least one concussion during their career (10,16,17). It is estimated that 68,860 concussions present to the emergency room yearly due to football, 21,714 due to soccer, and 4,820 due to ice hockey (6).

TABLE 24A.7

HEAD INJURY: TREND OF CONSCIOUSNESS, DIAGNOSTIC PROCEDURE AND TREATMENT

Trend of Consciousness	Diagnostic Procedure	Treatment
No LOC	C-spine and skull x-rays as indicated	Pain relief for headache if indicated
Transient LOC and improving	C-spine and skull x-rays	Consider admission to hospital if clinical or patient support system not satisfactory
Transient LOC and deteriorating (lucid intervals)	C-spine and skull x-rays (epidural hematoma); emergency CT scan	Admit; hyperventilate; furosemide 20–80 mg i.v.; mannitol if condition deteriorates
Prolonged unconsciousness with signs of brain herniation	C-spine and skull x-rays; emergency CT scan	Admit; hyperventilate; furosemide 40–80 mg i.v.; early ICP monitoring; manitol if needed to lower ICP
Rapidly deteriorating consciousness with signs of herniation	C-spine and skull x-rays; emergency craniotomy after CT-scan if there is surgical lesion	Admit; hyperventlate; furosemide 40–80 mg i.v.; mannitol 1 g/kg; consider emergency burr hole

LOC = loss of consciousness; CT = computed tomography; ICP = intracranial pressure.

A full discussion of concussions including presentation, physical examination findings, workup, return to play decision making, and postinjury sequelae can be found in Chapter 14.

Differential Diagnosis

Vasovagal Syncope

A syncopal episode may be the result of a substantial blow to the body without direct trauma to the head. In this circumstance, the vagus nerve is stimulated, causing a decreased pulse, hypotension, light-headedness, or possible unconsciousness. There is no associated amnesia but respiratory difficulty can occur while unconscious. Recovery is usually quick and no symptoms of concussion are present. This may be the mechanism in brief losses of consciousness not being associated with prolonged concussive symptoms so often seen in athletics (18).

Post-traumatic Migraine

Rarely, cerebral vasospasm caused by trauma has resulted in a migraine-like clinical picture. Symptoms do not occur at the time of impact but shortly afterward (19). Prodromal, visual, motor, or sensory-symptoms may be noted by the player. This may be the source of prolonged headaches seen in some athletes. A trial on migraine medications may be worthwhile.

SEVERE HEAD INJURY

Intracranial Lesions

Intracranial hemorrhage is responsible for most injury-related deaths due to head injury. It can also be the most amenable to surgery. Bleeding may be arterial, most commonly the middle meningeal artery, or venous (most commonly the longitudinal sinus or bridging cerebral veins). A general treatment protocol is outlined in Table 24A.7, placing emphasis on the level of consciousness over time. Figure 24A.6 presents common intracranial lesions schematically.

Classification

Epidural hematoma. Blood may collect in localized pockets within the epidural space after injury, usually as the result of a head-on collision. Most (75%) are due to fracture of the temporal bone with injury to the middle meningeal artery. The resultant space

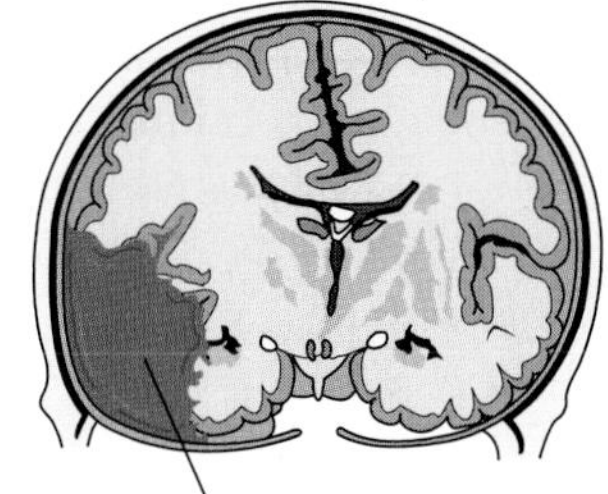

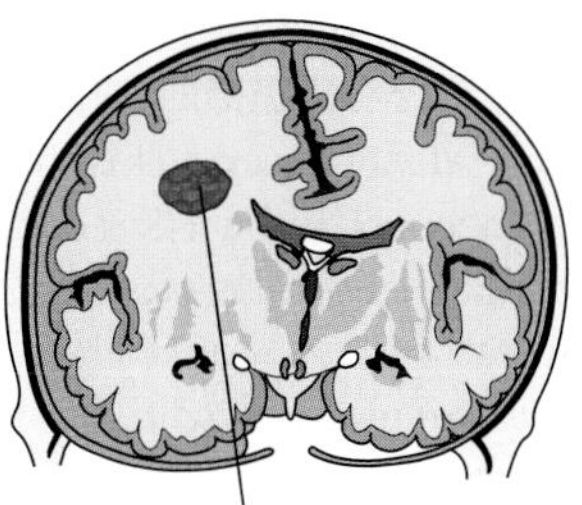

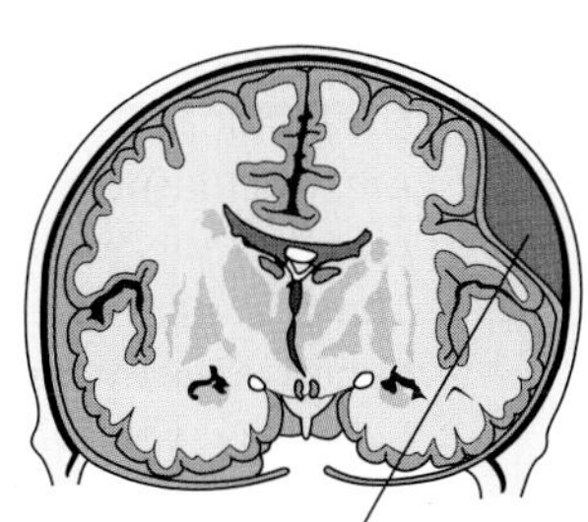

Figure 24A.6 Intracranial lesions. Epidural hematoma, subdural hematoma, and cerebral hemorrhage are shown here in their respective tissue planes. (*Source*: From Smeltzer SC, Bare BG. *Textbook of medical surgical nursing*, 9th ed. Philadelphia: Lippincott Williams & Wilkins, 2000.)

occupying mass can increase intracranial pressures and compress brain tissue. Fortunately, these injuries are rare in sports. They represent only 1% to 3% of all head injuries, but the mortality rate is unusually high (8%–50%). Be wary of this lesion as it is an easily treatable lesion that may occur with a relatively mild blow and may be easily overlooked. Clinical signs include the following:

- An initial period of unconsciousness, then followed by a lucid interval, drowsiness, headache, and vomiting. After 1 to 2 hours a progressive deterioration of consciousness, impaired respirations, and cardiopulmonary arrest can occur.
- Dilation and fixation of the ipsilateral pupil usually occurs. Mortality approaches 90% if both pupils are affected.
- Contralateral weakness or paralysis and attenuated deep tendon reflexes (DTRs) can also be seen.

Chronic epidermal hemorrhage. The source of the hemorrhage in *venous* and will result in vague neurological symptoms taking 2 to 7 days to appear.

Subdural hemorrhage/hematoma. Subdural hemorrhage is arbitrarily classified as acute, subacute, or chronic.

- *Acute subdural hemorrhage/hematoma.* Often caused by rotational or shearing forces and seen sometimes in whiplash injuries. Bleeding is due to tearing of the bridging veins in the space between the inner layer of the dura and the arachnoid space. It is usually present over roughened areas in the calvarian such as the frontal and temporal areas overlying the bony ridges of the skull, regardless of the area of impact (20). It is often a *countercoup* injury involving vessels opposite the area of impact. It can also be associated with skull fractures.

  Acute subdural hematoma is the most frequent cause of death due to athletic head injuries, having a 60% to 70% mortality rate (21) and accounting for approximately 75% of all vascular complications encountered in sports. Mortality correlates with the duration of loss of consciousness. In most cases, the patient is rendered unconscious by the cerebral contusion, which overshadows many of the symptoms of the expanding hemorrhage. The prognosis is favorable in those less common circumstances where there is not a concomitant brain contusion in addition to the hemorrhage. The onset of unconsciousness and rapid deterioration may not develop for hours or days after the injury (i.e., Talk And Die [TAD] presentation), although unconsciousness is not always seen. This injury may be one cause of second impact syndrome. The treatment is immediate surgical removal of the hemorrhage by craniotomy.
- *Subacute subdural hemorrhage/hematoma.* A subacute subdural hematoma occurs when the symptoms and signs appear 2 to 10 days after the injury (TAD). For several days after the injury, the patient is usually drowsy and disoriented. The presentation is similar to an acute hematoma once neurological deterioration begins. Treatment is the same as that for an acute hematoma.
- *Chronic subdural hemorrhage/hematoma.* Chronic subdural hematomas produce signs and symptoms 2 weeks or more after the initial injury. The symptoms are usually subtle and may include persistent headaches, personality changes, or other signs of cerebral irritation. These hematomas tend to develop as a result of bleeding from small fragile vessels (often veins) in the subdural space. This type of injury results in a slow increase in pressure due to venous bleeding. Their insidious onset highlights the necessity for close follow-up of any head injury.

Subarachnoid hemorrhage. Blood may collect in the space between the arachnoid and the pia mater owing to pia vessel injury, parenchymal injury, or extension from an intraventricular hemorrhage. This is uncommon in athletes, usually correlates to significant trauma, and is usually found in association with diffuse axonal injury. Surgery is not usually required if bleeding is superficial.

Cerebral hemorrhages and contusions. These represent brain parenchymal injury due to direct damage to the brain (coup or countercoup). The tips of the temporal and frontal lobes are most vulnerable. Contusions cause focal swelling and are best visualized with magnetic resonance imaging (MRI). Disruption of numerous small capillaries of the brain itself results in a hematoma, which tends to be located deeper in the brain substance than contusions. Hemorrhages are best seen by computed tomography (CT) early and MRI after several days. Symptoms are usually rapidly progressive and without a lucid period. Death can occur quickly in some instances.

SECTION B
FACE

EPIDEMIOLOGY

Injuries to the maxillofacial area of the body represent 2% to 3% of all sports injuries and sports activities account for 12% of all maxillofacial injuries. Despite the use of face guards, masks, and other protective equipment, facial trauma continues to present significant problems for sports physicians. Most injuries occur in one of the following three ways:

- A direct blow from fists, elbows, or objects such as pucks, baseballs, tennis balls, hockey sticks, rackets, or foreign objects from the stands.
- Direct contact with a playing surface such as ice, basketball courts, or turf.

- Injury from damaged or improperly fitting protective equipment.

GENERAL PRINCIPALS

There are several factors common in the management of maxillofacial injuries:

- Be aware of associated injuries. Additional, sometimes hidden, neurotrauma may be present in an athlete with maxillofacial injury. These nonfacial problems should take precedence.
- Infection must be prevented. The risk of possible contamination of the wound by oral flora or extrinsic agents is high. Irrigate, explore, and consider prophylactic antibiotics.
- Tetanus toxoid should be given if a previous immunization was more than 10 years ago; 5 years if the wound is deep and/or contaminated.
- Dental occlusion should be assessed when evaluating jaw fractures and dislocations (see Figure 24B.1). Deviation in occlusion may indicate malocclusion secondary to jaw fracture or pterygoid muscle spasm.
- Significant maxillofacial trauma may interfere with either the oral or nasotracheal airway. The following airway equipment is suggested: ambu-bag and mask, oral airway, laryngoscope, endotrachial tube, and suction tip. This equipment should be available for use on-site at competitions and practices.

CONTUSIONS/ABRASIONS

Contusions usually resolve spontaneously but they must be differentiated from facial edema associated with underlying fractures (see Figure 24B.2). Abrasions must be thoroughly cleansed and small foreign bodies removed to prevent permanent tattooing. A surgical scrub brush is helpful. Grease or oil can be dissolved and removed with small amounts of acetone.

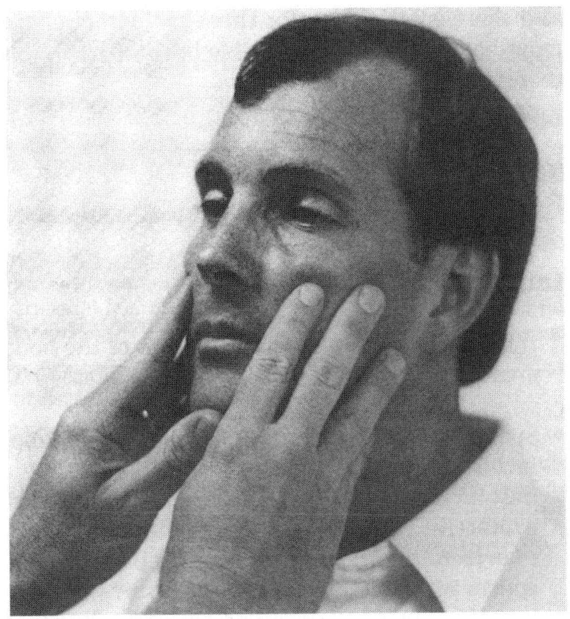

Figure 24B.1 Assesment of dental occlusion.

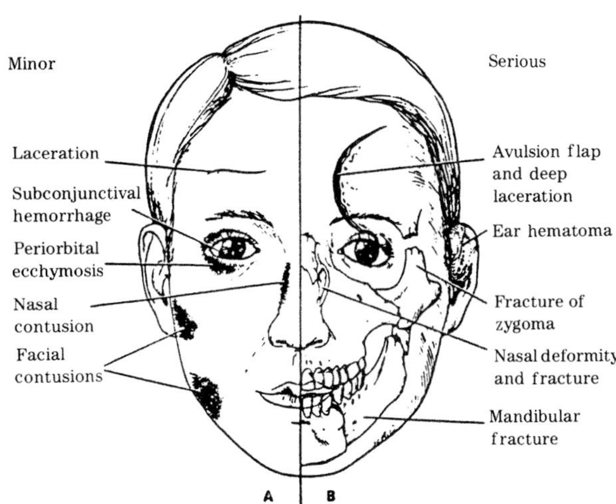

Figure 24B.2 Comparison of minor versus serious facial injuries. **A:** Simple lacerations, contusions, and ecchymosis. **B:** Complex lacerations, facial asymmetry, deformity, and malocclusion with underlying facial bone fractures. (*Source*: From Schultz RC, de Camara DL. Athletic facial injuries. *JAMA* 1984;252(24):3395–3398, 44.)

LACERATIONS

Treating facial lacerations is complicated by the increased vascularity of the face, and the necessity for acceptable cosmetic results. The absence of underlying damage to neural, vascular, muscular, and bony structures should be determined before closure of any wound. If there is damage, referral (without wound closure) to a surgeon is appropriate. If the patient is to be moved or referred, adequate hemostasis should be obtained, the wound covered with sterile gauze and any avulsed tissue preserved for possible use in the final repair.

Strive for cleanliness in repair to eliminate the possibility of infection. Skin approximation can be accomplished with Steri-Strips or skin glue if the laceration is small, superficial, or noncomplicated. Lacerations that are more extensive require the use of 5-0 or 6-0 nonabsorbable suture ((polydioxanone) [PDS] suture causes less foreign-body inflammation) although many of these more extensive lacerations can also be repaired with skin glue with good cosmetic result. If sutures are utilized, use a local anesthetic with epinephrine to control bleeding unless the area involves the pinna of the ear or the tip of the nose. The effects of epinephrine on the microcirculation of the digits, nose, penis or ear may cause ischemia and have detrimental effects on healing and the control of infection. If the wound is deep, a two-layer closure is necessary, using absorbable sutures to approximate deep structures before final closure. Cartilage must be very carefully approximated. Insertion of a rubber drain may be necessary to prevent hematoma formation in large, deep wounds (remember, overlying hematomas may cause cartilaginous resorption). If there are jagged edges to the laceration, the edge should be trimmed to leave an uninterrupted linear surface. After 3 to 4 days, every other suture can be removed to reduce local reaction and scarring with removal of the reminder at 6 to 7 days.

Points to consider with facial lacerations:

- Eyebrows should not be shaven.
- Use eyebrow shape and direction as landmarks for repair.
- Eyelid lacerations should be closed in layers (see section on Eye Injuries).
- Facial muscles should be repaired at the time of the initial closure.
- Deep cheek lacerations can involve either the parotid gland or the branches of the facial nerve.
- Interoral and tongue lacerations should be only loosely closed followed by prophylactic antibiotic therapy (see section on Mouth Injuries).

FACIAL FRACTURES

Facial fractures are not usually medical emergencies but reduction is necessary to restore form and function. Radiological evaluation can be unnecessary or special views required to visualize specific pathology. Table 24B.1 gives some specific recommendations and the best imaging method for the evaluation of the facial bone involved. Nasal bones are the most frequent facial fracture and are discussed in the section on Nose.

TABLE 24B.1
THIS TABLE PROVIDES APPROPRIATE IMAGING OPTIONS FOR VARIOUS FACIAL FRACTURES

Structure	Appropriate Imaging
Mandible	Panoramic (Panorex)[a]
	PA of mandible
	Townes' view (AP "from above")
	Lateral obliques
Nasal bones	No x-ray required—clinical[a]
	Diagnosis may do Waters' view and/or lateral
Zygomatic and orbital bones	CT scan*
	Waters' view (AP "from below")
	Caldwell's view (PA at 150 degrees)
	Submento vertex
Maxilla	CT scan—axial and coronal[a]
	Conventional x-rays of little value

PA = posteroanterior; AP = anteroposterior; CT = computed tomography
[a] Best imaging method.

Maxillary Fractures

Zygoma

Fractures of the zygomatic arch account for 10% of the sport-related maxillary fractures. They are typically caused by blunt trauma to the cheekbone. Deformity of the zygoma can be detected by looking at both cheeks from the top of the patient's head while palpating to determine the presence and degree of depression. A "step-off" deformity can be palpated at any one of three attachments (maxilla, frontal bone, temporal bone). All three attachments should always be palpated if the physician suspects a zygomatic fracture. Other signs include periorbital ecchymosis, enophthalmos, numbness in V2 distribution, and diplopia. The degree of displacement can be radiographically determined with the use of a Waters' view (see Figure 24B.3). An associated fracture of the maxillary sinus on the affected side is common and will be opacified with blood in this view if present. Further evaluation with CT scan is the imaging method of choice and may identify associated injuries or make a definitive diagnosis. Complications include restriction and entrapment of extraocular muscles and hyperesthesia of the infraorbital branch to the facial nerve.

Treatment of these injuries should include a thorough examination of the affected eye including all eye movements, and prophylactic antibiotics. Exploration of the fracture is necessary if deformity of the malar eminence exceeds 1 cm, or if enophthalmos or restricted ocular mobility exists. If the zygomatic arch is fractured at mid-point, it can impinge upon mandibular function, specifically jaw opening (trismus). Reduction may be necessary.

Orbital Blowout Fracture

Direct trauma to the eye can transmit a force that fractures the bony orbit. The fracture usually occurs in the orbital floor or, less commonly, the medial wall. Enophthalmos, diplopia, and extraoccular muscle restriction are common findings. Sports where this injury is likely to be seen include racket sports, handball and baseball. For further information, see the section on Eye.

Le Fort Fractures

High velocity impact to the mid-face can cause fractures of the maxilla that result in varying degrees of deformity. Le Fort fractures I–III are gradations of severity based on the pathological mobility of the maxilla (see Figure 24B.4 for a visual representation):

- Le Fort I: Palate separated from midface.
- Le Fort II: Maxilla separated from face by a fracture through inferior orbital rims and nose.
- Le Fort III: Facial bones separated from cranial bones by a fracture through the suture line between zygoma and frontal bones, across orbital floor and through the nasofrontal junction.

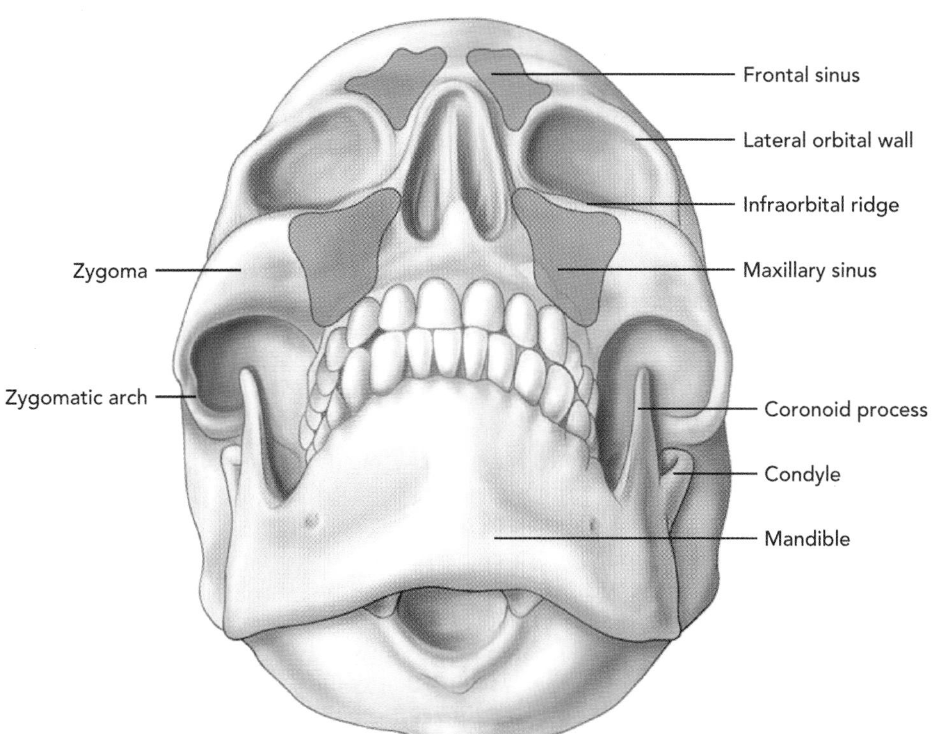

Figure 24B.3 Illustration of a Waters' view radiograph depicting the location of the sinuses, orbital wall, zygoma, and mandible.

Facial deformity, massive tissue edema, Battle's sign, raccoon eyes, malocclusion, intraoral bleeding (causing respiratory distress), and CSF rhinorrhea/otorrhea are common findings in these injuries. Fortunately, these injuries are uncommon in sports because the force needed to generate them is rarely found in athletics. Immediate referral is necessary for open reduction and internal fixation and/or intramaxillary fixation. Return to play may be accomplished anywhere from 6 weeks to many months after repair depending on the severity and the presence of secondary injuries. A face shield may be required initially, or permanently if instability remains.

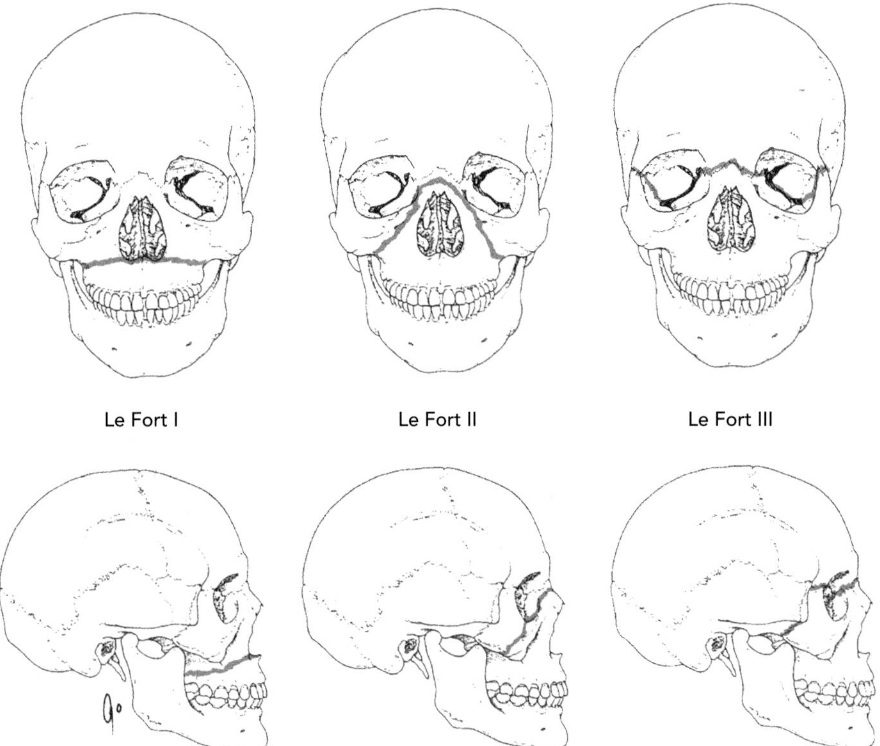

Figure 24B.4 Illustration of Le Fort classification of maxillary fractures grades I through III. (*Source*: From Snell MD. *Clinical anatomy*, 7th ed. Lippincott Williams & Wilkins, 2003.)

Sinus Fractures

Fractures of facial bones can be associated with extension into paranasal sinuses. Specifically, a maxillary sinus fracture may occur in association with a zygomatic arch or blowout fracture. A typical mechanism is by blunt force to the eyeball causing a sudden increase in intraorbital pressure such as seen with impact from a baseball. Alternatively, a direct blow to the anterior rim may transmit the force to the orbital wall with a resultant blowout fracture (see Figure 24B.5). Signs of a blowout fracture include periorbital and subconjunctival hemorrhage, enophthalmos, and diplopia. Fractures into the maxillary sinus are best seen on Waters' view although evaluation with a CT scan may show this fracture with improved sensitivity and further identify associated injuries. Sinus opacification secondary to the presence of blood will be the major finding on a plain film Waters' view. Air can sometimes be seen in the soft tissues of the cheek or orbit in these types of fractures. Treatment includes antibiotics to prevent infection in the blood filled sinus and close observation for signs of further swelling that could indicate development of a facial abscess. Athletes normally can resume workout activities within a week. Long-term complications occur rarely, but include chronic sinusitis or osteomyolitis of the maxilla.

Frontal sinus fractures secondary to blunt forehead trauma can present significant problems. There will be pain and swelling of the forehead. Immediate postinjury swelling may mask the depression normally seen with such fractures. Epistaxis as well as CSF rhinorrhea (secondary to disruption of the cribiform plate) frequently accompany such fractures. A fracture of the posterior wall of the frontal sinus should be treated as a compound skull fracture because there is communication between the sinus and anterior cranial fossa. Treatment includes hospitalization and prophylactic antibiotics. Close observation for developing meningitis should be continued until resolution.

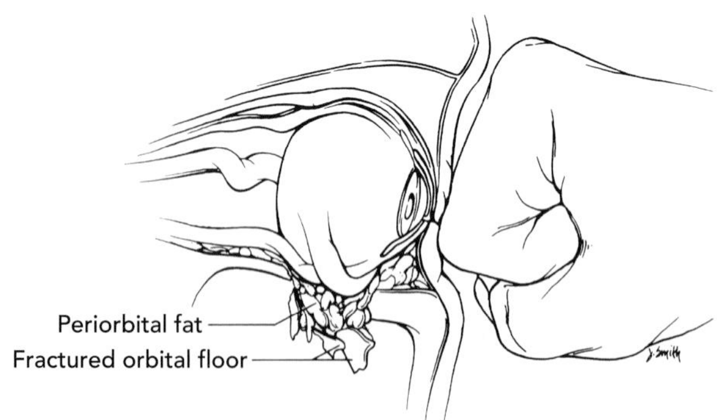

Figure 24B.5 Figure 24B.7. Blowout fracture. There are two theories on the mechanism. The *Buckling theory* maintains that an anterior force is transmitted back into the orbit. The *Retropulsion theory* refers to a fracture of the orbital floor caused by hydraulic forces in the closed orbital cavity. (*Source*: From Harwood-Nuss A, Wolfson AB, Linden CH, et al. *The clinical practice of emergency medicine*, 3rd ed. Philadelphia: Lippincott Williams & Wilkins, 2001.)

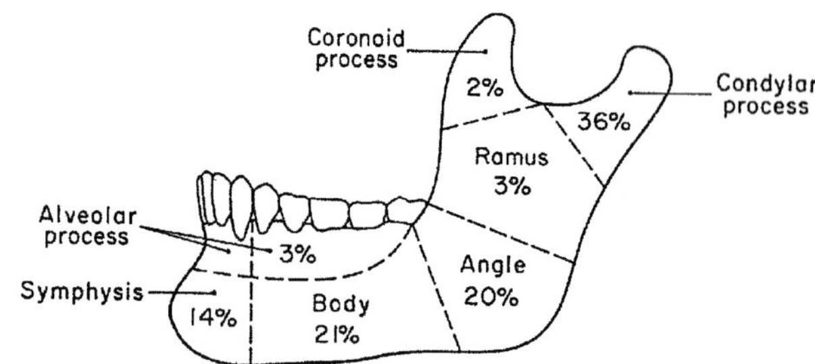

Figure 24B.6 Regions of the mandible with relative incidence of fractures.

The ethmoid sinuses can sometimes be involved, not as a result of direct trauma, but by forces transmitted through exposed structures such as the orbit and nasal bones. Presenting signs include swelling and palpable crepitus along the medial orbit. Treatment includes antibiotics, observation for infection, and restricted nose blowing for 5 to 7 days. Sports participation should be restricted for 7 to 10 days and contact for 6 to 8 weeks.

Mandibular Fractures

Mandibular fractures account for approximately 10% of all maxillofacial fractures seen in sports. Biomechanically, the mandible becomes involved when the athlete falls and strikes it against a hard playing surface, or when contact is made with another player or piece of equipment. An anterior force may result in a bilateral fracture. A lateral force may result in an ipsilateral subcondylar or contralateral angle or body fracture. The most frequently fractured parts of the mandible are shown in Figure 24B.6. Because of the semicircular structure of the mandible, fractures often occur at two sites (see Figure 24B.7). It

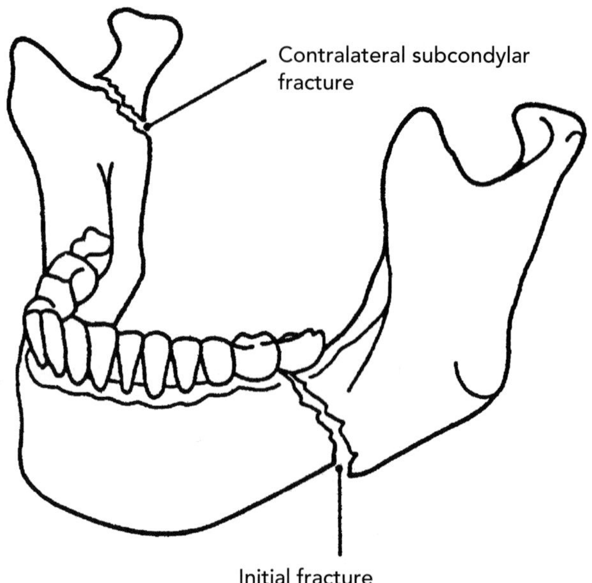

Figure 24B.7 Mandibular injuries.

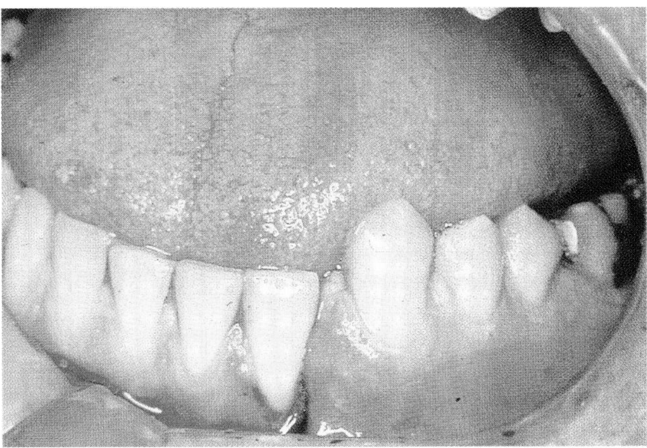

Figure 24B.8 Malocclusion due to mandibular fracture can be obvious on examination of the dentition. (*Source*: From Harries M. *Oxford textbook of sports medicine*. New York: Oxford University Press, 1998.)

is important to evaluate the athlete for a second fracture site after an initial fracture has been identified.

Most of these fractures extend through the intraoral mucosa and cause bleeding from the mouth. There is malocclusion of bite and abnormal mobility of the mandible (see Figure 24B.8). Drooling, caused by the athlete's inability to move his mandible without pain, can be present. Palpation shows irregularity in both the open and closed position of the jaw and may identify a step off at the site of fracture. There may be numbness in the V3 distribution. Mandibular trauma can transmit significant forces that may involve the external auditory canal and tympanomandibular joint, therefore careful examination should include these structures. Diagnosis of a mandibular fracture is usually verified with a plain film panoramic view.

Uncomplicated fractures can be treated conservatively by immobilization of the jaw with a Barton or barrel bandage if the fracture is uncomplicated (see Figure 24B.9). Complicated fractures require referral for intramaxillary fixation or open reduction and internal fixation. If the airway is not compromised, treatment consists of reduction and immobilization of fracture fragments and a liquid diet for 6 weeks, then a soft diet until the jaw can be moved without pain. If the oral mucosa or facial skin is broken prophylactic antibiotics should be instituted. If there is a malocclusion, surgical referral is indicated.

Mandibular Dislocation

Biomechanically, if the lower jaw is suddenly depressed during sports activity, dislocation of the mandible may occur. The mandibular condyle simply moves anterior to the temporomandibular joint. The chin deviates to the side opposite the dislocation and the patient is unable to close his/her mouth (open-bite deformity). Reduction of the dislocation should be attempted as soon as possible. The thumbs are placed supporting each side of the mandible as the hands pull in a downward and backward manner until

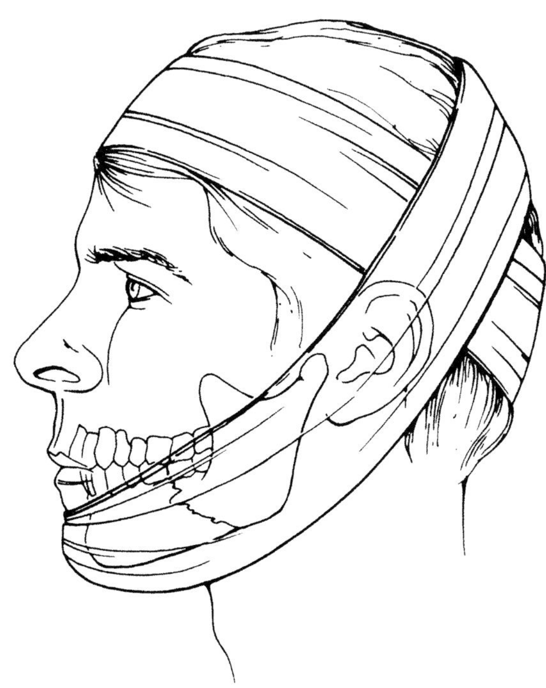

Figure 24B.9 Barton's bandage. Initial placement of the dressing is shown. Additional layers result in improved immobilization. (*Source*: From Harwood-Nuss A, Wolfson AB, Linden CH, et al. *The clinical practice of emergency medicine*, 3rd ed. Philadelphia: Lippincott Williams & Wilkins, 2001.)

the condyle is felt to slip into the joint. Do not force the reduction or a fracture or further damage may result.

PREVENTION OF FACIAL INJURIES

The use of improved protective equipment by athletes has had a significant impact on the prevention of facial injuries. Many factors influence the occurrence of facial injuries including the attitude, experience, and competence of coaches, players, and officials. In addition, the player's personal equipment, the playing surface, and structures on or nearby the playing surface may influence the risk of injury. The team physician should take an active role in making the playing area as safe as possible.

Football facemasks provide varying degrees of protection. The full cage facemask protects from most injuries including finger-induced facial lacerations. The half facemask will not prevent lacerations of the upper portion of the face or fractures of the cheek or nose. The mouth guard may protect against facial injuries by acting as a cushion against blows to the lower jaw.

The catcher's facemask in baseball and softball does not protect against possible injury to the throat (larynx and trachea). Requiring the use of throat guards by catchers and hockey goalies may remedy this situation.

Full facial clear plastic hockey shields, as well as cage-type facemasks have significantly reduced the incidence of facial injuries in nongoalie hockey players. Before this rule change, approximately 60% of all facial injuries in nongoalie players resulted from contact with the stick (22). Most hockey goalies now use a helmet with a wire or clear plastic facemask to keep the puck from making contact with facial bones. A throat protector that hangs below the facemask should always be utilized in order to prevent throat injuries.

SECTION C

EYE INJURIES AND ILLNESSES

PERSPECTIVE

Injuries to the eye are a major source of blindness or visual impairment in sports. Proper eye protection, regulations to limit dangerous exposure during athletic activity, and education are simple interventions that could prevent as many as 150,000 eye injuries a year (23). The National Society for the Prevention of Blindness estimates that more than 111,000 school age children suffer sports-related eye injuries each year. That is in addition to approximately 100,000 eye injuries in older athletes. Approximately 25% of persons with eye injuries develop serious complication and some lose their vision completely (24). Fortunately, 90% of all sports injuries are preventable with proper eye safety measures and protective eyewear (25).

ANATOMY

Anatomical features of the eye must be understood to properly diagnose and manage common eye injuries in sports. The orbit is made up of five or six different bones that form a socket that is open only anteriorly and posteriorly (see Figure 24C.1). The superior orbital ridge above, the infraorbital margins below, the malar bone on the temporal side, and the nasal bone on the medial side are designed to protect the eye within the recess they form. The eye is made up of three chambers separated by the iris and the lens. It is covered by the transparent cornea anteriorly, the remainder being encapsulated by the tough sclera. The posterior globe contains the retina, macula, fovea, and optic nerve. See Figure 24C.2 for details of the anatomy of the eye.

EPIDEMIOLOGY OF EYE INJURIES IN SPORTS

Ocular injuries are most common (in decreasing order) in baseball, basketball, tennis, football, biking, and soccer. Almost 20% of ocular trauma is sports related. Approximately 50% of the injuries occur in children under the age of 15 and 65% occur in individuals under the age of 31. There are more ocular injuries in recreational sports than in the work place (25). Several studies of ice hockey injuries have demonstrated significant reductions in eye injuries (>95%) when facemasks are used (26,27). Widespread use of facemasks in hockey has prevented an estimated 70,000 eye and face injuries in recent years.

ETIOLOGY

The eye and its surrounding structures are vulnerable to direct blows from objects less than or equal to 10 cm in diameter. Anything larger, the orbital rim absorbs much of the energy. The facial structures on the side of the head

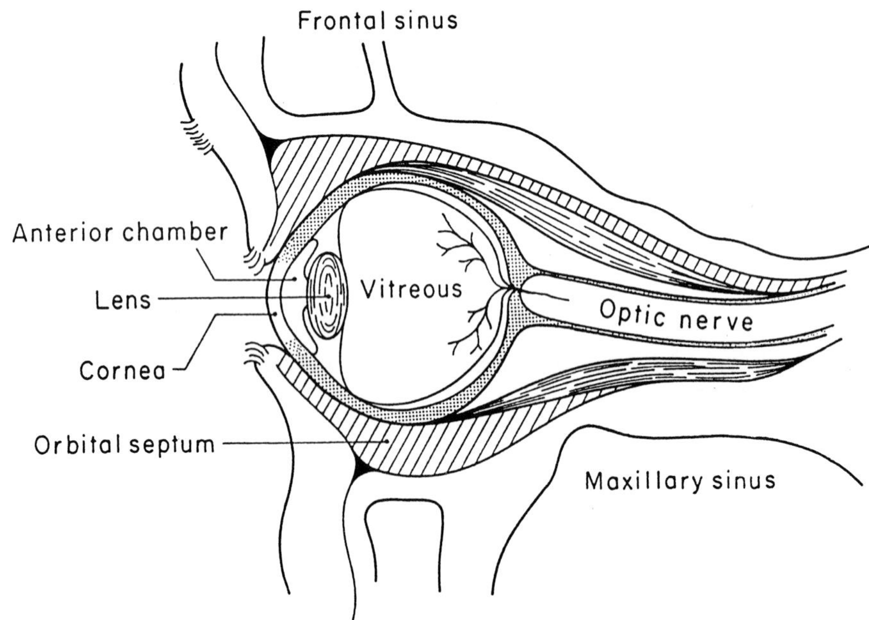

Figure 24C.1 Orbital anatomy.

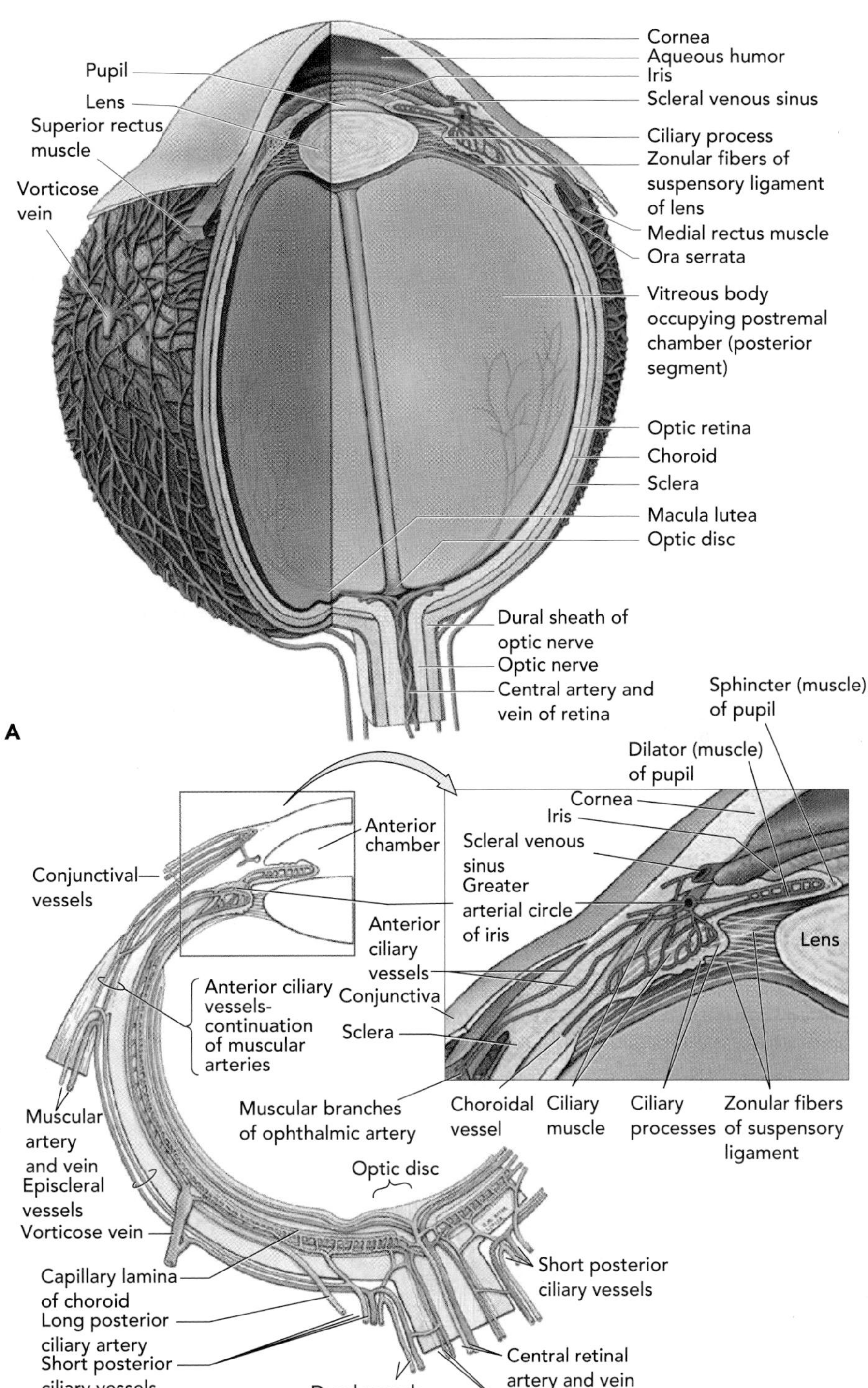

Figure 24C.2 Anatomy of the eye. Sagittal view of the human eye shows important anatomic structures including the retina, fovea, macula, optic nerve, lens, anterior and posterior chambers, conjunctiva, sclera and cornea. (*Source*: From Moore KL. *Clinically oriented anatomy*, 4th ed. Philadelphia: Lippincott Williams & Wilkins, 2000.)

offer much less protection to blows coming from the side, especially if the globe protrudes past the surrounding bone. Approximately 200 G of force is required to cause an orbital rim fracture.

Injury to the eye may occur from sharp objects (darts), objects less than 5 cm (fingers, BBs, hockey sticks, golf balls) and objects greater than 5 cm (softballs and baseballs). Objects greater than 5 cm may bring about injury by acting as a piston, pushing the eye tissue posteriorly and blowing out the floor of the orbit (see Figure 24B.5). Injury can also be caused by contact with other players, fixed structures around the playing area, or from foreign objects thrown by spectators.

Serious injuries that can lead to permanent loss of vision include hyphemas, corneal lacerations, retinal detachments, macular scarring, and secondary hemorrhages. Glaucoma and cataracts may develop much later and may also lead to permanent loss of vision. Serious eye trauma

TABLE 24C.1
POSSIBLE SIGNS OF SERIOUS EYE INJURIES IN SPORTS

Black eye
Red eye
A foreign object on the cornea
An eye that does not move as completely as the oppsite eye
One eye protruding compared with the opposite eye
Abnormal pupil size or shape compared with the opposite eye
A layer of blood between the cornea and iris
A cut or penetration of the eyelid or eyeball
A darkened subconjunctival mass that may indicate scleral rupture
Photophobia or ''flashing lights''

does not necessarily present with pain or visual disturbance at the time of injury. Blurred vision that does not clear with blinking, loss of all or part of the visual field of either eye, steady or deep throbbing pain, or double vision after the injury, should raise the suspicion that the eye has been seriously injured. Additional signs that a more detailed evaluation and treatment are needed are listed in Table 24C.1.

In evaluating an eye injury, check the patient's history for prior injury or diminished visual acuity. On examination, establish the current visual acuity immediately and then systematically examine the eye and its surrounding structures (see Table 24C.2). Separate the eyelids after instilling an anesthetic solution as necessary. Check the extra ocular movements (EOMs) and peripheral vision and completely view the conjunctiva and sclera. Restriction of EOMs may be secondary to a blowout fracture of the orbit or neuromuscular damage. Examine the lid for lacerations and foreign bodies and check the conjunctiva and anterior chamber for clarity. Evaluate the pupil size, reaction to light and accommodation, and shape. Finally, thoroughly evaluate the lens and retina, using a slit-lamp and ophthalmoscope. The athlete should be carefully evaluated for signs and symptoms of concussion. X-rays, including CT of the facial bones, may be needed to rule out fracture. Routine x-rays, often do not show orbital blowout fractures, see Figure 24B.4 for recommendations on radiological workup. If there is any doubt about the function of the eye or seriousness of the injury, referral is indicated.

TABLE 24C.2
OPHTHALMIC EXAMINATION

Thorough evaluation of sport-related eye injuries involves the following areas:
- Visual acuity
- External lids, conjunctiva
- Pupils
- EOM's
- Confrontation fields
- Anterior segment
- Fundus

Equipment needed:
- Acuity chart
- Penlight or flashlight
- Proparacaine
- Fluorescein strips
- Ophthalmoscope

EOM = extra ocular movements.

COMMON EYE INJURIES AND ILLNESSES

For a complete overview of common eye injuries in sports, see Table 24C.3.

Eyebrow and Eyelid Lacerations

Lacerations of the eyebrow are common and require careful repair. Even a simple contusion over the ridge of the eyebrow can sever the supraorbital nerve, therefore function must be assessed before treatment. Care must then be taken during the repair not to damage this nerve.

Lacerations of the medial canthus may involve the lacrimal system and should be referred for surgical repair. Prolapsed fatty tissue associated with a lid laceration may indicate a fracture of the orbital roof or involvement of the globe and should be evaluated by an ophthalmologist. If an eyelid laceration results in the avulsion of tissue, save the avulsed tissue for the best final repair.

Eyelid lacerations require accurate closure, particularly where they cross skin creases, otherwise an irregular scar may result. After local infiltration with 1% lidocaine with epinephrine an infraorbital nerve block may be given to patients with lower lid lacerations. Instilling topical ophthalmic anesthetic drops may improve patient comfort. Irrigate the wound with sterile saline to remove any debris. After sterile drapes are placed the laceration can be repaired. If the tarsus is lacerated repair with 6-0 absorbable suture taking 0.5 to 0.75 thickness bites with the needle. The obicularis muscle is then repaired with a 6-0 absorbable suture. If the lid margin is involved close with a nonabsorbable suture with eversion of the lid margin to prevent notching. The skin can then be closed using 6-0 or 5-0 nonabsorbable suture. Ensure adequate corneal lubrication, as needed. Patching patients is not preferred so acuity can be checked and undue pressure on the globe avoided. Head elevation, cold compresses, and antibiotic ointment are advisable. Cutaneous sutures are removed on day 5, and Steri-Strips are applied, if necessary. Removal of lid margin sutures at day 11 to 14 is a preferred method.

TABLE 24C.3
COMMON EYE INJURIES IN SPORTS

Problem	Usual Characteristics	Treatment
Blow-out fracture of orbit	Restricted ability to elevate the eye Hypesthesia—lower lid and cheek—due to damage to infra-orbital nerve X-ray-cloudy antrum with tissue herniation into maxillary sinus; laminogram may demonstrate break	Consultation with an ophthalmologist
Orbital Hemorrhage	Proptosis-forward bulging of eye Hematoma	Cold compresses Watch for signs of corneal exposure or retinal vascular compromise
Ptosis	Droopy upper eyelid due to trauma of levator palpebral superiorus muscle or its nerve	Consultation with an ophthalmologist
Lid Laceration	Lacerations requiring special consideration: Through and through lacerations involving the lid margin Lacrimal canalicular, ligament, or complete severance of the levator palpebral superiorus All other lacerations	For fear of lid margin notching, unless you are familiar with special techniques, seek ophthalmic consultation Ophthalmic consultation As with all periorbital lacerations examine the globe for injury The usual surgical repair is with 5-0 or 6-0 suture removed in 3 days

Orbital Injury

A direct blow to the anterior orbit may produce rapid passage of serum and blood into the soft tissue of the eyelid resulting in a periorbital hematoma or "black-eye." This may prevent the lid from opening altogether. A swollen eye should not be dismissed as minor as the blow may have caused other serious injury. If the lids are swollen shut or the eye is difficult to examine, do not force the lids open, and consult an ophthalmologist. The use of ice to reduce swelling may improve visualization of the globe.

Swelling from a black eye is usually self-limited and cold compresses should help during the first 24 to 48 hours. Do not use instant cold packs because they may rupture and cause caustic burns to the eye and surrounding structures. If hemorrhage occurs more posteriorly in the orbit significant proptosis and ophthalmoplegia (dilated, fixed pupil with paralysis of accommodation) may occur. Look for anesthesia above the orbital ridge to assess underlying nerve injury. Palpate for subcutaneous or subconjunctival emphysema, which can result from a sinus fracture, and may lead to osteomyelitis of the facial bones.

Corneal Abrasion

The cornea is the most exposed part of the eye. As a result, abrasions are common injuries. The patient usually has significant pain, photophobia, and the sensation of a foreign body in the eye.

Examination and Treatment

Use an anesthetic solution and examine the cornea with a bright light obliquely. If there is no foreign body, evert the upper lid and examine the tarsal conjunctiva. Use fluorescein stain on the cornea to visualize the extent of the abrasion (see Figure 24C.3). Treat with an antibiotic solution, and mydriatic drops. If significant photophobia is present, an eye patch may bring about relief. If quick improvement is not seen, refer to an ophthalmologist.

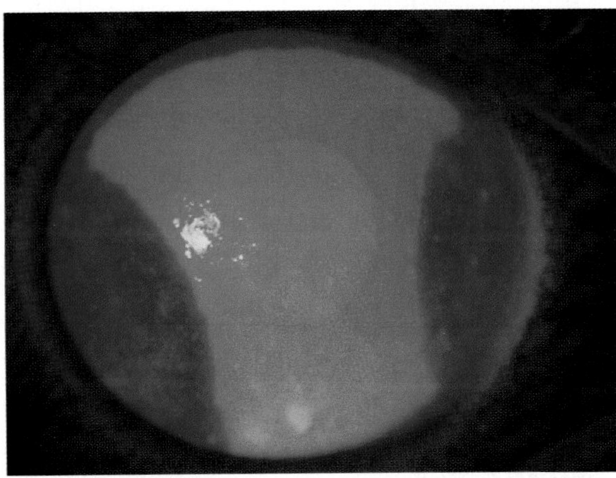

Figure 24C.3 Photo shows a diffuse corneal abrasion on slitlamp visualization after instillation of fluorescein dye. Note injected sclera and palpebral mucosa. (*Source*: From Tasman W, Jaeger EA. *The wills eye hospital atlas of clinical ophthalmology*, 2nd ed. Philadelphia: Lippincott Williams & Wilkins, 2001.)

A rupture or laceration of the cornea or sclera requires immediate ophthalmological evaluation. When this occurs, patch the eye and have the patient lie down until further evaluation can be done. If visual acuity is less than 20/30, suspect an intraocular foreign body. Never instill ointments where there is a full thickness corneal laceration.

Hyphema

Hyphema is a very common ocular injury that results from damage to the small vessels of the ciliary body causing hemorrhage into the anterior chamber (see Figure 24C.4). This injury is often associated with other severe intraocular injuries and requires immediate referral. Blunt trauma to the eye is usually followed by inflammation of the iris and ciliary body, producing dilation or constriction of the pupil that may persist for days to weeks. There may be increased lacrimation, blurred vision, photophobia, and severe eye pain. A blood-fluid level is often visible in the anterior chamber. Immediate treatment requires shielding the eye, bed rest, and evaluation by an ophthalmologist. It may be several days before an ophthalmologist can view the retina, and the patient must continue bed rest during this period. Typically, there is a 75% chance of good visual outcome in patients with hyphemas. Long-term complications include rebleeding, glaucoma, and the accumulation of white cells and protein in the anterior chamber. Because of the risk of rebleeding during the first week after injury, nonsteroidal anti-inflammatories should be avoided during this time. Most uncomplicated hyphema resolve within 5 or 6 days. Before return to play is allowed, clearance from an ophthalmologist is recommended to rule out glaucoma or other complications.

Snow Blindness

Excessive exposure to ultraviolet (UV) light reflected from the snow or water may produce a painful superficial inflammation of the cornea (keratitis) referred to as *snow blindness*. This is most often seen in outdoor winter sports and water sports such as water skiing. Symptoms include tearing, pain, redness, swollen eyelids, headache, a gritty feeling in the eyes, halos around lights, hazy vision, and temporary loss of vision. These symptoms may not appear until 6 to 12 hours after the exposure. Snowblindness is prevented by proper eye protection. It does not typically cause a permanent loss of vision. Pain and visual symptoms usually resolve with several days of rest in a dark room, cold compresses and pain medications.

Intraocular Foreign Bodies

Foreign bodies should be identified and removed as soon as possible (see Figure 24C.5). Copper or iron foreign bodies may produce degenerative changes and scarring in the eye. An orbital x-ray may be necessary to localize radio-opaque foreign bodies. Gentle removal with a sterile cotton tipped applicator moistened with sterile saline may be attempted after topical anesthetic is instilled. Refer promptly if the object is not easily removed.

Penetrating Eye Injuries

When evaluating an eye injury, examine the pupil and anterior chamber carefully. If the pupil is teardrop-shaped, or the anterior chamber is flat, there is almost always a penetrating injury of the cornea or limbus (see Figure 24C.6). Also evaluate the eye for hyphema, uveal prolapse or obvious lacerations of the eye structures. Always refer patients with penetrating wounds of the

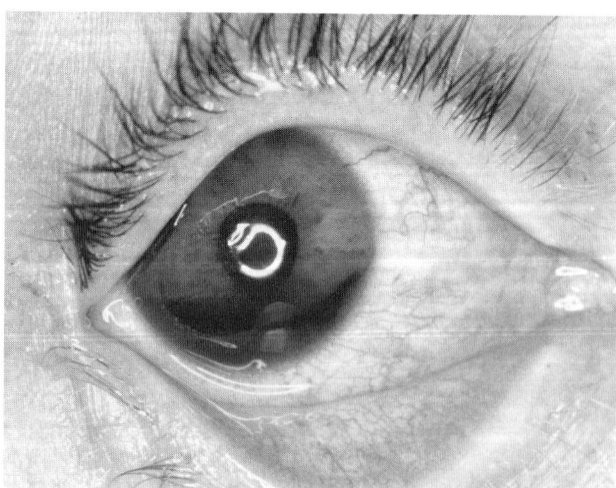

Figure 24C.4 Hyphema. Hyphema noted after blunt trauma to the eye, may be a sign of serious intraocular pathology and can lead to serious complications. Immediate ophthalmology referral is usually necessary. (*Source*: From Harwood-Nuss A, Wolfson AB, Linden CH, et al. *The clinical practice of emergency medicine*, 3rd ed. Philadelphia: Lippincott Williams & Wilkins, 2001.)

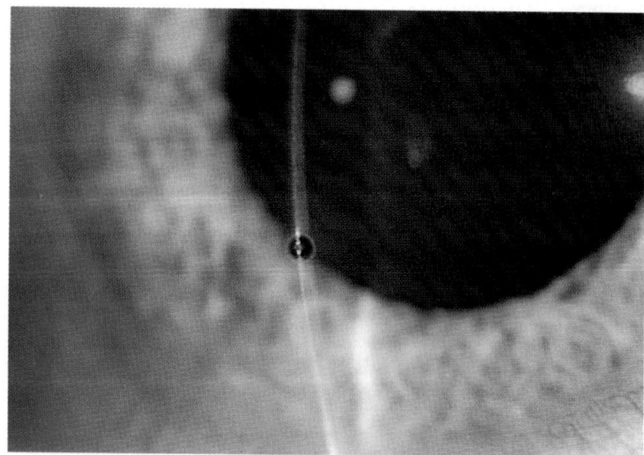

Figure 24C.5 Corneal rust ring A small reddish, brown circular opacity remains in the cornea after removal of an iron foreign body. Prompt removal of metal is necessary to prevent further injury and scarring. (*Source*: From Tasman W, Jaeger EA. *The wills eye hospital atlas of clinical ophthalmology*, 2nd ed. Philadelphia: Lippincott Williams & Wilkins, 2001.)

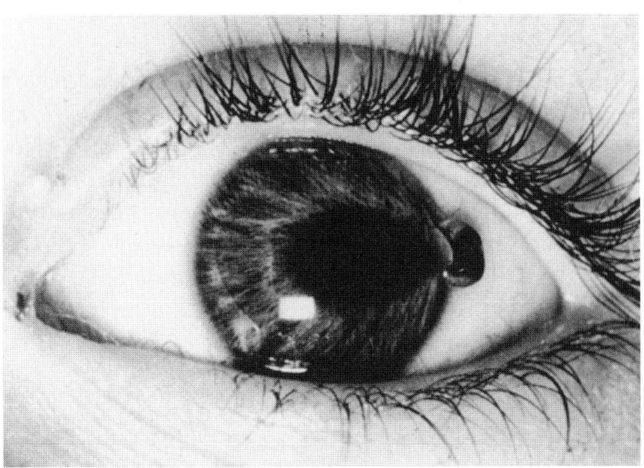

Figure 24C.6 Irregularity to the pupil as seen here or flatting of the anterior chamber usually signifies penetrating injury to the eye. Always evaluate the pupil after eye injuries. (*Source*: From Harwood-Nuss A, Wolfson AB, Linden CH, et al. *The clinical practice of emergency medicine*, 3rd ed. Philadelphia: Lippincott Williams & Wilkins, 2001.)

eye to an ophthalmologist for evaluation and treatment. Treat acutely with a noncompressive dressing and patch, prophylactic antibiotics, pain medications as needed, and relative rest. Proper tetanus prophylaxis should be administered.

Traumatic Cataract

Traumatic cataracts are a common secondary result of a metallic intraocular foreign body damaging the lens. The lens turns white soon after entry of the foreign body owing to laceration of the lens capsule and leakage of aqueous or vitreous humor into the lens (see Figure 24C.7). Posterior subcapsular cataracts are common in boxers who have sustained repeated trauma to the eye. Symptoms of a traumatic cataract include blurred vision, red eye, opaque lens, and intraocular hemorrhage. Complications include infection, uveitis, retinal detachment, and glaucoma. Traumatic cataracts are treated with antibiotics and corticosteroids, both systemically and locally, to decrease infection and the development of uveitis. Atropine sulfate 2%, two drops t.i.d. should be used to keep the pupil dilated until an ophthalmologist evaluates the injury. The cataract is usually removed after the inflammation has subsided. If the patient is under the age of 20, the lens material often absorbs on its own without surgery. An ophthalmologist should evaluate all traumatic cataracts.

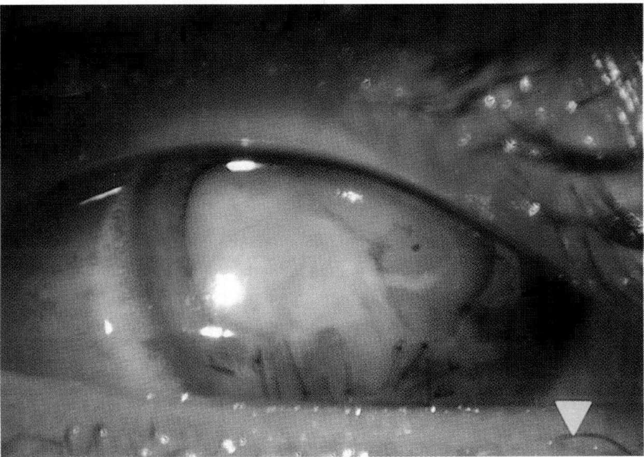

Figure 24C.7 Traumatic cataracts are often seen after penetrating injury from metallic foreign bodies or from repeated trauma. The lens opacifies due to exposure to vitreous humor. (*Source*: From Tasman W, Jaeger EA. *The wills eye hospital atlas of clinical ophthalmology*, 2nd ed. Philadelphia: Lippincott Williams & Wilkins, 2001.)

Retinal Detachment

Detachment of the retina is a very serious problem that usually causes blindness unless treated. Symptoms of flashing lights, floating objects, or a gray curtain moving across the field of vision are all indications of a retinal detachment. Retinal tears or detachments can occur after a blow to the eye, especially in athletes with a predisposing family history. Once a tear is present, vitreous fluid may collect between the retina and the choroids causing it to detach. Detachment is more likely in individuals with degenerative lesions of the retina. Retinal detachment may occur weeks or months after an injury. Diagnosis is made by visualization with an ophthalmoscope (see Figure 24C.8). An ophthalmologist should be consulted for a full assessment and appropriate treatment. Isolated

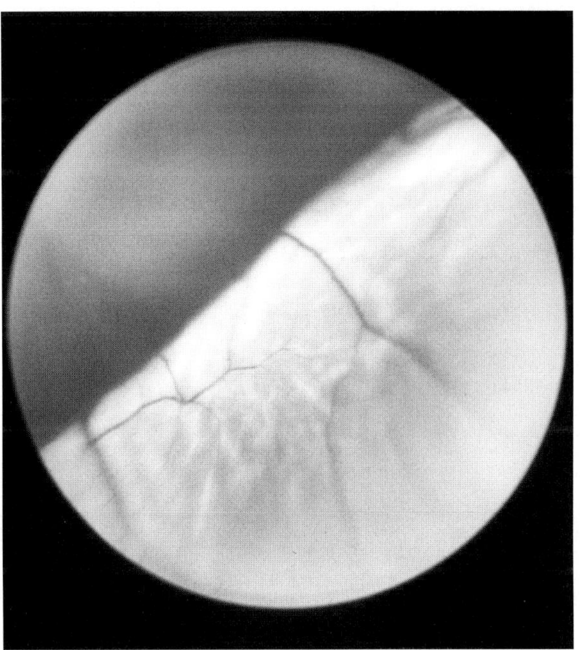

Figure 24C.8 Retinal detachment. The arrows outline the area of detachment as seen on ophthalmoscopic evaluation. (*Source*: From Harwood-Nuss A, Wolfson AB, Linden CH, et al. *The clinical practice of emergency medicine*, 3rd ed. Philadelphia: Lippincott Williams & Wilkins, 2001.)

retinal edema will usually resolve without problem unless it is located in the area of the macula.

Traumatic Optic Neuritis

Neuritis is usually a late development of traumatic eye injuries. A normal initial eye examination is common although decreased visual acuity is often seen. A pale optic nerve develops much later. Treatment includes systemic steroids and ophthalmological consultation. Disc edema usually results in some degree of permanent optic nerve atrophy.

Blow-out Fracture of the Orbit

Blunt trauma to the orbit may increase intraorbital hydrostatic pressure and fracture the weak bone of the orbital floor. The force of the blow may cause herniation of the orbital contents into the maxillary sinus with entrapment of the inferior rectus or inferior oblique muscle of the eye. An athlete with a blow-out fracture will have severe pain in the eye, periorbital edema and hemorrhage, nausea, limited movement of the eye, and diplopia while attempting to look up or down. The infraorbital rim may feel asymmetric on palpation. This is a difficult diagnosis and requires multiple x-ray views, either a Waters' view or a Caldwell's view. CT scanning is often required to make the diagnosis. Immediate surgical intervention is needed if there is a large fracture or severe muscle imbalance. Surgery may be delayed 10 to 14 days for less serious conditions. The eye should always be shielded and immediately evaluated by an ophthalmologist.

Conjunctivitis

Dust and dirt from playing surfaces may irritate an athlete's eyes. If the conjunctiva becomes inflamed, the physician should look for a corneal abrasion or foreign body. Infectious conjunctivitis may be caused by bacterial or viral infections. Allergic conjunctivitis and chemical irritations from smog, hairsprays, and deodorants should be considered in the differential diagnosis. Use of ophthalmic steroid solutions should be reserved for chemical or allergic conjunctivitis.

SECTION D
EARS

INJURIES/ILLNESSES OF THE EXTERNAL EAR

Important structures of the ear and their location are the pinna, tympanic membrane, ear ossicles, eustachian tube, and auditory nerve. Note that the middle ear is air filled and normally connects with the throat through the eustachian tube. See Figure 24D.1 for details.

Auricular Hematoma (Wrestler's Ear, Cauliflower Ear)

This injury is not seen in many athletes except boxers, rugby players, and wrestlers. Many wrestlers suffer ear contusions that can lead to chronic fibrous thickening called

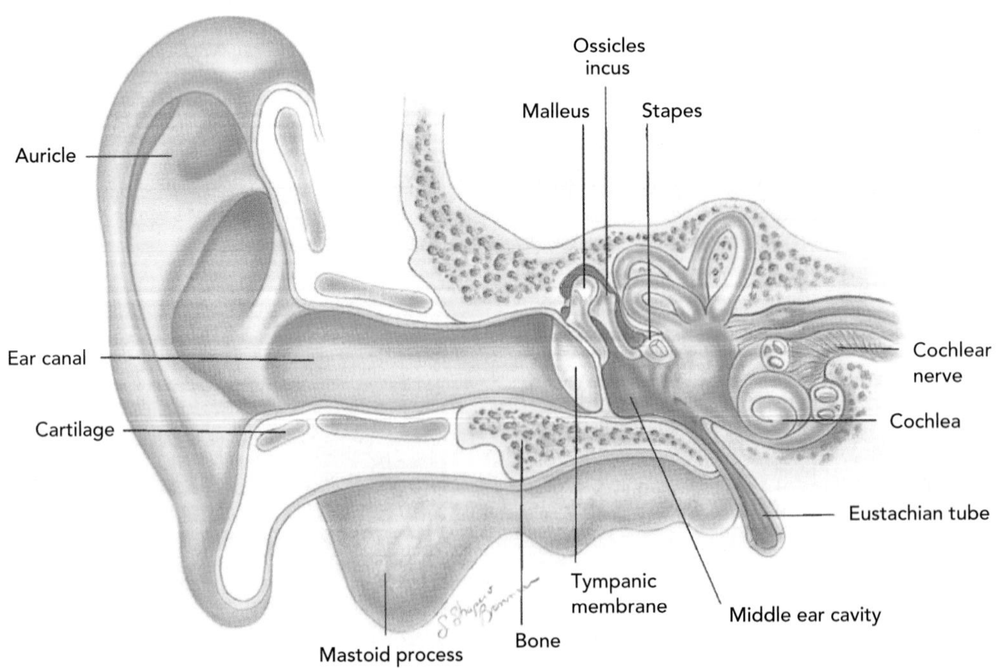

Figure 24D.1 Anatomy of the ear. (*Source*: From Bickley LS, Szilagyi P. *Bates' guide to physical examination and history taking*, 8th ed. Philadelphia: Lippincott Williams & Wilkins, 2003.)

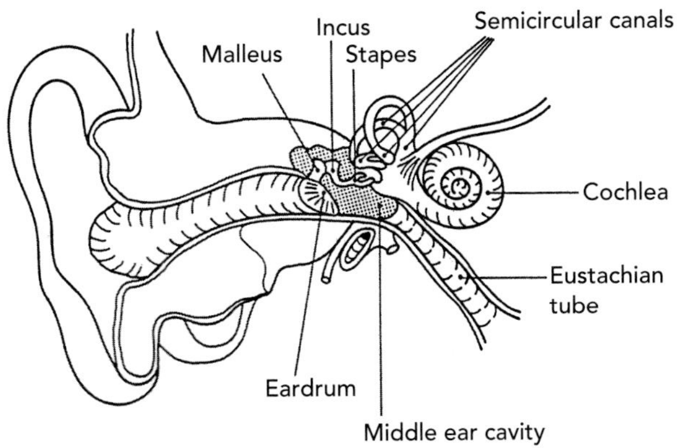

Figure 24D.2 External ear.

cauliflower ear (see Figure 24D.2). It is usually caused by repeated rubbing of the athlete's ear (friction) or by absorbing repetitive blows, both causing leakage of blood between the skin and perichondrium. The ear initially becomes swollen and painful, and a well-defined hematoma develops in the helix fossa within hours. If not treated initially, the ear develops the classic deformed, cauliflower-like appearance owing to chronic scarring after several weeks.

Initial treatment consists of the application of cold compressive dressings. Any hemorrhage present between the perichondrium and cartilage should be aspirated under sterile conditions. Failure to do so could lead to infection, chronic chondritis and collapse of the cartilage. After aspiration, the ear is compressed with a collodion pack, plaster of Paris cast, silicone mold, or a sterile button sutured through the ear. The collodion pack is made by layering cotton balls or strips of gauze soaked in flexible collodion over the affected ear and wrapping it with sterile gauze.

The ear is checked after 24 hours for reaccumulation of fluid, (which may require additional aspiration) and is then repacked. This treatment is continued as long as necessary (usually 3 days). Chronic deformity can be definitively repaired by plastic surgery but this is best done at the end of an athlete's sports career.

To prevent ear contusions and their complications, all wrestlers, rugby players, and amateur boxers should wear ear protectors during practices and matches. The headgear must be properly fitted and worn or it will be of little protection (see Figure 24D.3).

Ear Laceration

An ear laceration is usually secondary to injury from a sharp instrument, although avulsion injuries can occur. Partial avulsion or tearing away of the pinna is most common in the latter of these injuries. Avulsion injuries occur when the ear is forcibly pulled forward and the skin fold between the ear and the scalp is split. This injury could be missed when the ear falls back into its normal position unless the examination is careful. Untreated, this could lead to contamination and infection of the wound. Treatment consists of careful cleansing and suturing, paying attention to pertinent anatomical landmarks, especially if

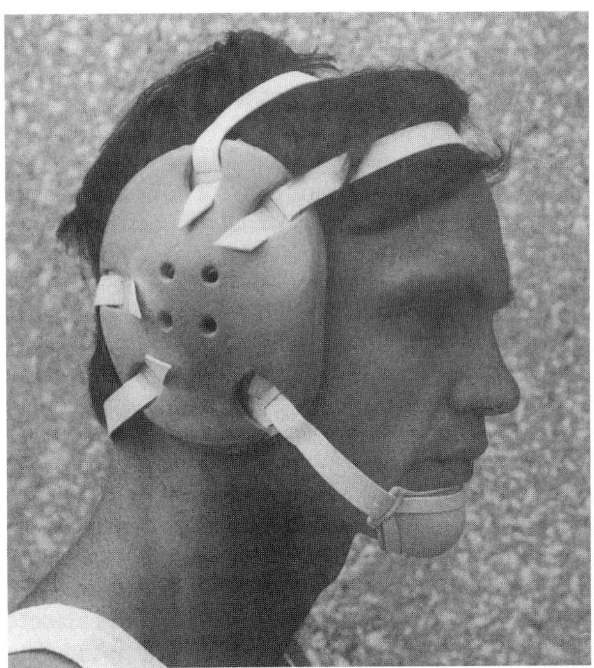

Figure 24D.3 Ear protector.

the auricular cartilage is torn. Use a lidocaine solution *without* epinephrine for anesthesia to avoid ischemia. Any cartilage tears should be repaired with an absorbable suture, taking care to realign to normal anatomy. When repairing the overlying skin take deep bites to include the skin and perichondrium in a single bite using nonabsorbable suture material. Meticulous closure is important to minimize scarring and to prevent chondritis. Consider prophylactic antibiotics and tetanus prophylaxis.

Otitis Externa (Swimmer's Ear)

By definition, otitis externa is an acute bacterial infection of the auditory canal caused predominantly by *Pseudomonas aeruginosa* and occasionally *Escherichia. coli, Proteus, Staphylococcus aureus*, or fungi *(Candida* or *Aspergillus)* (28). When the ear canal is exposed to water over time, the protective effect of the normally present cerumen is lost. The skin becomes irritated and itchy. If the athlete scratches it, the canal's epithelium is disrupted. The normal epithelium produces protective substances capable of inhibiting bacterial growth. When it is damaged, infection can occur and may spread to the middle ear, mastoid, or brain if not property treated. The external canal is swollen and tender and usually has a visible discharge when present. Cultures of the discharge should be obtained to ensure proper treatment.

Treatment of otitis externa involves reacidifying the ear with an acetic solution (1 tablespoon vinegar in 1 pint water). Antibiotic and cortisone combinations are useful after all debris is removed from the canal (polymyxin, neomycin, and hydrocortisone q.i.d.). An ear wick soaked in Burrow's solution (aluminum acetate) can be applied every 2 hours. Otitis externa can be prevented if the swimmer removes trapped water by vigorously shaking the head while it is tilted to one side, drying the ears by fanning or blowing dry with a hair dryer or by instilling four drops of acetic or boric acid solution to dry the canals before and after swimming. The use of pure vinegar, cotton tip applicators, and earplugs should be discouraged as they may aggravate the problem (29). Cases of otitis externa that are resistant to conservative measures will require the use of topical and/or oral antibiotics (dicloxacillin 500 mg PO q.i.d.) and possibly an otolaryngology consultation.

INJURIES/ILLNESSES OF THE MIDDLE EAR

Tympanic Membrane Rupture

Tympanic membrane rupture is caused by a blow to the ear or a fall and is common in surfing, water skiing, scuba diving, and water polo. The athlete will notice a "pop," decreased hearing acuity, and perhaps nausea and dizziness secondary to the caloric effect of cold water on the labyrinth. Fracture of the ossicular chain can occur in severe water skiing accidents and require evaluation and possible surgical repair by an otolaryngologist.

The usual treatment of a ruptured tympanic membrane is conservative, evaluating for infection daily until the rupture heals. If an infection occurs, antibiotic therapy is instituted. Some otolaryngologists recommend prophylactic antibiotics and surgical repair of the rupture, but this is usually not necessary. In sports where significant pressure changes occur, such as platform diving, scuba diving, and high altitude mountain climbing, athletes should not return to play until the membrane has healed. Athletes participating in water sports, such as swimming and water polo, should use custom-fabricated earplugs to ensure a dry ear canal. Dry-land athletes may return to play as soon as any vertigo has resolved (30). Using appropriate protective headgear and proper diving techniques can prevent this injury.

Barotrauma

Although divers may encounter serious systemic problems, such as air embolism, pneumothorax, or the "bends," significant barotrauma to the air-filled sinus cavities and especially middle ear is more common. Barotrauma results from inadequate pressure equalization between the middle ear or sinus and the external environment. During compression when the diver descends, continuous swallowing or nose plugging with a nasal Valsalva is necessary to keep the eustachian tube open.

Ear or sinus squeeze develops as pressure differentials cause localized inflammation and swelling and prevent further air pressure equalization. Eventually, bleeding may occur in the middle ear from blood vessel rupture in the tympanic membrane or round window. The diver notices the sensation of ear blockage; then as the descent continues, ear pain, conductive hearing loss, tinnitus, vertigo, and sometimes blood-tinged sputum.

Inexperienced divers may not be able to equalize pressure adequately, especially if they are still learning appropriate techniques. Because the greatest pressure changes are seen within the first 15 ft below the surface, barotrauma can occur even during shallow dives. Respiratory allergies, infection, rhinitis, large adenoids, or congenital obstruction of the eustachian tube may hamper a diver's ability to equalize pressure easily.

Treatment of barotrauma without perforation of the eardrum includes the use of systemic and nasal decongestants, systemic antibiotics, analgesics when necessary, and avoidance of further diving until resolution. Perforation of the eardrum may require referral to an otolaryngologist. Divers should be cautioned about using antihistamines that can cause drowsiness when diving because of the potentiating effect diving has on these drugs.

Prevention of ear squeeze and perforation is accomplished by the following:

- Removing impacted cerumen
- Using air-pressure equalization techniques frequently on descent
- Avoiding earplugs
- Not diving during acute sinusitis or seasonal allergy flare-ups.

Otosclerosis (Hearing Loss)

Otosclerosis is common in marksmen or sports officials who use starting guns. Repetitive noise from firearm explosions is usually worse in the ear closest to the gun. One hundred and fifty decibels and higher is the most damaging to the ear. Most weapons easily exceed this limit. The patient usually presents with a sensorineural hearing loss on audiogram with a characteristic "notching pattern" at high frequencies (usually between 2,000–4,000 Hz). Prevention of otosclerosis involves modification of the gun barrel, shooting on open terrain, and wearing ear protection (31,32).

Otitis Media and its Complications

Otitis media and its complications are handled as in the general population, with the same differential, complications, and treatment. Because of the risk of rupture, however, diving below 4 ft should be avoided until normal tympanic membrane mobility returns. Air travel should also be avoided until normal tympanic function returns. Be aware that some decongestants are banned by sports governing bodies.

SECTION E
NOSE

HEMATOMAS, CONTUSIONS AND ABRASIONS

Hematomas must be distinguished from simple ecchymosis and swelling due to contusions. Simple contusions are treated with ice and analgesics as needed. Most abrasions are superficial, result from friction, and are easily treated by cleansing with soap and water and using topical antibiotic ointments. Full thickness skin loss, however, requires skin grafting, usually with postauricular skin. All foreign material are cleansed from the skin, removing loose foreign bodies with a brush. Athletes may resume normal activities after the abrasion is appropriately dressed. Any secondary bacterial infection should be treated aggressively.

Septal Hematoma

A septal hematoma produces a characteristic bluish bulge on the septum. The mucoperichondrium may dissect off the underlying cartilaginous septum as a result of the hematoma and lead to resorption of the cartilage and loss of tip support. Because of this, incision, drainage, and nasal packing should be performed without delay. In some cases, cartilage is laid down as in the cauliflower ear, producing a mass that obstructs the airway. Formation of a septal abscess is also possible. The examiner should always check for evidence of significant head trauma or leakage of CSF with these injuries.

Lacerations

Lacerations are the most common facial injury (33) although nasal lacerations are relatively rare. Most should be cleansed and repaired with proper plastic technique within 24 hours. Anesthetize with 1% lidocaine without epinephrine to avoid ischemia. Lacerations that extend to or through the nasal cartilage require proper layer-by-layer closure. All cartilaginous lacerations should be meticulously reapproximated and given prophylactic antibiotics. All avulsed tissues should be saved for definitive repair. In complex lacerations and those needing skin grafting, referral may be necessary.

Nasal Fracture

Nasal fractures are the most frequent facial fracture, although they often do not receive proper attention (34). The patient may hear or feel a crack at the time of injury. Profuse epistaxis and a deformity are usually obvious on examination. Diagnosis is made by a careful history and examination of the nose.

The nose should be examined as soon as possible, before major swelling develops. The examiner should palpate the nasal area between the fingers while assessing for crepitation. Evaluate for depression of the nasal dorsum and deviation of the nasal septum. Tenderness and ecchymosis without crepitation suggest a soft tissue injury without fracture. The nose should be examined internally after suctioning clots. It may be helpful to use a vasoconstrictor medication to improve visualization of the nasal passage. Examine the nasal septum closely for development of a hematoma, which may cause obstruction (see preceding text).

Lateral and oblique radiographs of the nasal bones are usually not indicated to confirm a fracture but may show other facial bone fractures. These radiographs may be falsely negative, 60% of the time. An exaggerated Waters' view is necessary to properly evaluate the nasal arch. A CT scan may be needed for complex fractures or for a definitive diagnosis. The type and extent of the fracture is dependent upon the force and direction of the blow. Rule out orbital globe fractures if the history or examination is consistent with or equivocal to this injury.

The timing of nasal fracture reduction, when necessary, is controversial. It can be done under local or general anesthesia after the swelling has subsided, usually within 4 days for children and 10 to 12 days for adults. Intranasal packing and plaster splinting are usually necessary for injuries involving comminuted fractures or septal hematomas, but simpler fractures may be treated without these procedures. If there is displacement of the nose but minimal swelling, the injury may be splinted and referred to an ear, nose, and throat (ENT) specialist for closed reduction. When the swelling is severe, ice should be applied to the nose frequently and the injury re-evaluated in 2 to 3 days, at which time definitive treatment is usually administered. Delaying diagnosis of a nasal fracture over 2 weeks may make a closed reduction impossible. All nasal fractures should be managed to restore normal appearance and prevent problems associated with a deviated nasal septum or obstructed eustachian tube.

An athlete should not participate in contact sports for at least 1 week after a nasal fracture of any consequence. Before he/she returns, check that no significant swelling or bleeding recurs and that the fracture is stable and does not require external support. The athlete can be fitted with a protective device over the nose so that sports can be continued while the injury heals completely. The devise is usually required for at least 4 weeks after the fracture. Chronic deformity secondary to a nasal fracture may require reconstruction by an otolaryngologist.

Epistaxis

Profuse bleeding from the nose is common because of the abundant blood supply to nasal mucosa. Fortunately, most instances of bleeding are readily controlled. Bleeding usually originates from the Kiesselbach's plexus located on the anterior nasal septum. Generally, the younger the patient, the more anterior the bleeding site. Most nosebleeds come from septal blood vessels, but a significant nosebleed can be caused by injury to the anterior ethmoidal artery. Posterior epistaxis can be an ENT emergency. Epistaxis commonly presents as nasal hemorrhage alone, but if it is severe and uncontrolled it could lead to syncope, anemia, aspiration, and death.

Management of epistaxis depends on the type of injury, the sport involved, and whether bleeding occurs spontaneously or after physical contact. Prophylaxis is the best approach. Athletes who have recurrent nasal hemorrhage should coat each side of Kiesselbach's area with petroleum jelly at least twice a day. These precautions are also appropriate for skiers at high altitudes and for boxers or hockey players before practice or competition. The physician may use electrical or chemical cautery to help control epistaxis. Cautery should be used conservatively to avoid perforating the septum, especially if performed repeatedly.

If epistaxis occurs suddenly during an athletic event, the player should sit forward with his head down and gently blow one nostril at a time. This helps remove clots and allows the vessels to contract, retract, and facilitate stasis. The nose should then be gently pinched and the nosebleed usually stops quickly. The player or athlete can return to activity if there is no further bleeding.

When there is an associated fracture that prevents the patient from applying pressure to the nose, ice applied to the back of the neck will cause reflex vasoconstriction. Packing both sides of the nose also helps. Tampons cut to fit and with the wick intact, make excellent packing for acute epistaxis. They can also be soaked in neosynephrine to facilitate vasoconstriction.

If these simple measures are unsuccessful in controlling nosebleeds, the athlete should be seen at a medical office or hospital where the nose can be properly evaluated and packed if necessary. Anterior packs made of Iodoform or thrombin soaked gauze should be layered into the nose in an accordion-like manner, using 12 to 20 ft of gauze. Anterior–posterior nasal packs are used for severe epistaxis. This pack consists of a conventional tampon or the less reliable balloon or Foley catheter (35). Consultation with an otolaryngologist should be obtained immediately.

Patients with anterior nosebleeds that are controlled by the procedures mentioned in the preceding text may return to activity if there is no further bleeding. Nasal packing should be left in place for up to 3 to 5 days. Longer periods increase the risk of toxic shock syndrome and meningitis by way of the cribiform plate. All nasal packs should be removed carefully and prophylactic oral antibiotics should be administered. Athletes should be instructed to avoid chronic use of nasal decongestants that cause dryness and rebound swelling of the nasal mucosa, which increase the potential of epistaxis.

SECTION F
MOUTH INJURIES IN SPORTS

PERSPECTIVE

Injuries to the mouth are usually considered less serious than those to other regions, but serious morbidity does occur on rare occasions. Before face and mouth guards were introduced, oral injuries constituted 50% of all football injuries; and each player had a 10% chance of sustaining an oral injury during any playing season (36). The injury rate for basketball, without mouth guards, was equal to the rate in mouth-guarded football players. More recent pediatric data suggests a significantly lower rate at 0.39% of all athletic injuries. Boys soccer accounted for the highest percentage, 23%, followed by baseball and wrestling at 14%, football at 12%, boys basketball at 11%, girls soccer and softball at 5%, and girls basketball at 4% (37).

TOOTH INJURIES

A fractured tooth is a common sports injury and has less chance of healing normally than almost any other mouth injury. Most physicians see little importance in evaluating an injured baby tooth because it will eventually be replaced by a permanent tooth. However, the roots of the front teeth (most often injured) are not completely formed until age 12. An injury before this age can damage the root and prevent normal root and permanent tooth development.

The examiner should try to determine how the athlete was injured and examine for foreign and loose bodies, especially if there is a laceration of the mouth or lips. Irrigate the area with warm saline, using sterile swabs soaked in a solution of 2% iodine or benzalkonium chloride (Zephiran) 1:10,000 to debride the injured lip.

A broken tooth may or may not need emergency treatment. If the pulp is bleeding, the nerve may be exposed and immediate dental evaluation may be necessary. Avoid extremes of temperature (hot or cold drinks) and biting down. Make a temporary filling by covering a fractured tooth with calcium hydroxide [$Ca(OH)_2$] or Ravit, a temporary filling material. Early treatment of a pulp injury is preferable, especially in children. Apply external ice packs to control swelling and reduce bleeding. All imbedded teeth require referral to a dentist or an oral surgeon. Do not attempt to bring the tooth down into place. The tooth socket usually has been spread out during injury and grasping the imbedded tooth may dislodge it completely. Always check the teeth when a patient has a lip laceration.

Eighty-five to 90% of loose teeth can be saved with proper treatment and repositioning. There is a 35% to 40% chance of saving a tooth that is knocked out. Handle it by the crown only, place it in warm saline and have the patient see a dentist immediately. Oil of clove (Eugenol) may provide initial pain relief while in transit. Apply an ice pack to the face and have the athlete hold the tooth in its socket with his fingers or by closing his mouth. The athlete should have x-rays taken to rule out a mandibular or alveolar fracture after a severe mouth injury. Fracture of the mandibular condyle can affect the growth center in children. Obviously, loose fillings require the timely attention of a dentist.

LACERATION OF THE TONGUE

All tongue lacerations require proper evaluation and examination for foreign bodies that may be embedded in the tissues. Copious lavage with benzalkonium is suggested. Many tongue lacerations do not require repair if they are not deeper than 0.5 cm or if there is no gaping when the tongue is at rest. Because the tissue of the tongue is very soft, it is necessary to take a bigger bite when suturing and only leave the sutures in place for 2 or 3 days.

A severely bleeding tongue should be sutured after blocking the lingual nerve distal to the second or third molar, and approximately 0.5 in. above the plane of the molar. Use a 3-0 or 4-0 absorbable suture. Use crushed ice and a solution of one part hydrogen peroxide (H_2O_2) to three parts water or Amosan for 48 hours after repair for comfort and oral hygiene. The repair of all "through and through" lingual lacerations should be left to an oral surgeon. All lip lacerations should be carefully repaired, paying close attention to the proper alignment of the frenulum and underlying muscles.

JAW AND TEMPOROMANDIBULAR JOINT PROBLEMS

A temporomandibular joint (TMJ) injury or fracture/dislocation to the jaw may occur with any serious mouth injury. Refer these injuries to an oral surgeon. Taking office x-rays before referral is unnecessary and time consuming. The clinical diagnosis is straightforward. Ask the patient if he can open and close his jaw and if his teeth meet the way they did before injury. If not, you can be 95% certain that the jaw is fractured and/or dislocated (especially if the jaw is painful and cannot be closed). A fractured tooth is often associated with a TMJ dislocation. If the athlete has swelling of the cheek but no malocclusion, check for a fracture of the zygomatic arch. Check for numbness of the skin around the mouth, which would indicate injury to the infraorbital nerve.

TMJ sprains should be differentiated from a mandibular fracture, as the symptoms are similar. X-ray all questionable TMJ injuries to rule out a mandibular fracture. TMJ dysfunction is found by placing the index and middle fingers over the TMJ and feeling for irregular movement or subluxation while the patient opens and closes his mouth. Listen with a stethoscope for clicking or crepitation in the TMJ during range of motion. Also, test for spasm of the pterygoid muscles by palpating posterior to the affected side. This will produce exquisite pain if spasm is present. Arthrography, CT scan, or MRI of the TMJ may aid in the diagnosis. If the patient has TMJ dysfunction, a referral may be necessary.

COMMON ORAL CONDITIONS

Abscessed Tooth

A periapical abscess usually presents with sensitivity to hot liquids. Analgesics, such as aspirin, acetaminophen, ibuprofen or codeine may be necessary for adequate pain relief. Place the athlete on antibiotics, such as penicillin or erythromycin, for 5 to 6 days. Oral gargles of a hydrogen peroxide solution (one part H_2O_2 to three parts H_2O) may be helpful. Referral to an oral surgeon is usually necessary.

Wisdom Tooth Eruption

Treatment consists of gargling with a hydrogen peroxide solution (one part H_2O_2 to three parts H_2O) every 2 hours and an anti-inflammatory for pain. If pain lasts more than 24 hours, place the athlete on antibiotics (clindamycin 300 mg PO b.i.d. or amoxicillin clavulanate 875/125 mg PO b.i.d.). Dental referral may be necessary in more difficult cases.

Vincent's Stomatitis

This condition presents as red, painful gums with hemorrhages. Use of a hydrogen peroxide solution and Vitamin B complex appears helpful. Slowly increase the athlete's intraoral care (teeth brushing, flossing). If there is no improvement within 24 hours, start antibiotics (clindamycin 300 mg PO b.i.d. or amoxicillin clavulanate 875/125 mg PO b.i.d.).

PREVENTION: MOUTH PROTECTORS

Faceguards were first adopted for football during the early 1950s, with mouth guard use becoming mandatory in 1962 at the high school level and in 1973 for college athletes. Facemasks and mouth guards have eliminated most serious mouth injuries. Mouth guards were mandated for use in amateur ice hockey during the 1977 to 1978 season but the rule is not uniformly enforced. In the United States children under age 13 are not required to wear mouth guards, although there is a requirement for facemasks.

Mouth guards not only reduce the incidence of injury to the mouth, teeth, and lips but they are touted to help decrease concussions by absorbing the forces of a blow to the chin. However, evidence to this effect is lacking (38). All athletes, including youngsters, should wear acceptable mouth guards. This is also important during informal contact/collision sporting activities, where most mouth injuries occur in sports.

The three types of mouth protectors available in order of athlete preference are custom-made, mouth-formed, and stock-type. Custom-made mouth guards require a dental impression and are more expensive (see Figure 24F.1). Mouth-formed guards are bought off the shelf, boiled and then placed in the mouth for an individual fit. The stock-type rubber mouth guard fits poorly and is not as effective as the other types.

A properly fitted mouth guard is comfortable and does not interfere with breathing or speech. All mouth guards should be checked periodically for wear and replaced

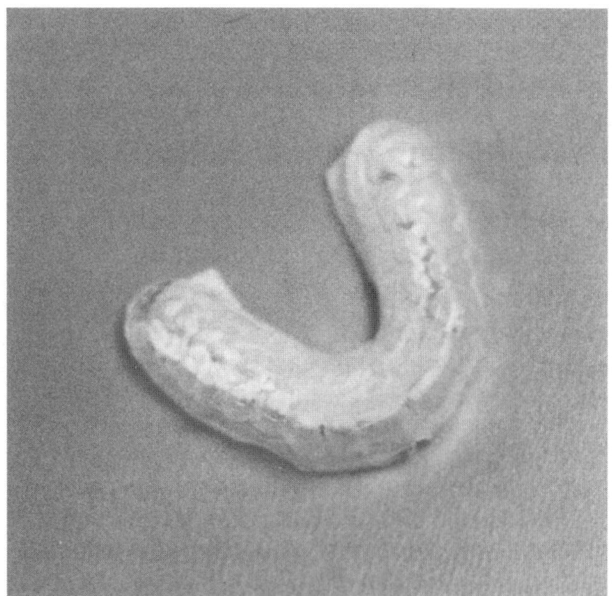

Figure 24F.1 Latex mouthguard.

if necessary. Be wary of the athlete who whittles the mouthpiece down to cover only the front teeth. Not only does this defeat the purpose of the guard, but it is now an aspiration risk as well.

SECTION G

THROAT INJURIES AND ILLNESSES

EPIDEMIOLOGY

Airway compromise secondary to laryngotracheal trauma ranks second only to intracranial injuries as the most common cause of death following head and neck trauma. A direct blow in football or other contact sports (boxing, karate, basketball) or from projectiles (ice hockey, baseball, lacrosse, and field hockey) can cause injury to the larynx. Occasionally trail bike riders or snowmobilers strike wires, ropes, or chains and sustain laryngeal injury. Any blow to the anterior neck can cause significant airway obstruction owing to glottic edema, vocal cord disarticulation, hemorrhage, laryngospasm, or a crushed larynx or trachea. Symptoms of airway obstruction may be insidious, therefore close monitoring of patients with anterior neck injuries is imperative.

LARYNGOTRACHEAL INJURY

A blow to the anterior neck may be serious and potentially life threatening. The athlete usually protects this area by dropping his chin before an impending blow. The structures most likely to be damaged are the larynx and trachea. Extreme agitation, dyspnea, and possible respiratory compromise are common after laryngeal injury. Injuries to the cartilaginous structures, connecting muscle and soft tissue, or the supporting nervous and vascular system may occur individually or in combination.

Cartilaginous fracture most often occurs to the thyroid and cricoid cartilages (see Figure 24G.1). Although hyoid, epiglottic, and tracheal rings can break, it is unlikely because these structures are very mobile. Cartilaginous fracture may result in a visible or palpable flattening of the laryngeal contour (Adam's apple). Thyroid cartilage fractures often occur in the region of the attachment of the two vocal cords. Dislocation of the arytenoids or corniculates may result in hoarseness or aphonia.

The athlete is initially speechless, struggles to breathe, and has a feeling of impending doom. Acute injury may cause swelling and spasm of the larynx, and the thyroid cartilage, hyoid bone, or trachea may be contused or fractured. Laryngeal spasm usually resolves quickly and the athlete can then breathe easier. The athlete may have stridorous breathing, dyspnea, and cyanosis if the airway is threatened. Crepitation may be noted on palpation of the anterior neck. Cough, hemoptosis, or hematemesis may occur with a mucosal tear of the larynx.

More severe cases present with hematoma either intrinsic to the larynx or in the muscles of the neck. This may lead to severe respiratory stridor, or complete airway obstruction and constitutes an obvious medical emergency. The possibility of a concomitant vertebral fracture with severe neck injuries must always be kept in mind. Fortunately, sports-related anterior neck injuries involve less force and cause cervical vertebral fractures less often than those from automobile crashes. If the athlete is unconscious, the injury should be managed as if a cervical fracture is present. The airway should be maintained with as little extension of the neck as possible.

Laryngeal trauma is not always obvious in the patient who has an uncompromised airway. Physical signs and symptoms are not highly correlated with the ultimate severity of the injury. An extensive injury may have little initial evidence of airway obstruction but can produce significant airway compromise as edema and hematoma formation progress. Consequently, indirect laryngoscopy and CT scanning should be considered on every patient with severe anterior neck trauma and ENT consultation sought.

The first consideration of treatment is ensuring the adequacy of the airway. If the patient does not have obvious signs of cartilaginous fracture, discontinuity of the airway, or vertebral trauma, reassure the patient and position the head in a chin-up position to straighten the airway. If the athlete's breathing is noisy but he/she can inflate the chest well, there is time to get the player to a hospital for proper examination and treatment. If the athlete's breathing is ineffective or if increasing subcutaneous emphysema confirms discontinuity of the airway, cardiopulmonary

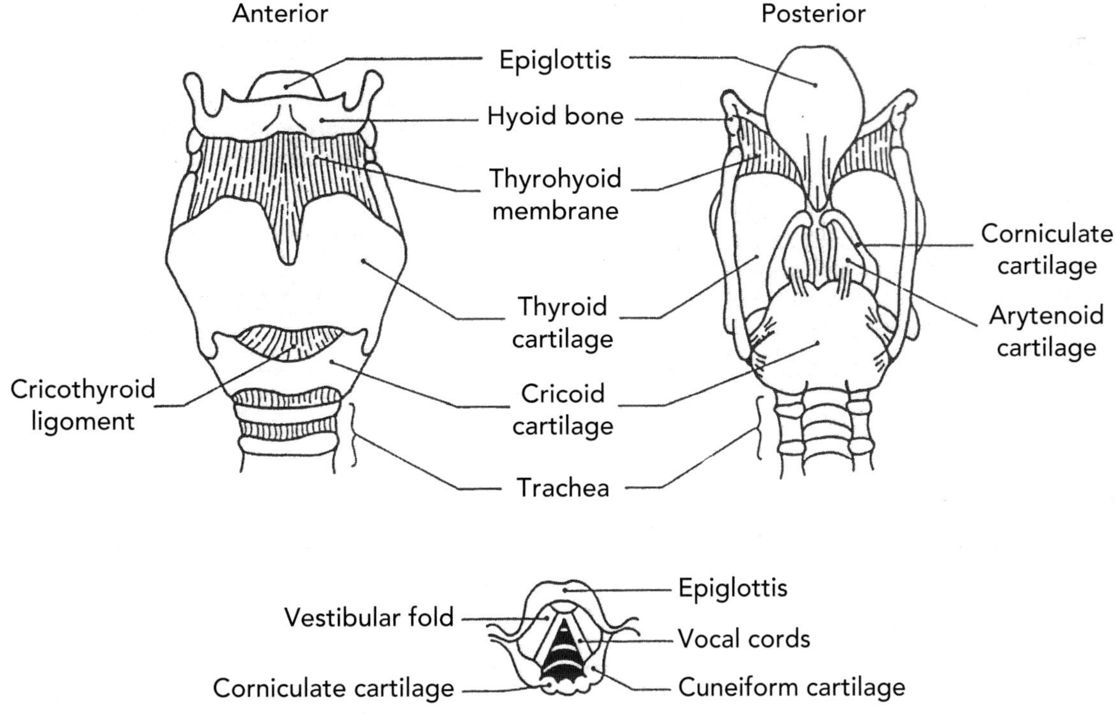

Figure 24G.1 Anatomy of the laryngeal area.

resuscitation (CPR) is instituted and an artificial airway must be established immediately.

Oral airways and oral screws are useless because the obstruction is below the oral cavity. An inexperienced examiner should not attempt to intubate an agitated athlete lying on the ice or playing field. An orderly tracheostomy, usually lower than the second tracheal ring, is most desirable. Fortunately, most laryngeal fractures involve the thyroid cartilage so placing an airway into the cricothyroid membrane alleviates most of the obstruction. Cricothyrotomy is a simpler, safer, and faster alternative for the team physician at the scene of the injury. It can be performed before a more permanent tracheostomy is done in the operating room or emergency room. The cricothyroid airway should be properly secured and the patient moved to the emergency room. Supplemental oxygen and assisted ventilation may be needed.

A player with a neck injury and any degree of airway obstruction should be sent to the nearest hospital for indirect laryngoscopy as soon as possible. The most common finding on laryngoscopy is some degree of laryngeal edema, with or without submucosal hemorrhage. Because the edema is likely to progress for 12 to 24 hours, the athlete should be kept under close observation in the hospital until the airway returns to normal. Most injuries do not require surgical intervention and subside with rest, steam, and reassurance. Sedatives are contraindicated because of their respiratory depression. Most athletes can leave the hospital within a few days.

The threat of a severe anterior neck injury is highest to baseball catchers and hockey goalies. Prevention is best accomplished by using protective headgear with a throat flap. An inexpensive flap can be made by attaching the spine pad from a football girdle to the catcher's mask with leather lacing (39). Many commercially available throat protectors are also available for a wide variety of sports.

LARYNGOSPASM

Laryngeal spasm is another type of upper airway obstruction resulting from anterior neck trauma. Closure of the larynx is caused by a spasm of the adductor muscle of the true vocal cords and pressing of the pre-epiglottic muscles against the upper surface of the false vocal cords. The athlete becomes agitated, often panic stricken, and may become cyanotic. Persistent laryngospasm may cause loss of consciousness. The athlete usually is aphonic and unable to cough. Contours of the thyroid and cricoid cartilages are normal and there is no palpable subcutaneous emphysema.

To treat laryngospasm, move the chin forward and place strong anterior pressure behind the angle of the jaw. This forward movement is transmitted to the hyoid bone, hypoepiglottis, and periglottis, which pulls these structures from the false cords and reopens the laryngeal passage. Spasm will begin to decrease within 45 to 60 seconds and a loud inspiratory crowing sound will be heard. Give the patient oxygen by venti-mask. Suctioning of the oropharynx should be avoided to prevent further laryngeal spasm.

After recovery, the athlete should be referred for immediate laryngoscopy to rule out other injuries. Observation for the development of subsequent edema or hematoma formation may be indicated. If dyspnea persists, voice rest and thorough evaluation of the neck and larynx by a specialist is indicated. Radiographs of the anterior neck should be obtained, with soft tissue and lateral views. If severe injury is suspected, hospitalize the patient for immediate laryngoscopy.

Following injury to the neck, the athlete with laryngospasm should be placed at bed rest with local ice application to the neck. Recovery may be complete in minutes but the athlete should be re-evaluated frequently. If injury is more severe, observe the athlete for subsequent development of a hematoma. If present, the athlete should be managed by the otolaryngologist.

RECURRENT TONSILLITIS

Upper respiratory infections and their complications are the most common illnesses in athletes of all ages. Proper evaluation should be performed, along with screening for group A beta-hemolytic streptococcus. Athletes with recurrent episodes of tonsillitis or otitis media should be referred to an otolaryngologist for possible tonsillectomy. Use of appropriate antibiotics for bacterial tonsillitis is advisable.

SECTION H
CERVICAL SPINE

The neck is not injured as often as some joints, but neck injuries can be associated with high rates of mortality and morbidity. It is estimated that approximately 114,000 neck injuries of all severities occur in football each year, 19,000 in soccer, and 5,000 in ice hockey (40). Water sports and football have the highest incidents of catastrophic neck injury. Rugby, wrestling, gymnastics, and competitive swimming also have significant rates of cervical spine injury. The frequency of cervical injuries is inversely proportionate to their severity.

Until recently, there were almost no comprehensive guidelines that set appropriate criteria for a safe return to contact sports after an injury to the cervical spine. The most recent guidelines have been outlined by Cantu (41).

In this section, a brief description of catastrophic neck injuries, including the mechanism of injury, role of equipment, impact of rule changes, and the possibility of injury prevention will be presented.

EPIDEMIOLOGY IN SPECIFIC SPORTS

The development of better protective football helmets, including the addition of the facemask, has led to a decrease in serious facial and intracranial injuries. The false security of the protective equipment thought to exist by some may have led to the use of the head and helmet as a blocking aid (spearing or head tackling). This practice may have been responsible for the significant increase in catastrophic head and neck injuries seen in football in the 1970s. Rule changes were made in 1976 outlawing spearing and head tackling, which is thought to be responsible for the decreased injury rate in the following years (see Table 24H.1) (42).

Since 1976 serious cervical injuries in hockey saw a dramatic increase (see Table 24H.2). All injuries studied involved axial loading of the cervical spine. A C5-6 fracture dislocation was the most common site of injury. Most of these athletes were wearing helmets with a facemask at the time of injury. The most common mechanism of injury was a push or check from behind causing the player to strike the boards with the crown of his helmet (43). Recent rule changes and increased enforcement will likely resolve this trend.

In wrestling, from 1976 to 1984, neck injuries were found to represent 12% of all injuries. Sprains/strain and brachial plexus injuries were by far the most common (87%). Wrestlers had a 20% chance of neck injury in a

TABLE 24H.1
SERIOUS CERVICAL SPINE INJURIES IN FOOTBALL

	1959–1963	1971–1975	1976[a]	1977	1978	1979	1980	1981	1982	1983	1984
C-spine fracture, dislocation, subluxation	56 (1.36)	259 (4.14)	110	96	51	51	62	67	57	69	42
permanent guard	30 (.73)	99 (1.58)	34	18	16	3	16	11	10	11	5

() = rate per 100,000 participants
[a]rate change penalizing spearing 1976
Source: From Torg JS, Vegso JJ, Sennett B. The national football head and neck injury registry: 14-year old report on cervical quadriplegia (1971–1984). *Clin Sports Med* 1987;6(1):67–72.

TABLE 24H.2
SERIOUS CERVICAL SPINE INJURIES IN HOCKEY

	1966	1976	1976–79	1980	1981	1982	1983	1984
Cervical spine dislocation, fracture with and without spinal cord injury	1	1	10	7	12	14	16	15

Source: From (Tator, 1987)

given year if they had no prior neck injury, compared with a 50% chance in those with a history of previous injury. Similar statistics seem to exist for other sports. No single mechanism for catastrophic injury in wrestling has been established. The most likely mechanism is throwing an opponent to the mat on the crown of the head (44), a highly illegal move.

Headfirst diving into shallow water (axial compression) is the most common mechanism of neck injury in water sports. Alcohol intake is often a factor in recreational diving injuries. Specific preventive measures for the prevention of recreational injuries to the cervical spine are presented in Table 24H.3:

Most serious cervical injuries resulting from rugby are from the hyperflexion sustained during the collapse of the scrum, the tackle, rucks and mauls. For details on the common mechanisms of injury and recommendations for prevention, refer the article by Scher (44).

TABLE 24H.3
RECOMMENDATIONS OR THE PREVENTION OF RECREATIONAL DIVING INJURIES TO THE SPINE

Do not dive into water that is shallower than twice your height
Do not dive into unfamiliar water
Do not assume that the water is deep enough or obstruction-free because even familiar swimming holes change
Do not dive near dredging or construction work
Do not dive until the area is clear of other swimmers
Do not drink and dive
Do not dive into the ocean surf or from lakefront beaches

Source: From Torg JS. Epidemiology, pathomechanics, and prevention of athletic injuries to the cervical spine. *Med Sci Sports Exerc* 1985;17:295–303; Torg JS, Vegso JJ, O'Neill MJ, et al. The epidemiologic, pathologic, biomechanical, and cinematographic analysis of football-induced cervical spine trauma. *Am J Sports Med* 1990;18:50–57, (42,45).

Methods that may aid in the prevention of catastrophic neck injuries in athletics are presented in Table 24H.4.

ANATOMY

The cervical spine has two main functions: supporting the head and neck while allowing a wide range of motion, and protecting the spinal cord and cervical nerve roots.

The first two cervical vertebrae have a unique structure designed to allow both rotational and flexion/extension movements. The anatomy of the cervical vertebra, discs, nerve roots, and significant ligaments is reviewed in Figure 24H.1. The brachial plexus anatomy and common injuries to this structure are discussed elsewhere in this chapter.

HISTORY AND PHYSICAL EXAMINATION

The proper diagnosis and management of neck injuries calls for knowledge of the mechanism of injury and appropriate

TABLE 24H.4
PREVENTION OF CATASTROPHIC NECK INJURIES IN ATHLETICS

Coaches/players
Awareness of the possibility of injury and avoidance of axial loading
Year round neck conditioning program
Properly fitted equipment
Coaches teaching proper tackling techniques
Sport leagues
Enforcement of current rules
Introduction of new rules as needed
Avoid small rinks (hockey)
Sportsmedicine staff
Promote reporting system for injuries
Research into mechanism of injury

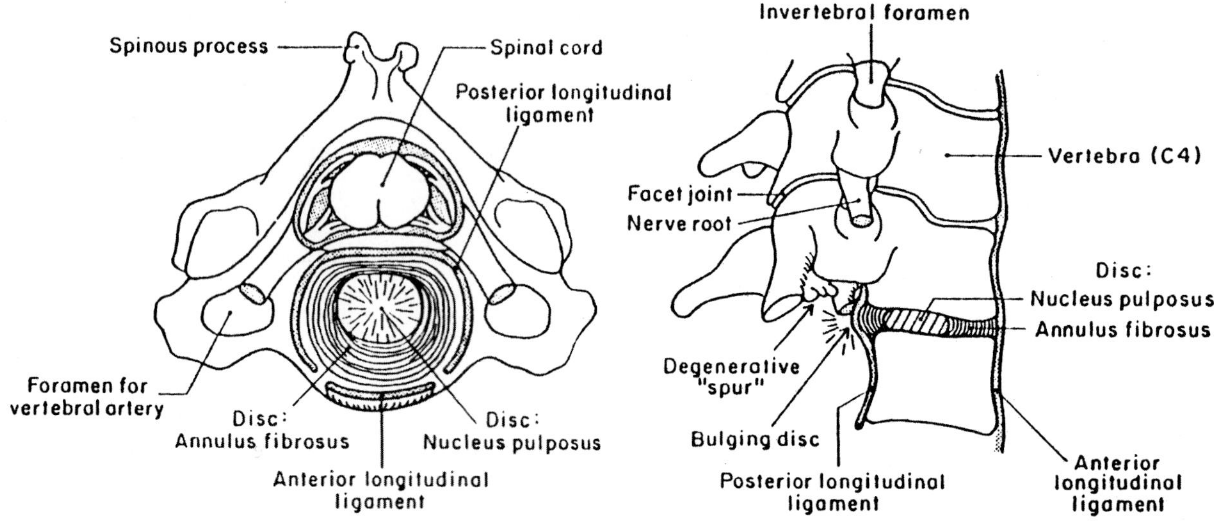

Figure 24H.1 Typical cervical vertebra C-C7.

questioning and physical examination skills. When dealing with a potentially serious cervical injury such as a fracture or dislocation, with or without spinal cord involvement, every precaution should be taken to prevent further injury during the initial evaluation and transportation of the athlete. Of injuries that resulted in permanent damage, up to 50% could be attributed to improper handling of an unstable injury **after** the initial trauma.

If the athlete is unconscious, assume a serious neck injury has occurred (see Table 24H.5). If not, proceed with appropriate questioning and perform the examination outlined in Table 24H.6. A more complete evaluation can be completed on the sideline, in the training room or clinic (see Table 24H.7).

TABLE 24H.5

ASSESSMENT OF THE UNCONSCIOUS ATHLETE

Evaluate airway and, if impaired, stabilize the head and neck and establish the airway by removing the face mask without removing the helmet.

Check pulses and, if absent, begin CPR. Check blood pressure and pupillary reflexes.

Athlete should be removed from field on a spine board using appropriate transportation techniques that stabilize the head and neck. Appropriate radiographs must then be taken.

CPR = Carchiopulmonary resuscitation

COMMON CERVICAL SPINE INJURIES

First and Second Degree Sprains and Strains

First- and second-degree cervical sprains (ligament) and strains (muscle or tendon) are the most common neck injuries. Complete third degree ruptures are rare. A strain results when a force exceeds the strength of the

TABLE 24H.6

ASSESSMENT OF THE CONSCIOUS ATHLETE

Determine the mechanism of injury.

Ask about neck pain; tingling, burning or numbness going down the arms or legs; or problems moving the arms or legs.

Physical examination should include:

1. A-B-C (basic CPR evaluation)
2. Palpation of c-spine for tenderness
3. Perform brief neurologic examination of all extremities.
4. Ask player to perform active range of motion of cervical spine if steps (a-c) are negative

If above history and physical are negative, the player can be allowed to walk off the field of play to complete a more detailed examination If any parts of the history and physical examination are positive, the player should not be allowed to move until the examination is completed. Transport the athelete using appropriate precautions to stabilize head and neck.

CPR = cardopulmonary resuscitation.

TABLE 24H.7
TABLE ASSESSMENT OF THE CERVICAL SPINE IN CLINIC OR TRAINING ROOM

Ask about neck pain; radiation, exacerbating factors
Ask about tingling, numbness or weakness of the extremities.
Palpate directly over c-spine, then along paracervical musculature.
Ask athlete to perform active range of motion including flexion, extension, lateral flexion and rotation. Repeat above against resistance. Brachial plexus symptoms may be elicited by either extreme passive lateral flexion to contralateral side or by active lateral flexion against resistance to ipsilateral side.
Spurling's test should be performed by placing the chin in the supraclavicular fossa and applying axial compression. A positive test reslts when pain radiates to the shoulder or arm, suggestive of nerve root impingement. Varying degrees of neck extension or flexion, while maintaining the chin in the supraclavicular fossa and applying axial compression, will increase the true positive result. In the presence of radicular pain, a distraction test is performed with the patient in the supine position and the examiner placing his hands on the occipital region and under the mandible. If the pain is diminished or relievd by appling traction, the test is positive and reinforces the probability of nerve root impingement.

muscles involved. The most common muscles involved are the trapezius, sternocleidomastoid, erector spinae, scalenus, levator scapulae, and the rhomboids. Forced extension, flexion, rotation, and side bending are common mechanisms of injury. A sprain to the anterior ligaments and capsule of the facet joint of the neck can result from a hyperextension injury, or to the interspinous and supraspinous ligaments from a hyperflexion injury. These injuries are commonly seen in wrestling, hockey, and football.

Neck pain and limited range of motion are the usual presenting complaints. The appearance of symptoms may be delayed in mild to moderate strains, but typically there will be weakness when resistance is applied to the affected muscle. The degree of pain and limitation of range of motion at 24 to 48 hours seems to be a reliable indication of the severity of the injury.

Typically point tenderness to palpation along the involved muscle or ligament, limited range of motion, negative neurological findings (except for tenderness) and a negative axial compression test are seen on initial examination. Movement toward the contralateral direction often produces tenderness. Active contraction toward the ipsilateral side will also cause discomfort.

If there is a history of significant trauma, past history of surgery or significant pathology, radicular symptoms, positive findings from a Spurling's test, midline tenderness, or severe symptoms or physical findings, a plain film evaluation is recommended. This should include at a minimum, AP, lateral, and bilateral oblique films. Odontoid views should be considered. Any abnormality may require further workup. See discussion on Radiologic workup later in this chapter for more details.

Treatment

Treatment may include a brief period of immobilization with a soft collar as needed, and nonsteroidal anti-inflammatory drugs (NSAIDs) or analgesics as needed. Isometric exercises are used as tolerated and proprioceptive neuromuscular facilitation may be utilized for the rehabilitation of strains. Sever sprain/strains may necessitate hospitalization.

Contusion

A contusion is caused by direct trauma to the cervical spine. It may result in a muscular contusion, soft tissue edema, spinous process fracture or injury to the spinal accessory or long thoracic nerve.

The mechanism of injury of the direct trauma includes a punch to the neck, a wayward elbow while rebounding a basketball, a knee during a wrestling match, or a blow from a recklessly handled hockey stick or racquet. The athlete may complain of localized neck pain (may be severe) and have restricted range of motion and weakness.

Physical findings may include localized tenderness, swelling, ecchymosis, restricted range of motion, pain with forward flexion (fractured spinous process), or weakness on shoulder deviation (injury to spinal accessory nerve), winging of scapula (injury to long thoracic nerve). Appropriateness of radiologic workup is similar to sprains and strains as mentioned in the preceding text.

Treatment for a muscle contusion includes ice, protection, stretching, and strengthening. Injury to the spinal accessory nerve may respond to heat, and superficial massage. Recovery for both occurs in days to weeks. Injury to long thoracic nerve may require restriction of activity for the first 2 to 3 weeks. The prognosis is variable; orthopedic referral may be necessary.

Brachial Plexus Neuropraxia and Nerve Root Impingement

Brachial plexus neuropraxia (stinger or burner) is typically caused by forced lateral flexion with resultant contralateral stretching of the cervical nerve roots or upper brachial plexus. A drawing of the pertinent anatomy is provided in Figure 24H.2. Additional mechanisms include a direct blow to the supraclavicular fossa and compression of the cervical

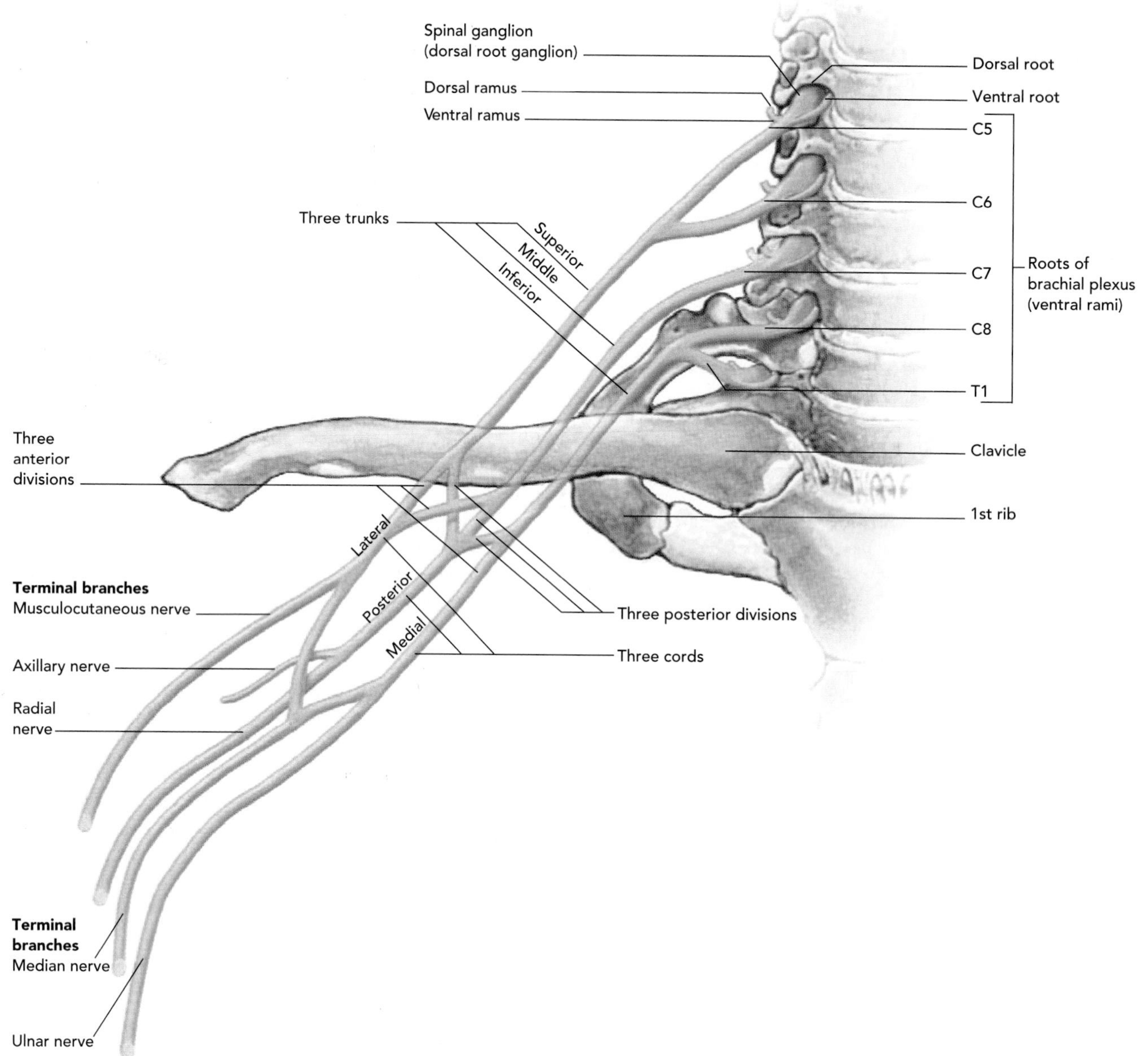

Figure 24H.2 The brachial plexus. Shown are the nerves, trunks, divisions, cords, and branches that make up the brachial plexus. Asset provided by Anatomical Chart Company.

roots when the head is forced toward the side of injury. The latter of these, compression injuries, tends to produce a more serious injury, therefore determining that exact mechanism is very important. Nerve root impingement secondary to compression is usually due to a pinching of the nerve roots on the ipsilateral side of pain typically as they exit the spine. Impingement is usually from a herniated disc or due to degenerative changes (stenosis or osteophytes), but can be from congenital abnormalities of the spine and cord. This injury is often seen in football, hockey, and wrestling.

Clinically, brachial plexus neuropraxia presents with a sharp burning pain in the neck on the opposite side of the forced flexion. It may radiate to the shoulder, arm and hand. The most commonly affected nerves are the axillary, musculocutaneous, suprascapular and thoracodorsal nerves. Pain lasts seconds to minutes, sometimes longer, but typically resolves within 30 minutes. If pain in ipsilateral to forced flexion consider nerve root compression as the cause. These often last longer and the injury is potentially more serious.

Physical Findings

With brachial plexus neuropraxia, pain is increased when the neck is flexed to the opposite side of the pain. Paresthesias may be present along with weakness and

TABLE 24H.8
SUMMARY OF NEUROLOGICAL EVALUATION OF CERVICAL NERVES BY NERVE BOOT

Disc	Root	Reflex	Muscles	Sensation
C4-5	C5	Biceps reflex	Deltoid biceps	Lateral arm Axillary nerve
C5-6	C6	Brachioradialis reflex	Wrist extension biceps	Lateral forearm Musculocutaneous nerve
C6-7	C7	Triceps reflex	Wrist flexors triceps	Middle finger Median nerve
C7-T1	C8	—	Hand intrinsics	Medial forearm Medial anterior branches Cutaneous nerve
T1-2	T1	—	Hand intrinsics	Medial arm Medial branches Cutaneous nerve

changes in the deep tendon reflexes of the upper extremity. Compression testing is typically negative.

In compression injuries, the pain is increased when the neck is flexed in the ipsilateral direction of pain. The symptoms are usually present in specific nerve roots rather than the entire extremity as seen in brachial plexus neuropraxia. Axial compression and distraction tests are usually positive. Nerve cord compression injuries may be complicated by peripheral degeneration. Tables 24H.8 and 24H.9 provide a functional summary of both cervical nerve roots and the peripheral nerves.

Evaluation may include a radiologic workup to rule out degenerative changes or narrowing of the nerve root outlet, particularly if symptoms or signs persist. Utilize MRI to rule out more significant injuries and to assess disc degenerative changes and stenosis.

Treatment

Treatment of brachial plexus neuropraxia is usually self-limited unless there are persistent symptoms or recurrent episodes. Restrict activity until full painless range of motion against resistance occurs. Use NSAIDs or oral corticosteroids for comfort and to reduce edema in the nerve tissue. Monitor neurological changes on a daily basis. Consider EMG and referral if neurological deficits continue longer than 3 weeks.

Cervical Neuropraxia with Transient Quadriplegia

Mechanism of Injury

Transient quadriplegia is seen with forced hyperextension, hyperflexion, or axial loading of the cervical spine in a patient with a decreased anteroposterior (AP) diameter of the cervical cord (cervical stenosis). This results in mechanical compression of the cord that causes transient but completely reversible motor or sensory changes. It has a similar presentation to brachial plexus neuropraxia but involving all four extremities.

Clinical Presentation

The athlete may experience burning pain, numbness, tingling or loss of sensation, weakness, or complete paralysis.

TABLE 24H.9
SUMMARY OF NEUROLOGICAL EVALUATION OF CERVICAL NERVES BY PERIPHERAL NERVE

Nerve	Motor Test	Sensation Test
Radial nerve	Wrist extension	Dorsal web space between thumb and index finger
Ulnar nerve	Adduction, abduction of fingers (interosseous muscles)	Distal ulnar aspect—little finger
Median nerve	Thumb pinch	Distal radial aspect—index finger
Axillary nerve	Abduction	Lateral Arm—deltoid patch on upper arm
Musculocutaneous nerve	Elbow flexion	Lateral forearm

TABLE 24H.10
FINDINGS THAT CONTRAINDICATE RETURN TO PLAY FOLLOWING AN EPISODE OF NEUROPRAXIA

Ligamentous instability
Intervertebral disc disease
Degenerative changes
Magnetic resonance imaging evidence of defects or swelling
Positive neurological findings lasting >36 hr
More than one occurrence

Source: From Torg JS, Glasgow S. Criteria for return to contact activities following cervical injuries. *Clin J Sports Med* 1991;1(1):12–26, (46).

Episodes are transient and usually last 10 to 15 minutes and rarely up to 36 to 48 hours. There is typically no neck pain at the time of injury. After resolution, there is full, pain free range of motion and normal motor-sensory function. X-rays and MRI of the cervical spine may show narrowing of the central canal.

Recommendations

There is no apparent risk of permanent spinal cord injury following a single episode. The risk of recurrence among football players with cervical stenosis who returned to play was 50%. Those with cervical spine instability or acute or chronic degenerative changes in the spine should not be allowed to participate in contact sports. Athletes who have cervical stenosis alone should be evaluated on an individual basis. See Table 24H.10 for contraindications to continued participation following a documented episode of neuropraxia.

Cervical Spine Fracture, Dislocation or Fracture/Dislocation

Mechanism of Injury

Typically forced hyperflexion, hyperextension, lateral rotation, lateral flexion, compression, and combinations of these mechanisms cause these injuries. The most serious injuries occur with axial compression in the flexed or extended position. Specific injuries are attributed to each mechanism obviating the need for close observation of on-field activities in order to obtain the proper mechanism of injury. The typical mechanisms will be addressed individually and their characteristic injuries discussed briefly.

Presenting Complaint

For most of these injuries, neck pain, tingling, weakness or numbness of the extremities is the usual presentation. In severe injuries, unconsciousness, severe neurological deficits, cardiopulmonary failure, and death can be seen.

Physical Findings

Midline cervical spine tenderness with or without neurological deficits is almost always seen. Do not force any

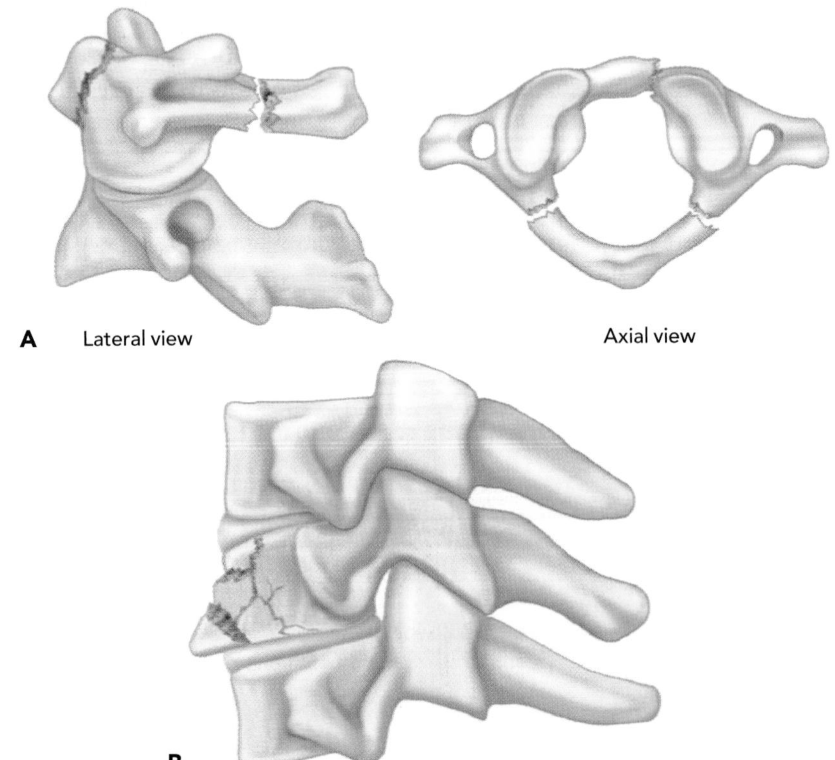

Figure 24H.3 Fractures of the cervical spine due to compression as a mechanism. **A:** Jefferson burst fracture of the atlas. **B:** Burst fracture of the cervical vertebra.

movement. Do not perform range of motion if a severe injury is possible.

Compression Injuries

This mechanism usually involves a direct axial force to the axis (C2) or the vertebral body. A Jefferson's fracture or explosion fracture of the vertebral body may occur (see Figure 24H.3). Clinically the athlete will present with localized neck pain and variable neurological symptoms. On examination, tenderness over the vertebral body, decreased range of motion, and possible instability may be noted. These injuries need immediate immobilization and transport.

Flexion Injuries

The mechanism of this injury is typically falling on the back of the head with the neck in a flexed position. The chin will usually come in contact with the sternum before a fracture occurs. Sprains of the supraspinous or interspinous ligaments are likely, although with intense flexion, dislocation is possible (see Figure 24H.4A and B). Continued flexion may produce a stable simple wedge fracture of the vertebral body (see Figure 24H.4C) or it may result in a fracture of the odontoid (see Figure 24H.5) and subsequent dislocation of the atlantoaxial joint. Clinically they may present with severe neurological deficit, pain, instability and even cardiopulmonary arrest. On examination, tenderness over cervical spine, decreased range of motion, instability, and variable neurological deficits may be present and/or the neck may be locked in one position. Radiographs may show an odontoid fracture by open mouth view, instability may be seen on flexion/extension views, or a dislocation may be noted. These injuries need immediate immobilization and transport.

Flexion-Compression Injuries

This mechanism is typically seen during spearing or head tackling in football. The athlete usually has his chin tucked and makes contact with the crown of his head. This position

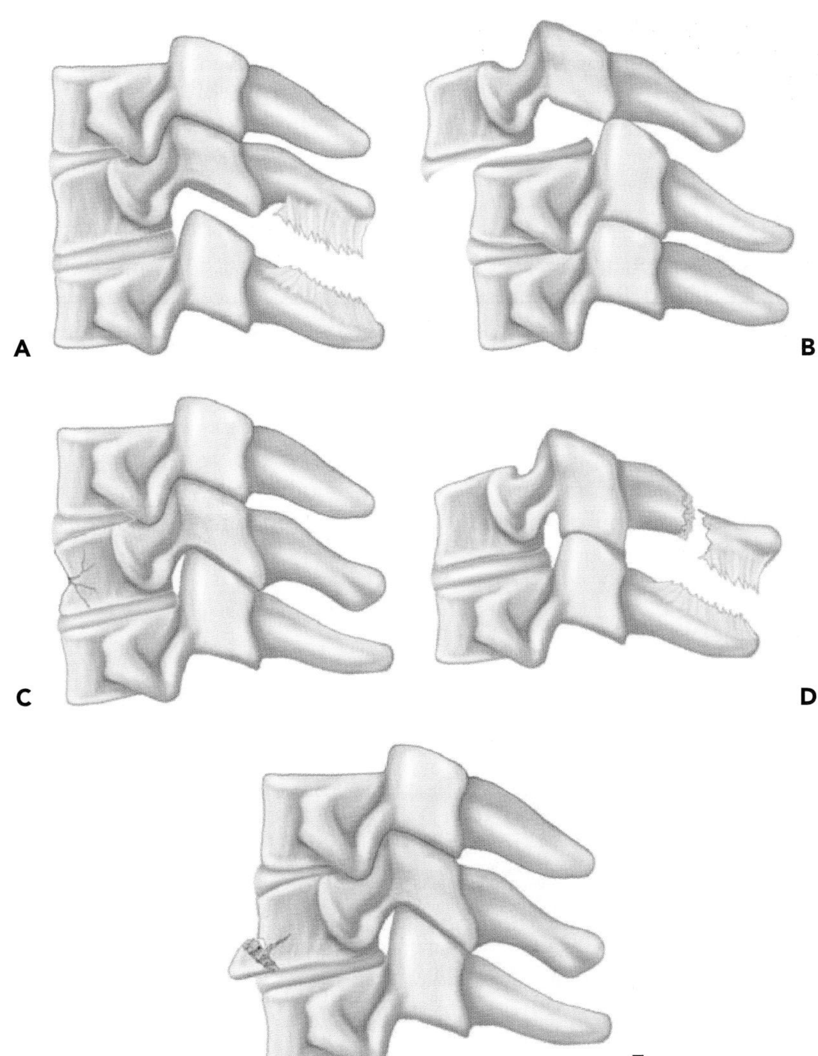

Figure 24H.4 Fractures of the cervical spine due to flexion as a mechanism. **A:** Anterior subluxation. **B:** Bilateral interfacetal dislocation. **C:** Simple wedge fracture. **D:** Clay shovelers fracture. **E:** Flexion teardrop fracture.

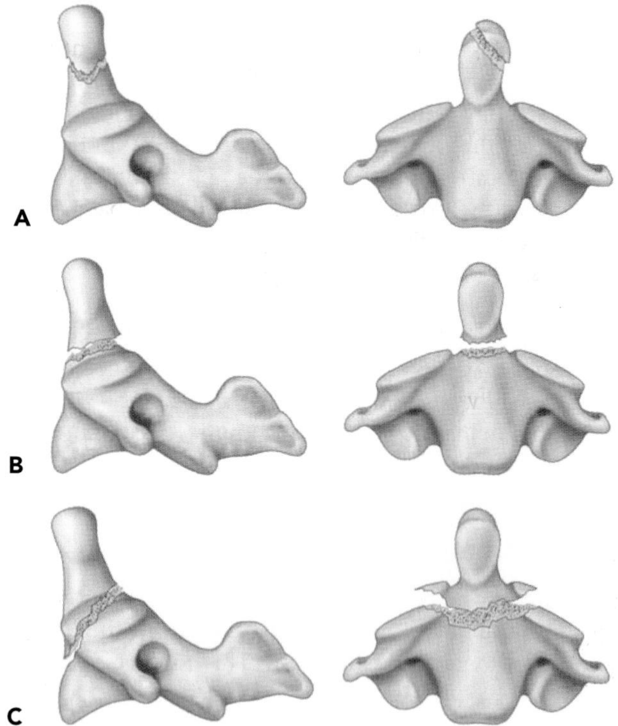

Figure 24H.5 Fractures of the odontoid process. **A:** Oblique fracture through the superior odontoid. **B:** Fracture at the junction of the odontoid and axis. **C:** Fracture with extension into the body of the axis.

causes some of the most catastrophic injuries seen in sports. Most stress occurs at the C5-6 level, which may produce a wedge-shaped fracture off the anterior lip of C5 (see Figure 24H.4E). This injury is unstable if the posterior elements are compromised. Clinically, the athlete may present the same as flexion injuries but there is a greater possibility of a transverse lesion of the cord. In this case, tetraplegia will be noted on examination and the athlete may be in cardiopulmonary arrest. These injuries need immediate immobilization and transport and possibly cardiopulmonary resuscitation.

Flexion-Rotational Injuries

This mechanism of injury usually occurs when landing on the temporal region of the head from a fall or a throw, such as in wrestling or martial arts. The athlete may dislocate one or both facet joints (see Figure 24H.6A) and excessive rotary force may fracture the facet completely (see Figure 24H.6B). Clinically, pain and decreased range of motion with variable neurological deficit may be seen. On examination, the athlete may have his head locked into one position. Radiographs may show a 25% subluxation in a unilateral dislocation and 50% subluxation in a bilateral dislocation. This injury requires gentle traction with immobilization and immediate transport. Do not force the neck into repose.

Hyperextension Injuries

This mechanism usually occurs by striking the athletes face with a knee or by grabbing a facemask and levering it backwards. The occiput may actually contact the thoracic spine. During the hyperextension, injury to the arteries of the spine may cause thrombosis in the vertebral arteries or spasm may occur in the spinal arteries with resultant ischemia of the spinal cord (see Figure 24A.2). Hyperextension is also the most common cause of cervical nerve root damage. Additionally, fractures of the lamina or pedicle of the axis or the odontoid may occur (see Figure 24H.7). In middle-aged athletes central cord syndrome may be seen (see Figure 24H.8). Clinically, the athlete may present with nerve root palsies, momentary paralysis, paresthesia or flaccid paralysis of the upper extremity with spasticity at the trunk and lower extremity. These injuries need immediate immobilization and transport.

Lateral Flexion Injuries

This mechanism results from contact at the level of the shoulder and lateral skull such as seen when being checked into the boards in hockey. This may cause fracture through

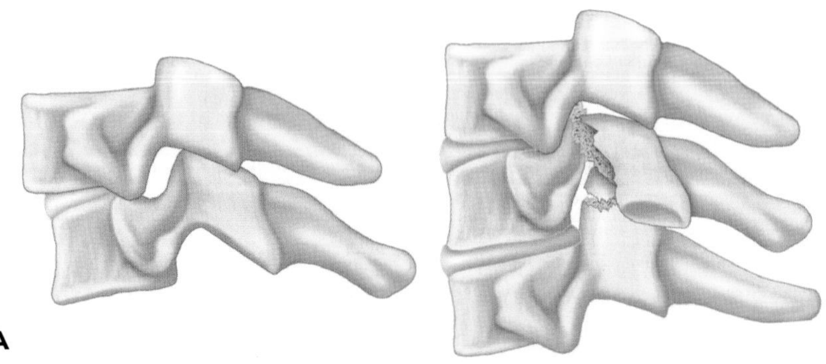

Figure 24H.6 Fractures of the cervical spine due to flexion-rotation and extension-rotation as a mechanism. **A:** Unilateral inter-facetal dislocation. **B:** Pillar fracture.

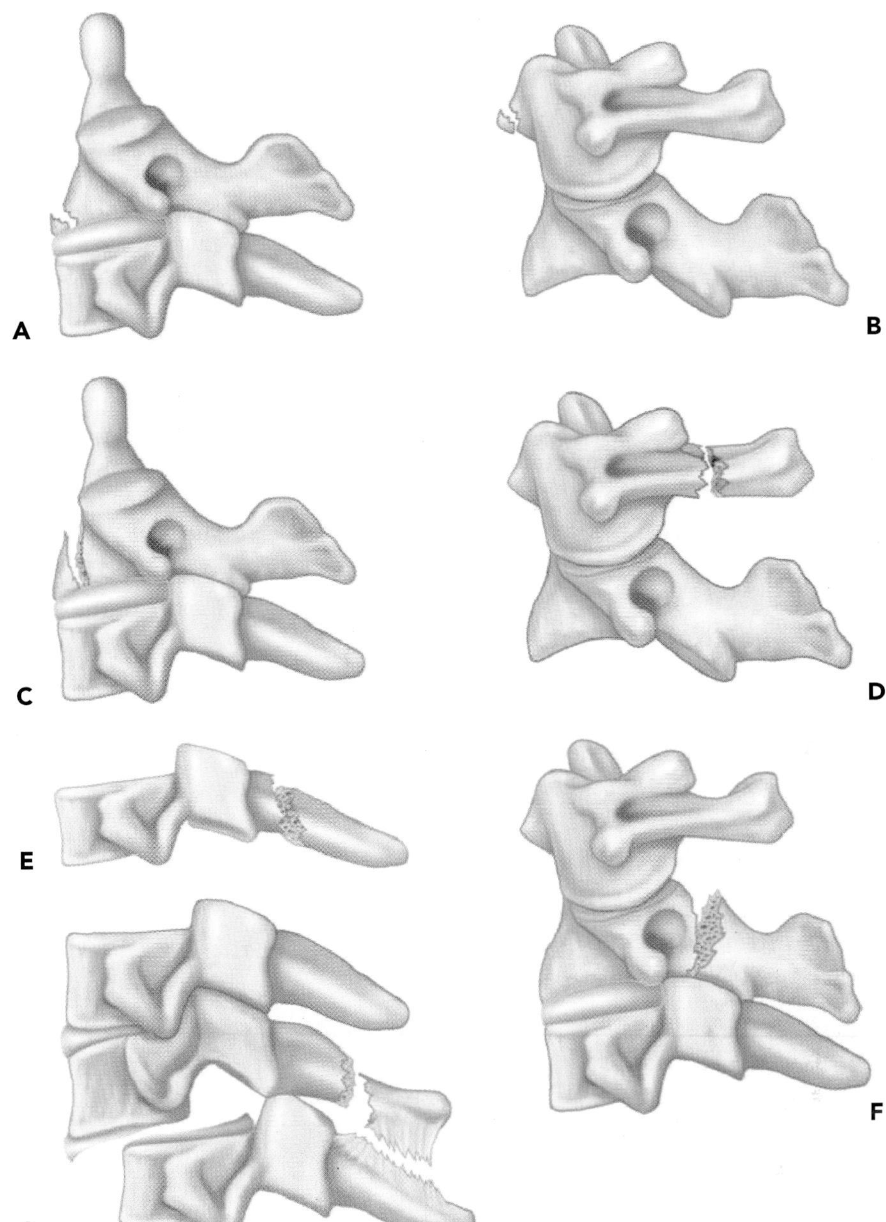

Figure 24H.7 Fractures of the cervical spine due to hyperextension as a mechanism. **A:** Hyperextension dislocation. **B:** Avulsion fracture of the anterior arch of the atlas. **C:** Extension teardrop fracture of the axis. **D:** Fracture of the posterior arch of the atlas. **E:** Laminar fracture. **F:** Traumatic spondylolisthesis (hangman's fracture). **G:** Hyperextension fracture dislocation.

the lateral mass of the pedicle, intervertebral foramen, or within a facet joint (see Figure 24H.9). Clinically they may present with Brown Sequard syndrome (Figure 24H.8). These injuries need immediate immobilization and transport.

ON FIELD CARE OF HEAD AND NECK INJURIES

The Conscious Athlete

A rapid neurological assessment should be performed while still on the field. The athlete should be able to give an accurate history of the injury and the play that led to it. He should be asked to report any paresthesia or paralysis. Ask him to move his fingers, toes and extremities while you perform a strength assessment. Any abnormality (even transiently) implies serious injury and proper immobilization, and transport should be initiated. If normal, examine the neck. If there is pain at rest, immobilization is necessary. If there is no pain at rest, go through gentle voluntary range of motion with support by the examiner's hand. If the pain is minimal or absent, try gentle active motion in all directions (nod head, touch chin to chest, chin to shoulder, ear to ipsilateral shoulder) without support. If there is minimal or no pain, the athlete

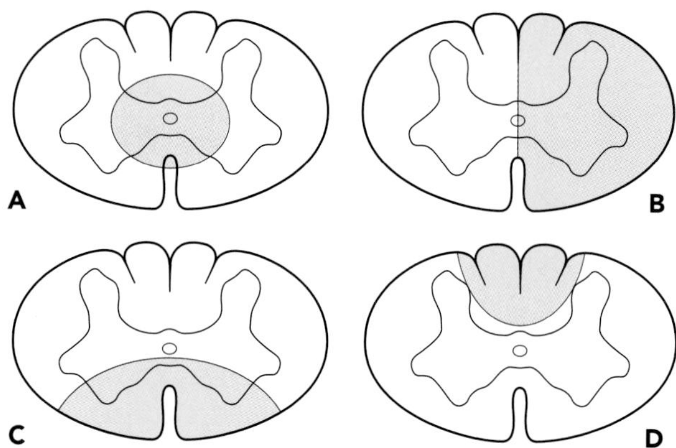

Figure 24H.8 Patterns of incomplete spinal cord injury are shown in the bottom four cross-sections. The tracts affected are shown in the top cross-section. (*Source*: From Bucholz RW, Heckman JD. *Rockwood and green's fractures in adults*, 5th ed. Lippincott Williams & Wilkins, 2001.)

may sit and then stand. If he still has full range of motion with no or mild pain at the extremes of motion, he may leave the field. At this point the athletes should remove their own helmet carefully and a more detailed examination should be performed on the sideline or in the training room (see Table 24A.4).

The Unconscious Athlete

The unconscious athletes should be assumed to have an unstable neck injury. DO NOT USE AMMONIA CAPSULES! Their use may cause a sudden jerking of the head away from the noxious stimuli. The head should be stabilized between the hands of an adult or with sandbags until a backboard and cervical collar can be properly placed. The football helmet should not be removed nor should the chinstrap be loosened (see section on Removal of the Helmetin the following text). Generally, the facemask should be removed before transport using a screwdriver, anvil pruner, Trainer's Angel, Face Mask Extractor (FME) knife, scissors, or nail clippers. The potential for the emergent need of an airway during transport requires that removal be accomplished before transport by personnel who have the proper tools required and who are familiar with the equipment. Prone athletes or those with their heads turned need repositioning with proper technique before immobilization. Do not force the neck into position. The front of the shoulder pads can be opened for CPR but keep the pads on until arrival at an emergency facility and a stiff collar is in place.

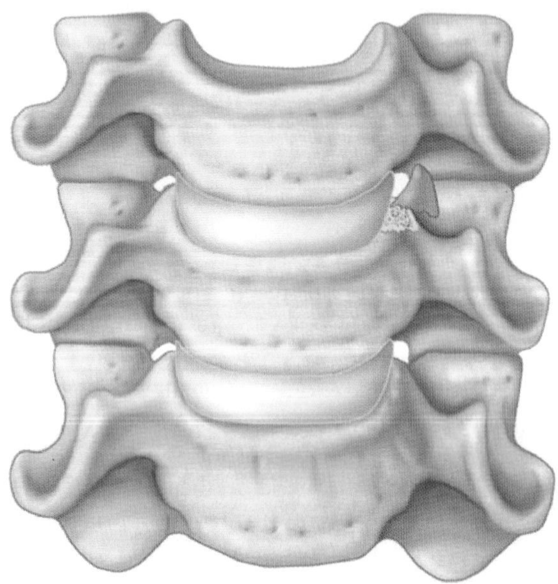

Figure 24H.9 Fractures of the cervical spine due to lateral flexion as a mechanism include fracture through the lateral mass of the pedicle, intervertebral foramen, or within a facet joint. Shown here is a uncinate process fracture.

Positioning and Transport

Use of the five-man transportation team is recommended for the following:

1. After evaluating the airway the leader immediately stabilizes the head and neck. The airway may become patent with just the removal of the mouth guard. If not, establish an airway and initiate CPR.
2. Prone athletes, or those with their heads turned, need repositioning. A log roll onto a spine board should be performed while stabilizing the neck.
3. Removal of the facemask should be performed in case CPR is necessary. Double- and single-barred masks are removed with bolt cutters. Cage-type masks are removed by cutting the plastic loops with a special tool, knife or nail clippers.

Removal of the Helmet

Removal of the helmet must not be taken lightly. There are numerous studies that indicate that removal of football, hockey, and lacrosse helmets submit the cervical spine to undue motion and potential trauma (47–50). Unlike motorcycle and race car helmets, it is best to leave the football, hockey, or lacrosse helmet, chin strap, and shoulder pads in place until the athlete can be transported to a experienced medical center unless the indications noted in Table 24H.11 are observed. The facemask should always be removed before transport in the event that an airway is needed in transit.

SPINAL ALIGNMENT MUST BE MAINTAINED! Remove the cheek padding and deflate the air bladder before attempting to remove the helmet. The team leader grasps the helmet by the ear guards while another rescuer maintains the neck alignment. The ear guards are pulled laterally and the helmet is removed with a posterior to anterior motion in order to free the occipital prominence

TABLE 24H.11
INDICATIONS FOR HELMET AND CHIN STRAP REMOVAL

If helmet and chin strap do not stabilize head/neck properly (i.e., too loose)
If an airway cannot be obtained despite removal of the face mask
If the face mask cannot be removed within a reasonable time period when an airway is necessary
If the helmet prevents proper immobilization of the neck
Padding may need to be place under head for proper alignment if the helmet is removed. This is particularly true with football helmets because the shoulder pads will force the neck into hyperextension if padding is not in place

See text for cautions.

from its position in the helmet. Again, padding must be placed under the head for proper alignment when removing football helmets.

Radiological Evaluation

Radiological evaluation is needed for persistent or significant pain, limitation of motion, or transient or persistent neurological symptoms (except transient brachial plexus neuropraxia). Minimal evaluation requires an AP, lateral and open-mouth views (three-view trauma series). It is important to visualize from C1-7 including the joint space between C7 and T1. Visualizing C7 can be difficult, especially in large, obese, or muscular patients. A swimmer's view may be needed to view poorly visualized areas. If a shoulder girdle injury or other contraindication exists, then fluoroscopy or a CT should be obtained. If a discrepancy exists between clinical findings and the three-view trauma series, then additional bilateral supine oblique films should be obtained (five-view trauma series). If these are normal, flexion and extension views are necessary to evaluate ligamentous integrity. If any doubt exists, CT scan, MRI or bone scans may be necessary.

The Cross-Table Lateral

A good mnemonic for systematic evaluation of the cross-table lateral view involves the ABCS of x-ray diagnosis: A = alignment, B = bony changes, C = cartilage space assessment and S = soft tissue changes.

A: *Alignment.* Lines drawn on the posterior and anterior margins of the vertebral bodies (anterior and posterior contour lines) and a third line along the base of spinous processes, should have a smooth, lordotic contour.

B: *Bony changes.* Assess for areas of decreased symmetry or obvious fracture sites. Areas of increased density may represent compression fractures.

C: *Cartilaginous space assessment.* Slight anterior or posterior widening of the intervertebral disc space or the interspinous spaces may be the only clues to an unstable dislocation. If widening of these spaces is present, oblique films should be obtained for proper evaluation of subluxations.

S: *Soft tissue changes.* Prevertebral swelling and hemorrhage may be the only radiographic findings in some cases of significant spinal injury. The retropharyngeal space at the level of C2 should not exceed 7 mm in adults or children (measured from the anterior inferior border of C2 to the posterior wall of the pharynx). At the level of C3 and C4, it should not exceed 5 mm, and at the level of C6 it should not exceed 22 mm in adults and 14 mm in children less than 15 years of age. Anterior bulging of the prevertebral fat stripe is an indirect sign of soft tissue or bony injury.

Odontoid View

If fracture or malalignment is noted, further evaluation of the area with CT scanning is required.

AP View

A straight line should connect a point bisecting the tips of the spinous processes seen at midline. Asymmetry of this line suggests fracture or dislocation. The laryngeal and tracheal air shadows should be midline. Deviation from their normal position suggests fracture, dislocation, soft tissue damage, edema, or hematoma formation. Fractures of the vertebral bodies and transverse processes are usually evident on this view.

Oblique Views

This view confirms posterior laminar fractures, unilateral facet dislocations, and subluxations. It also evaluates the lateral mass and the lateral foramen.

Computed Tomography Indications

Indications for further evaluation by CT scan include the following:

- Inadequate plain film survey
- Suspicious plain film findings
- Fracture or displacement demonstrated by standard radiography
- High clinical suspicion of injury despite normal plain film survey

Magnetic Resonance Imaging

Typically, MRI is reserved for fine resolution of perivertebral soft tissue, intervertebral discs, the spinal canal, nerve roots, and the presence of stenosis.

RETURN TO PLAY AFTER HEAD AND NECK INJURIES

Before an athlete is allowed to return to play, the following must be met:

- Examination must be normal
- Athlete must be asymptomatic
- Athlete/parents must agree
- Functionally test the athlete before returning to play
- Refer to scales for recommendations on return to play after concussion(s) (see Table 24A.7)
- In brachial plexus neuropraxia, return to play is possible if symptoms are absent within a few minutes after the injury
- Athletes with instability, or acute or chronic degenerative changes should avoid sports with a risk of neck injury
- Athletes with spinal stenosis may return to play if no symptoms are present, the follow-up examination is normal and no instability is seen on x-ray
- Disc ruptures, stable compression fractures, subluxation without fracture and those injuries resulting in cervical fusion should probably permanently avoid contact sports

For further discussion on this see reference (41).

PREVENTION

Many injuries are preventable with better conditioning of athletes, better coaching techniques, proper supervision by qualified individuals, stricter enforcement of safety rules, and the proper use of safety equipment (51) (see Table 24H.8). Since the implementation of helmet laws in football, fatalities have decreased by 74% and serious injury due to head injury by 16% (2). Mouth guards certainly prevent some injures to the structures of the mouth, and may help prevent some concussions. Face shields have similarly been shown to significantly reduce the incidence and severity of facial trauma and head injury (52). Conditioning should include a neck strengthening program (discussed in the following text) which may be helpful in preventing both neck and head injuries (including concussion). See Table 24H.7 for recommendations concerning the prevention of neck injuries due to recreational diving.

NECK STRENGTHENING PROGRAM

All athletes competing in high-risk sports should be involved in a year-round neck-strengthening program. Neck exercises should not be performed before practice, a game, or a match to avoid excessive muscle fatigue that may lead to injury. Isotonic exercises with variable resistance in flexion, extension, and lateral flexion (not rotation) are necessary. Optimal results can be achieved by using a buddy system with constant communication between partners and the supervising adult or coach. General instructions include the following:

- Begin each session with the exerciser relaxed and the spotter gently applying resistance to prestretch the muscles involved.
- Allow the exerciser to warm up the neck muscles by withholding maximum resistance for the first few repetitions.
- Perform 10 repetitions against near-maximal resistance. Each repetition should be performed for 6 to 8 seconds, with 3 to 4 seconds for the concentric contraction through the full muscle range of motion, a 1-second hold, and then a 3 to 4 second eccentric contraction (lengthening) while returning to the starting position. At the start of the eccentric phase, the spotter may increase resistance slightly as more weight can be handled in the eccentric than the concentric phase. As the exerciser approaches the starting position, resistance must be gradually decreased.

APPENDIX 24A.1
ESSENTIAL HEAD AND NECK CHECKLIST FOR THE SPORTS PHYSICIAN AT SPORTING EVENTS

Basic Medical Kit for Head Injuries

- Airways
- Injectable sedative for seizure (phenobarbital)
- Cervical Collar
- Ringer's Solution
- 20% mannitol
- Intravenous tubing and cannula

Name, Location, Transit Time to

- Nearest Hospital
- Neurosurgical Center

Facilities and Personnel Familiarization

- In-field first-aid personnel
- Intermediate transport (stretchers, ski patrol, etc.)
- Medical first-aid station
- Ambulance transport

Preset Communication Between

- Site of injury
- Intermediate transport team
- Organizers of the event
- Police and/or coroner
- Ambulance
- Relatives
- Press

APPENDIX 24B.1

RAPID NEUROLOGICAL EVALUATION OF CRANIAL NERVE FUNCTION

Nerve	Frequency	Sites of Involvement	Tests	Abnormal Findings
I Olfactory	Uncommon	Fracture of cribriform plate or in ethmoid area	Apply simple odors such as peppermint to one nostril at a time	Anosmia
II Optic	Common	Direct trauma to orbit or globe, or fracture involving optic foramen	Light flashed in affected eye Light flashed in normal eye	Loss of both direct and concensual pupillary constriction Direct and consensual pupillary constriction
	Common	Pressure on geniculocalcarine tract. Laceration or intracerebral clot in temporal, parietal, or ocipital lobes (rarely from subdural clot)	Bring hand suddenly toward eye from the side	Absence of the blink reflex indicates a visual field defect (always homonymous)
III Oculomotor	Very frequent	Pressure of herniating uncus on nerve just before it enters cavernous sinus or fracture involving cavernous sinus	Light flashed in affected eye Light flashed in normal eye	Dilated pupil, ptosis, eye turns down and out Direct pupil reflex absent. Consensual reflex present Direct pupil reflex present. Consensual reflex absent
IV Trochlear	Infrequent	Course of nerve around brain stem or fracture of orbit	Isolated involvement requires special equipment	Eye fails to mvoe down and out
V Trigeminal	Uncommon	Direct injury to terminal branches, particularly 2nd division in roof of maxillary sinus	Sensation: 1st division: Above eye and cornea 2nd division: Upper lip 3rd division: Lower lip and chin Motor function: "Bite down" or "Chew"	Loss of sensation of pain and touch. Paresthesias Palpated masseter and temporalis fail to contract
VI Abducens	Quite frequent	Base of brain as nerve enters clivus. Fracture involving cavernous sinus or orbit	"Look to the right—Look to the left"	Affected eye fails to move laterally. Diplopia on lateral gaze
VII Facial	Frequent	Peripheral: Laceration or contusion in parotid region		Paralysis of facial muscles. Eye remains open. Angle of mouth droops. Forehead fails to wrinkle
		Peripheral: Fracture of temporal bone		As above plus associated involvement of acoustic nerve (see below) and chorda tympani (dry cornea and loss of taste on ipsilateral 2/3 of tongue)

(continued)

APPENDIX 24B.1
(continued)

Nerve	Frequency	Sites of Involvement	Tests	Abnormal Findings
	Frequent	Supranuclear: Intracerebral clot	"Wrinkle your forehead"	Forehead wrinkles because of bilateral innervation of frontalis. Otherwise paralysis of facial muscles as above
VIII Acoustic	Common	Fractures of petrous portion of temporal bone. Seventh nerve also often involved	In children and uncooperative patients, slap hands close to ear Weber Test: Tuning fork middle of forehead	Startle reflex Sound not heard by involved ear
IX Glosso-pharyngeal	Rare	Brain stem or deep laceration of neck	Motor power of stylopharyngeus—impractical to test Cotton applicator to soft palate	Loss of taste posterior one-third of tongue Loss of sensation on affected side of soft palate
X Vagus	Rare	Brain stem or deep laceration of neck	Inspection of soft palate. Laryngoscopy	Sagging of soft palate; deviation of uvula to normal side. Hoarseness from paralysis of vocal cord
XI Spinal accessory	Rare	Laceration of neck	Hand on side of chin: "Push your chin against my hand" "Shrug your shoulders" "Stretch out your hands toward me"	Palpated sternocleidomastoid fails to contract Palpated upper fibers of trapezius fail to contract Affected arm seems longer (scapula not "anchored")
XII Hypoglossal	Rare	Neck laceration usually associated with major vessel damage	"Stick your tongue out"	Tongue protrudes toward affected side. Dysarthria

APPENDIX 24C.1
GENERAL OBSERVATIONS FOR HOME:

- Check on patient about every hour while he is awake.
- During the first night, patient should be awakened once to be certain that he is in a natural sleep and responds normally to the waking.
- Signs of danger:
  - Patient acts very "dopey" and with a reduction of response to questions and stimulation.
  - Very unsteady—poor coordination of arms and legs.
  - Marked difference in size of pupils (from baseline).
  - Increasingly severe or persistent headache or vomiting. (Patient may normally have a mild headache or an upset stomach after minor concussion.)
  - Development of weakness in arms or legs.
  - Convulsive movement of limbs or face.

Summary

- If the patient's alertness and appetite return quickly to normal, treatment may be limited to the above observations and gradual increase in activity.
- If *any* of the above signs appear, contact your physician *immediately*.
- Call your physician if you have any concern regarding the patient's condition.
- No matter the case, report to your physician on the next day.

REFERENCES

1. Newsome PR, Tran DC, Cooke MS. The role of the mouthguard in the prevention of sports-related dental injuries: a review. *Int J Paediatr Dent* 2001;11:396–404.
2. Levy ML, Ozgur BM, Berry C, et al. Birth and evolution of the football helmet. *Neurosurgery* 2004b;55(3):656–661.
3. Levy ML, Ozgur BM, Berry C, et al. Analysis and evolution of head injury in football. *Neurosurgery* 2004a;55(3):649–655.
4. Mueller FO, Blyth CS. Fatalities from head and cervical spine injuries occurring in tackle football: 40 years' experience. *Clin Sports Med* 1987;6:185–196.

5. Mueller F, Blyth C. Can we continue to improve injury statistics in football? *Phys Sportsmed* 1984;12:79–84.
6. Delaney JS. Head injuries presenting to emergency departments in the United States from 1990 to 1999 for ice hockey, soccer, and football. *Clin J Sports Med* 2004;14(2):80–87.
7. Grindel SH, Lovell MR, Collins MW. The assessment of sport-related concussion: the evidence behind neuropsychological testing and management. *Clin J Sport Med* 2001;11:134–143.
8. Ommaya AK, Gennarelli TA. Cerebral concussion and traumatic unconsciousness. Correlation of experimental and clinical observations of blunt head injuries. *Brain* 1974;97:633–654.
9. Alves WM, Rimel RW, Nelson WE. University of Virginia prospective study of football-induced minor head injury: status report. *Clin Sports Med* 1987;6:211–218.
10. Collins MW, Grindel SH, Lovell MR, et al. Relationship between concussion and neuropsychological performance in college football players. *JAMA* 1999;282:964–970.
11. Macciocchi SN, Barth JT, Alves W, et al. Neuropsychological functioning and recovery after mild head injury in collegiate athletes. *Neurosurgery* 1996; 39:510–514.
12. Cantu RC. Second-impact syndrome. *Clin Sports Med* 1998a;17:37–44.
13. Reid S. Brain trauma inside a football helmet. *Phys Sportsmed* 1974;8:32.
14. Rimel RW, Giordani B, Barth JT, et al. Moderate head injury: completing the clinical spectrum of brain trauma. *Neurosurgery* 1982;11:344–351.
15. Cantu RC. Guidelines for return to contact sports after a cerebral concussion. *Phys Sportsmed* 1986;14:75–83.
16. Barnes BC, Cooper L, Kirkendall DT, et al. Concussion history in elite male and female soccer players. *Am J Sports Med* 1998;26:433–438.
17. Gerberich SG, Priest JD, Boen JR, et al. Concussion incidences and severity in secondary school varsity football players. *Am J Public Health* 1983;73: 1370–1375.
18. Lovell MR, Iverson GL, Collins MW, et al. Does loss of consciousness predict neuropsychological decrements after concussion? *Clin J Sport Med* 1999;9:193–198.
19. Bennett DR, Fuenning SI, Sullivan G, et al. Migraine precipitated by head trauma in athletes. *Am J Sports Med* 1980;8:202–205.
20. Ommaya AK, Grubb RL Jr, Naumann RA. Coup and contre-coup injury: observations on the mechanics of visible brain injuries in the rhesus monkey. *J Neurosurg* 1971;35:503–516.
21. Gennarelli TA, Spielman GM, Langfitt TW, et al. Influence of the type of intracranial lesion on outcome from severe head injury. *J Neurosurg* 1982;56:26–32.
22. Wilson K, Cram B, Rontal E, et al. Facial injuries in hockey players. *Minn Med* 1977;60:13–19.
23. LaForge R. Preventing eye injuries. *Exec Health Report* 1990;3(26):7.
24. Rutherford G, Miles R. *Overview of sports related injuries to persons 5–14 years of age report.* U.S. Consumer Product Safty Commission, 1981;17–21.
25. Pine D. Preventing sports-related eye injuries. *Phys Sportsmed* 1991;19(2): 129.
26. Capillo J. Hockey masks go on, face injuries go down. *Phys Sportsmed* 1977;5:77.
27. Marton K, Wilson D, McKeag D. Ocular trauma in college varsity sports. *Med Sci Sports Exerc* 1987;19(2 Supp):553.
28. Gilbert DN, Moellering RC, Eliopoulos GM, et al. eds. *The Sanford guide to antimicrobial therapy*, 36th ed. Hyde Park, VT: Antimicrobial Therapy, Inc, 2006:6–7.
29. Strauss M. Swimmer's ear. *Phys Sportsmed* 1979;7:101.
30. Romeo SJ, Hawley CJ, Romeo MW, et al. Facial injuries in sports: a team physician's guide to diagnosis and treatment. *Phys Sportsmed* 2005;33(4):45–53.
31. Odess J. The hearing hazard of firearms. *Phys Sportsmed* 1974;2:65.
32. Taylor GD, Williams E. Acoustic trauma in the sports hunter. *Laryngoscope* 1966;76:863–879.
33. Schendel S. Sports-related nasal injuries. *Phys Sportsmed* 1990;18(10): 59–74.
34. Illum P. Long-term results after treatment of nasal fractures. *J Laryngol Otol* 1986;100:273–277.
35. Gottschalk GH. Epistaxis and the nasostat. *J Am Coll Emerg Physician* 1976;5:793–795.
36. Heintz WD. Mouth protectors: a progress report. *J Am Dental Assoc* 1968; 77:632.
37. Beachy G. Dental injuries in intermediate and high school athletes: a 15-year study at Punahou school. *J Athl Train* 2004;39(4):310–315.
38. McCrory P. Do mouthguards prevent concussion? *Br J Sports Med* 2001; 35:81–82.
39. Middleton J. Football spine pad protection for baseball catchers. *Athl Train* 1980;15:82.
40. Delaney JS, Al-Kashmiri A. Neck injuries presenting to emergency departments in the United States from 1990 to 1999 for ice hockey, soccer, and American football. *Br J Sports Med* 2005;39(4):e21.
41. Cantu RC, Bailes JE, Wilberger JE Jr. Guidelines for return to contact or collision sport after a cervical spine injury. *Clin Sports Med* 1998c;17: 137–146.
42. Torg JS, Vegso JJ, O'Neill MJ, et al. The epidemiologic, pathologic, biomechanical, and cinematographic analysis of football-induced cervical spine trauma. *Am J Sports Med* 1990;18:50–57.
43. Tator CH. Neck injuries in ice hockey: a recent, unsolved problem with many contributing factors. *Clin Sports Med* 1987;6:101–114.
44. Scher A. Rugby injuries of the spine and spinal cord. *Clin Sports Med* 1987; 6(1):87–100.
45. Torg JS. Epidemiology, pathomechanics, and prevention of athletic injuries to the cervical spine. *Med Sci Sports Exerc* 1985;17:295–303.
46. Torg JS, Glasgow S. Criteria for return to contact activities following cervical injuries. *Clin J Sports Med* 1991;1(1):12–26.
47. Laprade RF, Schnetzler KA, Broxterman RJ, et al. Cervical spine alignment in the immobilized ice hockey player. A computed tomographic analysis of the effects of helmet removal. *Am J Sports Med* 2000;28(6): 800–803.
48. Swenson TM, Lauerman WC, Blanc RO, et al. Cervical spine alignment in the immobilized football player. Radiographic analysis before and after helmet removal. *Am J Sports Med* 1997;25(2):226–230.
49. Waninger KN. On-field management of potential cervical spine injury in helmeted football players: leave the helmet on!. *Clin J Sports Med* 1998;8(2):124–129.
50. Waninger KN, Richards JG, Pan WT, et al. An evaluation of head movement in backboard immobilized helmeted football, lacrosse, and ice hockey players. *Clin J of Sports Med* 2001;11(2):82–86.
51. Biasco SW, Tegner T. The avoidability of head and neck injuries in ice hockey: an historical review. *Br J Sports Med* 2002;36:410–427.
52. Benson BW, Rose MS, Meeuwisse WH. The impact of face shield use on concussions in ice hockey: a multivariate analysis. *Br J Sports Med* 2002; 36:27–32.

The Shoulder and Upper Extremity

25

David J. Petron *Umar Khan*

SECTION A

THE SHOULDER

The shoulder is the most vulnerable joint in the human body. It is also one of the most complicated anatomical and biomechanical joints. Sports medicine specialists have begun to redirect their attention from the problems of the knee to the complexities of the shoulder. Advances in arthroscopy have changed treatment protocols and extended the competitive lives of athletes, especially throwing athletes. The shoulder is a site of major injury in competitive sports, including a variety of injuries ranging from those involving joints (e.g., glenohumeral [GH] dislocations, acromioclavicular [AC] separations), to those involving bones (e.g., fractures of the clavicle, upper humerus), to those involving muscles and tendons (e.g., rotator cuff injuries). In a study involving 336 elite college football players, approximately half had a history of shoulder injuries. The most common injuries were AC separation (41%), anterior instability (20%), rotator cuff injury (12%), clavicle fracture (4%), and posterior instability (4%). The most common surgeries performed were anterior instability reconstruction (48%), Mumford/Weaver-Dunn surgery (15%), posterior instability surgery (10%), and rotator cuff surgery (10%) (1).

ANATOMY/BIOMECHANICS

To put the anatomy of the shoulder in perspective, one needs to consider evolution. As we evolved from a quadruped to a biped, we ceased to use our upper extremity for weight bearing. The shoulder remains a ball and socket joint but the borders of the socket have fallen back to allow the greatest range of motion (ROM) of any body joint. In contrast, the hip joint maintains much of its stability because it is a deep ball and socket joint. To make up for a loss of dynamic stability, the shoulder relies heavily on the musculature of the rotator cuff. What the shoulder has given up in stability, it gains in ROM.

The shoulder exhibits the following three planes of motion:

- Sagittal—flexion, extension, and elevation
- Coronal—adduction and abduction
- Medial—internal and external rotation

The functional anatomy of the shoulder includes five articulations (see Figure 25A.1). From distal to proximal these are as follows:

1. *Glenohumeral.* The shoulder joint and major articulation of the upper extremity. This joint can be described as an incongruent joint that uses a gliding motion about a nonfixed axis of rotation. It is made up of the concave surface of the glenoid fossa and the more circular convex surface of the humeral head. During motion only a small portion of the humeral head is in contact with the fossa at any one time. Supporting soft tissue structures intimate to the joint include the glenoid labrum, joint capsule, and the anterior placed GH ligament. The joint capsule is normally loose, becoming taut only in extreme movements (the external rotation and abduction of throwing) beyond the normal ROM of the joint. Movement between the shoulder and elbow is coordinated by the long head of the biceps muscle. The long head of the bicep's proximal tendon runs intracapsularly but extrasynovially through the GH joint.
2. *Suprahumeral.* Not a true joint but a physiological one. This protective articulation is between the humeral

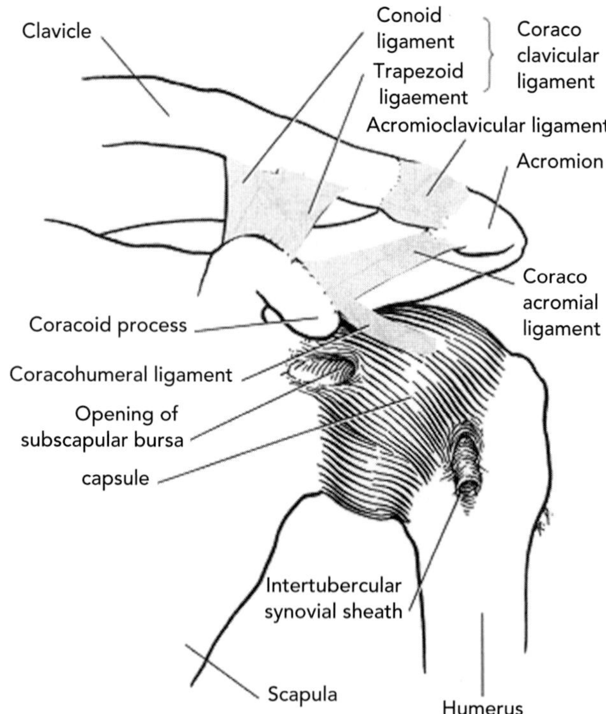

Figure 25A.1 Articulation and ligaments around the shoulder. (*Source:* Reproduced with permission from Jenkins DB, Hollinshead WH: *Hollinshead's functional anatomy of the limbs and back,* 8th ed. Philadelphia: WB Saunders, 2002.)

head and the coracoacromial ligament. It allows the greater tuberosity of the humerus to pass under the coracoacromial ligament without compression during abduction. This is the site where most shoulder impingement occurs.

3. *Scapulothoracic.* Another physiological joint. The motion of the scapula is to glide along the posterior thoracic wall when there is motion and rotation of the clavicle. This movement is produced by the coordinated movement of two muscles—the trapezius and serratus anterior muscles.
4. *Acromioclavicular.* A plane joint containing a meniscoid structure. This meniscoid structure rapidly degenerates and disappears by the fourth decade of life. The AC joint is stabilized by the AC and coracoclavicular (CC) ligaments. The physiological movement of the clavicle is by rotation when the arm is adducted or elevated.
5. *Sternoclavicular.* A plane joint that acts as a ball and socket joint. The anterior and posterior sternoclavicular ligaments reinforce a loose fibrous capsule making up the joint. Stability is aided by the costoclavicular and infraclavicular ligaments.

Bursae. There are usually a total of eight bursae present around the shoulder joint.

Only the large subacromial bursa is clinically significant (see Figure 25A.2B).

Glenoid labrum (Figure 25A.2A). The fibrocartilaginous labrum acts to expand depth and increase the area of the glenoid. It is triangular on cross section with a thin, free intra-articular apex and three sides that face the humeral head, the joint capsule, and the glenoid surface, respectively. The labrum is anchored to the glenoid at the periphery. The presence of an intact labrum increases humeral contact area by up to 75% in the vertical plane and 56% in the transverse plane. This additional contact area improves GH joint stability without compromising motion.

Joint capsule. Mobility is further enhanced by a thin joint capsule that has almost twice the surface area of the humeral head. This allows tremendous ROM. The passive stability is provided by selective tightening of various portions of the joint capsule depending on arm position. At rest, with the arm in a dependent position, the superior portion of

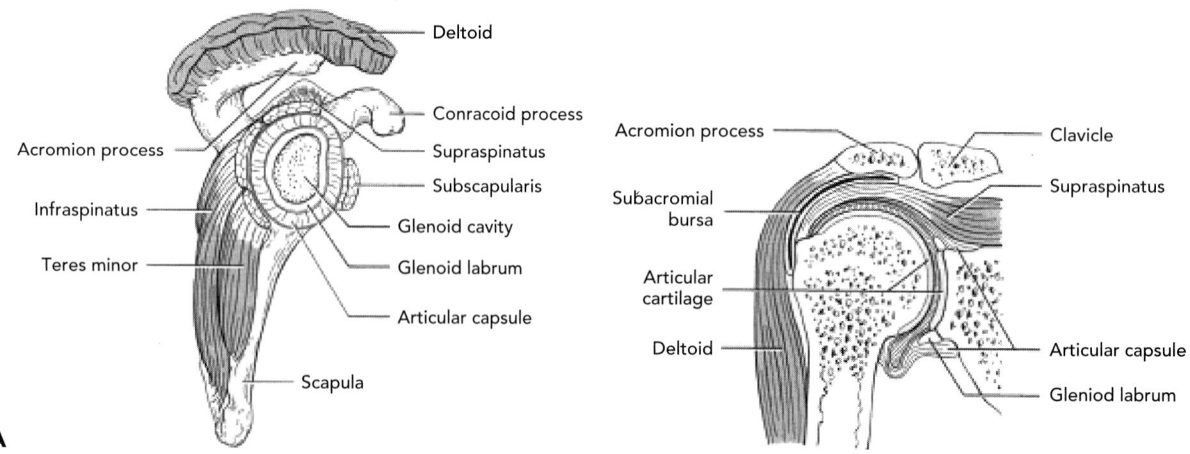

Figure 25A.2 **A:** Anatomy of the glenohumeral joint and surrounding structures. **B:** Lateral view showing a cross-sectional view of the subacromial bursae. (*Source:* Reproduced with permission from Jenkins DB, Hollinshead WH. *Hollinshead's functional anatomy of the limbs and back,* 8th ed. Philadelphia: WB Saunders, 2002.)

the capsule is taut and the inferior region is lax. With overhead elevation this relation is reversed. External rotation tightens the anterior and releases the posterior capsule whereas horizontal flexion does the opposite.

GH ligaments. Structural reinforcement of the anterior capsule is provided by folds in its inner wall that have been designated as the superior, middle, and inferior GH ligaments. The most significant of these structures is the inferior GH ligament. It is the primary restraint to external rotation at 90 degrees of shoulder abduction. Overhead athletes often place their arm in this position and risk injury of the inferior GH ligament.

IMPORTANT MUSCLES

Deltoid. Acts as an elevator of the arm. This is a superficial muscle that normally contributes the round, contoured look to the anterior and lateral profile of the shoulder. It initiates abduction.

Supraspinatus. Initiates arm elevation and primarily depresses the humerus during abduction. It passes under the acromion and coracoacromial ligament and can be easily "pinched" between these structures and a moving humeral head. This is the main tendon affected with impingement syndrome.

Subscapularis, infraspinatus, and the teres minor act synergistically as a conjoined tendon to compress the joint and displace the upper extremity downward: (a) *subscapularis*—responsible for internal rotation; (b) *infraspinatus and teres minor*—responsible for external rotation.

Note: The latter four muscle attachments to the humerus make up the rotator cuff of the shoulder (see Figure 25A.3).

GENERIC EXAMINATION

Because of the complexity of the shoulder, we will discuss the important subjective and objective aspects without relation to any specific shoulder diagnosis (see Table 25A.1).

History

When confronted with an undiagnosed shoulder injury, the physician must elucidate the exact mechanism of injury and position of the shoulder at the time of injury. The history should include the following:

Mechanism of injury. Did the patient fall on the outstretched hand? ("FOOSH" injury) This could indicate shoulder dislocation or fracture injury. Did the patient fall directly on the tip of the shoulder or did he/she land on the elbow, driving the humerus upward? This finding may indicate an AC disruption or subluxation. Did the shoulder feel loose or like it was "coming out?" This may indicate instability. Was the onset insidious and, now, the patient has pain only with overhead motion? This may be impingement syndrome. Please see Appendix 25A.1 for images.

- *Movements*. Are there movements that cause pain or problems? Cervical spine movements may cause pain in the shoulder. Abduction and external rotation of the shoulder may lead to apprehension, which indicates anterior instability. Pain during certain phases of throwing such as cocking or acceleration phases) may indicate anterior instability or internal impingement. Pain with simple overhead motion may indicate impingement syndrome. Instability and impingement frequently occur together. Night pain and resting pain are often associated with rotator cuff tears, subacromial

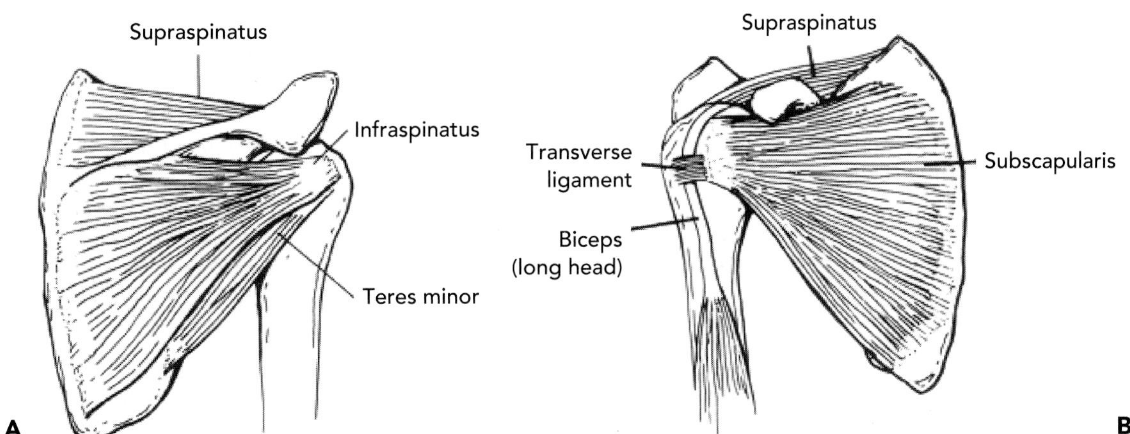

Figure 25A.3 **A:** Posterior view of shoulder. **B:** Anterior view of shoulder. Muscles of the Rotator Cuff. (*Source:* Reproduced with permission from DeLee JC, Drez D Jr. *Orthopaedic sports medicine principles and practice*, Vol. 1. 1st ed. Philadelphia: WB Saunders,1994:624.)

TABLE 25A.1

DIFFERENTIAL DIAGNOSIS OF ROTATOR CUFF DEGENERATION, FROZEN SHOULDER, ATRAUMATIC INSTABILITY, AND CERVICAL SPONDYLOSIS

	Rotator Cuff Lesions	Frozen Shoulder	Atraumatic Instability	Cervical Spondylosis
History	Age 30–50 yr Pain and weakness after eccentric load	Age 45+ (insidious type) Insidious onset or after trauma or surgery Functional restriction of lateral rotation, abduction, and medial rotation	Age 10–35 yr Pain and instability with activity No history of trauma	Age 50+ years acute or chronic
Observation	Normal bone and soft tissue outlines Protective shoulder hike may be seen	Normal bone and soft tissue outlines	Normal bone and soft tissue outlines	Minimal or no cervical spine movement Torticolis may be present
Active movement	Weakness of abduction or rotation, or both Crepitus may be present	Restricted ROM Shoulder hiking	Full or excessive ROM	Limited ROM with pain
Passive movement	Pain if impingement occurs	Limited ROM, especially in lateral, rotation, abduction, and medial rotation (capsular pattern)	Normal or excessive ROM	Limited ROM (symptoms may be exacerbated)
Restricted isometric movement	Pain and weakness on abduction and lateral rotation	Normal, when arm by side	Normal	Normal, except if nerve root compressed Myotome may be affected
Special tests	Drop-arm test positive Empty can test positive	None	Load and shift test(+) Apprehension test (+) Relocation test (+) Augmentation tests (+)	Spurling's test (+) Distraction test (+) ULTT (+) Shoulder abduction test (+)
Sensory function and reflexes	Not affected	Not affected		Dermatomes affected Reflexes affected
Palpation	Tender over rotator cuff	Not painful unless capsule is stretched	Anterior or posterior pain	Tender over appropriate vertebra or facet
Diagnostic Imaging	Radiography: Upward displacement of humeral head; acromial spurring MRI diagnostic	Radiography negative Arthrography decreased size	Negative	Radiography: narrowing osteophytes

ROM = range of motion; ULTT = upper limb tension test; MRI = magnetic resonance imaging.
Source: From Magee DJ, *Orthopedic physical assessment*, 4th ed. St. Louis, Missouri: WB Saunders/Elsevier, 2006.

bursa pain (impingement syndrome), and, on occasion, tumors.

- *Handedness.* A key element in the historical review. A conditioned athlete using his or her arm in sport (pitcher, volleyball player) will often have restriction in the ROM in their dominant as compared to the nondominant arm. The examiner should not attribute such alterations to a pathological state.
- *Occupation/position.* Certain positions played in sports lend themselves to certain injury. A baseball catcher throwing overhand may be at more risk than a shortstop for an overuse injury or impingement syndrome. Overhead activity, such as swimming, volleyball, and throwing sports are at particular risk for injury. In an older patient, a simple overhead activity such as painting may start the cycle of impingement type pain.
- *Review of systems.* Specific inquiry should be made of history of rheumatoid arthritis, diabetes mellitus, gout, or other systemic diseases. Also, the physician needs to know about previous surgery or trauma to the area.
- *Medication use.* A history of both oral and injected medications is useful.
- *Age.* Many problems of the shoulder are related to the patient's age. Rotator cuff degeneration usually occurs in patients between 40 and 70 years of age. Calcium deposits frequently occur between the ages of 20 and 40. Rotator cuff tears, in patients under the age of 40, are almost nonexistent unless

TABLE 25A.2
SHOULDER PAIN FROM OTHER DISEASE PROCESSES

Disease Process	Referred Pain
Pulmonary apical pathology	Pancoast's tumor: can cause shoulder pain radiating to the arm in an ulnar distribution
	Apical tuberculosis: shoulder pain on either shoulder depending on the side of the lesion
Diaphragmatic irritation	Gallbladder or hepatic disease affecting the right shoulder
	Splenic rupture/contusion affecting the left shoulder
	Increased respiration in a deconditioned athlete while running can affect either shoulder
Abdominal disease	Gastric or hepatic disorder can also be referred to the interscapular region
Tension myalgia	Localizes in the trapezius muscle
Cervical radiculitis	Result of a brachial plexus injury or cervical root nerve impingement affecting the shoulder and arm
Cardiac disease	Classical left shoulder pain

associated with trauma. Frozen shoulder is seen in persons between the ages of 40 and 60 years if it results from causes other than trauma.

- *Inherent ligamentous laxity*. Some individuals (and some sports) may possess generalized joint laxity (swimming). Do "loose joints" run in the family?
- *Pain*. The characterization of pain, onset, and specific biomechanical actions generating the pain are obviously important. Training habits in relation to pain should be asked. The specific character of the pain can vary as follows:
  - *Dull* pain may indicate a rotator cuff tear.
  - *Burning* pain may indicate cervical radiculopathy.
  - An audible *snap* may indicate subluxation of the GH joint or biceps tendon.
  - *Crepitation* with passive motion may indicate a passive bursitis or scapular dyskinesia.
  - *Referred pain* (see Table 25A.2).

Physical Examination

Specific and unique aspects of examination of the shoulder include the following:

- *Inspection*. Both shoulders should be exposed to allow comparison and to detect any signs of asymmetry. The authors recommend Y-style tank tops for female patients whenever possible. Also, an examination room mirror allows the physician to face the patient and still observe the posterior motion of the scapula on abduction and ROM testing. Look from both sides, back, and front especially noting muscle atrophy, erythema, swelling, or deformity.

  With the patient sitting, look for atrophy in three sites; the supraspinatus fossa, the infraspinatus fossa, and the deltoid. This demonstrates weakness due to either a rotator cuff tear, or neurological deficit.
- *Palpation*. The primary care physician should think of the topographical anatomy and, whenever possible, palpate both shoulders at the same time while the patient describes differences in sensation of tenderness. Feel for crepitation and spasm. The order of examination from proximal to distal on the upper extremity should be sternum, sternoclavicular joint, clavicle, AC joint, coracoacromial ligament, coracoid process, GH joint (passively abducting the upper extremity), biceps tendon and groove (passively performing external rotation), and scapula. The presence of pain, swelling, crepitation, muscle spasm, tenderness, or warmth may indicate underlying pathology (see Table 25A.3).

TABLE 25A.3
SUSPECTED INJURIES BASED ON ANATOMICAL LOCATION OF PAIN

Anatomic Area	Possible Pathology
Sternoclavicular joint	Strain, dislocation
Clavicle	Fracture
Acromioclavicular joint	Separation
	Contusion
	Arthritis
	Osteolysis of the lateral clavicle
Anterior shoulder with arm at side	
Anterior deltoid	Strain
Anterior capsule	Subluxation
Bicipital groove	Tendinitis
Anterior shoulder with arm held in full extension	
Subdeltoid bursa	Bursitis
Rotator cuff	Tendinitis, tear
Lateral shoulder with arm at side	
Middle deltoid	Strain, tear, supraspinatus tendonitis
Subdeltoid bursae	Bursitis, Impingement syndrome
Posterior shoulder with arm at side	
Posterior deltoid	Strain
Posterior capsule	Anterior subluxation/dislocation
Scapula	Neuropraxia, strain

- *Neurovascular examination.* This should include palpation of the pulses and a determination of the sensory and motor functioning, as well as of the deep tendon reflexes of the upper extremity. Test for deep tendon reflex and sensory perception (see Figure 25A.4 for dermatome distribution)
  - Axillary nerve—loss of sensation over the lateral aspect of the upper arm
  - Long thoracic nerve—winging of the scapula (serratus anterior muscle dysfunction).
- *Neck.* ROM should be examined for any shoulder pain and for alignment of cervical vertebrae. Note any pain or tenderness over the paracervical muscles or spinous process. Abnormal movement patterns of the head and neck should be examined closely. Spurling's test should be elicited to rule out cervical disc/nerve disease as a cause of shoulder pain.
- *Active range of shoulder motion.* Evaluate: (a) abduction—determined by raising the outstretched arm laterally overhead while observing from behind; (b) flexion—assessed by having the patient raise the arms forward until they touch overhead; (c) internal rotation—the patient places the thumb as high as possible on the opposite scapula; (d) external rotation—the patient places his/her

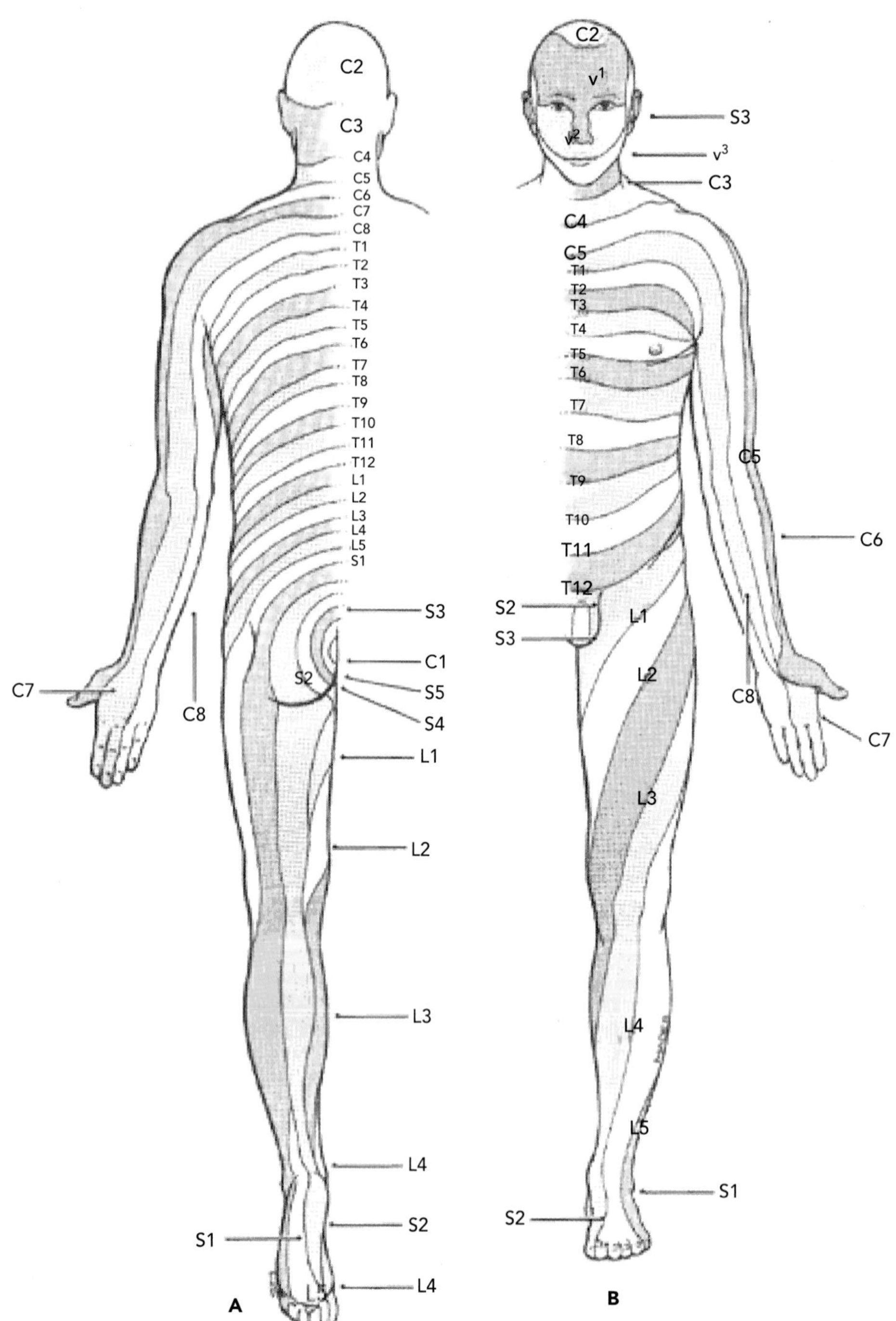

Figure 25A.4 Dermatomal distribution of the upper extremity. (*Source:* Reproduced with permission from Agur A, Lee M. *Grant's atlas of anatomy*, 10th ed. Philadelphia: Lippincott Williams & Wilkins, 1999.)

hand on the same shoulder; (e) AC and sternoclavicular joints—the patient places the hands across the chest on the opposite shoulder; (f) horizontal flexion with the arm in abduction—ask the athlete to place his/her arm on the opposite shoulder; (g) protraction and retraction (see discussion on scapular motion); (h) shrug the shoulders—testing the 11th cranial nerve innervating the trapezius) ask the athlete to perform movements that cause pain or those that are believed to be associated with the condition (tennis serve or baseball pitch) (see Table 25A.4).

- *Passive range of shoulder motion.* If the patient has difficulty performing any of the tests mentioned earlier in the active ROM segment, passively repeat each of the movements on the patient yourself.
- *Scapular motion.* It functions as a stable base to allow (a) appropriate positioning of the glenoid; (b) maximize rotator cuff function. Alterations in scapular position and/or motion can occur both as a result or as a cause of injury. There are six possible motions in three different planes. (a) anterior/posterior (A/P) tilt in the sagittal plane; (b) interior/exterior rotation in the transverse plane; (c) upward/downward rotation in the frontal plane. One should observe the dynamic scapula motion from behind a seated patient. During abduction, as the scapula elevates it should tilt posteriorly, externally rotate, and upwardly rotate. Scapular dysfunction occurs when there is alteration in position and/or motion that deviates from normal. Proper stabilization and movement of the scapula is critical to maintain healthy shoulder mechanics. Its role in the function of the shoulder cannot be over emphasized. Scapular dyskinesia is the abnormal movement pattern of the scapula. There are three general patterns/types of dyskinesia. Type 1—winging or prominence of the inferior angle. Type 2—winging/prominence of the entire medial border. Type 3—winging/prominence of the superior medial border. These different patterns will guide the rehabilitation of the shoulder. Scapular dyskinesia has clinical implications in all sports, especially pitching. A lack of scapular retraction in pitching will lead to an inability to achieve a full set position during the late cocking phase and will diminish eccentric control (protraction) during follow-through. This places both the shoulder and elbow at risk for injury. Loss of inferior force couple (inferior scapula winging) leads to a loss of control of elevation with a relatively protracted scapula which can lead to impingement problems. Scapular dysfunction must be addressed as a part of the patients' rehabilitation. Experienced physical therapists are helpful in retraining the scapula stabilizing muscles and returning normal scapular function. Scapula dyskinesia can be either a primary or secondary cause of dysfunction. Identification and treatment of causative factors is crucial to restoring proper scapulohumeral mechanics. Look beyond the shoulder complex as pain is often the symptom of dysfunction somewhere in the kinetic chain.
- *Muscle testing*
  - *Supraspinatus*—resistance to initiation of abduction. The athlete's arm should be placed at 90 degrees abduction, 60 degrees of horizontal flexion, and full internal rotation. The examiner directs the force downward with *two fingers*, not the whole hand (empty can sign).
  - *External rotators (infraspinatus and teres minor muscles act as a unit)*—arm should be adducted to the side, elbow at 90 degrees with the patient externally rotating against resistance.
  - *Internal rotator (subscapularis)*—with the arm still abducted to the side, the elbow at 90 degrees, and the forearm externally rotated, ask the patient to internally rotate against resistance. The Lift-Off test can also be performed. This involves having the patient place the

TABLE 25A.4
NORMAL RANGE OF MOTION AT THE SHOULDER JOINT AND MUSCLES INVOLVED

Movement of the Shoulder	Normal Range of Motion	Muscles Involved
Forward flexion	Approximately 90 degrees	Anterior fibers of the deltoid, pectoralis major, biceps, and coracobrachialis
Extension	Approximately 45 degrees	Posterior fibers of the deltoid, latissimus dorsi, and teres major
Abduction	Approximately 180 degrees	Middle fibers of the deltoid, supraspinatus (initiates), after 120 degrees, assisted by the trapezius, serratus anterior (by rotation of the scapula)
Adduction	Approximately 45 degrees	Pectoralis major, latissimus dorsi, teres major and teres minor
Lateral rotation	Approximately 40–45 degrees	Infraspinatus, teres minor, posterior fibers of the deltoid
Medial rotation	Approximately 55 degrees	Subscapularis, latissimus dorsi, teres major and the anterior fibers of the deltoid.
Circumduction	Combination of the above movements	

back of the hand against the lower back and attempt to move the hand away from the lower back. Failure to do so is a sign of subscapularis injury.
- *Palpate the long head of the biceps in the groove*—external rotation is necessary to find the groove (see discussion on Speed's test in the following text).
- *Deltoid*—resistance/tenderness to abduction past 30 degrees. The deltoid initiates abduction.
- *Scapula stabilizing muscles, such as the serratus anterior (protraction) lower trapezius and rhomboids*—essential to maintain normal scapular kinematics.

- *Tests*
  - *Apprehension*. To test the stability of the GH joint, the arm is abducted and externally rotated while an anterior force is applied. A positive sign is when the patient resists rotation in apprehension of the pain (see Figure 25A.5). This may be performed either seated or supine (referred to as the *crank test*).
  - *Load-and-shift test* (see Figure 25A.5). The patient should sit with no back support and with the hand of the test arm resting on the thigh. The examiner stands behind the patient and stabilizes the shoulder with one hand over the clavicle and scapula. With the other hand the examiner grasps the head of the humerus. The humerus is gently pushed into the glenoid to seat it properly in the glenoid fossa. This is the load portion of the test, and this "seating" of the humerus allows true translation to occur. The examiner then pushes the head anteriorly or posteriorly noting the amount of translation. This is the "shift" portion of the test.
  - *Sulcus sign*. The patient's arm is held at his side in a position of rest. The arm is gently pulled downwards while the examiner looks and palpates for a depression below the acromion.
  - *Impingement tests*. The arm is brought in extreme forward flexion with the humerus externally rotated (Neer's impingement sign see Figure 25A.6). The arm is forward flexed to 90 degrees and medially rotated (Hawkin's impingement sign—see Figure 25A.6) A positive sign is eliciting pain during movement (Painful arc see Figure 25A.6).
  - *Roos maneuver*. This test is used to assess for thoracic outlet syndrome. With this test the arms are abducted to 90 degrees laterally, the shoulder is rotated and the elbows are flexed to 90 degrees so the elbow is behind the frontal plane. Then the patient opens and closes the hands looking for ischemic pain on the affected side in less than 3 minutes.
  - Speed's test for bicipital tendonitis. The shoulder is flexed forward to 90 degrees with the arm extended at the elbow and palm facing up. Pain in the region of the bicipital groove on downward force against resistance suggests bicipital tendonitis.
  - *Hyperabduction*. A test for thoracic outlet syndrome. Abduction of the arm causes numbness.
  - *Crossover test*. A test that differentiates impingement from AC/sternoclavicular injury. This can be done by asking the patient to flex the arm at the shoulder at approximately 90 degrees and adduct across the chest to try to touch the opposite shoulder. A positive test isolates pain to the AC joint.
  - *Test for labral tears*. The tests generally lack both specificity and sensitivity. Various tests include Clunk test, compression rotation test, anterior slide test, and O'Brien's test.

The O'Brien's test (see Figure 25A.7) evaluates for AC joint and/or labral abnormalities. The patient's shoulder is flexed to 90 degrees with the elbow fully extended. The arm is then adducted 15 degrees and the shoulder is internally rotated so that the patient's thumb is pointing down (like pouring out a glass). Downward force is applied against the arm against the patient's resistance. The shoulder is then externally rotated so that the palm is facing up, and the examiner applies a downward force on the patient's arm, which the patient is instructed to resist. A positive test is indicated by pain during the first part of the maneuver with the patient's thumb pointing down, which is then lessened or eliminated when the patient resists a downward force with the palm facing up. Pain in the region of the AC joint is indicative of AC pathology, whereas pain or painful clicking deep inside the shoulder suggests labral pathology (2).

Diagnostic Injections

Occasionally, injection of an anesthetic agent (Xylocaine) into a painful area can assist in making a diagnosis (see Figure 25A.8). It may be possible to determine if the pain origin is the GH or AC joint, subacromial bursae, long head of the biceps tendon, or the result of the biomechanics of an impingement syndrome (Barth, 1989). This is a procedure that should only be done by a physician who is comfortable with the anatomy of the shoulder and who has experience with injections.

Radiographic Studies

Standard x-ray studies should include the following four views:

- *Anteroposterior views*. One is in internal rotation and one in external rotation (see Appendix 25.1.7).
- *Lateral view/scapular-Y view*. The Scapular-Y view is the best view for evaluating impingement and the type of acromion. The Hill/Sachs lesion (see Appendix 25.1.3) is also nicely evaluated. The Hill/Sachs lesion is caused when the humeral head is impacted against the glenoid of the shoulder. This lesion is an injury that causes damage to the head of the humerus. It is usually a complication of a shoulder dislocation. When the shoulder dislocates, the smooth cartilage surface of the humerus is impacted against the rim of the glenoid.

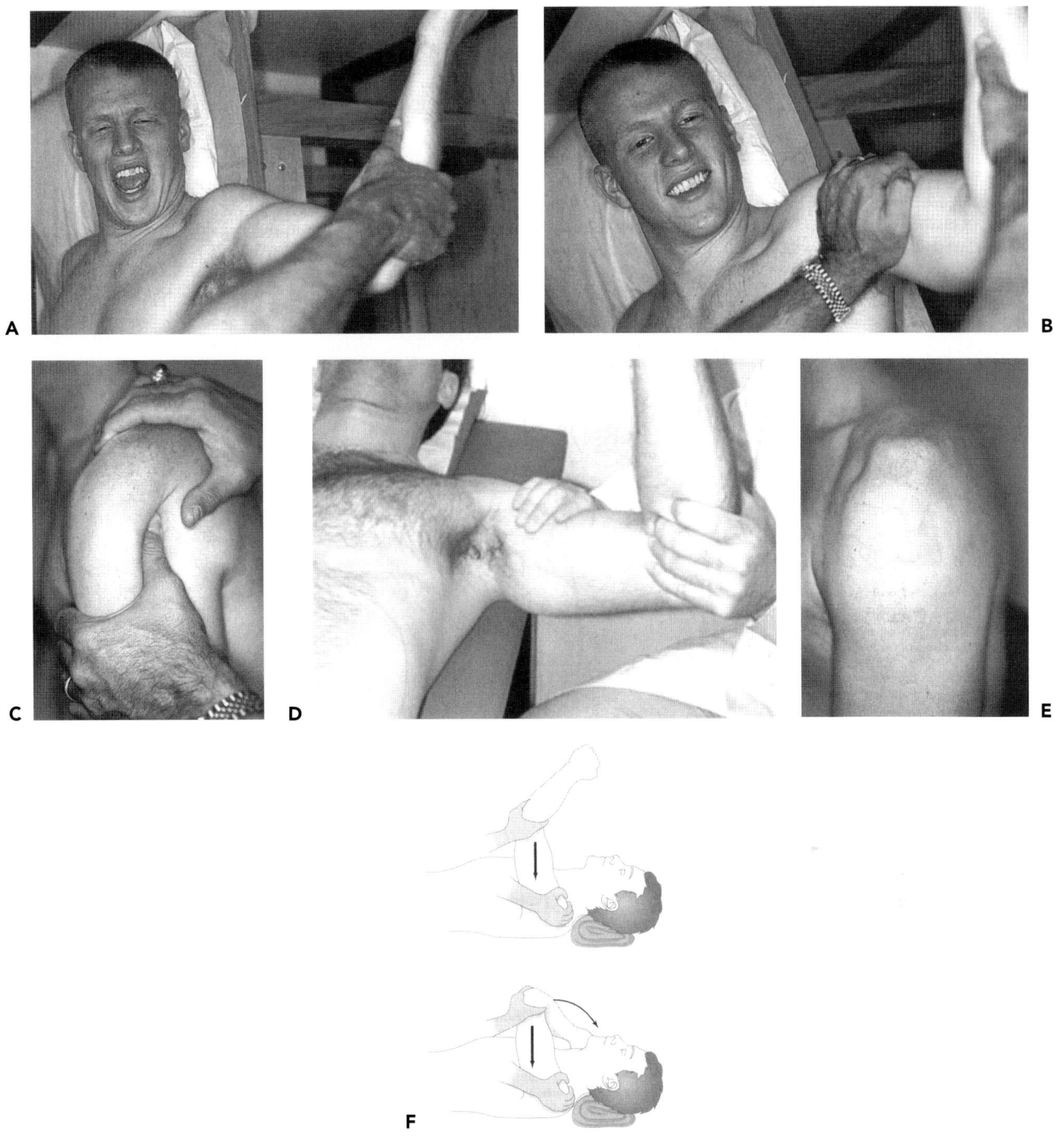

Figure 25A.5 Instability tests. **A:** Apprehension test. **B:** Relocation test. **C:** Load-and-shift test (seated). **D:** Load-and-shift test (supine). **E:** Sulcus sign. **F:** Jerk test. (*Source:* **A, B, C, and E** Reproduced with permission from Miller MD, Howard RF, Plancher KD. *Surgical atlas of sports medicine.* Philadelphia: WB Saunders, 2003, **D:** Reproduced with permission from Miller MD, Cooper DE, Warner JJP. *Review of sports medicine and arthroscopy.* Philadelphia: WB Saunders, 2002; **F** Reproduced with permission from Miller M, Sekiya JK. *Sports medicine: core knowledge in orthopaedics.* Mosby, 2006.)

Radiographically it demonstrates an impaction fracture on the posterior humeral head.

- *Axillary view.* Taken with the arm abducted and the radiographic beam passing inferiorly to superiorly through the axilla to the cassette placed on the superior aspect of the shoulder. This is another lateral view of the shoulder and is excellent for evaluating the position of a shoulder dislocation, as well as glenoid fractures, os acromial, Hill/Sachs lesions, and the lesser tuberosity of the humeral head.

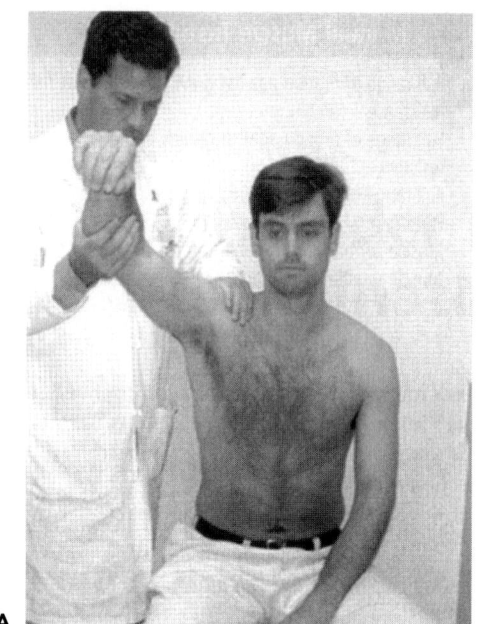

A

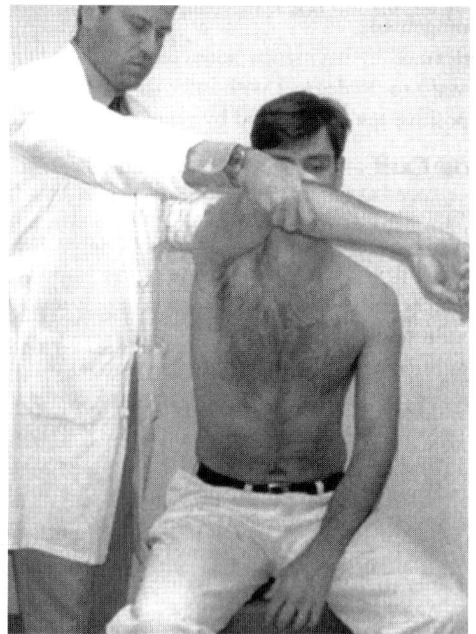

B

180°
170°
Acromioclavicular painful arc
120°
Painless
Glenohumeral painful arc
45°–60°
Painless

C

Figure 25A.6 Impingement tests. **A:** Neer's impingement sign. **B:** Hawkin's impingement sign. **C:** Painful arc. (*Source:* **A and B** Reproduced with permission from Miller MD, Cooper DE, Warner JJP. *Review of sports medicine and orthroscopy*. Philadelphia: WB Saunders, 2002; modified from Hawkins RJ, Hobeika PE. Impingement syndrome in the athletic shoulder. *Clin Sports Med* 1983;2:391 and Magee DJ. *Orthopedic physical assessment*, 4th ed. St. Louis: WB Saunders/Elsevier, 2006.)

Other Diagnostic Tests

Other diagnostic tests may be performed for specific indications and they include the following:

- *Arthrogram*—usually to show full thickness rotator cuff tears. It is invasive and has essentially been replaced with magnetic resonance imaging (MRI) or ultrasound.
- *MRI*—is proving to be most useful in diagnosing soft tissue injuries to the shoulder. It is the gold standard method for noninvasive assessment of the rotator cuff. It is possible to differentiate partial from full thickness rotator cuff tears. Sensitivity of the test increases with MRI arthrogram, which is the test of choice when looking for labral pathology.

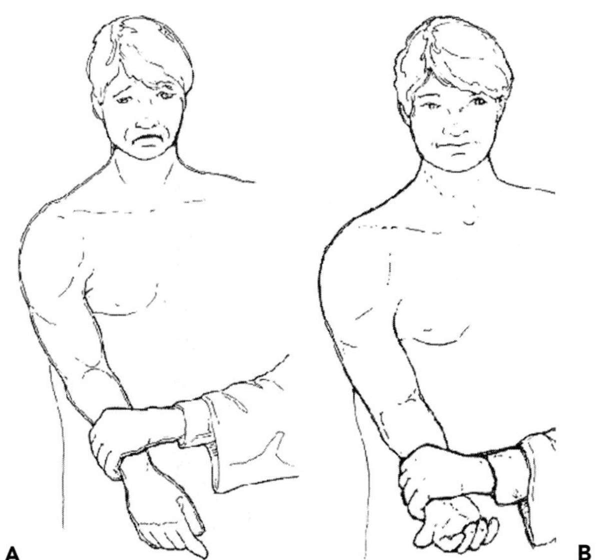

Figure 25A.7 O'Brien's test. Deep anterior pain with **(A)** resisted down force of the adducted 90 degree forward elevated and fully internally rotated arm that is in **(B)** relieved with external rotation. (*Source:* Reproduced with permission from Miller MD, Howard RF, Plancher KD. *Surgical atlas of sports medicine.* Philadelphia: WB Saunders, 2003. Seen in Miller MD, Sekiya J. *Sports medicine core knowledge in orthopaedics.* Philadelphia: Mosby/Elsevier, 2006.)

- *Ultrasound*—notably helpful for partial or full thickness rotator cuff tears. The test requires experience for accurate interpretation.

SPECIFIC INJURIES

Sternoclavicular injuries and clavicle fractures are discussed in detail in Chapter 28. This chapter will focus on injuries of the AC and GH joints, the distal clavicle and soft tissue injuries of the shoulder.

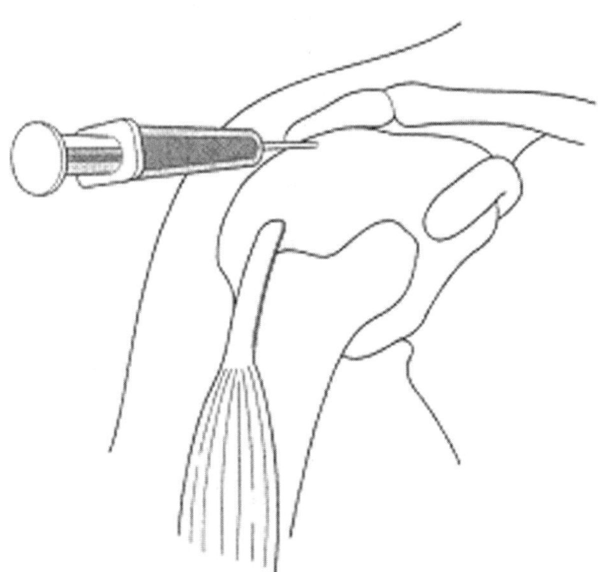

Figure 25A.8 Subacromial injection of 1% xylocaine.

Osteolysis of the Distal Clavicle

Osteolysis of the distal clavicle is usually caused by repetitive overload forces. The problem most likely begins as a stress fracture. Subsequent bone resorption causes cystic and erosive changes and bone remodeling cannot occur because of the continued stress on the joint (see Appendix 25.1.8 for radiology). This can be seen in athletes who perform activities that increase the stress load on the shoulder joint, (e.g., bench press and shoulder presses with a straight bar with improper technique). The patient's chief complaint is pain at the AC joint while performing the movement. Cross arm adduction, on physical examination, usually reproduces the pain. Radiographic examination shows distal clavicular subchondral bone loss and cystic changes. There may be widening of the AC joint during later stages. Bone scans can be helpful to confirm active disease, but is usually not necessary (3).

Nonoperative treatment of distal clavicular osteolysis involves avoiding activities that aggravate the injury. Nonsteroidal anti-inflammatory drugs (NSAIDs), ice and AC joint injections with corticosteroids may help in controlling the symptoms. The injection is diagnostic and will give immediate pain relief. For most athletes, lifestyle modification is not practical and does not lead to significant improvement in symptoms. In athletes who fail nonoperative measures or who cannot modify their activities, distal clavicular resection is the surgery of choice (4). This can be performed open or arthroscopically.

Acromioclavicular Separation

An AC separation accounts for roughly 40% of shoulder injuries in elite athletes participating in high-impact sports (1). An intra-articular meniscoid fibrocartilaginous disc is unique to the anatomy of this small joint. This disc may be absent in as many as half of all shoulders but it seems to be present in most children and young adults. The joint is stabilized by surrounding ligamentous and muscular structures, including trapezius muscles. The mechanism of injury in most AC separations is a fall on the top of the shoulder or a direct blow to it (see Figure 25A.9).

This is commonly seen in wrestling or football. The relatively weak AC ligaments rupture first, followed by the CC ligaments. There are six grades of AC sprains (see Figure 25A.10).

Grade I is by far the most common. There is no laxity of the AC joint or any gross deformity, with the possible exception of swelling over the joint. Radiographs appear normal. Physical examination reveals tenderness to palpation of the joint and pain with motion, especially abduction of the shoulder. Ice should be applied acutely and a sling worn for comfort. When there is no pain at rest, strength and ROM exercises (especially of the deltoid

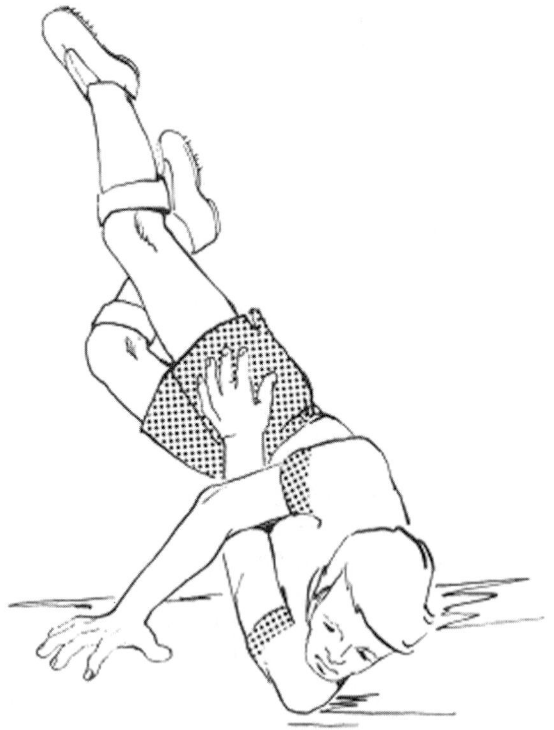

Figure 25A.9 Figure showing the most common mechanism of injury for an AC separation. (*Source:* Reproduced with permission from Rockwood CA, Green DP, ed. *Fractures in adults*, 2nd ed. Philadelphia: JB Lippincott Co, 1994.)

and trapezius muscles) should be begun and continued to the point pain begins. Ice should be applied after exercise. Return to competition is allowed when there is normal flexibility function and lack of symptoms. This takes approximately 1 to 2 weeks (5).

Grade II injuries involve rupture of the AC ligament and capsule, and possible tearing of the CC ligament. A gross defect may be present. Some cases may have little or no involvement of the CC ligament but this is unusual. Special care should be taken to palpate for posterior displacement of the clavicle. The physical examination generally reveals small gross deformity, swelling, tenderness to palpation, significant pain on motion and joint instability elicited by distal pull on the arm at the wrist. In the past, x-ray evaluation included an anteroposterior (AP) standing film of both shoulders with and without weights (10 lb) suspended from wrists (not held in hands). But a study published in 1994 showed that weight-bearing imaging had no benefit over non–weight-bearing imaging and the results do not change the treatment (6).

Elevation and displacement of the distal clavicle less than the width of the clavicle in comparison with the unaffected side is indicative of a grade II injury.

Treatment of grade II is similar to grade I injuries. Treatment includes rest, ice for the first 12 hours, and a sling for support. Encourage the patient to begin gentle ROM exercises and activities of daily living as soon as symptoms permit. This usually takes about a week (7). Return to athletics can be attempted assuming that the athlete has regained a pain-free ROM and demonstrates full strength. This usually takes 6 to 8 weeks. The use of a protective pad placed on the superior aspect of the AC joint to guard against a superior blow may be used to return patients to contact sports more quickly (7). Cosmetic concern over a "bump" over the AC joint should not be a signal for surgical intervention. The rest of the treatment is identical to that of a grade I injury.

Grade III (separation) injuries involve complete rupture of both the AC and CC ligaments. Physical examination reveals a gross deformity with distal clavicle elevation that usually creates a visual and palpable "shelf" or step-off deformity. The x-ray film reveals widening at the AC space as well as the CC space.

Grade III injuries can be divided into two groups: (a) marked prominence of the clavicle on examination indicates that there is a probable penetration of the overlying deltoid muscle, and (b) clavicular prominence demonstrated only by distal pull or weights is associated with spontaneous partial reduction.

Treatment has long been controversial. From a primary care perspective, conservative management appears appropriate. Several recent articles indicate that nonoperative versus operative treatment for type III AC injuries does not show much difference in outcome (8). There is little significant strength deficit in patients treated nonoperatively for complete AC dislocation. A sling for 1 to 2 weeks is recommended followed by early ROM. The Kenny-Howard sling has fallen out of favor because of neurovascular complications and skin breakdown (9). Newer percutaneous and arthroscopic techniques are being studied for acute surgical intervention with promising results. Use of steroids to reduce inflammation has been shown to prolong recovery and return to contact sports.

Grade IV results when the distal end of the clavicle is displaced posteriorly into or through the trapezius muscle. Treatment is usually surgical.

Grade V results when there is disruption of the AC, CC ligaments, as well as disruption of the muscular attachments. This results in separation that is so severe that surgical consultation is mandatory.

Grade VI is an inferior dislocation of the clavicle in which the clavicle is below the coracoid process and may end behind the conjoined tendon of the biceps and coracobrachialis. This requires surgery.

Glenohumeral Subluxation/Dislocation

Inherent instability of the shoulder joint appears to be far more prevalent than was once thought. The very nature and anatomy of this joint makes it a candidate for instability. GH dislocation is defined as complete separation of the articular surfaces without immediate spontaneous reduction. This injury is relatively easy to diagnose given signs, symptoms, and loss of function. However, GH subluxation defined as transient displacement of the joint

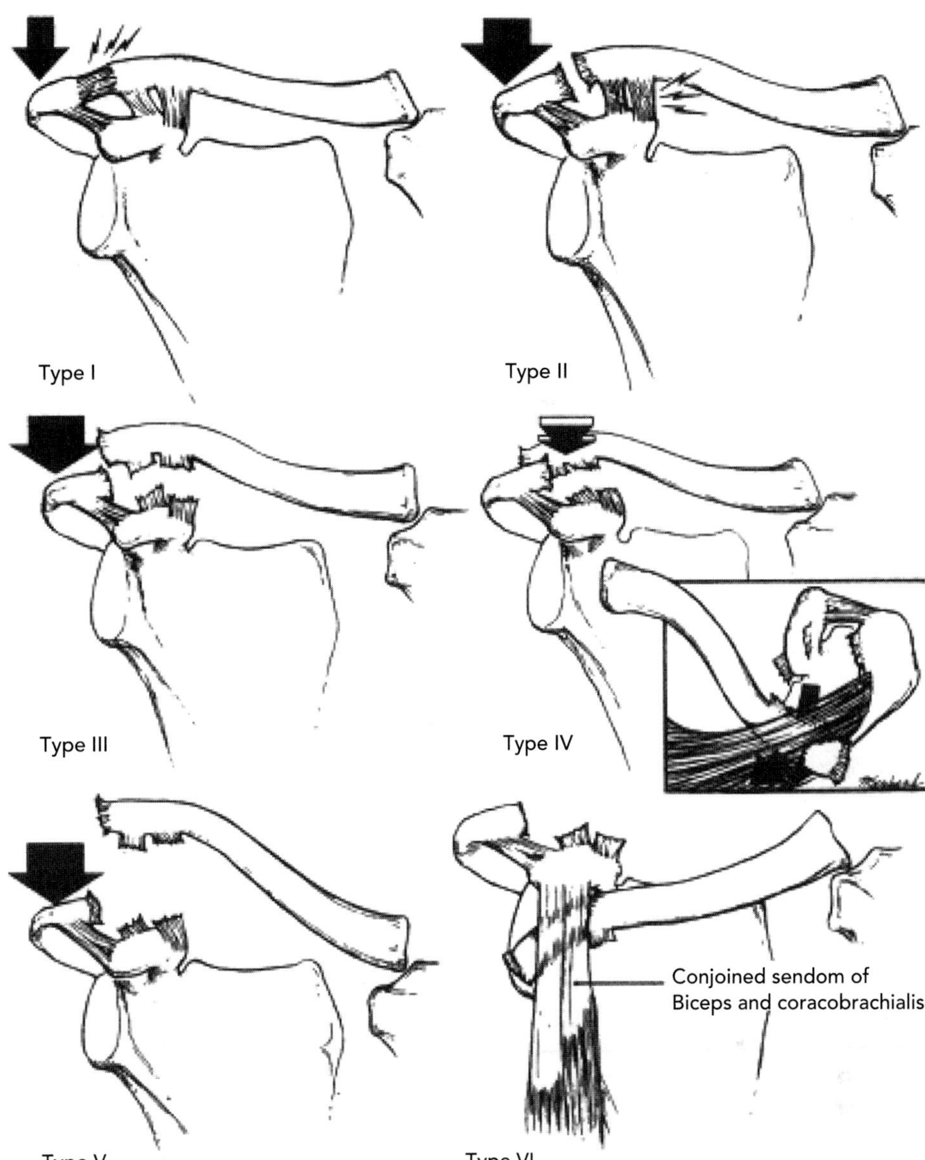

Figure 25A.10 Schematic drawings of the classification of acromioclavicular separation. (*Source:* Reproduced with permission from Rockwood CA, Williams GR, Young DC. Injuries to the acromioclavicular joint. In : Rockwood CR, Green DP, Bucholz R, et al., eds. *Fractures in adults*, 4th ed. Philadelphia: Lippincott–Raven, 1996:1354.)

where the humeral head extends to the edge of the glenoid fossa without dislocation is much more difficult to diagnose than dislocation. Microinstability is also a component of shoulder instability that consists of repetitive micro traumatic or congenital laxity of the GH ligaments and is usually multidirectional. Approximately 95% of all GH dislocations are anterior.

Etiology

Dislocation/subluxation in sports is usually caused by trauma. With a classic anterior dislocation, there is a sudden violent overload. An arm tackle in football, with the arm at 90 degrees abduction in forced external rotation and with extension of the arm, is an example. The humeral head, unstable in its normal relation to the GH fossa, is held into the shoulder joint only by the anterior soft tissue supporting structures. When these are overwhelmed, the shoulder is dislocated, or at least subluxated.

Posterior dislocation is usually associated with severe trauma. Motor vehicle accidents, seizures, and electroconvulsive therapy are the types of trauma most likely to cause posterior instability. Alcohol-associated accidents such as a FOOSH with the shoulder adducted, internally rotated, and the elbow extended will transmit stress to the posterior capsule. Some athletic activities that are capable of producing posterior dislocation include throwing, football, and skiing. Treatment is usually nonsurgical. In athletes with ongoing posterior instability the treatment is arthroscopic posterior labral repair.

Instabilities resulting from chronic stress on the shoulder joint occur in different sports. In the first phase of throwing, abduction and external rotation stress the anterior and inferior structures. In the follow-through (third) phase, stress is on the posterior and inferior shoulder capsule. Similarly, swimming stresses the anterior structures in backstroke and the posterior structures in freestyle. Tennis stresses the anterior structures during the serve and the posterior structures in backhand strokes. Chronic instability as a result of previous dislocation, subluxation, or overuse is considered to be more disabling than periodic recurrent dislocation. If there is atraumatic or recurrent dislocations, consider congenital disorders such as Ehlers-Danlos syndrome.

Symptoms

It is helpful to think of shoulder instability as a continuum, with dislocation at one end of the scale and minimal subluxation (slippage) at the other. The mechanisms and pathophysiology remain the same. Pain will be the only complaint in many patients, which makes diagnosis extremely difficult. Subluxation may start suddenly or have a gradual onset. With dislocations, there is always acute onset of pain and a lack of function which makes diagnosis easier. Where there is a gradual onset of subluxation, patients often complain of pain on the side of the shoulder that is opposite to the instability. In other words, a patient with anterior subluxation may complain of posterior pain. The physician must understand the patient's sport and know the biomechanical factors involved. It is also important to have the patient say which arm position produces pain. Many times, athletes with subluxation present with only apprehension or fear of shoulder instability. This, however, can be as disabling as recurrent dislocations and may require surgical intervention.

Signs

Accurate shoulder evaluation should include assessment of shoulder strength and stability. The position of the shoulder will be in moderate abduction with an anterior dislocation. The contour of the shoulder is flattened and the humeral head is usually palpable below the coracoid process. With a subluxation, the athlete will react when the arm is placed in certain positions. Apprehension suggests instability in that direction. Inferior subluxation can be tested by placing the traction on the wrist and examining the laxity of the GH joint beneath the acromion, the "sulcus sign." This type of laxity often exists in patients with multidirectional instability. Anterior instabilities are tested by having the physician stabilize the scapula and acromion while the arm is abducted and externally rotated. As the examiner pushes the humeral head anteriorly, pain, crepitation, and apprehension are elicited. To detect a posterior instability, the physician pushes the humeral head in a posterior direction while the humerus is adducted and internally rotated and pain and apprehension will be elicited.

The relocation test may add significant information to the instability examination. Initially the crank (apprehension) test should be performed, and if pain/apprehension is elicited, the patient should be placed supine and the test repeated. In the Jobe relocation test, the patient is supine. The patient's abducted arm is externally rotated until pain or apprehension is felt. A posterior force is then applied to the patient's arm and the symptoms of pain and apprehension will be relieved in cases of anterior instability.

Radiological Evaluation

Radiographs are necessary in the evaluation of any dislocation/subluxation. An AP and lateral shoulder view (axillary or scapular Y), are essential to confirm the position of the humerus in acute dislocation. The axillary view helps to rule out a fracture of the humeral head or glenoid labrum.

Please consult preceding text of this chapter for further description of diagnostic imaging techniques.

Types of Anterior Dislocations

There are basically three types of anterior dislocation: subcoracoid (anterior)—most common; subglenoid (inferior)—relatively common, and subclavicular (anteromedial)—rare.

Treatment

Reduction. Acute dislocations of the GH joint should be reduced as quickly as possible. Early reduction minimizes stretching of neuromuscular structures, decreases muscle spasm, and stops further damage to the humeral articular surface. Reduction should be attempted only after assessment of the neurovascular function of the affected extremity. Once the diagnosis of dislocation is made, especially on the field of play, it is not required that a prereduction x-ray be obtained. Ability to perform an on-field reduction depends on the expertise of the examiner. Radiographs should be taken when the physician is uncertain of dislocation or reduction. Prereduction films should be obtained in patients with blunt traumatic mechanism of injury because of the risk of fracture, and postreduction films in those who have fracture dislocation (10). Many reductions can be accomplished without anesthesia if performed shortly after the injury. The extent of anesthesia required for a gentle reduction depends upon the severity of the trauma that produced the dislocation, the number of previous dislocations, the extent of muscle spasm, the presence of "locking" in the dislocation. These factors are frequently associated with the amount of time that has transpired since the dislocation and attempted reduction. If performed immediately on the field, anesthetics are frequently not required. If there is access to lidocaine, an intra-articular injection in the locker room is helpful before the attempted reduction. For difficult dislocations, conscious sedation and rarely general anesthesia may be required.

Reduction of an anterior dislocation is usually performed by applying traction to the abducted, externally rotated, flexed arm along the line of the arm. The patient should be prone or supine with the body fixed. Slight counter traction by an assistant can be helpful. A rocking of the humerus from internal to external rotation can help unlock most dislocations and stretch out the anterior capsule to facilitate the reduction. If spontaneous reduction does not occur when dislocation is unlocked, the physician should internally rotate and adduct the arm. This is basically the modified Kocher method. The Snowbird method, developed at the Snowbird Emergency Clinic in Utah, is a nice way to reduce dislocations, usually without anesthesia. This method is performed with the patient seated in a chair with the chair used as countertraction. The physician applies traction to the affected shoulder using downward pressure on a loop of stockinette wrapped around the patient's forearm (11).

Other methods of anterior GH dislocation reduction include (a) the Simpson method. With this method the patient lies on a table with a weight or tension on the arm. If done gradually, gravity and/or the tension/weight with some muscle relaxation will spontaneously reduce the humerus; (b) the Milch method where the physician externally rotates and abducts the arm overhead, unlocking the head of the humerus, then pushes the humeral head posteriorly back into place and returns the arm to a normal relaxed position. Self-reduction can be taught to patients with recurrent dislocations. The patient is taught to wrap the arms around the knees with the uninjured hand grabbing the other at the wrist/forearm. The knee acts as a fulcrum while the patient leans back causing traction.

After any reduction, the physician should reassess neurovascular status and the integrity of the rotator cuff.

Reduction of rare posterior dislocations are preformed in the exact opposite manner, placing the arm in adduction and doing internal rotation as traction is applied.

Rehabilitation. The goal of rehabilitation for shoulder dislocation/subluxation is to optimize shoulder stability. Immobilization is the main stay of therapy. Immobilization has not been shown to reduce the incidence of recurrent dislocation. Reported recurrence rates of anterior dislocations, particularly in younger athletes who throw overhead, are as high as 90%. Symptoms of instability persist for as many as 50% to 60% (12,13). A newer method of immobilization with the arm externally rotated to approximately 10 degrees increases contact forces and may increase the healing rate. Recent studies with this method have shown promise in decreasing recurrent dislocation rates (14). Rehabilitation is begun following the immobilization period, emphasizing the muscles of internal rotation and adduction. Progressive isometric exercises should target the subscapular and infraspinatus muscles. Mild resistance exercises with rubber tubing can be used along with free weights. For the first 2 or 3 weeks of active rehabilitation, the athlete should use a sling during the day to rest the shoulder muscles and avoid overstress. After 4 to 5 weeks, the patient will progress to complete shoulder rehabilitation exercises on all aspects.

Treatment of the young athlete. Keep in mind that the young athlete with an anterior shoulder dislocation has such a high risk of redislocating that surgery is frequently required. Arthroscopic Bankart repair results in significantly less recovery than open repair and has led many orthopedic surgeons to elect surgery acutely in the young athlete.

Return to competition. This decision should be individualized, on the basis of the skill level of the athlete, the type of competition, and the intensity of the sport (15). Full ROM should be achieved before return to practice. Also, the athlete should be able to perform internal and external rotation against resistance equal to his/her body weight before being able to return to competition.

Associated Injuries

The following injuries are commonly associated with dislocation/subluxation of the GH joint and the physician should have a high index of suspicion for them during examination.

1. *General Injuries*
   (a) Joint capsule injury
   (b) Glenoid apophyseal avulsions in the young athlete
   (c) Capsular tear in older patients
   (d) SLAP (superior labrum anterior posterior) tears of the glenoid labrum.
2. *Fractures*
   (a) Greater tuberosity of the humerus—most common (but results in no chronic instability).
   (b) Glenoid rim (labrum) aka Bankart lesion—chronic instability results particularly if more than 25% of the rim is involved in the fracture.
   (c) Hill-Sachs defect caused by a compression fracture of the posterolateral aspect of the humeral head.
3. *Neurovascular injury*
   (a) Axillary nerve
   (b) Axillary artery

   Consider rotator cuff tears—especially in athletes above 40 years of age.

Keep in mind that recurrent GH instability may have many causes. There is no essential pathological lesion. Correct diagnosis is necessary for appropriate treatment.

OVERUSE INJURIES OF THE SHOULDER

Syndromes resulting from repeated use of the shoulder can be categorized according to the phase of motion during which symptoms appear. Overuse syndromes are a result of microtrauma rather than macrotrauma. Throwing is the most common shoulder action in sports and there are six phases: (a) wind-up, (b) stride, (c) arm cocking, (d) arm acceleration, (e) arm deceleration, and (f) follow-through (see Figure 25A.11).

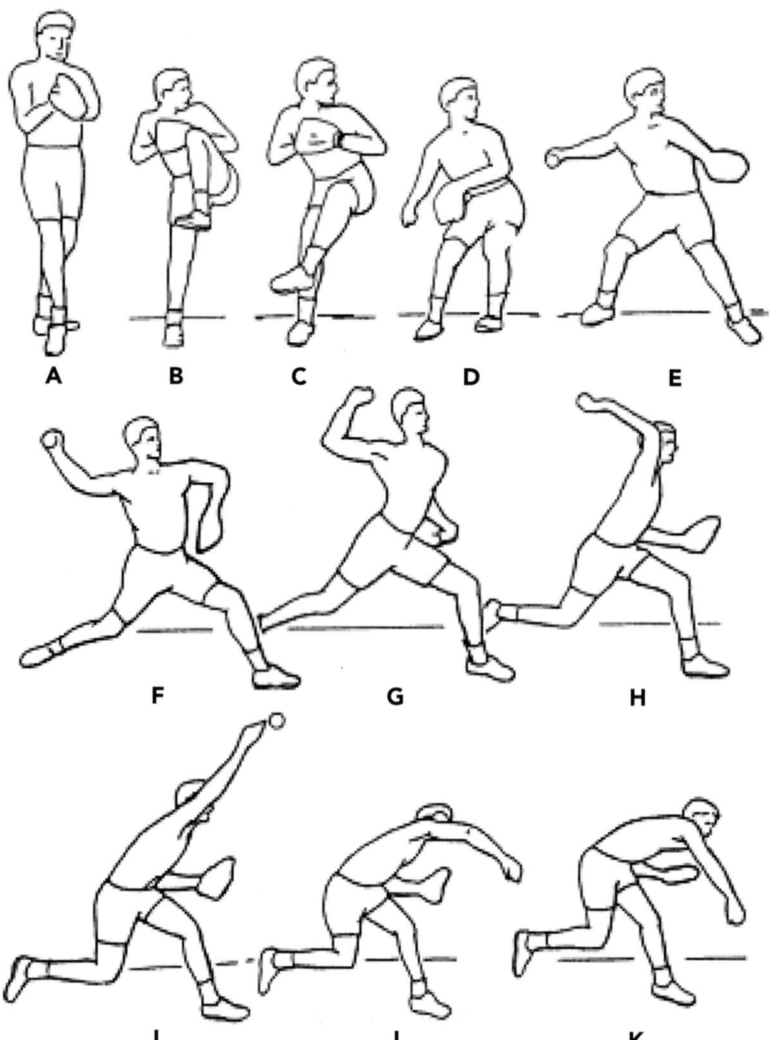

Figure 25A.11 The six phases of pitching: Wind-up **(A–C)**, stride **(C–F)**, arm cocking **(F–G)**, arm acceleration **(H–I)**, arm deceleration **(I–J)**, and follow-through **(J–K)**. (*Source:* Reproduced with permission from Dillman CJ, Fleisig GS, Andrews Jr. Biomechanics of pitching with emphasis upon shoulder kinematics. *J Orthop Sports Phys Ther* 1993;18:402–408.)

Wind-up. Starts with a two-legged stand and ends with maximum knee lift with the lead leg. The body's weight is shifted posteriorly, the lead leg is flexed, and the hands are in front of the chest. Forces on the shoulder are minimal in this early phase.

Stride. The upper extremity's energy is stored as both arms abduct and separate from each other. External rotation is initiated in the throwing shoulder. The active muscles include the deltoid, upper trapezius, supraspinatus, and serratus anterior. Kinetic energy builds as the lead leg moves towards the target. The stride ends when the forefoot hits the ground.

Arm cocking. Cocking begins when the lead foot hits the ground and ends with maximal external rotation at the shoulder. Upper extremity elastic energy accumulation continues during the arm-cocking phase. There is maximal external rotation of the humerus reaching between 150 and 180 degrees. There is extension of the elbow and the ball reaches its furthermost position behind the body, causing a peak in elastic energy. Once the lead foot plants, kinetic energy is incorporated. The pelvis and upper torso rotate causing more torque. The cocking phase consists of two phases, early and late cocking phases. In the early phase, the trapezius and serratus anterior position the glenoid through scapular protraction and upward rotation. The scapular stabilization forces work with the deltoids and supraspinatus to abduct the arm. In the late cocking phase, external rotation of the humerus reaches maximum levels. Eccentric activities by the subscapularis and pectoralis major and latissimus dorsi greatly increase. External rotation is also caused by the serratus anterior, infraspinatus, and teres minor. These muscles also counteract anterior translation of the humeral head. Biceps contraction peaks while the supraspinatus activity diminishes during this phase.

Arm acceleration. Arm acceleration begins with the humerus internally rotating and ending with the ball release. During acceleration, kinetic energy from the torso is passed to the upper extremity. Musculature of the shoulder not only transmits this energy but builds velocity as well. Extension of the elbow increases ball velocity by linear velocity as a result of elbow extension. Secondly, the angular velocity of internal rotation of the shoulder is augmented because extending the elbow reduces the amount of inertia resisting in internal rotation. Major muscle activity is seen in this phase through muscles, posterior deltoid and supraspinatus, pectoralis major, teres minor, the latissimus dorsi, and subscapularis.

Arm deceleration. This phase begins with ball release and ends with the humerus at maximal internal rotation. These muscle forces are eccentric. It has been shown that these eccentric loads generate the greatest tensile forces. It is the rapidly decreasing angular velocity that generates substantial torque at the shoulder. Scapular muscle activity is maximal during deceleration. The middle and posterior deltoid muscle is responsible for antagonism to the humeral head. The teres minor and latissimus dorsi continue with peak activity, while the pectoralis major decline.

Follow-through. This is the last phase of throwing. It consists of continued energy dissipation beginning with maximum internal rotation and ending when the thrower reaches a balanced position. There is low-grade eccentric loading of shoulder muscles that occurs during follow-through.

Some Causes of Shoulder Pain During the Throwing Phases

Cocking or Recovery Phase

Anterior shoulder pain can be caused by chronic inflammation of the anterior rotator cuff, including the subscapularis and supraspinatus muscles. Other muscles involved that can contribute to anterior shoulder pain include the pectoralis major, anterior deltoid, or the long head of the biceps. The latissimus dorsi can be involved. Generally speaking, anterior shoulder pain encountered in the cocking or recovery phase is due to a problem of eccentric muscle loading.

Acceleration Phase

Injuries in the acceleration phase have been categorized as those of friction or muscle fatigue (16).

Friction injuries. The prototypical friction injury is impingement syndrome. Inflammation of the bursa surrounding the shoulder, specifically the medial scapular bursae, falls into the category of friction injuries in the acceleration phase.

Fatigue injuries. The maximum muscle power of an athlete's throw, stroke, lift, or pull takes place in this phase so that muscles subjected to repeated heavy loading can fatigue. This results in stress fractures at muscle insertions or origins.

Because a great amount of torque is developed about the humerus during the acceleration phase, it is not surprising that stress fractures or even complete fractures of the proximal humerus have been seen (17). These are sometimes referred to as spontaneous ball-throwing fractures of the humerus. The muscles involved depend upon the sport and include the following:

- Insertion of the pectoralis muscle—ringman's shoulder (gymnastics)
- Subscapularis, coracobrachialis/short head of the biceps at the attachment on the elbow (swimming, gymnastics)
- Triceps and teres minor originating on the lateral border of the scapula (swimming)

Follow-through Phase

Characteristically the follow-through phase involves deceleration. Injuries in this phase are largely the result of the eccentric load placed on the posterior structures of the shoulder. Posterior lesions occur in throwing athletes as a result of rapid deceleration. The posterior rotator cuff may have varying degrees of inflammation in muscle insertions and the shoulder capsule. The rhomboid muscles can also be injured during this phase as acceleration is completed, with scapula rotation laterally and the rhomboids, levator scapulae, and inferior trapezius muscles acting to reverse that lateral rotation. Inflammation and tendinitis are the most common types of injury. Tendinitis of the rhomboid and levator scapulae muscles must be differentiated from the medial scapular bursitis often seen as a result of friction in the acceleration phase.

In the normal throwing shoulder, translation and rotary motion is a function of static capsular restraint and dynamic muscular action. The repetitive forces involved in throwing can eventually alter performance of one of the soft tissue components, leading to dysfunction. Jobe and Jobe (18) pointed out how repetitive microtrauma, also known as the "overuse" syndrome, in excess of normal physiological function causes injury in soft tissue. Stresses inflicted upon the anterior capsular structures overstrain these tissues, leading to fatigue and failure.

A common physical finding in the throwing shoulder is increased external rotation and decreased internal rotation. This implies relative laxity of the anterior inferior capsule.

Treatment of throwing injuries should lay emphasis on proper throwing mechanics. This frequently may involve the use of video and the expertise of a throwing coach. Emphasis on a return to the normal kinetic chain of throwing motion is essential to prevent further overuse injuries. Particular attention should be directed towards returning normal scapular stabilization and kinematics. Treatment should address the specific pathology (see Figure 25A.12). The most common lesions in the shoulder that result from throwing include superior labral tears or detachment and partial tearing of the rotator cuff.

ROTATOR CUFF INJURIES

Rotator cuff injuries refer to diagnoses specific to the tendinous attachments that make up the muscles of the rotator cuff. These injuries can be caused either by chronic

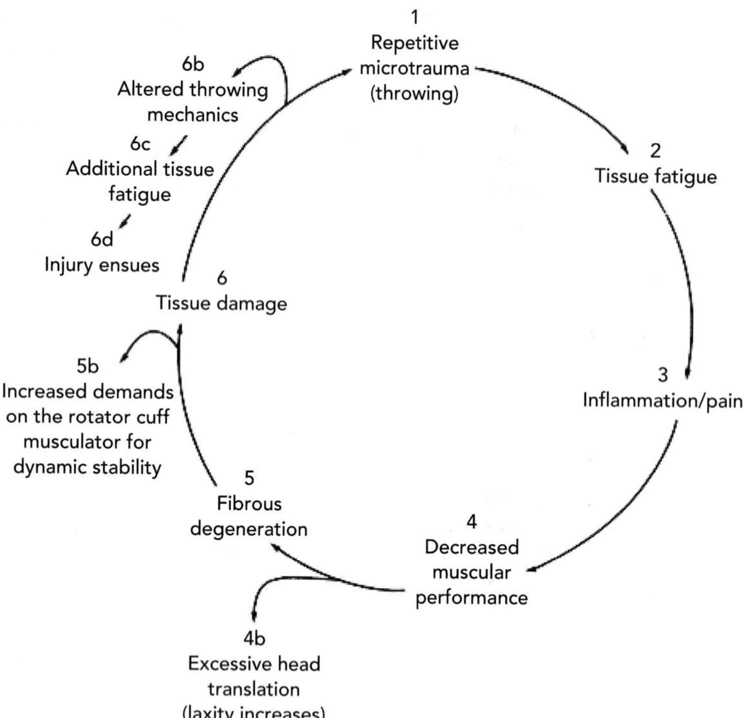

Figure 25A.12 Circular diagram of pathological forces involved in the throwing shoulder. (*Source:* Reproduced with permission from Andrews JR, Wilk KE. Shoulder injuries in baseball. In: Andrews JR, Wilk KE, eds. *The athlete's shoulder.* New York: Churchill Livingstone, 1994:369–389.)

repetitive microtrauma (as discussed in the preceding text), acute macrotrauma, or a combination of both. Rotator cuff injuries are the most common sports related to shoulder injury. The shoulder plays a major role in virtually all sports where activities involve repetitive use of the arm above the horizontal level of the shoulder and may create some of the most damaging injuries. Specifically, they can lead to impingement of any of the rotator cuff tendons.

Functional Anatomy

Four muscles form an inverted U-shaped reinforcement of the GH joint. They act in common, drawing the humeral head into the shallow glenoid fossa. These muscles, taken in order of attachment to the humeral head from anterior to superior to posterior aspect, are as follows:

Subscapularis the major attachment of the rotator cuff responsible for internal rotation of the humerus and downward rotation of the humeral head into the GH joint.

Supraspinatus forming the major superior attachment of the rotator cuff and lying underneath the coracoacromial ligament. This muscle and its tendinous attachment is responsible for elevation and abduction of the humerus and for upward traction of the humeral head into the GH joint. It is the major muscle affected in impingement syndrome.

Infraspinatus forms the posterior–superior attachment of the rotator cuff and is responsible for external rotation of the humerus and downward traction of the humeral head into the GH joint.

Teres Minor forms the posterior–inferior attachment of the rotator cuff. It is responsible for external rotation of the humerus in concert with the infraspinatus muscle and downward traction into the GH joint.

Impingement Syndrome

The space between the under surface of the acromion and the superior aspect of the humeral head is called the *impingement interval.* This space is normally narrow and is maximally narrowed when the arm is abducted. Any condition that further narrows the space may cause impingement.

The subacromial space is very limited and that predisposes the rotator cuff tendons to become mechanically impinged if any of these tendons are injured or swollen. Impingement can result from extrinsic compression (e.g., tendon edema/bone spurring) or as a result of loss of competency of the rotator cuff and/or scapula stabilizing muscles. The biceps tendon also passes within this space. Bigliani classified the curve of the acromion into three types (see Figure 25A.13).

He found a relation between the acromial shape and the presence of rotator cuff tears (19). The greater the curve the higher the incidence of rotator cuff tears and impingement.

Neer, Welsh and others such as Nirschl have postulated the basis for impingement injury to be the result of one of the following two mechanisms (20):

1. According to Neer, the vast majority of such cases are due to primary impingement of the rotator cuff muscles/tendons as a result of the anatomical restrictions of the subacromial space. The contents of this narrowed

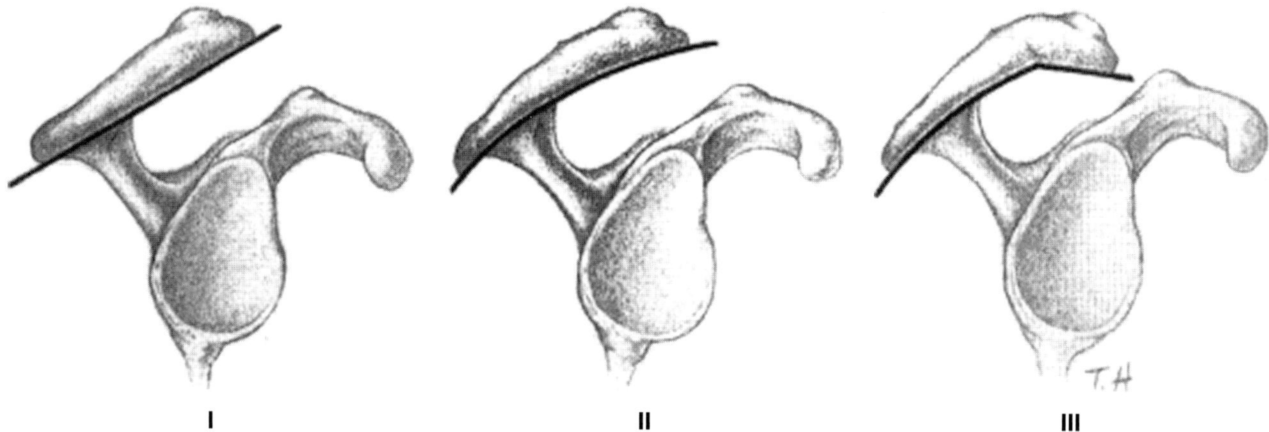

Figure 25A.13 Morphology of the acromion. Type I flat. Type II curved. Type III hooked. (*Source:* Reproduced with permission from Esch JC. *Op Tech Orthop* 1991;1:200; in Miller M, Sekiya J. *Sports medicine; core knowledge in orthopaedics.* Philadelphia: Mosby/Elsevier, 2006.)

space would rub against elements of the coracoacromial arch when repetitive shoulder action is performed, especially in elevation and internal rotation, which eventually leads to compressive tendonitis. The structure exposed to maximum impingement is the area of insertion of the supraspinatus tendon, but the biceps tendon, subacromial bursa, and even the acromialclavicular joint may be involved as well.

2. Nirschl argues that the primary cause is multiple repetitions of stretch injury under contractile load, or intrinsic overload of the musculotendinous unit, leading to tensile tendonitis. It is true that impingement does complicate the process, but it is due to the swelling of the subacromial bursa and/or inflammation of the muscle/tendon and is therefore secondary in nature. Secondary impingement may also result from pain, which causes reflex inhibition and weakness of the rotator cuff muscles, which in turn, fail in their function to center the humeral head in the glenoid. Subsequent translation superiorly then adds to the impingement by further decreasing the subacromial space. Other factors, such as poor scapular control, capsular laxity, instability and abnormal biomechanics may also contribute to secondary impingement.

History and Physical Examination

Pain, weakness and a loss of motion are the most common impingement symptoms reported.

The clinical picture of an athlete with rotator cuff problems can include a wide variability in signs and symptoms. These can range from minimal pain with activity without weakness or restricted ROM, to marked tendinitis accompanied by significant pain and decreased ROM, and/or pain with significant weakness that may signal a tear. Rotator cuff impingement syndrome is caused by repetitive microtrauma. Neer classically described impingement as consisting of three stages. Stage I involves edema and hemorrhage of the supraspinatus tendon and subacromial bursa. Stage II disease involves fibrosis and tendonitis. Stage III generally occurs in patients over 50 years of age and is a process of attrition and the culmination of fibrosis and tendinosis that have been present for many years. This can lead to full thickness cuff tears (21).

The physical examination should focus on the signs of impingement. This includes observing scapulothoracic motion while the patient abducts the shoulder. The affected side usually reveals early firing of the upper trapezius and weakness of the scapula stabilizing muscles leading to slight winging of the inferior medial scapula border. This usually produces a painful arc at approximately 90 to 120 degrees of abduction. The patient will also usually have a positive Neer's and/or Hawkin's impingement test.

Plain radiographs are useful in depicting anatomical variants or calcific deposits. The scapular-Y view is especially useful because it shows the subacromial space and can differentiate the three types of acromial processes. The AP view is helpful in assessing the GH joint, and sclerosis of the greater tuberosity.

Classically, diagnosis of stage III rotator cuff lesions involve arthrograms, however, MRI or ultrasound are becoming more popular procedures than the arthrogram. Shoulder arthroscopy has recently become a more definitive procedure in the workup. Differential diagnosis of rotator cuff pathology of the shoulder include the following:

- Acute bursitis
- Chronic shoulder instabilities
- Primary AC pathology
- Frozen shoulder syndrome (adhesive capsulitis)
- Suprascapular nerve injury
- Cervical radiculopathy

The approach to treatment of rotator cuff injuries should be conservative, avoiding surgery whenever possible. Impingement syndromes involving the supraspinatus and biceps tendons are by far the most common causes of stage I, II, and III injuries. The examiner should also distinguish between primary and secondary impingement. Initial treatment of both problems is conservative, but when this treatment fails the surgical approach to the two problems differs markedly. In the older patient the finding is usually supraspinatus degeneration and a decreased impingement interval. This is primary impingement and the surgical treatment is arthroscopic debridement and acromioplasty. In contrast the younger patient is more likely to have secondary impingement, with an underlying problem of instability. Therefore, the primary problem in athletes is instability with the secondary problem being impingement syndrome. Secondary impingement can occur when fatigue and dysfunction of the rotator cuff and scapula stabilizers cause the humeral head to migrate superiorly within the GH joint impinging the rotator cuff tendons under the coracoacromial arch. The main approach to this problem both conservatively and surgically is to address the instability as well as the impingement.

Not all cuff tears diagnosed by MRI, ultrasound or clinically require surgery. The age of the patient and the expected demands must be considered. Many elderly patients with cuff tears do well nonoperatively. Survey studies using MRI have shown a high incidence of rotator cuff tears in asymptomatic adults. Most participants younger than age 60 with full thickness cuff tears and impaired function usually require surgery. Most cuff tears in an experienced surgeon's hands can and should be repaired arthroscopically, whenever possible. Patients with an intact rotator cuff and ongoing impingement symptoms in spite of adequate conservative care usually do well with an arthroscopic debridement/acromioplasty.

Conservative medical management of lesser rotator cuff injuries involves the following:

- *Strengthening.* All shoulder muscles, in general, should be strengthened especially the external and internal rotators. Particular attention must be made to normalizing the scapula function/motion. The exercises should be pain free and useprogressive resistance (PRE).
- *Biomechanical and training changes.* As with any overuse injury, decreasing or changing the practice regimen is imperative. In swimming, this means decreasing yardage, changing biomechanics of the stroke, and paying specific attention to careful warm-up exercises. It may be necessary to temporarily change a swimmer from long distance training to sprinting to decrease the repetitive microtrauma. In baseball, it is usually necessary to change the throwing technique and perhaps the type of pitch. It is also important to decrease the number of pitches. With tennis, the stroke may need to be changed, with special emphasis on changing the position of the body or attempts to put "spin" on the ball. Decreasing the intensity of the serve is also important. Looking at the entire kinetic chain is crucial to returning athletes back to competition without reinjury. This is especially important in overuse sports, such as throwing or swimming. Adequate core strength is a vital part of the kinetic chain.
- *Ice.* Ice should be applied directly to the area after all exercise for 10 to 15 minutes.
- *Heat and deep muscle massage.* This therapy is impractical to increase the blood supply. However, if used, it should be done before exercise.
- *Electrical stimulation.* Temporary relief of pain can be achieved by using a muscle or nerve stimulator. Electrogalvanic stimulation is used where swelling is evident.
- *Medications.* NSAID medications can be used but only after an accurate clinical diagnosis has been made and masking of the pain in the individual is not a significant factor.
- *Corticosteroid injection.* Injected into the subacromial space may be helpful in resolving pain in an inflamed shoulder. Reducing pain is important so the patient may begin the rehabilitation exercises.
- *Rest.* Relative rest should be imposed. The activity producing the pain should be decreased and maintenance of cardiovascular fitness should be accomplished either with decreased regimen or by alternative exercise.
- *Prevention.* Stretching and strengthening exercises as well as warming up before activity.

Chronic rotator cuff tears with GH arthritis is becoming a more frequent problem with our aging population. Total shoulder arthroplasty is very successful for isolated severe GH arthritis. However, for GH arthritis along with chronic rotator cuff tears, there is a new procedure that has been approved by the USFDA in March of 2004 called the *reverse shoulder replacement surgery*. It consists of reversing the ball and socket of the shoulder. It is reserved for those patients who suffer rotator cuff tear arthropathy or irreparable rotator cuff injury, or those who suffer arthritis or failed shoulder replacement surgery. The reverse ball and socket total shoulder implant is designed to restore overhead shoulder function in the presence of irreparable rotator cuff deficiency by using the intact deltoid muscle and the stability provided by the prosthetic design. The purpose is to evaluate the clinical and radiographic results of this arthroplasty in a consecutive series of shoulders with painful pseudoparesis due to irreversible loss of rotator cuff function (22).

SUPERIOR LABRUM ANTERIOR TO POSTERIOR LESIONS

These lesions were first recognized by Andrews et al. in 1985 and later described as "SLAP" (superior labrum anterior to posterior) by Snyder and Walsh in 1991 when they saw pathological changes to the superior labrum during arthroscopic surgery. Different mechanisms have been proposed for SLAP lesions. Falling on the outstretched arm causing a traction or compression injury related to the fall (23). Overhead throwing motion in the deceleration phase causing traction on the superior labrum by the bicep muscle (24). The cocking phase of the overhead throw causes a torsional peeling-back stress to the glenoid

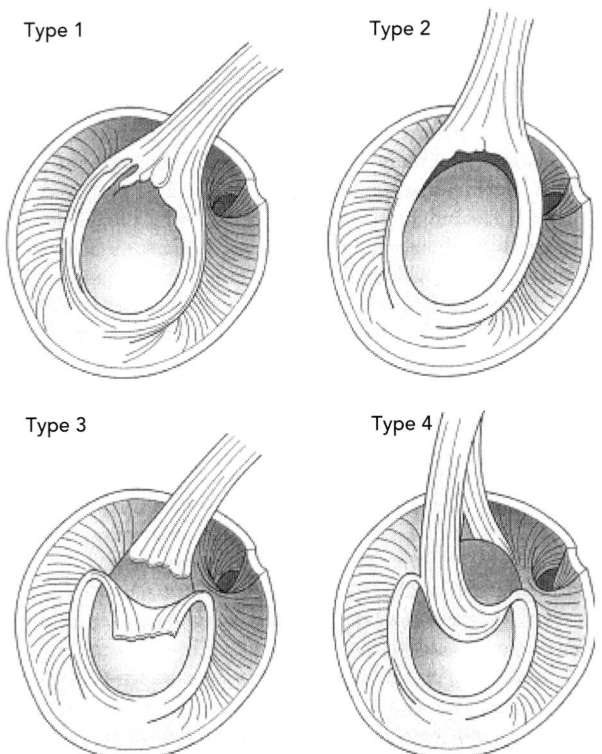

Figure 25A.14 Classification of superior labral anterior to posterior lesions.

labrum leading to a SLAP lesion (25). The (Snyder and Walsh) classification of SLAP lesions has been described in four types (23). Type 1 lesions involve fraying injury to the superior labrum without detachment of the biceps tendon. Type 2 lesions are seen when the biceps tendon is detached from the supraglenoid tubercle. Type 3 lesions are characterized by bucket handle tearing of the superior labrum without detachment of the biceps tendon. Type 4 lesions involve a tear of the superior labrum and extend into the biceps tendon (see Figure 25A.14).

Patients may complain of vague deep shoulder pain associated with a popping, catching or grinding sensation with overhead movements. Differentials can include impingement syndrome, AC joint pain, biceps tendon abnormalities, or GH instability.

Physical examination findings include tenderness at the rotator interval. The crank test causes pain or a click with varying positions while internally rotating. There is GH internal rotation deficit compared to their nondominant shoulder. Plain radiographs are not helpful in diagnosing SLAP lesions. The gold standard test is an MRI arthrogram with gadolinium. Treatment is surgical.

BICEPS TENDON INJURY

Biceps tendon injuries are common. This musculoskeletal soft tissue unit is anatomically and pathophysiologically involved with the shoulder but is unrelated to GH or "true" shoulder movement. The biceps brachii has two heads but only one common tendon insertion on the tuberosity of the radius. The short medial head originates from the coracoid process whereas the long head comes from the superior lip of the glenoid fossa traveling through the bicipital groove in the humeral head. This bicipital groove is covered by a transverse humeral ligament "roof". The biomechanical action of the biceps tendon is primarily supination of the forearm and elbow flexion. It should be pointed out that the biceps tendon does not move within the groove without movement of the GH joint.

There are three types of injuries to the biceps tendon: biceps tendinitis, dislocation of the biceps tendon, and biceps tendon rupture. Many biceps injuries are associated with rotator cuff stage II and impingement injuries. One third of all rotator cuff tears in older patients also involve the biceps. The etiology, biomechanics, presentation, and treatment of accompanied biceps tendon injuries are very similar to that of impingement syndrome.

Biceps Tendonitis

Inflammation of the biceps tendon involves the following one or two mechanisms:

- Trauma to the tendon is secondary to repetitive use or overuse, usually throwing or overhead occupational work, such as baseball or overhead carpentry. Pain and varying degrees of inflammation and edema are seen.
- Sudden violent extension of the elbow can produce bicipital trauma and pain, especially in the younger athlete. Activities where this may occur are basketball, bowling, or power lifting.

Examination reveals tenderness of the tendon when palpated in the groove, sometimes accompanied by crepitation and/or a snapping sensation on flexion of the elbow. The Speed's test or the Yergason's test (requesting the patient to flex the elbow to 90 degrees before the examiner extends the elbow while externally rotating the GH joint) will produce tenderness here.

Treatment consists of limiting activity until the patient is asymptomatic. Uses of NSAIDs, ultrasound and electromuscular stimulation (EMS), as well as ROM exercises are helpful. Once the patient is pain free, strength training is encouraged. Bicipital tendonitis can be associated with impingement syndrome and physical therapy for impingement syndrome is also beneficial for bicipital tendonitis. A word of caution about injecting corticosteroids into the bicipital tendon: they can contribute to further weakening of the tendon and increase the possibility of subsequent rupture, especially if they are repeated. This should be discouraged.

Dislocation of Biceps Tendon

Rarely, the biceps tendon can become dislocated if a tear occurs in the transverse humeral ligament or roof of the bicipital groove. The biomechanics include three types of injuries:

- Sudden interrupting force while the arm is abducted and externally rotated (football quarterback hit on his throwing arm while in the act of throwing).
- Chronic degradation of the soft tissue tendon from repetitive throwing or overhead use.
- A congenital, shallow medial wall of the bicipital groove can predispose the transverse humeral ligament to significant stress that causes subsequent rupture and dislocation. Surgery is rarely indicated in this situation.

Patients typically present with a popping or snapping in the anterior arm, usually associated with pain. Palpation of a subluxating biceps tendon or a snapping sensation is elicited on Yergason's test. Ultrasound or MRI can readily diagnose the biceps tendon dislocation. If the bicipital groove is empty with the tendon lying adjacent, this would be considered diagnostic of a bicipital tendon dislocation.

Surgical treatment includes relocating the tendon in the bicipital groove and repairing the transverse ligament, and sometimes deepening the bicipital groove.

Bicipital Tendon Rupture

Violent trauma may rarely result in complete interruption and tear of the biceps tendon, usually at the musculotendinous junction. This is usually seen in younger athletes. A similar type injury in the older athlete may result from chronic impingement that causes a complete tear. Physical examination reveals classic contraction of the distal muscle unit with balling up of the muscle at the attachment site (Popeye deformity). Surgical reattachment of a complete tear of the long head of the biceps tendon is rarely required. The major disadvantages of conservative treatment include 10% to 15% loss of strength and a cosmetic deformity.

Adhesive Capsulitis (Frozen Shoulder)

Adhesive capsulitis or frozen shoulder results from thickening and contraction of the capsule around the GH joint and causes loss of shoulder motion and pain.

Adhesive capsulitis usually occurs in middle age and is more common in women and diabetic patients. It is not a direct result of sports participation but exercise can unmask the problem. Onset often follows a period of prolonged shoulder immobilization and results in decreased ROM, leading to marked fibrosis and lesions surrounding the shoulder articulation. Another mechanism is that supraspinatus tendonitis spreads to the subacromial bursae causing subsequent bursitis. As the inflammation continues, fibrosis involves the soft tissue tendons, bursae and GH capsule, and synovium, causing subacute decreased ROM.

The syndrome may go through four distinct stages: (a) significant pain on movement of the GH joint without significant restriction in movement usually lasts 1 to 2 months; (b) severe limitation of both active and passive motion (frozen) with associated pain. This lasts usually 3 to 9 months: (c) minimal pain but continued restricted ROM, can last 9 to 15 months; (d) spontaneous recovery usually seen in months 15 to 24 (26). In addition to a painful, stiff shoulder, there may be nocturnal pain, often poorly localized, which frequently extends down the arm. Unique to this condition is a palpable mechanical block to the motion that is not pain related. On physical examination the GH joint motion should be isolated. This motion is severely restricted. The examiner may be fooled into thinking that the patient has fairly good overhead motion if the patient is allowed scapulothoracic movement. A decrease in volume about the GH joint is usually seen on arthrogram, however this is rarely needed as this is a clinical diagnosis. There is no need for further diagnostic studies.

Treatment may include physical therapy to improve ROM. NSAIDs and analgesics to control pain. Daily increasing ROM exercises should be encouraged, however, forced active or passive ROM should be discouraged and is frequently counter productive. A tincture of time is part of the treatment and patients should be informed that this is usually a self-limiting problem. Complete recovery including pain free ROM usually occurs with time. Occasionally, manipulation of the shoulder under general anesthesia followed immediately by physical therapy has proved effective. Rarely, surgical intervention for open release of adhesions is necessary.

Epiphyseal Injury

The preadolescent and adolescent shoulder contains epiphyseal plates, causing the shoulder injury pattern in young athletes to be different from adults. Ligamentous tissue surrounding the GH joint is much stronger than that of the epiphyseal plate. Therefore, an injury that might cause the sprain of a ligament in an adult might fracture a growth plate in an adolescent.

Tibone summarizes four adolescent shoulder injuries (27):

- *"Little League Shoulder"*. This is believed to be the result of a proximal humeral epiphyseal separation secondary to the considerable stresses placed upon the shoulder by throwing or pitching. This repetitive stress can lead to a fracture at the epiphysis of the proximal humerus. Treatment is obvious—total cessation of pitching and throwing. There should be no long-term sequelae if the athlete complies. If an appropriate preseason conditioning and strengthening program is followed, the athlete should be able to return the following season.
- *Acromioclavicular dislocation (grade III separation)*. Unlike the adult pattern of AC dislocation, injuries under the age of 13 are rare. Children most often suffer a fracture of the distal clavicle with rupture of the CC ligament. Surgery is not recommended.
- *GH shoulder dislocation*. Adolescents have a high incidence of GH dislocation. There is also a high incidence of recurrent shoulder dislocation in patients younger than 20 years. It is believed that surgical repair is not appropriate in the average adolescent athlete, but that

aggressive therapy should be advocated to decrease the incidence of recurrence.

- *Sternoclavicular dislocation.* In a sternoclavicular dislocation (SC) dislocation, adolescents usually suffer from fractures of the epiphyseal plate of the proximal clavicle. These fractures heal and remodel well and treatment is conservative.

Brachial Plexus Injuries

Although bony and musculotendinous injuries account for most shoulder injuries in athletes, neurological injury can be one of the most serious and permanent injuries encountered. Shoulder trauma can produce a variety of nerve injuries. There is disagreement in the literature about their nomenclature. Bergfield differentiates the various types of neurological injuries in the shoulder as follows:

Neck sprain. A mechanically induced injury to the neck which produces local pain and stiffness but is not accompanied by neurological symptoms or deficit. There is no fracture or dislocation.

Burner or Stinger phenomenon (cervical nerve pinch syndrome, pinched nerve). A neurological injury accompanied by burning paresthesia and transient neurological deficit probably due to instantaneous stress on a portion of the brachial plexus.

Brachial plexus injury symptoms are similar to Burner phenomenon but with persistent neurological deficit.

Most neurapraxia seen in the upper extremity falls into the category of cervical pinched nerve or Burner syndrome. Contact sports such as football, hockey, wrestling, and the riding sports account for most of the injuries seen in competition.

The brachial plexus is a collection of the ventral rami of spinal nerves C5-T1 (see Figure 25A.15). Injury to the brachial plexus can occur at any one of the following three anatomical levels:

- Cervical nerve root trunk
  a. Upper (superior) trunk—ventral rami of C5 and C6
  b. Middle—ventral ramus of C7
  c. Lower (inferior)—ventral rami of C8 and T1
- Nerve cords—portions of each nerve trunk divide and reform into three nerve cords named according to their relation to the axillary artery.
  a. Lateral—comes off the lateral root to the medial nerve and then becomes the musculocutaneous nerve
  b. Medial cord—gives off the medial root to the medial nerve and then continues as the ulnar nerve
  c. Posterior cord—terminates by dividing into the axillary and radial nerves
- Peripheral nerves—lesions proximal to the plexus occur either in the spinal cord or spinal nerve root and cause

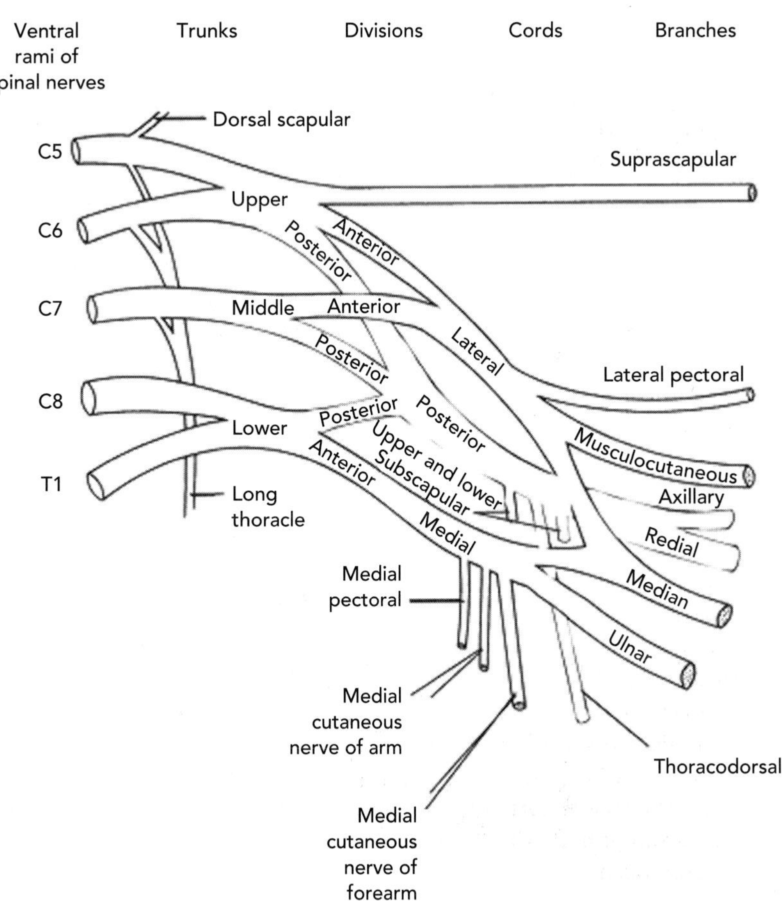

Figure 25A.15 Brachial plexus. (*Source:* Reproduced with permission from Jenkins DB, Hollinshead WH. *Hollinshead's functional anatomy of the limbs and back*, 8th ed. Philadelphia: WB Saunders, 2002.)

sensory and motor deficits on a segmental basis, similar to a cervical disc protrusion. Their sensory deficit follows this dermatome distribution of the upper extremity:

C4—shoulder pad area
C5—lateral aspect of the arm
C6—lateral aspect of the forearm, hand, and radial two digits
C7—middle finger
C8—ulnar two digits and medial aspects of the hand and wrist
T1—middle aspect of forearm
T2—medial aspect of arm

Lesions may involve the plexus itself. The plexus can be damaged by forcible adduction of the arm or any type of traction trauma of the upper extremity. Various segmental deficits may occur, depending upon whether rami trunks, cords, or peripheral nerves are involved.

Injuries may be distal to the brachial plexus and involve one or more peripheral nerves somewhere along their course. Most peripheral nerve injuries are in the super clavicular portion of the brachial plexus near the actual anatomical origin of the nerve. The injuries are sustained either from direct trauma or from traction of the head to the opposite shoulder while the injured shoulder is depressed. This creates a bowstring effect that increases the tightness of the nerve and plexus and predisposes the nerve to a stretch injury. Infraclavicular branches plexus can be involved if the shoulder girdle is elevated so that the axilla is injured.

Specific Injuries

Suprascapular nerve. The suprascapular nerve emerges from the upper trunk and innervates the supraspinatus and infraspinatus muscle. It is usually injured by direct trauma, which causes weakness in both muscles. There will be a loss of external rotation of the scapula. It must be differentiated from the rotator cuff tear in older athletes. Because of its high position in the plexus, it is usually the first to receive the brunt of a severe impact. It may also be entrapped and damaged by a spinoglenoid notch cyst. This cyst is frequently associated with other shoulder pathology such as labral tears. The problem is most frequently seen in overhead activity such as volleyball tennis and throwing sports. The cyst is easily seen on MRI and electromyelogram (EMG) and is also useful to localize the site of compression. Treatment consists of removing the cyst and addressing the underlying shoulder pathology arthroscopically.

Musculocutaneous nerve. This nerve is often injured by direct frontal trauma and is occasionally involved in shoulder dislocations. Weakness in the biceps and a decrease in sensation over the dorsal and lateral aspect of the forearm will be noticed. Fracture of the coracoid process with displacement can also infringe upon this nerve.

Axillary nerve. Axillary nerve injury may occur from direct trauma or from shoulder dislocation. There will be a loss of deltoid musculature and ability to abduct the shoulder. The pocket sign (inability to place hand in pocket) is positive.

Long thoracic nerve. The long thoracic nerve innervates the serratus anterior. Isolated paralysis of this muscle has been reported in weight lifting injuries when traction of the scalenus medius muscle entraps the nerve. This leads to the classic finding of a "winged scapula."

Spinal accessory nerve. This nerve does not directly originate from the cervical nerve roots (it is actually the 11th cranial nerve) but its anatomical course makes it vulnerable when there is trauma to the upper anterior border of the trapezius at the clavicle. This type of injury most often comes from stick contact to the body (field hockey, hockey, lacrosse). Paralysis of the trapezius may result with subsequent rotatory winging of the scapula.

We recommend that the upper thorax as well as major vessels involving the upper extremity be also examined when there is a suspected brachial plexus injury, the reason being that there may be associated thoracic and vascular injuries in these patients.

Initial treatment consists of rest and protection of the injury site while maintaining ROM to the affected joint. Careful repeated monitoring is important because brachial plexus injuries in initial stages can be dynamic, with the full extent of neurological loss not fully appreciated for up to 2 weeks after the initial trauma. Concurrent fractures (including the cervical spine) should be ruled out. If a brachial plexus injury is still a problem after 2 to 3 weeks, an EMG may help demonstrate the extent of the injury. Controversy continues about using electrical stimulation to maintain muscle tone and about the use of oral corticosteroids. A program to maintain cardiovascular fitness is indicated but it should not involve major use of the affected upper extremity.

Return to play should occur only after the individual has fully recovered at least 90% of his neurological status. Repeated examination will be necessary to fully appreciate postinjury muscle weakness. Too early a return to competition places the athlete at much greater risk for reinjury. Obtaining baseline measurements before the start of the season to see how much strength has been lost or gained will be useful.

Several important considerations for the prevention of these injuries include the following:

- Preseason isometric exercises
- Proper coaching technique for blocking and tackling
- Appropriate protective equipment such as properly fitted shoulder pads
- Additional protective equipment such as cervical collars for those individuals predisposed to this type of injury (usually past victims of neurapraxia)

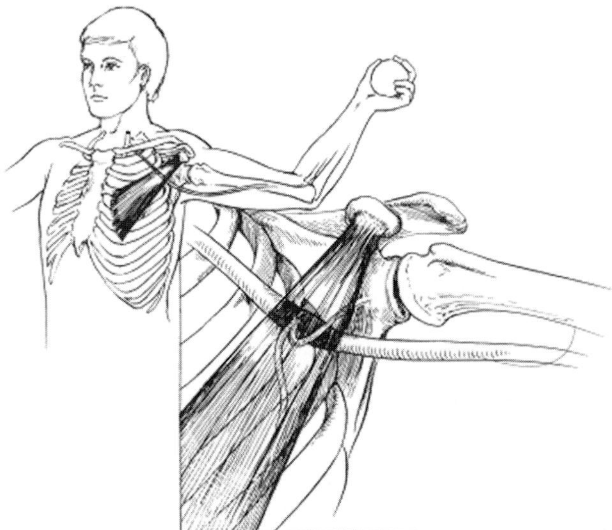

Figure 25A.16 Axillary artery compression by the pectoralis minor muscle at coracoid process insertion in the throwing athlete.

HYPERABDUCTION (WRIGHT'S SYNDROME)

Compression of the brachial plexus and vessels at the thoracic outlet by the pectoralis minor and the coracoid process can result in neurocirculatory signs and symptoms when the arm is hyperabducted. During abduction,. the brachial plexus and axillary vessels are pulled around the pectoralis tendon and coracoid process (see Figure 25A.16). Compression of the neurocirculatory structures (brachial plexus and axillary artery) results in the axillary pulse being dampened or obliterated. The symptoms can be reproduced on examination. Wright's criteria are as follows (28):

- Presence of neurovascular symptoms in one upper extremity
- Reproducible obliteration of pulse with abduction of upper extremity (or exaggeration of symptoms)
- Confirmation of occupation or habit patterns involving hyperabduction (overhead work, exercise, sleep position)
- Relief through avoidance of hyperabduction

SECTION B

UPPER ARM

Upper arm structures are continually exposed to athletic trauma. In football, blocking is taught with elbows protruding and the forearms and hands held protected close to the body. This technique often results in upper soft tissue injury. It can include the following forms (listed in increasing severity):

Contusion. This is the result of a direct blow to the upper arm that causes bruising of the skin, soft tissue edema, and inflammation. Treatment consists of application of ice, compression, rest, and protection from further injury through the use of donut padding.

Hematoma. A deeper contusion that injures blood vessels within the musculature causes hematoma formations in relatively small, restricted areas. Physical examination will often reveal fluctuance in the area. Treatment of a first time hematoma consists of ice, compression, and protection from further injury. Aspiration of a hematoma is controversial at present. We do not advise it because no useful purpose seems to be served.

Myositis ossificans. This results from ossification of encapsulated blood secondary to hematoma formation. It is usually the result of chronic, repeated trauma to the same lateral area of the forearm. A history often reveals continued use of the injured area without protection and a gradual loss of function of the underlying musculature (29). Physical examination will show a firm, mobile mass within the musculature, an increased forearm girth, and loss of ROM. Pain may not be present when the forearm is moved but it is present on palpation of the mass. Diagnostic x-rays will show heterotrophic calcification within the localized muscle area if there has been chronic trauma. Ossification is a time-related, severity-related process, so the x-ray findings may not be positive. Treatment is with ice and protection. Surgery may be necessary if the mass interferes with normal functioning of the upper arm. Surgical removal is usually at 6 months or later. Early removal may provoke recurrence of even greater growth of unwanted bone (30).

Blocker's (Tackler's) exostosis. This lesion is very similar in pathophysiology to myositis ossificans. It is usually present in the upper extremity, most often in the biceps muscle area and comes from repeated damage at the insertion of the deltoid or biceps brachialis muscles. Heterotrophic new bone forms after tearing of the periosteum of the bone secondary to trauma. Physical examination is similar to that in myositis ossificans. Confirmation by x-ray is possible 2 to 3 weeks postinjury. Remember, this exostosis is attached to normal bone. Treatment is as follows:

- Early recognition and follow-up
- Ice, compression, and rest
- If the arm is seen 2 weeks postinjury and new bone formation is noted, the arm should be rested in a splint due to the possibility of spontaneous resorption of the mass, and surgical excision may be necessary.

Differential diagnosis. Although the differential diagnosis between myositis ossificans and Blocker's exostosis is an academic exercise, it is important to rule out osteosarcoma in the upper arm from any heterotrophic bone formation.

APPENDIX 25A.1
RADIOGRAPHS OF SOME OF THE COMMON SHOULDER PROBLEMS

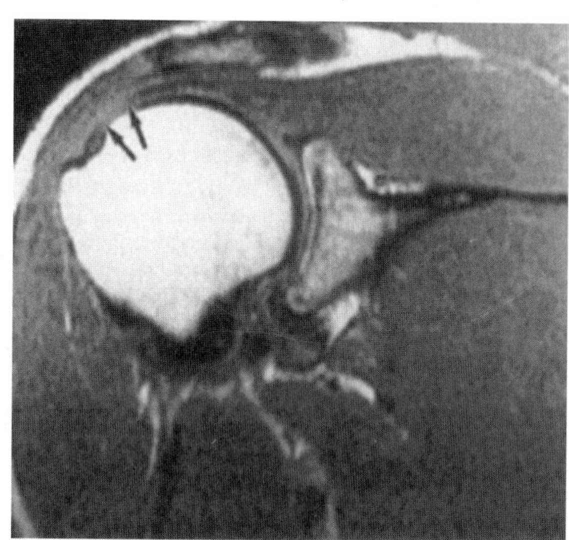

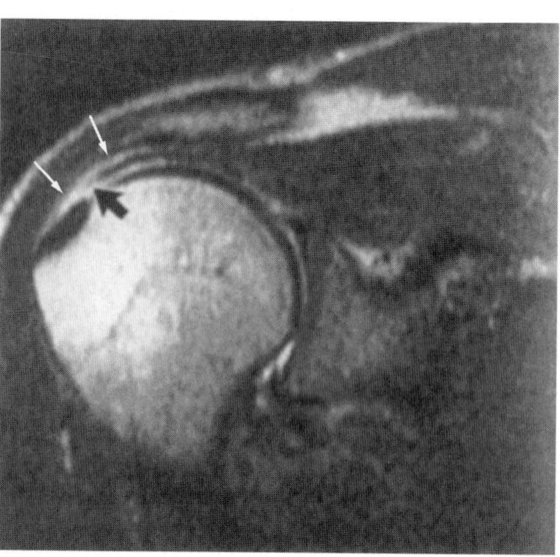

Appendix 25A.1.1 Midplain coronal oblique magnetic resonance images showing a small tear of the rotator cuff. **A:** Small tear seen in the supraspinatus tendon (*arrows*). **B:** Seen on image made with long repetition time and echo time. The intensity of the signal within the small region of discontinuity in the tendon is increased further (*black arrow*). High signal intensity fluid is seen in the subacromial–subdeltoid bursa (*white arrows*). (*Source:* reproduced with permission from Iannotti JP, Zlatkin MB, Esterhai JL, et al. Magnetic resonance imaging of the shoulder. *J Bone Joint Surg Am* 1991;73:20.)

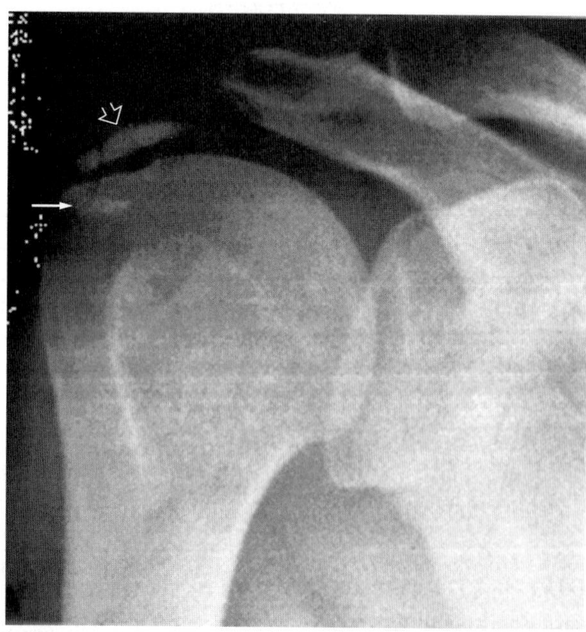

Appendix 25A.1.2 Calcific tendonitis. Lateral rotation view shows calcification projected over the base of the greater tuberosity (*white arrow*) and above the greater turberosity (*open arrow*). (*Source:* reproduced with permission from Weissman BNW, Sledge CB. *Orthopedic radiology*. Philadelphia: WB Saunders, 1986:227.)

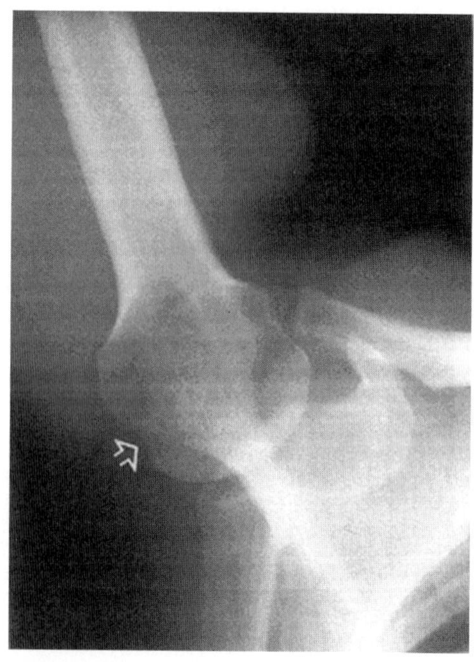

Appendix 25A.1.3 Hill-Sachs lesion (*arrow*). (*Source:* reproduced with permission from Magee DJ. *Orthopedic physical assessment*, 4th ed. St. Louis: WB Saunders/Elsevier, 2006.)

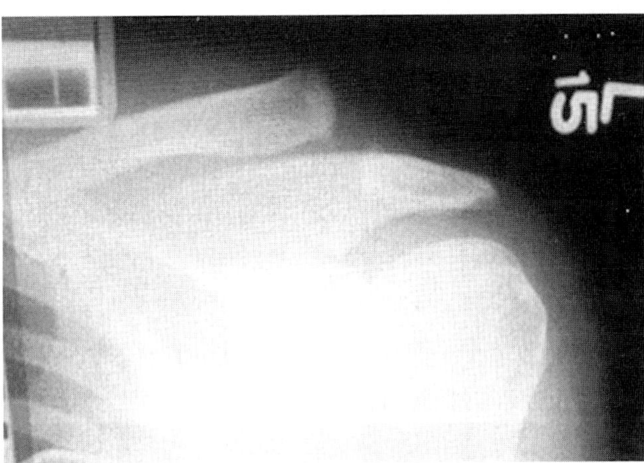

Appendix 25A.1.4 Acromioclavicular separation of left shoulder. (*Source:* reproduced with permission from Miller MD, Sekiya JK. *Sports medicine core knowledge in orthopaedics*. Philadelphia: Mosby/Elsevier, 2006.)

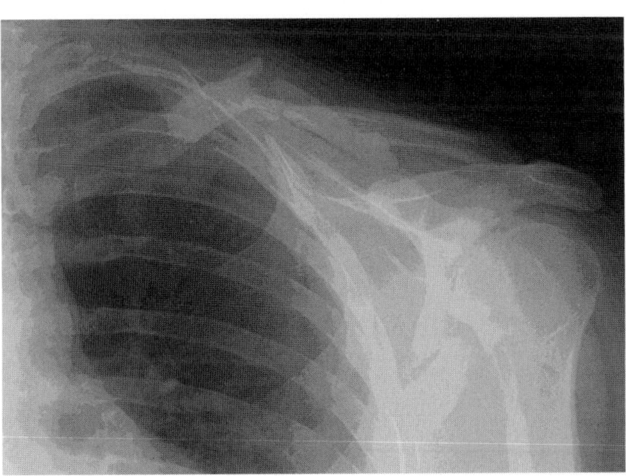

Appendix 25A.1.5 Frontal Radiograph of a typical midshaft clavicular fracture with apex-cranial angulation and subsequent inferior subluxation of the shoulder girdle. The accompanying scapular fracture is incompletely evaluated and involvement of the glenoid cannot be excluded.

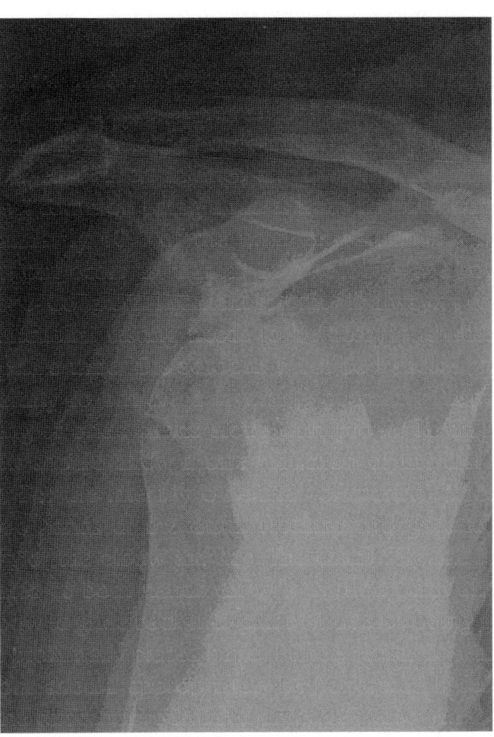

Appendix 25A.1.6 Frontal radiograph of a typical subcoracoid anterior dislocation. Small boney fragments above the humeral head suggest a fracture, although localization of the donor site cannot be determined.

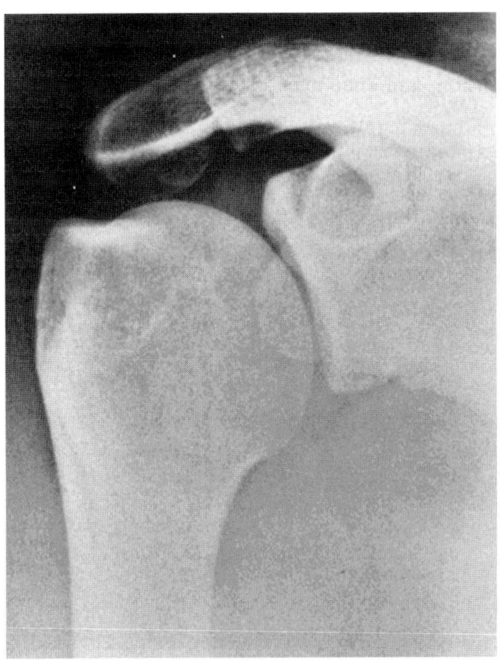

Appendix 25A.1.7 Normal posteroanterior view of the shoulder.

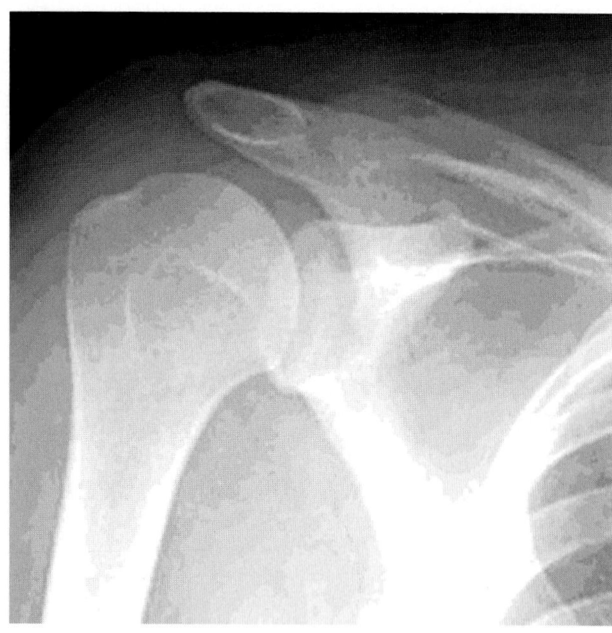

Appendix 25A.1.8 Osteolysis of the distal clavicle.

REFERENCES

1. Kaplan LD, Flanigan DC, Norwig J, et al. Prevalence and variance of shoulder injuries in elite collegiate football players. *Am J Sports Med* 2005;33:1142–1146.
2. O'Brien S, Pagnani MJ, Fealy S, et al. The active compression test: a new effective test for diagnosing labral tears and acromioclavicular joint abnormality. *Am J Sports Med* 1998;26:610–613.
3. Mazzocca A, Sellards R, Garretson R. Injuries to the acromioclavicular joint in adults and children. In: DeLee J, Drez D, Miler MD, et al. eds. *Orthopedic sports medicine practices and principles*. Philadelphia: WB Saunders, 2003:912–934.
4. Slawski D, Cahill B. Atraumatic osteolysis of the distal clavicle: results of open surgical excision. *Am J Sports Med* 1994;22:267–271.
5. DeLee JC, Drez D Jr. *Orthopaedic sports medicine: principles and Practice*, Vol. I. No. 15. Philadelphia: WB Saunders, 1994:504.
6. Vanarthos WJ, Ekman EF, Bohreer SP. Radiographic diagnosis of acromioclavicular joint separation without weight bearing: importance of internal rotation of the arm. *Am J Roentgenol* 1994;162:120–123.
7. DeLee JC, Drez D Jr. *Orthopaedic sports medicine : principles and Practice*, Vol. I. No. 15. Philadelphia: WB Saunders, 1994:505.
8. Philips AM, Smart C, Groom AFG. Acromioclavicular dislocation: conservative or surgical therapy. *Clin Orthop* 1998;353:10–17.
9. Swiontkowski MarcF, ed. *Manual of orthopaedics*, 5th ed, Vol. 14. Philadelphia: Lippincott Williams & Wilkins, 2001:190.
10. Hendley GW. Necessity of radiographs in the emergency department management of shoulder dislocations. *Ann Emerg Med* 2000;36:108–113.
11. Westin CD, Gill EA, Noyes ME, et al. Anterior shoulder silocation. A simple and rapid method for reduction. *Am J Sports Med* 1995;23:369–371.
12. Rowe CR, Sakellarieds HT. Factors related to recurrences of anterior dislocation of the shoulder. *Clin Orthop* 1961;20:40–48.
13. McLaughlin HL, MacLellan DJ. Recurrent anterior dislocation of the shoulder II. Comparative study. *J Trauma* 1967;7:191–201.
14. Itoi E, Hatakeyama Y, Kido T, et al. A new method of immobilization after traumatic anterior dislocation of the shoulder : a preliminary study. *J Shoulder Elbow Surg* 2003;12(5):413–415.
15. Puffer J, ed. *20 common problems in sports medicine*, Vol. 2. New York: McGraw-Hill, 2002:42.
16. Richardson AB. Overuse syndromes in baseball, tennis, gymnastics and swimming. *Clin Sports Med* 1983;2:379–390.
17. Tullos HS, King Jw. Throwing mechanism in sports. *Orthop Clin North Am* 1972;4:709–720.
18. Jobe FW, Jobe CM. Painful athletic injuries of the shoulder. *Clin Orthop* 1983;173:117–124.
19. Bigliani L, Morrison DS, April EW. The morphology of the acromion and its relationship to rotator cuff tears. *Ortho Trans* 1986;10:228.
20. Neer CS II, Welsh RP. The shoulder in sports. *Orthop Clin North Am* 1977;8:583–591.
21. Neer CS II. Impingement lesions. *Clin Orthop* 1983;173; 70; Puffer J, ed. *20 common problems in sports medicine*, Vol. 1. McGraw-Hill, 2002:15.
22. Werner CML, Steinmann PA, Gilbart M, et al. Treatment of painful pseudoparesis due to irreparable rotator cuff dysfunction with the delta III reverse-ball-and-socket total shoulder prosthesis. *J Bone Joint Surg Am* 2005;87:1476–1486.
23. Snyder S, Karzel RP, Del Pizzo W, et al. SLAP lesions of the shoulder. *Arthroscopy* 1990;6:274–279.
24. Andrews J, Carson WG, McLeod WD. Glenoid labrum tears related to the long head of the biceps. *Am J Sports Med* 1985;13:337–341.
25. Burkhart S, Morgan CD. The peel-back mechanism: its role in producing and extending posterior type II SLAP lesions and its effect on SLAP repair rehabilitation. *Arthroscopy* 1998;14:637–640.
26. Hannafin J, Chiai TA. Adhesive Capsulitis. *Clin Orthop* 2000;372:95–109.
27. Tibone JE. Shoulder problems of adolescents. How they differ from those of adults. *Clin Sports Med* 1983;2(2):423–427.
28. Wright IS. The neurovascular syndrome produced by hyper abduction of the arm. *Am Heart J* 1945;29:1.
29. Huss CD, Puhl JJ. Myositis ossificans of the upper arm. *AM J Sports Med* 1980;8:419–424.
30. DeLee JC, Drez D Jr. *Orthopaedic sports medicine : principles and Practice*, Vol. I. 16. Philadelphia: WB Saunders, 1994:788.
31. Puffer J, ed. *20 common problems in sports medicine*, Vol. 2. McGraw-Hill, 2002:21.

The Elbow

26

Roger L. McCoy, II *C. Edward Clark, III*

ANATOMY/BIOMECHANICS

The bony anatomy consists of the distal humerus, which has the trochlea medially and the capitellum laterally. The radial head articulates with the capitellum and the proximal ulna articulates with the trochlea. The humeroradial joint is a uniaxial diarthrodial joint that functions as a hinge for flexion and extension and as a pivot in the longitudinal axis to allow rotational motion. The medial humeral epicondyle serves as the origin of the flexor–pronator muscle (FPM) group and the medial ulnar collateral ligament (UCL) (see Figure 26.1, Table 26.1). The lateral epicondyle serves as the origin of the extensor–supinator muscle group and the radial and lateral UCL (see Figure 26.1, Table 26.2) (1,2).

The elbow joint comprises three articulations: the ulnohumeral, the radiocapitellar, and the proximal radioulnar joint. These allow the elbow two degrees of freedom: flexion–extension and pronation–supination. The normal elbow moves from 0 degree to 135–150 degrees of flexion and possesses approximately 70 to 90 degrees of pronation and 80 to 90 degrees of supination. The normal carrying angle of the extended elbow is approximately 15 degrees of valgus in relation to the humeral shaft (11–14 degrees in men, 13–16 degrees in women) (see Figure 26.2) (3,4).

The medial and radial collateral ligaments, the closely matching bony surfaces, the joint capsule, and the surrounding muscles provide stability to the elbow. The primary structure providing valgus stability is the medial collateral ligament complex, which consists of three portions: the anterior oblique, posterior oblique, and a transverse intervening portion. The anterior oblique portion of the medial collateral ligament is the primary valgus stabilizer of the elbow (see Figures 26.3 and 26.4) (1,4).

ELBOW INJURIES

Obtaining a thorough history is essential in arriving at the correct diagnosis in the athlete who presents with elbow pain. Determining the onset of pain, whether acute or chronic, the mechanism of injury, the exact location, exacerbating factors, and quality, intensity, and radiation of the patient's pain is important in establishing an accurate differential diagnosis. Associated symptoms, such as muscle weakness, numbness, clicking, catching, and locking of the joint, as well as neck, shoulder, wrist, and hand complaints, are also important in the history acquisition. The level and magnitude of competition of the athlete is also important to note; because this may direct modes and aggressiveness of treatment in the use of diagnostic studies. Earlier injuries and treatment protocols may also help in determining diagnostic and treatment strategies (2).

It may also help to organize the symptoms to coincide with a particular area of the elbow anatomy. Certain diagnoses are unique not only in their symptomatology, but also in their location. Not all conditions listed will be specifically addressed in this chapter as they may be readily found in many other texts (see Table 26.3) (5).

GENERAL PHYSICAL EXAMINATION

The physical examination of any joint is best done in the order of inspection, palpation, range of motion (ROM), and then stability/provocative maneuvers. This order minimizes patient discomfort early in the examination, which can minimize guarding. Inspection should preferably start with the patient standing, and any clothing covering the shoulder and arm should be removed. The examiner should observe the carrying angle (see section "Anatomy/Biomechanics"), color, size, and note

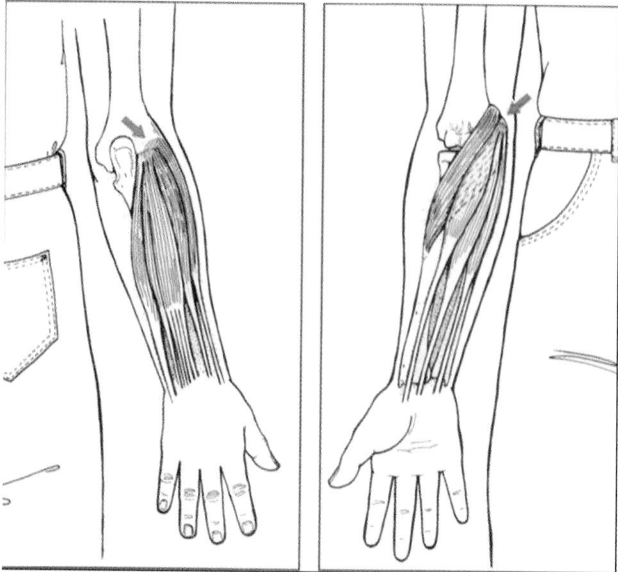

Figure 26.1 Origins of wrist extensors and flexors. Extensors originate from the lateral epicondyle (left half of figure), and the flexors from the medial epicondyle (right). Also locations of pain from medial and lateral epicondylosis. (*Source*: Reproduced with permission from Hannafin JA. How I manage tennis and Golfer's elbow. *Phys Sportsmed* 1996;24(2):63–68.)

any swelling, ecchymosis, or obvious signs of trauma. General size differences could be from normal muscle hypertrophy expected in certain athletes (pitchers, racquet sports), while atrophy should be considered abnormal. Posterior swelling could represent olecranon bursitis or joint effusion (2).

The examiner begins palpation away from the patient's reported point of maximal tenderness when possible, noting any pain, crepitus, or other deformity. Palpation should begin posteriorly over the distal humerus and move towards the olecranon, while addressing any tenderness of the supracondylar region and the triceps tendon. Olecranon palpation can be assisted by placing the joint in slight flexion to free it from the olecranon fossa. A chronically enlarged olecranon bursa is not usually tender, but may be tender if infected or acutely inflamed from an injury. Proceeding laterally from the olecranon one finds the lateral epicondyle, and 1 to 2 cm more distally is the radial head. The radial head articulation can be easily found by pronating and supinating the forearm while palpating just distal to the lateral epicondyle. An effusion can be palpated in an imaginary triangle defined by the olecranon tip, lateral epicondyle, and radial head while the elbow is flexed to 90 degrees. Next palpate the medial epicondyle. The ulnar nerve sits posterior to the medial epicondyle, between it and the olecranon in the groove for the ulnar nerve (2,6,7).

ROM should be first evaluated passively then actively, including flexion, extension, pronation and supination (see section "Anatomy/Biomechanics" for normal ranges). While checking the ROM one should note any ulnar nerve subluxation by flexing the elbow to 50 to 60 degrees, while placing the shoulder in slight external rotation and palpating over the ulnar nerve. During subluxation the nerve may "roll up" onto the epicondyle (2).

TABLE 26.1

FLEXOR–PRONATOR MUSCLE GROUP

Pronator teres
Flexor carpi radialis
Palmaris longus
Flexor carpi ulnaris

Source: Adapted from Data from Delee J, Drez D. *Orthopaedic sports medicine: principles and practice*, Vol. 1. WB Saunders, 1994.

TABLE 26.2

MOBILE WAD EXTENSORS (EXTENSOR–SUPINATOR GROUP)

Brachioradialis
Extensor carpi radialis longus
Extensor carpi radialis brevis
Supinator

Source: Adapted from Data from Delee J, Drez D. *Orthopaedic sports medicine:principles and practice*, Vol. 1. WB Saunders, 1994.

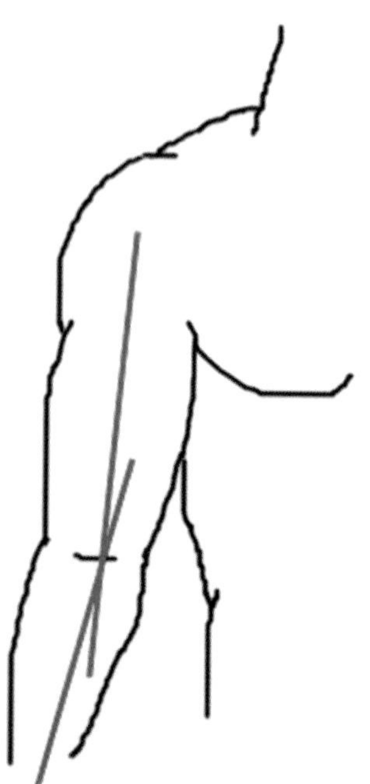

Figure 26.2 Normal carrying angle of the elbow.

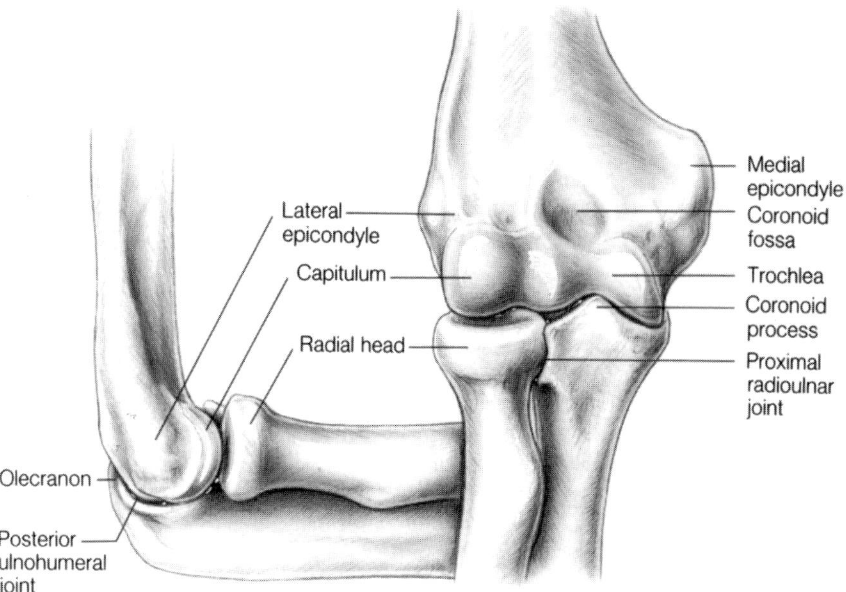

Figure 26.3 Bony anatomy of the elbow. (*Source*: Adapted from Chumbley E, O'Connor FG, Nirschl RP. Evaluation of overuse elbow injuries. *Am Fam Physician* 2000;61:691–700.)

Stability of the medial or UCL is assessed by placing a valgus stress to the elbow and is explained in detail later in this chapter (see Figure 26.5). Radial collateral ligament stability is assessed in a similar manner with varus stressing. These and other specific maneuvers is discussed later in the chapter (5).

GENERAL RADIOGRAPHIC PRINCIPLES

A standard elbow series includes an anteroposterior (AP) view in full extension (see Figure 26.6) and lateral view at 90 degrees (see Figure 26.7) of flexion. Two lines should be drawn in cases of trauma or when fracture is suspected. The anterior humeral line is drawn on the lateral view, parallel and along the anterior surface of the humeral cortex (see Figure 26.8). If the line does not transect the middle third of the mid capitellum, then a supracondylar fracture should be suspected. The radiocapitellar line can also be helpful in detecting pathology. It is drawn through the center of the radial head and neck and extended proximally (see Figure 26.8). Normally it extends in all views through the midcapitellum. Dislocation of the radial head is suspected if the line does not transect this region, or if there is relative movement of the capitellum from a supracondylar fracture (7,8).

The presence of two fat pads in the elbow are also helpful in detecting pathology. The anterior fat pad is located just anterior to the distal humeral diaphysis and can be seen in a normal elbow series as a small line or triangular radiolucency. The posterior fat pad is usually not visible because it lies in the olecranon fossa. Effusion from intra-articular bleeding or inflammation can elevate

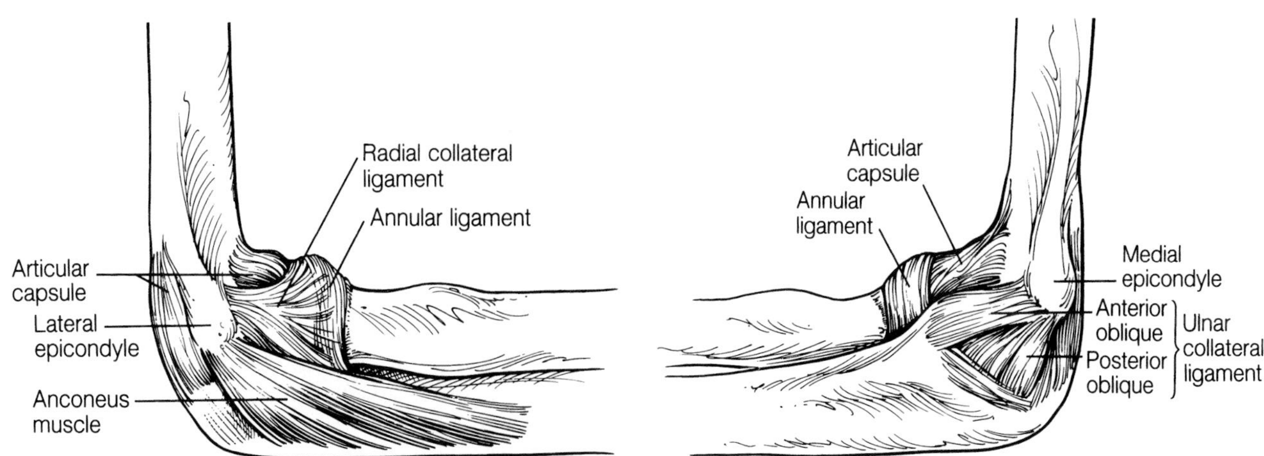

Figure 26.4 Ligamentous support of the elbow. (*Source*: Adapted from Chumbley E, O'Connor FG, Nirschl RP. Evaluation of overuse elbow injuries. *Am Fam Physician* 2000;61:691–700.)

TABLE 26.3
DIFFERENTIAL DIAGNOSIS OF ELBOW PAIN BY SYMPTOM LOCATION

Location	Possible Disorders
Anterior	Anterior capsular strain
	Biceps tendon rupture
	Biceps tendonitis
	Dislocation
	Median N compression (pronator syndrome)
Medial	Flexor–pronator muscle strain
	Fracture
	Medial epicondylitis
	Ulnar collateral ligament injury
	Ulnar neuritis (compression syndrome)
Posteromedial	Olecranon tip stress fracture
	Posterior (olecranon) impingement
	Trochlear chondromalacia
Posterior	Olecranon bursitis
	Olecranon process stress fracture
	Triceps tendonitis
	Triceps rupture
Lateral	Capitellum fracture
	Lateral epicondylitis
	Lateral ulnar collateral ligament injury
	Osteochondritis dessicans
	Posterior interosseous nerve syndrome
	Posterolateral rotatory instability
	Radial head fracture
	Radiocapitellar chondromalacia

Source: From Conway J. Clinical evaluation of elbow injuries in the athlete. *J Musculoskel Med* 1998;15(10):43–52.

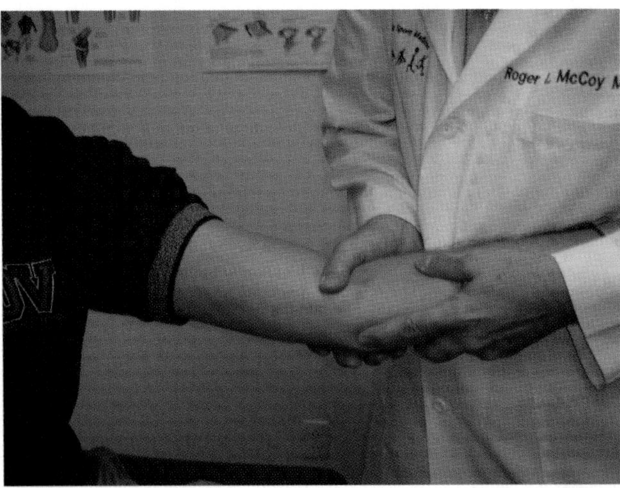

Figure 26.5 Valgus stress test to assess the ulnar collateral ligament.

these fat pads away from the cortex and either make them larger or visible. The anterior fat pad makes a "sail sign" when elevated (see Figure 26.9). Any presence of a posterior fat pad is abnormal and suggests fracture (see Figure 26.9) (7–9).

ACUTE TRAUMA

Any athlete presenting with significant pain around the elbow resulting from an acute event should be carefully evaluated to rule out a fracture or dislocation. The athlete should be removed from competition, and all equipment, tape, and padding from the shoulder to the hand should be removed so that an adequate examination can be performed. This is, of course, if it is safe and timely to do so. Tenderness, swelling, and ecchymosis should be noted. Any findings of bony crepitus or deformity warrants high suspicion of a fracture. The shoulder, forearm, wrist, and hand should be carefully and expediently examined. A thorough neurovascular examination of the median, ulnar, and radial nerves and pulses is essential. Sensory testing of peripheral nerves should include the first web space on the dorsum of the hand (radial nerve), volar tip of the index finger (median nerve), and volar tip of the small finger (ulnar nerve). Any deficiencies need to be noted and charted, as chronic sequelae may arise that may be directly related to the trauma as opposed to the physicians treatment (6,9,10).

Motor examination includes testing the extensor pollicis longus for interphalangeal joint extension of the thumb (radial nerve), the index flexor digitorum profundus for flexion at the distal interphalangeal joint (median nerve), and the dorsal interossei and abductor digiti quinti muscles

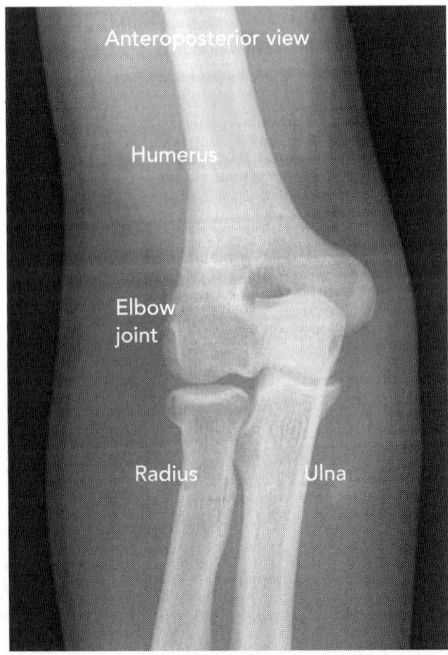

Figure 26.6 Normal anteroposterior radiograph.

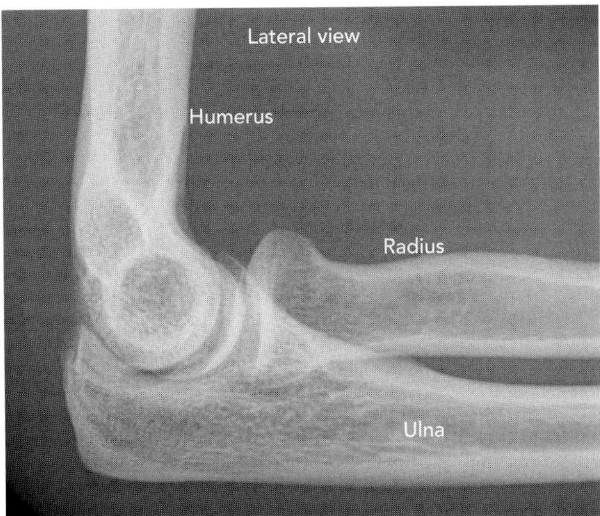

Figure 26.7 Normal lateral radiograph.

of the index and small fingers for abduction strength (ulnar nerve). The vascular examination is also essential in any trauma. Brachial, radial, and ulnar pulses need be checked immediately and any question of compromise considered an emergency situation. ROM at the elbow, including pronation and supination, should be carefully checked and recorded (6,7).

With an elbow trauma that is accompanied by any abnormal findings on physical examination, plain radiographs are warranted. Good quality AP and lateral radiographs are necessary to rule out occult fractures, especially those involving the radial head. A positive "fat pad" sign or "sail" sign (see Figure 26.9) on the posterior aspect of the humerus indicates an effusion within the joint and may be associated with a fracture. Any fracture should be appropriately immobilized with a well-padded posterior splint (6,7,11).

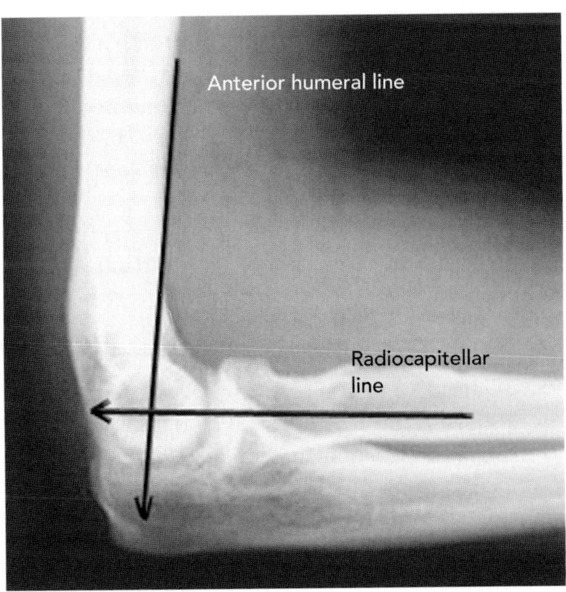

Figure 26.8 Positioning of the anterior humeral and radiocapitellar lines.

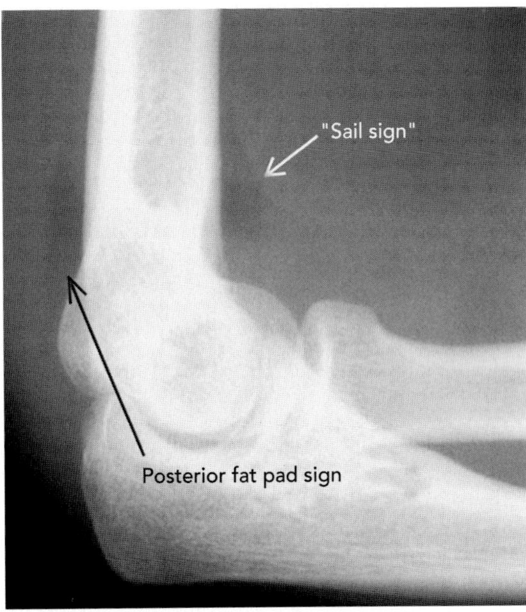

Figure 26.9 Elevation of anterior fat pad creating a "sail sign", and posterior fat pad sign.

FRACTURES AND DISLOCATIONS OF THE ELBOW

Fractures or dislocations of the elbow do occur during athletic competition, especially in contact sports, and knowledge of the initial evaluation and management of these injuries is essential for the team physician. Elbow trauma includes fractures of the distal humerus, radial head and neck fractures, olecranon fractures, simple elbow dislocations, and fracture-dislocations of the elbow. Generally, most fracture patients can start rehabilitation at 6 to 8 weeks postinjury if good callous formation is present, and can expect return to play at 12 weeks. Simple elbow dislocations need physical therapy early in the healing process to prevent loss of extension, and these patients can usually return to play in 1 to 3 months depending upon stability and ROM.

Distal Humeral Fractures

These fractures include supracondylar, transcondylar, intercondylar, T-condylar and medial/lateral condylar fractures.

Supracondylar fractures of the distal humerus commonly occur between 5 and 10 years of age, and they usually occur from a severe fall on an outstretched hand (see Figure 26.10). If displaced, supracondylar fractures need to be treated operatively, whereas nondisplaced fractures can be treated with a long-arm cast for 3 to 4 weeks (90 degrees

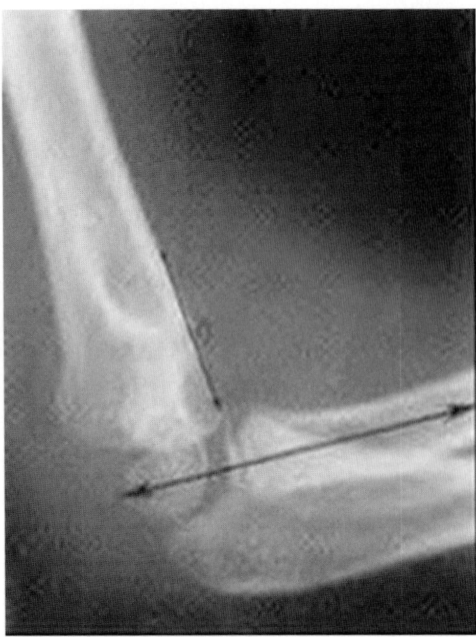

Figure 26.10 Supracondylar fracture. Note that the anterior humeral line does not cross the midportion of the capitellum, signifying supracondylar pathology (fracture).

flexion, neutral forearm rotation). If callous formation is confirmed at that time immobilization can be discontinued and active ROM exercises can be initiated. Supracondylar fractures in adults are best managed by an orthopedic surgeon unless nondisplaced or minimally displaced without neurovascular compromise. Nondisplaced fractures are placed in a long arm posterior splint at 90 degrees flexion with frequent re-examinations for neurovascular status in the early stages. At 2 weeks, gentle ROM exercises can begin, but splinting should continue for a total of 6 weeks, or until callus formation occurs. More vigorous rehabilitation can then be started to regain ROM and is usually best with the assistance of a physical therapist (6–8).

Fracture of the lateral condyle is the second most common pediatric elbow fracture and may also be caused by falling on an outstretched hand. These fractures are intra-articular, and open reduction is essential to avoid nonunion and malunion in displaced fractures. If nondisplaced, these fractures are initially placed in a posterior long arm splint, and if they remain nondisplaced over the first 10 to 14 days a long arm cast can be applied for 3 to 4 weeks, or until radiographic evidence of healing is seen. These fractures are also best managed by orthopedic surgeons due to the incidence of nonunion and growth arrest, which can cause cubitus varus or valgus deformity. Lateral condyle fractures in adults should also be evaluated by a surgeon (6,8,12).

Coronoid Fractures

There needs to be a high index of suspicion for coronoid fractures during dislocation injuries. If greater than 20% of the anterior coronoid (type II) is involved, reconstruction is necessary to preserve the attachment site for the anterior capsule and the brachialis muscle. Type I or small avulsion fractures will heal with conservative treatment. If most of the coronoid is involved (>50%), reconstruction must be performed to preserve the stabilizing effects brought about by the anterior oblique ligament. This would indicate a type III coronoid fracture and can occur in 80% of dislocations. Return to full function for the athlete is usually not obtained (6).

Olecranon Fractures

A direct blow to the elbow, a fall on the flexed elbow, or a fall on an outstretched arm with associated dislocation, can all result in a fracture of the olecranon. These fractures can be displaced or nondisplaced and can be transverse, oblique, or comminuted in nature. Olecranon fractures are uncommon in young children but can occur in adolescents from a direct blow to the posterior elbow (6,12).

Findings include global swelling around the elbow with very restrictive and guarded ROM. Fragments and point tenderness can be found if the fracture is either comminuted or displaced. AP and lateral views are usually sufficient to adequately see the fracture on radiographs.

Treatment of nondisplaced fractures is accomplished with a 90 degree posterior splint for 2 to 3 weeks. Wrist flexion and extension motion is accompanied by some mild grip strengthening during this immobilization. After immobilization, elbow ROM can be started, with triceps strength exercises initiated only after radiographic signs of healing are seen. Most displaced fractures should be referred for orthopedic surgery for internal surgical fixation. Physical therapy is essential as stiffness and occasional hardware irritation may hinder full rapid recovery (6,12).

Radial Head Fractures

Radial head fractures can occur either during a dislocation of the elbow or upon a fall on an outstretched arm with the arm and forearm rotated inward. Radial neck fractures or physeal fractures of the radial head in children above the age of 9 years usually occur from a valgus, axial load to the radiocapitellar joint. Findings usually consist of an inability to pronate or supinate the forearm, limited ability to flex or extend the elbow, and palpable tenderness laterally just inferior and posterior to the extensor muscle mass. Swelling is usually present but can be deceivingly mild on occasions (6,9).

Radial head fractures can be classified into three categories (see Table 26.4). Most type II and type III radial head fractures are adequately seen on AP and lateral films. Some type I fractures can be missed on initial films but later become evident in 2 to 3 weeks on follow-up radiographs. Type I fractures are splinted or placed in a sling for 3 to 7 days and early ROM is essential. Complete extension and supination are the most difficult rehabilitative goals to achieve and some residual loss of ROM can occur. Type II

TABLE 26.4
RADIAL HEAD FRACTURE TYPES

Type I:	Fractures with no displacement of the radial head
Type II:	Fractures with some displacement and not greater than 5 to 10 degrees of angulation. Oblique or horizontal neck fractures can occur
Type III:	Complete disruption of the radial head from its normal anatomical position, usually comminuted

fractures can also be treated this way unless the fragment occupies more than 30% of the head or is displaced more than 2 mm (see Figure 26.11). These type II fractures, as well as all type III fractures are best treated surgically, with excision being the choice for most type III fractures (6,9).

Monteggia's Fracture/Dislocation

This is a fracture of the proximal third of the ulna with an accompanying dislocation of the radial head. The most common mechanism is forced hyperpronation during a fall on an outstretched hand. On occasion either the fracture of the ulna or the dislocation of the radial head may be slight and, therefore, sometimes missed. This is more common in children in whom most Monteggia's fractures are often treated with closed reduction. Adults often require open reduction and internal fixation (6,9).

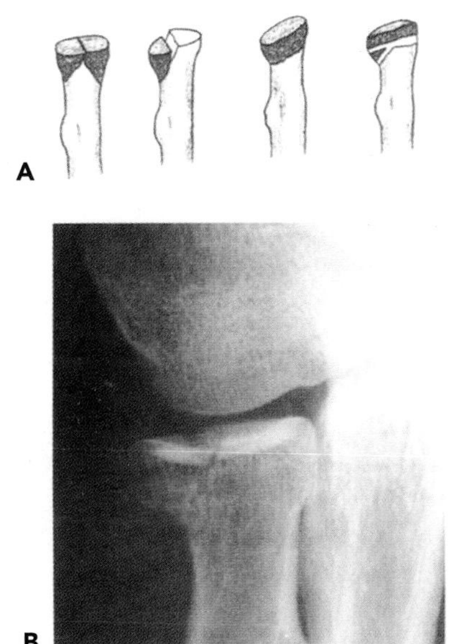

Figure 26.11 Variations of type I radial head fractures. (*Source*: Reproduced with permission from Mercier L, Pettid FJ, Tamisiea DF, Heieck JJ. The elbow. In: *Practical orthopedics*. Chapter 6. Mosby, 2000:75–85. On page 83.)

Dislocations of the Elbow

Most elbow dislocations occur posteriorly and are usually due to a fall on an outstretched hand/arm. By far, the most common posterior dislocation is the posterolateral position. Associated injuries are always a concern with the most common being a radial head fracture, occurring approximately 10% of the time. Associated fractures in general can occur as high as 25% to 50% in elbow dislocations. Collateral ligament stability is always a concern and functional testing needs to be accomplished at the appropriate time. Dislocations must be handled quickly and calmly to achieve a favorable outcome. Proper positioning of one's hands along with proper leverage and rotation should allow a safe reduction of the dislocated elbow. For the laterally dislocated olecranon, placement of one's hands at the distal forearm and posterolateral portion of the elbow are key. The distal forearm is then supinated as both hands direct a traction force allowing the elbow to glide back into place while also being guided by the proximally placed hand. Pulses, sensations, and inspections should appropriately be performed before and after the relocation. Medially dislocated elbows require a similar procedure with the exception of having the forearm pronated rather than supinated, and several techniques currently exist (Figure 26.12). After the neurovascular examination is completed, the elbow should be splinted at 90 degrees and the athlete transported to the medical center of choice for follow-up radiographs and further examination. If the neurovascular examination is normal upon evaluation on the field, and transport to the nearest medical center is readily available, the clinician should opt to immobilize the dislocated elbow until prereduction films can be obtained. Individual clinician experiences with the reduction of dislocations will direct the most appropriate choice. Any neurovascular compromise undoubtedly constitutes an emergency and on-field reduction becomes

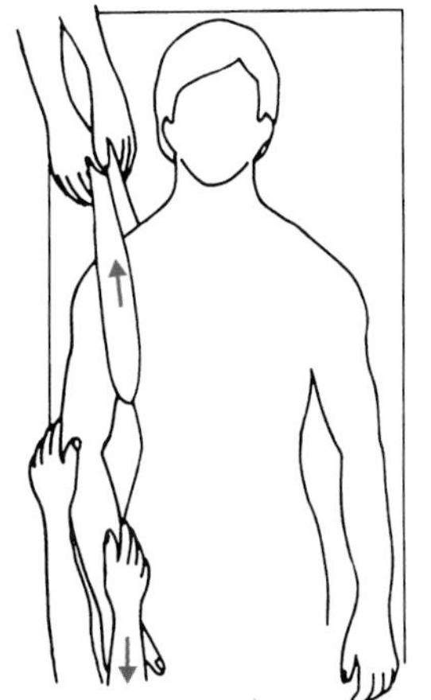

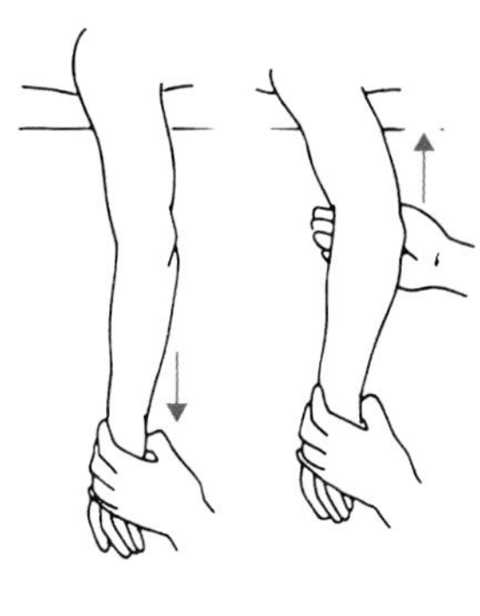

Figure 26.12 Reduction technique for medially dislocated elbow. (*Source*: Reproduced with permission from Mercier L, Pettid FJ, Tamisiea DF, Heieck JJ. The elbow. In: *Practical orthopedics*. Chapter 6. Mosby, 2000:75–85. On pg 81.)

a riskier option for the physician. Minimal repositioning may facilitate some return of the neurovascular compromise. Splinting in this position is then followed by rapid transport to the nearest medical facility (6,9,13).

OVERUSE AND CHRONIC ELBOW CONDITIONS

Overuse conditions can easily and quickly turn into chronic problems, as many athletes will tend to ignore early minor symptoms and only report to the team physician when their symptoms finally inhibit their play (see Table 26.5) (1).

Lateral Elbow Conditions

Lateral Epicondylitis (Tennis Elbow)

One of the more common injuries, that until recently was misunderstood as an inflammation problem, is lateral epicondylitis, also known as *tennis elbow* (see Figure 26.1). The condition in its early stages will have inflammatory responses to the tension overloads placed on the tendon–bone junction, yet, most lasting longer than a few weeks become more of a chronic change, called *tendinosis* (angiofibroblastic degeneration) and *epicondylosis*. The athlete will present with pain and tenderness over the lateral epicondyle as well as the extensor tendon and will have pain with resistance to wrist and third digit extension. Occasionally grip strength testing will also elicit pain (14).

Therapies are presently being researched with none taking a substantial lead as the single best treatment. Besides addressing the athlete's biomechanics and equipment (tennis racquet grip size, golf/tennis swing paths, etc.), the mainstay for recovery is physical therapy. NSAIDs, and modalities such as cryotherapy, phonophoresis, iontophoresis, and steroid injections have all shown to alleviate symptoms, yet do not resolve the underlying condition. There must be an awakening of the body's healing processes through some form of prescribed trauma to the tissue, followed by flexibility and functional eccentric exercises in physical therapy. Other newer modalities such as extracorporeal shock-wave therapy and nitrous oxide therapy, although showing some initial success, have not statistically been shown to be better than vigorous deep tissue massage (vigorous enough to cause bruising) followed by a functional rehabilitation program. One such system is called *Augmented Soft Tissue Manipulation* or ASTYM (see Figure 26.13) (14,15).

TABLE 26.5
ACTIVITIES COMMONLY ASSOCIATED WITH OVERUSE ELBOW INJURIES

Activity	Injuries
Bowling	Biceps tendinosis, radial tunnel syndrome
Boxing	Triceps tendinosis
Friction in football, wrestling, or basketball	Olecranon bursitis
Golf	Golfer's elbow (trailing arm), radial tunnel syndrome
Gymnastics	Biceps tendinosis, triceps tendinosis
Posterior dislocation	Posterolateral rotatory instability
Racquet sports	Pronator syndrome, triceps tendinosis, olecranon stress fracture, lateral tennis elbow, radial tunnel syndrome, golfer's elbow, ulnar nerve entrapment
Rowing	Radial tunnel syndrome
Skiing	Ulnar nerve entrapment
Swimming	Radial tunnel syndrome
Throwing	Pronator syndrome, triceps tendinosis, olecranon impingement, olecranon stress fracture, radiocapitellar chondromalacia, ulnar collateral ligament sprain, golfer's elbow, ulnar nerve entrapment
Weight lifting	Biceps tendinosis, triceps tendinosis, anterior capsule strain, radial tunnel syndrome, ulnar nerve entrapment

Source: From Chumbley E, O'Connor FG, Nirschl RP. Evaluation of overuse elbow injuries. *Amer Fam Phys* 2000;61:691–700.

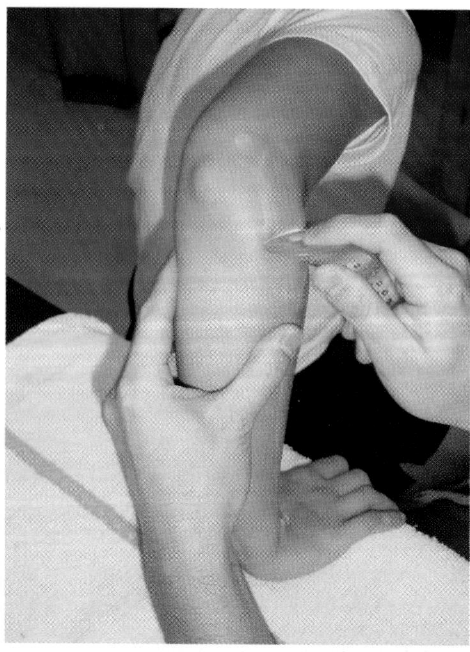

Figure 26.13 Demonstration of Augmented Soft Tissue Manipulation (ASTYM) technique for treatment of lateral epicondylosis and extensor tendonosis.

Posterior Interosseous Nerve Compression Syndrome (Radial Tunnel Syndrome)

Radial tunnel syndrome is a relatively uncommon disorder seen in golfers, batters, racquet sports, and, occasionally, throwers. This syndrome involves the compression of the posterior interosseous nerve, a deep branch of the radial nerve, most commonly compressed under the fibrous arch of the supinator (arcade of Frosche) or more distally in the body of the supinator. Pain is in the dorsal forearm and may also occur at night but is usually associated with and after activities involving repetitive pronation and supination. Transient weakness of dorsiflexion can occur especially just after activities (16).

Physical examination elicits palpable pain over the posterior interosseous nerve as it crosses over the radial head (see Figure 26.14). Tinel's sign may or may not be positive locally and/or distally. Pain may also be elicited with resisted supination, especially with the wrist in a flexed position. Electromyogram (EMG) studies are rarely helpful but may be positive if performed right after activity. A lidocaine block can aid in diagnosis. In cases of refractory tennis elbow, radial tunnel syndrome could be another possibility, as symptoms are similar. Time, relative rest, and rehabilitation are usually successful in treating this condition (16).

Other Lateral Conditions

Osteochondritis dissecans of the capitellum and radial head fractures also cause lateral symptoms and are covered elsewhere in this chapter.

Lateral Radial Collateral Ligament Injury (Posterolateral Rotatory Instability)

The radial collateral ligament is usually injured from a fall on an outstretched hand with the elbow slightly flexed

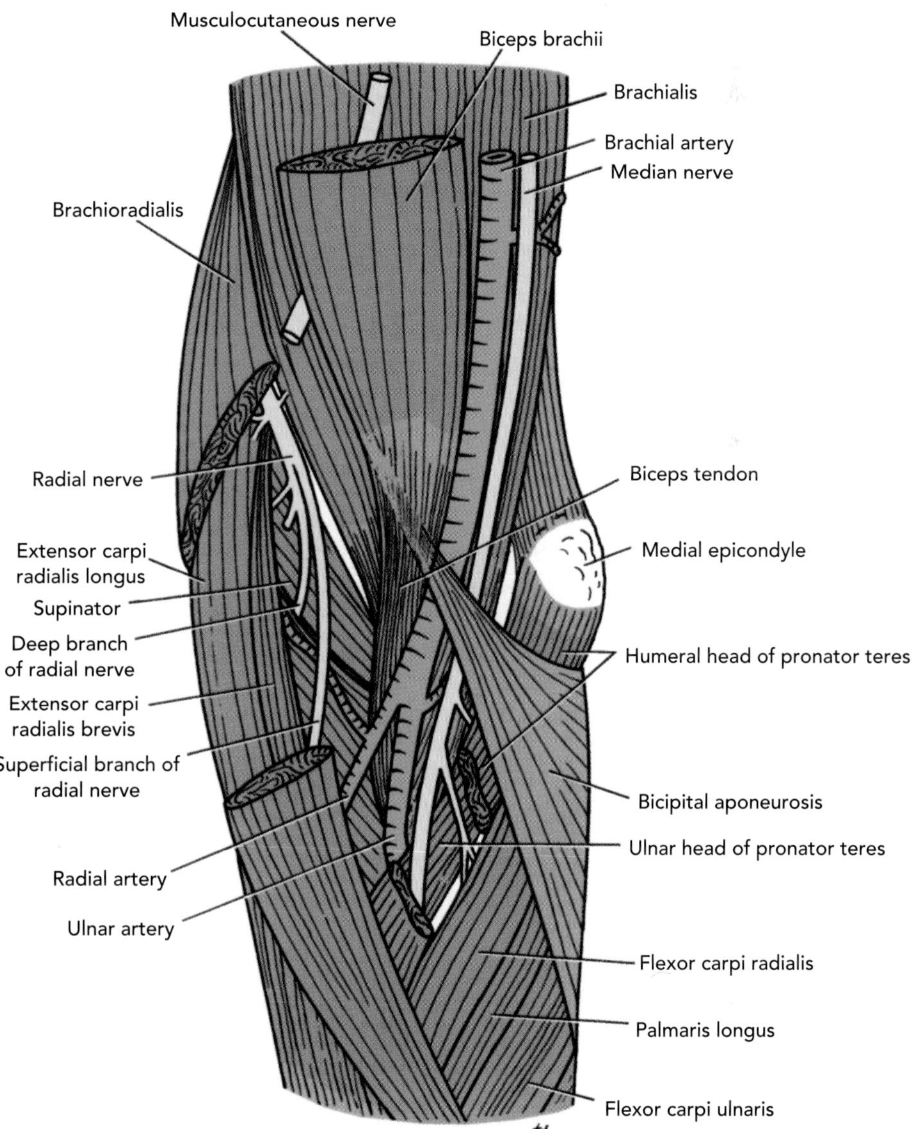

Figure 26.14 Location of the posterior interosseous nerve. (*Source*: Adapted from Chumbley E, O'Connor FG, Nirschl RP. Evaluation of overuse elbow injuries. *Am Fam Physician* 2000;61:691–700.)

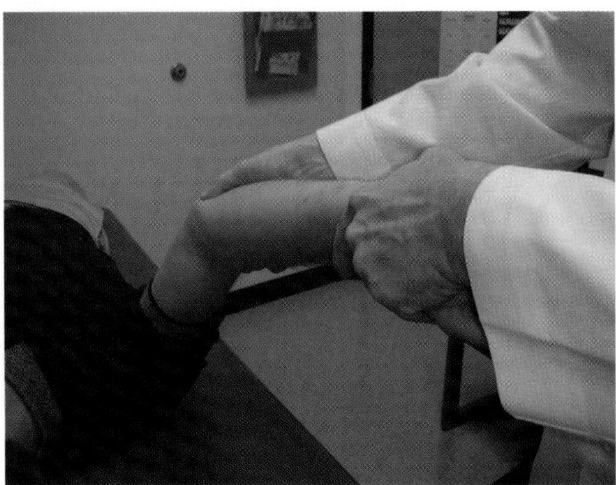

Figure 26.15 Hand positioning while performing the lateral pivot-shift test.

and the arm in a rotating forced supination. Whether the elbow subluxes or dislocates, the athlete will present with a chronically sore elbow and/or symptoms of subluxation and lateral elbow pain. The diagnosis can be difficult without a more specific test called the *Lateral Pivot-Shift test* (see Figure 26.15). The supine patient's arm is extended back over the patient's head with the shoulder externally rotated. The examiner then supinates the forearm and applies a valgus stress followed by axillary compression and flexion at the elbow. Apprehension from the patient and/or a shifting or clunk sensation constitutes a positive test. Surgical consult is usually necessary and radiographic findings are usually negative (17,18).

Medial Elbow Conditions

Medial Epicondylitis (Golfer's Elbow)

Medial epicondylitis can occur in many sports (golf, tennis, racquetball, archers, volleyball, etc.) and can have symptoms similar to a FPM strain (see Figure 26.1). On examination, however, palpable tenderness is over the epicondyle and pain can be elicited with resisted pronation, wrist flexion, and grip strength testing. Chronically, the same epicondylosis and tendinosis can occur here as well. Physical therapy is usually sufficient to resolve this condition, and radiographs are rarely needed and may only show some extra-articular calcifications (14,19).

Flexor–Pronator Muscle Strains and Ulnar Collateral Ligament Sprains

Although UCL sprains will be covered in the section, "The Elbow in the Throwing Athlete", FPM strains will usually precede them or be a forewarning for subtle UCL damage. Larger tears of the FPM will inevitably weaken the medial support of the elbow in a throwing athlete and if not already present, lead to UCL damage. Resisted wrist flexion, grip strength testing, and resisted pronation (if pronator involved) will elicit pain in the area. Relative rest and rehabilitation with attention paid to overall upper extremity and kinetic chain strength as well as biomechanics should suffice in resolving this condition (4,20,21).

Anterior Elbow Conditions

Elbow Dislocations and Fractures

Discussion on this was covered earlier in the section "Fractures and Dislocations of the Elbow"

Biceps Injuries

Biceps tendonitis/tendinosis is an overuse injury due to repetitive elbow flexion with supination. Examination is straightforward with palpable tenderness to the bicipital tendon and pain with resisted flexion and supination. Weeks of symptoms lead to more of a tendinosis condition. Conservative therapy is almost always successful for the acute biceps tendonitis (16,19).

Bicipital ruptures at the distal end of the elbow are less common and occur only in 3% of all biceps ruptures. Most will occur in athletes older than 30 years of age and may be accompanied by an avulsion fragment from the radial tuberosity. Treatment is almost always surgical, as opposed to the more common proximal ruptures which are generally treated conservatively (7,16).

Anterior Capsule Strains

The anterior capsule is most commonly strained (micro-tears) during a hyperextension-type injury mechanism. Usually the elbow experiences a force not great enough to cause dislocation. Pain is poorly localized with deep palpation resulting with pain across the antecubital area. Radiographic findings are usually normal but could show heterotopic ossifications in chronic situations. Limited immobilization followed by aggressive rehabilitation should return the athlete to full function, although flexion contractures may arise from chronic fibrosis formation (7,16).

Median Nerve Compression Syndrome (Pronator Syndrome)

This entrapment neuropathy is relatively uncommon in most sports but may be seen occasionally in rowers, kayakers, fast-pitch softball and overhead throwers, racquet sports players, and racecar drivers. Presenting symptom is a dull to occasionally sharp anterior elbow pain and sometimes a proximal forearm pain that is consistently relieved with rest from the athletes' activities. On occasion the distal volar forearm and/or radial $3\frac{1}{2}$ digits may experience numbness and tingling (22).

The entrapment/impingement of the median nerve occurs due to either a hypertrophied muscle or an aponeurotic fascia. Four areas are commonly attributed to being the site of entrapment with the pronator teres being the most common. Each area has a unique physical examination finding that may help elicit the exact location of the problem (see Table 26.6). Other

TABLE 26.6
SYMPTOM ELICITATION FOR DIFFERING MEDIAN NERVE ENTRAPMENTS

Site	Examination
Supracondylar process	Flexion of elbow 120–135 degrees
Lacertus fibrosus	Resisted forearm supination
Pronator teres	Resisted forearm pronation
Flexor digitorum superficialis arcade	Resisted flexion of long (middle) finger

Source: Adapted from data from Conway J. Clinical evaluation of elbow injuries in the athlete. *J Musculoskel Med* 1998;15(10):43–52.

physical examination findings include Tinel's sign positive proximally, with Tinel's and Phalen's signs negative at the wrist (22).

Confirmation may be made by an EMG or nerve conduction velocity (NCV) test but these are not always reliable. Treatment consists of relative rest with rehabilitation progressing gradually with strength and flexibility. Decompression is only necessary in rare recalcitrant cases (16,22).

Posterior and Posteromedial Conditions

Posterior conditions include triceps tendonitis, olecranon bursitis, and stress fractures. More rarely a triceps rupture may occur. All are found in athletes involved in heavy weight training or vigorous repetitive extension motions (e.g., canoeists). Most athletes are treated conservatively and the athlete returns to full function. Olecranon osteophytes may also contribute to symptoms and can be elicited utilizing the reverse axial projection method radiographically (see Figure 26.16). Olecranon stress fractures in young athletes usually affects the apophysis while in the adult a hairline stress fracture can be missed on plain films and require a bone scan/magnetic resonance imaging (MRI) confirmation (16,23).

Posteromedial pain can be specifically described and differentiated from the other posterior and ulnar nerve symptoms and conditions. When evaluating an overhead-throwing athlete with pain in this area, the examiner usually finds etiology due to valgus extension overload that can result in olecranon hypertrophy, olecranon fossa impingement, olecranon osteophyte formation, or posteromedial trochlear chondromalacia. The pitcher involved will notice pain during the acceleration phase of throwing and after a few innings, will lose control by releasing the ball early causing the pitch to be continuously high (21).

Physical examination will elicit palpable tenderness on the olecranon tip or medial portion of the olecranon fossa. A flexion contracture may also be found. Radiographs are used to identify any bone spurs or fractures. Care in distinguishing normal anatomy is essential as a spur

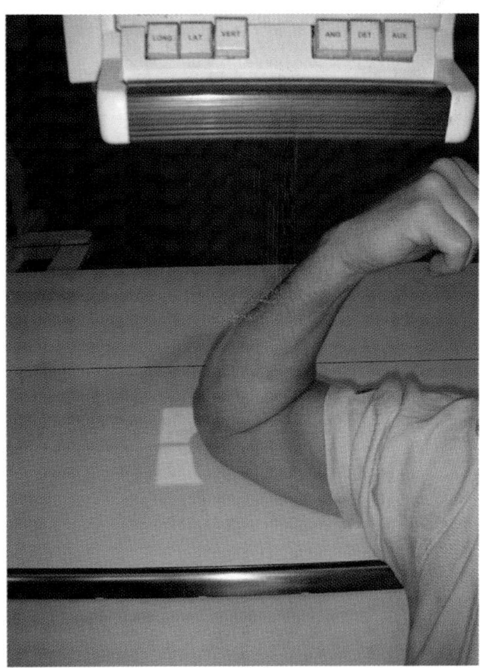

Figure 26.16 Reverse axial projection for assessing olecranon osteophytes.

located on the radial side of the olecranon tip can be mistaken for pathology. Computed tomography (CT) or MRI may also be used when appropriate or if the diagnosis is in question. Conservative therapy is often unsuccessful and surgical referral is necessary to remove any osteophytes, loose bodies, or impingements (4,21).

THE ELBOW IN THE THROWING ATHLETE

Elbow pain is a common entity at some point in many a throwing athlete's career. Younger throwers tend to see more injuries related to the epiphysis while older adolescents and adults tend to have more overuse and degenerative ligament and tendon injuries. Some studies have shown that although the incidence of elbow pain in Little League baseball was high as 45% to 78% only 1% to 5% ever had pain severe enough to stop pitching (4,20).

There are six stages of throwing and different injuries can be associated with the different stages. The six stages of throwing are the windup, early cocking, late cocking, acceleration, deceleration, and the follow-through (see Figure 26.17). More injuries occur during the late cocking and acceleration phases as high valgus forces are placed on the elbow causing the popularly phrased medial tension injuries. During these phases, lateral compression forces are also placed on the elbow inciting other possible injuries. Deceleration and follow-through require the proper firing of the biceps, brachialis, and brachioradialis or hyperextension can occur leading to posterior impaction injuries (17,20).

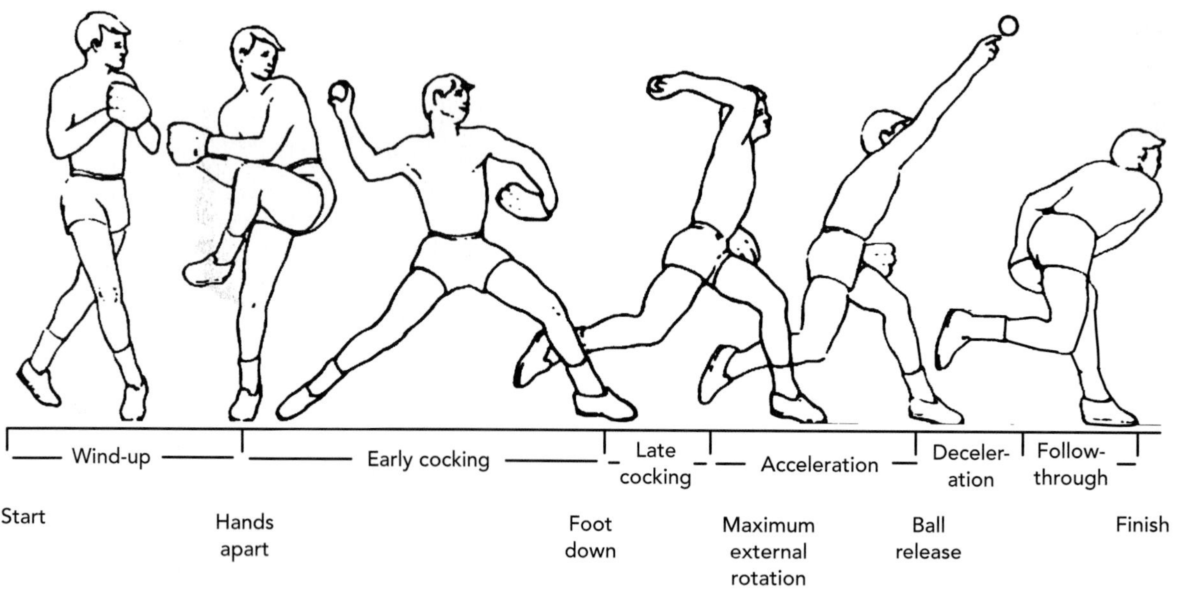

Figure 26.17 Six stages of the throwing motion.

ULNAR COLLATERAL LIGAMENT INJURY IN THROWERS

A history of pain medially during late cocking and acceleration phases of throwing are commonly seen in UCL injuries. The valgus torque experienced from repetitive throwing can create gradual or abrupt tearing of the UCL and hinders the throwers' ability either insidiously or acutely. Acute injuries are usually accompanied by a "pop" while chronic conditions progress through a series of changes characterized by edema, scarring, calcification, and ossification (24).

Physical examination elicits palpable tenderness diffusely over the medial elbow with more specific point tenderness over the ulnar attachment of the anterior band and the tubercle of the coronoid process. Neurological examination should also be performed, as ulnar nerve pathology can be present as well. The examiner then places a valgus stress on the elbow to test the stability of the UCL. The elbow is positioned at 30 degrees of flexion with the shoulder abducted and externally rotated (see Figure 26.5). The examiner tucks the wrist under his axilla and places one hand laterally with the medially placed hand under the ulna and the thumb or index finger over the UCL to palpate the medial joint line. This test is repeated on the contralateral side. Differences in pain and opening of the joint line can lead to the diagnosis of an UCL injury (4,24).

Two more recent examination techniques were added to this initial test; the milking maneuver (see Figure 26.18) and the O'Driscoll moving valgus stress test. The milking maneuver involves placing the affected elbow at 90 degrees of flexion with the shoulder at the side and 90 degrees of abduction. The examiner grabs the thumb and externally rotates the arm and supinates the forearm while applying a valgus force on the elbow. The thumb is pulled downward towards the floor as if "milking" the udder of a cow. The examiner places his other hand over the medial joint line to monitor pain and/or instability. The moving valgus stress test is performed by placing the elbow in maximum flexion, and applying a valgus force until maximum external rotation is reached. The elbow is extended rapidly to 30 degrees flexion while constantly under the valgus force. A positive examination recreates the patients medial elbow pain, and should be maximal between 120 and 70 degrees of

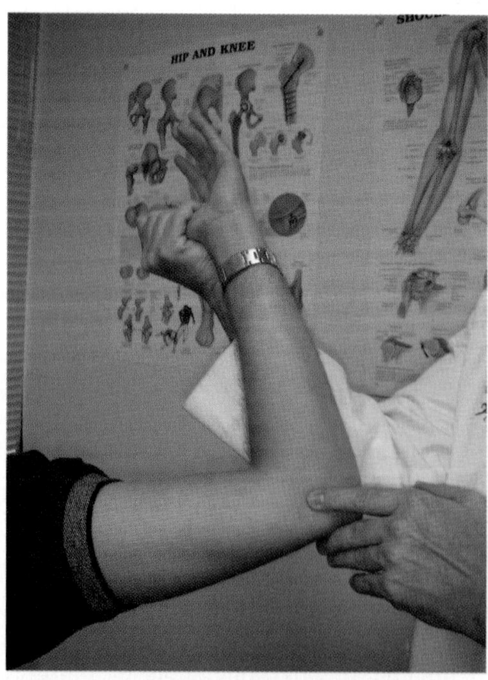

Figure 26.18 Positioning for performing the milking maneuver.

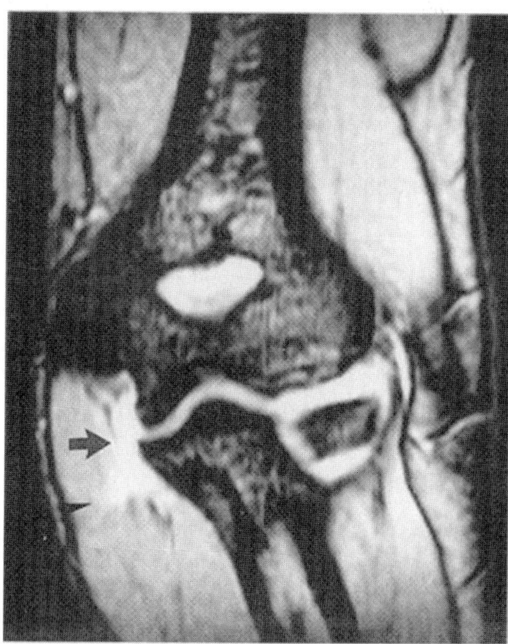

Figure 26.19 Elbow magnetic resonance imaging (MRI) with arthrogram. The large arrow points out the disruption of the ulnar collateral ligament (UCL), and the small arrow shows contrast leakage.

flexion as the elbow moves through the arc. These represent the flexion angles of the elbow during the throwing positions of late cocking and early acceleration, respectively. O'Driscoll reports a sensitivity of 100% and a specificity of 75% for diagnosing UCL injury when compared with surgical exploration or arthroscopic stressing (4,25,26).

Diagnostic studies are still being normalized for the throwing athlete with UCL pathology. In addition to the usual plain radiographs, most sports physicians will obtain amagnetic resonance (MR) arthrogram (see Figure 26.19). However, since a negative MR arthrogram does not eliminate the possibility for chronic laxity, most will augment a normal MR arthrogram with a valgus stress radiograph, if one was not obtained earlier. The amount of force applied, the angle of flexion, and the landmarks for measurement all determine the measured laxity. More studies are helping distinguish these numbers as compared to controls. Despite all the above imaging modalities, equivocal findings can still occur and the decision toward surgical reconstruction is still on a clinical basis (26–28).

Return to throwing competitively is determined by the severity and type of injury and whether surgical intervention was required. UCL sprains usually require relative rest and rehabilitation that includes a graduated throwing program. The entire process requires a minimum of 12 to 14 weeks before the athlete returns to competitive throwing. UCL reconstruction however, usually has most pitchers returning to competitive throwing in 12 months on average. It is this author's experience at the major league level that most pitchers postreconstruction do not "feel" as crisp and sharp as they felt until 18 months, preinjury (29).

ULNAR NEUROPATHY IN THE THROWING ATHLETE

The act of throwing causes a great deal of traction force on the medial aspect of the elbow and can lead to many conditions. Symptoms of tingling and numbness of the fourth and fifthdigits and/or forearm can indicate that those traction forces are causing damage to the ulnar nerve. The late cocking phase of throwing has the arm in abduction, the elbow flexed and the wrist extended, causing traction force medially and can cause a traction neuropathy. Dynamic compression forces can also add to the traction as the flexor carpi ulnaris (FCU) is activated and the FCU arcade impinges the ulnar nerve with active wrist flexion. Associated symptoms include subjective feelings of weakness at the elbow and possibly a popping sensation over the medial epicondyle (4,12,21).

Structural changes that may reduce the antecubital tunnel area and cause ulnar neuropathy include medial collateral ligament insufficiency, medial epicondylitis, medial compartment spurring, and synovitis. Physical examination may elicit a positive Tinel's sign over the antecubital tunnel and decreased two point tactile discrimination/sensory of the fifth digit. Atrophy of the intrinsic muscles of the hand is rare in athletes. Electromyographic and neurodiagnostic studies may be negative in the resting athlete. Therefore, all testing, including physical examination, should be performed after throwing (4,21).

Treatment consists of the restriction of activities and a review of the biomechanics of the throwing athlete. Conservative therapy consists of NSAIDs, night splinting, and cortisone injections. Conservative therapy should be employed for 3 to 6 months before surgery is considered. Surgical decompression has shown poor outcomes; so more surgeons opt for a transposition (either submuscular, intramuscular, or subcutaneous). Return to throwing is usually 6 to 9 months in the best circumstances (4,12,21).

ELBOW INJURIES/CONDITIONS IN THE YOUNG THROWING ATHLETE

Little Leaguer's Elbow

"Little Leaguer's Elbow" has been a broad term encompassing different diagnoses to differing professionals. Little league elbow (LLE) now includes a series of diagnoses including (a) medial epicondylar fragmentation and apophysitis (see Figure 26.20); (b) delayed or accelerated apophyseal growth of the medial epicondyle; (c) delayed closure of the medial epicondylar growth plate; (d) osteochondrosis and osteochondritis dissecans of the humeral capitellum; (e) deformation and osteochondritis of the radial head; (f) hypertrophy of the ulna, and (g) olecranon apophysitis. Two distinct entities, Panner's disease and Osteochondritis Dissecans, need to be differentiated while

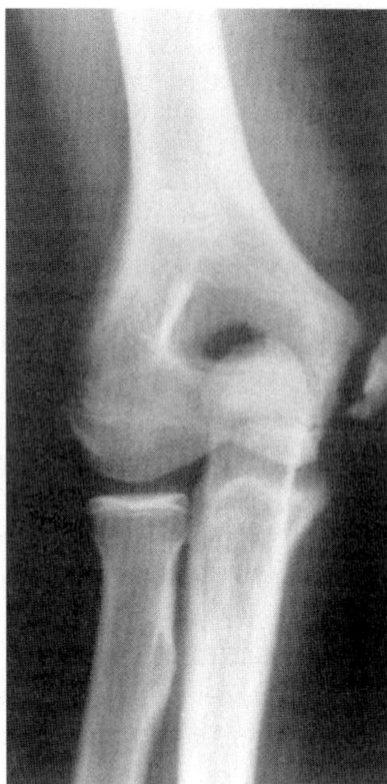

Figure 26.20 Medial epicondyle fragmentation and apophysitis in Little League Elbow.

diagnosing a young throwing athlete with elbow pain (see Table 26.7) (17,20,30).

Studies suggest that 20% of pitchers aged 10 to 14 years old suffer from elbow pain. Secondary ossification centers at the elbow appear at the capitellum at age 2, radial head at 5, medial epicondyle at 7, trochlea at 9, olecranon at 10, and lateral epicondyle at 11. Most fuse between 14 and 17 years of age (31).

LLE is usually defined as a set of conditions that lead to elbow pain from the act of throwing a baseball. Mechanisms of injury include both medial traction and lateral compression forces (see Figure 26.21). Common mistakes in the athlete's biomechanics or being allowed to overuse the pitching arm can lead to any of the above diagnoses. The American Academy of Pediatrics has set some guidelines regarding how often a young pitcher should be allowed to throw. Their recommendations include a maximum of 6 innings per week for ages 8 to 12 and definitely not more than 200 pitches per week or 90 pitches per outing. Many people have created guidelines, but one of the easiest recommendations is to limit pitches to 10 pitches times their age, per each 7-day period. More recent independent research suggests for all adolescents: (a) avoid pitching with arm pain and/or fatigue; (b) avoid pitching more than 80 pitches per game; (c) avoid pitching competitively more than 8 months per year and (d) avoid pitching more than 2500 pitches per year (4,17,32,33).

Olecranon Stress Fracture

Any widening of or persistence of the growth plate should be considered a stress lesion. Repeated extension loads or forceful traumatic displacement can lead to an acutely displaced fracture. Persistent lucency on radiographs after age 15 usually indicates an incomplete or nonhealing stress fracture. MRI confirms suspicions of a stress fracture. Physical examination often reveals 10 to 15 degrees of flexion contracture, pain with forced extension, and pain with resisted triceps extension. Treatment consists of rest with a temporary orthoplast posterior splint. This is followed by gradual rehabilitation up to 6 months before return to unrestricted activities. Radiographic findings need to be normal before complete clearance. Surgical fixation with a screw and/or wiring is indicated for failed conservative treatment or a completely displaced fragment (12,23).

With postoperative rehabilitation for surgical fixation, the athlete is allowed all the flexion/extension that the soft dressings allow. One week postoperatively, begins wrist and finger resistant exercises. The throwing program can usually begin at 6 weeks. Overall plan is to return to competition in 3 to 4 months. Open or closed procedures do not change the 10 to 12 weeks that a pitcher will be out. Re-evaluate the pitching mechanics along with any restrictions

TABLE 26.7
PANNER'S DISEASE VERSUS OSTEOCHONDRITIS DISSECANS

	Osteochondritis Dissecans	Panner's Disease
Age	Teens	~10 yr
Onset	Insidious	Acute
Radiography	Subchondral bone area demarcated by slightly dense linear zone	Fragmentation of capitellar ossific zone
Loose bodies	Present	Absent
Residual Capitellar deformity	Present	Minimal

Source: From Bennett J, Mehlhoff T. Immature skeletal lesions of the elbow. In: Drez D, DeLee J, eds. *Operative techniques in sports medicine*, Vol. 9. No. 4. WB Saunders, 2001:234–240.

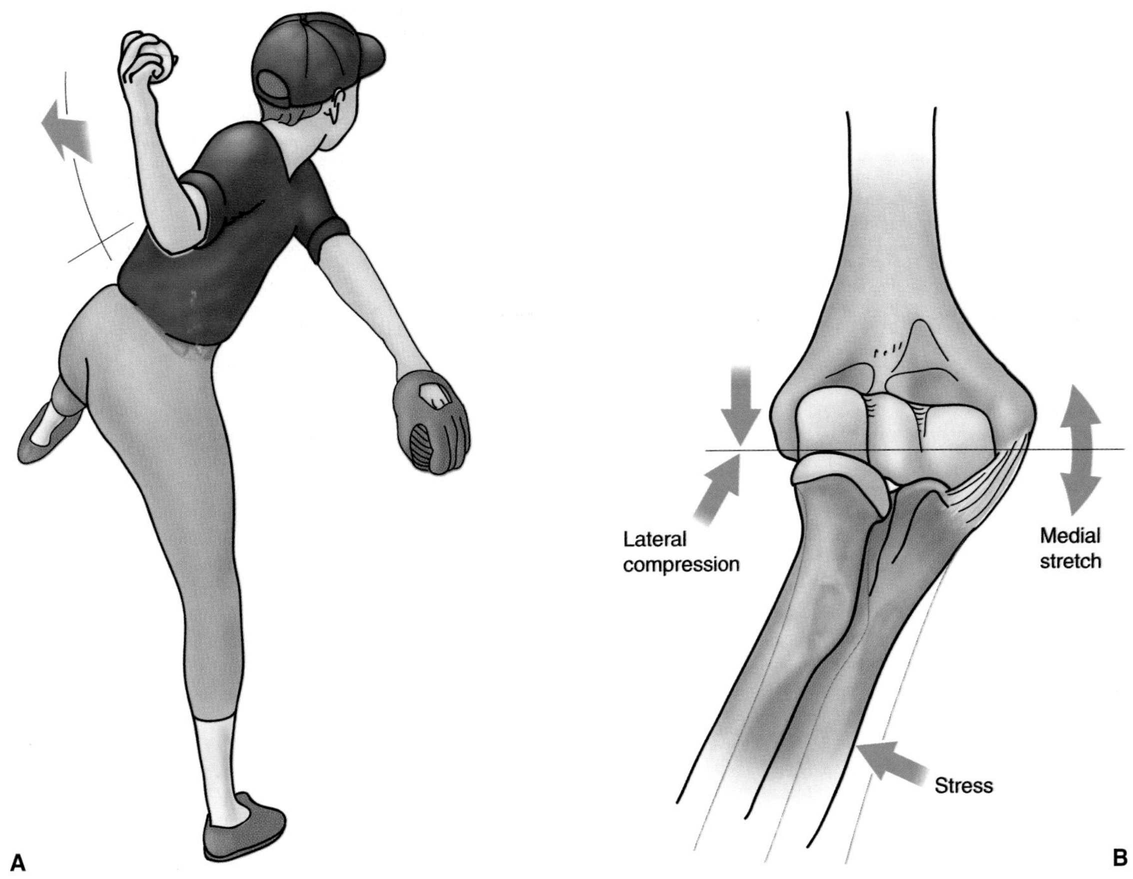

Figure 26.21 "Little League Elbow". The diagram on the right shows the direction of the medial traction and lateral compression forces. (*Source*: Adapted from Congeni J. Treating and preventing little league elbow. *Phys Sportsmed* 1994;22(3):54–64.)

or weaknesses in the entire kinetic chain. Preoperative care consists of several weeks of not throwing and conservative measures. Return to competition cannot be anticipated until complete healing of the fracture occurs, and only after the athlete regains his or her strength and ROM (17).

REHABILITATION OF THE THROWING ATHLETE

Rehabilitation of the throwing athlete after any elbow condition needs to focus not only on specific elbow ROM and strength issues, but also on the thrower's entire kinetic chain. Unpublished data at the major league level has demonstrated that lower body biomechanics and weaknesses can transpose themselves into upper extremity conditions in the throwing athlete. No longer can we just focus on the elbow, rotator cuff, and scapula when diagnosing the etiology of a thrower's injury. Although rehabilitation will be covered elsewhere in this book, the newer rehabilitation methods not published in general texts of yet, have demonstrated a superior success in dealing with athletic sports injuries. The rehabilitation needs to focus on functional strengthening in all three planes of motion, and most importantly in the *transverse plane.* It is recommended that one looks further down the kinetic chain as well as at the usual areas when dealing with injuries in a throwing athlete.

REFERENCES

1. Chumbley E, O'Connor FG, Nirschl RP. Evaluation of overuse elbow injuries. *Am Fam Physician* 2000;61:691–700.
2. Coleman WW. Physical examination of the elbow. *Orthop Clin North Am* 1999;30(1):15–20.
3. Timmerman LA. Elbow injuries. In: Garrett WE, Kirkendall DT, Speer KP, et al. ed. *Principles and practice of orthopaedic sports medicine.* Philadelphia: Lippincott Williams & Wilkins, 2000:307–327.
4. Ireland ML, Hutchinson MR. Elbow injuries. In: Andrews JR, Zarins B, Wilk KE, eds. *Injuries in baseball.* Philadelphia: Lippincott-Raven, 1998.
5. Conway John. Clinical evaluation of elbow injuries in the athlete. *J Musculoskel Med* 1998;15(10):43–52.
6. Kuntz DG, Baratz ME. Fractures of the elbow. *Orthop Clin North Am* 1999;30(1):37–61.
7. Rettig AC. Traumatic elbow injuries in the athlete. *Orthop Clin North Am* 2002;33(3):509–522.
8. Eiff MP, Hatch R, Calmbach WL. *Fracture management for primary care.* Philadelphia: Elsevier Science, 2003.
9. Mercier L, Pettid FJ, Tamisiea DF, Heieck JJ. The elbow. In: *Practical orthopedics.* Chapter 6. Mosby, 2000:75–85.
10. Behr CT, Altchek DW. The elbow. *Clin Sports Med* 1997;16(4):681–704.
11. Sofka CM, Potter HG. Imaging of elbow injuries in the child and adult athlete. *Radiol Clin North Am* 2002;40(2):251–265.
12. Bennett J, Mehlhoff T. Immature skeletal lesions of the elbow. In: Drez D, DeLee J, eds. *Operative techniques in sports medicine,* Vol. 9. No. 4. WB Saunders, 2001:234–240.
13. Nicholas JA, Hershman. *The upper extremity in sports medicine.* Mosby, 1990:273–306, 319–362.

14. Hannafin JA. How I manage tennis and Golfer's elbow. *Phys Sportsmed* 1996;24(2):63–68.
15. Melham TJ, Sevier TL, Malnofski MJ, et al. Chronic ankle pain and fibrosis successfully treated with a new non-invasive augmented soft tissue mobilization (ASTM). *Med Sci Sports Exerc* 1998;30(6):801–804.
16. Delee J, Drez D, Miller M. *Delee and Drez's orthopaedic sports medicine: principles and practice*, 2nd ed. WB Saunders, 2003.
17. Andrews JR, Zarins B, Wilk KE. *Injuries in baseball*. Lippincott-Raven, 1998.
18. Smith JP III, Savoie FH III, Field LD, et al. Posterolateral rotatory instability of the elbow. *Clin Sports Med* 2001;20(1):47–58.
19. Grana W. Medial epicondylitis and cubital tunnel syndrome in the throwing athlete. *Clin Sports Med* 2001;20(3):541–548.
20. Fleisig GS, Andrews JR, Dillman CJ, et al. Kinetics of baseball pitching with implications about injury mechanism. *Am J Sports Med* 1995;23:233.
21. Maloney MD, Mohr KJ, el Attrache NS, et al. Elbow injuries in the throwing athlete. *Clin Sports Med* 1999;18(4):795–809.
22. Rehak DC. Pronator syndrome. *Clin Sports Med* 2001;20(3):531–548.
23. Kourosh F, et al. Triceps tendonitis. In: Drez D, DeLee J, eds. *Operative techniques in sports medicine*, Vol. 9(4). WB Saunders, 2001:217–221.
24. Rettig AC, Sherrill C, Snead D, et al. Non-operative treatment of ulnar collateral ligament injuries in throwing athletes. *Am J Sports Med* 2001;29(1):15–17.
25. O'Driscoll SW, Lawton RL, Smith AM, et al. The "moving valgus stress test" for medial collateral ligament tears of the elbow. *Am J Sports Med* 2005;33(2):231–239.
26. Hyman J, Breazeale NM, Altechk DW. Valgus instability of the elbow in athletes. *Clin Sports Med* 2001;20(1):25–45.
27. Ellenbecker TS, Mattalino AJ, Elam EA, et al. Medial elbow joint laxity in professional baseball pitchers: a bilateral comparison using stress radiography. *Am J Sports Med* 1998;26(3):420–424.
28. Lee GA, Katz SD, Lazarus MD. Elbow valgus stress radiography in an uninjured population. *Am J Sports Med* 1998;26(3):425–427.
29. Wilk KE, Reinold MM, Andrews JR. Rehabilitation of the Thrower's elbow. *Clin Sports Med* 2004;23(4):765–801.
30. Bradley JP, Petrie RS. Osteochondritis dissecans of the humeral capitellum: diagnosis and treatment. *Clin Sports Med* 2001;20(3):565–590.
31. Patel DR, Nelson TL. Sports injuries in adolescents. *Med Clin North Am* 2000;84(4):983–1007.
32. Olsen SJ, Fleisig GS, Dun S, et al. Risk factors for shoulder and elbow injuries in adolescent baseball pitchers. *Am J Sports Med* 2006;34(6): 905–912.
33. American Academy of Pediatrics Committee on Sports Medicine and Fitness. Risk of injury from baseball and softball in children. *Pediatrics* 2001;107(4):782–784.

27

Wrist, Hand, and Finger Injuries

Wade A. Lillegard

The significance of wrist, hand, and finger injuries is often underestimated by the athlete and clinician because of their non–weight-bearing status, a tendency to consider this injury as a sprain, and the pressure to continue playing. These injuries are therefore considered "minor" and not often included in the statistical records. McGrew et al. reported that 11% of 1,286 injuries in a primary care sports medicine setting were to the fingers and hands (1). In Dobyn's series of 1,425 fractures, dislocations, and fracture–dislocations of the fingers and hands, the distribution was as follows: dislocations; 14 distal interphalangeal (DIP), 43 proximal interphalangeal (PIP), 19 metacarpophalangeal (MCP), 3 carpometacarpal (CMC), and 4 carpal (2). The remaining 1,342 fractures and fracture–dislocations were as follows: distal phalanx 133 (9%), DIP joint 160 (11%), middle phalanx (MP) 86 (5%), PIP joint 216 (14%), proximal phalanx 229 (15%), MP joint 88 (5%), metacarpalphalangeal (MC) joint 348 (24%), CMC joint 62 (4%), and carpal bones 217 (14%) (2).

The misdiagnosis of a sprain is potentially harmful as it may overlook an osseous, tendinous, or ligamentous injury, which could lead to chronic instability or pain.

WRIST ANATOMY

Functional Anatomy

No tendons originate from or insert into the carpal bones (except for the sesamoidal pisiform), rendering wrist motion purely passive, with the carpal bones functioning as an intercalated segment (3).

The scaphoid (navicular) is the only carpal bone to cross the proximal and distal carpal rows (see Figure 27.1). This position provides stability by preventing the proximal row from collapsing in a zigzag configuration under compressive loads. The position and function also places the scaphoid at the greatest risk of injury (3).

Ligamentous Anatomy

The general configuration of the ligaments in the volar wrist is a double inverted V (4). The distal inverted V is formed by the two components of the deltoid ligament (capitoscaphoid and capitotriquetral ligaments); these are intracapsular and intrinsic. The proximal inverted V is formed by two intracapsular extrinsic ligaments: the radiolunate and ulnolunate. Between these two Vs is an area frequently devoid of ligamentous support of the capitolunate articulation. This potentially weak space is called the *space of Porrier* and may predispose the wrist to perilunate instability in hyperextension injuries (5).

HAND ANATOMY

Tendons

The nine finger flexors and the median nerve pass into the hand through the carpal tunnel beneath the transverse carpal ligament in the wrist (6). Five of the nine are deep flexors that pass through a split in the superficialis tendons and course to the distal phalanx of each finger and thumb (see Figure 27.2). The other four are superficial flexors that insert on the MP of each finger. The flexor tendons pass beneath a series of unique anchoring ligaments between the distal palmar crease and the DIP joint. These annular ligaments create "pulleys" and prevent the tendons from bowstringing. Tendon repair in this so-called "surgical no

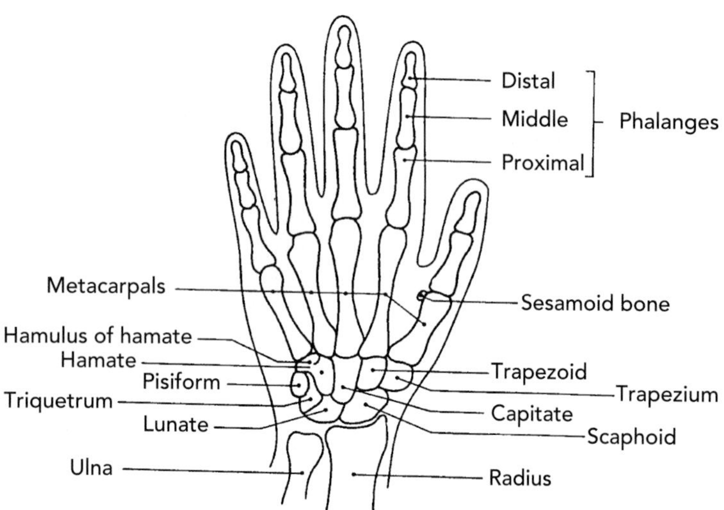

Figure 27.1 Bones of the hand and wrist.

man's land" is therefore often complicated due to adhesions that form between the lacerated tendon-ends and these ligaments.

The extensor tendons enter the dorsal extensor hood at the distal end of the MCs. Distal to the sagittal fibers of the extensor hood enter the transverse and oblique fibers from the interosseous and lumbrical muscles. These blend into the sides of the extensor hood over the proximal phalanx and flex the MCP joint by pulling on the extensor hood (7). The central portion of this extensor complex (central extensor tendon) travels distally over the PIP joint and inserts into the proximal dorsal aspect of the MP to extend the PIP. The lateral bands continue radially and ulnarly forming the terminal extensor tendon and insert onto the proximal dorsal aspect of the distal phalanx to extend the DIP (7) (see Figure 27.3).

Ligaments

The volar plate is a U-shaped thickened portion of the joint capsule on the volar aspect of the finger joints and is a static stabilizer against hyperextension forces. Disruption of this will lead to chronic deformities if not allowed to heal in its proper anatomic position.

The collateral ligaments afford medial and lateral stability and are at maximal tautness at 70 degrees flexion for the MCP, 30 degrees for the PIP, and 15 degrees for the DIP (7). When the hand is immobilized for any length of time, the collateral ligaments will contract, therefore the ligaments should be immobilized flexed at the above angles (collaterals maximally lengthened) to prevent permanent contractures.

Physical Examination Principles—Wrist

Significant pain and/or swelling after trauma to the wrist imply a significant injury. Osseous and ligamentous injury that may lead to instability must be carefully investigated and ruled out before the injury is classified as a wrist sprain (8). The history is generally similar for most of these injuries—the athlete falls on or strikes a dorsiflexed wrist (commonly referred to as a *foosh injury or fall on an*

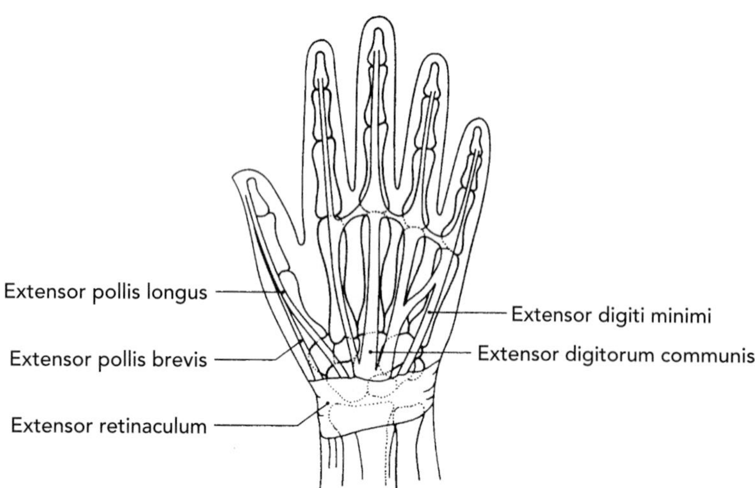

Figure 27.2 Tendons of the hand and wrist.

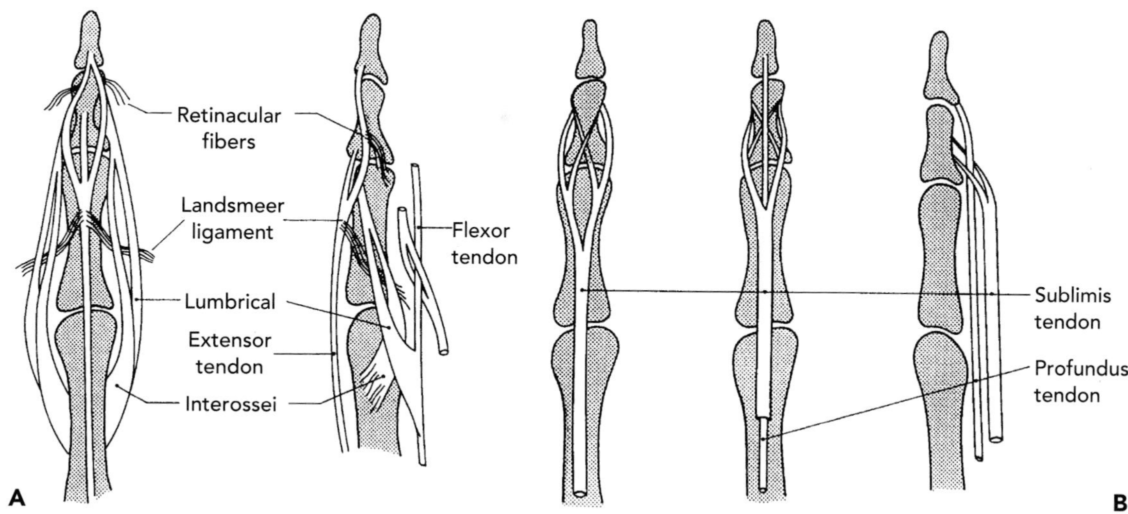

Figure 27.3 A: Digital extensor mechanism. B: Digital flexor mechanism.

out-stretched hand), has rotational stress, or the mechanism of occurrence is not remembered. Pain and/or swelling are often noted immediately.

On physical examination there may be a variable degree of swelling, with greater swelling indicating a more serious injury. Tenderness can be diffused or localized over the general area of injury, and range of motion (see Table 27.1) is limited by pain, swelling, or instability. The neurovascular status must be assessed on all injuries. Other specific tests and findings are mentioned under specific injuries.

Physical Examination Principles—Hand

Most injuries to the hand resulting in significant disability are caused by direct or indirect trauma, with subsequent disruption of a static (capsule, volar plate, collateral ligament, or bone) or dynamic (tendon, dorsal hood) stabilizer. Intricate interactions of the bones, ligaments, capsule, and tendons allow the exquisite functioning of the hand, and yet maintain its stability. Disruption of any of these may lead to significant functional disability (9). Central tendon rupture leads to "boutonniere" deformity, volar plate disruption leads to dorsal instability or a "swan-neck" deformity, angulated fractures lead to decreased grip function, and so on.

Clues to significant injuries can be any of the following: severe deformity on initial examination, incomplete reduction of the initial deformity, loss of normal alignment or joint motion (including catching, locking, or crepitus) during active or passive flexion and extension, an increase of more than 20% of the normal range of motion in any plane during passive testing, or pain or muscle contraction significant enough to inhibit testing (10).

With the wrist in mild dorsiflexion, the curve of the finger is noted. This is referred to as *the position of function* (see Figure 27.4). In the absence of obvious fracture or dislocation, deviation from the normal semiflexed position suggests a flexor (or less likely, extensor) tendon injury (11). The arm is then pronated with the wrist slightly flexed. An excessive drop may suggest an extensor tendon injury. The patient is then observed while actively flexing and extending the fingers, thumb, and wrist, looking for any deviation from the normal. With gentle flexion, all of the fingers

TABLE 27.1
NORMAL ROM OF THE WRIST AND HAND

	Direction of Motion	Normal Range (in degrees)
Wrist	Flexion	80
	Extension	70
	Radial deviation-	20
	Ulnar deviation-	30
	Forearm supination-	90
	Forearm pronation	90
Hand–finger MCP	Dorsiflexion	45
	Volarflexion	90
Hand–finger PIP	Extension	0
	Flexion	110
Hand–finger DIP	Extension 0 to	0
	Flexion	90
Hand–finger	Ab/adduction	20 arc
Hand–thumb MCP	Extension	0
	Flexion	70
Hand–thumb IP	Extension	30
	Flexion	90

MCP = metacarpophalangeal; PIP = proximal interphalangeal; DIP = distal interphalangeal; IP = interphalangeal

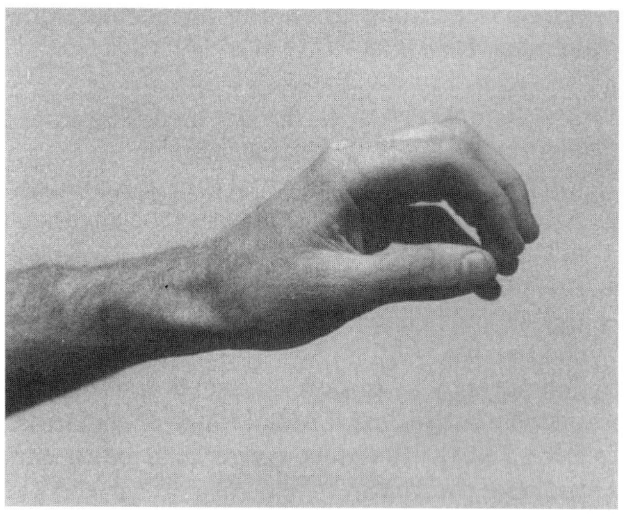
Figure 27.4 Position of function.

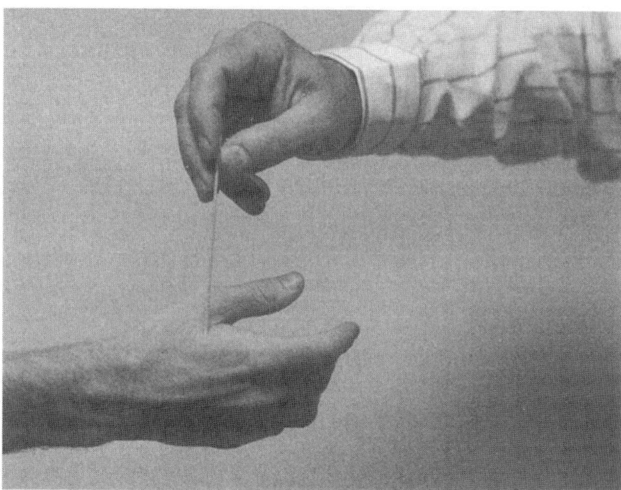
Figure 27.6 Radial nerve testing.

should generally point towards the scaphoid tuberosity (see Figure 27.5). Any deviation suggests a rotational deformity of a phalanx or MC (11). Active flexion and extension may be hampered by a disrupted tendon, ligament, or fracture, and an unstable joint may sublux. Sensation can be tested by asking the athlete to distinguish between the feel of the rough edge of a quarter and a smooth edged coin, or by two-point discrimination. Specific findings are discussed under individual injuries.

Neurological Examination of the Hand and Wrist

Because there are no distinguishable deep tendon reflexes in the wrists, hands, or fingers, the neurological examination concentrates on motor assessment and sensory testing (see Tables 27.2 and 27.3 and Figures 27.6–27.8).

IMAGING

Wrist

Initial radiographs for the acutely injured wrist should include at least a posteroanterior (PA) view of the wrist in neutral, and a true lateral view. Additional views, depending on the clinical indication, might involve PA in ulnar deviation and oblique and PA in 45 degrees pronation from neutral. Further imaging techniques may be necessary and are mentioned where indicated under specific injuries. Technetium 99 scintography (bone scan) is a useful study for evaluating suspected fractures not visualized on plain radiography. If there is focal increased uptake on the bone scan, computerized tomography (CT) or tomograms of the area should follow to define small fractures (12). Magnetic resonance imaging (MRI) of the wrist has a high rate of false-positive and false-negative results for many types of instabilities, but can be diagnostic in some cases. Wrist arthrography can be very useful, but decisions on this and other more detailed radiographic imaging techniques for suspected serious injuries are probably best left to the surgical consultant.

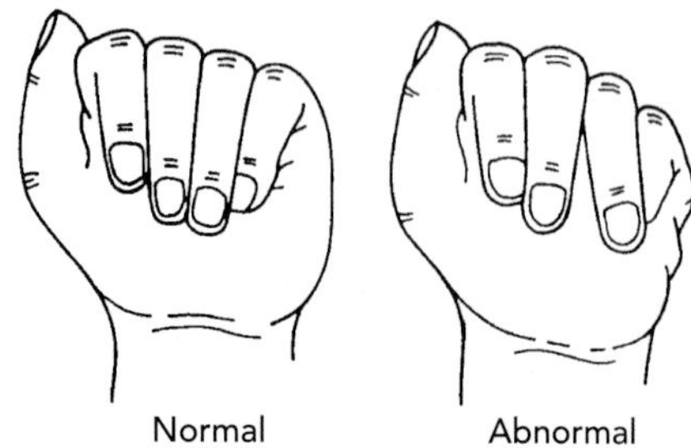

Figure 27.5 Position of fingers in flexion (malrotation test).

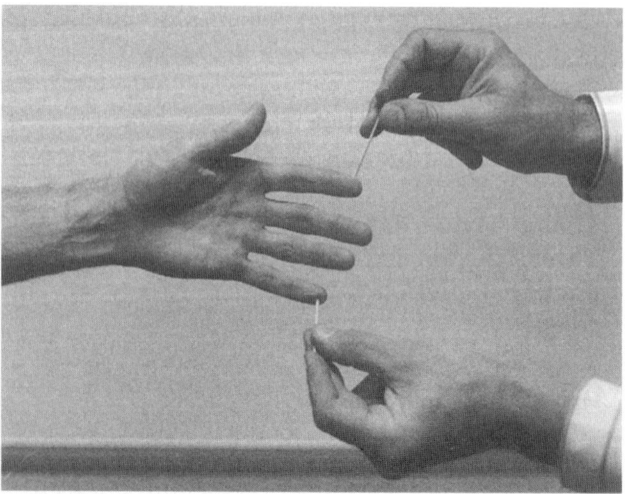
Figure 27.7 Medial and ulnar nerve testing.

TABLE 27.2
GUIDE TO NEUROLOGICAL ASSESSMENT OF THE HAND

Nerve	Sensation	Muscle Innervated	Test of Function
Ulnar	Ulnar aspect of hand and ulnar one and a half digits	Flexor digitorum profundus (ulnar two digits)	Stabilize MCP & PIP in extension (isolates superficialis), patient flexes isolated PIP
		Dorsal interossei DAB (Dorsal ABducts)	Patient fans extended fingers, examiner forces each pair together
		Palmar interossei PAD (Palmar ADucts)	Patient holds extended fingers together with paper interposed. examiner attempts to pull paper out longitudinally
		Adductor pollicus	Patient adducts thumb against resistance
		Abductor digiti mimimi	Patient abducts small finger against resistance (most specific for ulnar nerve)
Median	Radial side of palm, radial, palmer $3\frac{1}{2}$ digits, dorsal tips of index, middle, and radial 1/2 ring fingers	Flexor pollicus brevislateral portion of radial two lumbricals	Patient makes "O" with thumb and index finger, examiner attempts to break them apart.
		Opponens pollicus	Patient apposes small finger & thumb, examiner attempts to separate
		Abductor pollicus longus	Patient abducts thumb against resistance
		Flexor pollicus longus	Patient holds flexed thumb to hypothenar eminence, examiner attempts to pull thumb away
		Flexor digitorum superficialis	Fingers are held in extension to isolate superficialis patient flexes isolated PIP
Radial	Radial side of thumb, dorsal radial hand up tomi fingers of index middle and radial 1/2 of ring	Extensor carpi radialis, brevis, and ulnaris	Patient attempts to extend wrist against resistance
		Extensor pollicus longus and brevis	Patient estends thumb against examiners resistance
		Abductor pollicus longus	Patient abducts thumb against reisistance
		Extensor digitorum communis	Wrist is neutral. the patient extends the MCP with the PIP remaining flexed (to prevent use of intrinsics)

MCP = metacarpophalongeal; PIP = proximal interphalongeal

Hand

Radiographs should be taken for any injury with bony tenderness, angulation, rotation, or instability. Generally, PA and lateral (with splayed fingers) views will suffice.

TREATMENT PRINCIPLES

Injuries involving the hand and digits can be difficult problems to manage in athletes. Strict compliance with immobilization is often difficult to achieve with the athlete who perceives an urgent need to return to competition. A certain amount of risk is inherent in returning any athlete to play before complete healing. In the younger, skeletally immature athlete, the decision is easier because no risk should be taken and injuries should be allowed to heal fully. In a college or professional athlete the situation can be more complicated, requiring cooperation among the athlete, physician, trainer, therapist, and orthotist to agree on an acceptable solution. The ultimate decision to return to play is dictated by the individual's condition, specific sport and position played, and the ability to safely splint/protect the injury.

Three treatment principles apply in the management of most hand injuries: splinting, ice, and elevation. The hand has minimal space to accommodate swelling, and the treating clinician needs to be aware of the devastating consequences of compression injuries from compartment syndromes. Additionally, swelling contributes to increased

TABLE 27.3
MOTOR TESTING OF DISTAL UPPER EXTREMITY

Wrist: Muscle testing (by active or passive resistance)
1. Extensors: extensor carpi radialis longus and brevis extensor carpi ulnaris—radial nerve
2. Flexors: flexor carpi radialis—median nerve flexor carpi ulnaris—ulnar nerve

Digit
1. Extensors: extensor digitorum communis extensor digiti minimi—radial nerve
2. Flexors: DIP—deep digital flexor—ulnar nerve PIP—supervicial digital flexor—medial nerve MCP—lumbricals 2 and 3—ulnar nerve lumbricals 4 and 5—median nerve
3. Abduction: dorsal interossi abductor digiti minimi—ulnar nerve
4. Adduction: palmar interossi—ulnar nerve (test using piece of paper grasped between two fingers)
5. Thumb extension: IP—extensor pollicis longus—radial nerve MCP—extensor pollicis brevis—radial nerve
6. Thumb flexion: transpalmar abduction IP flexor pollicis longus—median nerve MCP flexor pollicis brevis—ulnar and median nerve
7. Thumb abduction: abductor pollicis longus—radial nerve abductor pollicis brevis—median nerve
8. Thumb adduction: adductor pollicis—ulnar nerve
9. Pinch test: joining thumb and each finger

DIP = distal interphalongeal; PIP = proximal interphalongeal; MCP = metacarpophalongeal; IP = interphalongeal

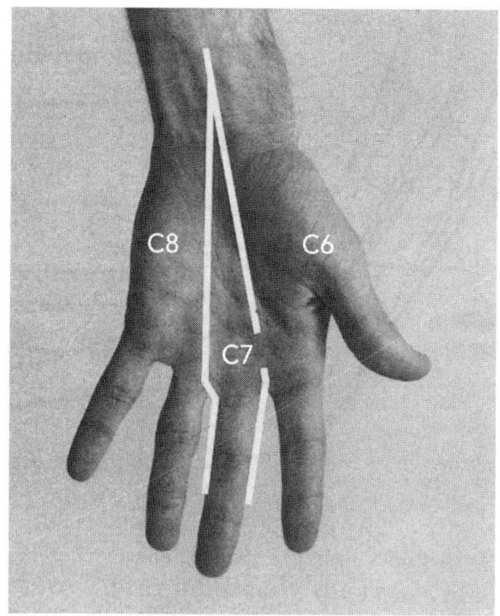

Figure 27.8 Dermatomes of the hand.

pain, and may interfere with fracture reduction or skin closure if open reduction is necessary. In acute cases, splinting or uni- or bivalved casts are acceptable for use instead of circumferential casts to allow further swelling to occur (10). These may be converted or changed to a cast in a week when the swelling has decreased.

Many fractures are nondisplaced and and show normal alignment. These fractures can usually be treated by closed methods as they are generally stable, and early, protected return to sports is usually achievable (13). Fractures that cannot be reduced, or are unstable after reduction, or those that involve displacement of the articular surface, should be referred to an orthopedic surgeon for management.

COMMON INJURIES

Wrist

Distal Radius Fractures

Distal radius fractures represent approximately 17% of all fractures seen in the emergency rooms. There are numerous classification schemes for these fractures, but the "universal" and "modified Mayo" classifications will classify most fractures well (11).

"Universal classification"

1. Type I: nonarticular, undisplaced
2. Type II: nonarticular, displaced
3. Type III: intra-articular, undisplaced
4. Type IV: intra-articular displaced (see Figure 27.9)
   a. Reducible (stable)
   b. Reducible (unstable)
   c. Irreducible (unstable)

Modified Mayo classification (used to identify distinct variants of intra-articular fractures)

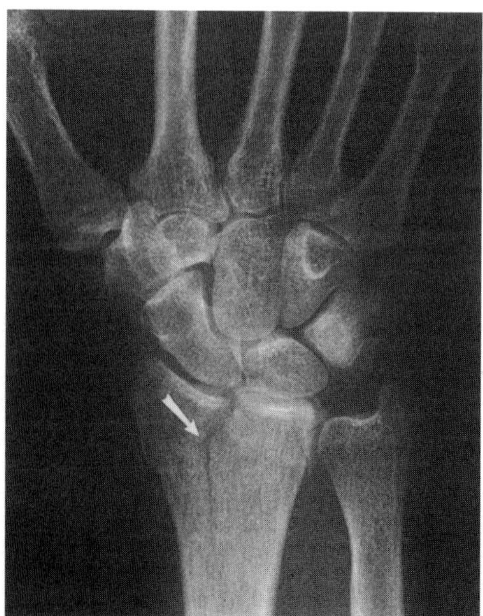

Figure 27.9 Radial styloid fracture.

1. Type I: intra-articular, undisplaced
2. Type II: intra-articular, displaced involving radioscaphoid joint ("Chauffeur's" fracture) (Figure 27.9)
   a. Associated with scapholunate tears
   b. Significant dorsal angulation and radial shortening
3. Type III: intra-articular, displaced involving radiolunate joint
   a. "Die-punch" or lunate load fracture
   b. Irreducible by traction alone
4. Type IV: intra-articular, displaced involving both radioscaphoid and radiolunate joints

When evaluating distal radius fractures, one should assess for characteristics that render the fracture pattern potentially unstable. These include radial shortening more than 1 cm, angulation (apex volar) more than 20 degrees, and metaphyseal comminution.

Treatment

Most intra-articular fractures should be referred to an orthopedic surgeon for consideration of surgical fixation. An exception may be a nondisplaced intra-articular fracture in a low-demand or arthritic wrist, generally an elderly athlete. The choice on whether to reduce or refer an angulated fracture depends on the comfort level and experience of the treating physician. General guidelines for treating injuries/fractures of the distal radius are discussed in the subsequent text (2).

Nonarticular, Undisplaced or Minimally Displaced (Universal Type I)

Treat with sugar tong splint for 2 to 4 days until swelling subsides and then place in a short-arm cast for 3 to 6 weeks, with weekly follow up. Six weeks in a cast is appropriate for most fractures; however the elderly or those with underlying radiocarpal arthritis should be mobilized earlier to minimize postimmobilization stiffness. A long-arm cast for 3 to 4 weeks should be considered in there is significant pain with forearm supination/pronation.

Nonarticular, Displaced/Angulated (Universal Type II)

After adequate reduction, these fractures should be treated with a long-arm cast for 3 to 4 weeks, followed up by a short-arm cast for 2 to 3 weeks. Weekly radiographs for 2 to 3 weeks should be taken to assure the fracture does not reangulate.

Intra-Articular, Undisplaced (Modified Mayo Type I)

Elderly patients or those with underlying radiocarpal arthritis can be treated with a long-arm cast for 3 to 4 weeks, followed up by a short-arm cast for 2 to 3 weeks. Younger patients should be referred to an orthopedic surgeon for consideration of anatomic reduction and surgical fixation (14).

Postcast Treatment

Cast immobilization invariably results in joint stiffness and hand/wrist weakness, which is directly proportional to the duration of casting. It generally takes as long as the joint was on cast to regain full range of motion. Weakness and discomfort generally takes as long as four times the duration of casting to resolve.

Home-based treatment with contrast baths for range of motion and theraputty for strength is quite effective (8). For contrast baths the patient draws two buckets of water, one at 100°F to 105°F and the other less than 50°F. Range of motion and stretching is performed in the warm water for 3 to 4 minutes, followed by soaking in the cold water for 1 minute. This cycle is performed four times, ending by bathing the joint in cold water.

Distal Radius Fractures in Children

Children have softer bones that frequently "buckle" rather than break (Torus or "buckle" fracture). A critical distinction must be made between this benign buckle fracture and the more concerning "greenstick fracture." The buckle fracture involves buckling of one cortex, with the opposite cortex remaining intact. A greenstick fracture involves flexible immature bone breaking like a tree sapling. The tension side splinters whereas the compression side (opposite) undergoes plastic deformation, leaving a permanent bend unless it is reduced. Simple reduction is often not effective and this "incomplete" fracture must be completed to allow for correct realignment.

A torus or buckle fracture can be treated with a short-arm cast for 3 to 4 weeks, followed up by splinting for at-risk activities for another 3 to 4 weeks. Greenstick fractures angulated more than 10 degrees should generally be reduced (14). A minimally angulated greenstick fracture should be treated with a long-arm cast in full supination for 4 weeks followed up by a short-arm cast until healed. Parents should be counseled at the onset that these have a propensity to angulate even in a cast and these should be followed up by weekly radiographs through the cast for 3 weeks.

Dorsal Compaction Epiphysitis is a common sports-related issue facing skeletally immature athletes. Gymnastics and related sports that involve weight-bearing while balancing on the upper extremity with the wrist in extreme extension can result in chronic wrist pain and insult to the distal radial epiphysis. The well-being of the young athlete by protecting the status of the distal radial epiphysis is paramount. Hand/wrist straps are commonly used to achieve some protection by limiting wrist extension. Control of inflammation with cold therapy, even prophylactic icing, is the mainstay of treatment. Relative rest from this weight-bearing activity is usually necessary. Because long bone growth is at stake here, the condition needs to be monitored after diagnosis until closure.

Scaphoid Fractures

Seventy percent of all carpal bone injuries are fractures of the scaphoid, probably because of the key stabilizing role it plays because it bridges the proximal and distal carpal rows (13). The fractured scaphoid is vulnerable to nonunion and avascular necrosis (AVN) due to its dependence on a single recurrent interosseous blood supply that enters distally and runs proximally. The more proximal the fracture, the more delayed the healing and higher the risk of AVN. Distal third fractures require an average of 8 weeks to heal, waist or isthmus fractures 3 months, and proximal third fractures require 4 months or longer (15).

Physical examination reveals pain and/or swelling in the "anatomic snuff box" formed by the tendons of the extensor pollicus brevis and abductor pollicis longus radially, and the extensor pollicus longus ulnarly. A fracture line may be visualized on scaphoid series radiographs and, if there is any question regarding displacement, a CT scan should be ordered (16). If no fracture line is visualized on radiographs but clinical suspicion persists (i.e., persistent "snuff box" tenderness), the wrist should be immobilized in a thumb spica cast (allowing for IP joint movement) and repeat radiographs taken in 10 days to 2 weeks, and even at 4 and 6 weeks if still symptomatic. If a more expedient diagnosis is desired, a technetium bone scan may be positive as early as 24 hours after injury. Fractures of the proximal third, displaced fractures, or fractures delayed in presentation (more than 2–3 weeks) are at high risk for AVN and nonunion and should be referred to an orthopedic surgeon (15,16). Nondisplaced (less than 1 mm displacement or one cortex intact) distal and waist scaphoid fractures can be treated in a long-arm thumb spica cast (with the MP joints of the fingers included) for 6 weeks, followed up by a short-arm thumb spica cast until there is radiographic evidence of healing. CT scan may be necessary to truly assess healing before discontinuing immobilization. Immobilization is then discontinued for activities of daily living and rehabilitation. The wrist needs to be protected from impact loading for an additional 3 months (15).

Other Carpal Fractures

Lunate

Acute fractures of the lunate are unusual, and include marginal chip, dorsal pole, sagittal and transverse body, and volar pole fractures. Fractures of the main body of the lunate may progress to carpal instability, nonunion, or AVN (15). Displaced volar pole and any body fractures should be referred for the consideration of open reduction and internal fixation (ORIF), as distraction by important volar stabilizing ligaments may interfere with healing. Marginal and dorsal fractures are inherently more stable and can be treated with casting for 4 to 6 weeks.

Kienbock's disease refers to idiopathic AVN of the lunate. This is generally atraumatic in origin, although trauma may precipitate symptoms. Patients present with wrist pain, stiffness, and variable swelling and tenderness localized over the dorsum of the lunate. The diagnosis is generally made radiographically. Plain radiographs frequently demonstrate a negative ulnar variance (the articular surface of the ulna aligns proximal to the articular surface of the radius). The lunate may appear normal in the early stages but will eventually progress to a linear compression fracture, increased sclerosis, and carpal collapse (2). If clinical suspicion is strong with normal radiographs, a bone scan or MRI should be considered. Patients with diagnosed or suspected Kienbock's disease should be referred because the treatment may involve complex joint leveling procedures, proximal row carpectomy or joint fusion.

Triquetral Fractures

Fractures of the triquetum can be to the body or, more commonly, a dorsal cortical chip fracture. Dorsal chip fractures are likely caused by the ulnar styloid impacting the dorsal triquetrum during forced dorsiflexion of the wrist (15). The fracture is best visualized on lateral and oblique views. The body fractures with direct trauma and is generally nondisplaced. Both dorsal chip fractures and nondisplaced body fractures can be treated with a short-arm cast for 4 to 6 weeks. Displaced body fractures should be referred for evaluation of associated ligamentous injury and consideration for surgery. Dorsal chip fractures that do not heal and are symptomatic can be treated with a local injection and possibly excision of the fragment.

Trapezium Fractures

The trapezium is fractured directly when the base of the thumb MC is axially driven into the articular surface, or indirectly from ligamentous or capsular avulsion. Isolated trapezial fractures are rare and can be one of three types: body, marginal trapeziometacarpal, and trapezial ridge (volar) (15). Trapezial ridge fractures are suspected with point tenderness just distal to the scaphoid tuberosity. Body fractures and trapeziometacarpal fractures are tender dorsally proximal to the thumb CMC joint. Thumb range of motion may be painless, but pinch strength is weak. Radiographic views should include PA, lateral, oblique, carpal tunnel, and Bett's view (thumb extended and abducted, wrist slightly pronated, hypothenar eminence on cassette, and the beam centered on the scaphotrapeziotrapezium joint).

Nondisplaced body, marginal trapeziometacarpal, and trapezial ridge fractures at the base (proximal) can be treated with a short-arm thumb spica cast for 4 weeks. Displaced body and distal trapezial ridge fractures should be referred for possible surgical treatment.

Capitate Fractures

Isolated capitate fractures are rare and predisposed to AVN or nonunion. PA and lateral radiographs may show a transverse fracture through the waist. If these views are

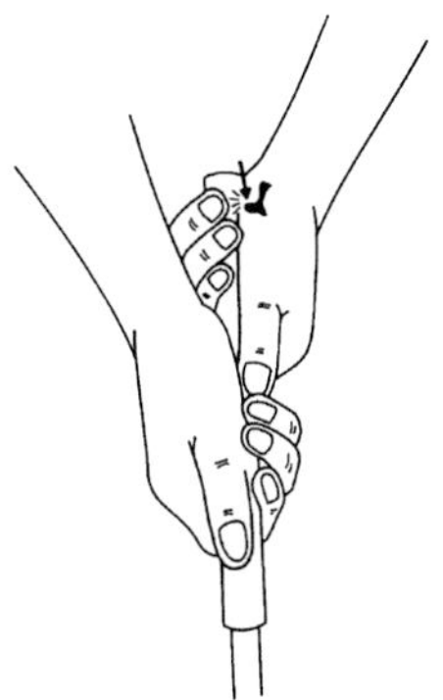

Figure 27.10 Fracture—hook of the hamate.

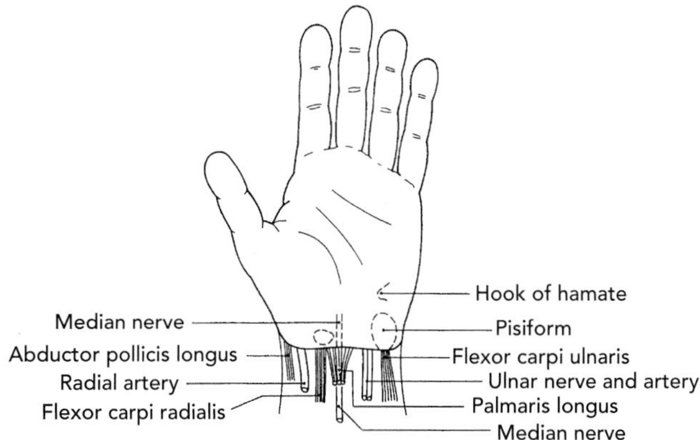

Figure 27.11 Palmar surface of the wrist.

normal and suspicion remains, a bone scan, CT, tomogram, or MRI should be ordered (8). These fractures should be splinted and referred for management due to the high complication rate.

Hamate Fractures

There are two main types of hamate fractures: body fractures and fractures of the hook of the hamate (hamulus). Body fractures occur with direct trauma, but hook fractures may be more insidious. The base of a bat, racquet, or golf club may abut the hook of the hamate at the end of a swing, causing a fracture (13) (see Figure 27.10). Hook fractures may be missed unless strongly suspected. Ulnar and palmar wrist pain is aggravated when the patient attempts to swing a club or racket. Deep palpation over the hook of the hamate in the base of the palm is painful and there may be tenderness over the dorsoulnar aspect of the hamate. Radiographs should include PA, lateral, carpal tunnel, and 45 degrees supinated oblique. Tomograms or CT may be necessary to demonstrate fractures at the base of the hook. Nondisplaced body fractures can be treated with a short-arm cast for 4 to 6 weeks and displaced body fractures should be referred for possible ORIF. The treatment for acute hook fractures is somewhat more controversial as only approximately 50% will heal with prolonged casting (6 weeks to 4 months or longer) (15). Adults with an acute injury can be given the option of a trial of casting (if they present within 2 weeks of injury) or early excision. Early excision and rehabilitation may be warranted as athletes can generally return to full, painless activity by 3 months. Fractures older than 2 weeks should undergo excision of the hook.

Pisiform Fractures

Pisiform fractures are uncommon, but can occur with a direct blow to the hypothenar eminence or repetitive microtrauma (15). Affected individuals will have tenderness over the pisiform on the proximal volar hypothenar eminence (see Figure 27.11). Radiographs should include 20 to 45 degrees supinated oblique and carpal tunnel views; however, a bone scan or CT may be necessary to confirm the fracture. Initial treatment is a short-arm cast for 4 to 6 weeks. Patients with symptomatic nonunions or subsequent pisotriquetral arthritis can be treated with a pisiform excision.

WRIST INSTABILITIES

Radial Ligamentous Injuries

Radial sided instabilities are the most common wrist instabilities and center around injuries to the ligaments surrounding the scaphoid (17). These include scapholunate dissociation (also called rotatory subluxation of the scaphoid), dorsal perilunate dislocation, and lunate dislocation.

Scapholunate Dissociation (Rotatory Subluxation of the Scaphoid)

Early diagnosis and treatment of this injury is imperative to prevent future static instabilities and degenerative changes. Normally, the scaphoid palmarflexes (becomes more vertical) with radial deviation of the wrist. The intact scapholunate ligament will force the lunate to move with the scaphoid, resulting in the lunate also palmarflexing with radial deviation. With a ruptured scapholunate ligament, the scaphoid will still palmarflex with radial deviation, but the lunate will now dorsiflex resulting in a vertical scaphoid (rotatory subluxation) and a dorsiflexed lunate. Because the lunate is essentially a passive intercalated segment, this is called a *dorsal intercalated segment instability* (DISI) pattern (17).

Physical examination of a patient with scapholunate dissociation will reveal a tender, swollen wrist with limited range of motion. A scaphoid click test may be positive and is performed as follows: the patient's hand is placed in ulnar deviation (making the scaphoid horizontal) and neutral. The examiner places his/her thumb on the scaphoid tuberosity and the four fingers of the same hand on the dorsal aspect of the distal radius. The thumb pushes on the scaphoid in an attempt to keep it from becoming vertical as the patients wrist is radially deviated. With rupture of the scapholunate ligaments, the thumb will effectively prevent the scaphoid from palmarflexing and force the proximal pole to rotate dorsally, causing pain and/or a painful click (5).

Posteroanterior radiographs will show the scapholunate space greater than 3 mm, or a space greater than that between the other carpal bones, and possibly a ring sign (the scaphoid appears short and the end-on projection of the rotated scaphoid gives a ringed appearance). If widening is seen, a contralateral wrist radiograph should be taken to make sure that the widening is not congenital (18). Lateral views may show the lunate in a dorsiflexed position with a capitolunate angle more than 15 degrees and/or the scapholunate angle greater than 65 to 70 degrees. If the plain PA and lateral views are normal but suspicion remains, a six view wrist trauma series should be ordered to include: PA, lateral, right and left oblique, and PA in radial and ulnar deviation with a clenched fist (5). These additional views may demonstrate subtle instabilities not readily seen on nonstressed views. Confirmed or suspected scapholunate instabilities should be referred to a hand surgeon.

Perilunate and Lunate Dislocations

A severe hyperextension injury to the wrist may result in rupture of the volar radioscaphoid and scapholunate ligaments, freeing the proximal pole of the scaphoid. Compressive forces then wedge the capitate between the scaphoid and lunate. A perilunate dislocation occurs when continued dorsiflexion forces the distal carpal row to "peel" away from the lunate and maintain a position dorsal to the lunate and radius (17). Further force will rupture the dorsal restraining radiocarpal ligament allowing the lunate to "flip" palmarward (spilled teacup sign) as the distal carpal bones relocate, resulting in a lunate dislocation.

Physical examination reveals a painful swollen wrist with marked limitation in range of motion. Particular attention must be paid to median nerve function after this injury. The lunate may appear three-sided rather than its normal trapezoidal configuration on PA radiographs. Lateral views show the distal carpal row dorsal to the lunate and radius in a perilunate dislocation, and a "spilled teacup sign" (the lunate faces palmarward and rests volar to the radius and distal carpal row) with a lunate dislocation (5). Confirmed or suspected carpal dislocations should be referred to an orthopedic surgeon for closed or open reduction.

Carpal Tunnel Syndrome

Carpal tunnel syndrome (CTS) (median neuropathy) is more common with sports involving repetitive wrist motion, such as rowing and racquet sports. This repetitive motion can lead to synovial hypertrophy around the flexor tendons leading to swelling in the rigid tunnel (19) (see Figure 27.12). This in turn can compress the median nerve and result in sensory and motor deficits. Diabetes and hypothyroidism are predisposing medical conditions, as well as pregnancy.

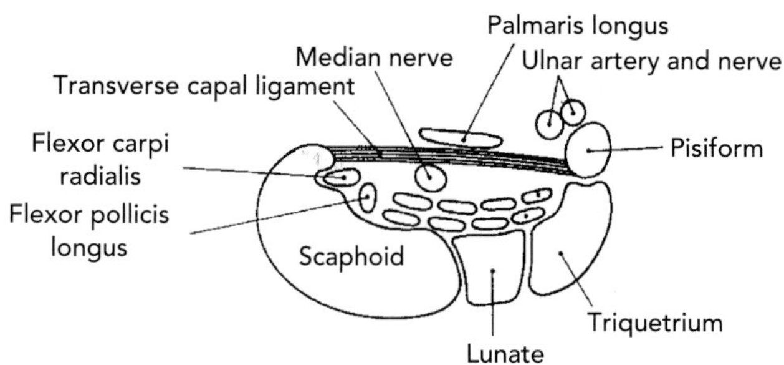

Figure 27.12 Contents of carpal tunnel.

The median nerve at the level of the carpal tunnel contains the sensory branches to the radial 3.5 digits and a motor branch to the thenar eminence. Symptoms of a median neuropathy are numbness in the radial 3 digits, variable pain in the hand, wrist and volar forearm, and occasional weakness.

Phalen's wrist flexion test reproduces the symptoms and Tinnel's test is positive in approximately 45% of the cases (19). Decreased vibratory sensation in the radial 3.5 digits is the first neurological finding followed by decreased two-point discrimination. Motor strength is assessed by having the patient oppose the thumb and small finger in an "O" position, with the examiner trying to break the ring with his/her finger. Thenar atrophy may be noted in severe or chronic cases. Electromyography and nerve conduction studies (EMG/NCS) can be useful to assess for other etiologies of neurogenic wrist pain, as well as to assess the severity of CTS. These studies can be normal in up to 20% to 25% of individuals with CTS and therefore cannot exclude the diagnosis. In such instances an MRI may be useful to look for tenosynovial edema and flattening of the median nerve (19).

Treatment is conservative consisting of splinting the wrist in 20 degrees to 30 degrees of dorsiflexion (especially at night), nonsteroidal anti-inflammatory drugs (NSAIDs), and relative rest for the wrist. A steroid injection may be given with persistent symptoms and is performed as follows: A No 25 needle is inserted just proximal to the distal flexion crease between the palmaris longus and flexor carpi radialis tendons and pierces the flexor retinaculum, and 1cc of a steroid preparation is instilled. Resistant cases, or electromyography/nerve conduction studies (EMG/NCS) showing moderate to severe median neuropathy, should be referred for a possible carpal tunnel release.

Ulnar Nerve Compression

The ulnar nerve traverses Guyon's canal between the pisiform and hamate (Figure 27.11) and is divided into the superficial terminal branch (supplying sensation to the ulnar palm, fifth digit, and ulnar side of the fourth digit) and the deep terminal branch (innervating the interossei, hypothenar muscles, third and fourth lumbricals, adductor pollicis brevis, and the deep head of the flexor pollicis brevis). The most common compression syndrome involves the deep terminal branch distal to the branch supplying the hypothenar muscles (13). The next syndrome involves both the deep and superficial branches proximal to Guyon's canal. This is most prevalent in sports such as cycling, weight lifting, and baseball (catchers) owing to chronic repetitive pressure on the hypothenar area (8).

Physical examination with the more common deep terminal ulnar nerve involvement reveals weakness in the interossei, third and fourth lumbricals, adductor pollicis brevis, and flexor pollicis brevis. The hypothenar muscles may be spared, because the compression is usually distal to this nerve branch. Proximal Guyon's canal involvement results in weakness in all of the ulnar innervated muscles plus numbness in the ulnar 1.5 digits.

Treatment involves protective padding over the hypothenar area and NSAIDs. Electromyography and nerve conduction studies should be considered if there is no improvement with initial intervention because these give useful information regarding chronicity, severity, and regeneration. Resistant cases or cases with evidence of motor loss should be referred to a hand surgeon.

Hypothenar Hammer Syndrome (Ulnar Artery Injury)

The ulnar artery traverses Guyon's canal and becomes relatively superficial for approximately 2 cm distal to the canal. It is covered at this point by the skin, the subcutaneous tissue, and the palmaris brevis muscle (Figure 27.11). A single blow or repetitive microtrauma in this vulnerable area (proximal ulnar palm) can cause spasm, thrombosis, or aneurysm of the ulnar artery (8). Patients may complain of numbness in the ulnar 1.5 digits, ischemic type pain, and possibly cold intolerance. Physical examination may reveal a mass in the hypothenar area, indicative of an ulnar artery aneurysm. An Allen's test will be positive if the ulnar artery is thrombosed, and intrinsic muscle cramping with repetitive finger flexion and extension suggests ischemia. Doppler ultrasonography may be helpful, and angiography is seldom needed but is diagnostic. Vascular surgery is the definitive treatment.

FINGER INJURIES

Mallet Finger

Mallet finger refers to an extensor lag at the DIP joint resulting from a loss of continuity of the terminal extensor digitorum tendon (EDT) at its insertion. Blunt axial trauma (a ball hitting the distal fingertip) to the slightly flexed DIP joint causes either a rupture of the EDT or an avulsion fracture (see Figure 27.13). After an acute injury, the patient will have tenderness over the dorsum of the DIP joint and cannot actively extend the distal phalanx, but passive extension is possible (20). Radiographs should be obtained to look for a bony avulsion from the dorsal proximal aspect of the distal phalanx and possible volar subluxation of the distal phalanx. Any subluxation of a Mallet deformity will result in eventual arthritis and dysfunction.

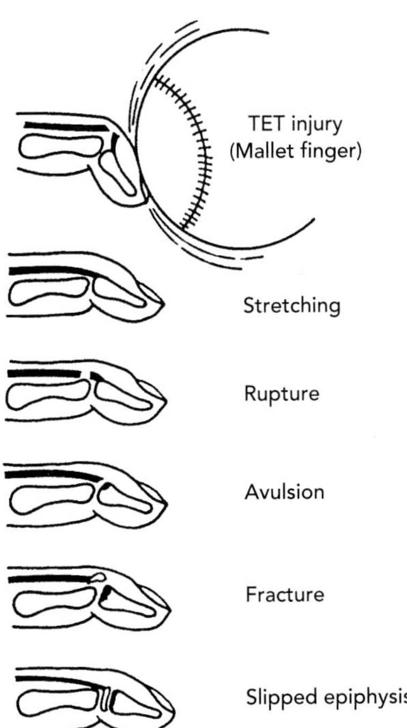

Figure 27.13 Mallet finger pathology. TET = terminal extensor tendon.

Bony avulsions should be treated with the DIP joint immobilized in full extension with a dorsal aluminum or stack splint for 4 weeks (see Figure 27.14). Patients should be counseled that they will likely have a residual bump over the dorsal DIP joint. If there is no bony avulsion, the splint should be worn for 8 to 10 weeks continuously and for an additional 6 to 8 weeks during athletic activities (20). Surgery is indicated with bony avulsions associated with volar subluxation of the distal phalanx.

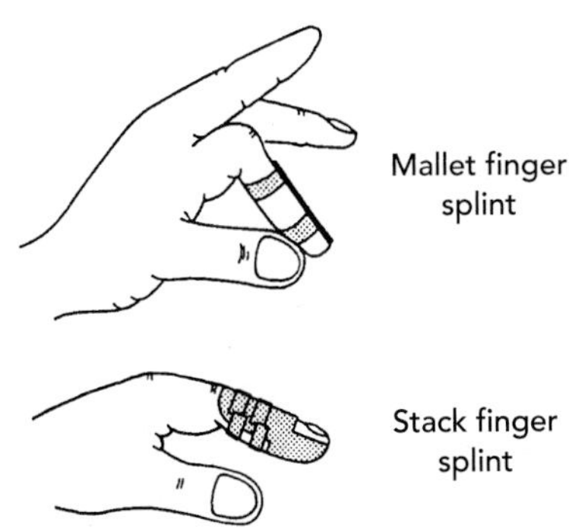

Figure 27.14 Mallet finger splint and stack finger splint.

Jersey Finger (Flexor Digitorum Profundus Avulsion)

A ligamentous rupture or bony avulsion at the insertion of the flexor digitorum profundus can occur as the actively flexed DIP joint is forcibly extended (e.g., an athlete grabs on to a jersey) or the ligament is forcibly overwhelmed, as is seen in rock climbing. Affected patients will have localized tenderness over the volar DIP joint and/or at the level of ligament retraction. The patient will have full passive range of motion but will be unable to actively flex the isolated DIP joint (see Figure 27.15). Radiographs should be obtained to assess for associated fractures and, if bone is avulsed, will help localize the level of retraction.

There are three different types of jersey finger, all requiring surgical repair and each with its own level of urgency for repair (21). A type III injury is an avulsion fracture of the volar lip of the distal phalanx. The bony fragment remains attached to the tendon, which limits retraction to just proximal to the DIP joint and enables repair by ORIF, generally within 6 weeks of injury. In a type II injury, the avulsed tendon retracts to the hiatus of the flexor digitorum superficialis (FDS) near the PIP joint and is held there by the intact vincula and can be surgically repaired up to 3 weeks postinjury. The avulsed tendon in a type I injury has retracted to the palm and its blood supply through the vinculum breve and longum has been severely compromised. Acute repair for these must be accomplished within 7 to 10 days as the repair becomes increasingly difficult until 3 to 4 weeks out, when its repair may be impossible (21). Reconstruction is necessary for late diagnosis because of joint and tendon contractures.

Proximal Interphalangeal Joint Injuries

The PIP joint is frequently injured due to its position between the long lever arms of the proximal and middle phalanges. Significant disability can result when this functionally important joint develops a fixed deformity from a missed diagnosis or inadequate treatment (22). Unfortunately, many of these injuries are difficult to diagnose. When a diagnosis is made, particular attention must be given to appropriate splinting and guided rehabilitation to allow the injured structure to heal, and yet maintain joint range of motion. Because of these concerns, it is advisable to refer patients with PIP joint injuries to an orthopedic surgeon if there is doubt as to the diagnosis or management.

Dorsal Dislocation of the PIP Joint

Dorsal dislocations result from a hyperextension injury to the PIP joint with resultant disruption of the volar plate at its attachment to the MP (see Figure 27.16). Without a volar stabilizing force, the MP rides dorsally on the proximal phalanx producing a bayonet deformity (23). Clinically, this is manifested by pain, swelling, and limited ability to move the PIP joint. Radiographs will show a dorsally displaced MP with some retraction and possibly a small avulsed segment of bone at the base of the MP. Reduction is performed by administering a MC block for anesthesia, stabilizing the MP, and slightly hyperextending the PIP joint. The thumb of the other hand then "pushes" the MP into reduction (22). Longitudinal traction of the MP must be avoided as this may allow the volar plate to become interposed in the PIP joint, making closed reduction impossible. A postreduction radiograph will confirm adequate reduction.

Treatment requires close supervision by a physician and/or therapist experienced in the management of hand injuries to ensure that the PIP joint does not become too stiff. If the PIP joint does not hyperextend when the digit is actively extended, the patient can be treated with buddy taping to the adjacent finger for 3 to 6 weeks. If the PIP joint hyperextends but does not redislocate, it should be treated with a dorsal extension block splint with the joint

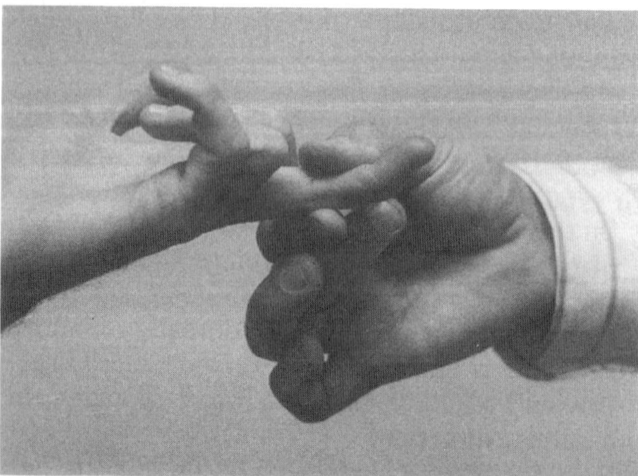

Figure 27.15 Deep digital flexor testing.

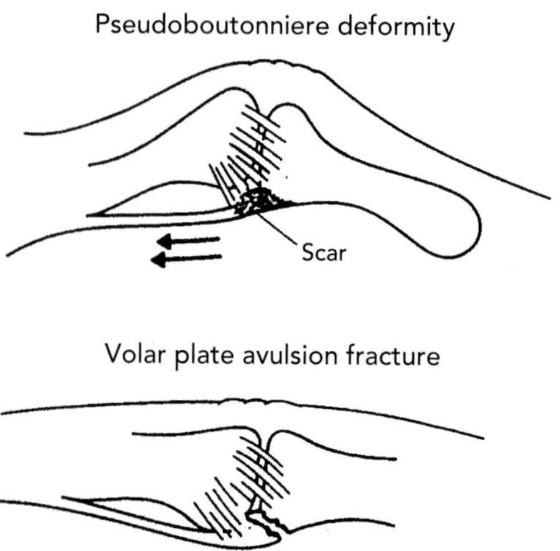

Figure 27.16 Pseudoboutonniere deformity and volar plate avulsion fracture.

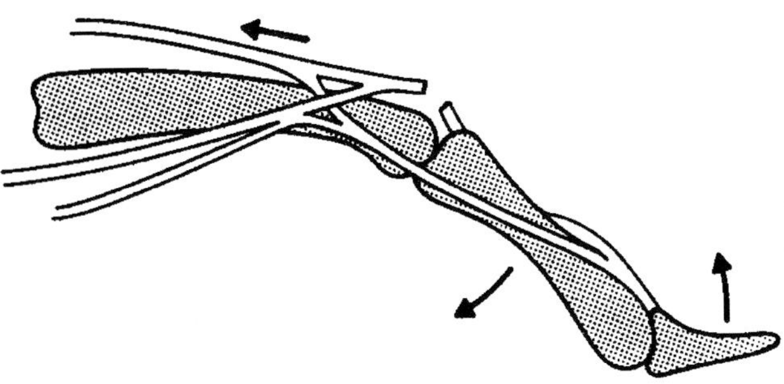

Figure 27.17 Boutonniere deformity.

blocked at 15 degrees to 20 degrees of flexion for 2 to 3 weeks, followed by buddy taping until the joint has full, pain-free range of motion (22). If the joint redislocates after reduction, volar plate interposition is likely and the patient should be referred to a surgeon.

Volar Plate Rupture (Without Dislocation)

A hyperextension injury to the PIP joint may cause the distal portion of the volar plate to rupture from its attachment to the MP (see Figure 27.17). This loss of the volar stabilizing force will allow the extensor tendon to gradually pull the PIP joint into a hyperextension deformity (reverse boutonniere) if untreated. After the acute injury, the PIP joint is in varying degrees of hyperextension and there is maximal tenderness along the volar aspect. Radiographs may show an avulsion fragment at the base of the MP. Acute injuries should be treated with an extension block splint for 3 weeks with the PIP joint blocked at 15 degrees to 20 degrees of flexion, or buddy taping for 3 to 6 weeks. Failure to diagnose and treat, preferably by an extension block splint, frequently results in a poor outcome (22). Patients with late presentations of a swan-neck deformity or flexion contracture of the PIP joint are difficult to manage and should be referred to a surgeon.

Proximal Interphalangeal Joint Fracture–Dislocation

This injury differs from dorsal dislocations (a hyperextension injury) in that the mechanism of injury is an axial load on a semiflexed finger. The MP shears dorsally, impacting the palmar articular surface of the MP with the condyles of the proximal phalanx. On physical examination there is a subtle dorsal prominence over the PIP joint with pain and swelling. Radiographs show the size of the volar impaction fracture. If there is only a small fragment, buddy taping is the only treatment necessary, whereas a larger fragment frequently requires closed reduction. An adequate reduction is confirmed by congruity of the intact articular surface of the MP with the head of the proximal phalanx. Reduction is followed up by an extension block splint with the joint blocked at 30 to 60 degrees of flexion for 1 to 3 weeks (2). This is followed up by buddy taping for 3 weeks or until the joint is pain-free with full range of motion. Weekly radiographs should be obtained to assess for maintenance of the reduction. If more than 35% to 40% of the joint surface is involved or the reduction is inadequate, surgical consultation is necessary for possible ORIF (22).

Central Slip of the Common Extensor Tendon Rupture

This tendon inserts on the dorsal base of the MP and may rupture with axial trauma to a semiflexed PIP joint (Figure 27.17). The common extensor tendon (CET) rupture and subsequent inability to fully extend the PIP joint allows the lateral bands to migrate volar to the axis of the joint. Over time, this leads to a flexion contracture of the PIP joint and hyperextension of the DIP joint (boutonniere deformity). Acutely, the PIP joint is in 15 to 30 degrees of flexion, there is point tenderness over the dorsal lip of the MP, the PIP joint is swollen, and the patient cannot actively fully extend the PIP joint (9). A radiograph may show an avulsion fracture at the dorsal base of the MP. Injuries less than 3 weeks old should be treated with the PIP joint splinted in full extension (see Figure 27.18) for 6 to 8 weeks and the digit should be further protected during sporting activity for and additional 6 to 8 weeks (22). While splinted, the patient should frequently and actively flex the DIP joint to help relocate the lateral bands back to there normal position (dorsal to the PIP joint) and maintain range of motion. If the avulsion fracture involves more than a third of the articular surface, the patient should be referred for possible surgical reduction.

Ulnar Collateral Ligament Injuries of the Thumb

"Skiers" or "Gamekeepers" thumb refers to damage to the ulnar collateral ligament (UCL) secondary to

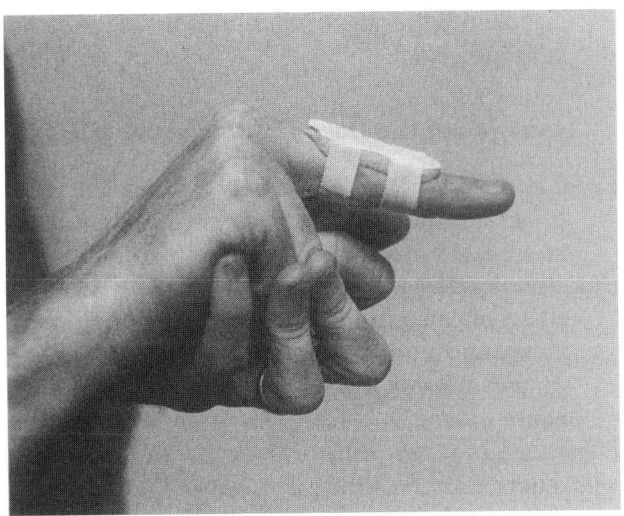

Figure 27.18 Boutonniere splint.

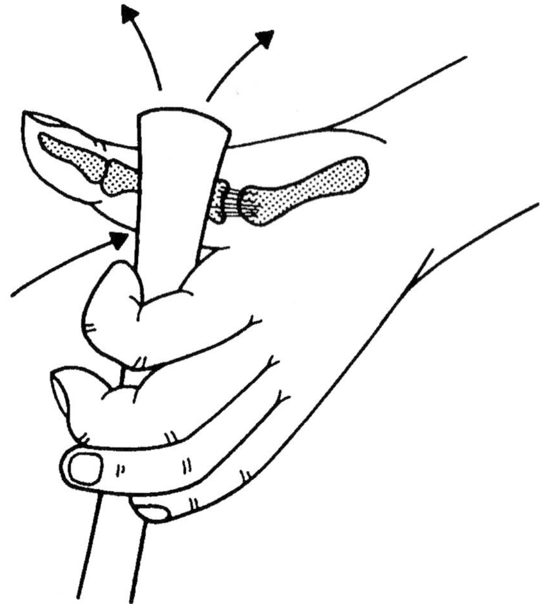

Figure 27.19 Ulnar collateral ligament sprain mechanism.

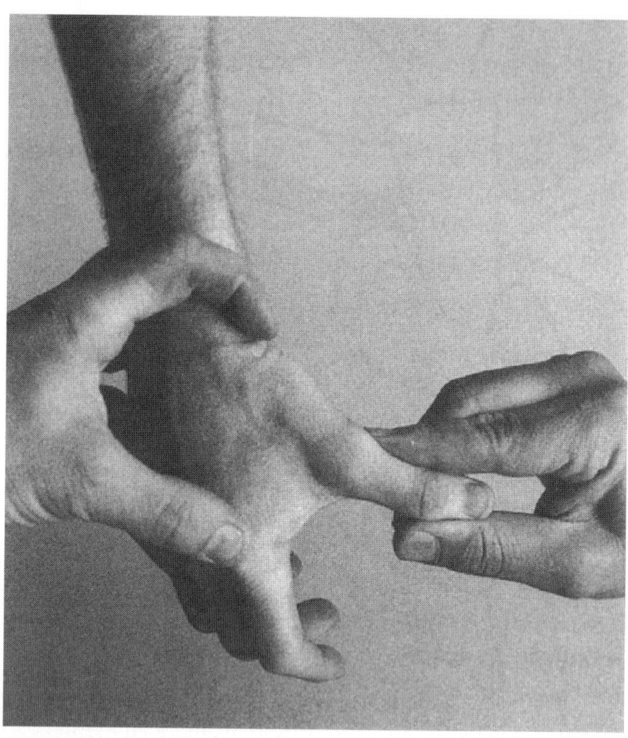

Figure 27.20 Ulnar collateral ligament stress test.

hyperabduction of the thumb MCP joint (see Figure 27.19). There are four types of injury as follows (22):

Type 1: avulsion fracture, nondisplaced
Type 2: avulsion fracture, displaced
Type 3: torn ligament, stable in flexion
Type 4: torn ligament, unstable in flexion

Type 1 and type 3 injuries can be successfully treated closed, and type 2 and type 4 injuries require surgical repair. Types 1 and 2 are readily identified on plain radiographs. The goal of the initial evaluation then is to determine which injuries are type 4 on the basis of physical examination and negative radiographs. The approach should be as follows: Injury to the UCL is suspected with an appropriate history and tenderness and swelling over the ulnar aspect of the MCP joint. Radiographs should be performed before stressing so as to not transform a nondisplaced avulsion fracture into a displaced one. If a fracture is not evident, stress testing is performed by stabilizing the thumb MC with one hand and applying valgus stress on the MCP joint with them both straight and at full flexion (see Figure 27.20). Accuracy is enhanced by infiltrating the site of injury with local anesthetic before stress testing (24). Testing is done in full flexion because at extension or slight flexion the joint is stabilized by the normal tautness of the volar plate. Complete rupture is suspected if there is angulation of 15 degrees more than the contralateral thumb or an absolute angulation of 35 degrees or more without a firm end point (11).

Treatment for a type 3 injury (partial tear with stable joint) is a thumb spica cast or splint for 3 weeks. A type 1 injury (nondisplaced avulsion fracture) should be treated with a thumb spica cast. Surgery is indicated for complete tears (type 4 injury), displaced fractures of more than 2 mm (type 2 injury), or rotated fractures.

Trigger Finger

Trigger finger is a nonspecific tenosynovitis of the flexor tendon sheath. In athletes, the most common cause is repetitive trauma that causes increased swelling within the tendon. The swollen tendon catches on the closely applied pulley system (usually the a1 pulley) causing the snapping sensation as the flexed finger is actively extended.

Early treatment may include splinting the finger straight at night, along with NSAIDs. More chronic injuries, especially with repetitive triggering, generally require injection of a local anesthetic and steroid into the tendon sheath (10). This is done through a midlateral approach at the level of the distal third of the proximal phalanx while the patient resists flexion. This may need to be repeated once or twice, and unresponsive cases require surgery to release the pulley. An important point of emphasis here is to make certain that steroids are never injected into the tendon substance itself.

Phalangeal Fractures

Bony "mallet finger" and management is covered in an earlier section. Other distal phalanx fractures are often caused by crush injuries, and ice and elevation are essential to prevent severe swelling. Unless they are severely displaced or angulated, a dorsal splint in extension, immobilizing the DIP joint for 2 to 3 weeks, is usually sufficient (11). Buddy taping may be used in conjunction with a splint with protective prolific padding when the patient is sent back to competition.

Fractures involving the MP are usually transverse and angulated with the apex dorsal. If they can be reduced and held in good alignment with the adjacent joints in slight flexion, closed management may be attempted. Maintaining reduction may be difficult because of the deforming forces of the flexor digitorum (FDS) or extensor mechanism. The dense cortical bone of the MP takes at least 12 weeks to heal radiographically, but is clinically stable much sooner (9). Range-of-motion exercises should begin at 4 to 6 weeks, but the fracture should be protected during competition for at least 3 to 4 months or the rest of that season, whichever is longer. If reduction cannot be maintained, referral should be made to a surgeon for probable closed reduction and percutaneous pinning.

Fractures of the proximal phalanx are the most disabling and challenging of finger fractures. These fractures are usually oblique or spiral fractures, which cause shortening and malrotation of the fragments. The reduction is difficult to maintain, even if the initial reduction is successful (11). Also, prolonged immobilization of this fracture often leads to stiffness and adhesions to the proximate flexor or extensor tendons. Because of these concerns, splinting, ice, and elevation, with consultation within 24 to 48 hours, are usually warranted.

Intra-articular fractures of the phalanges almost always should be referred to an orthopedic or hand surgeon. Anatomic reduction is desired, so only the perfectly nondisplaced fracture should be managed without internal stabilization. Small bony avulsions without subluxation of the joint may be managed as outlined in the section on Tendon Injuries.

METACARPAL FRACTURES

Boxer's Fractures

The most common fracture of the MC is at the fifth MC neck, which usually occurs after the patient strikes a hard object with a closed fist ("boxer's fracture") (see Figure 27.21). Fractures of the MC necks of the other fingers do occur, but with less frequency. These fractures angulate with the apex dorsal, leaving a prominence in the palm and a loss of the "knuckle" if allowed to heal without adequate reduction. Fractures of the fourth and fifth MC necks can functionally tolerate much more flexion than can the index and middle MCs (10). Up to 70 degrees of flexion may be acceptable with low morbidity after healing. However, most experts believe that a reduction to less than 30 degrees to 40 degrees is more acceptable to the patient (11). Fractures of the index and long MCs tolerate much less angulation because any remaining bony prominence is very tender and functionally limiting. A reduction to less than 10 degrees of angulation should be obtained. It is important to measure the angulation accurately: measure the angle between a line drawn along the longitudinal axis of the MC shaft and another line from the MC head to the fracture site using the true lateral view. Measuring on the oblique view consistently gives a falsely larger angle (25).

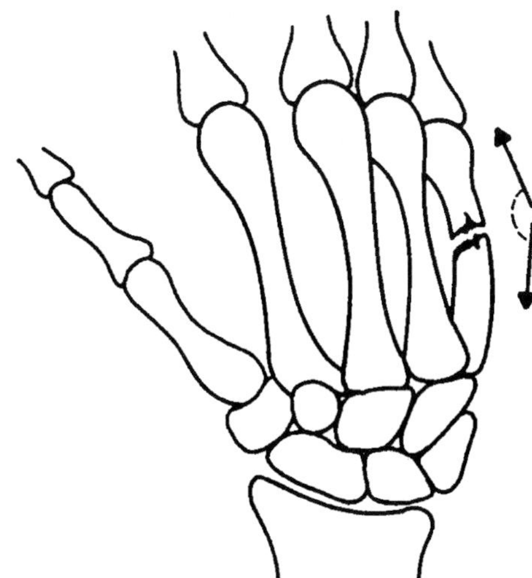

Figure 27.21 Boxer's fracture.

Treatment of these fractures can almost always be accomplished with closed reduction and casting. If the proper alignment cannot be maintained, then referral for additional treatment should be made. The reduction maneuver is done by putting pressure under the MC head with one hand and pressure over the dorsal MC shaft with the other, while maintaining flexion of approximately 90 degrees at the MCP joint (11). Once the reduction is obtained, the hand is placed in a splint or gauntlet cast with the MCP joints maintaining 50 degrees to 60 degrees of flexion. This helps maintain the reduction and prevents stiffness of the MCP joint. Radiographic confirmation of the reduction is then made. The fracture should be followed up with radiographs through the cast or splint for 2 weeks to assure maintenance of the reduction. The athlete should be maintained in the cast or splint for 4 or 5 weeks, or a molded orthotic may be made to allow participation in athletics at 3 weeks if adequate callus formation is apparent on radiographs.

Metacarpal Shaft Fractures

MC shaft fractures are generally spiral and sometimes complicated by shortening and malrotation. Any rotational deformity or shortening more than 5 mm is unacceptable and maintenance of these fractures is often difficult with casting (6). Therefore, unless the fracture is essentially nondisplaced, referral should be made to the orthopedic or hand surgeon for treatment and follow up. An undisplaced fracture may be treated in a short-arm cast for 4 to 6 weeks. For highly competitive athletes, return to competition may be expedited with the use of a molded and padded orthosis.

Metacarpal Base Fractures

MC base fractures usually occur at the base of the thumb MC (Bennett's or Rolando's fractures), and at the base of

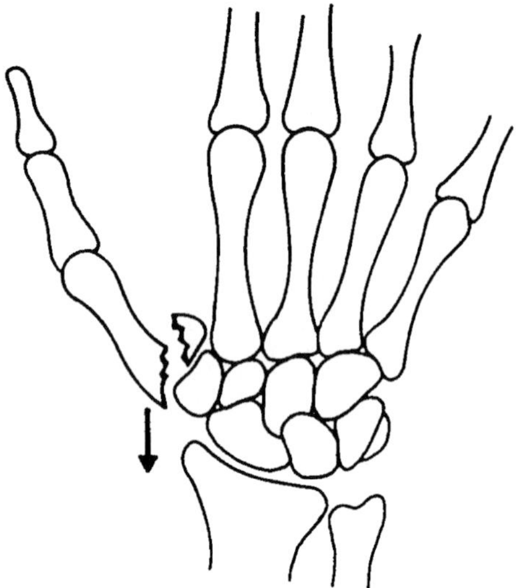

Figure 27.22 Bennett's fracture.

the fifth MC (see Figure 27.22). These fractures are often intra-articular and involve some subluxation at the CMC joint (11). Because anatomic reduction is necessary to reduce the long-term morbidity related to these fractures, referral to an orthopedic or hand surgeon is warranted.

LACERATIONS

Lacerations represent more significant injuries because of the potential of injury to deep structures including nerve, artery, and tendon. A thorough understanding of the subcutaneous anatomy of the hand is essential to recognize potential injury to these structures.

A thorough examination is needed to assess the neurovascular status before a local anesthetic is used for cleansing, debridement, or further examination. Testing of the flexor superficialis and profundus tendons is particularly important for lacerations on the volar surface of the hand or fingers (10).

Irrigation and debridement of the wound is crucial and is usually most successfully done under a local anesthetic nerve block (without epinephrine) and a tourniquet. If there is no nerve, artery, joint, or tendon involvement, simple closure with an interrupted 5-0 nonabsorbable suture is all that is necessary (10).

Antibiotics are usually not indicated if a thorough irrigation and debridement is performed. However, if the wound is particularly dirty or there is any question about the possibility of bacterial inoculation of deep soft tissue structures (especially if the palmar aponeurosis is involved), a first-generation cephalosporin provides appropriate prophylaxis for the usual gram-positive organisms (10). For any puncture wound, tetanus immunization status should be determined and tetanus toxoid given if necessary. These wounds must be followed up closely for deep-space infections (see section explaining Palmar Space Infections).

Lacerated Tendons

Diagnosis of an extensor tendon laceration is made by physical examination and/or direct visualization. With a complete laceration, the patient is unable to actively extend the digit at the PIP and DIP joints, but there is full passive range of motion. The lumbricals can also extend these joints, so the MCPs must be kept in full extension to block the action of these muscles (10). If the laceration is proximal to the MCP joints, finger extension may be possible through the extensor juncturae tendinum, which interconnect between adjacent tendons on the dorsum of the hand. When laceration is suspected, the hand is placed in a volar splint with the wrist extended to relieve tension on the injured tendon. The MCP joints should be flexed 30 degrees to 45 degrees to prevent contracture of the collateral ligaments. Referral should be made within 48 hours.

The flexor mechanism of the hand is much more complex than the extensor mechanism, because flexor tendons run through an intricate system of pulleys and tendon sheaths (21). These injured tendons should be evaluated by a hand surgeon and repaired in the operating room. These injuries are not emergencies, but referral should be made and the patient seen as soon as reasonably possible (within 48 hours).

The most important aspect of the initial treatment of flexor tendon injuries is the initial neural, vascular, and muscular examinations. Because of the proximity of the neurovascular bundle, the appearance of the fingertip, capillary refill, and two-point discrimination must be examined and recorded before treatment. Also, testing and differentiating between a laceration of the flexor superficialis and the flexor profundus will greatly assist the surgeon.

A thorough irrigation of the wound is indicated in the emergency room. Under no circumstances should a repair of the flexor tendon be attempted in the emergency room and the skin should be closed loosely with interrupted sutures of 5-0 nylon (10).

A dorsal splint should be applied with the wrist in 45 degrees of flexion, the MCP joints in 60 degrees to 80 degrees of flexion, and the IP joints in slight flexion.

Vascular Lacerations

A dual blood supply to the hand exists through the radial and ulnar arteries, and each digit has a dual blood supply through each digital artery. Therefore, even with a complete laceration, collateral flow is usually adequate to provide enough perfusion for the hand to survive (10). Pale, cool fingers with poor capillary refill are likely ischemic and should be referred to an orthopedic or hand surgeon for evaluation and treatment.

Vascular injuries of the hand can generally be managed with direct pressure and elevation. If this appears to be inadequate, a tourniquet may be applied with a blood pressure cuff. If a cuff is used, the hoses must be clamped off with a hemostat to avoid leakage and the development of a venous tourniquet. One should never attempt a blind stab with a hemostat in an attempt to control hemorrhage. Arteries in the hand are almost always accompanied by nerves, and blind stabs often result in nerve damage.

Nerve Lacerations

Nerve lacerations should be left for repair at a later date by a hand surgeon in an operating room with good lighting and appropriate instruments. Irrigation and closure appropriate for the laceration are indicated, with prompt referral to a hand surgeon.

Nail Lacerations

Badly lacerated nails should be trimmed or removed. If the laceration involves the nailbed, the nail must be removed and the nailbed repaired by an experienced physician with 5-0 or 6-0 absorbable suture (10).

Contusions beneath the nail are frequent because of its close proximity to bone and a painful subungual hematoma may develop. This can be relieved by drilling the nail at the center of the hematoma with the tip of a knife blade, a large-gauge needle, disposable electocautery unit, or a hot paperclip. Multiple holes (three to five) may be necessary to relieve all the pain.

Lacerations into a Joint

Lacerations involving a joint should be managed by an orthopedic or hand surgeon to avoid progression to a fulminant septic arthritis. If the laceration has obviously penetrated the joint, irrigation with normal saline and prompt referral are all that is needed. If there is a question as to whether the joint is involved, an injection of dilute methylene blue into the joint and extravasation out through the wound will confirm the diagnosis (10). This should be done only by someone who has had experience with injecting joints.

INFECTIONS

Serious hand infections are not common in athletes. Minor infections are more common and, if improperly treated, may develop into a more serious and devastating problem. Therefore, early recognition and treatment are of paramount importance.

Cellulitis

Cellulitis is the earliest manifestation of a hand infection and the most likely one to occur. The skin is inflamed, but without localization of pus or involvement of the joint. The treatment follows the basic principles of hand infections, which also apply to more serious infections. They are (a) splinting, (b) elevation, and (c) antibiotics.

Splinting is accomplished by a plaster or commercial volar splint or a bulky hand dressing that prohibits any movement of the fingers yet provides adequate immobilization.

The best method of elevation is to place the arm in a stockinette device hanging from an intravenous unit pole. The use of a plaster splint is helpful with this method, because it maintains the proper position of the hand in the stockinette. Other methods may be devised for the home. The use of pillows is less reliable for two reasons: (a) during sleep, the hand is more likely to fall off and move to a dependent position; (b) it is easier for the patient to be noncompliant and walk around with the hand in a dependent position. Warm compresses may be applied and are indeed helpful for minor infections; however, elevation is more important and should be maintained while moist heat is being applied.

Routine use of antibiotics in minor infections is contraindicated and may lead to superinfection (10). Most hand surgeons maintain that the proper treatment, whether it be splinting and elevation or incision and drainage, is enough to cure most minor hand infections. This is especially true of early, focal cellulitis. More extensive and severe cellulitis may require the use of antibiotics. The most common organism is Streptococcus and it responds well to first-generation cephalosporins.

Flexor Tenosynovitis

Flexor tenosynovitis is an infection of the flexor tendon sheath that normally provides a tight lubricated path for the tendon to glide within. When infected, this tight space fills with pus and rapidly progresses to a deep palmar space infection and/or necrosis and destruction of the flexor mechanism. These infections are emergent, and referral to an orthopedic or hand surgeon should be immediate (26). Treatment is incision and either open or closed irrigation of the tendon sheath.

Recognition of flexor tenosynovitis is of primary importance to the primary care person, and it can be confused with subcutaneous abscess and cellulitis. The four "cardinal signs" of flexor sheath infections (10) are as follows: (a) tenderness over the flexor tendon sheath, (b) symmetric swelling of the digit, (c) pain with passive extension of the finger, and (d) flexed posturing of the digit. If these signs are present, prompt referral should be made.

Clenched-Fist Lacerations and Septic Arthritis

Infections involving a joint in the hand should prompt emergent referral to a hand surgeon. Symptoms include swelling and erythema around a joint and severe pain with active or passive motion of the joint. At times this is difficult to distinguish from a cellulitis overlying a joint, as a cellulitis will also manifest the same symptoms. The most effective test for distinguishing them is axial compression of the joint. If axial compression produces intense pain, the joint is likely to be infected (10). Otherwise, the problem is more likely to be a cellulitis, but the joint should still be watched closely.

Clenched-fist injuries ("fight bites") almost always overlie the fourth or fifth MCP joint. When they do, it is very likely that the offending tooth entered the joint. These should be considered open, infected joints, and the patient should be referred to the appropriate surgeon. In wounds that involve human bites, one must consider *Eikenella corrodens* as a possible infecting organism. Staphylococcal and streptococcal organisms are still more common, but a first-generation cephalosporin will not be effective against Eikenella and other anaerobes (10). Consequently, either penicillin should be added, or a combination drug with the appropriate coverage should be used (i.e., ampicillin and clavulanic acid).

REFERENCES

1. McGrew C, Lillegard W, McKeag D, et al. Profile of patient care in a primary care sports medicine fellowship. *Clin J Sports Med* 1992;2:126–131.
2. Dobyns JH, Beckenbaugh RD, Bryan RS. Fractures of the hand and wrist. In: Flynn JE, ed. *Hand surgery*, 3rd ed. Baltimore: Williams & Wilkins, 1982:111–180.
3. Kauer JMG: Functional anatomy of the wrist. *Clin Orthop* 1980;149:9.
4. Taleisnik J. The ligaments of the wrist. *J Hand Surg* 1976;1:110–118.
5. Jennings JF, Peimer CA. Ligamentous injuries of the wrist in athletes. In: Nicholas JA, Hershman EB, eds. *The upper extremity in sports medicine*. Baltimore: CV Mosby, 1990:457–482.
6. Posner MA. Hand injuries. In: Nicholas JA, Hershman EB, eds. *The upper extremity in sports medicine*, Vol. 1. Baltimore: CV Mosby, 1990:445–596.
7. Rettig AC. Closed tendon injuries of the hand and wrist in the athlete. *Clin Sports Med* 1992;11(1):77–99.
8. Lillegard WA. Wrist injuries. In: Lillegard WA, Butcher JD, Rucker KS, eds. *Handbook of sports medicine: a symptom oriented approach*. Boston: Butterworth-Heinemann, 1999:159–180.
9. Strickland J, Rettig A. *Hand injuries in athletes*. Philadelphia: WB Saunders, 1992.
10. St. Pierre P. Hand injuries. In: Lillegard WA, Butcher JD, Rucker KS, eds. *Handbook of sports medicine: a symptom oriented approach*. Boston: Butterworth-Heinemann, 1999:181–193.
11. Green DP, Rowland SA. Fractures and dislocations in the hand. In: Rockwood CA, Green DP, eds. *Fractures in adults*, Vol. 1, 3rd ed. Philadelphia: JB Lippincott, 1991:441–563.
12. Culver JE, Anderson TE. Fractures of the hand and wrist in the athlete. *Clin Sports Med* 1992;11(1):101–128.
13. Rettig AC, Adsit WS. Athletic injuries of the hand and wrist. In: Griffin LY, ed. *Orthopaedic knowledge update: sports medicine*. Rosemont, IL: American Academy of Orthopaedic Surgeons, 1994:205–224.
14. O'Brien ET. Fractures of the hand and wrist region. In: Rockwood CA, Green DP, eds. *Fractures in children*, 2nd ed. Philadelphia: JB Lippincott, 1984:229–299.
15. Zemel NP, Stark HH. Fractures and dislocations of the carpal bones. *Clin Sports Med* 1986;5(4):707–724.
16. Mayer KB, Kitzinger HB, Frohner S, et al. Scaphoid fractures—operative or conservative treatment? A CT-based classification. *Handchir Mikrochir Plast Chir* 2005;37(4):260–264.
17. Mooney JF, Siegel DB, Koman LA. Ligamentous injuries of the wrist in athletes. *Clin Sports Med* 1992;11(1):129–139.
18. Vitello W, Gordon DA. Obvious radiographic scapholunate dissociation: X-ray the other wrist. *Am J Orthop* 2005;34(7):347–351.
19. Baker CL. Overuse injuries in the upper extremity. *Clin Sports Med* 2001;20(3):423–645.
20. McCue FC, Wooten L. Closed tendon injuries of the hand in athletics. *Clin Sports Med* 1986;5(4):741–755.
21. Strickland JW. Management of flexor tendon injuries. *Orthop Clin North Am* 1983;14:827–846.
22. Kahler DM, McCue FC. Metacarpophalangeal and proximal interphalangeal joint injuries of the hand including the thumb. *Clin Sports Med* 1992;11(1):57–76.
23. Bowers WH. Sprains and joint injuries in the hand. *Hand Clin* 1986;2:93–98.
24. Cooper JG, Johnstone AJ, Hider P, et al. Local anaesthetic infiltration increases the accuracy of assessment of ulnar collateral ligament injuries. *Emerg Med Australas* 2005;17(2):132–136.
25. Lamraski G, Monsaert A, De Maeseneer M, et al. Reliability and validity of plain radiographs to assess angulation of small finger metacarpal neck fractures: human cadaveric study. *J Orthop Res* 2006;24(1):37–45.
26. Gaar E. Occupational hand infections. *Clin Occup Environ Med* 2006;5(2):369–380.

Chest and Abdominal Wall

28

Sami F. Rifat

Injuries to the chest and abdominal wall can occur in any sport but are more common in contact or collision sports such as hockey, football, and soccer. It is important that the treating physician differentiates benign chest and abdominal wall injuries from those that are potentially life threatening. This chapter focuses on injuries to the chest and abdominal walls although it is important to recognize that there is often an overlap between these conditions and injury to the viscera and extremities. Injuries to the deep structures and viscera are discussed elsewhere.

CHEST

Blows to the chest are common in athletics. Blunt trauma can result in general injury to the chest wall or an injury to a specific structure, such as the sternum, sternoclavicular (SC) joint, clavicle, or ribs.

Chest Wall Contusion

Chest wall contusions usually result from blunt trauma. For all chest contusions, the physician should inspect the involved area to evaluate for gross deformity and abnormal, asymmetrical or paradoxical movement of the chest. Palpation for focal tenderness and crepitation should be performed. Auscultation of the heart and lungs for evidence of cardiac or pulmonary damage should be done. Severe blows to the chest can lead to comotio cordis, cardiac or pulmonary contusion, hemothorax, and pneumothorax. These entities are discussed elsewhere.

Treatment of minor, nonspecific chest wall contusions involves relative rest, ice, and consideration of an elastic bandage for support. Ace wraps should be used with caution because they may cause the athlete to take shallow breaths potentially leading to pulmonary atelectasis and pneumonia. Acetaminophen or a nonsteroidal anti-inflammatory agent may be used for analgesia. Large hematomas may require incision and drainage. Fortunately, most contusions heal after several days of conservative treatment. The athlete may return to competition when symptoms allow. Rib pads or a flak jacket may be required for protection in the short term.

Sternum Fractures

Sternal fractures are rare in sports. Although the fracture itself may not be that significant there is a high incidence of associated chest trauma such as cardiac and pulmonary contusions and injury to the internal mammary vessels. These injuries typically occur as a result of a direct high-impact blow, although a flexion-compression mechanism has also been reported (see Figure 28.1). Most commonly, a direct blow to the sternum causes a portion of the bone to displace inward resulting in fracture or sternomanubrial disruption. In the flexion-compression mechanism, flexion of the cervical spine drives the chin into the manubrium displacing it posteriorly.

Typically, the athlete presents with a history of trauma and localized pain over the sternum. A palpable defect is sometimes present. The pain is usually aggravated by deep inspiration. Plain radiographs, particularly a lateral chest film best demonstrate the fracture. Computed tomography (CT) is useful if the fracture is displaced and there is concern of damage to underlying structures.

Treatment of sternal fractures depends on whether displacement is present or not. Nondisplaced fractures

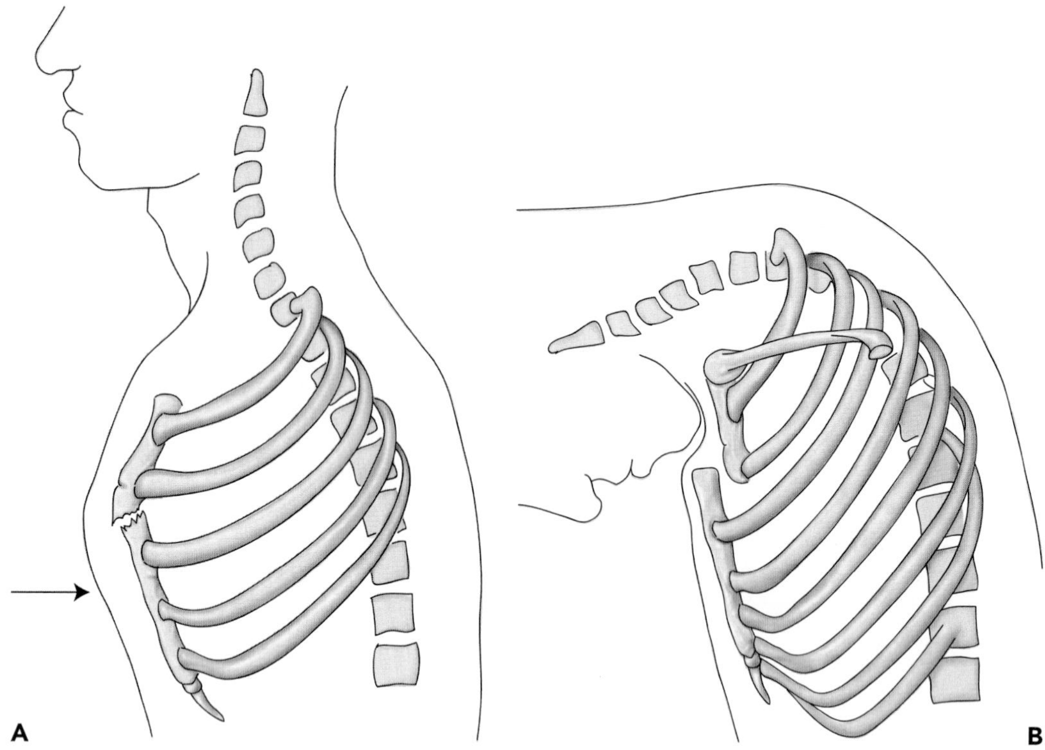

Figure 28.1 The mechanisms of sternal fracture; **(A)** direct blow and **(B)** flexion-compression.

are treated symptomatically with rest, ice, and analgesics. The athlete may return to noncontact participation once sufficient healing has been accomplished. Return to contact sports generally can occur in 6 to 12 weeks. Displaced fractures often need to be reduced. They may be reduced in a closed or open manner depending on the degree of displacement. Referral is indicated and close monitoring of the patient's cardiac and respiratory function is essential because of the high association with intrathoracic trauma.

Sternoclavicular Joint

SC joint injuries may be either traumatic or atraumatic. Symptoms arising from an inherent (atraumatic) instability of the joint are relatively rare and therefore most SC injures encountered in athletes are traumatic in nature. Acute SC joint injuries include subluxation, fracture, and dislocation. The medial clavicular physis is vulnerable to fracture in skeletally immature individuals. Dislocation of the proximal clavicle relative to the sternum may be in either the anterior or posterior direction. Anterior dislocation is much more common. Posterior dislocation is a medical emergency and requires immediate attention due to the potential involvement of the great vessels, trachea, and esophagus.

The mechanism of SC joint injury may be either direct or indirect. Direct blow to the joint can occur from another player, surface, stick, puck or ball. Indirect SC injury may occur when a compression or traction force is applied across the joint. In the compression mechanism the athlete often falls onto his lateral shoulder and another player lands on top of him or her. This (indirect) blow causes the SC joint to buckle. Alternatively, the joint may be injured by a traction mechanism in which the athlete's outstretched shoulder abducted to 90 degrees is forcibly extended.

Athletes suffering a SC injury usually complain of severe pain, especially with movement of the arm. The pain is usually worse with the individual in the supine position. Physical examination reveals swelling, deformity, and local tenderness. The physician should carefully assess the patients respiratory and neurovascular status to rule out pressure on the underlying vital structures. Specifically, the physician should evaluate for pulselessness of the ipsilateral arm, extremity swelling, claudication, and dysthesias. Hoarseness, dyspnea, and dysphagia are signs of tracheal or esophageal involvement. Plain x-rays including the serendipity view (see Figure 28.2) (Anteroposterior [AP] radiograph of the SC joints with a 40 degree cephalic tilt) should be obtained. A CT scan is the test of choice if x-rays are inconclusive or posterior displacement is suspected.

Anterior subluxation, dislocation, and nondisplaced fractures of the proximal clavicle are usually treated conservatively and do not require reduction or surgery.

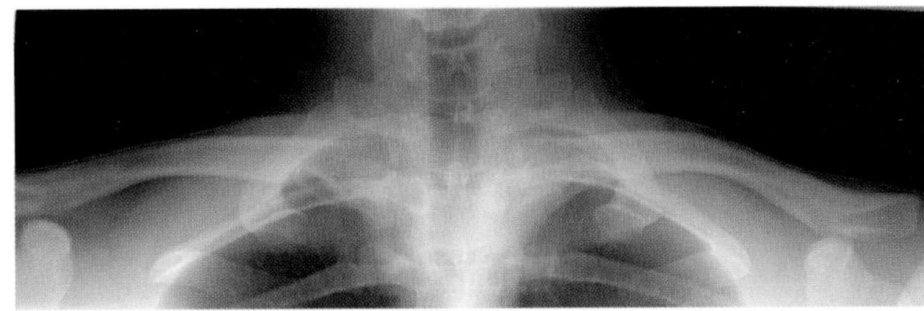

Figure 28.2 Serendipity view, anteroposterior (AP) radiograph of the sternoclavicular (SC) joints with a 40 degree cephalic tilt.

Generally a sling for comfort, ice, and analgesics are all that is required. Activity may be resumed as symptoms allow or once adequate bony healing takes place. Complete anterior dislocations usually require closed reduction. The patient is placed in the supine position and the shoulders are drawn backward while applying traction to the ipsilateral arm. A sandbag placed between the patient's shoulder blades is often helpful. A figure-of-eight bandage should be used post reduction for 4 to 6 weeks. The patient should be advised that there may be a persistent deformity of the joint.

Posterior dislocations of the SC joint should be evaluated in the emergency department. These are potentially serious injuries and any attempt at treatment should be performed in a setting where surgeons are available to address possible complications, such as injury to the great vessels. Closed reduction is performed in the manner discussed in the preceding text.

Clavicle Fractures

Clavicle fractures are common in sports. They can result from direct or indirect trauma. Individuals participating in stick sports such as hockey or lacrosse may sustain direct bony injury. Clavicle fractures can also occur from indirect trauma as a result of a fall or blow to the lateral shoulder or upper arm. Clavicle fractures can occur anywhere along the length of the bone with the midshaft being the most common location.

The patient usually recalls a clear history of trauma and complains of pain at the fractured site. The arm on the affected side is usually held in a guarded position. A deformity is often obvious. Evaluation involves palpation to assess for pain, deformity, and crepitance. A careful neurological and vascular examination is essential. Auscultation of the chest is important to evaluate for pulmonary injury. Clavicle radiographs should be obtained (see Figure 28.3) although proximal clavicle fractures are sometimes difficult to visualize with plain radiography and CT is sometimes required.

Treatment of midshaft clavicle fractures is relatively straightforward. Most midshaft clavicle fractures respond well to supportive treatment consisting of a sling or figure-of-eight bandage, analgesic medications, and ice. Figure-of-eight harness does not offer an advantage and the simple sling is often more comfortable (1). There is debate over the indications for surgical management of clavicle shaft fractures. Table 28.1 lists some potential indications for surgery (2).

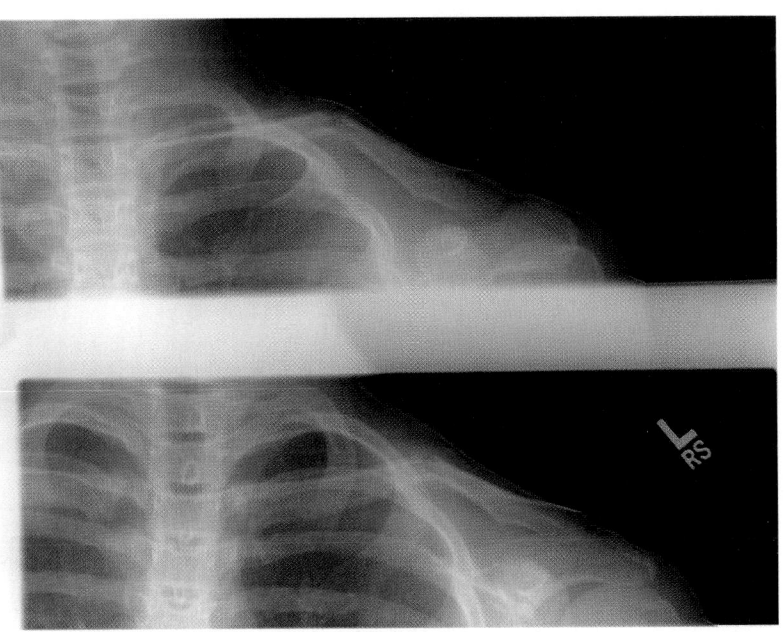

Figure 28.3 Midshaft clavicle fracture.

TABLE 28.1
SURGICAL INDICATIONS FOR ACUTE CLAVICLE FRACTURE

- Open fracture
- Multiple trauma
- Neurovascular compromise requiring exploration
- Displaced distal clavicle fractures
- Severely displaced or shortened shaft fractures
- Severe fracture with skin tension that fails closed reduction
- Nonunion after 3 mo

The treatment of proximal clavicle fractures is similar to SC joint injury and has been already discussed. Treatment of distal clavicle fractures is more controversial. Nondisplaced distal clavicle fractures can be treated conservatively similar to a shaft fracture. Displaced distal clavicle fractures may require surgical intervention and referral is indicated.

Rib Injuries

Rib fractures are one of the most common injuries to the chest wall (3). They typically occur with a blunt trauma to the chest. Diagnosis is generally straightforward and the individual usually presents with a history of trauma with localized pain and tenderness. There may be swelling, bruising, and pain with inspiration and cough. Chest radiographs can demonstrate the injury; however, fractures may not always be visible. Bone scan can confirm the diagnosis.

Treatment of stable rib fractures is symptomatic and consists of relative rest, ice, and analgesics. Rib belts and wrapping has been advocated, however, the author does not routinely recommend these measures because they often cause more pain and promote shallow breathing that can lead to pulmonary atelectasis. Intercostal nerve block can be a useful adjunct for pain control (see Figure 28.4). Ideally, healing should be advanced before the athlete is allowed to return to play due to the risk of the injured rib penetrating the lung, liver, or spleen.

Injury to the first rib has provoked a great deal of attention in the literature because of the possibility of serious underlying pulmonary or neurovascular damage (see Figure 28.5). Fortunately, this injury is rare in sports and when it does occur it usually does not occur as a result of major trauma. In athletics injury to the first rib has most often been described as a type of stress phenomenon (4).

The athlete may report a history of aching, but usually there is no warning sign before the fracture occurring suddenly during activity. A snap is sometimes audible and the

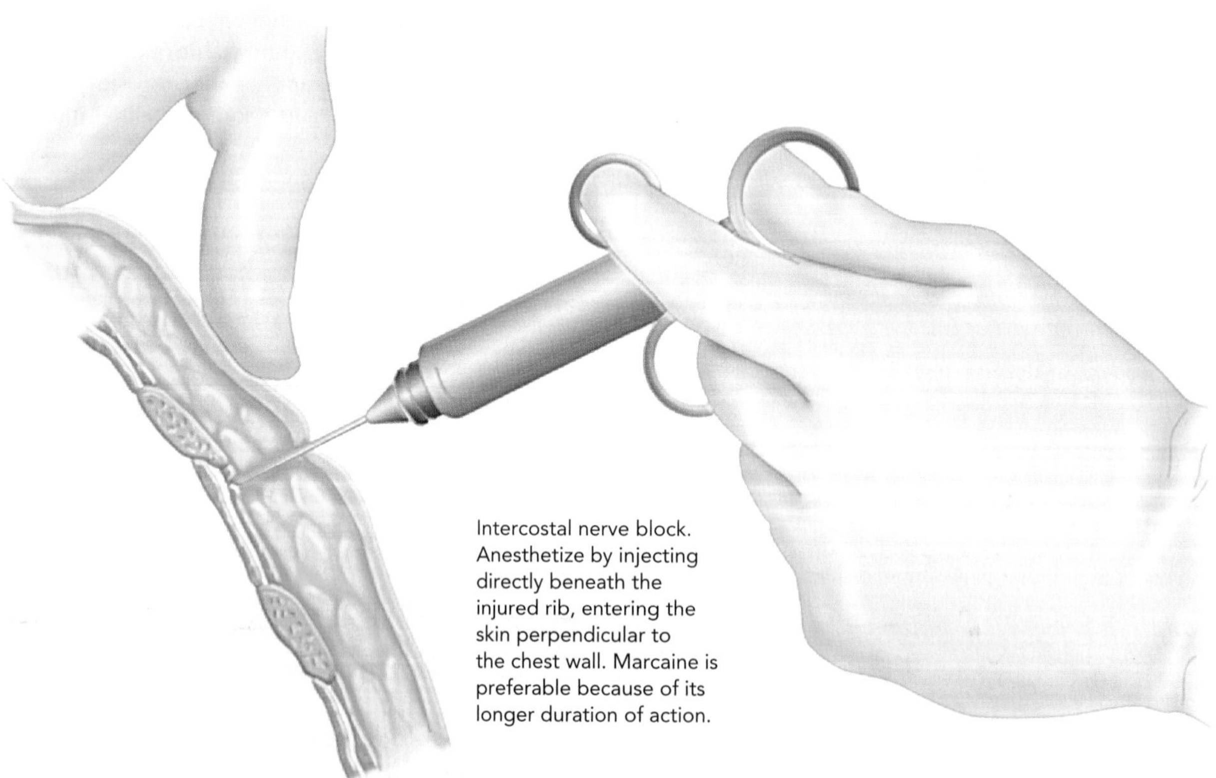
Intercostal nerve block. Anesthetize by injecting directly beneath the injured rib, entering the skin perpendicular to the chest wall. Marcaine is preferable because of its longer duration of action.

Figure 28.4 Intercostal nerve block. Anesthetize by injecting directly beneath the injured rib, entering the skin perpendicular to the chest wall. Marcaine is preferable because of its longer duration of action.

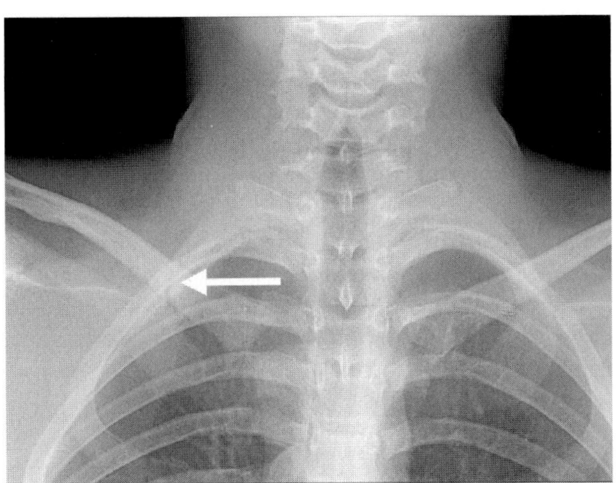

Figure 28.5 Radiograph of first-rib fracture.

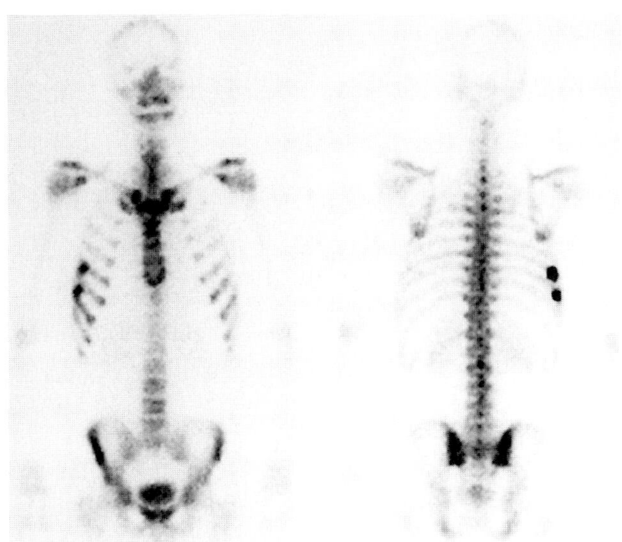

Figure 28.6 Rib stress fractures on bone scan.

initial pain can be quite severe. Symptoms are aggravated by deep inspiration and arm movement. Once the acute pain subsides, often there is little pain at rest. The patient is treated symptomatically and activity is resumed as symptoms allow. In those rare cases involving a direct trauma, the treatment of first-rib fractures is similar to SC injury, with great care taken to ensure that the underlying neurovascular structures are intact (5). These severe injuries necessitate referral.

Fracture of multiple ribs can lead to fail chest. This occurs when a portion of the thoracic rib cage separates from the rest of the chest wall. In order for this to occur there must be at least two fractures per rib in at least two ribs. This produces a freely moving segment that does not contribute to lung expansion. The segment moves paradoxically during inspiration and expiration. Large flail chests can significantly disrupt pulmonary mechanics and the patient may require mechanical ventilation. Flail chest is often associated with pulmonary contusion. This injury requires immediate transportation to an emergency center.

Stress fractures of the lower ribs have been reported in throwing, golf, rowing, canoeing, and swimming, whereas upper rib stress fractures have been reported in back packing (6). Though the exact mechanism of injury is unknown, rib stress fractures are believed to occur as a result of repetitive muscle action on the ribs associated with the high-risk sports. Usually the athlete presents with a localized rib/chest wall pain and palpable tenderness. There is often a history of increased activity before the onset of symptoms. As is typical of other stress fractures, plain radiographs are often negative and a bone scan is required to make the diagnosis (see Figure 28.6). Treatment involves relative rest, ice, and analgesics. The athlete may return to activity as symptoms allow.

Costochondral Separation and Sprain

Costochondral injury frequently occurs in contact sports such as football, ice hockey, and wrestling. In this injury, there is a separation of the costal cartilage as it attaches to the sternum or anterior rib. It most frequently occurs at the tenth rib, followed by the ninth and eighth. This injury is believed to occur by both direct and indirect mechanisms. Direct injury causing forced compression of the rib cage is common. Indirect twisting or stretching of the joint with vigorous forced movement of the arm has also been proposed as a mechanism.

The athlete often reports hearing or feeling a "pop" accompanied by a sharp discomfort at the site of injury. These symptoms often last for several days and then gradually begin to resolve. The symptoms can be aggravated with movement of the chest or arms. Sometimes a click is felt as the cartilage overrides the bone. Examination reveals localized swelling and tenderness of the involved joint. A visible and/or palpable deformity may also be present if the cartilage has been displaced. There may be radiation of the symptoms to the epigastrium or spine. Radiographs, although helpful in excluding fracture, are usually unremarkable.

Treatment of costochondral injury includes ice and analgesics. Lidocaine injection with or without corticosteroid at the site of the injury may help alleviate symptoms. Symptoms often take several weeks to resolve and are susceptible to reaggravation. Resection of the affected costochondral junction is sometimes needed in those individuals with intractable pain. The athlete may be allowed to return to play with extra padding (if applicable) (see Figure 28.7) when symptoms have resolved.

Pectoralis Muscle Injury

Pectoralis major muscle strains have been reported in weight lifting, football, wrestling, and rugby (7,8). They can be classified as complete or incomplete. Individuals with complete muscle or tendon ruptures usually present with a

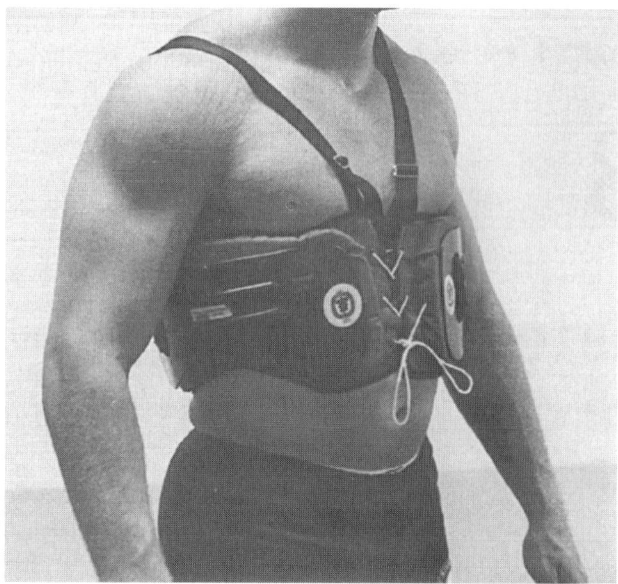

Figure 28.7 Flak Vest.

definite history of an injury with immediate severe pain at the site of the muscle or its attachments. Some individuals report an audible "pop". The individual presents with pain, supporting the affected extremity with the opposite arm. Deformity of the muscle may be visible or palpable although this may be obscured by swelling and bruising. Usually there is palpable tenderness, pain, and weakness with resisted adduction and internal rotation of the arm. The athlete will have difficulty performing a push-up. In the acute phase it may be difficult to distinguish between complete and incomplete injury. Magnetic resonance imaging (MRI) may help establish the extent of the injury. In chronic cases, there is an obvious asymmetry with a prominent "balling" of the retracted muscle belly.

Treatment depends on the extent of the injury (7). Simple strains respond to conservative treatment. Sling immobilization, ice, and analgesics may be used for comfort. Early range of motion exercises can be started in about a week and strengthening exercise in 3 to 4 weeks. Recovery from partial pectoralis major muscle rupture often takes several weeks. Complete ruptures usually require surgical repair. It is believed that prompt surgical repair of these injuries is optimal; however, recent studies suggest that late repair still yields good results.

Serratus Anterior

The serratus anterior is usually injured by a sudden pulling mechanism and is sometimes seen in rowers and weight lifters (performing a dead lift). The athlete will have difficulty protracting the scapula and is locally tender. A palpable swelling or lump may be present. Rib radiographs should be obtained to evaluate for avulsion fracture. These injuries usually respond to conservative treatment consisting of rest, ice, analgesics, and graded return to activity.

Breast Injuries

Runner's nipple is an irritating condition causing pain, chaffing, and occasional bleeding of the nipple. It occurs as a result of a mechanical irritation of the runners clothing against the nipple aggravated by sweat. The athlete should apply petroleum jelly and bandages before exercise. Nonabrasive materials and drying off after exercise can help prevent runner's nipple. Newer fabrics help wick out moisture from the skin and reduce the risk of developing this problem. Women should wear well fitting "sports bras" that are designed for comfort, breathability, and support with a minimum of mechanical irritation.

Breast contusions can affect both males and females. These injuries usually occur as a result of blunt trauma and are treated similar to other chest wall contusions. Occasionally a fibrous nodule may develop. These should be documented and observed, especially in women, and may be excised if painful.

ABDOMINAL WALL

The abdomen is largely unprotected and is at particular risk for injury in contact and collision sports. This section deals with conditions and injuries to the abdominal wall. Injury to the deep viscera is discussed elsewhere.

Transient Diaphragmatic Spasm

Transient diaphragmatic spasm or getting the "wind knocked out of you" is probably the most common abdominal injury in contact and collision sports. Typically, the injury occurs from a blow to the region of the epigastrium and solar plexus. This blunt trauma produces dyspnea secondary to temporary diaphragmatic muscle spasm. The athlete has difficulty breathing until the spasm has resolved. Symptoms last momentarily and are relieved by flexion of the knees towards the abdomen and loosening of any restrictive equipment or garments. The athlete may return to play once normal comfortable breathing has returned. If breathing does not return to normal, other more serious diagnoses should be considered, including xyphoid fracture, flail chest, avulsion of rectus abdominus muscle, or laceration of the abdominal viscera.

Abdominal Wall Musculature

The abdominal musculature is composed of the rectus abdominus, external oblique, internal oblique, and the transversus muscles (see Figure 28.8). These structures can be injured by direct or indirect means. A direct blow to the muscle can cause local injury and hematoma. Sudden violent muscle movements may also cause significant muscle injury or bony avulsion by an indirect mechanism.

Simple strains of the abdominal wall musculature usually present with acute or subacute symptoms. Typically,

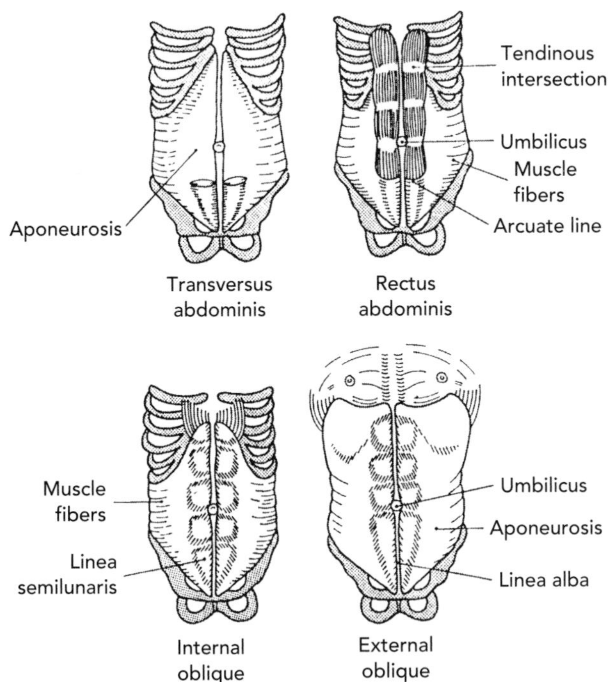

Figure 28.8 Abdominal anatomy.

the patient complains of pain with trunk flexion or rotation and local tenderness. These injuries are usually self-limited and may be treated with relative rest, ice, and analgesics. More significant abdominal wall muscle strains may be treated with rehabilitation in order to regain motion, strength, and endurance.

Injury to the rectus abdominus muscles may be complicated by concurrent injury to the epigastric or large intramuscular blood vessels causing hemorrhage and hematoma formation within the rectus sheath. Individuals with rectus sheath hematoma usually complain of sudden abdominal pain with rapid swelling. Occasionally, nausea and vomiting may be present. The individual is most comfortable with the trunk in the supported flexed position. Examination may reveal a tender palpable mass most often below the umbilicus. There may be guarding and rigidity of the abdomen. Flexion of the trunk will produce pain. The presence of a hematoma can be confirmed with ultrasound, CT scan, or MRI.

Treatment of rectus sheath hematomas includes, ice, relative rest, and analgesics. The athlete should avoid activities that require flexion and rotation of the trunk, and stretching of the abdominal musculature. Larger hematomas may require surgical evacuation and ligation of the epigastric artery. After the acute period, the athlete should begin rehabilitation with emphasis on regaining, flexibility, strength, and endurance.

Abdominal Hernia

Abdominal hernias are common in adults and are classified as inguinal, femoral, incisional, and umbilical. All hernias carry the potential for incarceration and strangulation of underlying bowel or soft tissue, which can lead to obstruction and/or toxicity. Most hernias result from repetitive heavy lifting activity that causes increased intra-abdominal pressure. Patients with a hernia complain of aching pain sometimes accompanied by local swelling.

Inguinal and femoral hernias occur in the groin (see Figure 28.9). Inguinal hernias are either direct or indirect. Indirect inguinal hernias can sometimes be distinguished from direct inguinal hernias by inspection. An indirect hernia, once it has entered into the inguinal canal, appears as an elliptical swelling descending toward or sometimes entering the scrotum. Direct hernias usually appear as an isolated oval swelling near the pubis and rarely enter the scrotum. If no abnormalities are visible, indirect hernias on physical examination are palpable with invagination of the scrotum into the inguinal canal using a finger. A bulge or impulse felt at the tip of the examiners finger with coughing or Valsalva is evidence of an indirect inguinal hernia. Herniography, ultrasound, CT, and MRI have all been used to study hernias, but most often the diagnosis is made on clinical grounds.

Almost all inguinal hernias should be repaired; however, the presence of asymptomatic hernias is not a contraindication to athletic participation (9). Athletes with hernias who are in the middle of their competitive season may defer repair until the end of the season, as long as they understand the potential complications of their condition and accept the risks. They should be monitored carefully throughout the season. Typically after surgery, the athlete may return to noncontact sports in 6 to 8 weeks and contact sports in 8 to 10 weeks in most cases.

A femoral hernia is a protrusion of the omentum and/or bowel through the femoral canal. Femoral hernias are palpable below the inguinal ligament and two fingerbreadths medial to the femoral artery. These become more prominent with increased intra-abdominal pressure or when the athlete stands. Femoral hernias should also be repaired. Management decisions and return to play is identical to the inguinal hernias discussed earlier.

Sports Hernia

Groin injuries comprise up to 5% of all sports injuries (10). They are more common in hockey, soccer, and Australian Rules football. The sports "hernia", also known as, athletic pubalgia, sportsman hernia, and Gilmore's groin, refers to an abnormality of the abdominal wall with disruption to the inguinal canal causing groin pain without a clinically detectable hernia (11,12). Gilmore first described a syndrome of chronic groin pain in individuals with a dilated superficial inguinal ring but no frank hernia. More recent operative studies have found an isolated tear of the external oblique aponeurosis together with separation of the conjoint tendon from the inguinal ligament and laxity of the transversalis fascia (see Figure 28.10). The exact mechanism of these injuries is not known, but researchers

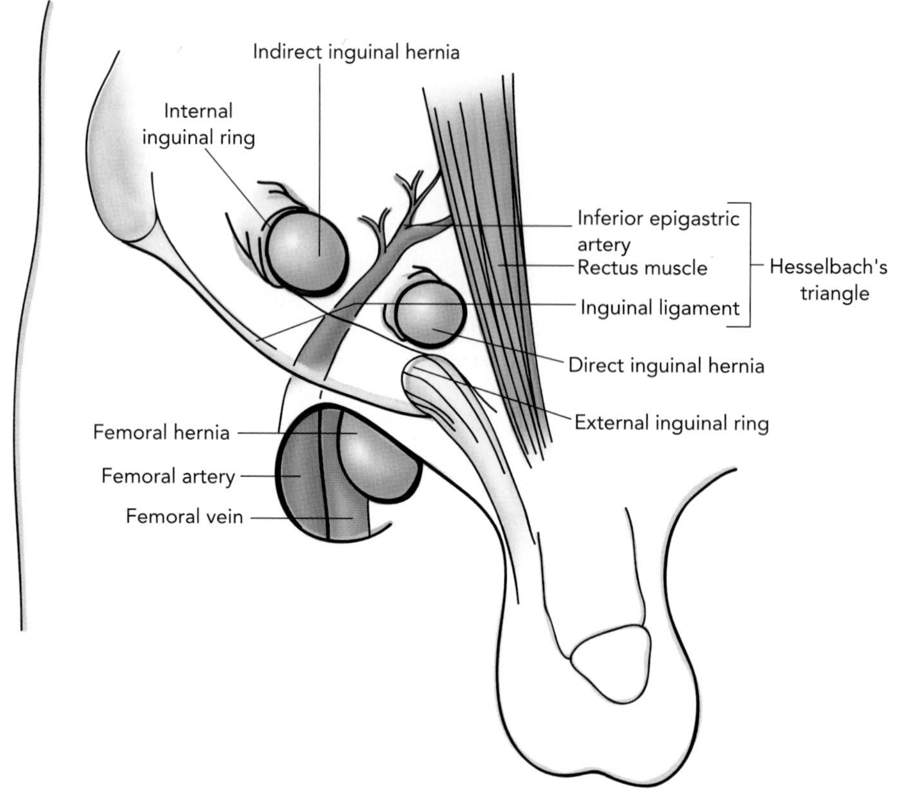

Figure 28.9 Abdominal wall hernias.

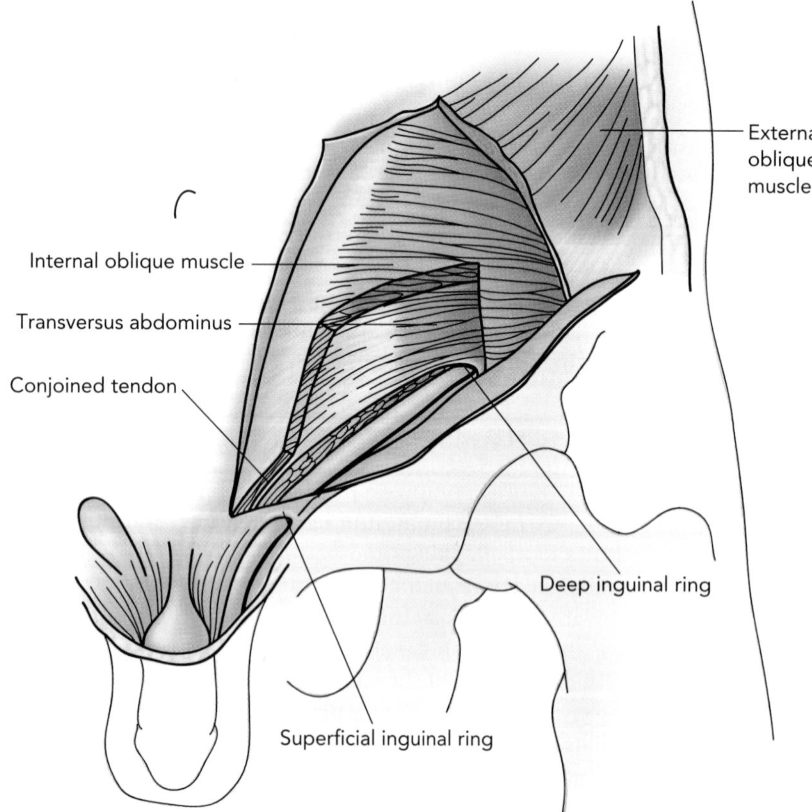

Figure 28.10 The sports hernia.

suggest that they occur because adductor action during certain sports activity creates shearing forces across the pubic symphysis that can stress the posterior inguinal wall. An intense sudden force or repetitive stretching can lead to separation of the conjoint tendon from the inguinal ligament.

Sports hernia is diagnosed by clinical means. The athlete often reports chronic pain around the pubic tubercle of the affected groin. Symptoms are usually worse after, and not during, activity. Symptoms are aggravated by coughing, straining, sneezing, and prolonged sitting. Sudden accelerations and movements such as, twisting, turning, cutting, and kicking can aggravate symptoms as well. Physical examination fails to demonstrate a frank hernia, but a dilated superficial inguinal ring is often present. Symptoms can often be reproduced by resisted sit-ups. An AP radiograph of the pelvis is helpful in excluding other pathologies such as, avulsion fracture, osteitis pubis, and hip osteoarthritis. A bone scan can identify active osteitis pubis, stress fractures, and avulsion fractures. Herniography, ultrasound, and MRI have also been advocated, but their effectiveness in diagnosing sports hernia has not been demonstrated.

The differential diagnosis includes, osteoarthritis of the hip, osteitis pubis, true inguinal hernia, adductor tendonopathy, stress fracture, and obturator neuropathy. Because of the lack easily identifiable physical examination findings and the absence of reliable diagnostic testing, surgery is considered only after a trial of nonoperative treatment. The author routinely places patients in a focused rehabilitation program for 6 to 8 weeks. A bone scan is ordered to rule out active osteitis pubis, stress, and avulsion fractures. If the patient does not respond to conservative treatment, the patient is then referred for surgery.

REFERENCES

1. Andersen K, Jensen PO, Lauritzen J. Treatment of clavicular fractures. Figure-of-eight bandage versus a simple sling. *Acta Orthop Scand* 1987;58(1):71–74.
2. Hill JM, McGurire MH, Crosby LA. Closed treatment of displaced middle-third fractures of the clavicle gives poor results. *J Bone Joint Surg Br* 1997;79(4):537–539.
3. Miles JW, Barret GR. Rib fractures in athletes. *Sports Med* 1991;12(1):66–69.
4. Gurtler R, Pavlov H, Torg JS. Stress fracture of the ipsilateral first rib in a pitcher. *Am J Sports Med* 1985;13(4):277–279.
5. Barret GR, Shelton WR, Miles JW. First rib fractures in football players. A case report and literature review. *Am J Sports Med* 1988;16(6):674–676.
6. Karlson KA. Rib stress fractures in elite rowers; a case series and proposed mechanism. *Am J Sports Med* 1998;26(4):516–519.
7. Hanna CM, Glenny SN, Stanley SN, et al. Pectoralis major tears: comparison of surgical and conservative treatment. *Br J Sports Med* 2001;35:202–206.
8. Kretzler HH, Richardson AB. Rupture of pectoralis major muscle. *Am J Sports Med* 1989;14:453–458.
9. Smith DM, Kovan JR, Rich BS, et al. *Preparticipation physical evaluation*, 2nd ed. Minneapolis, MN: American Academy of Family Physicians, American Academy of Pediatrics, American Medical Society for Sports Medicine, American Orthopedic Society for Sports Medicine, American Osteopathic Academy of Sports Medicine, The Physician and Sportsmedicine, 1997.
10. Renstrom P, Perterson L. Groin injuries in athletes. *Br J Sports Med* 1980;14(1):30–36.
11. Brannigan AE, Kerin MJ, McEntee GP. Gilmore's groin repair in athletes. *J Orthop Sports Phys Ther* 2000;30(6):329–332.
12. Gilmore OJ. Gilmore's groin. *Sportsmed Soft Tissue Trauma* 1992;3(3):12–14.

Thoracic and Lumbar Spine

29

Scott W. Eathorne

Back pain, specifically low back pain (LBP), is one of the most frequently encountered presenting symptoms in primary care and sports medicine offices. LBP is second only to the common cold as a reason for visiting the primary care physician (1). With a lifetime prevalence of 60% to 90%, annual incidence estimated at 5%, and estimated direct medical cost of treatment at $25 billion per year, LBP poses a significant challenge to the health care system and its providers (2). This challenge is made even more difficult by the fact that only 5% to 10% of individuals with LBP seek medical care for their symptoms. For the sports medicine provider, recognizing the prevalence of back pain in the overall community and preparing to recognize, diagnose, and effectively manage it in the athletic population is a matter of key competency.

Back pain is a symptom, not a diagnosis. Identifying its cause can be difficult given that potential etiologies include biomechanical, inflammatory, traumatic, infectious, developmental, neoplastic, metabolic, or emotional processes. Table 29.1 lists some of the diagnostic considerations for the athlete presenting with back pain. Considering such factors as the athlete's age, chosen sport, position played, onset and mechanism of injury, and vocation can provide clues to help narrow the differential diagnosis. Developing a systematic approach to evaluating the athlete with back pain will make the task of sorting out potential causes more manageable.

The U.S. Agency for Healthcare Research and Quality (AHRQ) clinical practice guideline for acute low back problems in adults provides a useful framework for approaching the athlete with LBP. Although the guideline, published in 1994, has undergone scrutiny and other evidence-based guidelines have been developed, it continues to provide a useful approach to evaluating and managing this common problem (3–5). It emphasizes stratification of clinical signs and presenting symptoms to focus on those most likely associated with more severe causes of LBP requiring urgent recognition and treatment. The guideline suggests various imaging and treatment modalities evaluated for proven value in establishing a diagnosis and improving outcomes, both short and long term. As the title implies, the guideline only applies to the evaluation of acute pain in adults. This is because adults tend toward a myofascial etiology for their pain, whereas children, adolescents and seniors are more susceptible to developmental, infectious, neoplastic, and inflammatory conditions.

Anticipating which athletes may be at greatest risk for developing a spine injury can assist providers in focusing on prevention through preparticipation evaluation, specific training protocols, rules modification, and protective equipment. Those involved in sports with repetitive hyperextension of the spine (gymnasts, football lineman, dancers) can experience injury to the posterior elements, including facet joint syndrome and stress fractures of the pars interarticularis. Athletes whose sport requires violent trunk rotation (golf, tennis, field events) may suffer disc-related or myofascial injury. Active children and adolescents are vulnerable to stress fractures through the pars interarticularis (traumatic spondylolysis, spondylolisthesis), with seniors susceptible to age-related illnesses that may present as back pain (metastatic disease, osteoporotic fractures, infectious, metabolic, and inflammatory processes). This chapter will focus on the key elements in the evaluation and treatment of back pain in athletes and active individuals and discuss a few specific problems encountered in this population.

TABLE 29.1
DIFFERENTIAL DIAGNOSIS OF LOW BACK PAIN

Structural/Mechanical	**Spondyloarthropathy**
Discogenic	Ankylosing spondylitis
Traumatic (acute, macro, repetitive, micro)	Reiter's syndrome
Fracture	Psoriatic arthritis
Sprain/Strain	Enteropathic arthropathies
Facet syndrome	Scheuermann's disease
Myofascial pain	Diffuse idiopathic skeletal hyperostosis (DISH)
Congenital/developmental	
Scoliosis	
Spondylolysis/spondylolisthesis	
Transitional vertebrae	
Spinal stenosis	
Metabolic Bone Disease	**Infection**
Osteoporosis	Osteomyelitis
Osteomalacia	Discitis
	Epidural abscess
Neoplasia	**Referred Pain**
Benign	Pelvic/Abdominal (kidney, aorta, pancreas, uterus, prostatitis, bowel, lymphatic)
Malignant	

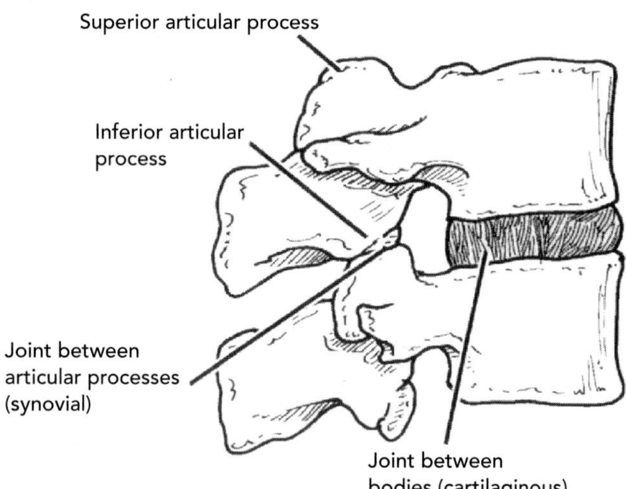

Figure 29.1 Functional unit—spine.

ANATOMY/BIOMECHANICS

Understanding the anatomy and biomechanics of the spine and its related structures is key to understanding patterns of injury and presenting findings in the athlete with back pain. The basic functional unit of the spine consists of two adjacent vertebrae and the interverterbral disc that separates them (see Figure 29.1). This functional unit is the building block for the entire spine, which as a whole can be further subdivided into anterior and posterior elements to gain a better appreciation of the key functional role that each plays.

The vertebrae of the thoracolumbar spine consist of an anteriorly oriented vertebral body, composed of both cortical and cancellous bone, and the posterior elements, which form the vertebral foramen or spinal canal. Posterior elements include the pedicles, lamina (including the pars interarticularis), superior and inferior articular processes, and the transverse and spinous processes. Vertebral body size and weight-bearing capacity increase with progression from the cervical to lumbar spine. Cancellous bone contributes most to the load-bearing capacity of the vertebrae (6). At the superior and inferior surface of each vertebral body is a cartilaginous endplate, which undergoes circumferential ossification to form a ring apophysis. Fibers of the outer intervertebral disc annulus attach to this apophysis, with the avascular nucleus pulposus receiving nourishment through the central endplate, an important factor in understanding certain injury patterns in the developing spine.

The intervertebral discs consist of an outer annulus fibrosis and inner nucleus pulposus. The fibrocartilaginous annulus, slightly thicker anteriorly than posteriorly, consists of a ring of concentrically aligned outer fibers attached to the vertebral endplate. It is composed of 60% to 70% water, which remains relatively constant with age, and receives sensory innervation posteriorly from the sinuvertebral nerves and laterally by branches of the ventral rami and grey rami communicans (7). The nucleus pulposus consists of a hydrophilic, proteoglycan matrix contained by the lamellar annulus, with a water content that approximates 90% in infancy and follows a linear decline into adult life (8). It possesses an inherent internal pressure that provides separation and shock absorption between the adjacent vertebrae. There is no direct blood supply to the nucleus in adults and no direct innervation. The intervertebral discs are susceptible to failure through desiccation associated with the aging process and exposure to acute and repetitive traumatic effects, including compression, rotation, and shear forces.

Posteriorly, the superior articular process of the vertebrae below and the inferior articular process of the vertebrae above join to form a facet joint. This zygapophyseal joint is a paired synovial joint surrounded by a redundant capsule that allows for flexion and extension movement while restricting lateral flexion and rotation. Between the articular processes lies a fibroadipose meniscus, or meniscal equivalent, that is well innervated with proprioceptive and nociceptive fibers. The vertebral arch, formed by the lamina, the pedicles, and posterior aspect of the vertebral body form the vertebral canal, containing the spinal cord. The spinal cord terminates at the level of the first lumbar vertebra, becoming the conus medullaris.

The intervertebral foramen is formed by the pedicles above and below, the intervertebral disc and vertebral body anteriorly, and the lamina and anterior facet joint posteriorly. It contains the associated spinal nerve (see Table 29.2 for level) that occupies approximately 35% to 40% of the area, connective tissue, ligamentum flavum, arteries and veins, lymphatic vessels, and the sinuvertebral nerve. The L1-2 foramen has the largest cross-sectional diameter with L5-S1 having the smallest, while housing the largest nerve root (L5). This creates a level of vulnerability to injury from any relative change in the surrounding structures, such as disc protrusion, facet arthropathy, and local soft tissue swelling and edema.

The spinal nerve roots, carrying motor, sensory, and sympathetic fibers, are enclosed in a dural sheath that provides protection and nourishment to the root. The segmental organization of the spinal elements allows a "pattern" recognition of injury to a given level. Table 29.2 lists the more commonly affected lumbar nerve roots and the associated sensory, motor, and reflex changes. It is important to remember that a given nerve root may cross one to two vertebral levels before exiting the intervertebral foramen and may therefore be affected by pathology at a different level than predicted.

In addition to the elements of the columnar functional units, the static, erect spine is stabilized by a variety of other soft tissue structures, including muscular, ligamentous, and fascial supports. The intact spine consists of four physiological curves, a cervical and lumbar lordosis and thoracic and sacral kyphosis, which provide a spring-like mechanism to absorb shock and improve load bearing. Four muscle groups, the erector spinae, multifidus, intersegmental, and quadratus lumborum, compose the thoracolumbar paraspinal muscle mass. The erector spinae group, the predominant extensors of the lumbar spine, lies lateral to the multifidi, consists of longissimus, iliocostalis, and spinalis groups, and attaches from the pelvis to the thoracic and lumbar spinal elements and ribs. The more medial multifidae originate at the lumbar lamina and spinous processes and attach at the sacrum, acting to extend the spine, rotate to the opposite side, and control deceleration of forceful spinal flexion. The intersegmental muscles, intertransversalis and interspinalis, attach to adjacent transverse and spinous processes, and laterally bend to the ipsilateral side and extend the spine, respectively. The quadratus lumborum, a powerful lateral trunk flexor, attaches to the 12th rib, iliac crest, and transverse processes of the lumbar vertebrae.

In addition, various other muscle groups exert effects on the thoracolumbar spine, and include the glutei, hamstrings, quadriceps, latissimus dorsi, iliopsoas, and the anterior abdominals—rectus abdominus and abdominal obliques. Further support is provided by the thoracolumbar fascia that encloses the erector spinae and quadratus lumborum muscles. Additional stability is afforded by the ligaments acting on the bony spine, including the ligamentum flavum, supraspinatus ligament, interspinous ligament, and the anterior and posterior longitudinal ligament (see Figure 29.2).

Coordinating the various structural elements of the spine to produce a functional outcome is a complex, highly integrated system of neurophysiological and biomechanical processes. A three-system theory, consisting of neural, passive, and active components, has been proposed to help explain this complex interaction (9). The neural component initiates the precise movement and coordinates all motion factors. The passive component consists of the static structures discussed previously, including discs, facet joints and capsules, and ligaments. The active component

TABLE 29.2
LUMBAR NERVE ROOTS AND ASSOCIATED SENSORY, MOTOR, AND REFLEX DISTRIBUTION

Root Level	Most Common Disc	Sensory	Motor	Reflex
L3	L2-3	Buttock Lower anterior thigh Medial lower leg	Hip Flexor Psoas muscle, quadriceps	Patellar
L4	L3-4	Lateral thigh/knee Anterior leg Dorsal foot, great toe	Leg extension Foot dorsiflexion	Patellar
L5	L4-5	Posterior thigh Lateral thigh Dorsum foot	Ankle dorsiflexors Great toe (ehl)	Medial hamstring Posterior tibial
S1	L5-S1	Post thigh Lateral leg Lateral/plantar foot	Leg flexion Ankle plantarflexion	Achilles

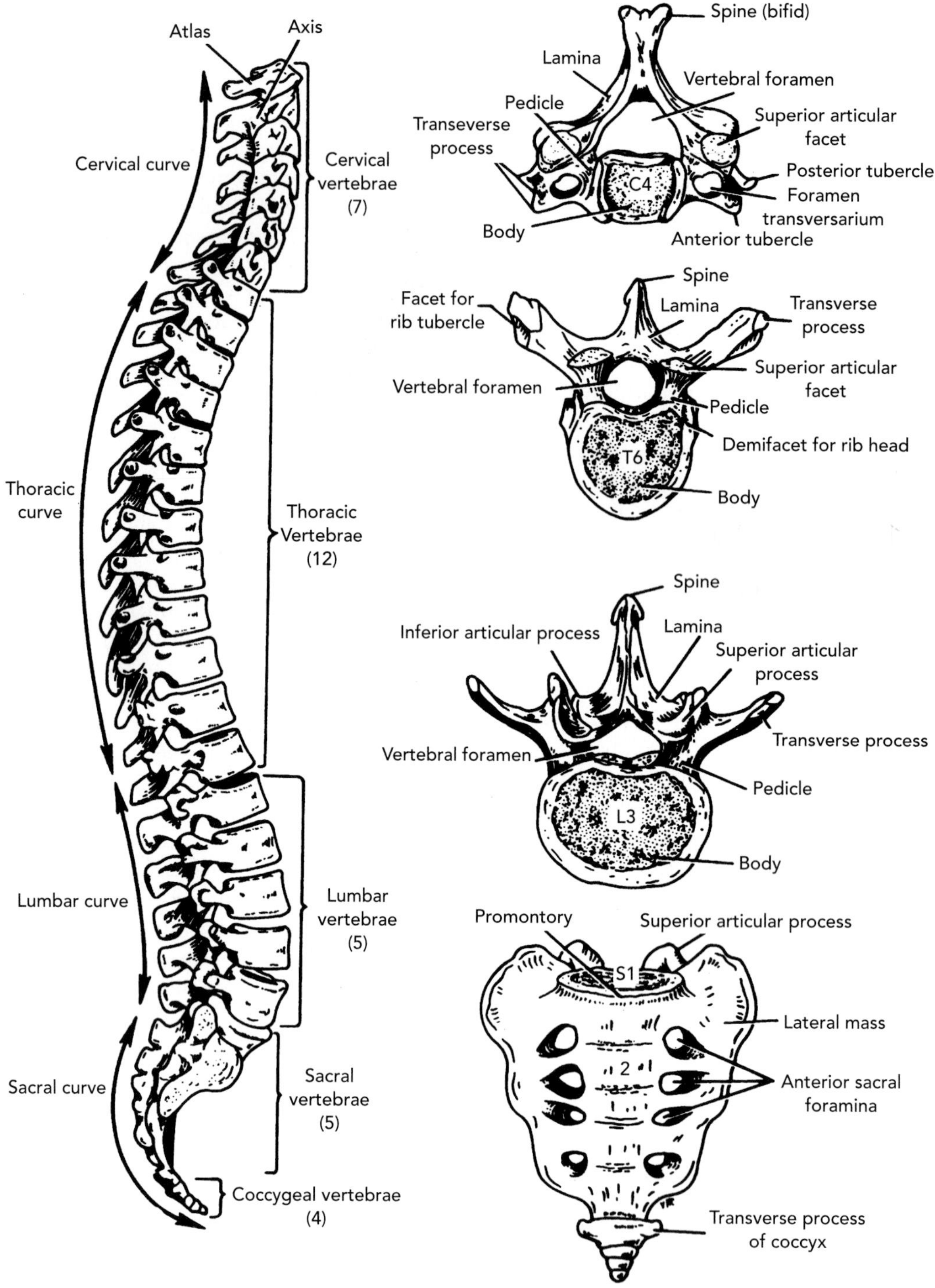

Figure 29.2 Lumbar myofascial anatomy: (A) osseous and ligamentous structures, (B) myofascial anatomy.

includes the various muscles and ligaments acting on the passive structures. The effective interaction of the three components constitutes the kinetic or dynamic spine. Any breakdown in the function of one or more components can produce a mechanical irritation that triggers a pain response and altered function.

Pain is generated when nociceptive fibers are stimulated by mechanical or chemical means. A number of structures in the back possess such fibers and are therefore potential pain generators. These include the disc annulus, anterior and posterior longitudinal ligaments, facet joint capsule, and various other muscular and other ligamentous groups. Trauma, either micro or macro, activates a cascade of events leading to the release of the chemical mediators of pain, including bradykinins, prostaglandins, leukotrienes, and histamines. In addition, there are psychosocial factors that

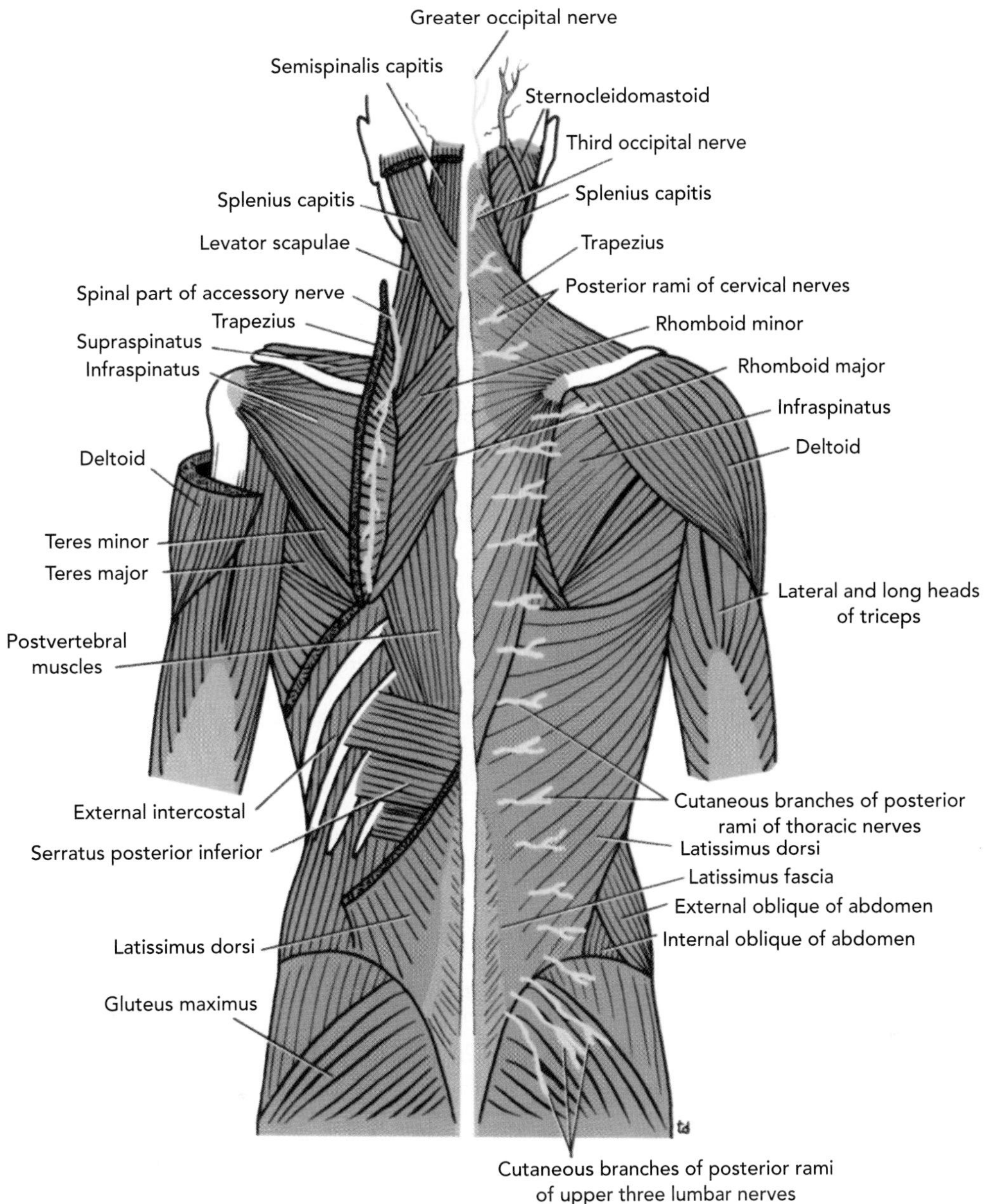

Figure 29.2 *(continued)*

impact an individual's subjective pain experience and may play a significant role in the athlete with back pain.

APPROACH TO DIAGNOSIS

A directed history and physical examination, cognizant of key elements needed to rule in or out specific disorders, is key to developing an accurate differential diagnosis and selecting appropriate further diagnostics and treatment interventions. The AHRQ guidelines for acute low back problems in adults provides a useful starting point for developing an initial approach to the athlete with LBP, recognizing the limitations inherent in the guideline, including age restriction and chronicity.

History

Important demographical factors include athlete's age, sex, sport and position played, skill level, vocation, and other recreational or training activities that may be relevant to their presenting complaint. In evaluating the complaint of back pain, it is imperative to gather information on its onset, duration, nature, location, and severity, as well as any palliative or provocative factors that relate to the pain. Understanding a specific mechanism of injury can target the likely structures injured. Any history of previous back pain episodes and earlier or current interventions is also helpful in establishing a chronic or recurrent pattern of injury and success of treatment. Past medical and surgical history, tobacco and alcohol use, and family history may reveal clues helpful in assessing the current pain. One of the key aspects of gathering history in acute LBP is the ability to begin differentiating axial back pain from back pain associated with leg pain, an important step in developing an accurate differential diagnosis. Table 29.3 lists various potential etiologies for LBP and associated key features or symptoms.

Key "red flag" historical factors include the presence of fever, chills, night pain and other constitutional symptoms, a history of cancer, recent urinary tract infection, intravenous drug use, age over 50 or under 20 (infection, tumor), saddle anesthesia, recent onset bladder or bowel dysfunction, severe or progressive neurological deficit in the lower extremity (cauda equina syndrome), and major trauma such as motor vehicle accident (MVA) or fall or minor trauma in an osteoporotic individual (fracture) (4). The presence of such factors should warrant timely investigation aimed at ruling out the listed underlying etiology (see Table 29.4).

TABLE 29.3
POTENTIAL PAIN SYNDROMES AND THEIR ASSOCIATED SYMPTOMS

Syndrome	Key Features/Symptoms
Myofascial pain	Exacerbated by activity Relieved by rest Gradual onset, periods of intensity Localized to low back
Discogenic pain	Worse with prolonged sitting/standing Often radicular pain, parasthesias Intermittent, often incapacitating pain Aggravated by Valsalva (cough, sneeze)
Neoplastic/ infectious	Night pain or supine pain Fever, chills, night sweats, wt loss Recent urinary tract infection, IV drug use, immunocompromise Constant, unremitting pain
Spondylytic	Adolescent onset History of extension mechanism of injury Localized, often unilateral pain Exacerbated by extension
Cauda equina	1%–2% of disc herniations Usually above L4 Bilateral radicular symptoms, weakness Back/perianal pain Onset impotence, urinary frequency, incontinence, more commonly retention Decrease anal sphincter tone. Saddle anesthesia
Neurogenic claudication	Vague leg pain with ambulation ±back pain Symptoms progress proximal to distal Pain in anterior/posterior thighs and calves Intact pulses Worse with postures that decrease spinal canal diameter (extension) Improved with rest, flexion

TABLE 29.4
RED FLAG SIGNS AND SYMPTOMS

Sign/Symptom	Diagnostic Consideration
Recent significant trauma	Fracture
Mild trauma w/age >50 yr	Acute disc herniation
Unexplained weight loss	Neoplasm
Unrelenting night pain or pain at rest	
History of cancer	
Pain with distal numbness	Disc herniation with radiculopathy
Leg weakness	
Loss of bowel or bladder control (retention or incontinence)	Cauda equina Large disc herniation
Unexplained fever (38°C or 110.4°F >48 hr)	Infection
Hx recent or remote IV drug use	
Prolonged use of corticosteroids	
Osteoporosis	Compression fracture

A nutritional history may be of value, particularly in the young, female athlete. Decreased caloric intake can be associated with decreased calcium stores and place the adolescent female at risk for osteopenia and stress fractures (pars interarticularis, sacrum) (10,11). Surveying for recent growth spurts in the young athlete may also be of diagnostic value. Athletes should be questioned regarding the use of assistive devices, both for management of back symptoms as well as those used for other purposes as they may impact spine mechanics. The use of patient- or parent-completed questionnaires and pain diagrams can be helpful in gathering historical data and understanding the athlete's reaction to their symptoms.

Physical Examination

The physical examination of the athlete with back pain should be systematic and driven by historical findings. An overall assessment of the athlete's appearance, including posture, facial expression, and position when encountered (sitting, standing, supine), is a key step in understanding the severity of pain and degree of disability. Observing gait, sit-to-stand, ease of movement, and ability to perform active and sport-specific tasks provide further clues as to the level of functional impairment. Inspection continues with the evaluation of the physiological curves and normal landmarks, evidence of muscle atrophy, and asymmetry of posture, both static and active. Range of motion should be assessed in flexion, extension, lateral flexion or sidebending, and rotation. Although there is variability in lumbar spine range of motion for the lumbar spine, typical ranges include flexion of 40 to 60 degrees, extension of 20 to 35 degrees, lateral flexion of 15 to 20 degrees, and rotation of 3 to 18 degrees (12). Schober's Test, a method of assessing the amount of flexion in the lumbar spine, measures the difference between three static points in neutral and forward flexion, the difference being the amount of lumbar flexion. Normal flexion is reflected by greater than a 5 cm increase, with movement less than 5 cm suggestive of decreased lumbar range of motion (see Figure 29.3).

Palpation should include the accessible bony structures and landmarks of the spine and pelvis, including individual spinous and transverse processes, posterior ribs, sciatic notches, greater trochanters, sacroiliac joints, and iliac crests and spines. The relevant muscle groups of the spine (erector spinae, thoracolumbar fascia, and quadratus lumborum) as well as the gluteals, piriformis, abdominal wall, and hip flexors should be evaluated for tender spots, tone, and general character. A thorough abdominal and genitourinary examination should be included as indicated. Skin color, temperature, and texture of the low back and lower extremity may reveal changes reflecting an infectious or inflammatory process. The One-leg Standing Lumbar Extension Test (Stork Test) places a stress on the posterior elements and may cause pain in the athlete with a pars interarticularis defect or facet joint arthropathy (see Figure 29.4).

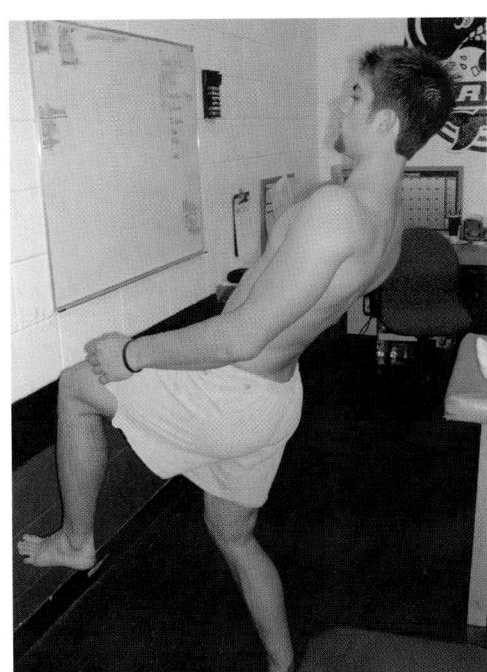

Figure 29.4 Stork test.

A neurological assessment should include strength testing of myotomal muscle groups using manual muscle testing and functional assessments, such as heel and toe raises and walking, squats, and sit-to-stand. Sensory testing, including light touch and pin-prick evaluation, and reflex testing of hamstring, patellar and Achilles reflexes, can aid

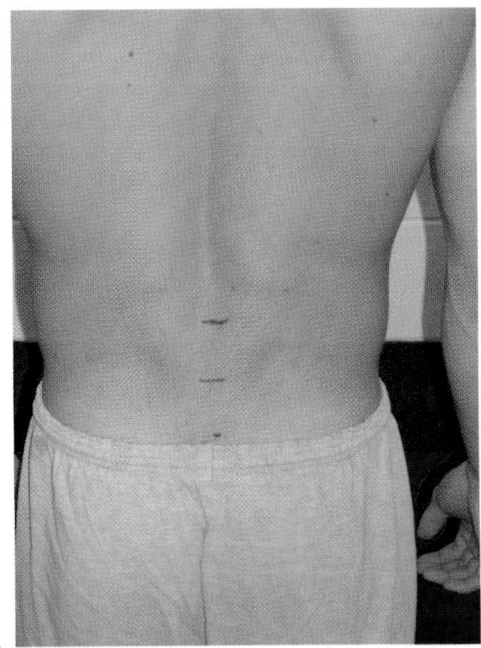

A

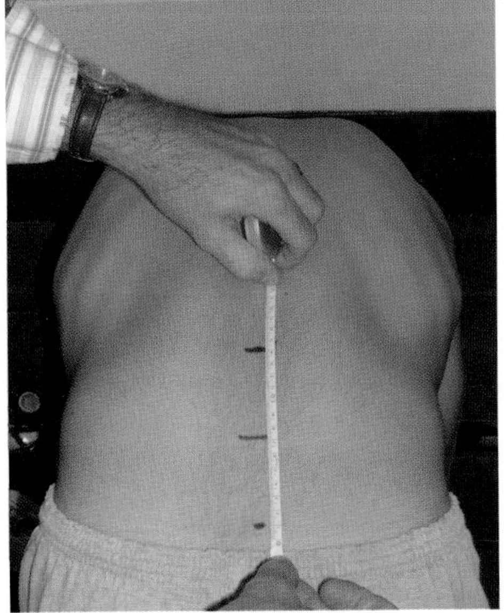

B

Figure 29.3 Schober's test.

in the identification of radicular patterns of injury. Straight leg raise (SLR) testing (Lasegue's Test), performed passively on a supine, relaxed patient, is generally considered positive with re-creation of radicular pain down the leg being tested, between 30 to 70 degrees of hip flexion. This is confirmed by including dorsiflexion of the ankle (Braggard's Test) or neck flexion (Brudzinski's sign). Back pain during testing does not constitute a positive SLR. If pain occurs beyond 70 degrees of hip flexion, the etiology of pain may be hamstring pathology or lumbosacral or sacroiliac joint dysfunction. Positive cross-over testing (Lhermitt's Test) of the asymptomatic side is typically associated with a large lumbar disc herniation. Babinski testing should be included to rule out upper motor neuron lesions. Simple log rolling, hip scour, or Flexion, ABduction, and External Rotation (FABER) testing of the hip are useful in helping to identify potential hip pathology in the patient with back pain.

In addition to range of motion testing, further functional testing of the lumbar spine, including trunk strength and lifting capacity, is available. Isokinetic testing devices are available in select settings and can provide objective measurement of an athlete's trunk strength and range of motion. Further study is needed to determine the relationship between these measures and a patient's subjective experience of pain and normal muscle function in athletic and daily activities. Its use in the athletic population is limited to specific situations at this time.

Diagnostics

The use of further diagnostics, beyond the history and physical examination, is driven by the presence of suspicious signs and symptoms suggestive of a potentially serious underlying condition. Most adult athletes, lacking such "red flag" findings (see Table 29.4), are not likely to need routine testing in the first 4 weeks of management of their acute back pain symptoms. Alternatively, those athletes considered high risk based on initial assessment may require one or more further diagnostic studies. To aid the clinician in this decision making, the American College of Radiology has developed appropriateness criteria for imaging patients with LBP (13).

Plain film radiographs, including standing anteroposterior (AP), lateral and oblique views, are typically obtained to evaluate bony structures of the spine and derive any indirect evidence of associated disease. Knowledge of normal bony anatomy on each view is essential to recognize subtle changes such as vertebral wedging or compression (fracture) (see Figure 29.5), loss of disc space height (disc disease), pars defect or "scotty dog" sign (spondylolysis) (see Figure 29.6), osteophyte formation (degenerative disease) (see Figure 29.7), spina bifida occulta (6–10% of the population) (see Figure 29.8), and intervertebral foramina changes. Flexion–extension views may be added to evaluate for instability, while a pelvis study can reveal hip joint pathology presenting as back pain.

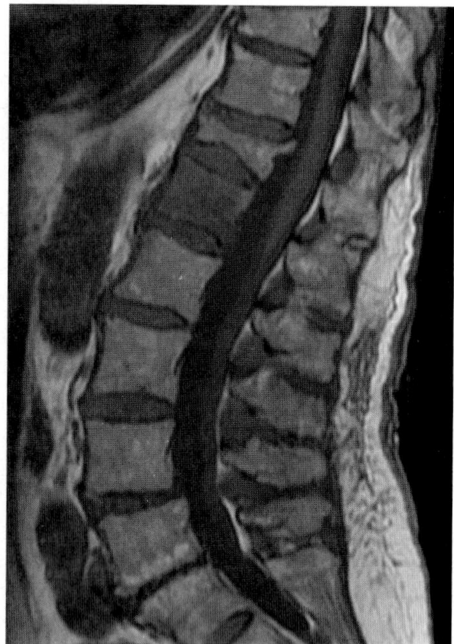

Figure 29.5 Vertebral compression fracture.

Computed tomographic (CT) scanning provides better bony detail than plain film radiography, although less soft tissue detail thanmagnetic resonance imaging (MRI). It is most helpful in delineating bony pathology including vertebral, facet joint, sacroiliac joint, and pars pathology. When performed with myelography, it provides a more accurate assessment of disc disease, although this role has generally been replaced by MRI.

MRI is more expensive than CT, but provides significantly better soft tissue evaluation. In the assessment of back pain, it is often used for preinjection or presurgical evaluation, or for evaluating suspicious findings from other studies. Claustrophobia may require sedation to obtain an accurate study. As with any imaging, correlation of the findings from the study must be done with the patient's clinical presentation. Studies have shown that patients without symptomatic complaints of back pain may have abnormalities on imaging of their lumbar spine, including disc bulging, protrusion, extrusion, facet arthropathy, and disc annulus defects (14). It is important to realize that these asymptomatic abnormalities increase with age, and should be a reminder that MRI is a part of the diagnostic algorithm but should not be relied upon solely for diagnosis and treatment.

Bone scanning provides a noninvasive means of assessing bone function and metabolism. It is useful in the evaluation of athletes suspected of having a metastatic, infectious (septic arthritis), traumatic (stress fracture), or metabolic (primary hyperparathyroidism, renal osteodystrophy, osteomalacia) etiology for their symptoms. Adding single photon emission computed tomography (SPECT) to bone scanning improves diagnostic accuracy in evaluating for stress injuries such as spondylolysis (see Figure 29.9).

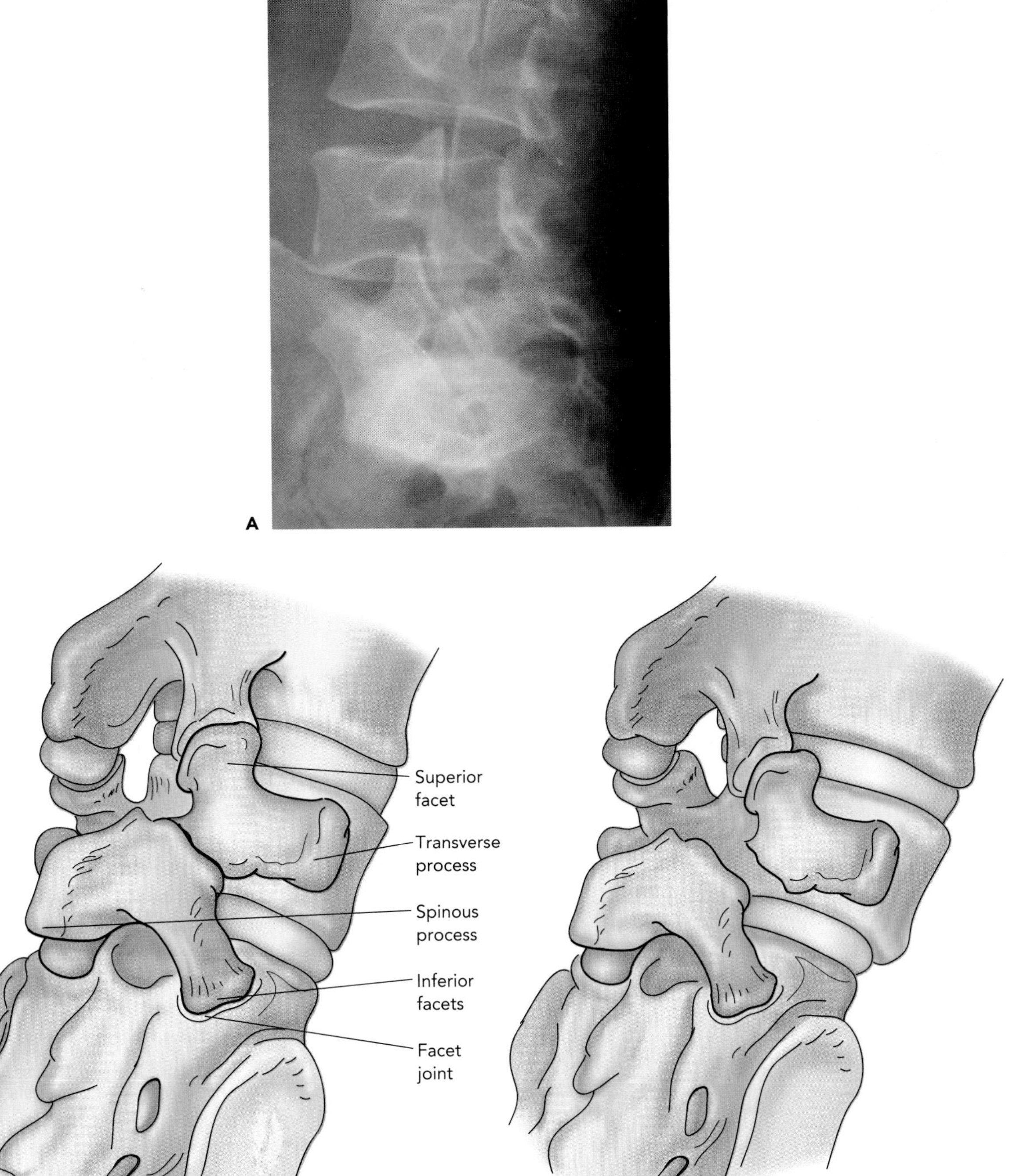

Figure 29.6 Scotty dog sign: (A) oblique view showing defect through pars interarticularis, (B) illustration of anatomic defect.

Bone densitometry may be indicated in the evaluation of the senior athlete or adolescent female suspected of having an underlying osteoporosis complicating their injury.

Employing other nonimaging diagnostic modalities may be indicated in the evaluation of back pain. The complete blood count (CBC) with differential and erythrocyte sedimentation rate (ESR) are useful in identifying infectious and inflammatory conditions. Additional chemistries and immunological testing (human leukocyte antigen [HLA] typing, rheumatoid factor) are obtained based on clinical suspicion. Electromyelogram (EMG) and nerve conduction studies (NCS) serve as an extension of the clinical

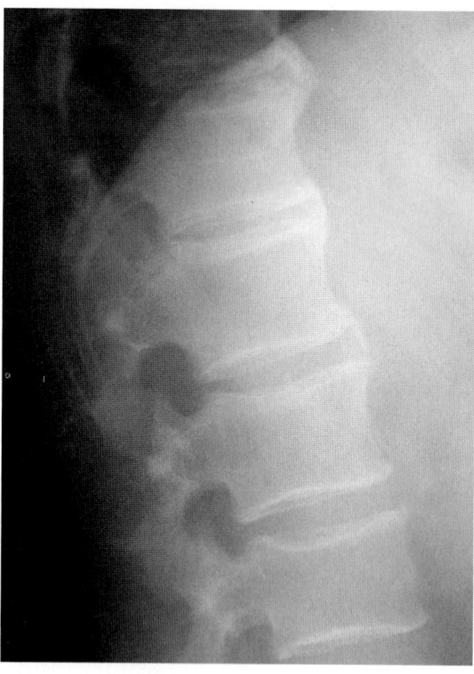

Figure 29.7 Osteophyte formation—anterior vertebral osteophyte bridging on lateral view.

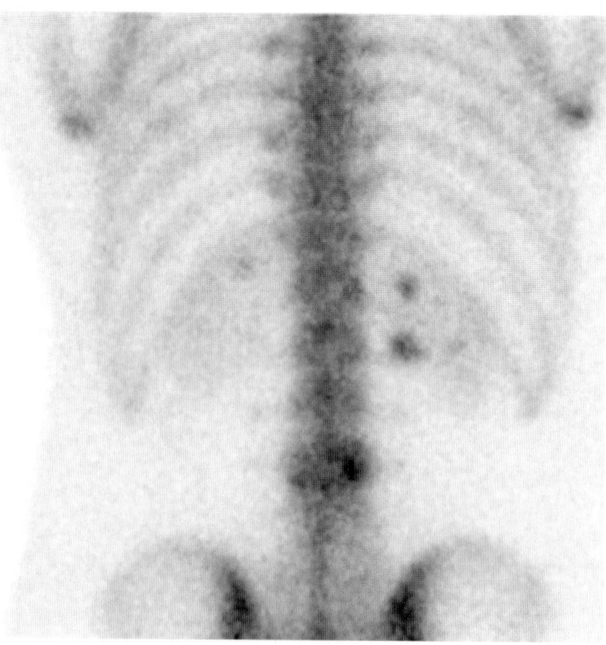

Figure 29.9 Bone scan with single photon emission computed tomography (SPECT) demonstrating pars defect.

neurological examination and provide a means of objectively documenting muscle and nerve damage. Timing of the study is important in that electrophysiological signs of damage may not be evident for 2 to 3 weeks after the initial injury. Biopsy of suspicious lesions identified on imaging or examination may be required to obtain tissue diagnosis.

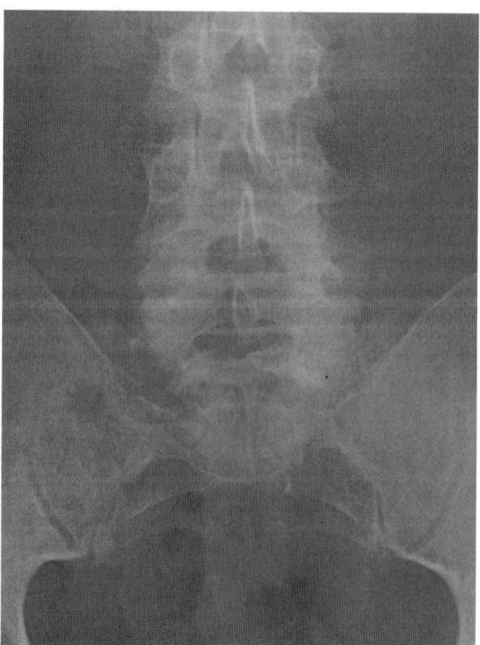

Figure 29.8 Spina bifida occulta.

SPECIFIC DISORDERS

Myofascial Strain

It has been estimated that 30% of athletes will experience acute LBP at some point, directly related to their activity, and most often due to a soft tissue injury (15,16). Although clearly the most common cause of back pain presenting in the adult population, it is prudent to consider myofascial strain a diagnosis of exclusion made only after ruling out more potentially serious etiologies. This is most easily achieved through a thorough history and physical examination and use of select diagnostic tests. In the case of myofascial strain, a mechanism of repetitive overload or acute, traumatic event may be identified as causative. There is typically localized, persistent, aching back pain, short in duration, and related to the inciting event. It may radiate to the buttock or posterior thigh, not usually more distal. Mobility is limited in all directions and spasms may be debilitating. Symptoms are relieved in the recumbent position, with hips and knees flexed providing the most comfort. Radicular symptoms are uncommon, the neurological examination is normal, and plain films are rarely of use in establishing the diagnosis.

Treatment of myofascial strain is directed at decreasing pain while maintaining mobility, strength, and aerobic conditioning. Prolonged bed rest is to be avoided, as it has not been shown to improve outcomes and is associated with deconditioning. Instead, relative rest through activity modification (avoiding those movements that aggravate symptoms) is combined with local cold application and selective use of analgesic medications, including nonsteroidal anti-inflammatory medications.

Gentle, pain-free stretching exercises are started as tolerated, with progressive range of motion, strengthening, and spine stabilizing exercises initiated as pain improves. Use of local heat may be of benefit in the subacute phase. Physical therapy modalities and chiropractic treatment may provide short-term relief, but do not impact long-term outcomes. Trigger point injection, in the appropriate setting, may help reduce acute pain symptoms and facilitate progression with therapeutic activities. Return-to-play decisions are supported by demonstration of painless range of motion and sport-specific task performance, normal strength, and lack of development of any other suspicious signs or symptoms.

Recovery from myofascial strains is highly variable, lasting from a few days to 6 to 8 weeks. Athletes with pain lasting longer than 6 weeks and a working diagnosis of myofascial strain should be re-evaluated for another etiology. Recurrence rates are high and warrant a thorough assessment of the athlete for predisposing factors. Risk factors for lumbar myofascial strain include sport and position played, past history of back injury, flexibility and strength deficits, poor aerobic conditioning, leg length discrepancies and other biomechanical abnormalities, and improper technique. Prevention should be emphasized by addressing risk factors in a preseason program, or before return to play.

Facet syndrome is a diagnostic consideration in the athlete with LBP. It is typically the result of repetitive hyperextension activity and presents with pain that is localized to the lateral structures, worse with hyperextension and movement, and relieved with rest. The neurological examination is normal, x-ray may show degenerative changes of the facet joints, and therapeutic exercises are designed to avoid hyperextension in the acute and subacute phase. In the adolescent athlete, back pain associated with hyperextension should prompt an evaluation for spondylolysis.

Sacroiliac joint dysfunction (SIJD) is another potential cause of mechanical LBP that should be considered in the athletic population, particularly in certain higher incidence sports, such as rowing and cross country skiing (17). Affected athletes often present with pain in the area of the sacroiliac (SI) joint, which is often unilateral, dull in nature, and radiating to the buttock, posterior thigh, or groin. Examination should include observation of the athlete both statically and dynamically, with attention to asymmetries and restricted motion segments. Restrictions in forward flexion of the lumbosacral spine, asymmetric tight hamstrings, unilateral restriction of pelvic mobility, and functional leg lengths may be noted. In addition to more traditional modalities, such as ice, heat, and anti-inflammatory agents, physical therapeutic interventions aimed at correcting biomechanical restrictions may be of benefit. Osteopathic manipulative therapy can be particularly useful at helping to address the athlete with SIJD.

Lumbar Disc Disease

LBP may be the common end point of distinctly separate pathological conditions involving the intervertebral disc. A tear in the annulus fibrosis, usually secondary to age-related desiccation, may result from repetitive microtrauma or acute macrotrauma. Herniation of the nucleus pulposus through the annulus may also occur, producing pain and associated radicular symptoms. Herniated nucleus pulposus (HNP) is most common in the third and fourth decade, with most herniations occurring at the L5-S1 level, followed by L4-L5 in terms of frequency. It is important for the clinician to differentiate localized LBP, from that associated with leg pain, and recognize that some athletes with HNP may present with radicular signs and symptoms only, without LBP. Athletes with lumbar disc disease and radiculopathy typically present with sharp, shooting, or burning pain radiating to the lower extremity, often associated with paresthesias and involving the lower extremity. Symptoms may be insidious or sudden in onset, often related to a specific inciting event. Pain is often worse with trunk flexion, Valsalva maneuvers (cough, sneeze, straining), or prolonged sitting (driving), and improved in extension. The athlete typically presents with an antalgic gait, unilateral lumbar paraspinal tenderness, a lateral shift away from the side of the pain, and spasm, and when radiculopathy is present, positive SLR test, weakness, and with myelopathy asymmetric reflexes based on the nerve root affected (see Table 29.2).

Decisions to image the athlete with suspected lumbar disc disease follow the same principles discussed in the preceding text. Plain film radiographs, although generally negative in this setting, may show decreased disc space height or vertebral end-plate changes suggestive of disc disease. CT scanning and MRI may be indicated in select populations to rule out other causes of pain, with MRI of value in presurgical planning of those athletes with lumbar disc disease and clinical indications for operative intervention. Electrodiagnostic studies may be beneficial in clarifying specific radicular patterns in situations where the clinical findings and imaging studies are less than definitive and where surgical intervention may be considered. They should not be performed earlier than 2 to 3 weeks from the onset of symptoms, as electrodiagnostic findings may not be evident early on in the disease process.

Conservative treatment of acute lumbar disc herniation follows much the same principles as discussed for myofascial strain. Anti-inflammatory pain medications, relative rest, activity modification, gentle stretching, ice, and in some cases, use of narcotic analgesics are indicated in the management of acute symptoms. A brief period of bed rest (<48 hours) may be indicated in athletes incapacitated by their symptoms. Some clinicians employ short courses of oral corticosteroids for relief of neuropathic pain characteristic of acute radiculopathy. Specific physical therapy protocols (McKenzie extensions) and modalities are initiated as the athlete's pain symptoms warrant. The athlete who develops increasing pain with McKenzie extension exercises and relief with Williams flexion exercise suggests a mechanical etiology to pain. Radicular symptoms refractory to this initial intervention may benefit in the short term from a trial of epidural steroid injections or selective nerve root blocks. Bilateral radicular leg symptoms, progressive pain and/or neurological deficits, or refractory symptoms (LBP with radiculopathy) after 4 to 6 weeks of conservative intervention for acute lumbar disc herniation warrants further evaluation for possible surgical intervention. Bowel or bladder symptoms, specifically loss of control or acute urinary retention, suggests acute cauda equina syndrome, and requires urgent surgical evaluation as delay in intervention beyond 24 hours significantly worsens recovery. Return-to-play decisions are supported by demonstration of normal neurological examination, full range of lumbosacral motion, correction of strength and flexibility deficits, and the ability to perform sport-specific skills without pain.

Cauda equina syndrome, resulting from a large central disc herniation and producing central cord compression, often presents with LBP, bilateral lower extremity pain, paresthesias, or weakness, and bowel or bladder dysfunction. Clinical suspicion for this entity should prompt urgent referral for possible surgical decompression. Spinal stenosis of the lumbar spine, either congenital or acquired, frequently presents with activity-related unilateral or bilateral buttock, thigh, or leg pain, worsens with standing or walking, and is relieved by rest and flexion. Nerve tension tests are usually negative at rest. This pseudoclaudication occurs in the setting of adequate vascular supply and, when recognized, warrants further imaging with MRI to confirm the diagnosis. Standing lateral radiographs are important, as the supine positioning in the MRI may dramatically underestimate the degree of degenerative spondylolisthesis, which can cause further significant canal narrowing. In the setting of a stable neurological examination, spinal stenosis is managed conservatively with close observation for evidence of progression.

Spondylolysis/Spondylolisthesis

Diagnostic considerations for the athlete with LBP vary significantly based on age. Young athletes, in whom an estimated 10% to 15% will experience a back injury (18), have a higher incidence of injuries to the pars interarticularis compared with adults, who more often present with a myofascial or discogenic cause for their pain (19). Chief among the potential causes of back pain in the adolescent athlete is spondylolysis, a stress-related injury to the ossification center on each side of the neural arch, the pars interarticularis. Its incidence is more common in sports and positions characterized by repetitive hyperextension, with a suspected familial association (20). When bilateral pars defects occur at a given vertebral level, the adjacent vertebrae are vulnerable to forward slippage of one vertebra over another, or spondylolisthesis (see Figure 29.10). Depending on the degree of slippage, the typical back pain symptoms may be accompanied by those of spinal stenosis or neurological impingement.

The adolescent athlete with extension-aggravated LBP should be suspected of having spondylolysis until proved

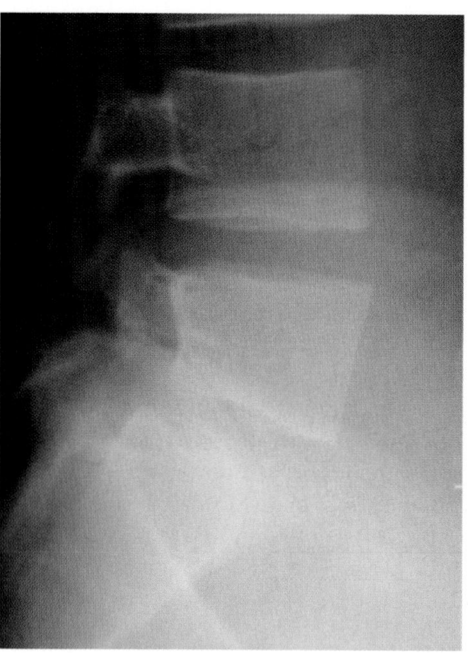

Figure 29.10 Spondylolisthesis L5-S1.

otherwise. Typical presenting symptoms include the gradual onset of unilateral, nonradicular LBP, worsening with trunk extension and/or rotation, and relieving with rest. With progression, pain may become constant with activity, present at rest, and quite disabling. The history of participation in a high-risk sport or position, such as gymnastics, figure skating, or football lineman, should raise further suspicion for the presence of a spondylitic defect. Physical examination findings may include focal spinal tenderness, limited lumbosacral range of motion, hamstring inflexibility, a positive stork test, a palpable step-off at a given spinal level, and a wide-based, short-stride gait.

Imaging studies are indicated in the evaluation of the adolescent with LBP and typically begin with plain film radiographs, to include at least an AP and lateral view. Standing studies, with flexion–extension views, may be needed to demonstrate subtle degrees of slip or segmental instability. Depending on the clinician, clinical situation, and concerns regarding ionizing radiation exposure, oblique studies may be of benefit in demonstrating the spondylitic defect. If not evident on initial radiographs and in the presence of high clinical suspicion, bone scan with SPECT can be obtained to improve detection and localize lesions (21). It is important to be aware that 6% of the normal nonpainful population will have radiographic evidence of a spondylolytic defect, so that the mere presence of radiographic defects does not prove that the lesion is the source of the patient's pain. Confirmation with SPECT or MRI is often needed. On the basis of the results of the SPECT bone scan, further diagnosis and treatment can be determined. Scans indicating focal uptake are followed by CT scanning to confirm the presence of fracture and determine the need for bracing. Diffuse uptake indicates a stress reaction and can be managed expectantly (22). An algorithm to assist the clinician in the rational management of back pain in the child and adolescent athlete has been developed (23). Using lumbar radiographs and bone scan with SPECT results, athletes are stratified into either acute or progressive pars defects or terminal pars defects, and prescribed a stepwise treatment plan progressing over a 2- to 7-month period.

Spondylolisthesis is generally diagnosed on the lateral plain film view and classified using the Meyerding system: grade I (0–25%), grade II (25–50%), grade III (50–75%), grade IV (>75%). However, it is preferable to classify these injuries as a simple percentage slip (24), allowing for a more precise method of monitoring slip progression than the Meyerding system. Athletes appear to be at a lower risk for progression of their spondylolisthesis (25). Spondylolisthesis may progress rapidly during the adolescent growth spurt, so immature athletes should be monitored carefully.

Treatment of the athlete with symptomatic spondylolysis is based on the results of the imaging studies that help predict the likelihood of healing of the defect. In the acute phase, athletic participation is restricted, pain management measures implemented, antilordotic bracing considered, and physical therapy initiated. Although bracing may be helpful in managing the athlete with pain that is refractory to initial management, no studies have definitively shown improved long-term outcomes of spondylolysis management as compared to non-bracing (23). If bracing is initiated, specific protocols have been devised to assist the clinician in management (22,23). Bracing at 0 degrees of extension is initiated, in conjunction with physical therapy, and continued for 4 months. At that time, limited CT scanning is repeated to establish evidence of healing and weaning begun if healing demonstrated. Physical therapy is directed at improving flexibility and lumbar stabilization, while avoiding hyperextension activity.

Athletes may be eligible for return to play when they are pain free with full range of trunk motion and have progressed rehabilitation to being pain free with sport-specific activity. It should be noted that not all pars defects will demonstrate radiographic healing and that a pars nonunion does not disqualify an athlete from returning to play. Those athletes with diffuse uptake on bone scan consistent with a stress reaction or grade I spondylolisthesis follow a modified protocol with consideration of limited bracing and return to play when pain free. Any adolescent athlete with a symptomatic pars fracture refractory to conservative treatment after 9 to 12 months or spondylolisthesis greater than 50% warrants evaluation for possible surgical intervention.

Scheuermann's Disease and Atypical Scheuermann's

Adolescent athletes with thoracic or lumbar back pain aggravated by repetitive trunk flexion should be evaluated for the presence of Scheuermann's disease. Diagnostic criteria for the "classic" thoracic variant include the radiographic presence of anterior vertebral wedging of at least 5 degrees for each of three consecutive vertebrae (see Figure 29.11). Additional diagnostic signs include vertebral end-plate changes, the presence of Schmorl's nodes, and disc space narrowing (26). A Schmorl's node, recognized on lateral radiographs as an end-plate depression of 3 mm or more, represents the loss of nuclear material through the growth plate and end plate and into the vertebral body. Anterior or marginal Schmorl's nodes represent loss of material through the annulus fibrosis. Blumenthal et al. (27) have proposed a classification system that may provide the clinician with a useful system for approaching this entity (see Table 29.5).

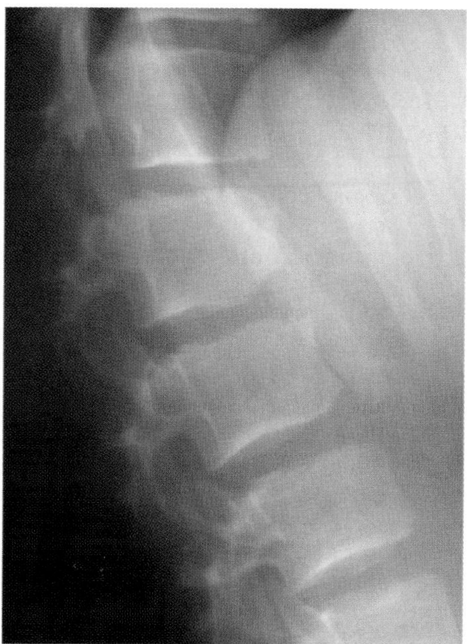

Figure 29.11 Scheuermann's anterior wedging.

High-risk sports for developing Scheuermann's disease include diving, gymnastics, wrestling, and butterfly swimming. In addition to back pain, which is often disabling and aggravated by forward flexion, these athletes tend to present with a "flat back" (thoracic hypokyphosis and lumbar hypolordosis) and thoracolumbar and hamstring tightness (28). Treatment consists of relative rest, activity modification to avoid the offending movement, and physical therapy aimed at spine stabilization, exercises, and flexibility training. Hyperextension bracing (15–30 degrees) may be required. With timely treatment, the athlete may be asymptomatic within 4 to 6 weeks, and return to play considered when the athlete is pain free with sport-specific activity and able to demonstrate improvement in biomechanical deficits, usually in 3 to 6 months.

Scoliosis

Clinicians caring for child and adolescent populations will inevitably encounter the athlete with scoliosis or the parent

TABLE 29.5
SCHEUERMANN'S DISEASE CLINICAL CLASSIFICATION

Type I	"Classic" Scheuermann's—3 or more consecutive vertebra each wedged 5 degrees or more
Type IIa	"Atypical" Scheuermann's—vertebral end-plate irregularities Anterior Schmorl's nodes Disc space narrowing
Type IIb	Acute traumatic intraosseous disc herniation—History of acute vertical compression injury resulting in severe back pain and evidence of end-plate fracture (anterior Schmorl's node)

Source: From: Greenan TL. Diagnostic imaging of sports-related spinal disorders. *Clin Sports Med* 1993;12(3):487–505.

concerned about its presence. Adults with the remnants of childhood idiopathic scoliosis may present for recommendations on managing back pain symptoms, or counseling about starting an exercise program. Defined as an abnormal lateral curvature of the spine, scoliosis is typically classified as idiopathic or secondary to either a congenital or other condition (spasm, tumor, infection). Although the U.S. Preventive Services Task Force (USPSTF) recommends against the screening of asymptomatic adolescents for idiopathic scoliosis (29), it is still commonly performed in many preschool and preparticipation examinations. Developing a consistent approach to the evaluation and management of the athlete with scoliosis is key.

Initial classification of the athlete with scoliosis will include consideration of their age, assessment of skeletal maturity, type of curve, and chosen sport or activity. Idiopathic scoliosis in the childhood population, either juvenile (3–10 years of age) or adolescent (10 years to skeletal maturity), tends to be more common in women, is typically non-painful, and should not alone be a contraindication to participation in sports or physical activity. Detailed history and physical examination to rule out other causes of scoliosis (infection, tumor, disc herniation, spondylolysis, syringomyelia, or tethered cord) should be performed in every case. There is no evidence to suggest that sports participation is a causative factor for idiopathic scoliosis. However, the repetitive movements inherent in some sports may lead to the development of a functional scoliosis, which should be considered in the initial evaluation of the athlete with an abnormal spinal curve.

Curves up to 25 degrees are generally managed with observation and repeat x-ray in 4 to 6 months to monitor for progression. Scoliotic curves in idiopathic, skeletally immature cases ranging from 25 to 40 degrees may benefit from bracing (Milwaukee, Boston) and warrant evaluation by a pediatric spinal surgeon for monitoring. Skeletally immature athletes with curves greater than 40 degrees, or the skeletally mature with curves greater than 50 degrees should be assessed for possible surgical intervention (30,31). Therapeutic exercise may be of benefit to the patient with idiopathic scoliosis and should be considered an adjunct treatment, but not expected to correct or improve the degree of curve in idiopathic scoliosis. Decisions regarding participation in select sports in the face of idiopathic scoliosis requiring bracing should be made on an individual basis. More severe degrees of curve in both the adolescent and adult population may compromise respiratory function and should be considered when making recommendations for participation. Patients with scoliosis treated surgically require special consideration and consultation, given the change in spine mechanics, rotational forces generated in certain sports (volleyball, gymnastics), and the subsequent risk for injury.

Fractures

The differential diagnosis for thoracolumbar back pain in the athletic population should include acute, traumatic fractures. The forces required to sustain a fracture of the thoracic or lumbar vertebrae, in the absence of an underlying pathology (tumor, infection, osteoporosis) are significant and should be readily identifiable by history. Falls from heights or at high rates of speed, direct trauma, or violent rotational or sidebending forces with localized spine or paraspinal tenderness, should raise suspicion for fracture. Plain film x-ray will often reveal the injury, with CT reserved for equivocal cases and MRI utilized when associated neurological involvement is suspected. Acute compression fractures, in the nonosteoporotic patient, can be managed conservatively in the absence of neurological signs and symptoms and when there is less than 50% loss of vertebral height or 20 degrees of angulation, facet joint involvement, or widening of the space between spinous processes (32). Neurosurgical consultation is warranted for acute compression fractures suspicious for instability, or any evidence of a vertebral burst fracture, which is inherently unstable with risk of cord compromise. Spinous and transverse process fractures may be seen following a violent or forceful trunk flexion, rotation, or side-bend, or from a direct blow. Typically benign injuries, they are usually confirmed on plain film x-ray and are managed conservatively. Symptoms will often resolve in 4 to 6 weeks, although nonunion may be seen on follow-up imaging. Athletes with either spinous or transverse process injuries from direct blows should also be evaluated for the potential of an associated renal injury.

Another diagnostic consideration for thoracolumbar spine pain in the absence of acute trauma is the osteoporotic fracture. Fortunately, the characteristics of the active, older athlete are typically contrary to the risk factors for osteoporotic compression fractures: smoking, history of increased alcohol consumption, low calcium and vitamin D intake, inactivity, and chronic corticosteroid use. However, in the older, small framed, female athlete, perhaps with a history of premature menopause or hyperparathyroidism, presenting with atraumatic mid to low back pain and point tenderness, this diagnosis should be considered. Plain film radiographs typically establish the diagnosis, although CT may be of further benefit in equivocal cases with a high index of suspicion. MRI will show marrow edema in acute injuries and is useful to determine whether a fracture is old or acute. Due to the high degree of morbidity associated with these injuries, the focus should be on prevention through early recognition of risk factors, detection of osteopenia (Dual energy x-ray Absortiometry [DEXA] scan), and appropriate, individualized management through diet, calcium and vitamin D supplementation, weight-bearing exercise, smoking cessation, and medications (bisphosphonates, selective estrogen receptor modulators, estrogen/progesterone therapy, calcitonin, etc.).

CONCLUSIONS

Back pain is a common symptomatic complaint in the active and athletic population. Recognizing the potential causes in various populations, understanding the relevant anatomy, physiology and biomechanics, and appreciating the natural histories of the more common entities leading to back pain will assist the clinician in providing timely diagnosis, treatment, and return to play for these individuals. Applying this knowledge and experience in a preventative setting such as preparticipation evaluations, may allow the clinician to positively impact the development of these often debilitating injuries through prevention.

REFERENCES

1. Biering-Sorenson F. Physical measurements as risk indicators for low-back trouble over a one-year period. *Spine* 1984;9(2):106–119.
2. Frymoyer JW, Cats-Baril WL. An overview of the incidences and costs of low back pain. *Orthop Clin North Am* 1991;22(2):263–271.
3. Shekelle PG, Ortiz E, Rhodes S, et al. Validity of the agency for healthcare research and quality clinical practice guidelines. How quickly do guidelines become outdated? *JAMA* 2001;286(12):1461–1467.
4. Bigos S, Bowyer O, Braen G, et al. *Acute low back problems in adults. Clinical practice guideline, quick reference guide number 14*. Rockville, MD: U.S. Department of Health and Human Services, Public Health Service, Agency for Health Care Policy and Research, AHCPR Pub. No. 95-0643. December 1994.
5. van Tulder Maurits W, Tuut M, Pennick V, et al. Quality of primary care guidelines for acute low back pain. *Spine* 2004;29(17):E357–E362.
6. White A, Panjabi M. *Clinical biomechanics of the spine*, 2nd ed. Philadelphia: JB Lippincott, 1990:38–79.
7. Borenstein DG, Wiesel SW, Boden SD. *Low back pain. Medical diagnosis and comprehensive management*, 2nd ed. Philadelphia: WB Saunders, 1995:1–21.
8. Gower WE, Pedrini V. Age-related variations in protein-polysaccharides from human nucleus pulposus, annulus fibrosus, and costal cartilage. *J Bone Joint Surg* 1969;51A:1154.
9. Macintosh JE, Bogduk N. The attachments of the lumbar erector spinae. *Spine* 1991;16:783.
10. Cann CE, Martin MC, Genant HK. Decreased spinal mineral content in amenorrheic women. *JAMA* 1984;251:626–629.
11. Drinkwater BL, Breumner B, Chestnut CH, et al. Menstrual history as a determinant to current bone density in the young athlete. *JAMA* 1990;263:545–548.
12. Magee DJ. *Orthopedic physical assessment*, 2nd ed. Philadelphia: WB Saunders, 1992:247–307.
13. Bradley WJ Jr, Seidenwurm DJ, Brunberg JA, et al. *Low back pain. Expert panel on neurologic imaging: appropriateness criteria*. Available at www.acr.org. 2005.
14. Jensen MC, Brant-Zawadzki MN, Obuchowski N, et al. Magnetic resonance imaging of the lumbar spine in people without back pain. *N Engl J Med* 1994;331(2):69–73.
15. Dreisinger TE, Nelson B. Management of back pain in athletes. *Injury Clin* 1996;21:313–320.
16. Nachemson A. Newest knowledge of low back pain. A critical look. *Clin Orthop* 1992;279:8–20.
17. Brolinson PG, Kozar AJ, Cibor G. Sacroiliac joint dysfunction in athletes. *Curr Sports Med Rep* 2003;2:47–56.
18. Hubbard DD. Injuries to the spine in children and adolescents. *Clin Orthop* 1974;100:56–65.
19. Micheli L, Wood R. Back pain in young athletes. *Arch Pediatr Adolesc Med* 1995;149:15–18.
20. Stewart T. The age and incidence of neural arch defects in Alaskan natives. *J Bone Joint Surg Am* 1983;35:937.
21. Bellah RD, Summerville DA, Treves ST, et al. Low back pain in adolescent athletes: detection of stress injury to the pars intra-articularis with SPECT. *Radio* 1991;180:509–512.
22. d'Hemecourt PA, Gerbino PG, Micheli LJ. Back injuries in the young athlete. *Clin Sports Med* 2000;19(4):663–679.
23. Standaert CJ. Spondylolysis in the adolescent athlete. Practical management. *Clin J Sports Med* 2002;12:119–122.
24. Myerding HW. Low backache and sciatic pain associated with spondylolisthesis and protruded intervertebral disc. *J Bone Joint Surg Am* 1941;23:461–470.
25. Muschik M. Competitive sports and the progression of spondylolisthesis. *J Pediatr Orthop* 1996;16:364–369.
26. Greenan TL. Diagnostic imaging of sports-related spinal disorders. *Clin Sports Med* 1993;12(3):487–505.
27. Blumenthal SL, Roach J, Herring JA. Lumbar Scheuermann's. A clinical series and classification. *Spine* 1987;12(9):929–932.
28. Gerbino PG II, Micheli LJ. Back injuries in the young athlete. *Clin Sports Med* 1995;14(3):580–582.
29. U.S. Preventive Services Task Force. Agency for Healthcare Research and Quality. Screening for idiopathic scoliosis in adolescents: update of the evidence for the U.S. Preventive Services Task Force. Agency for Healthcare Research and Quality, Available at www.preventiveservices.ahrq.gov. 2003.
30. Omey ML, Micheli LJ, Gerbino PG. Idiopathic scoliosis and spondylolysis in the female athlete. Tips for treatment. *Clin Ortho Rel Res* 2000;372:74–84.
31. McClure SK, Adams JE, Dahm DL. Common musculoskeletal disorders in women. *Mayo Clin Proc* 2005;80(6):796–802.
32. Eiff MP, Hatch RL, Calmbach WL. *Fracture management for primary care*, 1st ed. Philadelphia: WB Saunders, 1998:154–161.

SUGGESTED READINGS

Back

Deyo RA, Rainville J, Kentr DL. What can the history and physical examination tell us about low back pain? *JAMA* 1992;268(6):760–765.

Drezner JA, Herring SA. Managing low-back pain. Steps to optimize function and hasten return to activity. *Phys Sportsmed* 2001;29(8):37–43.

Frymoyer JW, Pope MH, Constanza MC, et al. Epidemiologic studies of low back pain. *Spine* 1980;5:419.

Garry JP, McShane J. Lumbar spondylolysis in adolescent athletes. *J Fam Pract* 1998;46:145–149; 1991;8(8):14–24.

Goldman S, Merritt JL. Using the pain drawing in evaluating low back disorder. *J Musculoskel Med* 1991;8(8):14–24.

Herman MJ, Pizzutillo PD. Spondylolysis and spondylolisthesis in the child and adolescent. A new classification. *Clin Ortho Relat Res* 2005;434:46–54.

Lahad A, Malter AD, Berg AO, et al. The effectiveness of four interventions for the prevention of low back pain. *JAMA* 1994;272:1286–1291.

Malmivaara A, Hakkinen U, Aro T, et al. The treatment of acute low back pain—bed rest, exercises, or ordinary activity? *N Engl J Med* 1995;332:351–355.

Micheli LJ, Wood R. Back pain in young athletes. Significant differences from adults in causes and patterns. *Arch Pediatr Adolesc Med* 1995;149:15–18.

Mooney V, Saal JA, Saal JS. *Evaluation and treatment of low back pain. Ciba clinical symposia*. Summit, NJ: Ciba Pharmaceutical Co., 1996.

Saal JA. Rehabilitation of football players with lumbar spine injury (part 1 of 2). *Phys Sportsmed* 1988;16(9):61–68.

Saal JA. Rehabilitation of football players with lumbar spine injury (part 2 of 2). *Phys Sportsmed* 1988;16(10):119–123.

Saal JA, Saal JS. Nonoperative treatment of herniated lumbar intervertebral disc with radiculopathy. An outcome study. *Spine* 1989;14(4):431–437.

Saal JA, Saal JS, Herzog RJ. The natural history of lumbar intervertebral disc extrusions treated nonoperatively. *Spine* 1990;15(7):683–686.

Stinson JT, Wiesel SW. Spine problems in the athlete. *Clin Sports Med* 1993;12(3):419–621.

U.S. Preventive Services Task Force (USPSTF). Primary care interventions to prevent low back pain in adults. *Am Fam Physician* 2005;17(12):2337–2338.

Weinert AM Jr, Rizzo TD Jr. Nonoperative management of multilevel lumbar disc herniation is an adolescent athlete. *Mayo Clin Proc* 1992;67:137–141

Pelvis, Hip, and Upper Leg

30

David M. Peck

SECTION A

PELVIS AND HIP

The pelvis functions as a connection between the trunk and the lower extremities as well as to provide protection to the internal organs (1,2). The hip joint is a deep ball and socket joint in which the functional stability mainly comes from the acetabular labrum shape and three thick capsular ligaments. The three ligaments run in a spiral course from their different sites on the pelvis to the femur (3). They are relaxed during flexion and lateral rotation of the hip joint, which is the position that the hip is most susceptible to dislocation.

Readily palpable landmarks of the pelvis region include the iliac crest with the anterior superior iliac spine and the pubic tubercle, which together are the attachment points of the inguinal ligament, and the posterior superior iliac spine. Four to six inches below this area the ischial tuberosity is palpable. The greater trochanter of the femur forms a bony landmark approximately 4 inches lateral and superior to the ischial tuberosity.

The muscles of the hip and pelvic area function to maintain stability of the weight-bearing joint and to propel the athletes' body forward (see Figures 30A.1 and 30A.2). The major muscles of the hip and thigh can be grouped by the main motions that they exert on the thigh or lower extremity (3). The abductor muscles are vital to counteract the body weight's forced adduction in the one-legged stance, which puts them under great force and places them at risk for wear and tear (3). They also function to move the thigh away from the midline. The abductors are made up of the Gluteus medius and minimus and the tensor fascia latae and they insert on the greater trochanter of the femur. The hip flexors are important to initiate the swing phase during ambulating and to pull the thigh towards the trunk (3). They are made up of the iliopsoas, rectus femoris, and to a lesser degree the pectineus and tensor fascia latae. The flexors generally insert on the lesser trochanter of the femur. The adductor muscles move the thigh to the midline and assist in hip flexion in the stance phase. They are made up of the adductor longus, brevis, magnus, the gracilis, and the pectineus, and insert along the medial border of the femur at the linea aspera. The extensors of the hip are the Gluteus maximus, long head of the biceps femoris, semimembranosus, and semitendinosus. They function to prevent hip and trunk flexion during the gait phase of ambulating and are responsible for climbing. The piriformis, superior and inferior gemelli, obturator externus and internus, and quadratus femoris all function as external rotators of the hip. The piriformis muscle is in intimate contact with the sciatic nerve. There are no true internal rotators of the hip, but several sections of hip muscle help in this function such as the anterior fibers of the gluteus minimus.

Three major nerves innervate the hip and the surrounding structures; the sciatic nerve, the femoral nerve, and the obturator nerve, which lie posteriorly, anteriorly, and medially, respectively (4). Knowledge of the muscle actions, locations and their innervations and the soft tissue structures about the hip is essential for proper diagnosis and treatment of most disorders that affect the pelvis and hip. Although this section concentrates on the orthopedic aspects of hip and pelvis disorders, it is paramount for the clinician to rule out other causes of

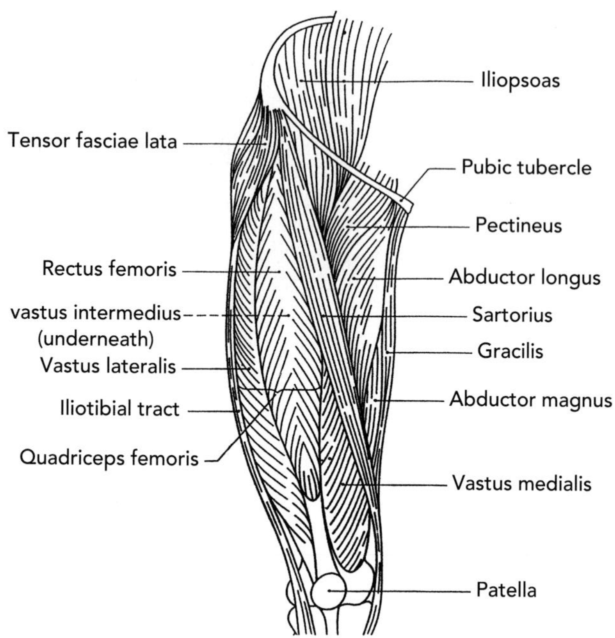

Figure 30A.1 Anterior muscles of the pelvis, hip, and thigh.

referred pain such as lumbar disc disease, gastrointestinal and genitourinary disorders, or other nonorthopedic conditions.

PHYSICAL EXAMINATION

After taking a thorough history of the hip or thigh problem, a physical examination should be undertaken. The examination should include inspection of the area, with adequate exposure, palpation of the area, assessment of the patient's gait, and examination of the biomechanics of the foot. Next a thorough neurovascular assessment, and an evaluation of muscle strength and flexibility, as well as a sensory examination should be performed. There are several provocative tests specific for the hip, pelvis, and thigh, and several will be reviewed (5,6).

Trendelenberg Test

With the patient standing, he/she lifts one leg flexing at the hip. The hip of the stance leg should remain level. If the stance hip elevates, the test is positive for abductor weakness. This can be a sign of hip arthritis, slipped capital femoral epiphysis (SCFE), peripheral nerve lesion, or fracture (see Figure 30A.3).

Patrick's Test

This test is also known as the *faber test*, which stands for flexion, abduction, and external rotation of the hip. The supine patient is asked to place the ankle of one leg on the opposite knee and externally rotate the bent leg. The inability to maintain this position is positive for either hip joint pathology or sacroiliac dysfunction (see Figure 30A.4).

Thomas Test

This test assesses the hip flexibility by having the supine patient maximally flex one hip while the opposite hip is maintained in extension. Inability to maintain the contra

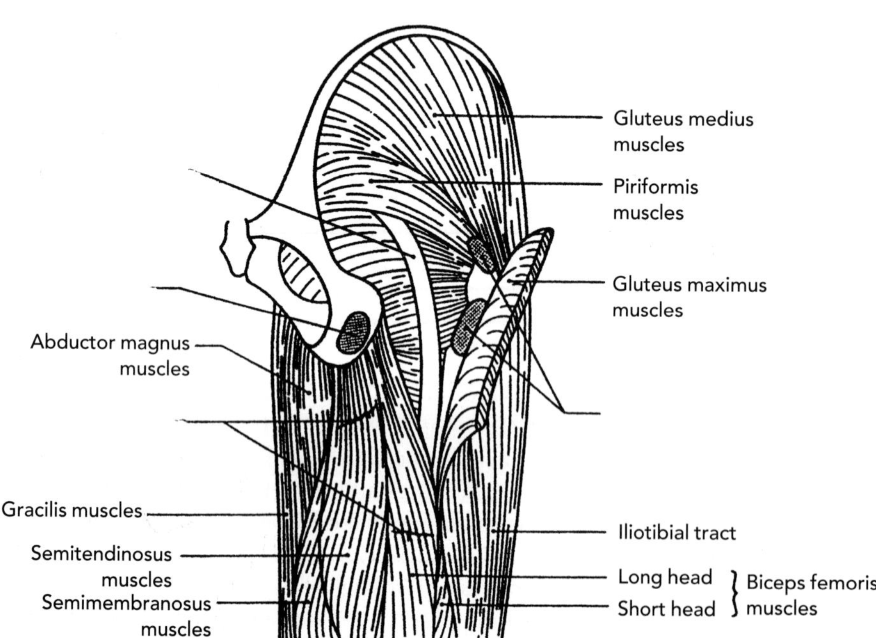

Figure 30A.2 Deep posterior muscles of the pelvis, hip, and thigh.

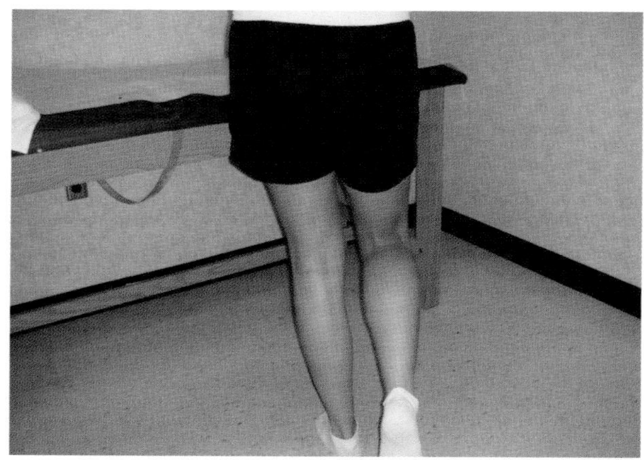

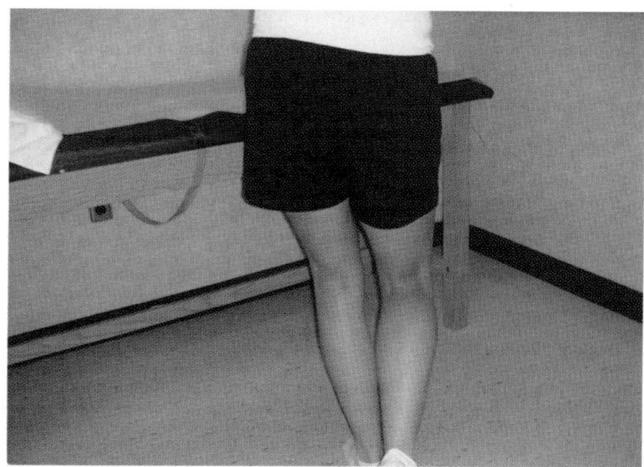

Figure 30A.3 A and B: Trendelenberg's test (A: normal test; B: positive test).

lateral knee or hip in extension is a sign of hip flexor contracture (see Figure 30A.5).

Ober Test

The ober test is a test for iliotibial band (ITB) tightness and is performed with the patient lying on one side. The hip and knee are flexed. The examiner abducts the hip and brings it into neutral. Then the hip is released and if no ITB tightness is present the leg should adduct freely to gravity (see Figure 30A.6).

Ely's Test

The patient is placed in the prone position and the knee is flexed to ninety degrees. The test is positive for rectus femoris tightness if the ipsilateral hip flexes.

It is important to test both legs for all of these tests (see Figure 30A.7).

Log Roll Test

The patient is supine and by holding the foot the hip is moved fully from internal rotation and external rotation. Reproduction of pain signifies a possible intra-articular infection, fracture, or synovitis (see Figure 30A.8).

Femoral Nerve Stretch Test

The patient is in the prone position and the knee is flexed to ninety degrees and the ipsilateral hip is extended. Reproduction of pain or numbness in the anterior thigh signifies either lateral femoral nerve dysfunction or nerve root pathology (see Figure 30A.9).

SOFT TISSUE CONTUSIONS

Contusions about the pelvis and hip are some of the most common injuries in athletics, especially in football, ice

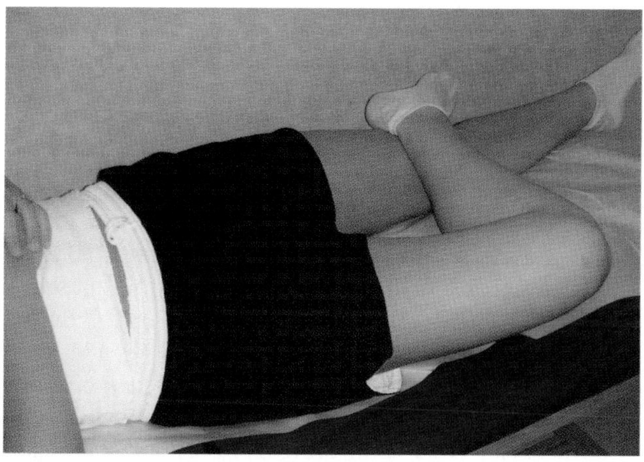

Figure 30A.4 Patrick's test.

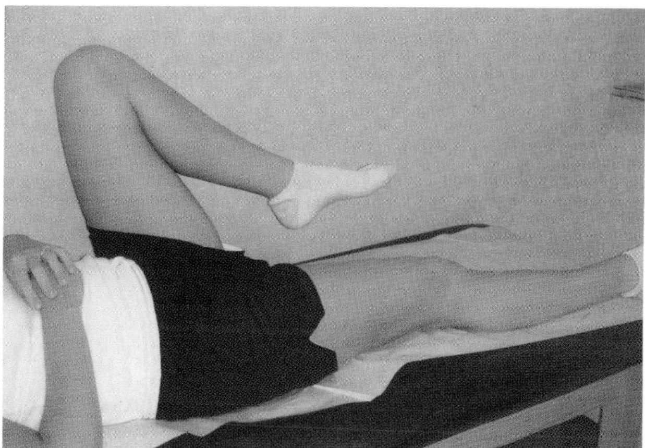

Figure 30A.5 Thomas's test.

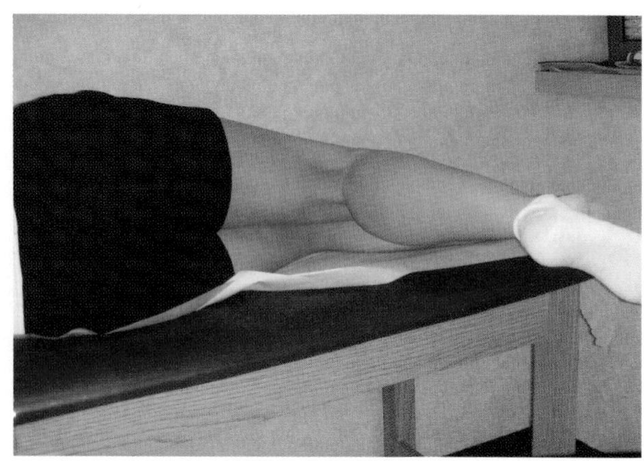
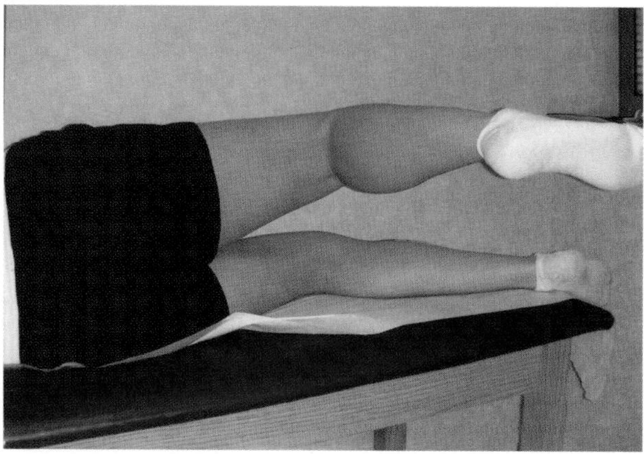

Figure 30A.6 A and B: Ober's test (A: normal test; B: positive test).

hockey, gymnastics, basketball, and volleyball (1,2). Injury is usually caused by contact with another player, another player's equipment (helmet), or the playing surface (floor, field, or boards) (2). Bony or soft tissue prominences are the most common sites of contusion including the iliac crest (hip pointer), ischial tuberosity, greater trochanter, pubic rami, and sciatic nerve.

The athlete will usually present with localized pain over the area in question, which can progress to loss of range of motion (ROM) and decrease in function. With iliac crest contusion (hip pointer), the athlete may be unable to straighten the trunk or rotate the trunk away from the site. With time, swelling and bruising may develop and in severe cases may lead to prolonged disability such as myositis ossificans (2). A full neuromuscular examination should be performed to rule out a complete avulsion.

Plain film radiological evaluation is essential to rule out an avulsion fracture and should be obtained in at least two planes. Treatment begins with immediate application of ice, compression with a wrap, and rest from painful activities to avoid prolonged disability. An attempt at aspiration of the hematoma may be considered, but the practice has met with limited success (1). Avoidance of heat modalities (hot packs, ultrasound, and electrical stimulation) and vigorous massage should be followed in the first 48 hours to limit the amount of bleeding into the area. Rehabilitation is aimed at maintenance of pain-free ROM, gentle stretching, and progressing to trunk flexion and strengthening for the iliac crest contusion. An injection with 1% to 2% Lidocaine and long acting cortisone into the area of maximal tenderness may shorten the course of the condition, but should be held off until after the acute phase (48 to 72 hours) (2).

Return to play may be considered when the athlete shows full pain-free ROM, full motor function, and ability to perform sports-specific activities without pain (1). The area should be padded with an elongated donut pad underneath any required equipment to prevent recurrence. A common practice to be avoided is altering (cutting part of the pad) or not using the hip pads in contact sports such as ice hockey and football.

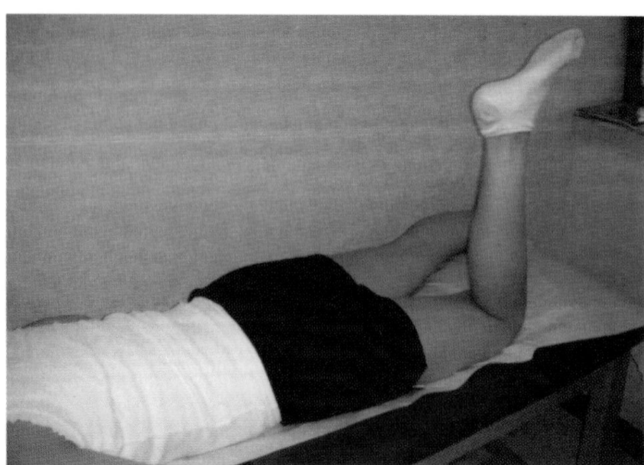

Figure 30A.7 Ely's test.

HIP APOPHYSITIS

Apophysitis is an inflammation at the site of a major tendinous insertion onto a bony prominence that is undergoing growth (7). Growth is a predisposing factor in this group of injuries in that it leads to muscle–tendon imbalance (inflexibility). This inflexibility combined with repetitive activity leads to this inflammatory condition (8). Apophysitis about the hip occurs at the origin or insertions of some of the major muscle groups including the iliac crest, (abdominal muscles) the ischial tuberosity (hamstring muscles), the anterior superior iliac spine (sartorius muscle), the anterior inferior iliac spine (quadriceps muscle), the lesser trochanter (iliopsoas muscle), and the greater trochanter (gluteus medius and minimus) (see Figure 30A.10). This condition can occur until the growth centers completely ossify. The following is a list of the relative ages of fusion of the apophyses: iliac crest (15 to 17 years), ischial

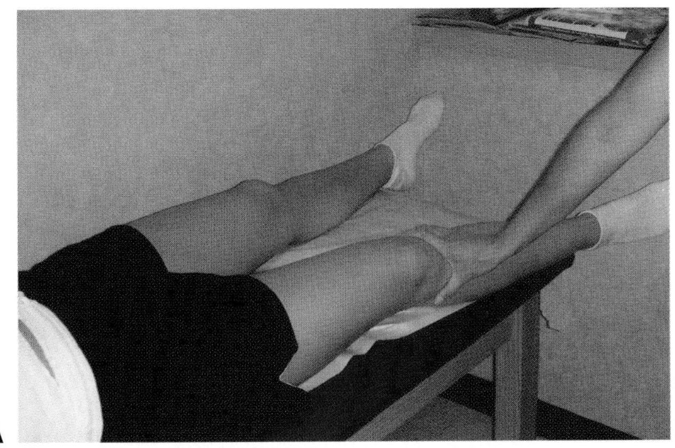
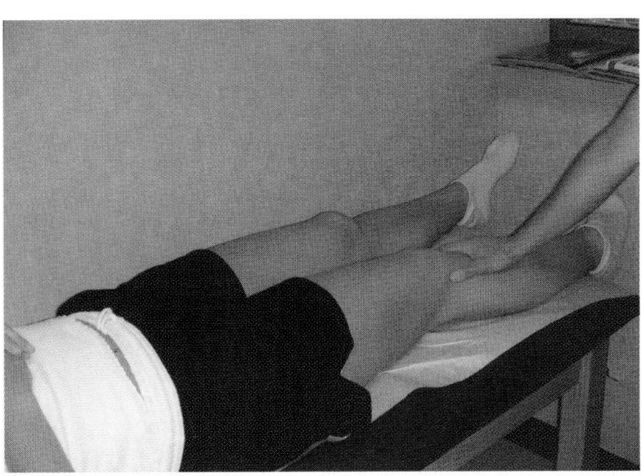
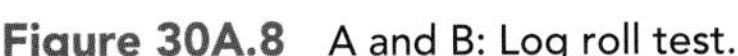

Figure 30A.8 A and B: Log roll test.

tuberosity (19 to 25 years), anterior superior iliac spine (21 to 25 years), anterior inferior iliac spine (16 to 18 years), lesser trochanter (16 to 18 years), and the greater trochanter (16 to 18 years) (1).

Iliac crest apophysitis is the most common of this group of injuries and usually presents with anterior and superior hip pain with activity. The iliac crest ossification center closes between the ages 16 and 20 in males and 14 and 18 in females and closes from anterior to posterior. Long distance runners and dancers often develop this condition. On examination, the athlete may have tenderness over the anterior half of the iliac crest and pain may be reproduced with hip abduction against resistance or trunk rotation. Plain film x-rays should be ordered to rule out an avulsion fracture.

Apophysitis about the hip, as with all apophysitis', has a very favorable prognosis and usually responds to a conservative treatment program (7). The mainstay of treatment is relative rest from pain-producing activities. The athlete may participate in his/her activity at a level that does not induce pain. In some cases, the athlete must rest from all activities and in rare cases must crutch-walk until pain-free. Rest, ice application, anti-inflammatory medications, and cross training are followed by a slow progression of activities over a 4- to 6-week period. An aggressive program of abdominal and hip flexibility is essential for return to pain-free activity.

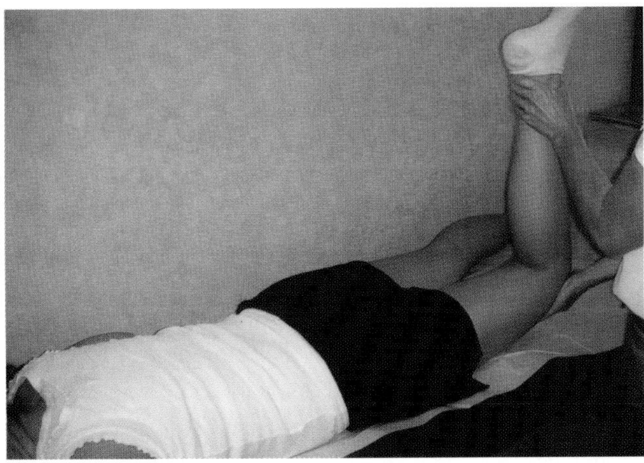

Figure 30A.9 Femoral nerve stretch test.

OSTEITIS PUBIS

Osteitis pubis in the athlete is a cause of chronic groin pain usually seen in distance runners, weight lifters, fencers, football, soccer, and basketball players (2,6). There are several etiologies for this condition including acute trauma to the area, but it is generally felt to be caused by repetitive trauma to the pubic symphysis from muscle strain of the gracilis or abdominal muscles. This sets up an inflammatory response. It has been postulated that this pathophysiology is similar to that seen in shin splint syndrome (2).

The athlete will usually complain of a slow insidious onset of dull groin pain which becomes worse with activity and which can be chronic and incapacitating. The pain may radiate into the lower abdomen, proximal medial thigh or inguinal area and is relieved by rest. The patient walks with an antalgic or waddling gait. Tenderness to palpation over the pubic tubercle and pubic symphysis is noted. Pain may be noted over the pubic symphysis on passive abduction or adduction against resistance. On examination, a one-legged hop test may reproduce the groin pain.

X-rays are important to rule out avulsion fractures, unstable symphysis, or other bony pathology. Radiographic changes can lag 2 to 4 weeks behind the Clinical findings. Harris and Murray studied 38 patients with osteitis pubis and found three characteristic findings on x-rays: (a) symmetrical bone resorption in the medial ends of the pubic bone, (b) widening of the pubic symphysis, (c) rarefaction or sclerosis along the pubic ramus (9). Bone scan shows diffuse uptake early in the course of the condition.

This condition is generally self-limited; hence rest from painful activity is the mainstay of treatment. Anti-inflammatory medications and modalities may speed the healing process, but it may take from 2 to 3 months up to 2 years. Cross training with swimming or other partial weight-bearing activities to maintain cardiovascular fitness can be performed. Severe cases of osteitis pubis may require a trial of cortisone injections. Chronic cases that don't respond to an exhaustive trial of conservative therapy may need surgical debridement and arthrodesis of the pubic symphysis.

AVULSION FRACTURES OF THE HIP AND PELVIS

Avulsion fractures of the hip and pelvis occur in the skeletally immature athlete, especially Tanner stage 3, when the relatively weak apophysis is subjected to a sudden violent contraction of one of the large muscle groups that attach here (10). Sprinters, jumpers, soccer players, gymnasts, dancers, and football players are at risk for this type of injury and this type of fracture accounts for 11% to 40% of all hip and pelvis fractures in children. The sites involved are as follows: (a) ischial tuberosity—hamstring muscles, (b) anterior inferior iliac spine—rectus femoris muscle, (c) anterior superior iliac spine—sartorius muscle, (d) iliac crest—abdominal muscles, (e) lesser trochanter of femur—iliopsoas muscle, and (f) greater trochanter of femur—gluteus medius and minimus (6,10) (see Figures 30A.10–30A.13). A study from 2003 in Italy, reviewed 1,238 radiographs of the pelvis in adolescent competitive athletes taken for traumatic symptoms and found 203 avulsion fractures of the pelvic apophyses. The most common site was the ischial tuberosity in 109 cases, anterior inferior iliac spine in 45 cases, and the anterior superior iliac spine in 39 cases, the most common sports involved in this study were soccer and gymnastics (11).

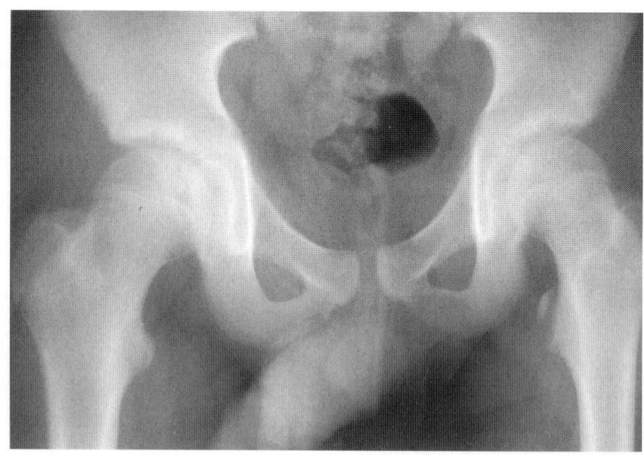

Figure 30A.11 X-ray of an avulsion fracture of the lesser trochanter of the hip.

The athlete will present with a history of sudden pull or pop while competing and will have localized pain and swelling over the bony attachment, and loss of motion in the involved area. X-rays are essential to diagnose this condition and comparison views of the uninvolved side should be obtained (2). Metzmaker and Pappas outlined a five stage progressive rehabilitation program for avulsion fractures, which includes the following: (a) rest in a position of comfort, ice, and anti-inflammatory medications, (b) gentle ROM exercises both passive and active, (c) progressive resistance exercise program when 75% of ROM and 50% of strength are reached, (d) stretching and strengthening combined with patterned motions, and (e) return to competition when there is pain-free ROM and the strength is 80% of the uninvolved side (12).

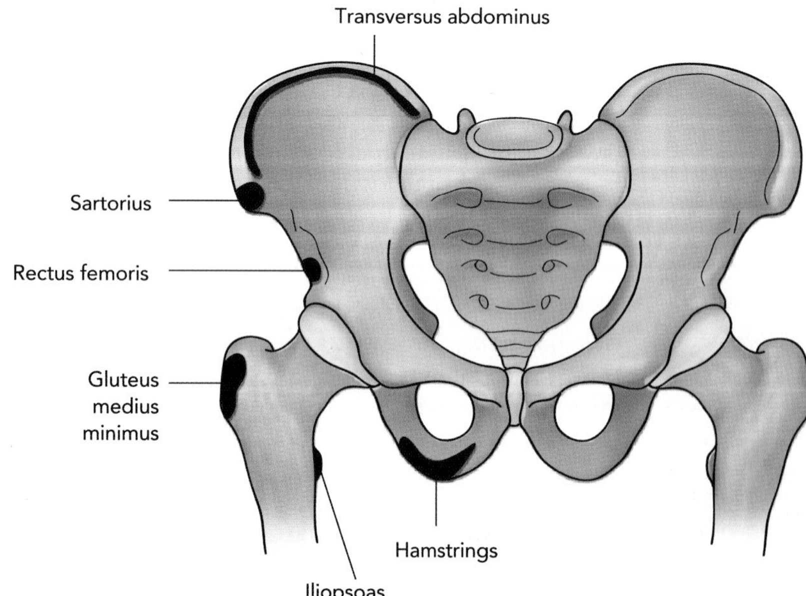

Figure 30A.10 Apophysitis of the hip.

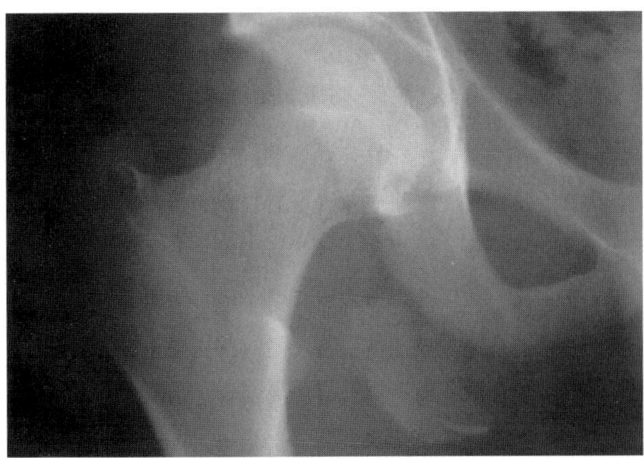

Figure 30A.12 X-ray of an avulsion fracture of the ischial tuberosity.

The general consensus on surgical intervention is that it should be considered only in rare cases with significant displacement of the avulsed fragment or recalcitrant cases. The surgical intervention is usually open reduction and internal fixation if the fragment is of a sufficient size to contain hardware and the displacement is 2 cm or greater (13). Most cases will respond to conservative therapy over a 5- to 6-week period. Ischial tuberosity avulsions generally take longer to heal than those at other sites and may heal with exuberant bony exostosis.

BURSITIS OF THE HIP

Bursae are fluid-filled sacs or cavities located throughout the body over bony prominences and joints, and help pad the area and aid in smooth motion of the tendons (1).

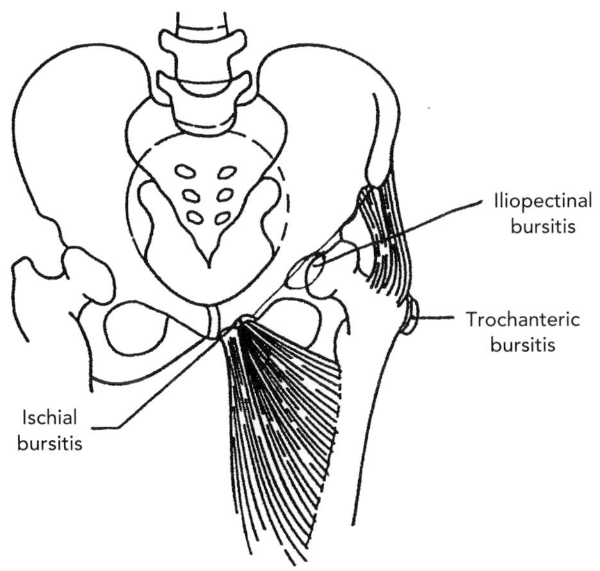

Figure 30A.13 Bursas of the hip.

Bursitis is inflammation of these structures caused either by repetitive overuse or through post-trauma after a blow to the area (2). The three most common bursa about the hip are the trochanteric bursa, ischial bursa, and iliopectineal bursa (Figure 30A.13).

Trochanteric Bursitis

Trochanteric bursitis presents as pain over the greater trochanter worsened by hip flexion and extension (3). This condition is associated with muscle imbalance between hip abductors and adductors, leg-length discrepancy, excessive training, and foot hyperpronation. External factors (hard surface, banked track, shoes) may also play a role.

Treatment consists of rest from painful activities, ice massage, and anti-inflammatory medications. Injection of steroids and local anesthetic into the point of maximal tenderness may speed the healing process. A stretching program addressing the ITB and adductor muscles, as well as addressing any internal causes (leg-length discrepancy, foot hyperpronation) should be undertaken. This is followed by a slow progression of activities as tolerated and, finally return to sport activities. Surgical release of a tight ITB or removal of the inflamed bursa is rarely indicted and only after an exhaustive trial of conservative therapy.

Ischial Bursitis

Ischial bursitis usually follows a blow to the ischial tuberosity, which leads to hematoma formation, scaring, and eventually palpatory tenderness (2). Pain is usually worsened with prolonged sitting and it is important to rule out avulsion fracture, apophysitis, or hamstring tendonitis.

Treatment involves ice, padding the area while seated, and anti-inflammatory medications. If no improvement is noted with conservative therapy, an aspiration and injection of steroids and local anesthetic should be performed. In rare cases, surgical excision of the bursa and removal of the bone spurs are needed.

Iliopectineal Bursitis

The iliopectineal bursa lies posterior to the inguinal ligament and between the iliopsoas muscle and the pelvis proximally. This condition presents with debilitating anterior hip pain. The pain is worsened with passive hip extension and the athlete will try to maintain the hip in flexion and external rotation to lessen pain (2). On examination, there may be tenderness to deep palpation.

Treatment centers on rest from offending activities, ice, anti-inflammatory medications, stretching of the iliopsoas muscle, and in rare cases, a steroid injection into the area of maximal tenderness.

PIRIFORMIS SYNDROME

Piriformis syndrome presents as a dull, achy pain in the buttocks that sometimes radiates into the posterior thigh or lower leg (14). This condition is commonly confused with lumbar disc disease. Piriformis syndrome can be caused by trauma, prolonged sitting, or overuse, commonly during the stance phase of running or trunk rotation in tennis. It is found that 15% to 20% of the population has an aberrant peroneal branch of the sciatic nerve that exits through the muscle instead of below it (1).

Examination reveals tenderness over the mid-buttock between the ischium and greater trochanter. The pain is worsened with passive internal rotation of the hip or external rotation against resistance. Bone scan or electromyogram may be needed to rule out other conditions.

Treatment centers on rest from offending activity and an aggressive stretching program for the external rotators of the hip (14). Spray and stretch with fluoromethane spray and in recalcitrant cases a steroid injection to the point of maximal tenderness may be needed. Rarely, surgical division of the piriformis muscle is required to treat a chronic case.

GROIN STRAIN

Groin strains or adductor muscle strains are common injuries seen in activities involving forcefully twisting or pivoting of the lower extremity. Football, ice hockey, soccer, baseball, karate, gymnastics, and track sports are sports that have a high rate of groin injury. The mechanism is usually forceful contraction of an overstretched adductor muscle commonly against another player, the ground, or a ball (2). Risk factors for the development of this condition include older athlete, muscle imbalance, inflexibility, inadequately warmed-up muscles, and early in the season. This type of injury has a high rate of chronicity usually due to premature return to activity; this needs to be considered in rehabilitation progression and return to sport questions.

Groin strain usually occurs at the musculotendinous junction, which is close to the origin of the adductor muscle group (longus, brevis, magnus, and minimus), along the inferior pubic ramus, pubic symphysis, and ischial tuberosity.

There is usually a history of a sudden onset of groin pain after overloading the muscles or, in rare cases, from direct blunt trauma. The pain may be dull or sharp, localized or diffuse, with radiation into the scrotum, hip, medial thigh, or deep pelvis. The pain may be worsened by activities involving forced adduction of the hip. Examination of the area may show palpatory tenderness over the pubic bone with discomfort on passive abduction of the thigh and resisted adduction of the thigh. In severe cases, a palpable gap may be felt in the adductor muscles. The differential diagnosis for groin pain is quite lengthy and should include inguinal hernia, femoral hernia, sport's hernia, hip dysfunction, lower back dysfunction, gastrointestinal disorders, genitourinary disorders, other soft tissue injury, and bony disruption of the hip. X-ray should be obtained to rule out avulsion fractures. Bone scan or magnetic resonance imaging (MRI) should be reserved for suspected stress fracture or severe muscle disruption.

Treatments begin with the RICE protocol (Rest, Ice, Compression, and Elevation) involving rest from painful activity, (and in some severe cases, crutch walking), ice application to the area, compression applied with ace wrap or neoprene sleeve, and elevation of the extremity. Progression of treatment is dependent on the initial severity and progression of symptoms with time. Matzenmayer developed a five-phase system for rehabilitation of avulsion fractures and which has been modified for adductor strains (2). Phase one involves reduction of pain, inflammation, and bleeding, which was outlined in the preceding text and lasts from 2 to 3 days. This is followed by phase 2 in which ROM is regained by the use of passive stretching and physical therapy modalities including ultrasound, heat, and electrical stimulation for up to 1 week. Strengthening, as well as flexibility and cardiovascular fitness is addressed in phase 3 by the use of isometrics and cycling or walking. Phase 4 continues to improve strength and begins to address coordination by weight lifting and a closed chain functional training. Finally in phase 5, the athlete is slowly progressed to sports with sports-specific training and continued cardiovascular training. It may take anywhere from 4 to 6 weeks up to several months (even years) to completely recover from a groin strain.

Return to sports may be attempted safely when the athlete attains full pain-free ROM, 90% to 95% of preinjury strength as compared to the noninvolved leg, and completion of all sports-specific activities. It is advised that the athletes use a pair of compression shorts or neoprene wrap when they return to sports. Their use has been shown to be beneficial by supplying support, warmth, and proprioceptive assistance.

LEGG-CALVE-PERTHES' DISEASE

Legg-Calve-Perthes' disease (LCP) is a disease of unknown etiology, but it is felt to be related to an interruption of the blood supply to the femoral epiphysis (2,15). It is most prevalent between 4 and 9 years of age and has a 4:1 male predominance. Athletes present with intermittent deep hip pain that may radiate to the groin, anteromedial thigh, or knee. It is found bilaterally 20% of the time, but rarely simultaneously. The athlete may ambulate with a limp, and symptoms are generally worse with activity. Examination of the involved hip may show decreased internal rotation; in chronic cases may show thigh atrophy.

X-rays are usually diagnostic for LCP disease (see Figure 30A.14), but if suspected early in the course of the disease, MRI or bone scan may be needed to show bone

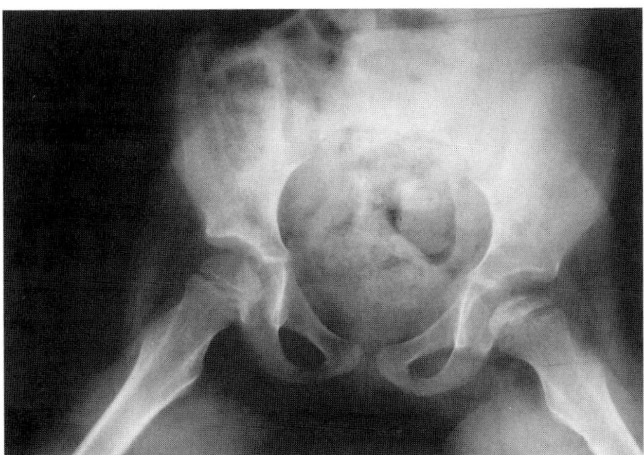

Figure 30A.14 X-ray of Legg-Calve-Perthes' disease.

edema of the femoral epiphysis (6). Plain films include AP and frog-leg views and show the typical cascade of changes with sclerosis of the epiphysis, fragmentation, apparent collapse of the bony epiphysis and finally reossification of the epiphysis.

Treatment is based on the principle that containment of the femoral head within the acetabulum will lead to the best chance of healing of the infarcted femoral head. Containment can be brought about by bracing, casting, or in some cases osteotomy.

Referral to an orthopedic surgeon with experience in LCP is the first step in treatment. To control symptoms, crutch walking or even bed rest as well as anti-inflammatory medications should be prescribed.. Further treatment of LCP is controversial and is dependent on the age at diagnosis, amount of femoral head involvement, and sex of the patient. Age less than 6 years and less than 50% involvement of the femoral head are both good prognostic signs (1). Return to play can be considered when the epiphysis shows healing on x-ray and the athlete is pain-free.

Acute transient synovitis is the most common cause of nontraumatic hip pain in kids under 10 years of age (2). This condition is usually self-limited and presents with hip pain on walking, low-grade fever, and normal complete blood count and sedimentation rate (3). This condition should be distinguished from acute septic arthritis, which presents as high fever, hip pain, increased white blood cells and sedimentation rate. If this condition is suspected, then urgent orthopedic consultation for joint aspiration and definitive treatment are required. MRI and ultrasound may be beneficial in differentiation between acute transient synovitis and acute septic arthritis.

SLIPPED CAPITAL FEMORAL EPIPHYSIS

SCFE is the one of the most common hip conditions in the adolescent population, but it is also one of the most poorly diagnosed conditions in adolescents. One of the most important points to remember about SCFE is that any child between the ages of 8 and 15 years presenting with pain between the pelvis and knee should have a thorough evaluation of the hip with strong consideration for getting x-rays of the hip. The earlier in the course of the disease that the diagnosis is made the better the long-term prognosis. During periods of rapid growth, shear forces across the proximal femoral physis may lead to posterior and medial slippage of the capital femoral epiphysis, which is felt to be the cause of this condition. Hormonal imbalance (sex and growth), genetic factors, and mechanical factors (growth, obesity, ipsilateral SCFE) may play a role in the development of SCFE (2). SCFE occurs generally between the ages of 9 and 15 years, and is seen most commonly in boys older than 11 and girls older than 9. The condition can be bilateral in up to 50% of the cases, usually in chronic cases due to the increased forces on the contralateral growth plate caused by the limp (15). It is common in obese males and during periods of growth. The onset is usually insidious with groin, hip, thigh, or knee pain with or without a limp. Physical examination will show limited internal rotation of the hip, and if the hip is flexed it will fall into external rotation. In chronic cases, muscle atrophy of the thigh and leg-length discrepancy may be noted. The diagnosis is confirmed by AP and frog-leg lateral radiographs, which will show widening or irregularity of the physis early on, which may lead to posterior and medial tilting of the epiphysis (looks like ice cream slipping off a cone) (see Figure 30A.15).

SCFE is classified by acuity as acute, chronic (most common), and acute on chronic (2). It is further classified by the severity of the slippage. The initial treatment should be non–weight-bearing and referral to an orthopedic surgeon with expertise in this condition. The epiphysis is usually stabilized to prevent further slippage by screw or pin, and more severe slippage may need stabilization as well as realignment to prevent development of avascular necrosis of the femoral head, osteoarthritis of the hip as an adult, and destruction of the articular cartilage (1).

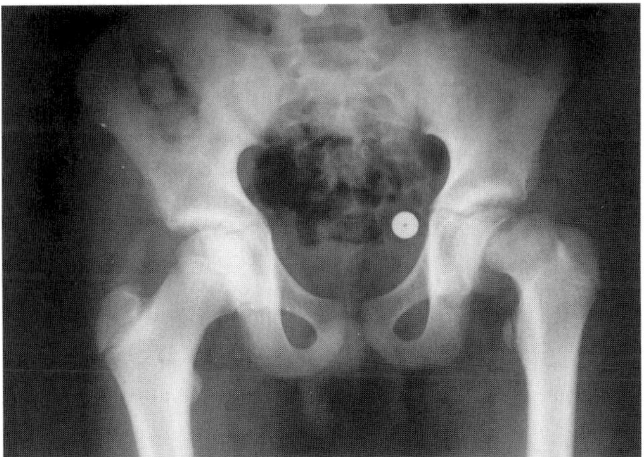

Figure 30A.15 X-ray of slipped-capital-femoral-epiphysis.

All athletes between the ages of 8 and 15 years with complaints of hip, thigh, and knee pain should have both hips evaluated for SCFE.

SECTION B

UPPER LEG

ANATOMICAL CONSIDERATIONS

The thigh consists of the femur, which is surrounded by large muscles in three compartments (4). The anteromedial or adductor compartment was discussed in the previous section. The anterior compartment is made up of the quadriceps femoris and the sartorius muscle (see Figure 30A.1). The quadriceps muscle is a large muscle mass covering the anterior thigh that is made up of the rectus femoris, the vastus medialis, the vastus intermedius, and the vastus lateralis. The rectus femoris, which is the only part that crosses the hip, originates at the anterior inferior iliac crest and inserts with the other quadriceps muscles onto the tibial tuberosity through the patella. It functions to flex the thigh at the hip and extend the knee. The vastus medialis, vastus intermedius, and vastus lateralis originate from different aspects of the anterior femur and have a common insertion with the rectus femoris. These muscles don't cross the hip joint, so they function to extend the knee. The sartorius muscle (tailor muscle), is a long thin muscle that originates at the anterior superior iliac spine, crosses the anterior and medial thigh and inserts with the medial hamstrings on the anterior medial surface of the tibia and is located in both the anterior and posterior compartments (4). The sartorius muscle functions as a flexor of the hip, flexor of the knee, weak abductor of the thigh, and external rotator of the thigh, which all function to assume the cross-legged seated position of a tailor. The femoral nerve innervates the muscles of the anterior compartment.

The posterior compartment of the thigh is made up of the hamstring muscles, gracilis muscle, and sartorius muscle (see Figure 30A.2). The semitendinosus originates at the ischial tuberosity, travels over the medial side of the thigh, and inserts on the anterior medial aspect of the tibia with the gracilis and sartorius muscles (4). The semimembranosus originates from the lateral aspect of the ischial tuberosity, crosses the medial thigh deep to the other hamstring muscles, and inserts on the posterior medial aspect of the tibia. The biceps femoris has two heads; the long head originates at the ischial tuberosity, and the short head originates from the posterior femur. The two heads form a conjoined tendon that passes on the lateral aspect of the thigh and inserts on the head of the fibula. The hamstring muscles function to extend the thigh at the hip and flex the knee. Except the short head of the biceps femoris which is innervated by the peroneal branch of the sciatic nerve, they are innervated by tibial branches of the sciatic nerve (16). This innervation inconsistency may become important in the development of hamstring strains.

THIGH CONTUSION

Thigh contusions commonly occur due to direct trauma to the anterior or lateral thigh in such contact sports as football or ice hockey. A seemingly innocuous thigh contusion may lead to severe complications such as anterior compartment syndrome or myositis ossificans if not treated appropriately in a timely manner. On a cellular level, the response to the compressive force on the muscle is initially vascular rupture, edema, inflammation, and bleeding (17). The severity of the injury is felt to be related to the extent of blood vessel damage and bleeding. Some theorize that quadriceps muscle contraction at the time of injury can minimize the severity of the injury.

The condition is diagnosed by history of trauma to the area, tenderness, swelling, possibly a palpable mass, and in some cases a limp. Thigh contusions are graded by the amount of knee flexion 12 to 24 hours after the injury. In a grade 1 or mild injury the knee flexion is greater than 90 degrees, in grade 2 or moderate injury the knee flexion is between 45 and 90 degrees, and a grade 3 or severe injury the knee flexion is less than 45 degrees.

Compartment syndrome is a severe complication of thigh contusions and femoral fractures, and presents with significant swelling in the thigh, pain out of proportion to the injury, as well as sensory changes (late) to the anterior knee, medial lower leg, and foot (18). To aid in diagnosis of this condition, serial thigh measurements and intracompartmental pressure measurements are required to avoid the ominous late signs of motor deficits and decreased pulses. Acute compartment syndrome is a surgical emergency and should be treated aggressively with surgical fasciotomy to prevent permanent muscle damage.

The most important aspects of the initial treatment of thigh contusion are to minimize the amount of hematoma formation by the RICE protocol and to wrap the area with the knee in maximal flexion (17) (see Figure 30B.1). It is generally felt that anti-inflammatory medications should be avoided in the first 24 hours and, the use of modalities such as local massage, local heat application, and ultrasound should be avoided to decrease the risk of myositis ossificans. Hematoma aspiration, injection of steroids, oral use of proteolytic enzymes, and local anesthetic injection have not been shown to be safe or effective and should be avoided under most circumstances.

Treatment should progress slowly with only ROM exercises performed until the athlete has pain-free ROM. The athlete may begin cross training when pain-free and then progress to isometric exercises followed by open chain strengthening. The athlete may then progress to closed chain multi-joint exercises and sports specific activities.

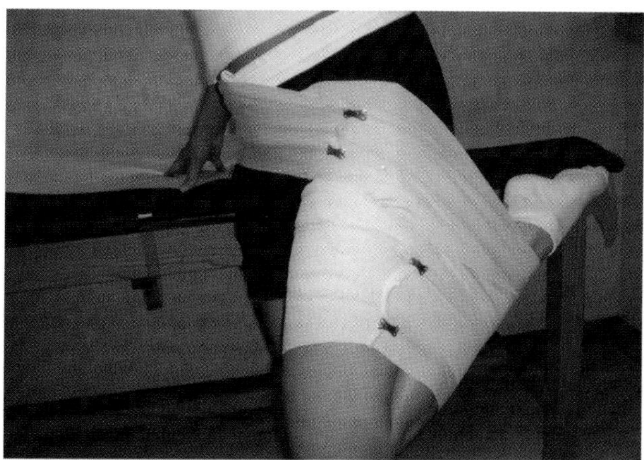

Figure 30B.1 Knee held in maximal flexion.

Return to sports may be attempted when ROM is full, strength is 90% to 95% of the uninvolved leg, and sports-specific activities are performed without pain. The athlete should wear a thermoplastic pad applied under the standard thigh pads.

MYOSITIS OSSIFICANS

Myositis ossificans is the deposition of calcium into the hematoma of a severe thigh contusion (see Figure 30B.2). Studies have shown the incidence of myositis ossificans in thigh contusion anywhere from 7% to 20% (16). Severe contusion to the thigh, continued participation after the contusion, initially aggressive rehabilitation (massage, heat, and ultrasound), forceful stretching of the contused quadriceps muscle, premature return to sports, reinjury, and a predisposition to heterotrophic bone development all have been shown to be risk factors for development of myositis ossificans.

The athlete usually presents with localized pain, warmth, tenderness, and a slowly expanding palpable mass after a thigh contusion (2). The initial x-ray changes are seen between 3 and 4 weeks, and include fluffy calcifications and periosteal reaction (17). The calcification process continues, and by 3 to 6 months, the bony mass stabilizes and usually shrinks. Before 3 to 4 weeks, bone scan or ultrasound may be needed to diagnose this condition. The lesion of myositis ossificans shows three different types: (a) a stalk connected to the bone, (b) a broad-based periosteal connection, and (c) unattached to the bone (17). It is important that osteosarcoma is differentiated from myositis ossificans, which is characterized by a history of trauma, x-ray stabilization by 3 to 4 months, age younger than 30 years, anterior thigh location, and negative alkaline phosphatase levels. In some cases, an MRI or bone scan is needed to differentiate myositis ossificans from osteosarcoma.

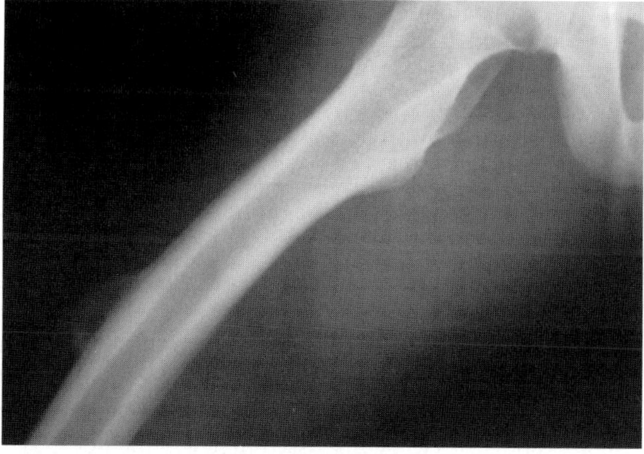

Figure 30B.2 X-ray of myositis ossificans.

The natural history of myositis ossificans is stabilization and shrinkage, and should be kept in mind in treatment decisions (16). Conservative treatment after diagnosis of this bony lesion should include discontinuance of heat, ultrasound, massage, and anti-inflammatory medications, gentle active ROM when the lesion is stable, and slow progression to activity with adequate protection of the thigh. Surgery is rarely indicated and is reserved for unresponsive cases after 6 to 12 months with significant pain and loss of motion, after a normal bone scan. The excision is undertaken with meticulous hemostasis and atraumatic dissection. The most important aspect of this condition is prevention by proper diagnosis and treatment of thigh contusion and use of protection and proper return to sport guidelines.

QUADRICEPS AND HAMSTRING MUSCLE STRAINS

Strains of the quadriceps and hamstring muscles are the most common sports injury of the thigh (with the hamstring as the most common). There are generally three mechanisms for quadriceps strain: (a) sudden deceleration of the leg, such as when a soccer player kicks the ball and hits another player, (b) violent contraction of the quadriceps, such as when an athlete tries to accelerate his body, (c) rapid deceleration of an overstretched muscle, such as when a player tries to change direction quickly (6). The mechanism of injury for a hamstring strain is usually an opposite force applied to a fully stretched hamstring, or a sudden stretch applied to the muscle, such as when a sprinter tries to accelerate. One of the most common risk factors for development of quadriceps or hamstring stain is muscle imbalance between the quadriceps and hamstrings. A study showed that when the ratio of quadriceps to hamstring strength is 0.55 or less, there is a 33% risk of reinjury (19). Other risk factors include inadequate flexibility, inadequate warm-up, strength imbalance between legs, history of previous injury, fatigue of muscles, and poor running form (16,20).

Quadriceps strains most commonly occur through the mid substance or musculotendinous junction of the rectus femoris. They may be found in the vastus lateralis and vastus medialis and rarely, a complete mid substance tear occurs. The most common hamstring strain is to the short head of the biceps femoris, which is theorized to occur because it has a different innervation than the other three hamstring muscles and this asynchronous contraction pattern leads to injury (20). It is also the only hamstring that originates on the posterior femur. Muscle strains are graded as mild (grade 1), in which the muscle is overstretched with minimal disruption, moderate (grade 2), in which partial muscle disruption occurs, and severe (grade 3), in which complete or near complete muscle tear develops (17).

Strains are diagnosed by a history of a force applied to the muscle and in some cases an audible pop will be heard or felt. On examination, there is tenderness over the muscle injury site sometimes with ecchymosis, swelling, and in more severe injures, a palpable gap is present in the muscle. A quadriceps muscle strain will present with exacerbation of pain with passive flexion of the knee or resisted extension of the knee. A rectus femoris injury can be isolated by the Ely test. A hamstring strain will present with exacerbation of pain with passive extension of the knee and flexion of the hip, and resisted flexion of the knee and extension of the hip. Plain x-rays are necessary to rule out avulsion fractures, myositis ossificans, or other osseous abnormalities, but are generally normal. MRI of the muscle, especially T2 weighted images, may be necessary to differentiate a grade 2 strain from a grade 3, but the study has not been shown it to be cost effective (16,20).

The initial treatment should follow the RICE protocol for the first 24 to 48 hours in order to minimize the amount of initial bleeding and hence inflammation. Crutch walking may be important in the first few days to weeks until pain-free ambulating is possible. The athlete is slowly progressed to gentle passive stretching and gentle active ROM in a pain-free zone (17). Isometric strengthening is slowly added as tolerated, and advanced to isokinetic exercises at slow speed, and finally when all phases of rehabilitation are pain-free, sports-specific activities are added. Cross training is started when tolerated to maintain cardiovascular fitness. After the initial phase of ice applications, physical therapy modalities (ultrasound, electrical stimulation, and deep massage) may be instituted to speed up the healing process. The general recommendations for steroid injections are that they are not advisable. Surgical intervention is rarely necessary, and only so in cases of complete muscle tears or widely avulsed fractures.

The athlete may be returned to sport when full pain-free ROM is obtained, quadriceps to hamstring strength ratio is 0.60 or more, strength is 90% to 95% of the uninvolved side, and sports-specific activities can be completed satisfactorily. The average time frame to return to sports is 1 to 2 weeks for grade 1, 3 to 4 weeks for grade 2, and 8 to 12 weeks for grade 3. A compression sleeve or shorts along with adequate warm-up, stretching, and proper rehabilitation from the original injury has been shown to decrease recurrences.

FRACTURES OF THE FEMUR AND PELVIS

The femur is the longest and strongest long bone in the body and the forces required to cause femur fracture are not generally encountered in sports activities (16). A femoral fracture may occur in older athletes with minor trauma due to the osteopenic nature of the senescent bone (3). The patient with a femoral fracture will present with an obvious bony deformity and immediate significant disability. There may be shortening and external rotation of the affected limb.

ACUTE FRACTURE OF THE FEMUR

If a femoral fracture is suspected, the athlete needs to be assessed, stabilized, and transported to a facility for definitive care. The complications of the fracture are related to loss of vascularity to the femoral head and the subsequent development of avascular necrosis of the femoral head. In the skeletally immature athlete, fracture may lead to partial growth arrest of the proximal femur, which may lead to a varus deformity to the leg. Some early complications of an acute fracture of the femur are fat emboli and internal bleeding.

HIP DISLOCATIONS

Acute dislocation of the hip is a true orthopedic emergency, which fortunately is a rare occurrence on the athletic field. The most common type of dislocation is a posterior dislocation in approximately 90% of cases. The patient will present with the leg held in flexion, adduction, and external rotation.

The treatment is to get the patient to an orthopedic surgeon as soon as possible for urgent reduction. The sooner reduction is performed, the better the prognosis generally. A further discussion of hip dislocations is beyond the scope of this chapter.

STRESS FRACTURE

Stress fractures are presumed to be caused by repetitive microtraumatic forces to the bone, which disrupt the cycle of bone resorption and bone repair (6,16). This bone resorption leads to weakness and eventually a stress fracture. Stress fractures of the pelvis and hip are commonly seen in military recruits and endurance athletes. Several factors predispose the athlete to stress fractures including training errors, change in running surface, inadequate footwear, and intrinsic factors (osteopenia, pes planus). The stress fractures to be discussed here will include pelvic, femoral neck, and femoral shaft stress fractures.

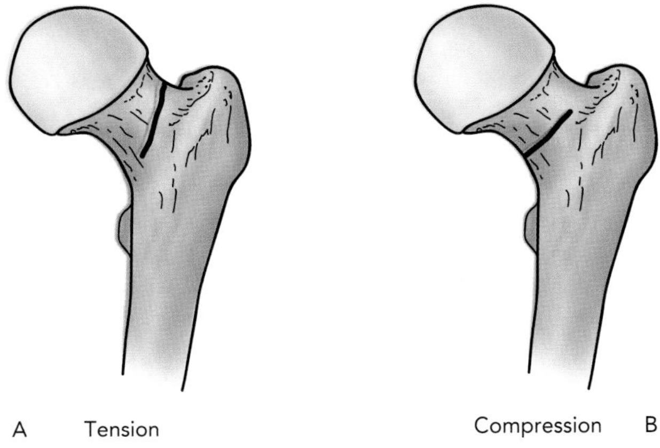

Figure 30B.3 Types of femoral neck stress fractures.

Stress fractures of the pelvis, femoral neck, and femoral shaft present as groin or thigh pain with activity. The athlete may have tenderness to palpation of the affected area with decreased ROM of the hip to internal rotation. They may have an antalgic gait and a positive one-legged standing test (2). The patient may be able to recall a consistent time or distance in their run when pain develops. With cessation of running the pain will cease.

In the first 2 to 4 weeks, plain x-rays will usually be negative for a stress fracture, due to the fact that plain films only show changes during the reparative phase (19). If a stress fracture is suspected in this area, a bone scan or MRI should be ordered and the patient should be put on strict non–weight-bearing crutch walking, pending the results of the imaging. It is imperative that the clinician differentiates between a femoral neck stress fracture and a femoral shaft or a pelvic stress fracture, because the former has a high likelihood of going on to displacement. A tension, or transverse, side femoral neck stress fracture, which will show as a crack in the superior cortex of the femoral neck, should be referred to an orthopedic surgeon for internal fixation. A compression side femoral neck stress fracture presents as a fracture line or bone changes on MRI or bone scan to the medial aspect of the neck and should also be referred to an orthopedic surgeon, owing to the possibility of progression to a transverse stress fracture and subsequent possible displacement although they are usually treated conservatively (see Figure 30B.3). Generally, a compression side femoral neck stress fracture has a more favorable prognosis than a transverse side femoral neck stress fracture, which has a poor prognosis and can progress to a displaced fracture.

Once the diagnosis is made of a pelvic or femoral shaft stress fracture, the patient should be treated with full rest until pain-free. The athlete is then allowed to crutch-walk and slowly progress to full weight-bearing when pain-free. After at least 6 weeks, the patient may begin partial weight-bearing cross training with biking or swimming, as tolerated. Studies have shown that athletes can safely return to their sport anywhere from 8 to 12 weeks after injury (16). This is dependent on age, sex, bone density, and other factors that affect healing. It is essential that the practitioner address any intrinsic or extrinsic factors that predispose the athlete to the stress fracture. X-rays are usually followed monthly for the first 3 months, and then less frequently until complete bony union is evident. It may take up to 2 years for complete healing of this type of stress fracture.

REFERENCES

1. Boyd KT, Pierce NS, Batt ME. Common hip injuries in sports. *Sports Med* 1997;24(4):273–288.
2. Gross ML, Nasser S, Finerman GA. Hip and pelvis injuries. In: Delee JC, Drez D, eds. *Orthopedic sports medicine,* Vol. 2. Philadelphia: WB Saunders 1994:1063–1085.
3. Steinberg GG, Akins CM, Baran DT. *Pelvis, hip, and proximal thigh. Ramamurtis' orthopedics in primary care,* 2nd ed. Williams & Wilkins, 1992:159–197.
4. Jenkins DB. *The bony pelvis, femur, and hip joint. Thigh and knee. Hollingsheads functional anatomy of the limbs and back,* 7th ed. WB Saunders, 1998:239–297.
5. Browning KH. Hip and pelvis injuries in runners. *Phys Sportsmed* 1995;29(1):23–34.
6. Mares SC. Hip, pelvis, and thigh injuries and disorders in the adolescent athlete. *Adolesc Med: State Art Rev* 1998;9(3):551–568.
7. Peck DM. Apophyseal injuries in the young athlete. *Am Fam Physician* 1995;51(8):1891.
8. Micheli LJ. The traction apophysitis. *Clin Sports Med* 1987;6(12):389–404.
9. Harris NH, Murray RO. Lesions of the symphysis in athletes. *Br Med J* 1974;4:211.
10. El-Khoury GY, Daniel WW, Kathol MH. Acute and chronic avulsive injuries. *Radiol Clin North Am* 1997;35(3):747–766.
11. Rossi F, Dragoni S. Acute avulsion fractures of the pelvis in adolescent competitive athletes: prevalence, location, and sports distribution of 203 cases collected. *Skeletal Radiol* 2001;30(3):127–131.
12. Metzmaker JN, Pappas AM. Avulsive fractures of the pelvis. *Am J Sports Med* 1985;13:349–358.
13. Anderson K, Strickland S, Warren R. Hip and groin injuries in athletes. *Am J Sports Med* 2001;29(4):521–533.
14. Rich BS, McKeag DB. When sciatica is not disc disease: detecting piriformis Syndrome in active patients. *Phys Sportsmed* 1992;20(10):104–115.
15. Waters PM, Millis MB. Hip and pelvic injuries in the young athlete. In: Staniski C, Delee J, Drez D, eds. *Pediatric and adolescent sports medicine,* Vol. 3. Philadelphia: WB Saunders, 1994:279–297.
16. Young JL, Laskowski ER, Rock MG. Thigh injuries in athletes. *Mayo Clin Proc* 1993;68:1099–1106.
17. Colosimo AJ, Ireland ML. Thigh compartment syndrome in a football athlete: a case report and review of the literature. *Med Sci Sports Exerc* 1992;24(9):958–963.
18. Agre JC. Hamstring injuries: proposed aetiological factors, prevention, and treatment. *Sports Med* 1987;2:21–33.
19. Brunet ME, Hontas RB. The thigh. In Delee JC, Drez D Jr. eds. *Orthopedic Sports Medicine,* Vol. 2. Philadelphia: WB Saunders, 1994:1086–1112.
20. Kneeland JB. MRI imaging of sports injuries of the hip. *MRI Clin North Am* 1999;7(1):105–115.

Knee Injuries

31

E. James Swenson, Jr.

The most often injured joint in sports participation is the knee (1–10). The keys to diagnosis and management are the following: (a) knowledge of the functional anatomy, (b) understanding the mechanisms of injury in traumatic events, (c) identifying training errors in overuse injuries, (d) familiarity with the more common knee injuries in sport, (e) knowledge of previous injury and rehabilitation of either knee, (f) a precise, thorough physical examination and (g) a meticulous and accurate evidence-based differential diagnosis.

This chapter begins with the diagnosis and management of traumatic and atraumatic knee emergencies. Sections on anatomy, history taking skills, physical examination skills, radiographic evaluation, and technique for aspiration/injection follow. The diagnosis and management of common traumatic and overuse injuries completes the chapter (see Table 31.1 for abbreviations used throughout this chapter).

EMERGENCIES

Traumatic

Acute Knee Dislocation

Clinical Features (11–15)

This injury is uncommon, but with the potential for catastrophic consequences including loss of limb or limb function (11). An acute knee dislocation involves a complete separation of the femoral condyles from the tibial plateau with associated disruption of most of the knee ligaments that results in global laxity of the joint. The condition may present "dislocated" on the field or a spontaneous reduction may occur. An anterior dislocation is most common (40%) followed by posterior dislocation (33%). The most common mechanism for anterior knee dislocation is forced hyperextension. Associated vascular and neurological injury can occur and must be documented. The popliteal artery can be damaged by traction or direct trauma and occurs in up to 40% of injuries. The incidence of neurological injury is reported to be 16% to 40%. The peroneal nerve is more commonly injured than the posterior tibial nerve.

Management (16–18)

The role of the team physician is to appreciate the severity of the injury. If the injury is evaluated on the field, an anterior dislocation will present with a very prominent tibial plateau. The tibia may be rotated but the patella/patellar tendon will be in line with the tibial shaft in contrast to a frank patellar dislocation where the tibiofemoral joint is aligned but the patella is laterally displaced. In a posterior dislocation the patella is dislocated laterally and the tibia posteriorly, with the femoral condyles very prominent. To limit excessive, prolonged traction on the neurovascular structures, a reduction should be attempted. Reduction for an anterior dislocation is accomplished by gentle traction coupled with extension of the knee when a single "clunk" will be felt. A posterior dislocation is reduced by applying a gentle traction coupled with an "anterior drawer force" as the knee is gently extended. The first "clunk" will be the reduction of the tibiofemoral joint and the second "clunk" occurs with the reduction of the patellar into the femoral trochlea (groove). A displaced meniscus may prevent reduction of a knee dislocation (19). Vascular and neurological function must be evaluated and noted followed by immediate transfer for appropriate consultation. The orthopedic and vascular surgeon's consultants will utilize imaging studies to document damage to capsule/ligaments (magnetic resonance imaging [MRI]) and vessels (magnetic resonance angiography [MRA] or arteriogram). To avoid confusion following the spontaneous reduction of a frank patellar dislocation, the examiner may note the presence of an immediate effusion, negative Lachman, negative collateral ligament testing but positive for a tender medial retinaculum coupled with a positive apprehension sign.

TABLE 31.1
ABBREVIATIONS USED THROUGHOUT THIS CHAPTER

Evaluation
MOI: mechanism of injury
ROM: range of motion
Anatomy
ITB: iliotibial band
Quad: quadriceps muscle
HS: hamstring
Ligaments
ACL: anterior cruciate ligament
PCL: posterior cruciate ligament
MCL: medial collateral ligament
LCL: lateral collateral ligament
Diagnosis
PFP: patellofemoral pain
ITBS: ITB syndrome
OCD: osteochondritis dessicans
OA: osteoarthritis
DJD: degenerative joint disease
Treatment
PT: physical therapy
PRE: progressive resistance exercise

Nontraumatic

Septic Arthritis (20)

Clinical Features

Pyogenic arthritis is characterized by an atraumatic severe joint pain, with limited range of motion (ROM) and a warm, swollen and markedly tender joint. A septic joint may present without warmth and only a minor effusion early in the course. Involvement is most often monoarticular but can involve more than one joint. The most commonly involved joint is the knee followed by the hip. In the initial 24 to 72 hours there may be no systemic manifestations. Eventually, systemic signs include fever, chills and an elevated white blood cell (WBC) count. Septic arthritis most often results from direct hematogenous seeding of the synovium. An extra-articular focus of infection can be identified approximately 25% of the time and is useful in deciding on appropriate antibiotic therapy.

Diagnosis and identification of the organism is critical and is made by needle aspiration and examination of the synovial fluid. The leukocyte count is usually over 100,000 per mL with over 90% neutrophils. Approximately 75% of nongonococcal infections are due to gram-positive cocci. Cases involving methicillin resistant *Staphylococcus aureus* (MRSA) have been documented and must be considered (21). Gonococcal infections are common in young adults and a presumptive diagnosis can be made if *Neisseria gonorrhoeae* is isolated from a primary source.

Management

Prompt arthroscopic irrigation and drainage, and initiation of appropriate antibiotic therapy are essential to minimize destruction of the articular cartilage thereby avoiding significant permanent consequences.

ANATOMY

The knee anatomy relevant to the sports medicine physician is presented in Figure 31.1 and in other select diagrams throughout this chapter. The knee joint is supported by a muscular tripod; the quadriceps/patella/patellar tendon anteriorly and the hamstrings (HSs); semitendinosis, semimembranosis at the posteromedial corner and the biceps femoris at the posterolateral corner. This joint is further protected by a thick fibrous capsule and strong ligaments that prevent anterior (anterior cruciate ligament [ACL]), posterior (posterior cruciate ligament [PCL]), medial (medial collateral ligament [MCL]), lateral (lateral collateral ligament [LCL]), and rotatory displacement. In the immature skeleton, the distal femoral physis or the proximal tibial physis may be the weak links and subject to Salter-Harris fractures with sufficient varus and/or valgus force to the knee.

The thick fibrous capsule surrounds the joint and is well outlined when a major effusion is present (inverted U). There is a thin synovial lining inside of the capsule. Multiple compartments are present during the embryonic development of the knee. The compartments join together but with incomplete reabsorption of the connecting walls. The remaining "walls" are known as *plica* (a shelf). The clinically relevant medial plica originates from the suprapatellar plica (that extends in a transverse plane proximal to the superior pole of the patella) and extends medially to the anterior fat pad (see Figure 31.2).

The cruciate ligaments cross one another from their point of origin on the femur to the point of insertion on the tibial plateau. The MCL is a broad, long ligament extending from the medial femoral condyle to the medial tibia plateau at the level of the tibial tubercle. The shorter LCL originates from the lateral femoral condyle and inserts onto the head of the fibula. Significant injury to any of these ligaments may result in laxity and clinical instability.

The patellofemoral (PF) joint is the most common site for anterior knee pain among all ages, fitness levels and sporting activities. The quadriceps control patellar tracking keeping the patella centered within the femoral trochlea with knee flexion and extension. Quadricep fatigue or inhibition may disrupt PF joint mechanics.

The iliotibial band (ITB) acts to provide dynamic lateral stability as the band crosses the joint line and inserts

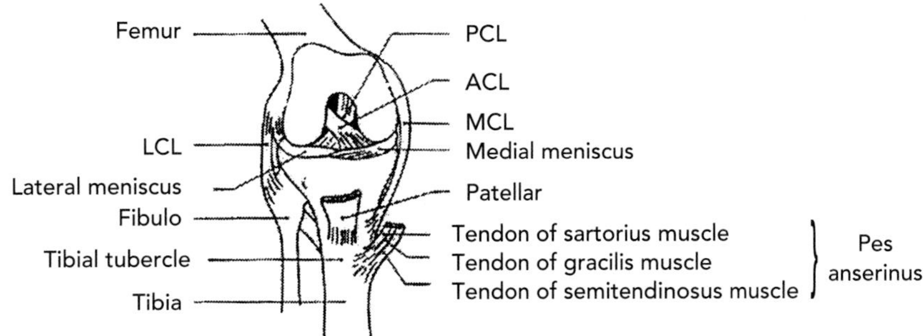

A. Anterior Aspect

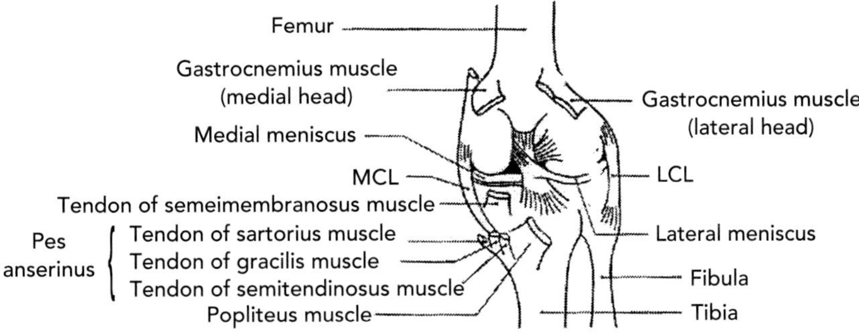

B. Posterior Aspect

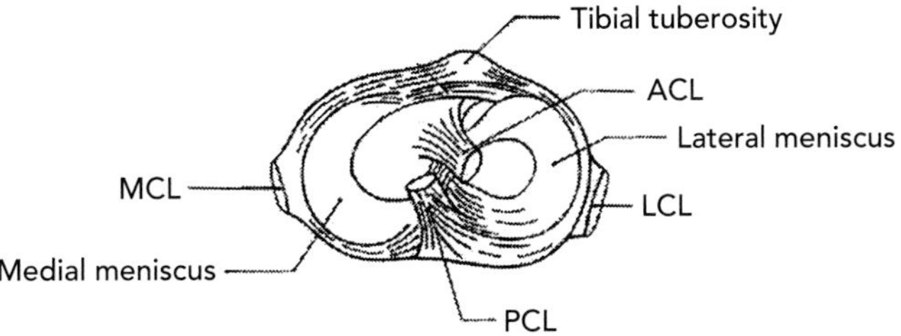

C. Cross-sectional caudal Aspect

Figure 31.1 Anatomy of the knee. PCL = posterior cruciate ligament; ACL = anterior cruciate ligament; MCL = medial cruciate ligament; LCL = lateral cruciate ligament.

into Gerdy's tubercle. A group of three muscles, the semitendinosis, gracilis, and sartorius insert medial to the tibia tubercle, and are collectively known as the *pes anserine tendons*. Both the ITB and the pes anserine tendons are common sites of overuse injury. The popliteus muscle originates from the posteriomedial tibia, forms a tendon that crosses underneath the LCL and inserts into the lateral femoral condyle anterior to the LCL. This tendon is an infrequent site of overuse injury or rupture.

There are many bursae that surround the knee. The prepatellar bursa located directly over the patella and the suprapatellar bursa located superior to the suprapatellar pouch of the capsule can become inflamed and swollen following blunt trauma. Bursae associated with the ITB, pes anserine tendons, patellar tendon, LCL, MCL, and semimembranosis muscle may become inflamed as a result of overuse injury.

The menisci (22,23) are composed of a C-shaped (medial meniscus) and an O-shaped (lateral meniscus) that act as shock absorbers and distribute body weight evenly through the femoral condyles onto the articular surface of the tibia. Complete removal of a meniscus will in time result in severe degenerative arthritis due to an asymmetrical redistribution of forces. The medial meniscus is attached to the MCL and joint capsule and is sometimes involved in knee injury involving a valgus force. The lateral meniscus is not attached to the LCL and is less frequently torn. Wrestling is the only sport where an equal number of injuries to both menisci occur (24,25).

HISTORY (26)

A precise and accurate history is essential to formulate a thorough differential diagnosis. Site of pain diagrams correlate the anatomical site with the most likely sources of pain in traumatic (see Figure 31.3) and overuse injury (see Figure 31.4). It is not uncommon to identify incomplete rehabilitation as a factor in a knee injury. The mechanism of injury (MOI) provides insight into the

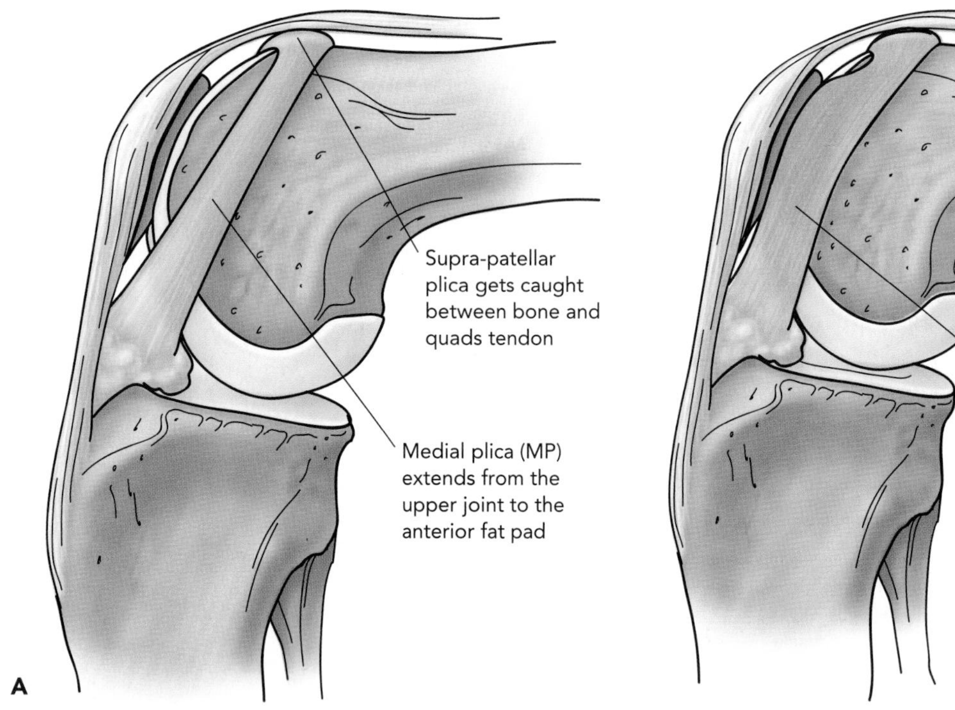
Supra-patellar
plica gets caught
between bone and
quads tendon
Medial plica (MP)
extends from the
upper joint to the
anterior fat pad
A
MP tightens as knee
extends and 'catching'
or pseudo-locking may
occur at 30 degrees as
the MP chaffs across the
medial femoral condyle
B

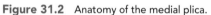

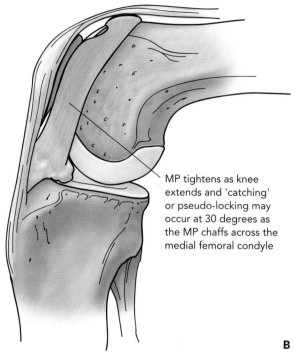

Figure 31.2 Anatomy of the medial plica.

anatomical structures at risk as a result of the trauma and the physical examination confirms the extent of injury. Table 31.2 identifies the direction of force and the supporting ligaments and other structures at risk. Most overuse injuries result from training errors that must be identified and modified in order to prevent recurrence.

Take the opportunity to gather precise information and direct the conversation as needed by asking specific questions about the following: (a) MOI or training errors; (b) site and nature of pain felt and determine the current limitations to participation (often a 10-point pain scale can be effective in quantifying the pain); (c) previous injury, surgery, and rehabilitation to date; (d) upcoming events and how important it is for the athlete patient. (For the in-season athlete the goal will be symptoms control, strength maintenance, and return to play [RTP], whereas for the out of season athlete or a low priority sport, the goal will be to control symptoms by limiting activity with a major emphasis on strengthening to expedite full recovery), and (e) ask the athlete if there is anything else that should be noted.

Presenting knee problems may be **atraumatic**, with the absence of any known trauma or overuse, a **result of a traumatic event**, or the result of **overuse**. Different information is needed to form a differential diagnosis for each category.

1. Atraumatic
   a. *Describe for me what happened to your knee(s)?*
   b. *Where do you feel the pain or discomfort?* (See Figure 31.4)
   c. *When was the first time you felt the pain?* If there is no history of trauma or overuse, it is still important to assume there may be an overuse component. Consider asking questions related to overuse.
   d. *Have you experienced any swelling?* If yes ask, How much swelling is there at this time compared to what there has been? (This question is asked without looking at the knee, it is nonjudgmental and allows you to gain insight as to the point of reference of the athlete.) If the athlete answers yes to swelling ask, **Has there been any recurrent swelling?** If yes find out how much and how often. **Have you noticed swelling, redness or stiffness in any other joints? Do you have any family history of arthritis?** If yes ask about which family member, age and type and severity of arthritis. If index of suspicion is present, follow an arthritis work-up (osteoarthritis [OA], gout, pseudogout, rheumatoid arthritis [RA], juvenile rheumatoid arthritis [JRA], etc.) (see Table 31.3)
   e. *How intense is the pain?* If the pain is moderate to severe at rest and the patient states that any movement of the knee causes intense pain, one must consider a septic joint (see section Emergencies)
   f. *Anything else you would like me to write down?*
2. Traumatic (see Table 31.4)
   a. *Describe for me what happened to your knee(s)?* Make sure you have a clear understanding of the MOI.
   b. *Was there a "pop" felt or heard?* If yes, think ACL until proved otherwise, but realize there may also be a patellar instability issue. With a frank patellar dislocation, there is a "pop" felt when the patella relocates over the lateral femoral condyle. Less often,

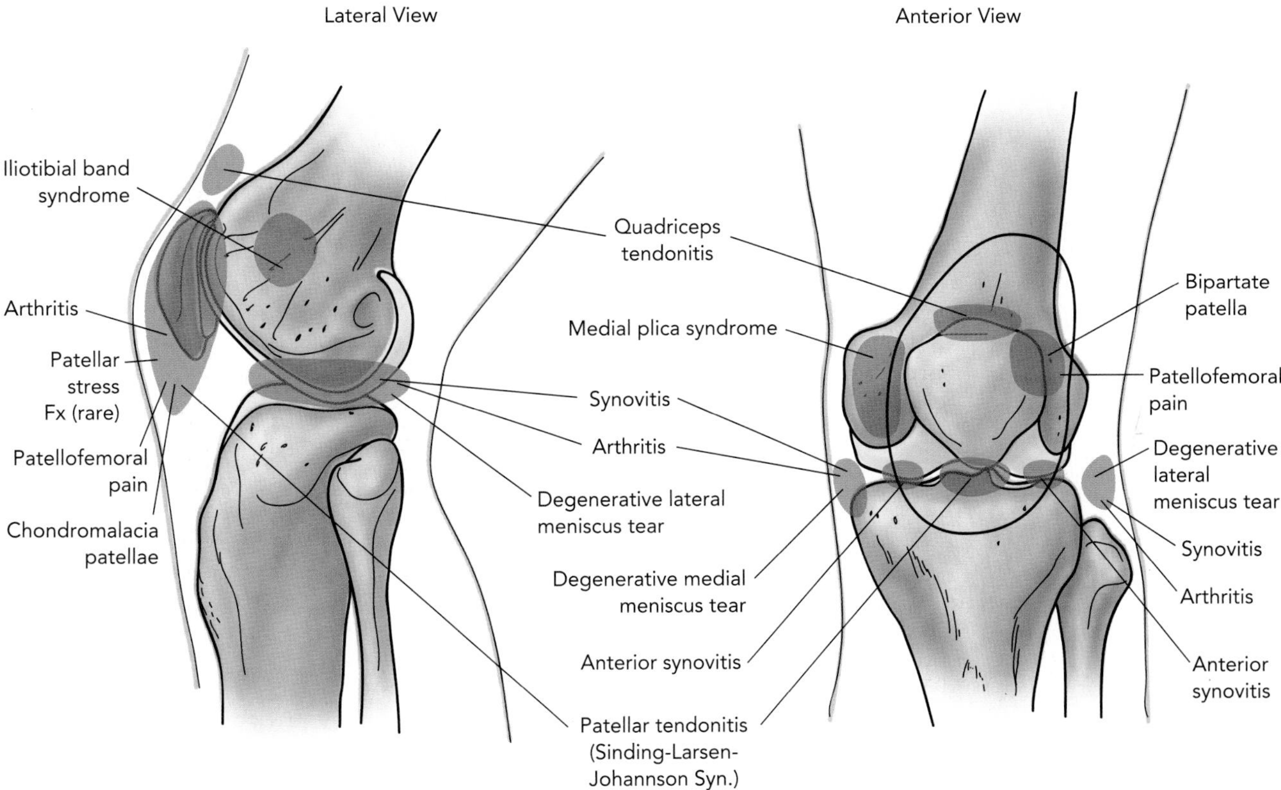

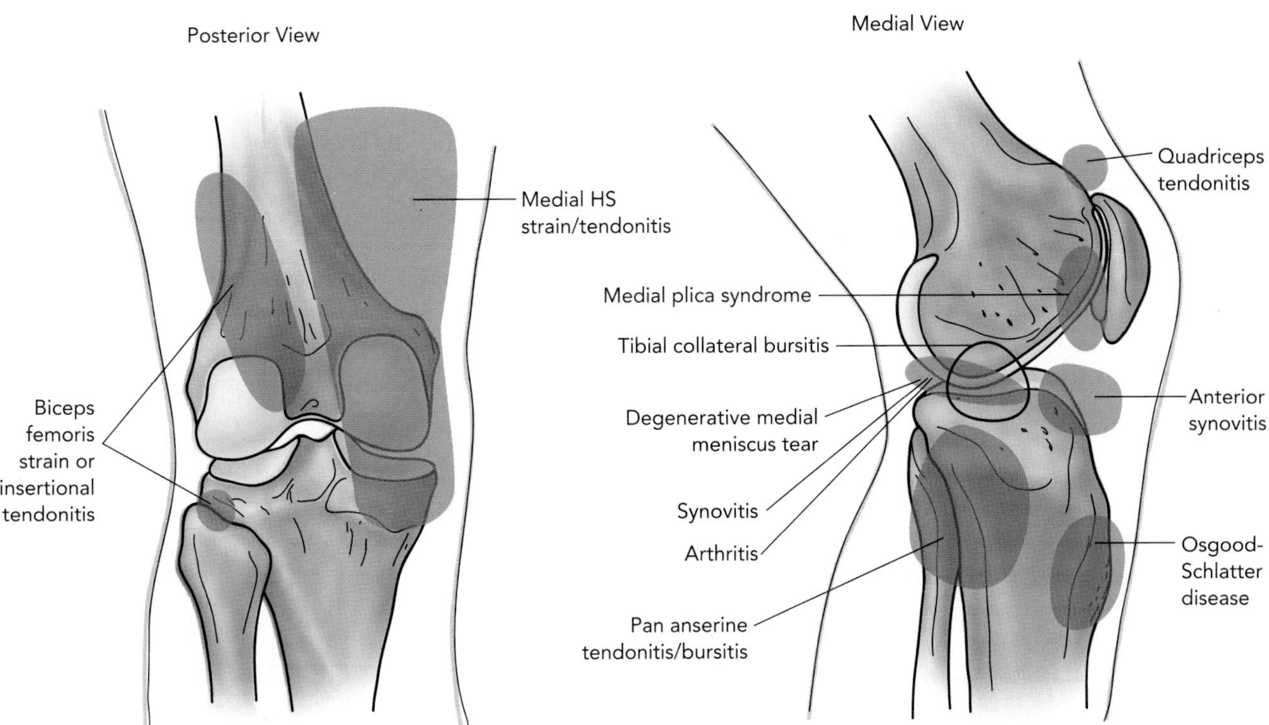

Figure 31.3 Differential diagnosis based on site of pain following traumatic injury. HS = hamstring.

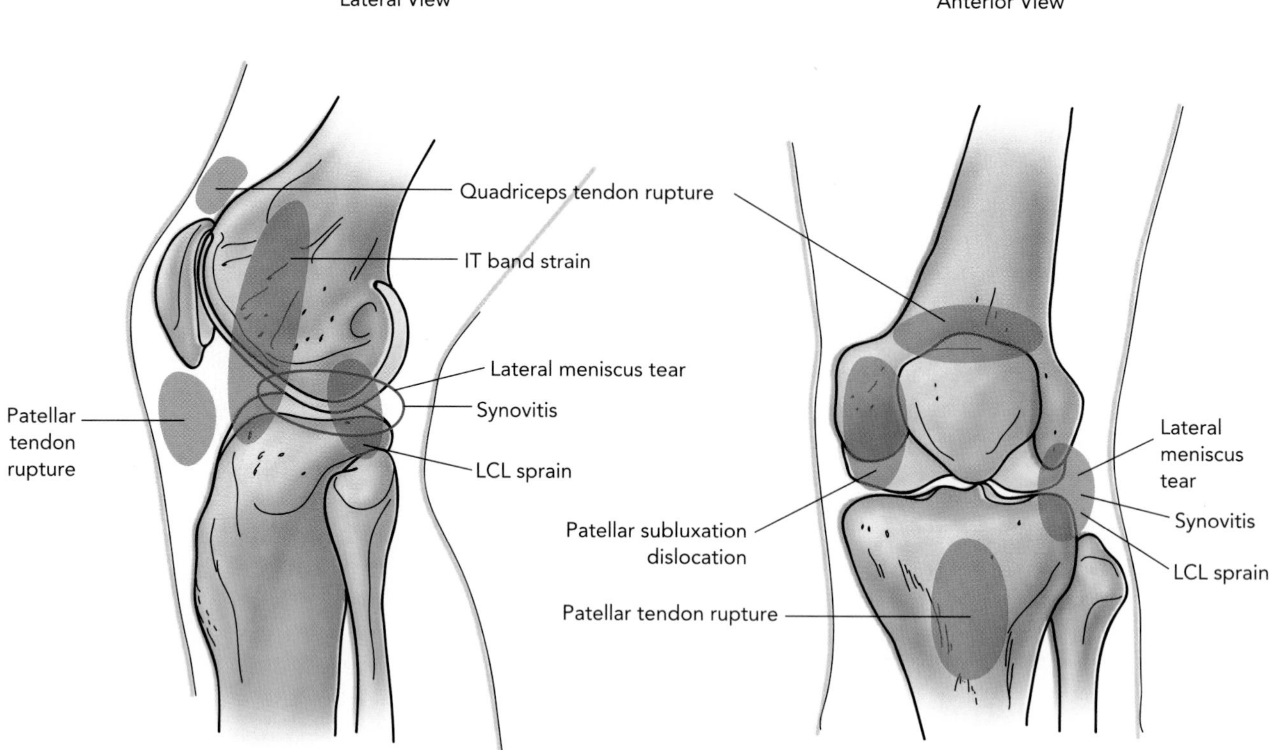

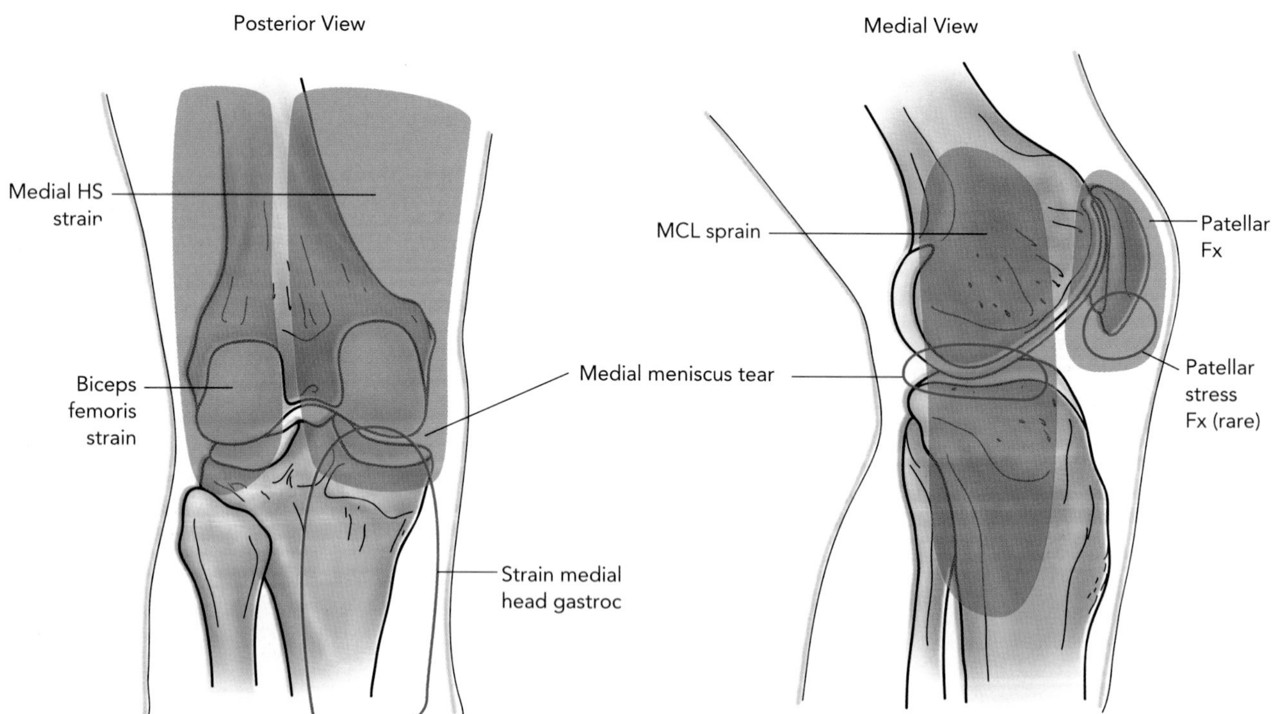

Figure 31.4 Differential diagnosis based on site of pain following overuse injury. HS = hamstring; PFP = patellofemoral pain; IT = iliotibial; LCL = lateral cruciate ligament.

TABLE 31.2

PREDICTING KNEE INJURY USING TRAUMATIC MECHANISM OF INJURY

Contact vs. Noncontact	Example in Sport	Structures Injured	Differential Diagnosis
		Contact: Foot Planted	
Valgus stress (force from outside knee that results in knee bent inward)	"Clip" in football	Soft tissue Bone: immature skeleton Bone: mature skeleton MCL Medial meniscus ACL	Contusion Saltar Harris fracture (distal femoral epiphysis) Fracture distal tibia or avulsion MCL MCL sprain grade I—III Possible torn meniscus Possible ACL sprain grade I–III
Varus stress (uncommon, force directed from inside of the knee toward the outside)	Player "blind sided" and unaware that opponent was coming; hit on the inside of the knee	Soft tissue LCL ITB	Contusion LCL sprain grade I—III ITB strain
Hyperextension force	Blow to anterior knee	Soft tissue Posterior capsule ACL Possible PCL if force persists	Contusion Posterior capsular sprain ACL sprain PCL sprain
Forced flexion	Landing in flexed position; skiing	PCL	PCL sprain grade I–III
Posterolateral directed force in extended knee	Football	Soft tissue Popliteal tendon	Contusion Popliteal tendon rupture
Anterior force at the level of tibial tubercle or anterior tibia.	Catcher blocking the plate in baseball or softball	Soft tissue PCL	Contusion PCL Sprain grade I–III
Anterior, medial or lateral force directed at quadriceps	Soccer or rugby knee to quadriceps	Soft tissue	Quadriceps contusion, mild to severe, myositis ossificans
		Noncontact Foot Planted	
Weight bearing, rotation toward planted foot ACL deficient knee	Ackward movement, but may occur in soccer, basketball, and football	ACL Possible meniscus Chondral surface Possible meniscus Chondral surface	ACL sprain Gr I—III Torn meniscus 50% in acute injury grade III ACL, 4:1 ratio lateral to medial 4:1 ratio, medial to lateral Osteochondral or chondral fracture
Weight bearing, rotation away from planted foot	Common movement in many agility sports	Patellar instability Chondral surface	Patellar dislocation or subluxation Osteochondral or chondral fracture
Any weight bearing with rotation	Common movement in many agility sports	Meniscus Chondral surface	Torn medial or lateral meniscus Osteochondral or chondral fracture
Jumping or landing	Jump shot in basketball	Quadriceps or patellar tendon	Complete rupture of quadriceps or patellar tendon
Falling with knee flexed landing on tibial tubercle	Soccer, football	PCL	PCL sprain grade I–III

MCL = medial collateral ligament; ACL = anterior cruciate ligament; LCL = lateral collateral ligament; ITB = iliotibial band; PCL = posterior cruciate ligament.

TABLE 31.3

EVALUATION AND SIGNIFICANCE OF KNEE SWELLING

Effusion/Swelling	Timing	Anatomical Structures	Differential Diagnosis
Intra-articular swelling = effusion (see Table 31.5) Most often post traumatic and associated with "pop"	Immediate (onset 2–6 hr) Hemarthrosis Most often 3–4+ effusion	Ligament injury, patellar instability, fracture, meniscus, synovial lining	ACL, patellar dislocation, osteochondral or tibial plateau fracture, tear in vascular portion of the meniscus, synovial contusion (if multiple ligaments are involved, suspect knee dislocation [emergencies])
Atraumatic effusion	Delayed	Capsule/synovial lining	Pigmented villonodular synovitis If pain is excessive, consider septic joint (emergencies)
Posttraumatic Effusion	Delayed (over 24 h) Synovial fluid Most often minor 1-2+ effusion	Meniscus, synovial lining, patellar instability, arthritis,	Torn Meniscus, reactive synovitis, patellar subluxation, OA
Most often activity related	Recurrent Most often minor	Arthritis, meniscus, chondral surface	Degenerative meniscus, OA, chondromalacia patellae, possible old ligament injury
Extra-articular swelling Post-traumatic	Immediate quadriceps trauma Valgus stress	Result of trauma to quadriceps MCL	Quadriceps contusion (may be difficult initially to distinguish from a major effusion) MCL grade II–III
Extra-articular swelling; may be post-traumatic	Delayed	Difficult to distinguish outline of patella	Prepatellar bursitis
Extra-articular swelling Overuse	Delayed	Various bursa Site specific	Pes anserine, ITP, deep infrapatellar, stress fracture medial tibial plateau
Extra-articular swelling Posterior knee	Delayed	Posterior capsule, bursa	Bakers cyst, lipoma, ganglion, semimembranosis bursitis

ACL = anterior cruciate ligament; OA = osteoarthritis; MCL = medial collateral ligament; ITP =.

there is a "pop" with a nondisplaced tibial plateau fracture or an osteochondral fracture. Rarely a torn meniscus will result in a "pop." All of the above will most often result in an immediate swelling because of the bleeding into the joint.

c. *Was there any swelling? How long was it before it began to swell?* Any immediate swelling represents a hemarthrosis with consideration of the differential in B. *Was there swelling by the next morning?* A delayed swelling (over 24 hours) represents synovial fluid and may represent a torn meniscus, synovitis, OA, or a true chondromalacia patella. *How much swelling is there at this time compared to what there has been?* (This question is asked without looking at the knee, it is nonjudgmental and allows you to gain insight as to the point of reference of the athlete.) Also, when there is swelling, it may be intra-articular (effusion) or extra-articular such as with a Grade II MCL sprain (see Table 31.3).

d. *Have you had any limitations in motion?* (Your ability to fully bend and straighten out the knee.)

e. *Have you experienced any catching, locking up or giving way of the knee (mechanical symptoms)?* Catching or locking up (inability to fully extend the knee) suggest a loose body or unstable meniscus. If the athlete is currently unable to extend the knee ask, *Have you been able to straighten your knee even once since the injury?* If the answer is no, suspect a displaced bucket-handle tear of the medial meniscus. If the athlete has experienced any giving way episodes, it is important to ask, *How many times has the knee given way? Did you experience any giving way episodes before the injury?* If yes, suspect a previous injury. Also ask, *When your knee gives way, is the sequence giving way followed by pain or is there pain felt before a giving way episode?* If it is the former, suspect a chronic ligamentous injury. If the latter suspect a patellofemoral pain (PFP), iliotibial band syndrome (ITBS), medial plica, meniscus, tendonitis, or any overuse injury that can cause pain with quadriceps muscle inhibition and giving way.

f. *Where are you feeling the pain?* (See Figure 31.3)

TABLE 31.4
DIFFERENTIAL DIAGNOSIS TO CONSIDER IN SEATED POSITION

Palpation

Numbers 1–10 should be considered in most examinations as it will provide information on PFP, medial plica syndrome, ITBS and patellar tendonitis, the most common overuse injuries. An effusion can be better identified in the supine position. Begin will less symptomatic or asymptomatic knee. It is helpful to consider a differential diagnosis as the examination is performed. The following is a suggested sequence to follow.

(a) **Tibial tubercle** (immature skeleton; Osgood Schlatter's disease, mature skeleton; ossicle within tendon, insertional patellar tendonitis, stress fracture of tibial tubercle.
(b) **Patellar tendon mid-body** (superficial or deep infrapatellar bursitis)
(c) **Anterior joint lines** (anterior synovitis found in 50% severe PFP, fat pad inflammation)
(d) **Medial joint line distal 2/3** (medial meniscus, reactive synovitis, MCL sprain, tibial collateral bursitis, DJD medial compartment)
(e) **Lateral joint line distal 2/3** (lateral meniscus, reactive synovitis, DJD lateral compartment)
(f) **Medial plica** (medial plica syndrome)
(g) **Medial femoral condyle** (friction rub from medial plica syndrome)
(h) **Lateral femoral epicondyle** (ITB syndrome friction rub)
(i) **Medial and lateral patellar facets** (PFP, patellar subluxation)
(j) **Inferior pole of the patella** (patellar tendonitis, Sinding-Larsen-Johansson syndrome, patellar stress fracture if involves distal 25%)

The following structures to be palpated as appropriate based on history

(k) **Patella** (symptomatic bipartite patella, stress fracture, prepatellar bursitis)
(l) **Superior pole of patella** (quadriceps tendonitis)
(m) **MCL** (mid portion—same as no. 4, distal portion—same as no. 11)
(n) **LCL isolated by placing patient's foot on opposite knee (figure 31.4 position) and palpating ligament** (LCL sprain, popliteus tendonitis; insertion anterior to LCL)
(o) **Head of fibula** (biceps femoris insertional tendonitis)
(p) **Neck of fibula** (Common peroneal nerve injury, sprain of proximal tibiofibular joint)
(q) **Pes anserine insertion** (tendonitis, bursitis, stress fracture of medial tibial plateau)
(r) **Posterior knee** (capsular sprain, Bakers cyst vs. semimembranosis bursitis, hamstring strain, head of gastro strain)
(s) **Superior pole of patella** (quadriceps tendonitis)

PFP = patellofemoral pain; MCL = medial collateral ligament; DJD = degenerative joint disease; ITB = iliotibial band; LCL = lateral collateral ligament.

g. *Have you experienced any prior significant injury to either knee? What type of treatment did you have? Was your rehabilitation complete?*

h. *Anything else you would like me to write down?*

3. **Overuse Injury**

a. *When did you first feel any pain? At what point did it become a disabling pain with activity that interfered with your ability to practice, participate in games or even in routine daily activities? Has there been any change in the character of the pain over time?* The pain may begin as a shin splint but progress to a tibial stress fracture.

b. *Where they any changes in your training 4 to 6 weeks before the onset of your pain? Any change in the duration or intensity of workouts? More interval workouts or hills? Any change in shoes or surface? Do you always run on the same side of the road?* Down leg will supinate and up leg will pronate leading to ITBS or PFP.

c. *Have you noticed any swelling?* (See Table 31.3)

d. *Please point out where you are feeling your pain?* (See Figure 31.4)

e. *Is your pain felt during and/or following activity?* If pain is felt with activity ask, *Is there a disabling pain with activity that prevents full participation?* If there is only pain felt following activity with or without a nondisabling pain felt with activity, it will respond much differently that a disabling pain felt with and following activity.

f. *Have you had any treatments to date? Have you made any modifications in your training?* Important to document response or lack there of to any treatments to date.

g. *What is on your schedule for the next 2 weeks?* Important to find out about any upcoming events that the athlete is preparing for.

h. *Describe a typical day for me? What do you feel like when you first wake up in the morning? How about going up or down stairs at school? Do you feel any symptoms by lunchtime? Are symptoms related to how active you are on a given day?* These questions can be helpful in defining the extant and severity of the symptoms.

i. *Anything else you would like me to write down?*

PHYSICAL EXAMINATION (27)

A variety of techniques and sequences are used to examine the knee. Each examiner may choose those techniques and sequences that fit one's style. It is important to be thorough and realize that competence results from practice. Never be afraid to adopt a new or different technique if it will improve your ability as a clinician. Never be afraid to leave something out if it is redundant. The following are some techniques that have been proved to have clinical value.

The knee examination should be modified to accommodate the patient's clinical presentation. For an **acute severe injury**, the examination should be carried out with the patient in the **supine position**; otherwise, if the **sitting position is comfortable** for the patient, identification of relevant landmarks will be facilitated for the examiner.

Many traumatic injuries and overuse syndromes affect very localized structures, which emphasizes the importance of knowing the functional anatomy and performing a precise examination (see Figures 31.3 and 31.4).

The biomechanical alignment and Q angle (if desired) can be noted in the standing position and throughout the examination as needed.

Biomechanical alignment. Note gait, genu varum or valgus, tibia varum, femoral anteversion, tibial torsion, arch type and heel forefoot alignment (forefoot varus or valgus). All of these factors may impact on knee mechanics.

Q angle. This is represented by the angle formed from the anterior superior iliac spine (ASIS) to the center of the patella from above, transected with a second line originating from the tibial tubercle to the center of the patella from below. Those individuals with an increased Q angle (females) or with the so-called miserable malalignment syndrome (femoral anteversion, tibial torsion, genu valgum, pes planus with a significant forefoot varus) are theoretically at higher risk for developing PFP. In clinical practice however, there are many other variables that contribute so that the role that an increased Q angle plays, is not a major predictive factor. The risk suggested by the Q angle, can be used to motivate compliance with rehabilitation. As opposed to PFP, the Q angle is more critical in the evaluation of patellar instability.

The knee examination in the **seated position** will include the following: (a) inspection looking for any bony or soft tissue swelling, bruising or muscle atrophy and (b) palpation (see Table 31.4).

TABLE 31.5
EVALUATION OF EFFUSION

Graded on a scale 0–4+
4+ = Tense effusion (entire inverted U-shaped capsule outlined)
3+ = Less tense effusion of entire capsule
2+ = No fluid identified within suprapatellar pouch. Obvious medial bulge on inspection enhanced with compression of suprapatellar pouch and lateral capsule
1+ = Less obvious but distinct small medial bulge with compression of supra-patellar pouch and lateral capsule
0 = No effusion
*Intermediate grades such as 1–2+ or 3–4+ can be implemented as needed.
Major effusion >2–3+ (most often 3–4+)
Minor effusion <2+ (most often 2+)

Steps included in the **supine position** include: (a) inspection, (b) palpation, (c) ligament testing, (d) apprehension testing, (e) meniscal testing, (f) muscle testing, and (g) functional testing.

Inspection in supine position. Note effusion (see Table 31.5), swelling, soft tissue or bony deformity, muscle atrophy, ecchymosis, erythema, abrasion, or surgical scares.

Bony and Soft Tissue Palpation

Examination in Supine Position allows for evaluation of thigh muscle atrophy or swelling.

Thigh Muscle Atrophy or Swelling

Pen marks can be placed mid thigh 5 and 15 cm above superior pole of patella to measure thigh circumference. The measurement is most accurate when thigh muscles contract. Ask the athlete to tighten the quadriceps and lift the leg off the table. An atrophy or swelling that is equal to or greater than 1 to 2 cm is felt to be relevant.

Ligamentous Evaluation

Table 31.6 gives the details of the evaluation of the laxity of ligaments.

Anterior/Posterior Stability Evaluation

ACL evaluation/Lachman (28). The ACL can be evaluated with the Lachman, Pivot Shift Test and the Anterior Drawer. The **Lachman** is the most reliable test for isolated ACL tears. It is performed by grasping the distal femur and proximal tibia (see Figure 31.5). With the knee in 15 to 20 degrees flexion, gently increase the anterior force applied to the tibia while

TABLE 31.6
LIGAMENTOUS LAXITY ASSESSMENT

mm Movement[a]	Grade
5	1+
10	2+
>10	3+

[a]Laxity is relative, based on the laxity found in the control knee (i.e., control 6-mm movement compared with 10-mm movement on the injured side). Difference would be 4mm = 1+ laxity. While there may be a difference in the laxity of ligaments between individuals, comparing the same ligament in knees of the same individual should be symmetrical.

stabilizing the femur. The force is directed in a pure anteroposterior (AP) plane. It is important to encourage the athlete to relax the HSs or the Lachman cannot be effectively done. The amount of anterior excursion, as well as the quality of the end point, should be noted. Any movement more than 3.5 to 5 mm (1–2+) is consistent with a complete rupture of the ACL. A "soft end-point" even without excessive excursion is consistent with a complete rupture of the ACL (HSs must be relaxed). Following the Lachman test and before additional testing, it can be very effective to perform the Apprehension test.

Patellar stability testing (the Apprehension test). To test for patella instability, the examiner following Lachman testing can make a slight adjustment of both thumbs. They are placed along the medial patellar border at the 1:30/4:30 positions for the right knee and 10:30/7:30 for the left knee (see Figure 31.6). A direct lateral force is applied and the knee is gently flexed from 0 to 30 degrees while continuing the lateral force to the medial border. At 30 degrees, the lateral femoral condyle is at its shallowest point. A positive apprehension sign occurs when the patient senses impending subluxation and simultaneously contracts the quadriceps, sits up, grasps the knee and has eyes the size of baseballs staring at you.

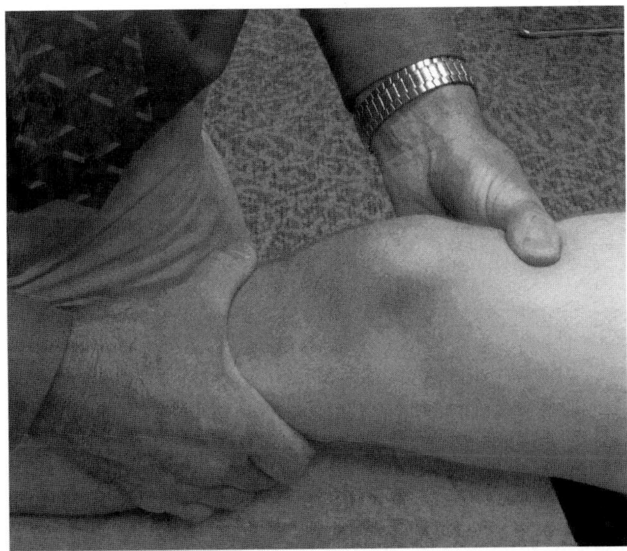

Figure 31.5 Technique for Lachman testing.

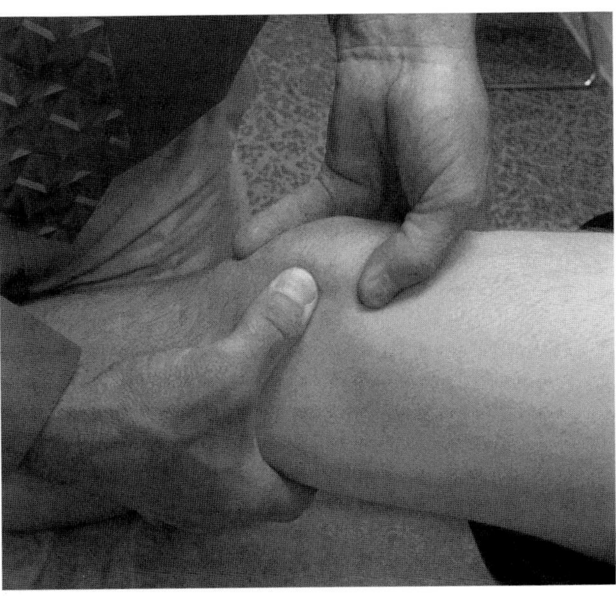

Figure 31.6 Technique for apprehension testing.

ACL evaluation/pivot shift. The **Pivot Shift Test** identifies anterolateral rotary instability, only present in the ACL deficient knee. The test reproduces the exact mechanism of instability that the patient experiences with giving way episodes. This test is performed by internally rotating the tibia (to keep the tibia in a reduced position), placing a valgus stress and an axial load on the knee (to accentuate subluxation) (see Figure 31.7). The knee begins in full extension

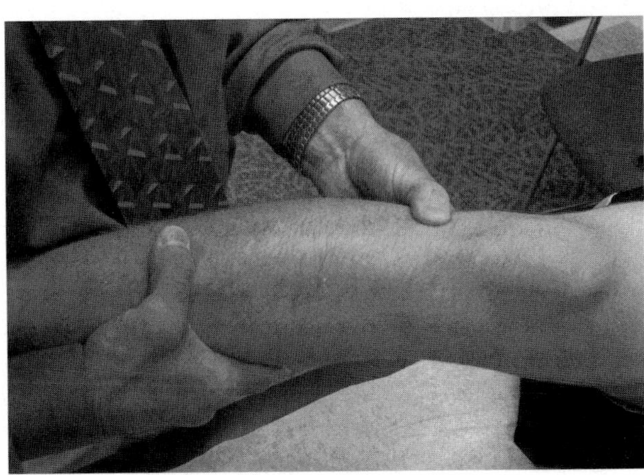

Figure 31.7 Technique for lateral pivot shift testing.

and is gently flexed. Anterolateral subluxation of the lateral tibial plateau is documented by the examiner and recognized by the patient as what happens when the knee gives way. The Pivot Shift is technically more difficult to master and is recommended only for sports medicine physicians. Primary care physicians should focus on the Lachman test.

PCL evaluation/posterior drawer. There may be a negative reverse Lachman test (the Lachman test can seem to be completely normal with solid end points in both anterior and posterior directions), hence the **gold standard for a PCL sprain** is the **posterior drawer test**. In a chronic injury with excessive laxity, it can be difficult to distinguish between PCL and ACL involvement. In both instances, there is a significant amount of anterior excursion. The PCL-deficient knee begins from an abnormal posterior position and moves forward to the normal position whereas the opposite is true with a chronic ACL starting in a normal position and moving to an abnormal forward position. The MOI if known may help indicate which ligament is involved but a careful physical examination is the key to diagnosis.

Drawer testing. The **Anterior Drawer** is much less sensitive than the Lachman or Pivot Shift test for confirming the diagnosis of an acute or chronic ACL injury. The **Posterior Drawer** as mentioned earlier is the **gold standard for PCL evaluation** and is performed with the patient in the supine position, with the hip flexed to 45 degrees and the knee to 90 degrees and the examiner sitting on the patient's foot to stabilize the tibia (see Figure 31.8). A view from the side may demonstrate a "**posterior sag sign**" with a posterior sagging of the tibial tubercle on the injured side. The hands are placed behind the proximal tibia and the tibia is pulled toward the examiner. It is important to check for relaxation of the HS muscles, as the examination is difficult to perform in the presence of contracting HSs. The test is performed with the foot pointing straight ahead. The thumbs are placed over the anterior tibial shelf and amount of shelf is appreciated. Forward movement is consistent with ACL laxity (comparison is relative to the uninjured knee). Backward movement, loss of tibial shelf (anterior tibia becomes flush with the femoral condyles) is consistent with PCL laxity. The technique for evaluation of the posterolateral corner at times associated with a PCL injury is discussed in the section on PCL Injuries.

Medial/Lateral Stability Evaluation

Medial stability. Valgus stress is applied to the knee in full extension to test the integrity of the MCL and cruciate ligaments. Valgus stress applied to the knee at 30 degrees flexion (see Figure 31.9) isolates the MCL as cruciate ligaments are relaxed. Laxity greater than that of the control knee indicates a sprain of the MCL. It is important to identify the quality of the end point when stressing the knee. Increased laxity but with a solid, abrupt end point indicates a partial tear of the MCL, while a soft, mushy end point and 3+ laxity indicates a complete rupture of the MCL. Splinting by contraction of the HSs or adductors may make the examination difficult. It is also important to note the presence of pain during the examination. Absence of pain may indicate laxity from a previous injury or a complete rupture of the MCL. Isolated Grade III sprains of the MCL are uncommon but may be less painful than the common Grade II sprains.

Lateral stability. A varus stress is applied to the knee in full extension to test the integrity of the LCL, ITB, popliteus muscle, lateral capsule, and cruciate ligaments. As in the preceding text, increased laxity as compared to the uninjured knee indicates injury. Varus stress applied to the knee at 30 degrees flexion isolates the LCL (see Figure 31.10). It is important to note that most people have a degree of physiological laxity in this position. By gently placing the lateral

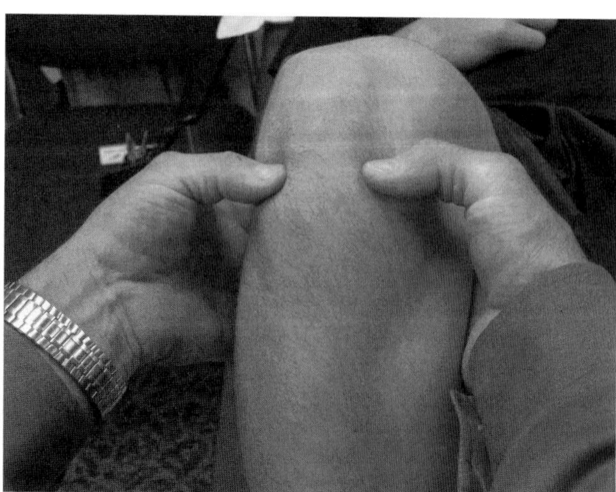

Figure 31.8 Technique for posterior drawer testing.

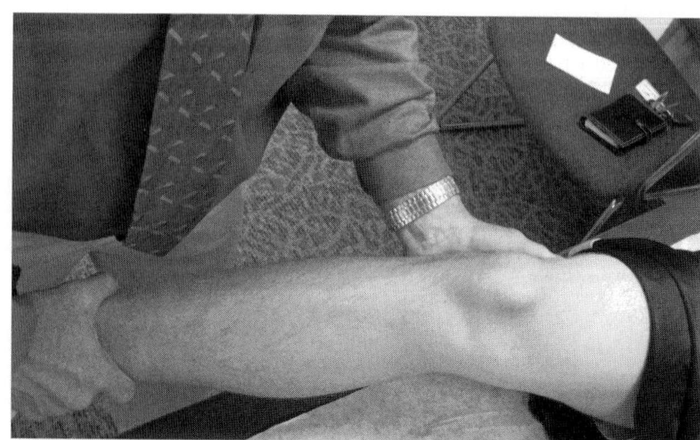

Figure 31.9 Technique for medial instability testing.

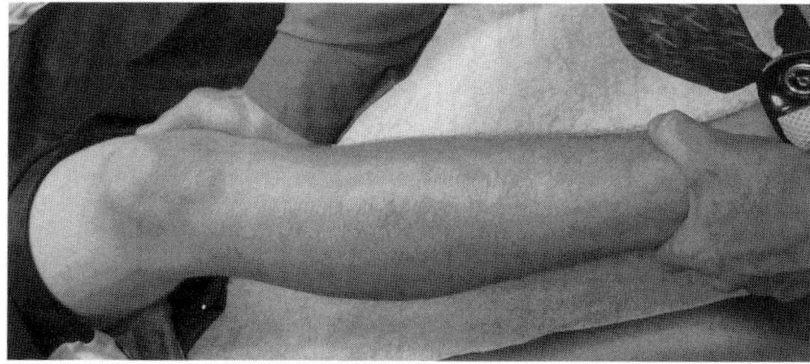

Figure 31.10 Technique for lateral instability testing.

ankle of the injured knee onto the opposite knee, "Figure of 4 position" (see Figure 31.11), the LCL can be readily palpated.

Meniscal Evaluation

Meniscus evaluation. A simple yet very effective way to assess a knee for a possible meniscal injury is to fully flex the knee (see Figure 31.12). The vast majority of torn menisci occur in the posterior horn and/or body of the meniscus and full flexion of the knee produces pain as the menisci are compressed. The McMurray Test can be used to localize the site of the tear. The knee is fully flexed and the heel is pointed in the direction of the meniscus to be tested, external rotation for the medial meniscus and internal rotation for the lateral meniscus (see Figures 31.13 and 31.14). The index or middle finger and thumb are then placed on the joint lines and the knee extended. A positive test results when a painful click or pain alone is felt and is recognized as "the pain" by the athlete. A painless click is not significant. It is not uncommon for there to be medial joint line tenderness coupled with a positive lateral McMurray and a lateral joint line tenderness coupled with a positive medial McMurray (29). Additional tests do not seem to increase the sensitivity of testing. Remember that a localized synovitis may present as a torn meniscus.

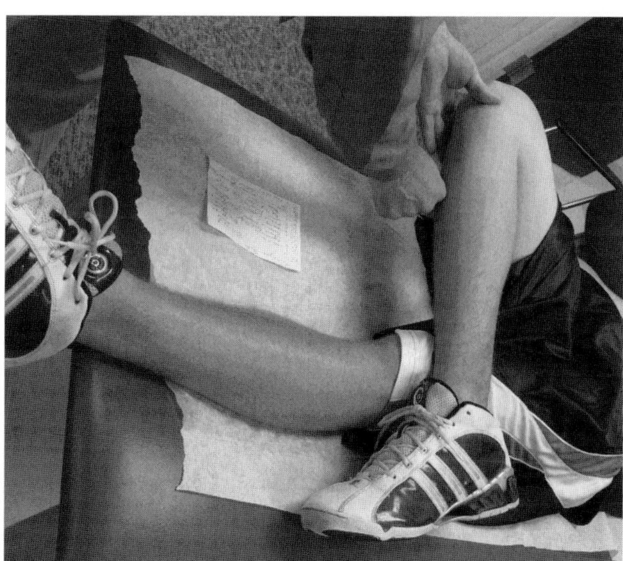

Figure 31.11 Utilization of "figure 31.4 position."

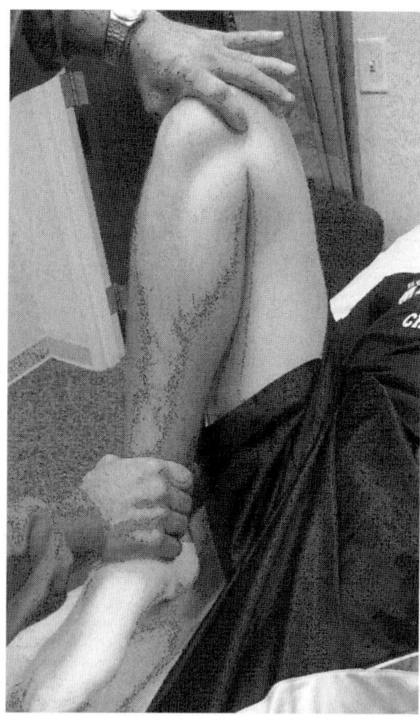

Figure 31.12 Meniscal testing—full knee flexion.

ITB Flexibility Evaluation

Ober test. The Ober test is used to evaluate ITB inflexibility in an ITB syndrome. The athlete is placed on his/her side with the injured knee up. The examiner stands behind the patient and places one hand on the hip and grasps the ipsilateral ankle with the other hand. The knee is flexed to 45 degrees and the hip extended (see Figure 31.15). The expectation is that the knee will fall toward the table by a few inches if there is adequate flexibility present. A tight ITB will remain in the same plane.

Radiographic Studies (30–38)

Routine radiographs are not necessary in the evaluation of every knee injury. Indications may include: (a) Severe pain following blunt trauma, (b) Presence of a minor, major or recurrent effusion, (c) Pain out of proportion to the apparent pathology present, and (d) Ongoing symptoms for more than 4 to 6 weeks duration.

Radiographic Evaluation for Mechanical Symptoms

If the history and examination are consistent with "mechanical symptoms", four views of the knee (AP, lateral, tunnel, and Merchant) are needed to try and identify a

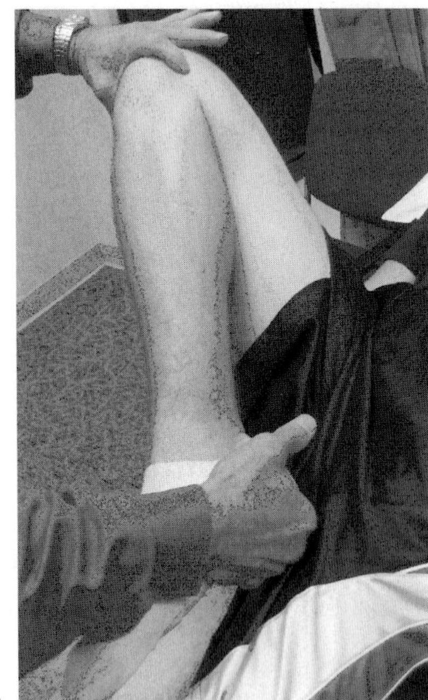

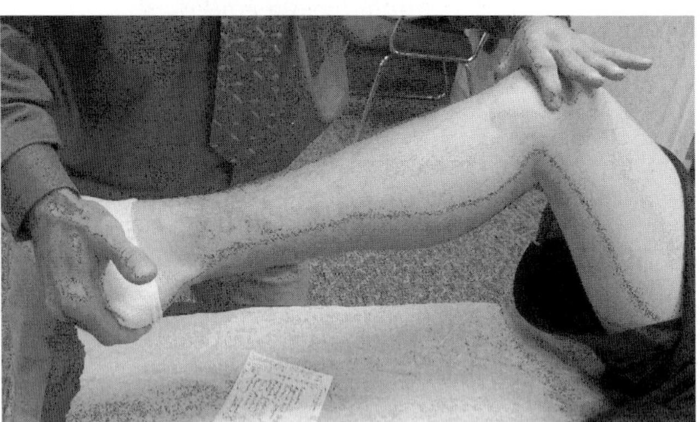

A B

Figure 31.13 **A and B:** McMurray testing—medial meniscus.

"loose body" and donor site. If the history is consistent with **osteochondritis dessicans(OCD)** the same four views are again needed. Of note, an **OCD** may be an incidental finding and therefore must be correlated with the clinical presentation (see Figures 31.16 and 31.17). Another incidental finding in the long bones at the knee is a "fibrous cortical defect" which does not compromise the integrity of the bone and may be ignored.

Complete Evaluation for Saltar Harris, Tibial Plateau, and Stress Fractures

Initial radiographs for certain injuries may be negative. Saltar Harris type fractures of the distal femoral epiphysis may require stress views or an MRI. Tibial plateau fractures on occasion present with a "pop," an immediate effusion but an otherwise unremarkable examination. A traumatic nondisplaced tibial plateau fracture may require oblique

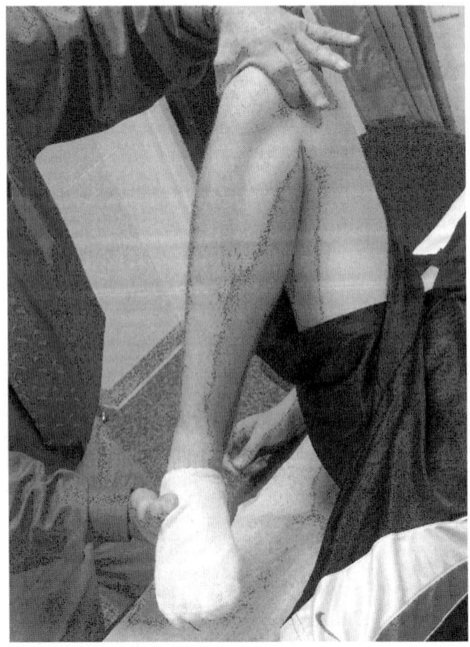

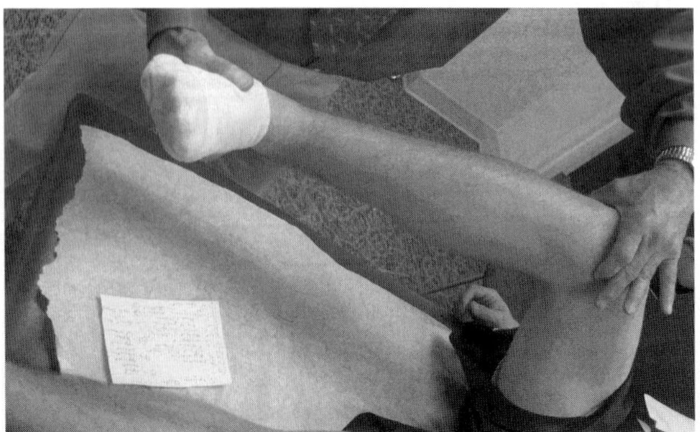

A B

Figure 31.14 **A and B:** McMurray testing—lateral meniscus.

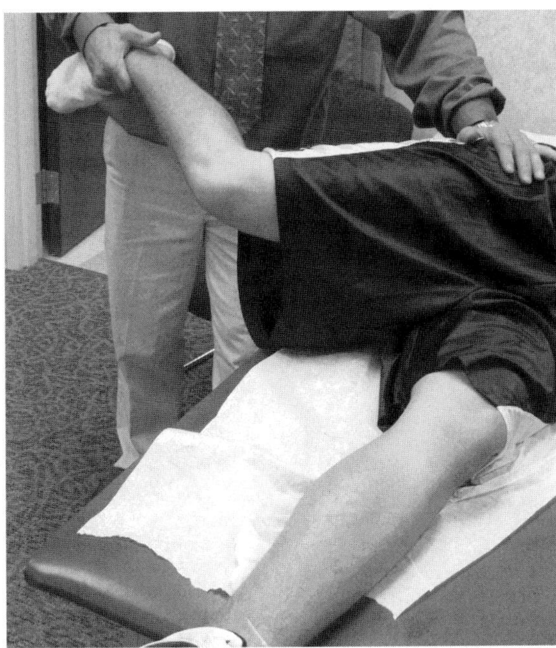

Figure 31.15 Technique for Ober test.

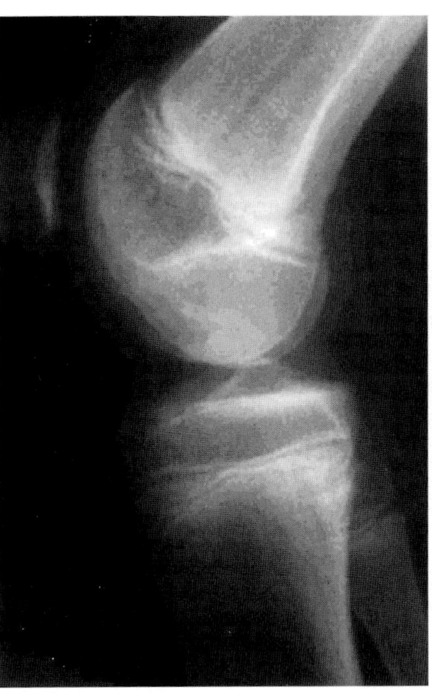

Figure 31.17 Osteochondritis dessicans (lateral view).

views or a MRI or computed tomography (CT) for confirmation.

Stress fractures include: (a) rare patellar stress fracture (PSF) involving distal quarter (must not confuse with a transverse fibrous union as seen with a secondary center of ossification), (b) medial tibial plateau and (c) the tibial tubercle (rare). All may require an MRI for an early diagnosis. A common proximal tibial shaft/tibial stress fracture may have a negative initial radiograph and require an MRI or bone scan.

Pathognomonic Findings

Certain findings can be pathognomonic such as the "Lateral' Segond Fracture" where there is a chip fracture/avulsion of the lateral capsule off the tibia is seen only with ACL rupture (see Figure 31.18). Of note a small avulsion of the

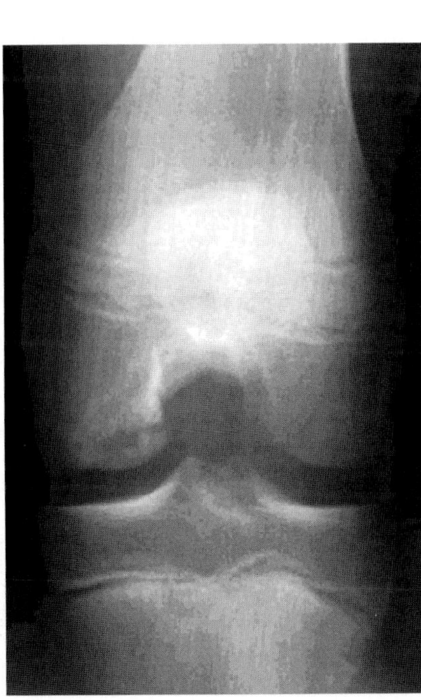

Figure 31.16 Osteochondritis dessicans (anteroposterior view).

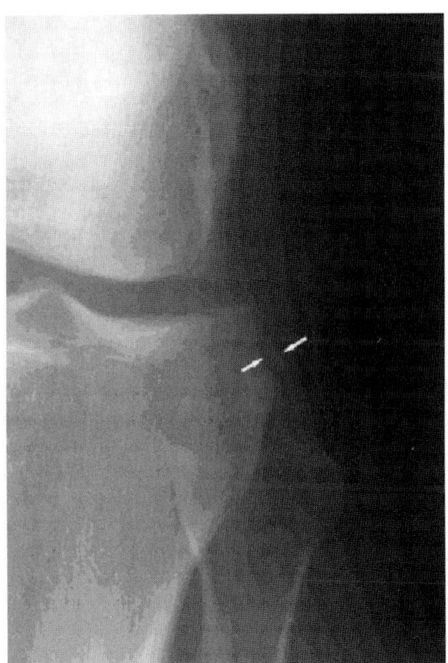

Figure 31.18 Segond fracture.

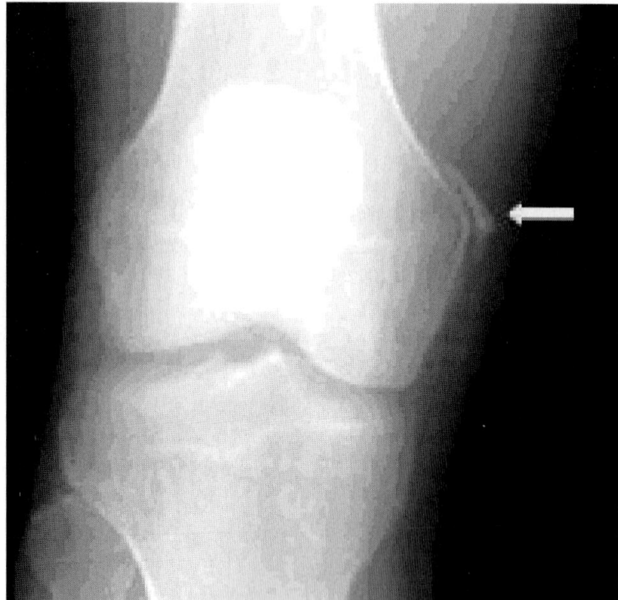

Figure 31.19 Pelligrini-Stieda sign.

lateral femoral condyle, while similar is relatively benign. A second type of " 'Medial' Segond Fracture" has recently been described that occurs over the medial side as a result of a medial capsular avulsion seen only with a complete PCL tear (39). Pellegrini-Stieda disease (calcification within the MCL, suggestive of old injury) (see Figure 31.19) or chondrocalcinosis (see Figure 31.20) can also be identified with the diffuse calcification within the synovium and meniscus.

BONE CYSTS AND TUMORS

Bone Cysts

Occasionally there can be "bone cysts" which are benign but may predispose to pathological fracture depending on size and location. The aneurysmal bone cyst (ABC) is the most common followed by uni- and multicameral bone cysts. Each case must be individualized and an orthopedic surgeon or orthopedic oncologist if available should be consulted regarding the risk of pathological fracture and whether bone grafting would be recommended.

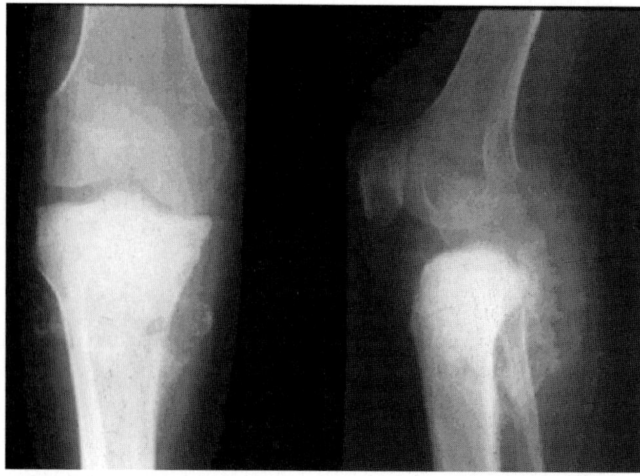

Figure 31.21 Osteogenic sarcoma.

Tumors

Fifty percent of osteogenic sarcomas involve the knee at the distal femoral or proximal tibial metaphyses (see Figure 31.21). Peak age of incidence is 20 and they are rarely seen in those older than 40, with a slight male predominance. Diffuse pain is gradually progressive with local heat and variable swelling. Tenderness is found over the involved site. Radiographic findings include periosteal elevation with extension into the soft tissues. Giant cell tumors occur in the long bones around the knee (see Figure 31.22). Radiologists and orthopedic surgeons

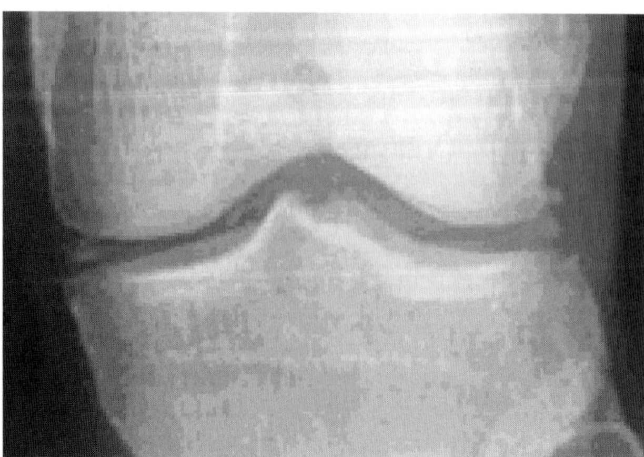

Figure 31.20 Chondrocalcinosis.

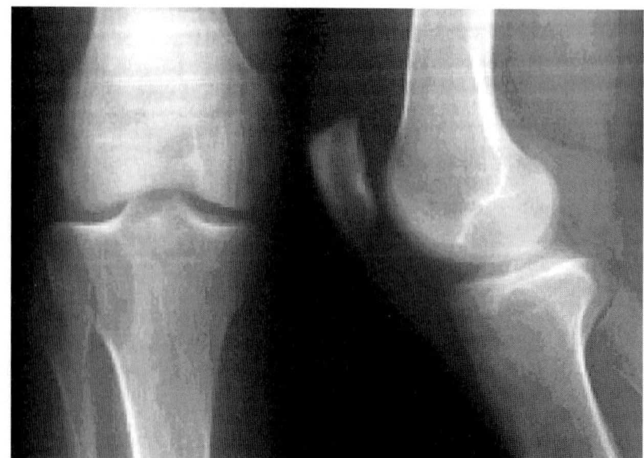

Figure 31.22 Giant cell tumor.

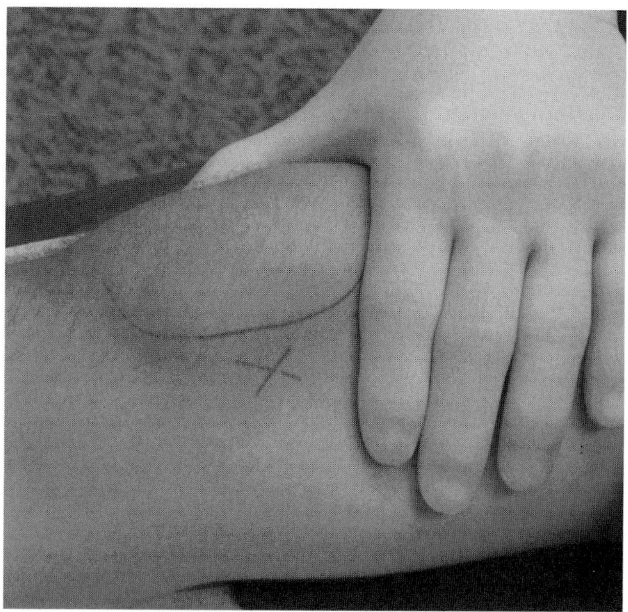

Figure 31.23 Technique for medial approach aspiration of minor effusion.

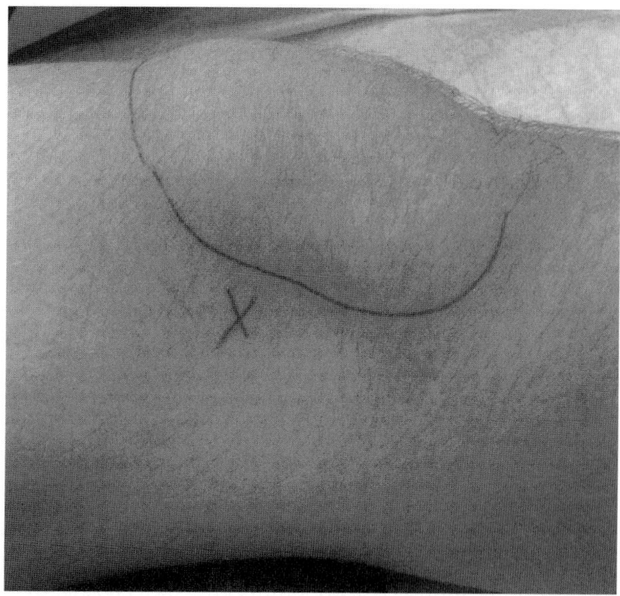

Figure 31.24 Technique for lateral approach for injection or aspiration.

should be consulted on any questionable finding on radiographs.

Technique and Role of Joint Fluid Aspiration

A therapeutic aspiration to control symptoms is rarely indicated. Using ice and proper immobilization can best control acute symptoms. A diagnostic tap can assist if history and MOI are unclear. Most often a minor effusion is clear synovial fluid while a major effusion is bloody. Aspiration would be indicated in a work-up for arthritis. With suspicion of a septic joint, joint aspiration is essential (see section on Emergency). A medial or lateral approach is suggested. With the patient in the supine position a medial patellar approach can be attempted. An assistant can facilitate the procedure by applying pressure over the suprapatellar pouch and the lateral capsule with a minor effusion (see Figure 31.23). A lateral approach at the level of the proximal quartile of the patella is usually well tolerated (see Figure 31.24). It is very important that the patient remain relaxed as a quadriceps contraction can narrow the joint space. Be gentle and careful with either approach. Local anesthesia may or may not be necessary. If in doubt use local anesthesia.

KNEE EXTENSOR MECHANISM INJURIES

Patellofemoral Pain (40–46)

Etiology—Overuse injury. The quadriceps muscle is responsible for the control of the patella as it glides in the femoral groove with each flexion/extension cycle of the knee. Control can be lost with (a) quadriceps fatigue or (b) quadriceps inhibition from any source of pain around the knee. As control is lost, instead of remaining centered in the "groove", the patella glides to one side or the other and produces abnormal pressure points that the individual feels as pain. This pain can further inhibit the quadriceps causing more abnormal tracking, more pain, more inhibition and the "rut" becomes deeper. Although females may have an increased predisposition because of a greater Q angle, the Q angle is not strongly predictive of PFP and does not need to be measured routinely.

Presenting complaint. The patient presents with anterior or lateral knee pain that may be random or associated with activity. May have a positive "theater sign", that is pain with prolonged sitting. May have multiple sites of pain because of associated involvement of the ITB, medial plica, and patellar tendon. It seems that the most common cause of lateral knee pain is not the ITB friction rub over the lateral femoral epicondyle but rather PFP with a tight lateral retinaculum and a tender lateral patellar facet.

Physical examination findings. Minor effusions are uncommon. Tenderness with direct palpation of the medial and/or lateral patellar facets. A tight lateral retinaculum and lateral facet tenderness that the individual recognizes as the pain felt is consistent with a lateral compression syndrome. Loading of the joint as such can be accomplished with the patient in the supine position. The examiners arm is placed behind the flexed knee and the opposite hand around the ankle to provide resistance as the patient attempts to extend the knee. If by history the pain is felt following activity and/or if it has been some time since the pain was last felt then the examination may be benign and a presumptive diagnosis will have to be made on the history alone. It should be possible on examination to exclude patellar instability as a concern with negative Apprehension Testing.

Differential diagnosis. Chondromalacia patellae especially with a history of recurrent effusion, also consider that the PFP may be secondary to an underlying condition such as an occult meniscal tear. Altered gait mechanics for any reason including any overuse or wearing a knee immobilizer may result in PFP.

Treatment. The first objective of treatment is to be as precise as possible with the diagnosis. In the opinion of this author, the associated presence of a medial plica syndrome is the most common cause for failure of a PFP rehabilitation program. The PF component of the pain is addressed with activity modification to control symptoms. Short-term crutch use is helpful if the patient cannot walk without disabling pain or a limp. Quadriceps exercises must be adequate to provide a strength stimulus but cannot cause excessive pain. If only quadriceps isometrics, straight leg raises (SLR) or terminal knee extension (TKE) exercises are done then the exercise must be done frequently. As the intensity of the quadriceps work increases, the recovery time will also increase meaning the exercises need be done less frequently that is, 2 to 3 times/day progressing to 1 time/day to every other day. Medication is not routinely used as there is no inflammatory component to the PFP. However to control the pain in the case of an in-season athlete or to control symptoms while establishing a strengthening program, NSAIDS or acetaminophen may be used short term. For Recalcitrant PFP, McConnell taping can be beneficial.

For an in-season athlete, the goal is to: (a) control symptoms in order allow continued participation and (b) maintain quadriceps strength. A PF brace often increases the threshold of activity before pain is felt and should be strongly considered with the in-season athlete.

Surgery is at times indicated for patellar instability but rarely indicated for PFP. The rare exception would be a consideration of a "lateral release" for the lateral compression type of PFP (very tight lateral retinaculum) that has failed an intense 3- to 6- month rehabilitation program. Most lateral compression type PFPs recover and return to full activity without such a procedure.

Radiographic findings. Routine radiographs for PFP will have a low yield. Indications could include: (a) failure of an adequate 2- to 3-month rehabilitation program, (b) suspicion of PF arthritis, (c) presence of an effusion, or (d) an atypical pain especially if duration of symptoms exceeds 4 to 6 weeks. AP, lateral and Merchant views are suggested.

Return to play guidelines

1. Full ROM
2. Adequate quadriceps strength; 80% to 85% strength of uninvolved side or if bilateral involvement consider using computerized isokinetic testing using body weight to peak torque ratio to confirm strength level. Important to maintain quadriceps strength.
3. Must complete functional testing at 70% capacity before returning to sport specific drills (This level is thought to allow participation in majority of drills.)
4. Must complete functional testing at 85% to 90% capacity before returning to full practice and competition. Athlete is phased into full practice or games using the 25% rule (participating at full intensity but limiting duration to 25% of game or practice and if no pain following play to include the next morning, athlete will progress to 50% duration for the next game or practice and so on, thus taking 4 days to complete the return.) This final phase should be individualized to meet the needs of the particular athlete.

Chondromalacia Patellae

At one time CP was a "waste basket" term used to describe any anterior knee pain. Today this term represents an arthroscopic diagnosis describing the state of the articular surface of the patella. There are four pathological stages progressing from mild fissuring to ulceration extending all the way to the bone. Clinically CP may present as a PFP but often with an effusion and history of recurrent effusions following physical activity. Significant crepitus may be present. Failure to improve after 2 to 4 months of rehabilitation in the presence of a recurrent effusion should prompt surgical consultation to investigate the role of arthroscopy. Radiographs and MRI may not demonstrate significant findings.

Return to play guidelines

1. No more than a minor effusion
2. See discussion on RTP guidelines under section on PFP

Medial Plica Syndrome (47–52)

The medial plica represents an infolding of the synovial lining that proceeds from the suprapatella plica to the anterior fat pad. Although there are multiple plica described in the knee, the medial plica is the only one of common clinical consequence.

Etiology. (a) Most symptomatic plica are a result of overuse injury. (b) Direct trauma can result in immediate disability, inflammation and thickening of the plica. If a plica becomes chronic, scarring may lead to a friction run and eventual "groove" within the medial femoral condyle.

Most common sports. Any sport or activity that can lead to PFP.

Presenting complaint. The presenting complaints are pain, snapping, or clicking over the medial knee (pseudolocking) or giving way.

Physical examination findings. The medial plica can be palpated over the medial femoral condyle, a finger breath medial at the two o'clock position on the patella. By gently rolling the index finger back and forth a clicking sensation can be appreciated. The medial plica is readily palpable in almost all athletes and should be a routine part of every knee examination. The plica may develop a painful click from a friction rub over the medial femoral condyle that is referred to as *pseudolocking* and occurs with knee extension against resistance at 30 degrees (see Figure 31.2). There may be tenderness over the medial femoral condyle.

Differential diagnosis. The differential diagnosis is PFP, torn medial meniscus, synovitis, tibial collateral bursitis.

Treatment. (a) Icing (b) nonsteroidal anti-inflammatory drugs (NSAIDs)—Most respond within 2 to 3 weeks. (c) Modification of activities to control symptoms and (d) consideration of modalities (i.e., iontophoresis) or injection before referral to orthopedics for possible surgical resection. Minimum 4 to 6 months of treatment should pass before serious consideration of surgical referral as almost all will respond without surgery. Of note, it is the opinion of this author that a symptomatic medial plica is the most common reason for failure of a PFP rehabilitation program

Return to play guidelines. See discussion on RTP guidelines under section on PFP.

Patellar Tendonitis (53–57)

This condition is often seen in jumping and leaping sports. Although commonly described as a tendonitis it is now appreciated that in truth it is a "tendinosis" representing a degenerative change or partial tearing of the tendon. True apophysitis of inferior pole of patella seen in 8- to 13-year olds (Sinding/Larsen/Johannsen Syndrome) may have a similar presentation.

Etiology. Injury results from overuse of the limb.

Most common sports. The most common are jumping and leaping sports.

Presenting complaint. The patient presents with gradual or abrupt onset of anterior knee pain, exacerbated by running or jumping sports.

Physical examination findings. There is point tenderness over the inferior pole of the patella. (It is helpful to apply pressure to the superior pole of the patella to better expose the inferior pole to direct palpation.) Rarely, there will be tenderness over the main body or insertion onto the tibial tubercle. There is pain with resistance to knee extension. Often HS inflexibility is present. There may be isolated findings or may be associated with PFP and medial plica syndrome.

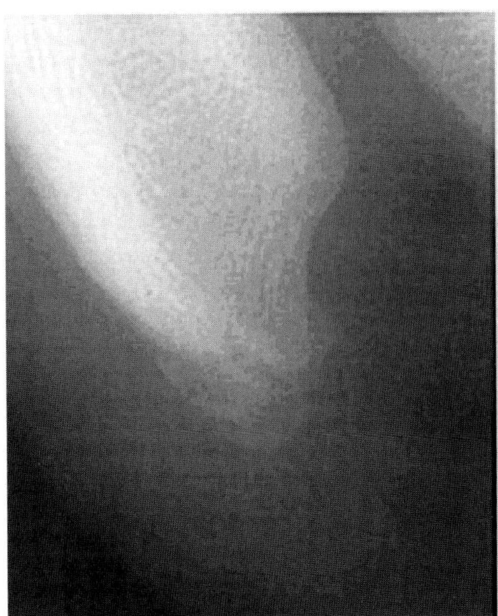

Figure 31.25 Sinding Larsen Johansen syndrome.

Radiographic findings. Fragmentation of inferior pole of the patella is seen in Sinding/Larsen/Johannsen Syndrome (see Figure 31.25). May see spurring at inferior pole in chronic patellar tendonitis.

Treatment. (a) Activity modification to minimize symptoms, use cross training, (b) HS flexibility is key part of plan, (c) quadriceps progressive resistance exercise (PRE) must be done with minimal to moderate pain, (d) trial with infrapatellar strap (e) diagnostic ultrasound coupled with color doppler can be very useful to define the extent of tendonosis (hypoechoic area within tendon and the vascular change). If the tendon is "normal" on ultra sound one can expect 2 to 3 months of treatment for symptoms to resolve. The more the injury within the tendon, the longer the treatment time to full recovery. Severe patellar tendonitis can take 8 to 10 months or more to recover and the more the abnormality, the greater the chance that surgery may be a necessary part of the treatment plan. The good news is that two thirds of the severe cases recovery without surgery. Surgical consultation should be considered after a minimum of 4 months of rehabilitation. Surgery consists of curetting out the degenerative area within the tendon as identified by MRI.

Return to play guidelines. See discussion on RTP guidelines under section on PFP.

QUADRICEPS TENDONITIS

Etiology. Injury results from overuse of the limb.

Most common sports. These are the same as for patellar tendonitis.

Presenting complaint. The patient presents with pain over the quadriceps tendon/superior pole of the patella. Onset of pain is similar to that seen in patellar tendonitis although it occurs less often than patellar tendonitis.

Physical examination findings. There is point tenderness over the superior pole of the patella or may be point tenderness within the tendon proper. Most often there is pain with resistance to knee extension. The patient may have HS inflexibility. Important to identify associated conditions such as PFP, medial plica syndrome, and ITB syndrome to formulate a complete treatment plan.

Treatment. (a) Use activity modification to minimize symptoms, use cross training, (b) HS flexibility is key part of plan, (c) quadriceps PRE must be done with minimal to moderate pain, (d) periodic functional testing with return to advancing of activities as tolerated. Quadriceps tendonitis tends to resolve more quickly than a patellar tendonitis. Bracing, does not seem to play a significant role.

Return to play guidelines. See discussion on RTP guidelines under section on PFP.

Bipartite Patella (58,59)

Etiology. The incidence is 0.5% to 2%; involves secondary center of ossification: (a) superolateral quadrant of the patella (see Figure 31.26), (b) transverse fragment at the distal quarter of the patella (may be confused with a PSF), and (c) longitudinal fragment at the lateral third of the patella. Each represents a fibrocartilaginous union that is subject to pain from direct trauma or overuse.

Presenting complaint. The patient presents with anterior knee pain with activity.

Physical examination findings. There is point tenderness over the fibrous union and pain with resistance to knee extension.

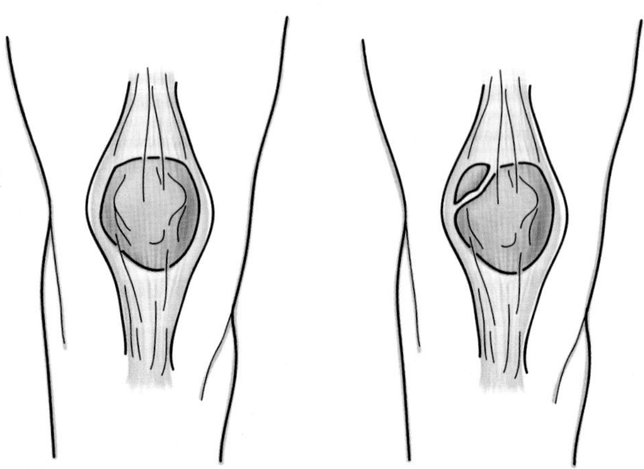

Figure 31.26 Bipartite patella (superolateral corner).

Radiograph findings. AP view demonstrates bipartite patella. Radiographs are ordered when point tenderness is seen over the above described sites or with significant trauma and an associated traumatic effusion.

Differential diagnosis. (a) The diagnosis may be an incidental finding without tenderness over the fibrous union. Other causes of anterior knee pain should then be considered, (b) PFP, (c) Quadriceps tendonitis and (d) Acute fracture which could have a similar finding on radiograph but would have an associated major effusion.

Treatment. (a) Use activity modification to control symptoms. May benefit from short term use of crutches. (b) There should be functional return to activity in 3 to 6 weeks. For persistent symptoms consider excision of bone fragment (rare).

Return to play guidelines. See discussion on RTP guidelines under section on PFP. Time should not exceed 3 weeks from time of onset.

Osgood-Schlatter Disease (60,61)

Osteochondrosis at the tibial tubercle is probably associated with repetitive microtrauma in predisposed preadolescents. This represents the most common form of traction apophysitis. Age of onset and duration of symptoms are 8 to 13 in females and 11 to 15 in males. Symptoms may be unilateral or bilateral.

Etiology. Injury results from overuse in the genetically predisposed.

Most common sports. Any that involves running, jumping, agility, such as football, soccer, and basketball.

Presenting complaint. There is pain at the enlarged and swollen tibial tubercle and inability to participate in sports without pain.

Physical examination findings. There is swelling and tenderness over the tibial tubercle, which may be bilateral. There is pain with resistance to knee extension and often HS inflexibility as may occur at a time of growth spurt.

Treatment. (a) Reassure patient that in spite of the name, the condition does not represent a disease but rather an abnormality in the growth plate that resolves as the growth plate closes, (b) share with patient and parents that in spite of a "self limiting" condition there are definite steps that can be taken to help control symptoms but that the potential for symptoms to be exacerbated persists until the growth plate closes, (c) suggest HS and quadriceps flexibility exercises and (d) quadriceps PRE that minimize pain, (e) recommend activity modification to control symptoms, which often requires a period of trial and error to determine and must be repeated as symptoms improve, (f) advise use of ice for symptomatic relief, and (g) consider an infrapatellar strap for reducing symptoms.

Return to play guidelines. See discussion on RTP guidelines under section on PFP. Realistic expectation is that some symptoms will persist until closure of the growth plate.

Osgood-Schlatter Disease and Complications

In the immature skeleton with a history and examination consistent with **Osgood-Schlatter disease** the x-ray will not be diagnostic. If there is a persistence of pain and tenderness over the tibial tubercle more than 1 to 2 years after expected closure of the physis (boys age >15, girls age >13), the index of suspicion for an ossicle within the patellar tendon must be high. Bilateral lateral radiographs of the knee can identify the ossicle. It is useful to compare with the asymptomatic side. Although modification of activities and time may result in temporary relief, most cases that present to a sports medicine clinic will require surgical excision of the ossicle to allow a return to full, unrestricted activity.

Quadriceps/patellar Tendon Rupture

Uncommon injury that most often occurs in weekend warrior or athletes who have used anabolic steroids.

Etiology. Complete rupture occurs with a forceful contraction of the quadriceps muscle such as in jumping or landing from a jump shot in basketball or heavy squats in power lifting. Most often occurs in athletes over 30.

Presenting complaint. Acute injury that has resulted in knee pain and swelling and difficulty with ambulation.

Physical examination findings. There is major effusion with inability to perform a SLR and palpable gap at the site of rupture.

Radiographic findings. AP and lateral views are negative for a fracture.

Treatment. Urgent orthopedic referral for surgical repair is required.

Distal Quadriceps Contusion

Etiology. Blunt trauma to the distal quadriceps muscle causes massive extra-articular swelling that can be confused with a major effusion.

Presenting complaint. The patient presents with anterior knee pain, which increases with attempts to extend the quadriceps, There is limited ROM, swelling and inability to ambulate.

Physical examination findings. There is extra-articular swelling in the absence of an effusion, tenderness over the injury site, limited ROM, and pain with attempts to extend the knee. Absence of positive Lachman, Apprehension Testing.

Differential diagnosis. The diagnosis is (a) major effusion, (b) quadriceps strain and (c) with mid-thigh contusion must consider myositis ossificans.

Treatment. (a) RICE, (b) crutches, (c) quadriceps PRE as tolerated, (d) ROM, (e) wean from crutches as tolerated, and (f) functional progression with full return to sport.

Return to play guidelines

1. Full ROM at knee
2. No quadriceps tenderness
3. See discussion on RTP guidelines under section on PFP.

Traumatic Patellar Fracture (62)

This is an uncommon sports injury most often caused by severe trauma directly to the patella. This type of force could be produced in a snowmobile accident. There is a case described of a weight lifter that sustained a patellar fracture while lifting. There is limited ROM, pain, and swelling over the anterior knee. Radiographs (AP and lateral views) will reveal the fracture, which may be comminuted. Orthopedic referral often needed. Initial treatment includes RICE, immobilization, and crutches.

Patellar Stress Fracture (63,64)

Infrequent but underdiagnosed condition.

Etiology. The patient may have an inflexible HS and significant overuse history with typical PFP symptoms that are severe enough to cause an involuntary decrease in activity. Most often a minor incident such as participating at 50% effort in an agility activity will cause a "pop" and giving way of the knee. Most often the patellar stress fracture (PSF) is diagnosed only after the complete fracture.

Physical examination findings. There is swelling at lower quadrant of patella/patellar tendon, may have effusion. There is marked point tenderness and inability to extend the knee without severe pain.

Radiographic findings AP and lateral views demonstrate a transverse fracture. This may be confused with the transverse secondary center of ossification.

Treatment. (a) Most often treatment is nonoperative in supportive brace. If fracture displaced more than 3 mm may require surgical intervention. Seek orthopedic consultation if in question. (b) If fracture; crutches for 4 to 6 weeks (c) cross training using upper body ergometer, (d) quadriceps isometrics after 2 to 4 weeks as tolerated and (e) more aggressive PRE and functional progression after 4 to 6 weeks as tolerated.

Return to play guidelines. After 6 to 8 weeks see discussion on RTP guidelines under section on PFP.

PATELLAR INSTABILITY

Patellar Subluxation/Dislocation (65,66)

Etiology. Weight bearing happens with rotation away from the planted foot. This usually occurs with the knee in slight flexion. A "pop" is felt as the patella relocates over the lateral femoral condyle, most often a spontaneous reduction occurs.

Most common sports. The common sports activity is agility sports.

Presenting complaint. There is immediate effusion, a "pop" is felt or heard with frank dislocation, there is inability to continue playing, and often with history of giving way. Less swelling and disability are noted if the condition is recurrent.

Physical examination findings. Dislocation (major effusion), subluxation (minor effusion). Diffuse point tenderness over the medial retinaculum and with localized tenderness over the adductor tubercle (attachment of patellar ligament), positive apprehension test, negative Lachman.

Differential diagnosis. (a) ACL sprain, (b) MCL sprain, (c) Osteochondral Fx.

Radiographic findings. If the examination is consistent with a patellar dislocation, bilateral AP, lateral and Merchant (PF) views are needed. An avulsion fracture off the medial patella border (from medial retinaculum) may be identified and any patellar asymmetry on the Merchant views, requires further MRI evaluation and orthopedic consultation (see Figure 31.27). Subacute or chronic patellar instability should be evaluated with same views. Noting on the Merchant view the depth of the femoral groove (more shallow more risk for recurrence), height of the lateral femoral condyle (loss of height more risk) and the shape of the patella (more off center the central ridge the greater risk). Patella alta can be assessed on the lateral views. Distance more than 1.2 times the length of patella from the inferior pole to the tibial tubercle equals patella alta with increased risk of recurrence as the patella rides in the more proximal, shallow portion of the groove.

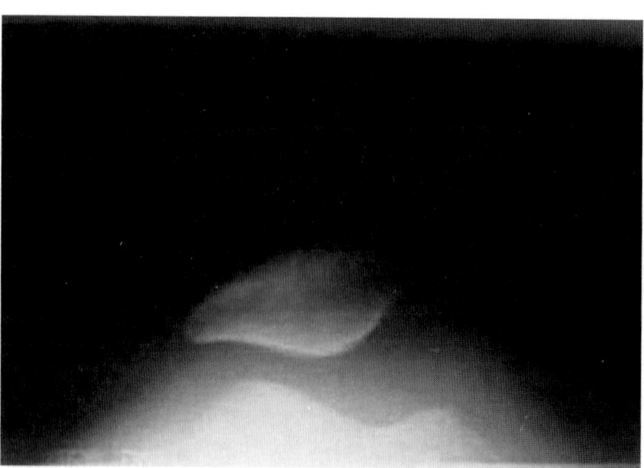

Figure 31.27 Patellar asymmetry on the Merchant view.

Treatment. (a) RICE and crutches, (b) consider knee immobilization with ROM brace locked at 30 degrees for 1 to 2 weeks with additional protection but increased ROM for 4 weeks for dislocation. Subluxation usually requires 1 to 2 weeks of protection. Avoid any prolonged use of a straight leg immobilizer, (c) Rehabilitation to begin with quadriceps isometrics after 1 week, (d) cross- training, (e) gentle ROM 3 to 4 weeks for dislocation and immediate for subluxation,(f) regain full ROM and strength, (g) functional progression with PF brace. Full return to sport in 8 to 12 weeks from injury with dislocation and 2 to 3 weeks with subluxation, (h) Long-term goal to maintain quadriceps strength and wear PF brace for high risk activities.

Recurrent subluxation/dislocation: For any recurrent instability episode, very important to note: (a) If the individual was wearing PF brace, (b) If good quadriceps strength maintained, and (c) did recurrence occur with a routine activity or was there excessive force in an atypical activity. Each episode must be evaluated as above, also considering predisposing factors identified on x-ray. Treatment as above, but expect more rapid resolution with recurrent episodes. Consider orthopedic referral to assess role of surgery. Options include proximal and/or distal realignment. The least intervention to accomplish stabilization is desirable. Surgery tends to be very successful.

Return to play guidelines. After 1 to 2 weeks following subluxation and after 6 to 8 weeks following dislocation see discussion on RTP guidelines under section on PFP.

Osteochondral Fractures (67–76)

Etiology. May be associated with subluxation or dislocation of the patella. It may result from direct trauma to the patella, medial, or lateral condyles. Direction rather than magnitude of force is the most important variable that results in an osteochondral fracture. An osteochondral fracture can result from the same MOI that causes intra-articular ligamentous or meniscal injury.

Most common sports. The common sports are agility sports (i.e., football, basketball).

Presenting complaint. The patient may experience an audible "pop", swelling, pain often is out of proportion to the known injury. Catching or locking up are possible if loose body is present. Recurrent swelling happens with activity.

Physical examination findings. There is major effusion, point tender at site of fracture, negative Lachman, may have positive Apprehension.

Differential diagnosis. ACL sprain, patellar dislocation/subluxation, torn meniscus.

Radiographic findings. There are four views: AP, lateral, tunnel and Merchant looking for a loose body and a donor site. Remember that chondral defects are not seen on radiograph and require a high index of suspicion and an MRI evaluation.

Treatment. (a) RICE and crutches; (b) if there is a high index of suspicion for chondral injury consider MRI; (c) orthopedic referral for reattachment or excision of fragments.

Return to play guidelines. This is dependant on MRI findings, otherwise see discussion on RTP guidelines under section on PFP.

LIGAMENTS/CAPSULE INJURY

MCL Sprains

Etiology. (a) Valgus force is applied to the knee. Limited force can result in isolated MCL involvement, whereas greater force can result in capsular as well as ACL rupture; (b) overuse.

Most common sports. The common sports are agility sports (i.e., football, wrestling, basketball).

Radiographic findings. These are indicated for any significant swelling or effusion in grade II–III sprains to rule out avulsion fracture. The Pelligrini-Stieda sign (see Figure 31.25) represents chronic injury to the MCL.

Etiology. **Grade I MCL sprain**: stretching of MCL fibers without an increase in joint laxity.

Presenting complaint. The patient presents with pain over medial aspect of knee.

Physical examination findings. There is point tenderness at any site along MCL, no swelling, no increased laxity with valgus stressing.

Differential diagnosis. The diagnosis is medial meniscus tear, medial plica syndrome, tibial collateral bursitis or pes anserine tendinitis.

Treatment. (a) Ice, (b) NSAID for less than 1 week PRN pain, (c) activity modification to control symptoms, crosstraining as needed, and (d) functional progression as tolerated, usually for less than 1 week.

Grade II MCL Sprain: partial tearing of MCL fibers with increased laxity on valgus stressing. Grade II can involve from 5% to 95% of the fibers.

Presenting complaint. The patient presents with pain and swelling over medial aspect of knee, which often prevents athlete from continued sports participation.

Physical examination findings. Swelling is localized to medial aspect of knee, with point tenderness at site of injury along MCL. There is pain and increased laxity with valgus stressing (1–2+) at 30 degrees but with distinct end point. If there is a trace to 1+ laxity (<5 mm) the term *Grade II Stage I MCL Sprain* may be used suggesting the injury is closer to a grade I than a grade III whereas if there is a laxity greater or equal to 1-2+ (>5–10 mm) the term *Grade II Stage II MCL Sprain* may be used suggesting the injury is closer to a grade III than a grade I MCL sprain. If there is any effusion present, it represents intra-articular damage. An effusion may represent a simple synovitis, ligament sprain, meniscal injury, chondral or osteochondral injury, or a patellar subluxation. It is somewhat common to encounter the combination of a grade II MCL and an acute complete rupture of the ACL or to have some MCL involvement with a patellar subluxation/dislocation.

Treatment. (a) Ice PRN pain (20 minutes every 2 hours), (b) immobilization as needed to control symptoms. Getting the athlete into the functional varus/valgus brace ASAP will enhance recovery time but if symptoms warrant, use of a ROM brace will be helpful. Brace may be locked in position or comfortable ROM allowed, (c) crutches should be used until the athlete can walk with a normal gait albeit slow, (d) maintenance of quadriceps PRE, (e) gentle ROM to begin after 1 to 2 weeks as tolerated. Each case must be individualized, (f) cross-training should begin ASAP, (g) once the diagnosis has been made it will be detrimental to the process of recovery to apply a valgus force to the injured and recovering MCL, (h) under the direction of the ATC or PT staff, the athlete can proceed with the functional rehabilitation.

Return to play guidelines. As part of step (h) see discussion on return to play guidelines under section on PFP.

Grade III MCL Sprain. complete disruption of MCL fibers. Uncommon injury as opposed to a severe Grade II Stage II as described in the preceding text which is much more common.

Presenting complaint. The complaint is the same as second degree, may experience less pain as nerve fibers are torn.

Physical examination findings There is swelling over medial aspect, point tender over MCL, increased laxity (3+) with soft end with valgus stressing at 30 degrees flexion. May open up like a gate greater than 45 degrees to 60 degrees. Any increased laxity at 0 degree with valgus stressing represents an ACL injury

Treatment (a) The combination of an acute grade III ACL and grade III MCL injury necessitates immediate orthopedic referral (surgery most successful if completed <10–14 days following injury.) (b) Otherwise, isolated grade III MCL sprains are treated conservatively with a variable ROM brace for 6 weeks using quadriceps isometrics as maintenance exercise and adjusting the brace to allow for increased ROM as tolerated while protecting against an valgus force (77). The same criteria must be met for return to full unrestricted activity as for a grade II Stage II MCL sprain. Full recovery may take 12 weeks or longer. Most isolated MCL sprains allow complete return to activities.

The Pelligrini-Stieda sign (see Figure 31.25) represents chronic injury to the MCL.

ACL Sprains (78–89)

The ACL is the key stabilizer of the knee. Complete rupture of this ligament will limit full participation in high-risk agility sports for most people.

Etiology. (a) The most frequent mechanism is noncontact and includes deceleration while pivoting toward the planted foot, the injury can also occur when pivoting away from the planted foot,(b) hyperextension force or (c) part of multiple ligament injury (severe valgus or varus force). The incidence of partial tears of the ACL is difficult to assess because there is no significant disability. Most injuries that present on the playing field or in the office represent mid substance full thickness tears where there is a "pop" felt or heard and followed by an immediate effusion. With a complete rupture of the ACL, there is a 50% incidence of a meniscal tear. (4:1 lateral vs. medial).

Gender Difference. An increased incidence of ACL rupture among adolescent female athletes is now appreciated. Successful intervention programs are now available.

Most common sports. The common sports are football, soccer, basketball, gymnastics. This may occur in any agility sport.

Presenting complaint. Most often this is an audible or palpable "pop" associated with an immediate effusion (usually within hours after injury). While on rare occasion there may be a small or no effusion it would be prudent to inquire regarding prior unrecognized injury with a subsequent "giving way" episode. In this instance an MRI may identify an acute injury with the characteristic bone bruise pattern involving the lateral femoral condyle.

Differential diagnosis. The differential diagnosis may be patellar dislocation, tibial plateau fracture, meniscal injury, or osteochondral fracture.

Physical examination findings/diagnosis. Effusion 3–4+ (less if seen immediately), Apprehension negative, Lachman positive (1–2+) with a soft endpoint. Approximately 20% of time there may be a minimal amount of excursion but with the soft endpoint. It is critical that the HS be checked to make sure they are not being contracted or there may be a false "soft" endpoint. The HS are checked by direct palpation of the medial and lateral HS tendons with the index fingers of the examining hands. The Lachman, Lateral Pivot Shift and Anterior Drawer tests have been the traditional tests to access ACL laxity. The Lachman is the test of choice as it is both sensitive and athlete friendly. The Lateral Pivot Shift test is sensitive but more difficult to master and can be uncomfortable for the athlete. See Lachman and Lateral Pivot Shift tests under physical examination. The Anterior Drawer test is specific but so insensitive that it is not a necessary part of a routine assessment. The posterior drawer however does play a key role in the assessment of PCL injury and should be a part of any routine examination to assess the integrity of that ligament.

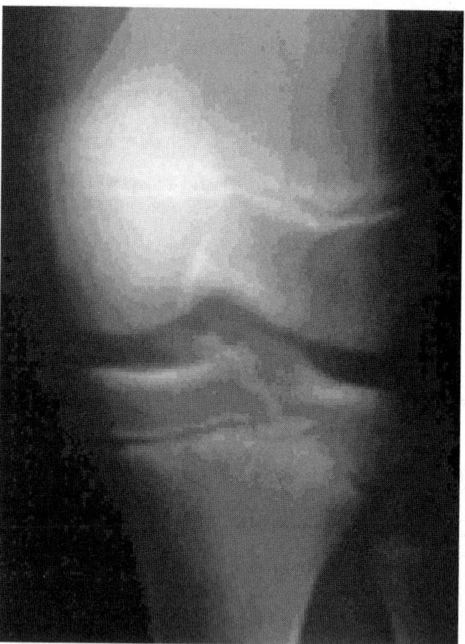

Figure 31.28 Avulsion tibial spine (anteroposterior view).

Radiographic findings. Routine radiographs should include AP and lateral views to rule out tibial spine avulsion; incidence 1% to 2% (see Figures 31.28) or the Segond fracture (see Figure 31.18), avulsion of lateral capsule with the lateral capsular sign (pathoneumonic for an ACL rupture). Open growth plates in the immature skeleton will factor into surgical planning. The history and physical examination are key elements in making the diagnosis and an MRI is not often needed and should never be part of a routine work up for an ACL injury. At times the athlete is unable to relax or there is suspicion of a more complicated injury and an MRI is beneficial.

Treatment. Isolated grade III sprain of ACL or with possible meniscal involvement; (a) Following the discussion of the diagnosis, the patient should be allowed to react and be heard and then told that the first weeks will be devoted to the recovery process and it will be important for the patient to prioritize sport of choice for the subsequent visit. If it is obvious that the patient wants to continue participation in a high-risk sport, the athlete can be told that he or she would be an excellent candidate for reconstructive surgery. Each case should be individualized as to further discussion depending on the athlete. High-risk activities involve quick stops, starts, and cutting such as football, soccer, rugby, full court tennis, volleyball, hockey and related sports. Low-risk activities include activities of daily living

(ADLs), walking, running straight ahead, biking, swimming, baseball or softball, most skiing and similar activities. The orthopedic referral should be made for reconstructive surgery if the athlete chooses to engage in high risk sports, (b) knee brace as needed for comfort, ice, crutches; (c) begin ROM as tolerated after 0 to 2 weeks, (d) cocontractions for the quadriceps/HS to preserve muscle mass along with heel pumps (25 repetitions three times/day) to prevent deep vein thrombosis (DVT).

The nonoperative treatment of acute grade III ACL injury is as above initially. After 3 to 5 weeks, aggressive treatment may begin. Emphasis is on regaining (a) full ROM, (b) strength (must avoid full range quadriceps lift PRE but may use 90 to 60 range and/or the leg press, both of which will protect joint from additional stress leading to instability), (c) propioception (6- to 8-week program of functional progression, agilities beginning with 50% for a week and progressing to 60% for 1 to 2 weeks and so on, until patient has accomplished desired level), (d) use of appropriate bracing and stressing the importance of limiting activities to those of low risk.

Return to play guidelines

1. Dependant on the surgeon following reconstructive surgery
2. For nonoperative RTP see preceding text and see discussion on RTP guidelines under section on PFP.

Note that if the athlete desires a nonsurgical treatment for high-risk activities it must be stressed that the chances are slim and none, that there can be participation in a high-risk sport without giving way episodes. It must be emphasized that giving way episodes cannot be tolerated because of potential damage to both meniscus and articular cartilage which will lead to early osteoarthritis. It must be acknowledged however that there are a small number of athletes (impossible to identify ahead of time) that may engage in high-risk sports without incident. They are referred to as *Copers*. Before an athlete can be considered a successful "coper" 2 full years must be completed in a high risk sport at full intensity without any giving way episodes.

PCL Sprains (90–93)

The incidence of PCL sprains is not known because the injury is not always appreciated when it occurs and there may be minimal to no disability following the injury.

Etiology. (a) Direct force against the fixed anterior tibia (i.e., baseball catcher blocking plate as the incoming runner collides with the planted anterior tibia), (b) a fall onto the flexed knee with the point of impact the tibial tubercle and (c) multiple ligament injury involving a sustained hyperextension, varus, valgus or rotational force.

Present complaint. The patient presents with a knee injury without a "pop" and immediate effusion. Athlete will seldom complain of instability but may have a significant swelling.

Physical examination findings. There may be a minor to major effusion. Reverse Lachman may be negative (Lachman may seem to have a solid endpoint in both directions and is not reliable to rule out injury to the PCL.) The gold standard is the Posterior Drawer test (see Figure 31.8) where there will be a disappearance of the tibial shelf. This is also a positive "sag sign". It is very important to check for posterolateral joint line tenderness and then with the athlete in the prone position and the knees flexed to 90 degrees look for pain and/or increased external rotation (>5 degrees) on the injured side (see Figure 31.29). Most often in athletes there is an isolated injury to the PCL with a 1 to 2+ positive posterior drawer test without lateral joint line tenderness or pain with increased external rotation. If the latter test is positive an orthopedic referral is appropriate to assess for injury to the posterolateral corner. Partial PCL injuries can occur and are identified by an abrupt endpoint but with increased laxity as compared to the control side.

Radiographic findings. AP and lateral views to identify bony pathology.

Differential diagnosis. In chronic ligament injury it can be a challenge to distinguish between injury to the PCL versus the ACL. It is very important to determine the neutral position. It is then possible with the Lachman and Posterior Drawer test to determine which

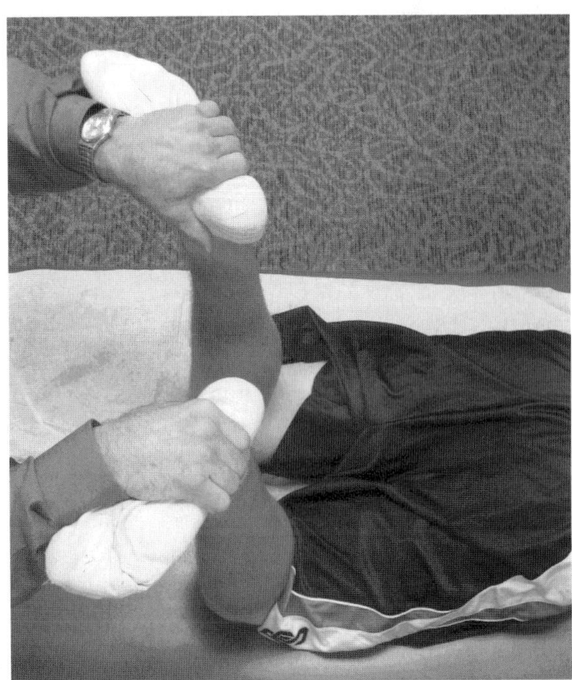

Figure 31.29 Technique for testing posterolateral corner in posterior cruciate ligament injuries.

ligament has been injured. Also keep in mind that a PCL injury may be part of a multiligament injury including a frank knee dislocation and all ligaments should be evaluated. Also remember that associated meniscal and osteochondral injury can occur.

Treatment. **Isolated PCL injury with positive posterior drawer less than or equal to 1–2+ and no posterolateral corner involvement:** (a) supportive; with a brace, crutches and icing as needed, (b) gentle ROM progressing to full ROM, (c) symmetrical strength in quadriceps and HSs, (d) Propioceptive/agility training, (e) Functional progression to ADL's then to full unrestricted activity will often take 3 to 4 months total time, (f) Functional bracing is optional but at least a PF type brace should be considered to increase propioception and (g) With persistent instability after 3 to 4 months one must consider the surgical option or modification of activities. Recurrent giving way episodes may result in meniscal or osteochondral injury and can never be tolerated.

Return to play guidelines. See discussion on RTP guidelines under section on PFP after step 6 in the preceding text **Isolated PCL injury with positive posterior drawer greater than 2+ or with posterolateral corner involvement or concern about associated injury** (a) Same as above initially and (b) Consider MRI and referral to orthopedics for management strategy. **LCL Sprains** Uncommon injury—less than 1% of acute knee injuries. LCL is a static stabilizer that is protected by the ITB which is the dynamic stabilizer.

Etiology. Varus force

Most common sports: The common sports are football, wrestling, gymnastics.

Presenting complaint The patient presents with lateral knee pain. Grade I may continue playing, grades II and III may have swelling and may be associated with a "pop" and most often not able to continue playing.

Physical examination findings. There is point tenderness over LCL (see Figure 31.4 position allows for most definitive palpation) (see Figure 31.11). Grades II and III have localized swelling and varus laxity noted when tested at 30 degrees. Grade II with solid end point.

Differential diagnosis The diagnosis is ITB strain, Biceps Femoris Strain/Insertional Tendonitis, Torn Lateral Meniscus, Synovitis, or Ruptured Popliteus Tendon.

Treatment. (a) Grades I, II–same as MCL, (b) Grade III–immobilize, ice and immediate referral for surgical repair.

Return to play guidelines

1. LCL grades I, II same as MCL Grade I, II
2. Grade III dependant on surgical consultant

Meniscal Injury (22,23,94–98)

Etiology. Meniscal tears may be traumatic (oblique, radial, longitudinal or complex) or degenerative (horizontal cleavage) (see Figure 31.30). Traumatic tears may occur at the periphery (red zone) or within the central portion of the meniscus (white zone). These tears may be complete or partial thickness. Traumatic tears are more frequent in the medial than lateral meniscus. Degenerative tears are atraumatic and may occur in anyone over the age of 30. Often asymptomatic until repetitive rotational loading forces set off the symptoms.

An important but little discussed cause of meniscal-like symptoms is a localized synovitis resulting from the same forces that cause traumatic or degenerative tears in the meniscus. The presentation is identical; effusion found in 50% of each group, joint line tenderness, pain with flexion and limitation with functional activities. Although a small percentage of the localized synovitis group may require arthroscopic excision, the majority respond to a 2- to 3-week course of NSAIDs. Repeat examination following the course of NSAIDs results in a dramatic improvement in signs, symptoms and functional ability.

(a) **Traumatic tears** result from single event weight bearing, deceleration/rotational forces. It may also be associated with intra-articular ligament injury.

(b) **Degenerative tears** are the result of a process. Repetitive, loaded weight bearing combined with rotational forces (lifting heavy boxes of books, rotating and carrying them from one location to another or sports such as basketball or racquetball) exacerbate these tears.

Most common sports. Any sport or activity that causes single event or repetitive weight bearing rotational forces such as football, basketball, skiing, wrestling (50% lateral), baseball, gymnastics.

Presenting complaint. Knee pain, with a limited ROM, particularly flexion. May have delayed swelling and mechanical symptoms such as catching or giving way but rarely will have a true locking of the knee (inability to fully extend). If initial injury was more remote and there has been a partial recovery, athlete may notice recurrent swelling with activity, inability to fully flex the knee without pain and limited functional ability.

Physical examination findings. May have 1 to 2+ effusion, joint line tenderness, some limitation in flexion associated with pain and an exacerbation of pain with forced flexion (see Figure 31.12) and McMurray testing (see Figures 31.13 and 31.14). At times McMurray testing can suggest paradoxical contralateral side involvement from the joint line tenderness. The same history and physical findings can be consistent with a localized synovitis mentioned in the preceding text. Locking of the knee suggests a displaced bucket handle tear of the medial meniscus or a lodged loose body. When accessible a functional assessment may add valuable objective data.

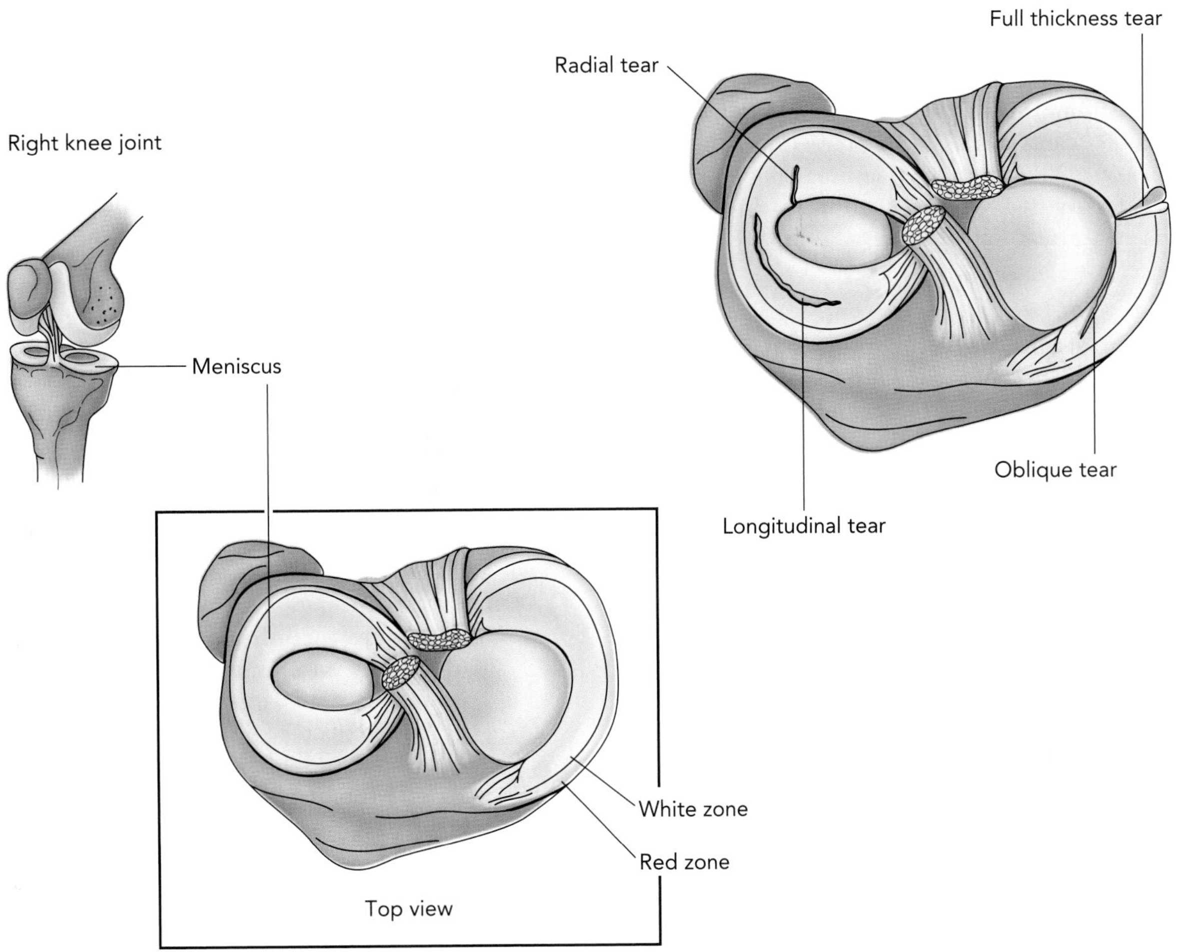

Figure 31.30 Types of meniscus tears.

Differential diagnosis. (a) Medial or lateral compartment DJD, (b) osteochondral or chondral fracture and (c) localized synovitis.

Note that it is not uncommon with a degenerative meniscus or a unicompartment at DJD to an associated PFP. At times, symptoms from the former two subside and the latter predominates. Quadriceps strengthening is a key to success in all three conditions.

Radiographic findings. (a) Standard AP and lateral views, (b) if concerned about possible DJD then bilateral weight bearing AP and 45 degree views, (c) if history of mechanical symptoms consider possible osteochondral fracture—four views (see section on Radiographic Studies).

Treatment. Immediate orthopedic referral for a locked knee is appropriate. Otherwise (a) RICE, crutches as needed with progression to walking as tolerated, (b) NSAID for 2- to 3-week duration, (c) gentle ROM, quadriceps isometrics and functional progression as tolerated and (d) RTC 2 1/2 to 3 weeks at which time examination will be repeated and functional testing performed as appropriate.

Return to play guidelines

1. In the competitive athlete population, it may be prudent to consider MRI imaging earlier in the course as compared to the noncompetitive recreational athlete.
2. With or without a documented torn meniscus, if the athlete has no more than a minor effusion (nor a recurrent effusion following activity), a functional arc of motion (0–120 degrees), equivalent bilateral strength, no history of mechanical symptoms and is able to complete functional testing at 85% to 90% without more than mild discomfort it is considered safe to allow a RTP.

With persistence of mild symptoms appropriate guidelines for physical activity based on functional testing can be given along with PRE and RTC in 2 to 3 weeks for further evaluation. Continuation of the NSAID should be considered. In the case of persistent or worsened symptoms there should be a heightened index of suspicion for a torn meniscus. An MRI should be considered to document the traumatic tear. If there is suspicion of a degenerative tear, consider noting the response to a quadriceps PRE program before ordering an MRI. Recurrent mechanical symptoms also require orthopedic consultation. If the MRI reveals an isolated degenerative horizontal cleavage tear, a prolonged course of quadriceps PRE and functional progression as tolerated will most often allow the patient to return to a vigorous lifestyle. May be a long process 6 to 10 months to full recovery but most often arthroscopic intervention is not necessary. It is important to maintain quadriceps strength and regular activity level.

Osteoarthritis

Etiology. This may occur following a partial or total meniscectomy, more common in overweight individuals, and greater incidence with aging. Once present will likely progress in proportion to amount and intensity of impact activity.

Presenting complaint. The patient presents with knee pain, swelling, limitations with ROM, pain with impact activity, pain going up or down stairs, difficulty flexing the knee when bending down.

Physical examination findings. The patient may have quadriceps atrophy, effusion, joint line tenderness, pain with flexion of the knee and possible limited ROM. May have PF findings.

Differential diagnosis. The diagnosis is torn meniscus, localized synovitis, Tibial collateral bursitis, or medial plica syndrome.

Radiographic findings: OA may be diffuse or limited to one of the three knee compartments. Radiographic evaluation of the medial and lateral compartments consists of bilateral standing AP and 45 degree views. The standing AP view accounts for that portion of the articular surface used in standing and walking. The standing 45 degree view accounts for that portion of the articular surface used in brisk walking, running and sport. It is critical that the tibial plateau be parallel to the ground with the more sensitive 45-degree view. Note joint space narrowing, osteophyte formation and subchondral sclerosis. If the menisci were both removed the joint space would be totally maintained. A standard joint space is approximately 5 mm. Narrowing of 1 to 3 mm may be symptom free but more than 3 mm is often symptomatic. (Never forget that we treat the patient not the radiograph.)

AP, lateral and Merchant views are indicated in the evaluation of PF compartment OA.

Treatment. (a) PT for instruction on ROM, PRE for quadriceps/HSs and hip musculature, (b) discussion on appropriate low and not impact activities, (c) consideration of pain control with glucosamine, acetaminophen, NSAID, (d) consideration of synovial type fluid injection for persistent symptoms, (e) consideration of unicompartmental replacement with bone on bone and persistent symptoms or (f) total knee replacement if multicompartmental DJD with persistent severe symptoms, (g) consideration of repeating radiographs at 1- to 5-year interval dependent on symptoms.

BURSITIS

Prepatellar Bursitis

A 3-year Iowa wrestling study (99) found 6 of 15 cases with septic bursitis; 50% were asymptomatic. Gram's stain and culture should be done on all aspirations in high-risk athletes. Must also consider risk of MRSA infection.

Etiology. It is caused by direct trauma, or repetitive friction, as in wrestling or in doing grass drills.

Most common sports. The common sports are those like wrestling, football, and soccer.

Presenting complaint: The patient presents with anterior knee pain and/or pain-free swelling.

Physical examination findings. There is prepatellar swelling, often crepitation, tenderness, pain-free ROM except in full flexion.

Differential diagnosis. PFP, contusion with hematoma.

Treatment. (a) Aspiration of bursa using sterile technique (may be hemorrhagic). Gram stain and culture should be done on all aspirations in high risk athletes, (b) compression bandage for 2 to 3 days, (c) injection of corticosteroids may be indicated with tenderness and if pain is disabling after infection has been ruled out, (d) protection with a knee pad important as recurrent episodes are likely with any repetitive trauma.

Suprapatellar Bursitis

Etiology. It is caused by direct trauma over suprapatellar bursa.

Most common sports. The common sports are those like football, wrestling, and rugby.

Presenting complaint. The patient presents with pain over distal, anterior quadricep muscle.

Physical examination findings. Point tenderness over suprapatellar bursa, may have crepitus; will often have pain with resistance to extension.

Differential diagnosis. Quadriceps strain, contusion (consider myositis ossificans as history dictates)

Treatment. (a) NSAID (consider 7—10-day course of Indomethacin), (b) activity as tolerated, must have full ROM, must complete functional progression before return to full activity, (c) protection with pad

Superficial and Deep Infrapatellar Bursitis

Etiology. Direct trauma or overuse.

Most common sports No specific sports.

Presenting complaint. The patient presents with pain or swelling over patellar tendon.

Physical examination findings. The patient may have significant swelling over or deep to patellar tendon but without a joint effusion. May be tender adjacent to patellar tendon.

Differential diagnosis. The diagnosis is anterior synovitis or fat pad inflammation.

Treatment. (a) NSAID, (b) activity as tolerated, (c) protection as appropriate and (d) consider aspiration only if swelling is affecting play.

Tibial Collateral Bursitis 100

Etiology. Unknown

Most common sports. No specific sports or activities.

Presenting complaint. The patient presents with pain over medial aspect of knee.

Physical examination findings. There is tenderness over 1.5 to 2 cm circumferential over medial joint line where bursa is located.

Diagnosis is one of exclusion. Must exclude: (a) MCL sprain, (b) medial compartment DJD, (c) torn meniscus, (d) localized synovitis, and (e) pes anserine tendon involvement.

Differential diagnosis. (See preceding text.)

Treatment. Dramatic response to steroid injection within 10 days. Remember the tibial collateral bursa is extra- articular. It is often useful to mark the area of tenderness with a pen before injection. Using a 25 gauge needle, one may pinch skin to facilitate needle puncture and then proceed gently to the bone, then slight withdrawal followed by injection of combination of 1 mL steroid of choice and 1 to 2 mL xylocaine into the bursa. Relative rest for 10 days is desirable but the athlete can return to activity immediately may be required. May use ice and NSAID post activity to control symptoms.

ATYPICAL KNEE PAIN; REFERRED PAIN, NEUROGENIC PAIN, REGIONAL COMPLEX PAIN SYNDROME AND TUMORS

It is important to recognize referred pain to the knee that originates from a distant source principally the hip. A full and painfree ROM of the hip eliminates the concern for a slipped femoral epiphysis, Legg-Calve-Perthes disease, or DJD as a primary source of pain. A limited ROM and/or pain at the extremes of motion should prompt further investigation.

Other possible causes of nonorthopedic pain in the knee area include (a) sciatica, (b) obturator nerve entrapment, (c) regional complex pain syndrome (RCPS), and (d) tumors, that is, osteogenic sarcoma, giant cell tumors.

REFERENCES

1. Ebstrup JF, Bojsen-Moller F. ACL injury in indoor ball games. *Scand J Med Sci Sports* 2000;10(2):114–116.
2. Delfico AJ, Garrrett WE Jr. Mechanisms of injury of the ACL in soccer players. *Clin Sports Med* 1998;17(4):779–785, vii.
3. Metzl JD, Micheli LJ. Youth soccer: an epidemiological perspective. *Clin Sports Med* 1998;17(4):663–673, v.
4. Harmon KG, Dick R. The relationship of skill level to ACL injury. *Clin Sports Med* 1998;8(4):260–265.
5. Jarret GJ, Orwin JF, Dick RW. Injuries in collegiate wrestling. *Am J Sports Med* 1998;26(5):674–680.
6. Seo R, Rupp S, Tempelhof S, et al. Sports injuries in team handball. A one-year prospective study of sixteen men's senior teams of a superior nonprofessional level. *Am J Sports Med* 1998;26(5):681–687.
7. Briner WW, Kacmar L. Common injuries in volleyball. Mechanisms of injury, prevention and rehabilitation. *Sports Med* 1997;24(1):65–71.
8. Fadale PD, Hulstyn MJ. Common athletic knee injuries. *Clin Sports Med* 1997;16(3):479–499.
9. Levy AS, Wetzler MJ, Lewars M, et al. Knee injuries in women collegiate rugby players. *Am J Sports Med* 1997;25(3):360–362.
10. Tucker AM. Common soccer injuries. Diagnosis, treatment and rehabilitation. *Sports Med* 1997;23(1):21–32.
11. Brautigan B, Johnson DL. The epidemiology of knee dislocations. *Clin Sports Med* 2000;19(3):387–397.
12. Miranda FE, Dennis JW, Veldenz HC, et al. Confirmation of the safety and accuracy of physical examination in the evaluation of knee dislocation for injury of the popliteal artery: a prospective study. Discussion 251–252. *J Trauma-Inj Infect Crit Care* 2002;52(2):247–251.
13. Martinez D, Sweatman K, Thompson EC. Popliteal artery injury associated with knee dislocations. *Am Surg* 2001;67(2):165–167.
14. Barnes CJ, Pietrobon R, Higgins LD. Does the pulse examination in patients with traumatic knee dislocation predict a surgical arterial injury? A meta-analysis. *J Trauma-Inj Infect Crit Care* 2002;53(6):1109–1114.
15. Tomaino M, Day C, Papageorgiou C, et al. Peroneal nerve palsy following knee dislocation: pathoanatomy and implications for treatment. *Knee Surg Sports Traumatol Arthrosc* 2000;8(3):163–165.
16. Noyes FR, Barber-Westin SD. Reconstruction of the anterior and posterior cruciate ligaments after knee dislocation. Use of early protected postoperative motion to decrease arthrofibrosis. *Am J Sports Med* 1997;25(6): 769–778.
17. Shelbourne KD, Klootwyk TE. Low-velocity knee dislocation with sports injuries. Treatment principles. *Clin Sports Med* 2000;19(3):443–456.
18. Mills WJ, Nowinski RJ. Dislocation of the knee with lateral dislocation of the patella. A report of four cases. *J Bone Joint Surg Am* 2001;83(4):530–532.
19. Baxamusa TH, Galloway MT. Irreducible knee dislocations secondary to interposed menisci. *Am J Orthop* 2001;30(2):141–143.
20. Rotrosen D. Infectious arthritis. In: Wilson JD, Braunwald AB, Isselbacher AB, eds. *Harrisons principles of internal medicine,* 12th ed. New York: McGraw-Hill, 1991:544–548.
21. Personal Case. September 2006.
22. Greis PE, Bardana DD, Holmstrom MC, et al. Meniscal injury: I. Basic science and evaluation. *J Am Acad Orthop Surg* 2002;10(3):168–176.
23. Rodkey WG. Basic biology of the meniscus and response to injury. *Instr Course Lect* 2000;49:189–193.
24. Pasque CB, Hewett TE. A prospective study of high school wrestling injuries. *Am J Sports Med* 2000;28:509–515.
25. Jarrett GJ, Orwin JF, Dick RW. Injuries in collegiate wrestling. *Am J Sports Med* 1998;26:674–680.
26. O'Shea KJ, Murphy KP, Heeking RD, et al. The diagnostic accuracy of history, physical examination and radiographs in the evaluation of the traumatic knee disorders. *Am J Sports Med* 1996;24(2):164–167.
27. Hoppenfield S. Physical examination of the knee. In: Hoppenfield S, ed. *Physical examination of the spine and the extremities.* New York, NY, Appleton-Century-Crofts, 1976:171–196.
28. Torg JS, Conrad W, Dalen V. Clinical diagnosis of ACL instability in the athlete. *Am J Sports Med* 1976;4(1):84–93.
29. Kim SJ, Min BH, Han DY. Paradoxical phenomena of the McMurray test. An arthroscopic investigation. *Am J Sports Med* 1996;24(1):83–87.
30. Oei Eh, Hikken JJ, Berstijnen AC, et al. MR imaging of the menisci and cruciate ligaments: a systematic review. *Radiology* 2003;226(3):837–848.
31. Munshi M, Davidson M, MacDonald PB, et al. The efficacy of MRI in the acute knee injuries. *Clin J Sports Med* 2000;10(1):34–39.
32. Alioto RJ, Browne JE, Barnthouse CD, et al. The influence of MRI on treatment decisions regarding knee injuries. *Am J Knee Surg* 1999;12(2):91–97.
33. Suarez-Almazor ME, Daul P, Kendall CJ, et al. The cost-effectiveness of MR imaging for patients with internal derangement of the knee. *Int J Technol Assess Health Care* 1999;15(2):3920405.
34. Elvenes J, Jerome CP, Reideras O, et al. MR Imaging as a screening procedure to avoid arthroscopy for meniscal tears. *Arch Orthop Trauma Surg* 2000;120(1–2):14–16.
35. Matava MJ, Eck K, Totty W, et al. MR Imaging as a tool to predict meniscal reparability. *Am J Sports Med* 1999;27(4):436–443.
36. Major NM, Helms CA. MR Imaging of the knee: findings in asymptomatic collegiate basketball players. *Am J Raentgenol* 2002;179(3):641–644.
37. Shepard MF, Hunter DM, Davies MR, et al. The clinical significance of anterior horn meniscal tears diagnosed on MRI. *Am J Sports Med* 2002; 30(2):189–192.
38. McNally EG, Nasser KN, Dawson S, et al. Role of MRI in the clinical management of acutely locked knee. *Skeletal Radiol* 2002;31(10):570–573.
39. Hall FM, Hochman MG. Medial segond-type fracture: cortical avulsion off the medial tibial plateau associated with tears of the PCL and medial meniscus. *Skeletal Radiol* 1997;26(9):553–555.

40. Fulkerson JP. Diagnosis and treatment of patients with patellofemoral pain. *Am J Sports Med* 2002;30(3):447–456.
41. Holmes SW, Clancy WG. Clinical classification of patellofemoral pain and dysfunction. *J Orthop Sports Phys Ther* 1998;28(5):299–306.
42. Witvrouw E, Lysens R, Bellemans J. Intrinsic risk factors for the development of anterior knee pain in an athletic population. A two-year prospective study. *Am J Sports Med* 2000;28(4):480–489.
43. Post WR. Clinical evaluation of patients with patellofemoral disorders. *Arthroscopy* 1999;15(8):841–851.
44. Mirzabeigi E, Jordan C, Gronley JK, et al. Isolation of the vastus medialis oblique muscle during exercise. *Am J Sports Med* 1999;27(1):50–53.
45. Gilleard W, McConnell J, Parsons D. The effect of patellar taping on the onset of vastus medialis obliquus and vastus lateralis muscle activity in persons with patellofemoral pain. *Phys Ther* 1998;78(1):25–32.
46. McConnell J. The physical therapist's approach to patellofemoral disorders. *Clin Sports Med* 2002;21(3):363–387.
47. Nottage WM, Sprague NF, Auerback BJ, et al. The medial Plica syndrome. *Am J Sports Med* 1983;11(4):211–214.
48. Broom HJ, Fulkerson JP. The Plica syndrome: a new perspective. *Orthop Clin North Am* 1986;17:279–281.
49. Sherman RM, Jackson RW. The pathological medial plica: criteria for diagnosis and prognosis,. *J Bone Joint Surg* 1989;71B:351.
50. Dorchak JD, Barrack RL, Kneisl JS, et al. Arthroscopic treatment of symptomatic synovial plica of the knee Long-term followup. *Am J Sports Med* 1991;19(5):503–507.
51. Johnson DP, Eastwood DM, Witherow PH. Symptomatic synovial plicae of the knee. *J Bone Joint Surg* 1993;75A:1485–1496.
52. Dupont Jy. Synovial plicae of the knee. Controversies and review. *Clin Sports Med* 1997;16(1):87–122.
53. Cook JL, Khan KM, Harcourt PR, et al. A cross sectional study of 100 athletes with jumperâ's knee managed conservatively and surgically. The Victorian Institute of Sport Tendon study Group. *Br J Sports Med* 1997;31(4):332–336.
54. Al-Duri ZA, Aichroth PM, Wilkins R, et al. Patellar tendonitis and anterior knee pain. *Am J Knee Surg* 1999;12(2):99–108.
55. Khan KM, Bonar F, Demond PM, et al. Patellar tendonitis (jumperâ's knee): findings at histopathologic examination, US and MR imaging. Victorian Institute of Sport Tendon Study Group. *Radiology* 1996;200(3): 83–87.
56. Weinberg EP, Adams MJ, Hollenberg GM. Color doppler sonography of patellar tendinosis. *Am J Roentgenol* 1998;171:743–744.
57. Al-Duri ZA, Aichroth PM. Surgical aspects of patellar tendonitis: technique and results. *Am J Knee Surg* 2001;14(1):43–50.
58. Singer KM, Henry J. Knee problems in children and adolescents. *Clin Sports Med* 1985;4(2):385–398.
59. Bourn MH, Bianco AJ. Bipartite patella in the adolescent: results of surgical excision. *J Pediatr Orthop* 1990;10(1):69–73.
60. Kujala UM, Kvist M, Heinonen O. Osgood-schatterâ's disease in adolescent athletes. *Am J Sports Med* 1985;13(4):236–241.
61. Schmidt DR, Henry JH. Stress injuries of the adolescent extensor mechanism. *Clin Sports Med* 1989;8(2):343–355.
62. Mayers LB, Khabie V, Castorina R, et al. Acute transverse patellar fracture associated with weightlifting. Case report and literature review. *Am J Sports Med* 2001;29(2):232–233.
63. Mason RW, Moore TE, Walker CW, et al. Patellar fatigue fractures. *Skeletal Radiol* 1996;25(4):329–332.
64. Brogle PH, Eswar S, Denton JR. Propagation of a patellar stress fracture in a basketball player. *Am J Orthop* 1997;26(11):782–784.
65. Arendt EA, Fithian DC, Cohen E. Current concepts of lateral patella dislocation. *Clin Sports Med* 2002;21(3):499–519.
66. Sanchis-Alfonso V, Rosello-Sastre E, Martinex-Sanjual V. Pathogenesis of anterior knee pain syndrome and functional patellofemoral instability in the active young. *Am J Knee Surg* 1999;12(1):29–40.
67. Hunt N, Sanchrez-Ballester J, Pandit R, et al. Chondral lesions of the knee: a new localization method and correlation with associated pathology. *Arthroscopy* 2001;17(5):481–490.
68. Rubin DA, Harner CD, Costello JM. Treatable chondral injuries in the knee: frequency of associated focal subchondral edema. *Am J Roentgenol* 2000;174(4):1099–1106.
69. Irrgang JJ, Pezzullo D. Rehabilitation following surgical procedures to address articular cartilage lesions in the knee. *J Orthop Sports Phys Ther* 1998;28(4):232–240.
70. Birk GT, DeLee JC. Osteochondral injuries. Clinical findings. *Clin Sports Med* 2001;20(2):279–286.
71. Loredo R, Sanders TG. Imaging of osteochondral injuries. *Clin Sports Med* 2001;20(2):249–278.
72. Wright RW, Phaneuf MA, Limbird TJ, et al. Clinical outcome of isolated subcortical trabecular fractures (bone bruise) detected on MRI in knees. *Am J Sports Med* 2000;28(5):663–667.
73. Lahm A, Erggelet C, Steinwachs M, et al. Articular and osseous lesions in recent ligament tears: arthroscopic changes compared with magnet resonance imaging findings. *Arthroscopy* 1998;14(6):597–604.
74. Levy AS, Lohnes J, Sculley S, et al. Chondral delamination of the knee in soccer players. *Am J Sports Med* 1996;24(5):634–639.
75. Sellards RA, Nho SJ, Cole BJ. Chrondral injuries. *Curr Opin Rheumatol* 2002;14(2):134–141.
76. Hinshaw MH, Tuite MJ, De Smet AA. Osteochondral injuries of the knee. *MRI Clin North Am* 2000;8(2):335–348.
77. Indelicado PA. Non-operative treatment of complete tears of the MCL of the knee. *J Bone Joint Surg* 1983;64A(3):313–329.
78. Andrish JT. ACL injuries in the skeletally immature patient. *Am J Ortho* 2001;30(2):103–110.
79. Lo IK, Kirkley A, Fowler PJ, et al. The outcome of operatively treated ACL disruptions in the skeletally immature chilled. *Arthroscopy* 1997;13(5):627–634.
80. Kocher MS, Micheili LJ, Zurakowski D. Partial tears of the ACL in children and adolescents. *Am J Sports Med* 2002;30(5):697–703.
81. Fritschy D, Panoussoupoulos A, Wallensten R, et al. Can we predict the outcome of a partial rupture of the ACL? A prospective study of 43 cases. *Knee Surg Sports Traumatol Arthrosc* 1997;5(1):2–5.
82. Murrell GA, Maddali S, Horovitz L, et al. The effects of time course after ACL injury in correlation with meniscal and cartilage loss. *Am J Sports Med* 2001;29(1):9–14.
83. Ireland ML. The female ACL: why is it more prone to injury? *Orthop Clin North Am* 2002;33(4):637–651.
84. Toth AP, Cordasco FA. ACL injuries in the female athlete. *J Gend Specif Med* 2001;4(4):25–344.
85. Griffin LY, Agel J, Albohm MJ, et al. Noncontact ACL injuries: risk factors and prevention strategies. *J Am Acad Orthop Surg* 2000;8(3):141–150.
86. Fitzgerald GK, Axe MJ, Snyder-Mackler L. The efficacy of perturbation training in nonoperative ACL rehabilitation programs for physical active individuals. *Phys Ther* 2000;80(2):128–140.
87. Lephart SM, Abt JP, Ferris CM. Neuromuscular contributions to ACL injuries in females. *Curr Opin Rheumatol* 2002;14(2):168–173.
88. Moller E, Forssblad M, Hansson L, et al. Bracing versus nonbracing in rehabilitation after ACL reconstruction: a randomized prospective study with 2-year follow-up. *Knee Surg Sports Traumatol Arthrosc* 2001;9(2):102–108.
89. Paluska SA, McKeag DB. Knee braces: current evidence and clinical recommendations for their use. *Am Fam Physician* 2000;61(2):411–418, 423–424.
90. St. Pierre P, Miller MD. Posterior cruciate ligament injuries. *Clin Sports Med* 1999;18(1):199–221, vii.
91. Duri ZA, Aichroth PM, Zorrilla P. The posterior cruciate ligament: a review. *Am J Knee Surg* 1997;10(3):149–164. discussion 164–165.
92. Ross G, Chapman AW, Newberg AR, et al. MRI for the evaluation of acute posterolateral complex injuries of the knee. *Am J Sports Med* 1997; 25(4):444–448.
93. Hamada M, Shino K, Mitsuoka T, et al. Chondral injury associated with acute isolated posterior cruciate ligament injury. *Arthroscopy* 2000;16(1): 59–63.
94. Muellner T, Weinstabl R, Schabus R, et al. The diagnosis of meniscal tears in athletes. A comparison of clinical and MR imaging investigations. *Am J Sports Med* 1997;25(1):7–12.
95. Petrosini AV, Sherman OH. A historical perspective on meniscal repair. *Clin Sports Med* 1996;15(3):445–453.
96. Steenvrugge F, Verdonk R, Verstraete K. Long-term assessment of arthroscopic meniscus repair: a 13- year follow-up study. *Knee* 2002;9(3): 181–187.
97. Wheatley WB, Krome J, Martin DF, et al. Rehabilitation programs following arthroscopic meniscectomy in athletes. *Sports Med* 1996;21(6):447–456.
98. Shelbourne KD, Patel DV, Adsit WS, et al. Rehabilitation after meniscal repair. *Clin Sports Med* 1996;15(3):595–612.
99. Iowa 1998.

Lower Leg and Ankle

32

Neeru Jayanthi

LOWER LEG

The lower leg—that portion of the body between the knee and ankle but not inclusive of those two joints—is the site of frequent injury. Injuries to the lower leg make up 3% to 5% of all reported sports injuries. If only those sports in which running is a major component are counted, the injury rate increases to 30% of all injuries.

Anatomy

The proximal lower leg serves as the insertion for muscles originating from the thigh. The distal portion of the lower leg is intimately involved in the function of the ankle joint. The cortical surfaces of the tibia and fibula are the origin of muscles that move the ankle, foot, and toes (see Figure 32.1). The tibia is the main weight-bearing bone of the lower leg. It is triangular in shape, with its anterior border and anterior medial surface primarily subcutaneous. The fibula is situated posterolaterally in the lower leg. Although not directly involved with the knee joint, it does form the distal attachment of the lateral collateral ligament (LCL). In addition, it forms the vital lateral border of the ankle mortise. Connecting the tibia and fibula is an interosseous membrane that serves as the floor of the anterior compartment of the leg. On cross-section, the lower leg (see Figure 32.2) consists of four muscular compartments separated by intermuscular septa or fascial sheaths and possibly another subcompartment. The anterior and lateral compartments permit little flexibility or expansion of the muscles contained within. Conversely, the posterior compartment is a loosely contained space not subject to the same constriction that might result from expansion due to injury. The muscles and neuromuscular bundles of the various compartments are as follows:

Anterior compartment. This consists of tibialis anterior, extensor digitorum longus, extensor hallicus longus, and peroneus tertius muscles; deep peroneal nerve.

Lateral compartment. This consists of peroneus longus and peroneus brevis muscles; superficial peroneal nerve.

Posterior compartment. This compartment is subdivided into the following:

a. *superficial posterior*—gastrocnemius, soleus and plantaris muscles, sural nerve.
b. *deep posterior*—flexor digitorum longus and flexor hallicus longus muscles, posterior tibial vessels and nerves (including the peroneal vessels)
c. *subcompartments of deep posterior*—fibular origin of flexor digitorum longus muscle, sometimes tibialis posterior muscle

Contusions

Contusions of the lower leg are extremely common because of the exposed anatomy of the lower leg. Sports in which contusions occur regularly include the following:

- *Soccer, rugby, football*—blow from an opponent's kick, usually to anterior lower leg
- *Field hockey*—blow from an opponent's stick to the anterior or posterior lower leg
- *Baseball*—two common mechanisms are a blow from a batted ball or laceration and contusion resulting from being "spiked" by a sliding opponent

Biomechanics. Acute trauma to the exposed lower leg usually occurs anteriorly and results in a contusion and/or hematoma of the underlying structures. These injuries are treated as bruises.

Signs and symptoms. Pain at impact, disability secondary to guarding, and swelling are associated with most soft tissue trauma. Swelling comes from extravasation of blood. Subsequent discoloration of the skin progresses within hours of injury. Assessment should

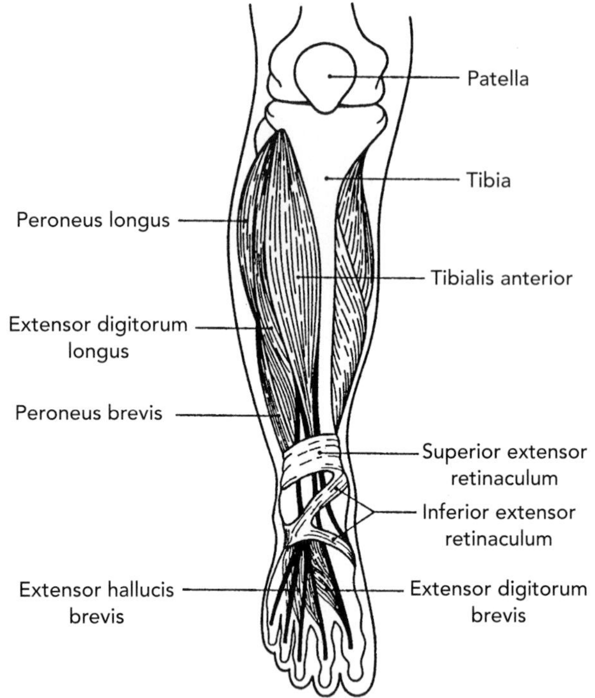

Figure 32.1 Lower leg muscle origins and attachments.

include evaluation of the neurovascular bundles examined distally, as well as muscle group testing using active and passive resistance.

Differential diagnosis. Although a contusion to the lower leg is considered a straightforward injury, several complications can develop. Consider these specific injuries in the differential diagnosis:

1. *Subperiosteal hematoma.* Commonly seen in the lower leg because of the subcutaneous nature of the tibia. This injury is suspected when the degree of debilitation and pain is severe and out of proportion to the relatively negative physical examination. X-rays are necessary to confirm the diagnosis and reveal periosteal elevation and/or thickening. Magnetic resonance imaging (MRI) can demonstrate edema in the bone and any hematoma formation with reasonable accuracy. Initial treatment includes close observation and continued ice therapy, long after the normal contusion treatment guidelines.
2. *Tibial or fibular fracture.* Fractures as a result of blunt trauma are unusual, but should be suspected when considering a diagnosis of a subperiosteal hematoma (see preceding text). Pain is elicited on palpation over the fracture. In addition, percussion at the ankle can produce pain over the fracture site. Most of these fractures involve the weight-bearing tibia and usually prevent the athlete from walking. If the history of trauma is to the lateral side of the leg, fracture to the fibula should be suspected. Examination of the fibula is difficult except at its most proximal and distal margins, so a fracture should be considered if palpation at these margins produces pain anywhere along the fibula. Remember, as a relatively non–weight-bearing bone, the fractured fibula will allow ambulation without much pain. If pain is present, the fibular fracture is usually more proximal in nature as a result of muscle spasm along the insertion of the upper leg muscles. Special note—a proximal fibular fracture can also mimic laxity in the LCL.
3. *Hematomas.* These usually occur in the anterior and lateral compartments and are present in most contusions of the lower leg. A severe hematoma in the anterior or lateral compartment may rarely lead to a compartment syndrome and eventual ischemia or necrosis of muscles, if not watched and controlled. Although uncommon, a hematoma to the posterior calf can cause damage to the venous outflow system and cause stasis of blood flow and possibly even a deep vein thrombophlebitis. Suspect such a complication 36 to 48 hours following an injury if an athlete complains of increasing dull ache in the posterior calf aggravated by ambulation or attempted exercise. Signs include observation of a red streak proximal to the tender calf (lymphangitis) and palpation of a tender "cord" (thrombosed vein). The classic "Homan's sign" has not been proven to be a reliable predictor of deep venous thrombosis (DVT). Treatment of DVT includes bedrest, elevation, and anticoagulation.
4. *Peroneal nerve palsy.* This injury is secondary to direct trauma of the peroneal nerve as it courses superficially over the proximal lateral surface of the lower leg, usually at the point of the head of the fibula. The injury will vary greatly according to its severity, but usually results in a transient period of pain, numbness, and paresthesia in the distribution of the common peroneal nerve. The patient usually describes a sharp shock-like pain that shoots to the lateral side of the leg and foot.

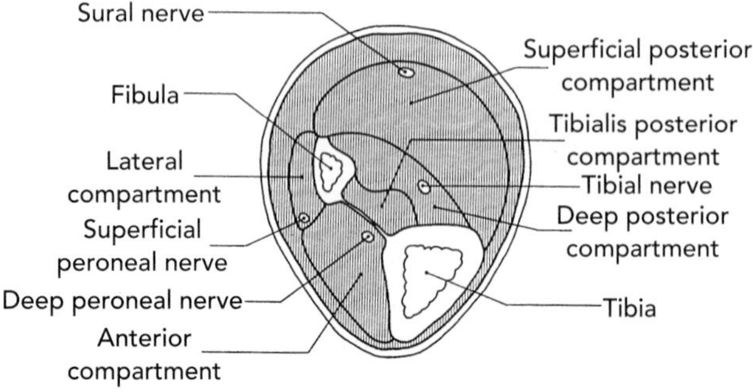

Figure 32.2 Cross-section of lower leg showing 5 fascial compartments.

Most of these cases need no specific treatment except for control of the resultant contusion. The presence of continued neurapraxia should eliminate the athlete from competition. Presence of a foot drop should be an indication for further investigation such as electromyography (EMG) and nerve conduction studies, as well as possible referral. There are multiple case reports of peroneal nerve palsy induced by nontraumatic situations including ice application to the lateral knee due to its relative lack of insulation in this region (1). It is important to remember this point when treating lateral knee injuries.

Treatment. Most minor contusions and/or hematomas are treated with ice, elevation, and judicious use of nonsteroidal anti-inflammatory drugs (NSAIDs) to control inflammation and prevent serious complications. Rest and reduced or limited weight-bearing should be advised if the contusion limits or affects the function of the leg. This may prevent further injury or extension of injury.

Return to play. With the resumption of the full function of the leg, an athlete can return to play so long as there is protective padding over the injured area. Rarely, aspiration of fluid from the hematoma can be considered in the acute setting, because of its inherent risks. Laceration, hematoma, and contusion (such as those seen in baseball injuries) should be appropriately cleaned, repaired, and sometimes treated with prophylactic antibiotics for a 1-week period. Any breakage of skin should be accompanied by tetanus prophylaxis unless immunization is up-to-date (within 10 years for adults; within 5 years for children).

Prevention. Sports in which lower leg injury is a common threat, have adopted standard equipments for their prevention (shin guards in soccer, ice hockey, and for baseball catchers). A patient with a past history of serious injury should be protected by a rigid shin guard.

Medial Tibial Stress Syndrome

Medial tibial stress syndrome (MTSS), sometimes referred to as *shin splints* is typically painful at the posteromedial border of the tibia generally because of an increase in the volume of impact exercises. Running generates many of these injuries and shin splints make up 15% of all running injuries, whereas stress fractures of the lower leg accounted for another 15%. Rapid increase in training regimens by either intensity, duration, or frequency, as well as running more than 40 miles per week and for 7 days a week are all considered as risk factors for the development of this type of overuse injury (2). Theories regarding the pathogenesis include a periostitis of the posteromedial tibia as well as a traction injury of the attachment of the tibialis posterior, flexor digitorum longus, or soleus muscles to the tibia.

Biomechanics and etiology. MTSS results from any number of the following factors. Poor conditioning, inappropriate training, improper footwear, running on inconsistent surfaces, running on sloped or banked surfaces, running on unbanked tracks, or any situation that allow for excessive foot pronation or excessive external rotation of the hip. Malalignment such as increased navicular drop and pronated foot or tibial varus may place undue stress on the posteromedial muscle-bone interface. This stress takes place at midstance with the foot pronated.

Diagnostic aids. After 3 to 4 weeks, x-rays may show irregularity of the bony cortex and new bone formation along a portion of the wide attachment of the tibialis posterior tendon to the proximal midshaft of the fibula and tibia. Bone scans may reveal increased uptake in a longitudinal pattern in the same area when compared with the localized, usually transverse, uptake seen in a stress fracture.

Treatment. In addition to treatment, in accordance with grades 2 and 3 of the overuse guidelines, proper support and possible orthotic devices should be considered to prevent hyperpronation and excessive tibial rotation. Some trainers will attempt taping to reduce the traction forces, as well as modalities for symptomatic relief.

Prevention. The best way to treat MTSS, like many overuse injuries, is to prevent it from happening. Some suggestions include careful training programs not exceeding 40 miles per week, and at least one rest day each week. A significant taper is necessary prior to distance events for injury prevention as well as for performance. Advanced runners will be careful to use running shoes with a good midsole cushion, and even consider alternating two pairs of the same type of shoes, to allow the return to normal cushion size on "off days". Also limiting mileage of one pair of shoes to 200 to 400 miles is advisable.

Stress Fractures

Epidemiology. Stress fractures occur most often in the lower leg, usually from a rapid or significant change in the volume of running or jumping activities, or because other factors are overloading the tibia and less commonly the fibula. Location varies but most of them occur in the distal third of the tibia, and occasionally in more high-risk areas such as the proximal tibia, anterior tibial cortex or medial malleolus. Less common proximal and distal fibular stress fractures also occur. Prognostically, stress fractures occurring proximally may be a greater cause for concern. Anterior tibial cortex stress fractures are notorious for protracted healing and progression to nonunion. Other high-risk stress fractures include the femoral neck (particularly tension-sided), patella, fifth metatarsal, tarsal navicular, talus, and first toe sesamoid. Early recognition of these stress fractures that have a propensity for delayed or nonunion may help prevent some long-term complications.

Biomechanics and etiology. Lower extremity stress fractures have many of the same predisposing risk factors as MTSS, which was discussed earlier. However, these stress fractures typically involve an abnormal balance between osteoblast and osteoclast activity. Osteoclasts, which aid in bony breakdown, may have increased activity in a stress reaction. Without appropriate rest to allow reduction in overload to the bone, a stress fracture may occur. Use of ankle braces may increase the risk of fibular stress fractures. Footwear required for particular sports (e.g., the rigid boots worn by figure skaters) may also increase the risk of fibular stress fracture.

Signs and symptoms. Consistent with Grade 4 overuse. The primary complaint is pain that gets worse with activity and initially relieved by rest. Later in the process, the athlete may complain of pain due to normal daily activities. They may also complain of swelling in the area of the stress fracture and may have painful limp.

Differential diagnosis.

- MTSS—pain consistent with Grade 2 or 3 overuse.
- Exertional compartment syndrome—pain worsens as exercise continues, but decreases with cessation of activity.
- Popliteal artery entrapment syndrome—immediate pain with exercise, followed by numbing and tingling.
- Peroneal nerve entrapment.
- Tenosynovitis of the dorsiflexors of the foot—superficial pain located directly over the dorsal-anterior portion of the lower leg with elicitation of pain on dorsiflexion.

Diagnostic aids. A complete tibia/fibula x-ray can be helpful but may be effective only after at least 3 to 4 weeks of symptoms. Periosteal bony reaction or sclerosis may be seen in the area of tenderness. Anterior cortex tibial stress fractures will have the "dreaded black line" and will often need clarification with a computed tomography (CT) scan. Bone scans can be ordered for confirmation of a diagnosis, which is often important, because (except for the cases in which a fracture line is seen) one cannot determine the age or metabolic activity of an injury based on x-ray changes alone, that is, the changes seen on x-ray may be due to an old injury and may not be the cause of current pain. MRI may demonstrate stress fractures well with edema on T2 weighted images and low intensity signal on T1 or proton density images (see Figure 32.3), but often is not cost-effective. Limited MRI has become a diagnostic option in some regions utilizing primarily short tau inversion recovery (STIR) images to evaluate edema patterns.

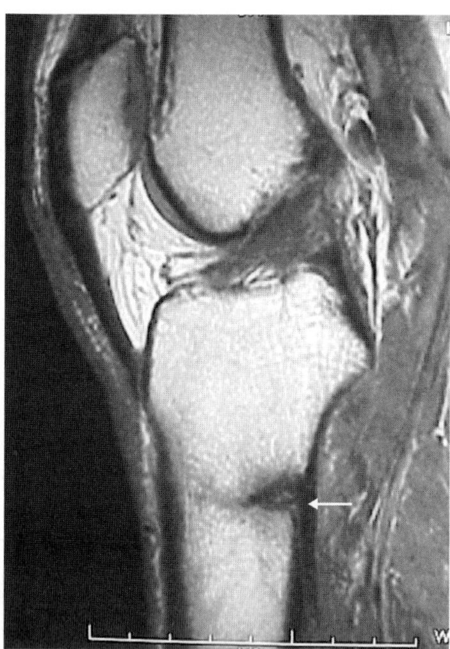

Figure 32.3 Magnetic resonance imaging (MRI) Tibial stress fracture: MRI (sagittal proton density) demonstrating proximal tibial stress fracture (see red arrow). (*Source*: Figure courtesy of Laurie Lomasney, MD, Dept. of Radiology, Loyola University Medical Center.)

Initial treatment. A significant reduction in impact volume is often adequate to treat straightforward distal tibia stress fractures in approximately 4 to 6 weeks. Higher-level athletes and those who are interested in earlier return to activity may be interested in pneumatic walking boots. Leg length ankle stirrup braces are available, and may allow for earlier low-impact activities for athletes with tibial stress fractures. To maintain conditioning, alternative non–weight-bearing sports such as swimming, running in water, or bicycling are appropriate. Once the individual is able to walk without pain, light intensity training (LIT) guidelines are applied. Return to activity should follow gradual increase in intensity, duration, and frequency, as well as sport-specific functional progression. Fibular stress fractures may often be treated similarly to distal tibia stress fractures, and also returned to activity in a graded manner.

Proximal tibial stress fractures and medial malleolus stress fractures usually require longer periods of immobilization. In medial malleolus stress fractures, Shelbourne et al. recommend internal fixation if a fracture line is present (3).

Anterior tibial cortex stress fractures have a poor prognosis, and will need a combination of rest, non–weight bearing and immobilization for at least 4 to 6 months. Use of a pneumatic lower leg brace and modified rest allowed return to unrestricted activity at an average of 12 months from presentation (4). None of the four patients in the study required surgery. Rest and pulsed electromagnetic therapy for at least 3 to 6 months has also been shown to return athletes to competition at an average of 8.7 months of treatment and 12.5 months from initial symptoms (5). In this study, only one of eight patients needed bone grafting procedure, whereas all of them demonstrated complete healing. If healing is not achieved, intramedullary rod placement in the tibial shaft should be considered. In one series, 9 of 17 patients failed conservative treatment at 6 months, progressed to delayed nonunion and required intramedullary rod placement (6). All five patients had good or excellent results after intramedullary nailing in patients who failed nonoperative therapy for more than 1 year (7).

Prevention. Although it would seem that certain people are prone to develop stress fractures, such a hypothesis has not been consistently proven. Many of the prevention studies discussed with MTSS apply with lower extremity stress fractures as well. Repeated stress fractures are certainly a cause of concern and causes of osteopenia/osteoporosis should be considered, particularly in the female athlete. Prolonged amenorrhea secondary to hypoestrogenism may be a factor. Dietary (low calcium and/or vitamin D intake) and eating pattern (anorexia nervosa and bulimia nervosa) problems may also play a role. Careful clinical monitoring of the progression from overuse injury to stress fracture in athletes should be done by medical personnel who are comfortable in evaluating such injuries. The most important preventative measure may simply be adopting a "start low, go slow" attitude to changes in training regimens.

Compartment Syndrome

Epidemiology. Theoretically, the signs and symptoms that make up a compartment syndrome could happen in any of the four major muscle compartments located in the lower leg. The most commonly involved compartment is the anterior compartment. Next in order of frequency is the lateral compartment.

Biomechanics. These syndromes can be either acute (trauma) or more commonly chronic (overuse), and are the result of intrinsic swelling followed by compression of vascular and muscular structures. The initial swelling is the result of overload on the muscles comprising the compartment.

Symptoms. The onset of pain over the compartment begins within the first 5 to 10 minutes of exercise, and is usually relieved when the activity ceases. This differentiates compartment involvement from that of generalized overuse (MTSS), where pain usually begins later during the exercise and may continue well after exercise. Numbing or tingling of the distal lower extremity may be present and reflects involvement of the neurovascular bundle, but this is often a late finding. There is controversy surrounding the deep posterior compartment incorporating the flexor muscles of the foot and the posterior tibial neurovascular bundle.

Signs. In the ambulatory setting, swelling and possible edema of the compartment may be noted. Compartment musculature will be painful to touch, possibly weak, but seldom is neurovascular compromise clinically evident. Passive stretching of the compartment muscles will cause pain. Clinical signs are usually historical, and it may be worthwhile to have the athlete formally note the timing of his/her symptoms with exercise.

Diagnostic aids. Compartment testing is the gold standard for diagnosis of this condition. Normal resting compartment pressures are 0 to 8 mmHg. Exertional compartment syndrome can be diagnosed with resting compartment pressure greater than 15 mmHg; 1-minute postexercise pressure greater than 30 mmHg; or 5-minute postexercise pressure greater than 20 mmHg (8). This test should only be performed by physicians who are experienced and comfortable with the procedure because of the possible risks involved, which includes inducing acute compartment syndrome.

Differential diagnosis. In addition to MTSS and tibial/fibular stress fracture, consider thrombophlebitis, osteomyelitis, cellulitis, tumor, nerve entrapment, and intermittent claudication.

Treatment. Correction of biomechanics, especially those mechanics that isolate the muscle group(s) involved. In the case of chronic exertional compartment syndrome, rest, stretching exercises, massage, and ice may be helpful. Because of the risk of formal compartment pressure testing, these conservative treatments may be instituted when the diagnosis is suspected. If these treatments fail, formal testing should be considered. Fasciotomy is required in the acute setting and is often required because of failure of conservative measures in the chronic exertional setting (9).

Medial Gastrocnemius Strain

Anatomy. The gastrocnemius (from the superficial posterior compartment) is injured most often in its medial belly when the foot is dorsiflexed and the knees are forcibly extended in an eccentric manner. When this happens, the medial head of the gastrocnemius near its musculotendinous junction can strain or tear. The gastrocnemius is vulnerable because it works across two joints and is a muscle of short action.

Epidemiology. The middle-aged athlete (usually between 35 and 45 years of age) appears most at risk. Racquet sports are most commonly implicated so that this condition is sometimes termed *tennis leg*.

Treatment. Following the standard RICE (rest, ice, compression, and elevation) regimen along with passive stretching exercises are done initially. Ultrasound can be used but should be avoided if a large hematoma is suspected as the deep heat generated may induce further bleeding. Active stretching and strengthening exercises can usually be started within a week. A calf sleeve may provide some warmth to the area to facilitate stretching. If a partial tear has taken place, a brief period of immobilization may be considered along with RICE protocol. A night splint to keep a passive stretch on the gastrocnemius during sleep may be very helpful initially as well. Advancement to active rehabilitation may take 1 to 2 weeks, even longer for higher-grade injuries. The prognosis for injuries to this muscle is good if treated early and appropriately.

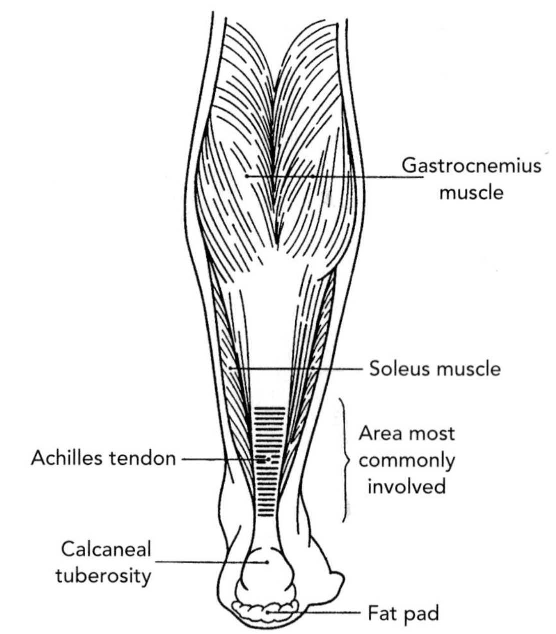

Figure 32.4 Achilles Tendinitis.

Achilles Tendon Injuries

Anatomy. The Achilles tendon represents the conjoined tendon of the gastrocnemius and soleus muscles, the latter a major contributor to the plantar flexion strength of the foot. The extreme distal portion of the Achilles tendon appears to have a poor blood supply, especially in the region 2 to 6 cm above the insertion on the calcaneus. A normal tendon is extremely strong and able to withstand forces up to 2,000 pounds during fast running.

Epidemiology. Three clinical entities will be discussed here:

- *Achilles tendinitis*—usually seen in repetitive overload overuse, common in running.
- *Complete tear or Achilles tendon rupture*—seen in sports such as basketball, tennis, or skiing that involve sudden maximal contraction of the musculotendinous unit.
- *Partial tear*—represents a crossover variant, with etiology representing either overuse and/or acute overload.

Achilles Tendinitis

This can be divided into two clinical presentations:

- *Acute*—involving just the peritenon (tendon sheath), not the tendon itself. The peritenon is not a true synovial sheath as seen with other tendons in the body.
- *Chronic*—the result of prolonged mucoid degeneration of the tendon substance itself. In the chronic condition, active inflammation may not be present, leading to the term *Achilles tendinosis*.

Biomechanics. The usual mechanism of injury is chronic, repetitive overload on the musculotendinous unit (see Figure 32.4). Biomechanical risk factors include tibia varus, tight hamstring muscles, tight calf muscles, and cavus foot. In addition, several training errors can cause this injury: constant hill running, shoes with rigid soles or soft heel counter, shifting from high heel dress shoes to low heel training shoes, changing from cross country running on uneven surfaces to more consistent elastic track surfaces, "ankling" too much in cycling. Repetitive eccentric loading of the Achilles tendon through jumping or running may contribute to injury of the tendon. Each of these situations results in increased pull and tension on the Achilles. Furthermore, the presence of other injuries such as plantar fascitis can cause the foot to land in excessive supination causing the ankle to dorsiflex to avoid pronating the foot. The Achilles tendon can move laterally or medially in response to such running biomechanics.

Signs and symptoms. As with any soft tissue overuse injury, signs and symptoms are consistent with those outlined in the earlier discussion of overuse syndromes.

Differential diagnosis. Although rarely a problem in running, partial rupture of the Achilles tendon should be ruled out.

Diagnostic aids. The work-up of severe or chronic tendinitis, especially if the examination has been accompanied by palpation and thickening of the Achilles tendon, may include x-ray evaluation of Kager's triangle (seen in the lateral view of the affected ankle). This triangle is bound anteriorly by the flexor tendons of the foot, posteriorly by the Achilles tendon unit, and inferiorly by the os calcis. The radiolucent area will become more dense and less radiolucent in cases of severe tendinitis or partial rupture. Failure of conservative treatment of chronic Achilles tendonitis after a dedicated eccentric load tendon strengthening program for typically 6 months or longer may necessitate further imaging, and possibly surgical referral. In these less common, recalcitrant cases, ultrasound images may demonstrate tendon pathology well. MRI can also be helpful in identifying abnormal Achilles tendon pathology, or particularly if there are other associated injuries.

Treatment. Initial treatment should consist of ice, initial stretching before exercise, use of NSAIDs, decreased mileage, avoiding banked roads and hills, and reassessing shoes, making sure that the following exist: flexible sole, molded heel pad. A heel lift at least 1/2 inch high has been shown to reduce the relative stress on the Achilles tendon, that is, the microtrauma throughout the day. It is imperative that this be done in conjunction with aggressive heel cord stretches, as wearing the heel lift functionally shortens the Achilles tendon. A walking-boot or ankle–foot orthoses (AFO) may be considered for temporary unloading of the tendon, in more severe cases. For recalcitrant cases, surgical debridement is rarely necessary. Ultrasound has some anecdotal success in these injuries. Rehabilitation should consist of stretching and eccentric strengthening exercises for the Achilles tendon. Eccentric tendon strengthening can show structural improvement of the tendon as well as clinical improvement within 3 to 6 months.

Prevention. Address any preexisting injury or deformity and attempt to correct before resuming exercise.

Special considerations. At no point in the therapy of Achilles tendinitis should steroid injections be used. The potential compromise to the vascular system of the Achilles tendon, as well as the weakening and possible necrosis stimulated by such an injection precludes this form of therapy for this injury.

Achilles Tendon Rupture

Epidemiology. Rupture occurs predominantly in male athletes in their third to fifth decade of life, in sports of sudden extreme movement such as basketball, tennis, long jumping, and skiing. Most ruptures occur 2 to 6 cm above the insertion of the Achilles tendon on the os calcis in the area of decreased vascularity. The left Achilles tendon is ruptured significantly more often than the right. Predisposing factors: (a) nonspecific degeneration perhaps secondary to vascular impairment produced by the particular repetitious form of exercise; (b) history of corticosteroid injections into the Achilles tendon; (c) repeated subclinical injury leading to necrosis and weakening of the tendon unit, and (d) normal tendon physiology that has undergone extreme pathomechanical stress.

Symptoms. Most published theories on acute tendon rupture include the statement that misdiagnoses can be as high as 20% to 25%. Usual symptoms include a sudden forced movement followed by a loud audible snap. The athlete will classically feel as if he/she has been struck on the back of his/her calf. Often, the initial pain will diminish and walking is possible. There is a weakness in plantar flexion and, at times, a feeling of the foot penetrating through the floor as if in plantar flexion.

Signs. The affected tendon may be thicker and a palpable gap may be felt. However, blood in the form of a hematoma may often collect underneath the peritenon and fill the gap, making it difficult to palpate the defect. The plantaris tendon may be palpable in this area leading the examiner to believe that the Achilles is only partially torn. Bruising and swelling is often apparent. The patient demonstrates a notable weakness in plantar flexion (although active plantar flexion is still possible because of intact secondary muscles of plantar flexion) and an inability to stand on tiptoe. Whether this inability is due to pain or actual loss of function must be determined. Careful palpation usually can show a difference between an entrapped hematoma and an intact tendon. On occasion, there may be a slight increase in dorsiflexion in the position of rest. The Thompson test should be done with the athlete prone, knee bent, and foot hanging. The calf should be squeezed with the examiner's hand distal to the apex of the soleus muscle. If plantar flexion cannot be elicited, it is a strong (but not an absolute) evidence for complete tendon rupture and the test is positive (see Figure 32.5).

Diagnostic aids. MRI can depict rupture and partial rupture of the Achilles tendon in excellent detail, but is often not necessary in diagnosing this condition. The merits of MR imaging with regard to the decision-making process are not usually cost-effective and therefore are not always necessary as a routine part of the work-up unless diagnosis is in question. Ultrasound is a less-expensive alternative to MR that also shows the Achilles tendon in nice detail and can differentiate between partial and complete Achilles tendon disruption (see Figure 32.6).

Initial treatment. Immediate ice, immobilization in slight plantar flexion, crutches, pain relief, if necessary.

Definitive treatment. There are three treatment options: open surgery, percutaneous repair, and closed repair (nonsurgical). A good deal of controversy exists about which is the most appropriate treatment. Recent studies suggest that there may be equivalent results in nonoperative treatment with cast immobilization in plantar flexion versus operative repair (10,11). Patients return to competitive sports without restriction in approximately 6 months in either group. A recent meta-analysis of studies involving these treatment options concluded that open operative treatment was associated with a lower risk of rerupture compared with nonoperative treatment (12). Operative treatment in general has more risks such as infection, adhesions, and disturbed skin sensibility. Operative risks may be modified by performing surgery percutaneously. It also appears that postoperative

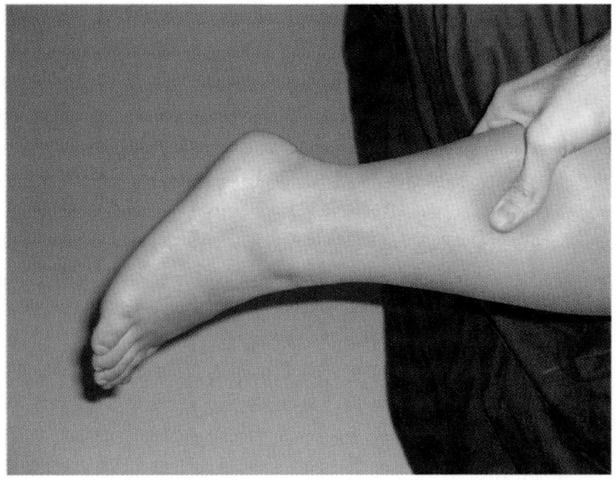

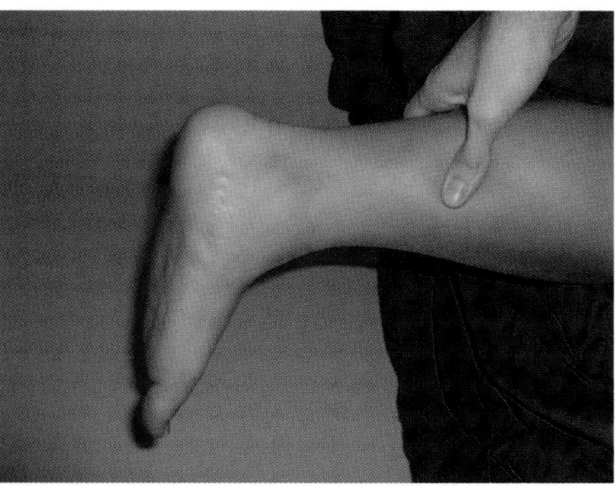

Figure 32.5 Positive Thompson test: Notice plantar flexion on unaffected leg and lack of plantar flexion on affected leg with compression of posterior calf.

splinting with functional brace reduces the overall complication rate. Nonoperative cast immobilization appears to have a higher rate of rerupture than functional bracing in this meta-analysis (12). From the primary care sports medicine standpoint, clinical evidence of a ruptured Achilles tendon should be followed up by referral to an orthopedic surgeon.

Postoperative rehabilitation. Although recommendations vary somewhat, the affected leg should be placed in plantar flexion in a long leg cast with slight knee flexion for 3 weeks. Note that, to prevent atrophy of the soleus muscle, place the foot in as much dorsi flexion as possible without straining the integrity of the tendon repair. Then a short leg cast or an AFO should be used for three more weeks. After immobilization, both legs should be fitted with an elevated heel and weight bearing begun until there is normal heel to toe gait. Heel elevation can then be decreased and stretching exercises begun. Strengthening should take place beginning with simple plantar flexion and gradually increasing the resistance until standing on toes can be done without

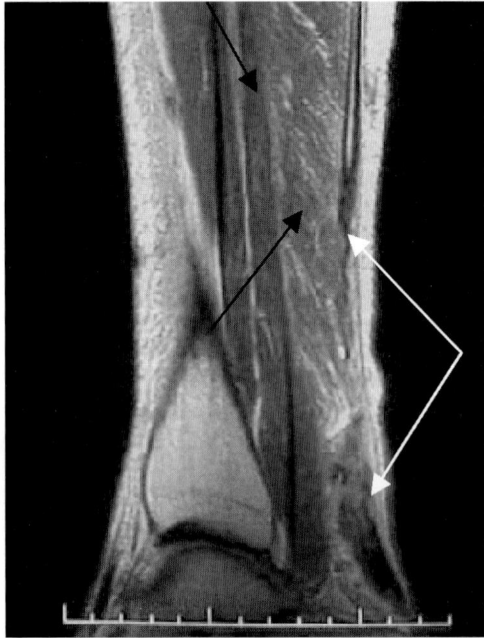

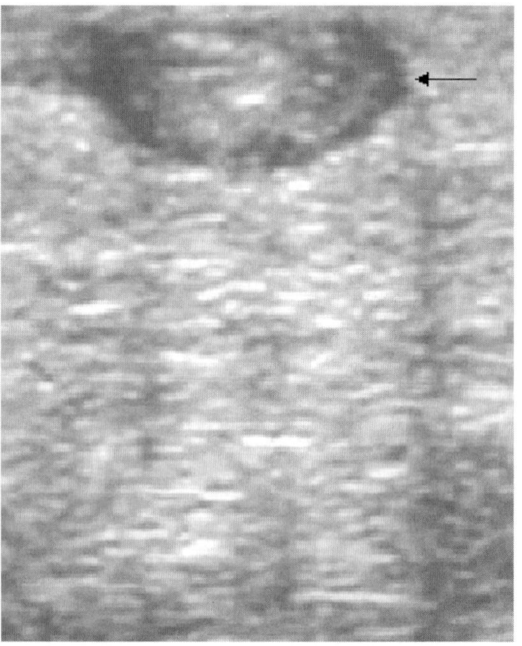

Figure 32.6 A: Magnetic resonance image (MRI) Achilles Tendon Rupture: MRI (sagittal Proton Density) demonstrating complete rupture Achilles tendon (see arrow). B: Ultrasound of high grade partial tear of Achilles tendon (see arrow). (*Source*: Figures courtesy of Laurie Lomasney, MD, Dept. of Radiology, Loyola University Medical Center.)

pain. Achilles tendon stretching using an incline board should follow. The prognosis is guarded and seems to be dependent upon the delay of initial treatment. A tendon graft may be necessary if there is a significant delay or misdiagnosis.

In one study, early mobilization in postoperative rehabilitation of Achilles tendon repair did not increase the rerupture rate and overall, all 64 patients returned to normal activities in an average of 3.3 months (13). The program consisted of wearing a moveable ankle brace for 4 to 6 weeks in 0 to 15 degrees of dorsiflexion and 10 weeks of regular exercises. Conservatively treated patients with early immediate weight-bearing program did not show any evidence of a functional benefit from immediate weight-bearing mobilization, without increase in rerupture rate even in postoperative group (14). Such early weight bearing and immediate mobilization programs seem to be effective in most cases, but caution should be taken in those athletes younger than 30 years (15).

Partial Rupture of Achilles Tendon

Epidemiology. Partial rupture usually occurs in the young athlete (20–30 years of age) at his/her highest level of performance.

Biomechanics. Biomechanics are similar to those seen with tendon rupture as well as tendinitis.

Symptoms. Symptoms can present either as a tendinitis-like picture except that symptoms do not clear with standard tendinitis treatment, or there can be a sudden onset, but with a negative Thompson test.

Signs. Classic signs include nodular or fusiform swelling, pain with motion, decreased function, possible crepitus, localized tenderness on palpation, pain on forced passive dorsiflexion, as well as resistance to active plantar flexion. A partial rupture can become chronic and result in calf muscle atrophy, as well as possible passive dorsiflexion of the ankle. A "hop" test (patient hops on bended affected leg) can help identify this complication.

Diagnostic aids. A soft tissue x-ray of the lateral aspect of the ankle may show a loss of radiolucence of Kagar's triangle, but no distortion. MRI may assist in determining the integrity of the tendon, in complex cases.

Treatment. Initial treatment consists of ice, strapping, heel lift, NSAIDs, and short-term immobilization. Steroid injections are discouraged for the reasons stated previously. If conservative treatment is not effective, the patient should be referred to an orthopedic surgeon.

Retrocalcaneal Bursitis

Epidemiology. Running or any sport involving the possibility of an ill-fitting shoe. Commonly referred to as a *pump bump*.

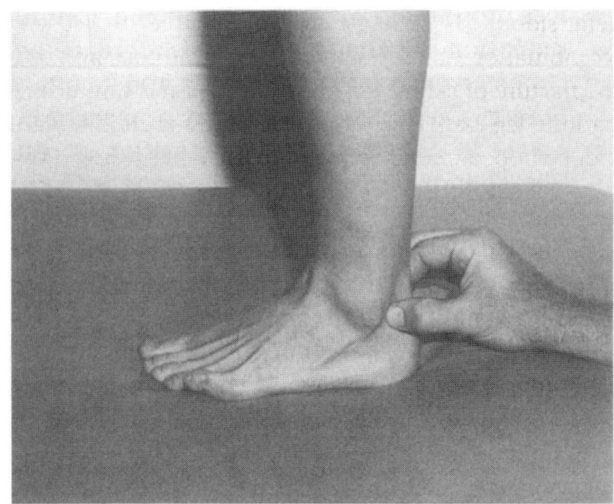

Figure 32.7 Retrocalcaneal bursitis.

Biomechanics. Irritation of the posterior calcaneal prominence by the heel counter causing swelling of the retrocalcaneal bursa.

Symptoms. Localized pain.

Signs. Palpation of the bursa elicits tenderness anterior to the attachment of the tendon on the os calcis (see Figures 32.7 and 32.8).

Diagnostic aids. X-rays may reveal increased bony deposition on the posterior superior calcaneus (Haglund's deformity)

Differential diagnosis Achilles tendonitis, calcaneus stress fracture.

Treatment. Correction of ill-fitting shoe with a higher (or lower) heel counter or pad, and ice. NSAIDs or analgesics may be helpful.

Acute Fracture

In the lower leg, athletes can fracture the tibia, fibula or both. Mid-shaft and proximal tibial fractures must be immobilized with a long leg cast following reduction. Fibular fractures (because the bone is essentially non–weight bearing) can often be treated with a short leg cast or walking-boot. Unstable fractures involving the medial or

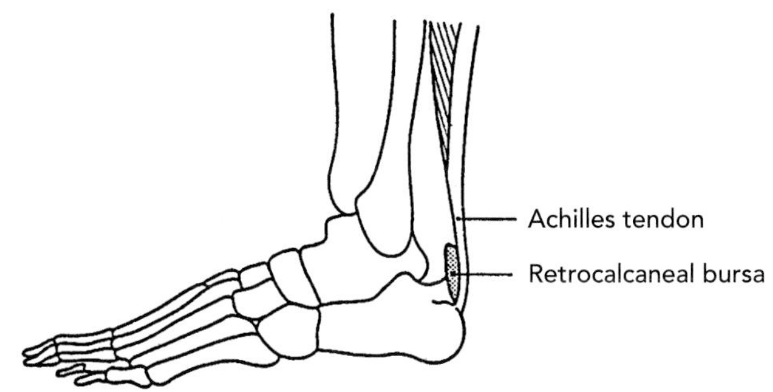

Figure 32.8 Retrocalcaneal bursitis.

lateral side of the ankle should be referred to a surgeon. A combination tibia/fibula fracture, or the common "boot top" fracture of skiing, must be reduced and immobilized in a long leg cast. This serious fracture should be referred to an orthopedic surgeon for possible open reduction and internal fixation.

ANKLE

The ankle is the most frequently injured joint in the body. It accounts for 30% to 50% of all reported athletic injuries and 20% to 25% of all time-loss athletic injuries. Although some believe it is a relatively simple joint to understand, ankle injury is often misdiagnosed and inadequately treated. Unfortunately, longstanding sequelae from inappropriate treatment are considerable. The chronically unstable, painful ankle accounts for significant disability, as well as premature osteoarthritis in the older athletes.

Anatomy

The ankle is a synovial hinge joint that functions basically in flexion and extension (see Figure 32.9). The ankle mortise has the shape of an inverted U with the lateral border formed by the distal fibula and the dorsal–medial border by the distal tibia. The talus, upon which these long bones sit, is a trapezoid-shaped, thick bone with flat lateral and dorsal surfaces for stability.

Ligaments

A protective shield of ligaments and tendons overlies the joint capsule (see Figure 32.10). The main ligaments involved in ankle stability include the following:

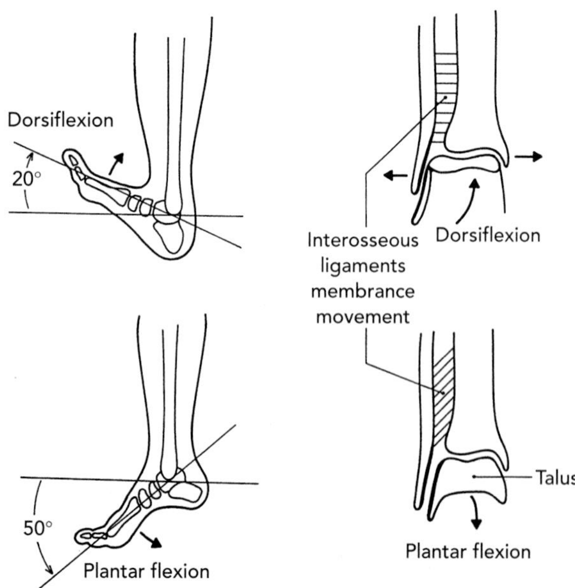

Figure 32.9 Ankle joint anatomy.

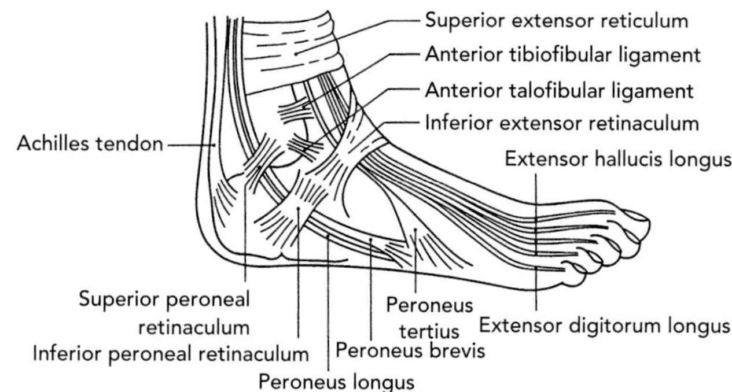

Figure 32.10 Tendons and ligaments of ankle.

- *Internal Stability*—the distal tibiofibular ligament, a thickened extension of the interosseous membrane maintains the anatomical relationship between the tibia and fibula.
- *Medial Stability*—the thick deltoid ligament, made up of superficial and deep components, prevents eversion.
- *Lateral Stability*—achieved by three major ligaments (anterior to posterior): (a) anterior talofibular; (b) calcaneofibular; (c) posterior talofibular, as well as inherent bony stability from the longer distal fibula (lateral malleolus).

Muscles

Further stabilizing the joint are the following muscle tendons that overlie the ligaments (see Figure 32.10):

- *Anterior and Medial Stability*—extensor tendons of the toes; tibialis anterior tendon.
- *Lateral Stability*—peroneus longus and brevis muscles, evertors of the foot.
- *Posterior Stability*—flexor tendons of the toes; posterior tibial muscle; gastrocnemius, and soleus muscles (Achilles complex).

Special Notes

The anterior and posterior tibial muscles coordinate to cause inversion, balancing the effect of the peroneal muscles. Joint forces generated in the ankle are a function of externally applied forces and the internal forces from muscles and ligaments around the joint. The common pathophysiological insult in soft tissue ankle injuries is an applied force that exceeds soft tissue strength. Therefore, more injuries are seen in areas where there are relatively weak bony interrelationships and soft tissue stabilizing structures.

Ankle Evaluation

History

There are six important facets of the history involved in any ankle injury, which are as follows:

1. *Biomechanics*. An understanding of the biomechanical action that produce an injury is the most important part of the history of an ankle injury.

2. *Weight bearing*. Was the athlete able to bear weight upon the injured extremity after injury?
3. *Sounds*: Were any sounds (pop, snap) heard at the time of injury? Although perhaps not as sensitive a measurement as similar sounds with knee injuries, their presence may help the physician in his differential diagnosis.
4. *Onset of Swelling*: The timing of swelling after injury is also not as sensitive as it is with knee injuries, but it gives a general idea of the seriousness of an ankle injury.

   Late ecchymoses, particularly near the base of the foot, may sometimes be extravasation of bleeding through the subtalar joint to the opposite side.

   Special Note— recurrent ankle soft tissue injury is common and it appears that scar tissue may actually serve to impede ankle swelling. Relatively mild swelling should not mislead the examiner into considering a diagnosis of minor ankle injury.
5. *Treatment*: Has any treatment been given for the injury before the examination? The misguided application of heat instead of ice can significantly change the presentation of ankle injuries.
6. *Past Medical History*: Many people have recurrent ankle injuries. This must be taken into account in assessing the current signs and symptoms.

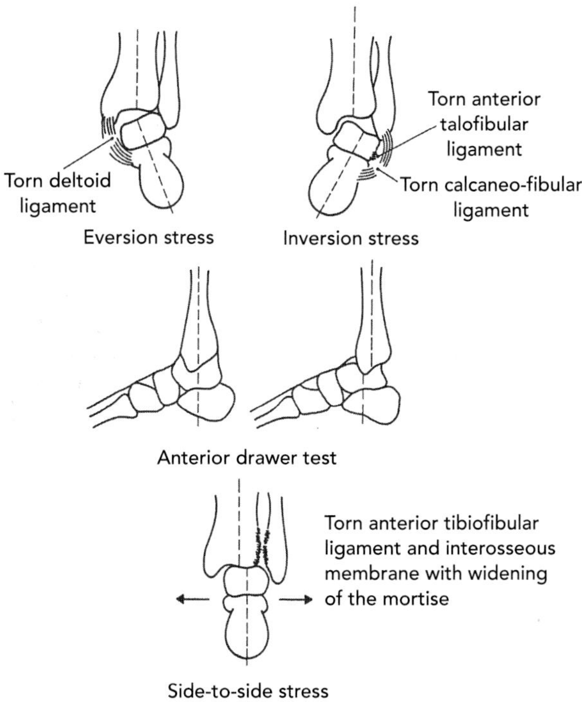

Figure 32.11 Ankle stress test.

Physical Examination

As with any other impaired extremity, always use the uninjured ankle as a reference and examine it first. Important points in the approach to examination of an injured ankle are:

- *Observation*. First, assess general disability by weight-bearing status, and gait. Assessment of foot cavus or pronation deformities, as well as observing if heels go into varus when double and single toe raise are performed. Observe the ankle at rest for bruising, swelling, or deformity that may be present.
- *Palpation*. Begin palpation proximal to the injury. A complete ankle examination begins at the knee and ends at the tips of the toes. Assess for bony tenderness. Important bony landmarks are medial/lateral malleoli, base of the fifth metatarsal, midfoot (navicular bone, Lisfranc joint) and proximal fibula. Assess for soft tissue tenderness. Important soft tissue landmarks include all three lateral ligaments, deltoid ligament, syndesmotic area (distal tibiofibular ligament), Achilles tendon, peroneal tendon, and posterior tibialis tendons. Palpate both the dorsalis pedis and tibialis posterior pulses.
- *Range of Motion*. Both passive and active range of motion (ROM) surrounding the four major movements of the ankle (dorsiflexion, plantar flexion, inversion, and eversion) should be assessed. Subtalar motion should also be assessed. Crepitus during ROM may indicate tenosynovitis, tendonitis or bony injury.
- *Stress Testing*. The following tests should be assessed in relation to the uninjured side (see Figure 32.11).

a. *Thompson Test*. To assess integrity of the Achilles tendon (see description in the preceding text).
b. *Syndesmotic tests*. The Squeeze sign involves compression of the tibia and fibula in the proximal leg to elicit distal pain (sign for distal syndesmotic injury). Dorsiflexion–compression test, with additional eversion if necessary typically elicits pain in syndesmotic injuries as well.
c. *Anterior Drawer*. Anterior translation of the talus within the ankle mortise with foot in slight plantar flexion (to isolate the anterior talofibular ligament). Depending upon comparison with the other side, the anterior drawer may have a normal shift of up to 3 mm.
d. *Talar Tilt (Inversion stress test)*. With the ankle at 90 degrees, the tibiotalar joint is inverted to assess the stability of the calcaneofibular ligament.
e. *Eversion Stress Test*. This test is done to check for stability of the medial compartment of the ankle. Any give at all, especially a tilt of more than 5 degrees, should be considered abnormal.
f. *Side-to-Side Test*. This maneuver assesses widening of the ankle mortise caused by instability of the tibiofibular ligament. If the examiner hears a "thud" or elicits pain on a side-to-side test, it is considered positive.
g. *External Rotation Test*. This is carried out with the patient seated, ankle and knee at 90 degrees, and foot externally rotated. This is usually painful in the setting of a stable or especially unstable syndesmotic injury.
h. *Strength testing*. Resisted ankle motion in all planes including planter flexion and inversion (tests tibialis posterior muscle) should be performed.

X-ray

Not every ankle injury requires ankle x-rays. As many as 75% to 85% of all ankle injuries involve no fractures and are essentially soft tissue trauma. The "Ottawa Ankle Rules" were developed to reduce the number of unnecessary x-rays in the emergency room (ER) setting, and have been shown to be clinically sensitive for not missing significant fractures (16). Anteroposterior (AP), lateral, and oblique x-rays (weight bearing if possible) should be considered in patients who (a) cannot bear weight after injury, (b) are tender over medial malleolus, talus, calcaneus, or posterior half of lateral malleolus, (b) are unable to ambulate four steps in ER (or office), (c) have prolonged pain or swelling, (d) are skeletally immature or over the age of 55 (16). Stress films can be performed but are not typically necessary to make an accurate diagnosis. This is an uncomfortable test for an injured athlete, therefore anesthetic block should be considered before testing.

Mechanisms known to cause ankle injury may produce fractures in bones around the knee and foot. Careful palpation will direct the clinician towards ordering the correct diagnostic study. Pain at the proximal fibula may indicate a Maisonneuve fracture that can be seen on knee or tibia/fibula x-rays. Pain at the base of the fifth metatarsal or navicular bone should direct the clinician to obtain foot radiographs instead of ankle films.

Common Injuries

Sprains

There are three major biomechanical types of ankle sprains: lateral inversion sprains, medial eversion sprains, and syndesmotic (dorsiflexion, abduction, external rotation) sprain.

Lateral Inversion Sprain

The lateral inversion sprains account for 80% to 85% of all ankle sprains.

Biomechanics. Plantar flexion, inversion, and internal rotation of the ankle results in isolation and stretching (followed by tearing) of the three lateral stabilizing ligaments of the ankle. These ligaments usually are torn in the same order. As stress is placed on the lateral compartment, the medial malleolus acts as a fulcrum for the talus so that the anterior talofibular ligament is injured. If the stress is enough, the calcaneofibular ligament and, finally the posterior talofibular ligament will give way. Occasionally, with the torque forces of rotation, the calcaneofibular ligament can be isolated and injured. Associated with the lateral inversion sprain is compression of the medial malleolar tip or avulsion of the distal fibula. Additional etiological factors that contribute to inversion injury include a tight Achilles tendon and an irregular playing surface.

Epidemiology. Of all inversion injuries, 85% involve an isolated tear of the anterior talofibular ligament. This injury is most frequently seen in sports such as football, basketball, baseball, and soccer.

Symptoms. Sudden onset of lateral ankle pain as a result of misstep and/or "turning-over" of the ankle.

Signs. Ankle sprains usually begin with immediate swelling, localized tenderness, signs of hemorrhage, varying degrees of weight-bearing intolerance, and joint laxity. Joint laxity and stability is best assessed by stress tests (see Figure 32.11). It should be first determined whether or not an ankle is stable. A general rule is that early motion and rehabilitation is suggested for stable lateral ankle injuries. Meanwhile initial immobilization to maintain the ligament in anatomic neutral position, followed by motion and appropriate rehabilitation is recommended for unstable lateral ankle injuries. Primary surgical repair of unstable lateral ankle sprains without fracture or syndesmotic injury is not usually recommended. The degree of swelling, sometimes, does not necessarily correlate with the severity of the injury. Swelling can be pronounced in a "virgin" uninjured ankle with a minimal injury and be minimal in a recurrent serious ankle sprain.

Treatment. Treatment of a stable lateral ankle sprain should follow a basic six-step program: 1) Protection of the joint with control of pain and swelling, 2) Regain/maintain motion, 3) Regain/maintain strength, 4) Proprioception training, 5) Advancement of sport-specific activities, and 6) Eventual return to sport.

Step 1 can be accomplished by a combination of RICE maneuvers, immobilization in a pneumatic walking-boot or stirrup splint, crutches or other assistive devices, electrical stimulation and analgesic and/or NSAIDs. Prolonged immobilization may result in faster pain relief, but often leads to prolonged rehabilitation because of joint stiffness and weakness.

Steps 2 to 4 can be accomplished by instituting a home exercise program of ROME (range of motion exercises), resistance strength exercises, and proprioceptive training drills such as one-foot standing (eyes open and eyes closed), standing on uneven surfaces (rocker boards, pillows, mini-trampolines) and one-foot squats. Most athletes can perform these therapeutic exercises on their own or under the supervision of an athletic trainer. In some cases, formal therapy may be appropriate.

Step 5 should only be instituted after good pain control has been achieved, motion is full and strength is within 85% of the uninjured side. Agility drills such as one-foot hop, lateral jumping, ladder drills, and lateral crossover running can be advanced into sport-specific activities at a low intensity. Intensity and difficulty of these drills can be advanced until the athlete is ready to return to full play. The speed of advancement is based on athlete response to lower levels of activity. There is no good way to predict how long it will take an athlete to return to the field after a lateral ankle sprain. Sometimes the seemingly mild injury may take months to improve, whereas the initially significant injury may progress much more rapidly. In view of this, each case must be approached individually.

There is much debate concerning which type of external ankle support should be used after injury or for prophylaxis. The three general types most commonly utilized are functional ankle taping, functional semirigid ankle support, and lace-up ankle braces. The use of ankle braces as part of the rehabilitation program is indicated to give the injured athlete some degree of protection. Initial return to activity after functional progression with some external support is generally recommended. Assessment of the various protective devices involves their comfort to the athlete and how restricted the ankle ROM will be after exercise.

- *Taping*. In the hands of a knowledgeable athletic trainer, ankle taping remains an effective means of restricting ROM. It takes knowledge and time and does have undesirable aspects such as skin and soft tissue irritations. Sweat and time may reduce tape's restrictive capabilities.
- *Semirigid-orthosis (e.g., Aircast, Active-Ankle)*. This brace restricts inversion and eversion while permitting plantar and dorsiflexion (see Figure 32.12).
- *Lace-up (e.g., Swede-O, Mueller)*. A laceable, cloth brace reinforced by medial and lateral plastic inserts. This brace is comfortable and functional and also holds restricted ROM as well as the above braces.

Conclusions. A systematic review of external ankle supports was recently performed examining joint kinematics as well as performance (17). Semirigid braces restricted inversion and eversion more than tape and lace-up braces before and after exercise, while the latter two provided similar protection. With regards to functional performance, external bracing did not seem to negatively affect sprint time or vertical jump, whereas the effects on agility were equivocal. Additionally, in stable first-time lateral ankle sprains, external bracing with elastic wrap and Air-Stirrup brace provides earlier return to preinjury function than either of these alone or even a walking cast for 10 days (18).

Author's preference. Any external bracing used to prevent further ankle injuries in a person with chronic, recurrent ankle sprains that is relatively comfortable is appropriate. Economics and convenience, as well as comfort and functional performance are factors to consider in choosing an appropriate brace. Information regarding the different types of braces can be provided by the physician, however the eventual decision is made by the athlete.

Medial Eversion Sprains

Epidemiology. This injury is commonly seen in wrestlers or football players who push off the inside or medial component of their ankle. The mechanism represents less than 10% of all ankle sprains, but more than 75% of all ankle fracture.

Biomechanics. External rotation of the leg, dorsiflexion, and pronation lead to isolation of and injury to the deltoid ligament. Medial compartment injury is more likely to cause bony damage than lateral compartment injury. The deltoid ligament is such a strong support structure that the medial malleolar bony substance will often avulse before a tear occurs in the deltoid ligament. Common extensions of this injury include the following (see Figure 32.13): (a) deltoid ligament tear and/or medial malleolar avulsion fracture; (b) extension to the tibiofibular ligament (usually anterior); (c) further extension to involve fracture of the distal fibular shaft; or (d) extension to the interosseous membrane.

Signs and symptoms. These are similar to those seen in the lateral ankle sprain.

Diagnostic aids. X-rays (possibly augmented by stress views) are indicated in medial compartment injuries. They may show a medial malleolar fracture creating an unstable joint, or a widening of the ankle mortise between the talus and medial malleolus

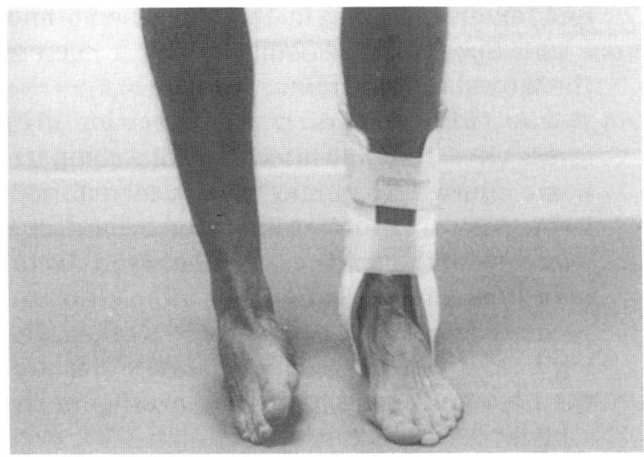

A

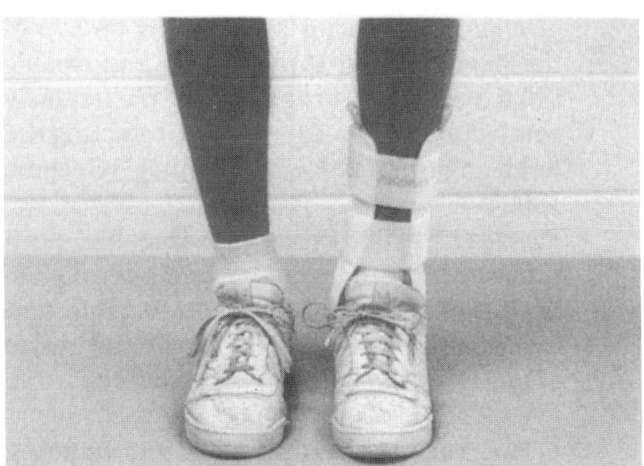

B

Figure 32.12 Functional Semirigid Bracing. A: Brace permits dorsi and plantar flexion but prevents excessive inversion. B: Can be readily accommodated by an ordinary athletic shoe.

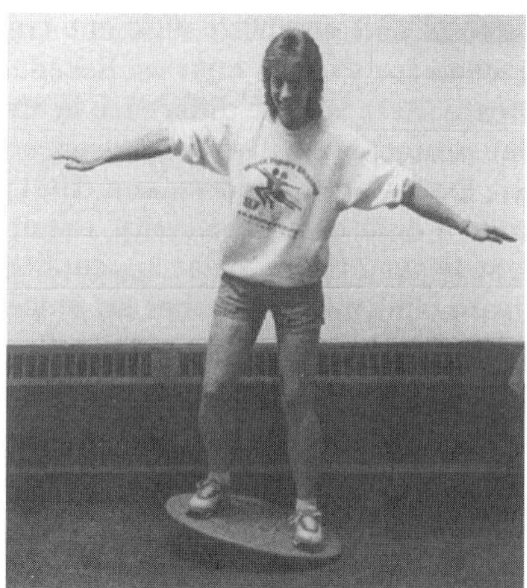

Figure 32.13 Injury of the Distal Tibiofibular Ligament.

(see Figure 32.14). Sometimes this is not appreciated unless an oblique view (or mortise view) is taken, giving a clear view of the ankle mortise, because the tibia and fibula frequently overlap in the straight AP view. If the patient can tolerate, weight-bearing ankle views can give more accurate representation of the ankle mortise.

Treatment. Similar treatment protocols as outlined for the lateral ankle sprains. In general, medial sprains take longer to heal than a lateral sprain, as it usually requires more force to injure the medial ankle ligaments. Surgery may be indicated if any of the four extensions outlined in the preceding text have occurred, primarily because of side-to-side instability that does not respond well to rehabilitation.

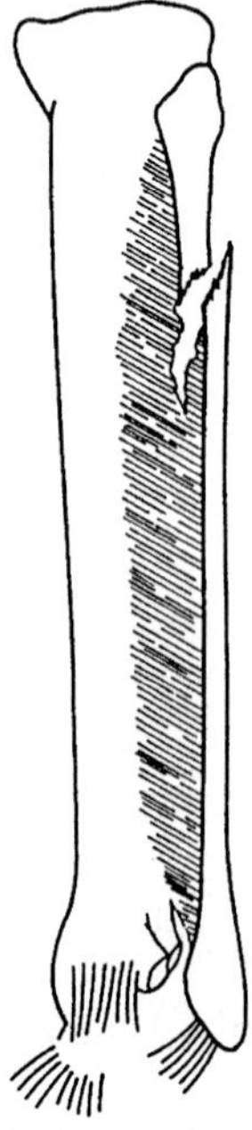

Figure 32.14 Widening of the ankle mortise.

Syndesmotic Injuries (High Ankle Sprain)

Epidemiology. This injury is caused by trauma or forced dorsiflexion with abduction and external rotation of the foot such as those seen in soccer, gymnastics, tennis, skiing, basketball, running backs in football, or sliding in baseball. True syndesmotic injuries are uncommon and are quite disabling with return to competition generally in 5 to 10 weeks (19).

Biomechanics. External rotation is felt to be the primary mechanism of injury. Extreme dorsiflexion after the normal ROM may also cause tearing of the extensor retinaculum and anterior tibiofibular ligament as the wider, anterior portion of the talus is forced into the ankle mortise. Fractures are commonly associated with syndesmotic injuries.

Diagnosis. Physical examination of an athlete with a syndesmotic injury differs significantly from the normal findings of lateral ankle sprain.

- Significant swelling and bruising in the anterolateral ankle, proximal to the joint.
- Tenderness elicited in the anterior tibiofibular ligament. Associated deltoid ligament injury is common. Be sure to palpate the proximal fibula as extreme forced external rotation may lead to Maisonneuve fracture.
- Radiation of the pain may occur proximally along syndesmosis.
- There is typically less tenderness over the lateral compartment (if there is no associated fracture).
- Pain can be reproduced either by passively rotating the foot externally or dorsiflexing the foot.

X-ray. X-rays of patients with syndesmotic injuries may initially be negative. Sometimes small associated fibular fractures, as well as medial malleolar fractures may be noted. Widening of the ankle mortise may also be seen and may need to be clarified with stress views.

Treatment. These injuries take much longer to heal than the more common lateral inversion injury. Return to a normal level of activity may take from 5 to 10 weeks, depending on the severity of the injury. A stable syndesmotic sprain may be treated with prolonged boot immobilization (up to 8 weeks or longer if needed) to allow appropriate healing of the syndesmosis as well as the deltoid ligament. Rehabilitation exercises, as described previously (with attention to tibialis posterior strengthening for medial stability), can be performed out of the boot. Unstable syndesmotic injuries with or without fracture should be referred to a surgeon. Surgical stabilization may be performed in some of these patients.

Heterotopic ossification of the interosseous membrane occurs in 25% to 90% of cases (20). This condition may or may not cause pain symptoms. If pain persists for several months, it is advisable to obtain a follow-up x-ray (once again in the oblique view) to discover whether ossification of the interosseous membrane or anterior inferior tibiofibular ligament has occurred. Surgical excision may be required if pain cannot be controlled with conservative measures.

Fractures

In the simplest of terms, there are two types of ankle fractures: stable and unstable.

1. *Stable.* These fractures that do not involve the articular surface or disrupt the stability of the joint. Treatment is closed reduction and immobilization with pneumatic walking-boot or casting. Immobilize the ankle at neutral (90 degrees) in most cases. Postreduction x-ray may help establish the correct position. Consider referral for those fractures with less than adequate anatomic alignment.
2. *Unstable.* These fractures involve much of the articular surface and cause significant instability in the ankle joint. The primary care physician must be able to recognize these fractures and refer appropriately.

Differentiating between stable and unstable ankle fractures is difficult but crucial for the team physician. For the purpose of discussion, consider the ankle as a horizontal ring comprised of the deltoid ligament and medial malleolus on the medial side, the lateral malleolus and lateral supporting ligaments on the lateral side, and the anterior and posterior lips of the tibia. This ring encloses and supports the talus. The talus bears more weight per unit area than any other bone in the body and a lateral shift of as little as 1 mm can reduce the contact area of the talus by 40%. Such a reduction in contact area greatly increases the force per unit area on the talus and enhances the development of osteoarthritis.

The Danis-Weber Classification system is a relatively simple method based on the location of distal fibula fractures with relation to the syndesmosis.

- Type A: Fibula fracture below the syndesmosis.
- Type B: Fracture at the level of the syndesmosis.
- Type C: Fracture above the syndesmosis.

There is more inherent instability, the higher the fracture is in relation to the syndesmosis. These three classes are further subdivided into locations of associated fractures. Type C fractures typically involve the syndesmosis as well as the medial side, and are subsequently quite unstable. Meanwhile a Type A that is isolated is typically more stable. This system has some correlation with the commonly used Lauge-Hansen Classification that is based mostly on mechanism of injury (21).

Epiphyseal Fractures

Epiphyseal fractures in the adolescent athlete that break through the distal epiphyses of the fibula and tibia are of some concern. See Figure 32.15 for examples of the Salter-Harris classification. Without comparison films or stress views, both Salter I (separation along the epiphysis) and Salter V (crush injury) can sometimes be missed. However, Salter I fractures through the epiphysis can be routinely diagnosed with clinical tenderness over the physes. Because the bony epiphysis is the "weak link" in the musculoskeletal chain in the skeletally immature, these injuries should be suspected in young individuals with ankle sprains. Careful clinical examination of the lateral or medial compartment will show tenderness over the substance of the malleoli and not at its distal border, the common site of ligamentous pain.

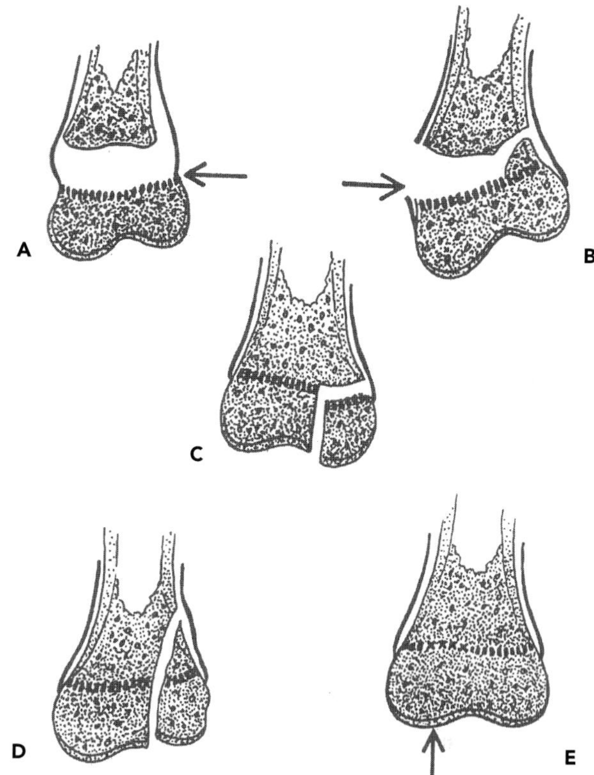

Figure 32.15 Salter-Harris Classification of Epiphyseal Injury. **A:** type I-separation of epiphysis; **B:** type II-Fracture–separation of epiphysis; **C:** type III-Fracture of part of Epiphysis; **D:** fracture of Epiphysis and Epiphyseal Plate; **E:** crush injury to epiphyseal plate.

Treatment involves immobilization, with a longer period of non–weight bearing than normally would be done for a typical ankle fracture. Salter III and IV fractures should be referred to surgeons due to the higher incidences of growth disturbances and potential for malunion. Salter V crush injuries should be suspected in individuals jumping from heights (playground equipment, skiing, cliffs). They should also be suspected when no fracture is found on x-ray, pain continues on weight bearing, and symptoms do not resolve over the normal recovery time for ankle sprains or strains. Once again, non–weight-bearing immobilization becomes an important part of the treatment and referral is advised.

Osteochondral Fractures

Osteochondral fracture of the dome of the talus may follow a compression injury to the subchondral bone. Lesions are often small and difficult to appreciate clinically. This

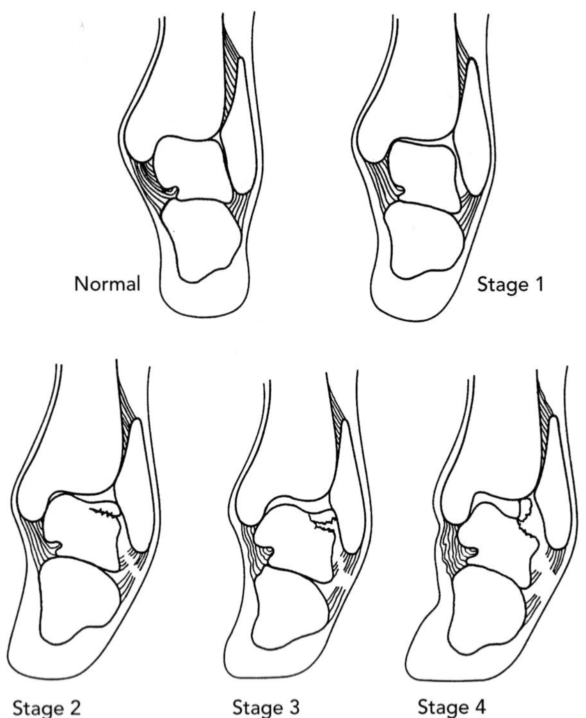

Figure 32.16 Talar dome osteochondral Fracture.

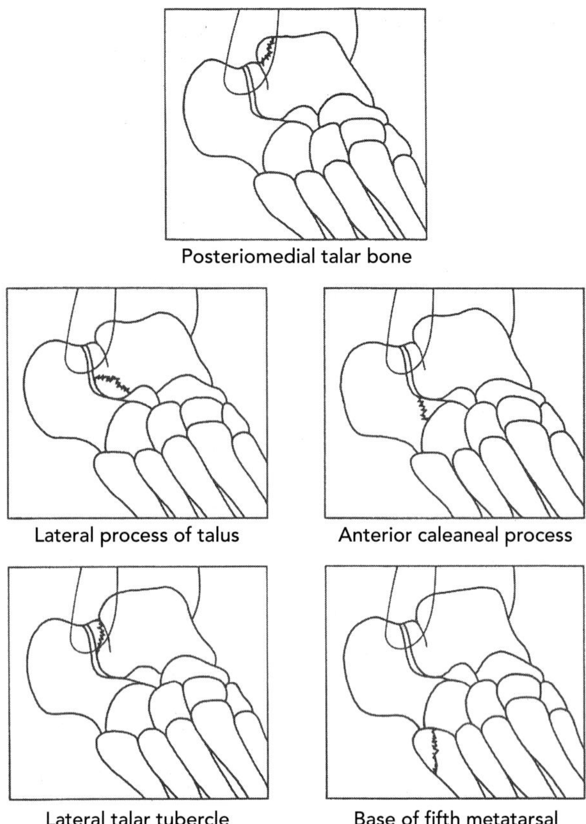

Figure 32.17 Occult fractures producing lateral compartment ankle tenderness.

fracture might be seen in a runner who missteps and later develops a weak ankle with deep pain, recurrent swelling, and crepitation. The lesion is usually found on the lateral dome of the talus and is caused by shearing forces produced by the accompanying inversion injury (see Figure 32.16) when the foot is dorsiflexed. Less common medial talar dome fractures occur with the foot plantar flexed.

Diagnostic aids. CT scans are needed if the lesions cannot be detected on a straight AP plantar-flexed view. MRI can also be used and may be able to differentiate stable versus unstable fragments. Grade 0 implies normal cartilage, grade 1 is abnormal signal but intact cartilage. Grade 2 has fibrillation or fissures not extending to the bone, and in grade 3 there may be flap present or bone exposed. Grade 4 has a loose undisplaced fragment, and a Grade 5 has displaced fragment (22). Grade 1, 2, or 3 lesions that are asymptomatic should initially be treated conservatively with immobilization for 4 to 6 weeks along with routine ankle rehabilitation. Symptomatic grade 3 to 4 lesions or grade 1 to 2 lesions that fail conservative immobilization should be referred for arthroscopy. Obviously unstable Grade 5 lesions are operative as well. Drilling of the lesion, pinning the lesion, removal of the fragment, and debridement are some of the surgical options.

Occult Fractures

Some fractures are particularly difficult to detect and are often missed on initial evaluation, even by the most experienced physician. Occult fractures (see Figure 32.17) can mimic the tenderness of the lateral ankle sprain. Many can be seen on standard x-ray views of the ankle, especially in the oblique position. However CT scan, and MRI can augment a questionable ankle x-ray. Some of the occult fractures to bear in mind are as follows:

- Anterior process of the calcaneus
- Lateral tubercle (posterior process of the talus—Shepherd's fracture)
- Lateral aspect of the cuboid
- Lateral process of the talus
- Base of the fifth metatarsal

Tendon Injury

Peroneal Tendons

Laterally, the peroneal tendons pass posterior to the distal aspect of the lateral malleolus in a shallow grove covered by a retinacular "roof." The peroneus longus is the major lateral tendon of the ankle. It is a strong everter and weak plantar flexor. Injuries to these structures include the following:

- Tendinitis secondary to overuse related to the pulley action of the tendon and analogous to the avascularity and blanching induced by the supraspinatus tendon of the shoulder (impingement syndrome).

- Subluxation/dislocation.
- Rupture.

Epidemiology. Sports most frequently involved are skiing and ballet dancing. However, Hamilton (23) suggests that peroneal tendon injuries (tendinitis) may not be as common in dancers as they are in other athletes. He feels that tenderness found behind the lateral malleolus in dancers is really a posterior impingement syndrome involving chronic irritation of an os trigonum or Stieda's Process (trigonal process).

Peroneal Tendinitis

Biomechanics. Injuries to the peroneal tendons are often incorrectly diagnosed and treated as sprains. These tendons are subject both to overuse and acute/chronic dislocation. Injury is caused by acute dorsiflexion coupled with internal rotation that isolates the tendons and produces stress, resulting in either strain of the musculotendinous unit or dislocation across the lateral malleolus.

Signs and symptoms. There is increased pain with passive plantar flexion and inversion, as well as active resistance to dorsiflexion and eversion (see Figure 32.18). Careful clinical examination will show the point of pain located posteriorly and laterally to the malleolus. Swelling may be present. This injury should be differentiated from a lateral ligament injury that is most often anterior and/or inferior to the malleolus.

Treatment. Decreasing the causal biomechanics (acute dorsiflexion) must be recommended. Ice, NSAIDs, and eccentric strengthening of the peroneal tendons may be helpful in the treatment of this condition. Steroid injection into the sheath of the peroneal tendons is acceptable in recalcitrant cases and administered by experienced hands only, with caution for risk of rupture of the tendon. Lateral ankle strapping may decrease the strain on the unit.

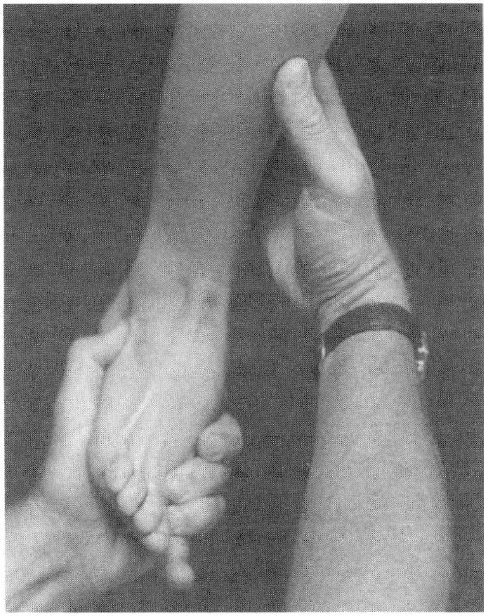

Figure 32.18 Testing of peroneal muscles.

Subluxation/Dislocation of Peroneal Tendon

Biomechanics. Forceful passive dorsiflexion with the ankle in slight eversion, which creates a violent reflex contracture of the tendons and disruption of the peroneal retinaculum or "roof". Injury to the lateral compartment of the ankle is normally associated with inversion stress. A history of lateral pain with eversion should raise suspicion about a peroneal tendon subluxation/dislocation. Some believe that the depth of the groove may be a factor.

Signs. This condition can be demonstrated by performing a stress test with active dorsiflexion and eversion of the foot and ankle that will reproduce the pain over the peroneal tendons and possibly subluxation, which may be visible and audible.

Treatment. Use of a U-shaped felt pad incorporated into ankle taping to discourage dislocation is recommended for a primary dislocation. Severe cases may require immobilization in a cast for 10 to 12 days, then use of an ankle stirrup splint for 4 weeks. With elite athletes, a case can be made for surgical repair, if only to prevent chronic dislocation, eventual rupture, ankle instability, and chronic pain. In others, surgery is recommended if the patient continues to have pain, swelling, decreased function or recurrent instability despite appropriate conservative measures.

Rupture

This is rare, and may be caused by iatrogenic injections of corticosteroids into the tendon substance. Classic absence of ability to evert the foot should lead the physician to the diagnosis. It requires immediate referral and surgical reconstruction.

Posterior Tibialis Tendon

Biomechanics. Medially, the posterior tibial tendon is important in assisting in stabilizing the longitudinal arch, as it has a broad insertion at the base of the navicular bone. Acute injuries and ruptures are rare, but over time the medial malleolus serves as a fulcrum for this tendon, predisposing it to tendinitis and tenosynovitis.

Signs and symptoms. Inflammation of this tendon is seen mostly in the 40- to 60-year old individual. Active plantar flexion and inversion as well as single toe raise will reproduce the symptoms. Patients may develop hyperpronation deformities and that may progress into more serious foot deformities if posterior tibialis dysfunction persists and is left untreated.

Treatment. Initial treatment can consist of typical overuse guidelines, orthotics with semirigid medial support and posterior tibialis strengthening. AFO for at least 6 to 12 months may be needed to treat higher-grade tendon dysfunction. MRI or ultrasound can document tears, and surgical referral is indicated with progressive foot deformity or recalcitrant cases.

Chronic Lateral Ankle Instability

Signs and symptoms. Untreated, poorly rehabilitated, or recurrent ankle sprains may result in chronic instability with or without pain. These injuries often lead to numerous recurrent mild sprains with occasional more serious sprains. Some of these injuries may happen with minimal force (e.g., walking on uneven surfaces). Physical examination will demonstrate significant laxity (greater than 3 mm) on anterior drawer testing with soft endpoint, as well as possible increased talar tilt (greater than 10 degrees). X-rays should be obtained to rule out causes of chronic ankle pain (described at the end of the chapter). Stress views may demonstrate this laxity, but are not necessary.

Treatment. Typically a long course (at least 6 months) of rigorous rehabilitation with peroneal tendon strengthening, as well as activities with external ankle support should be attempted. Continued instability should be referred for lateral ankle reconstruction.

Anterior Tibialis Tendon

The anterior tibialis tendon accounts for 80% of the dorsiflexion power of the ankle (see Figure 32.19). The following two injuries should be considered:

- *Tenosynovitis.* This is rare but may occur in people running for long periods of time, hiking, or running downhill. Inappropriate shoelace pressure may be a contributing factor. The resulting inflammation may lead to swelling and the development of an anterior compartment syndrome. Such swelling is usually short-lived because the tendon has no bony fulcrum or pulley-like action and has an excellent vascular supply.
- *Rupture.* Rupture may present with minimal pain but a "foot-drop" gait. It usually is an injury of the nonathlete and also relatively uncommon.

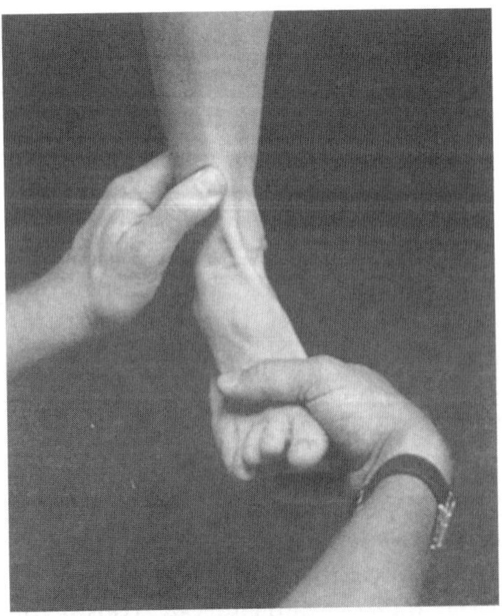

Figure 32.19 Testing of anterior tibial muscles.

Tarsal Tunnel Syndrome

Epidemiology. This is seen infrequently but tends to occur in jogging, walking, tennis, and basketball.

Biomechanics. The jarring action of these sports causes nerve compression, specifically to the posterior tibial nerve as it passes through the tarsal tunnel with the flexor tendons of the foot on the medial side of the foot. Improperly fitted shoes appear to be a major contributing factor. The biomechanics of tarsal tunnel syndrome are similar to those of the carpal tunnel syndrome with edema secondary to repeated trauma and tendinitis of those tendons coursing through the "tunnel."

Anatomy. The tarsal tunnel is bordered across its roof by the lacunate ligament coursing from the medial malleolus to the calcaneus. The plantar surfaces of the tarsal bones and the proximal metatarsals form the floor of the tunnel. The tunnel contents include: posterior tibial tendon, flexor digitorum longus tendon, flexor hallicus longus tendon, and the posterior tibial neurovascular bundle. After emerging through the tunnel, the posterior tibial nerve splits into three branches: the medial calcaneal nerve (sensory to the heel), the medial plantar nerve (motor and sensory to the medial foot), and the lateral plantar nerve (motor and sensory to the lateral foot).

Symptoms. Medial posterior foot pain accompanied by burning and tingling characterizes the syndrome. The foot may become numb over the medial aspect with toe flexors becoming weak. Pain is increased by standing and may be exacerbated at night, similar to that of carpal tunnel syndrome.

Signs. Tinel's sign (percussion over the posterior tibial nerve recreating the pain) should be positive.

Differential diagnosis. Tendinitis of any of the tendons coursing through this area; sprain of some of the underlying medial ligaments.

Diagnostic aids. EMG shows a prolonged nerve conduction of the medial plantar nerve (branch of the posterior tibial nerve).

Treatment. Begins with correctly fitting arch supports and a medial heel wedge to prevent eversion. Local injection of corticosteroids can be attempted in severe cases, or cast immobilization for 3 weeks may be done. Surgical decompression is considered if conservative treatment fails.

Sequelae. If undiagnosed or improperly or unsuccessfully treated, atrophy of the intrinsic foot muscles and the development of hammer toe deformities can develop.

Other Entities

Because ankle sprains are so common and diagnosis potentially so evasive, the primary care physician should consider the following when *conservative treatment of routine ankle sprains has failed*:

- *Bifurcate ligament sprain.* These athletes typically have a more forceful plantar flexion/inversion mechanism, with forces transmitted axially and more distally to the usual lateral ankle sprain. A small "ball" of effusion/ecchymoses with tenderness will be noted just distal to the region of the anterior talofibular ligament. The lateral calcaneonavicular and calcaneocuboid ligaments are most commonly injured, and this may be associated with a fracture of the anterior process of the calcaneus (where these ligaments originate). Typically the injury is quite painful, and may require boot immobilization for 1 to 3 weeks. Routine ankle rehabilitation protocol as described in the preceding text can be used. Recalcitrant cases may be due to a nonunion of the anterior process of the calcaneus, and occasionally need surgical excision.
- *Talar dome osteochondral defects.* A lesion that should always be considered in ankle sprains, and particularly those that are not improving as per routine treatment protocols (see section "Ankle Fracture").
- *Tarsal coalition.* Repeated ankle sprains in an adolescent or young adult is a common presentation of this condition. A tarsal coalition is a developed fibrous or bony connection between the calcaneus with either the navicular or talus. The patient may complain of a vague pain near the sinus tarsi and may have limited subtalar motion, therefore sometimes walking with an abnormal gait. Calcaneonavicular coalitions can be seen on oblique foot radiographs, but either can be confirmed with a CT scan. Selective injections in the subtalar joint may provide temporary relief, but definitive treatment is a surgical resection of the coalition.
- *Synovial pinch syndrome/anterior impingement.* This condition develops when a piece of hypertrophic synovium (the result of recurrent ankle sprains) becomes entrapped in the anterior aspect of the talofibular articulation. Arthroscopy can demonstrate the problem definitively but manual realignment of the synovium is usually all that is needed. Occasionally a trial injection of a local anesthetic is helpful. Occasionally, surgery may be needed to correct the entrapment.
- *Posterior Impingement Syndrome.* A small bony prominence (os trigonum), located posterior to the talus, can be fractured or pinched off during plantar flexion injuries to the ankle (seen frequently in ballet dancers).
- *Occult fractures.* These fractures are shown in Figure 32.17.
- *Traction Neurapraxia of the Peroneal Nerve.* Overstretching of the lateral compartment and the peroneal nerve can result from an initial ankle sprain.

REFERENCES

1. Moeller JL, Monroe J, McKeag DB. Cryotherapy-induced common peroneal nerve palsy. *Clin J Sport Med* 1997;7(3):212–216.
2. Bennett JE, Reinking MF, Pluemer B, et al. Factors contributing to the development of medial tibial stress syndrome in high school runners. *J Orthop Sports Phys Ther* 2001;31(9):504–510.
3. Shelbourne KD, Fisher DA, Rettig AC, et al. Stress fractures of the medial malleolus. *Am J Sports Med* 1988;16:60–63.
4. Batt ME, Kemp S, Kerslake R. Delayed union stress fractures of the anterior tibia: conservative Management. *Br J Sports Med* 2001;35(1):74–77.
5. Rettig AC, Shelbourne KD, McCarroll JR, et al. The natural history and treatment of delayed union stress fractures of the anterior cortex of the tibia. *Am J Sports Med* 1988;16:250–255.
6. Orava S, Karpakka J, Hullko A, et al. Diagnosis and treatment of stress fractures located at the mid-tibial shaft in athletes. *Int J Sports Med* 1991;12(4):419–422.
7. Chang PS, Harris RM. Intramedullary nailing for chronic tibial stress fractures. A review of five cases. *Am J Sports Med* 1996;24(5):688–692.
8. Hislop M, Tierney P, Murray P, et al. Chronic exertional compartment syndrome. *Am J Sports Med* 2003;31:770–776.
9. Pedowitz RA, Hargens AR, Mubarak SJ, et al. Management of chronic exertional anterior compartment syndrome of the leg. *Am J Sports Med* 1990;18:35–40.
10. Weber M, Niemann M, Lanz R, et al. Nonoperative treatment of acute rupture of the Achilles tendon. *Am J Sports Med* 2003;31:685–691.
11. McConis G, Nawoczenski DA, Dehaven KE, et al. Functional bracing for rupture of the Achilles tendon. *J Bone Joint Surg* 1997;79:1799–1808.
12. Khan RJ, Fick D, Keogh A, et al. Treatment of acute Achilles tendon ruptures: a meta-analysis of randomized, controlled trials. *J Bone Joint Surg* 2005;87(10):2202–2210.
13. Sorrenti SJ. Achilles tendon rupture: effect of early mobilization in rehabilitation after surgical repair. *Foot Ankle Int* 2006;27(6):407–410.
14. Costa ML, MacMillan K, Halliday D, et al. Randomised controlled trials of immediate weight-bearing mobilization for rupture of the tendo Achilles. *J Bone Joint Surg Br* 2006;88(1):69–77.
15. Rettig AC, Liotta FJ, Klootwyk TE, et al. Potential risk of rerupture in primary Achilles tendon repair in athletes younger than 30 years of age. *Am J Sports Med* 2005;33(1):119–123.
16. Pigman EC, Klug RK, Sanford S, et al. Evaluation of the Ottawa clinical decision rules for the use of radiography in acute ankle and midfoot injuries in the emergency department: an independent site assessment. *Ann Emerg Med* 1994;24:41–45.
17. Cordova ML, Ingersoll CD, Palmieri PL, et al. Efficacy of prophylactic ankle support: an experimental perspective. *J Athl Train* 2002;37(4):446–457.
18. Beynnon BD, Renstrom PA, Haugh L, et al. A prospective, randomized clinical investigation of the treatment of first-time ankle sprains. *Am J Sports Med* 2006;34(9):1401–1412.
19. Hopkinson WJ, St. Pierre P, Ryan JB, et al. Syndesmosis sprains of the ankle. *Foot Ankle* 1990;10(6):325–330.
20. Taylor DC, Englehardt DL, Bassett FH III. Syndesmosis sprains of the ankle: the influence of heterotopic ossification. *Am J Sports Med* 1992;20:146–150.
21. Lauge N. Fractures of the ankle: analytic historic survey as the basis of new experimental, roentgenologic, and clinical investigations. *Arch Surg* 1948;56:259–317.
22. Mintz DN, Tashjian GS, Connel DA, et al. Osteochondral lesions of the talus: a new magnetic resonance grading system with arthroscopic correlation. *Arthroscopy* 2003;19(4):353–359.
23. Hamilton WG, Geppert MJ, Thompson FM, et al. Pain in the posterior aspect of the ankle in dancers. Differential diagnosis and operative treatment. *J bone Joint Surg Am* 1996;78(10):1491–1500.

Foot and Toes

33

Katherine L. Dec

Foot and toe injuries can limit the functions of the athlete in any weight-bearing sport. True incidence in the athletic population can be difficult to ascertain because of the tendency to self-treat and minimize the injury. Incidence of injury in the foot appears to be greater in older athletes than in younger athletes (1). In this study, a greater number of plantar fasciitis and metatarsalgia injuries were noted compared to all other foot injuries reviewed. Interestingly, this particular anatomical area of the body is treated and advice administered by both medical and allied health providers. Sports medicine physicians, podiatrists, orthopedic surgeons with subspecialty training in foot and ankle and shoe salespeople all treat the foot.

The foot forms the base of support for the entire body in any gravity-controlled situation. Standing, walking, running, or cycling requires the foot to transfer the mechanical power of the legs to the ground for locomotion and to dissipate the forces generated by ground–body interaction (see Figure 33.1). Forces dissipate at three sites with three different actions: knee flexion, ankle dorsiflexion, and subtalar pronation. The foot is adaptable, being both rigid and flexible in different parts of the gait cycle. It is rigid with transfer of power from the lower extremity to the surface, and flexible when responding to changing surface characteristics. There are many demands upon the foot: (a) it must absorb shear loads with sudden stops/starts, (b) absorb the shock with the push-off and landing impact sustained in jumping, (c) bear continuous loads with lifting and standing, and (d) assume repetitive loads when walking or running.

During running, the foot sustains approximately 1.6 to 2.3 times body weight impact in the stance phase (2). On landing from a jump, usually on the forefoot, it is estimated that 4.1 times body weight impact is sustained (3). Nigg (4) has suggested that impact force factor is more of an issue in the muscle tuning/balancing of effort in effecting a change in the foot than the amount of the force. Waller (5) has proposed that the foot and structures deep within it are merely part of a chain linkage system and that a problem with any link in the system can cause imbalance in another segment. The secondarily affected system may actually be more symptomatic than the primary site of involvement. Most sports require running, either in conditioning or as an integral part of the sport. Jogging and running generate the most stress to the foot (6). Garrick and Requa (7) have also taken a good epidemiological look at foot injuries caused by sport, differentiating between acute versus overuse types (see Figure 33.2).

ANATOMY

The foot is made up of 28 bones and 57 joints. The bones are distributed in three segments (see Figure 33.3): (a) hindfoot or heel—talus and calcaneus; (b) midfoot—navicular, cuboid, and cuneiform bones; and (c) forefoot—metatarsals, phalangeal bones, and a pair of sesamoid bones. The joint between the hindfoot and midfoot is also called *Chopart's joint;* the joint between midfoot and forefoot is Lisfranc's joint. The medial portion of the calcaneus has a shelf-like piece called the *sustentaculum tali.* Innervation of the foot comes from the tibial, saphenous, sural, superficial and deep peroneal nerves. There can also be accessory bones, typically termed *os,* in the foot without biomechanical significance.

The foot has several planes of motion due to the structure of the ankle joint and talus. Typical range of motion (ROM) in a "normal" foot is 45 degrees plantar flexion, 20 degrees dorsiflexion, 30 degrees inversion, 20 degrees eversion, 20 degrees internal rotation, and 10 degrees external rotation.

X-rays. Typically three views are necessary to adequately see foot fractures/dislocations. Standard views are anteroposterior (AP), lateral, and oblique.

Consultation/evaluation. Please see an example protocol in Appendix 1 (8) that can be used as an office note.

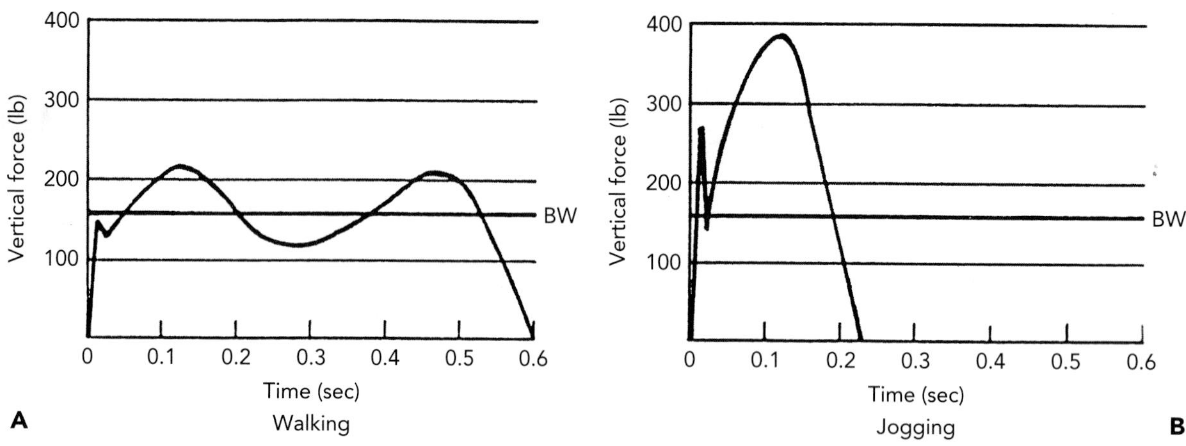

Figure 33.1 Vertical force measured by force plate in a 160-lb athlete. **A:** At time of initial ground contact, vertical force is equal to approximately 90% of body weight (BW). Force then drops slightly before rising above BW. During midportion of stance phase, force decreases to less than BW as center of gravity reaches peak elevation. This is followed by a second period in which ground reaction is greater than BW as center of gravity falls. Force then goes to zero as foot is lifted off ground. **B:** In jogging, foot is on ground for 0.25 second, compared with 0.6 second in walking. Force has increased significantly over that recorded during walking.

Aspects of the history and physical examination are summarized here:

History

- Date of injury—acute or gradual in onset?
- What activity/sports causes symptoms?
- Location of symptoms?
- Any previous treatment, including change in footwear and orthotics (off the shelf or prescriptive)?
- Training factors. Surface, intensity, and frequency, time during training when symptoms occur, incline or decline of surface.
- Medical history. Any prior foot surgeries, injections, osteoporosis, (in females, the female athlete triad) or rheumatoid disease involving the foot (i.e., gout, Reiter's syndrome, rheumatoid arthritis).
- Further questions addressing the lower kinetic chain include the following:
  - Any surgeries or injuries to the ankle, leg, knee, hip or back? (When mechanics are considered for the lower extremity, the lumbosacral junction through the foot is considered as one unit, as adaptations are made in muscles/joints to maintain stability of the extremity during weight bearing.)
  - Family history of rheumatoid disease, neuromuscular disorder (i.e., hereditary motor sensory neuropathy [HMSN]), or osteoporosis are important.

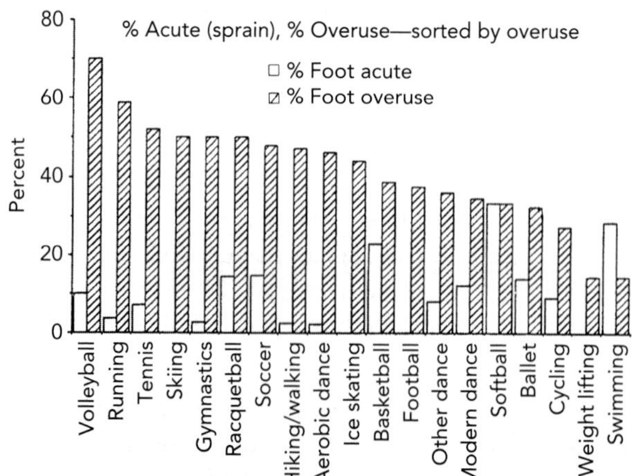

Figure 33.2 Percentage of foot injuries by sport: acute versus overuse.

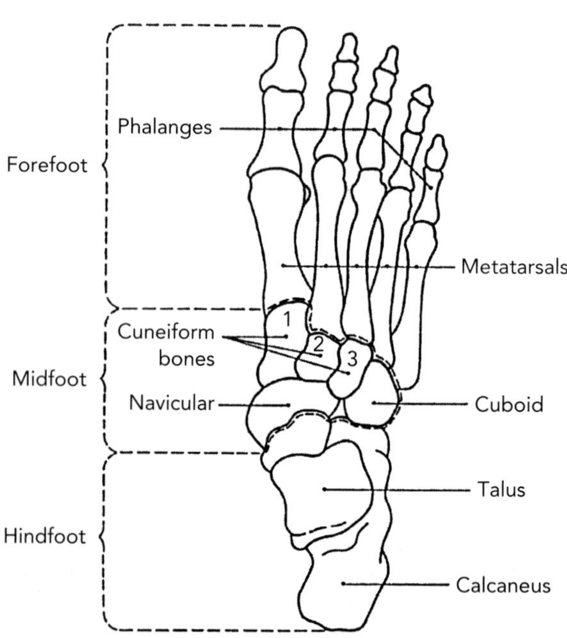

Figure 33.3 Foot anatomy (dorsal view).

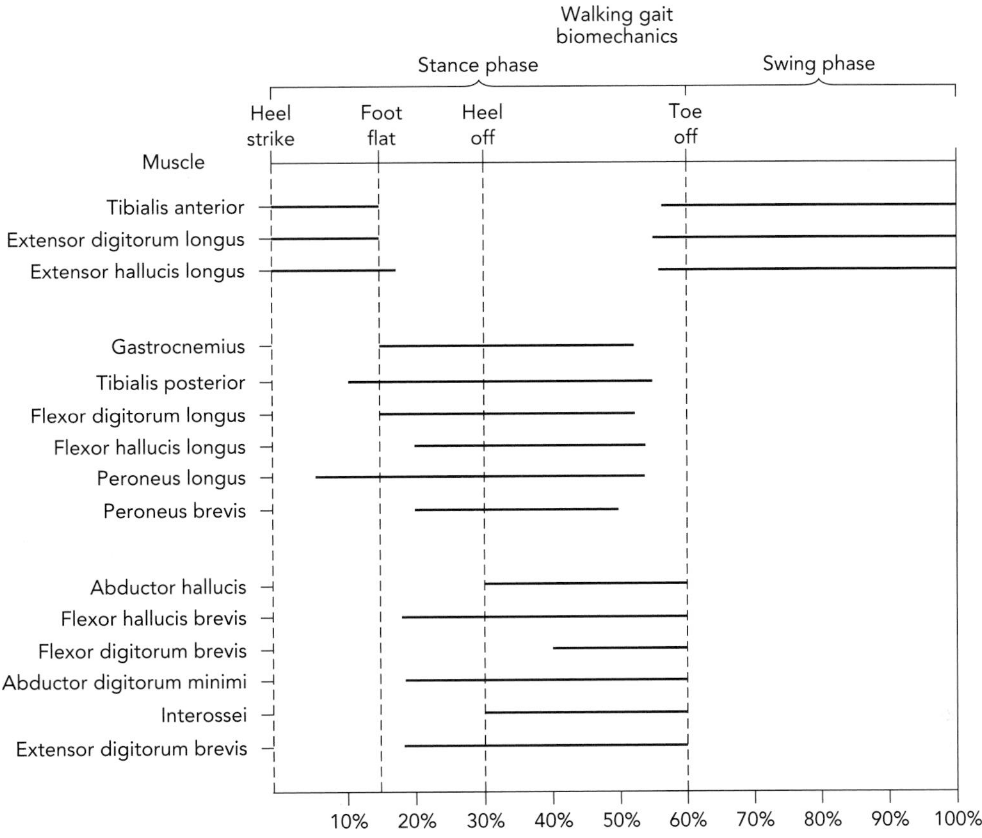

Figure 33.4 Electromyography of the foot during walking.

Physical examination (done in non–weight bearing and weight bearing includes) the following:

- Inspection of the foot. Effusion, ecchymosis, callus pattern, corn, wart, blisters; deformity (i.e., hammer toe); posture, foot position.
- If shoes present, inspection of shoes. Check wear pattern; and if orthotics used, how they fit in weight bearing.
- Gait pattern (see Figure 33.4). Lengthy discussions on clinical biomechanics for lower extremity exist in other texts. Focus primarily on movement of the foot, ankle, knee, hip, and pelvis during the heel strike to toe-off part of the cycle. This includes observing the pelvic rotation and list (4 degrees and 5 degrees respectively, on each side), knee flexion moment at stance, and displacement of trunk at toe-off and midstance.
- Pelvic/spinal abnormalities. Static testing in standing and supine/prone.
- Lower limb abnormalities. Static testing in supine/prone.
- Leg length measurement.
- ROM. Including first metatarsal-phalangeal (MTP) in ankle dorsiflexion and at rest; also passive midfoot and rearfoot ROM.
- Heel examination.
- Midfoot examination.
- Forefoot examination.
- Sensory examination, including assessment for upper motor neuron findings (i.e., clonus and Babinski test).
- Biomechanics are important in foot/toe injuries both in how their injury affects the rest of the leg and how the resultant healing affects the rest of the leg. Figures 33.4 and 33.5 outline muscle involvement during walking and running cycle (for foot and lower leg musculature). For example, at heel strike there is eccentric contraction of the quadriceps and anterior tibialis; treatment for tendinitis of the anterior tibialis considers function of the quadriceps, ROM of the foot and ankle, and positioning of the calcaneus.
- Any treatment that involves the proximal joints of the lower extremity can affect the biomechanics of the foot (10). Core trunk and proximal lower extremity muscles and joints can be more important as speed of gait changes. Neptune et al. (11) note that the gluteus muscles are critical in body support before plantar flexors become active in early stance phase. It is important to consider this relationship, between the foot and the rest of the body biomechanics, when formulating rehabilitation programs for resuming the sport.

HINDFOOT

Anatomy. The talus sits on top of the calcaneus and forms the subtalar joint. This joint contributes to

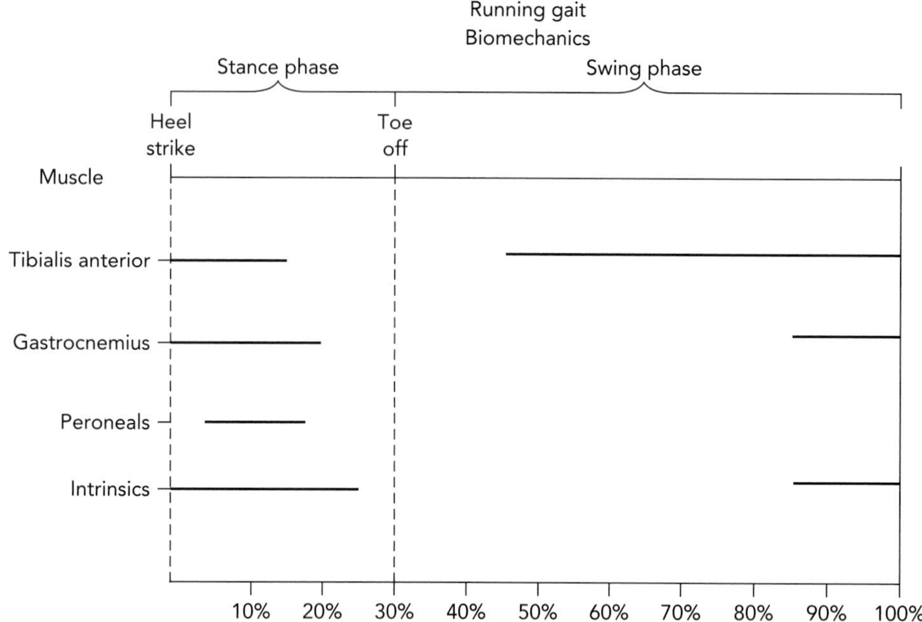

Figure 33.5 Electromyography of the foot during running. (*Source*: Adapted from Mann RA, Moran GT, Daugherty SE. Comparative electromyography of the lower extremities in jogging, running and sprinting. *Am J Sports Med* 1986;14:501, (9).)

the ROM in the hind foot. The joint is stabilized by the extrinsic lower leg muscles and intrinsic foot muscles. Anteriorly, the border between the hindfoot and midfoot is the transverse tarsal joint. This joint allows the midfoot to rotate for terrain adaptation. The subtalar joint is flexible in pronation but rigid in supination. Note that the biomechanics may explain why a pronated foot is better tolerated in running than a supinated one. Posteriorly, the Achilles tendon inserts on the posterior aspect of the calcaneus, at which point it becomes thinner, with its fibers sweeping underneath the posterior inferior aspect of the heel, and then continuing forward as the plantar fascia to insert on the metatarsal heads and proximal toes. Two bursae are at the insertion of the Achilles tendon, one in front of the tendon (subcutaneous, retro-Achilles bursa) and one between the tendon and the calcaneus (retrocalcaneal bursa).

Biomechanics. As expected, most foot problems are caused by overuse or repeated microtrauma. Although congenital defects may predispose a foot to injury, the initial etiological factor is almost always overuse.

PAINFUL HEEL

A painful heel can be caused by any one of the following (depending upon location of pain and structure involved): bone contusion, bursitis, plantar fasciitis, plantar tear, heel spur, apophysitis, exostosis, Achilles tenosynovitis, calcaneal stress fracture, calcaneal fracture, os trigonum pain, black-dot heel, and bruised or torn fat pad. Talus issues are covered in Chapter 32.

Plantar Calcaneal Pain

Plantar Fasciitis

Epidemiology. This is the most common cause of heel pain in sports. Graham (12) contends that most of the pathology is seen around the calcaneal attachment of the plantar fascia and flexor digitorum brevis muscle. In fact, these two structures attach inferior to calcaneal spur and not at its leading edge. Inflammation and/or microtearing near the origin of the plantar fascia is usually involved. The mechanics of the plantar fascia are illustrated in Figure 33.6.

Biomechanics. Normal gait cycle requires the foot to pronate from heel strike to toe-off in order to dissipate the force sustained on the foot during stance phase of gait. Excessive pronation results in abnormal stretching of the plantar fascia in midstance (13) with depression of the longitudinal arch. The presence of an arch is important with gait as it allows a rigid lever for push off, and is called the *windlass* function of the plantar fascia. As a continuum with the Achilles tendon, tightness in the Achilles tendon may result

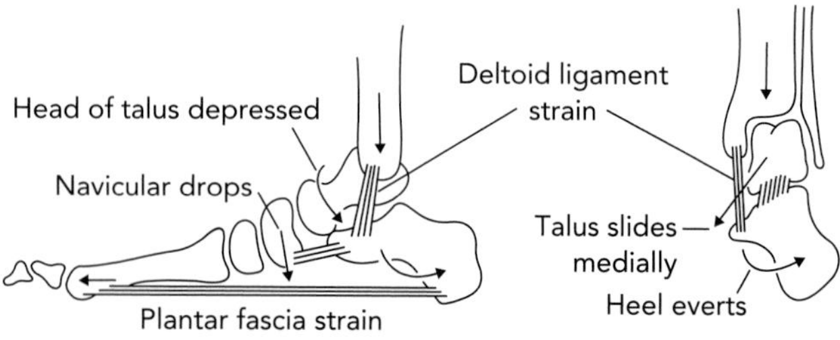

Figure 33.6 Biomechanics of the plantar fascia.

in further pronation of the forefoot as dorsiflexion of the foot is limited (14).

Predisposing factors. Pronated foot with high longitudinal arch or a tight Achilles tendon mechanism and related reduced dorsiflexion (15). Associated conditions include pes cavus, pronated foot with forefoot varus, or hypermobile pes planus.

Signs and symptoms. Pain on palpation of the anterior medial calcaneus or arch. Gradual onset of pain, usually located in the medial heel radiating toward the longitudinal arch of the foot. Pain on taking the first few steps in the morning (secondary to shortening of the fascia during sleep) and then a second episode, usually following exercise.

Diagnostic aids. X-ray is typically negative unless there is a traction spur—which is present 60% of the time but is not responsible for the patient's pain (16). Test passive dorsiflexion of the ankle (there should be 10 to 15 degrees of dorsiflexion). If dorsiflexion is less limited, a tight Achilles mechanism is presumed. Test with knee extended to test gastrocnemius and knee flexed to isolate soleus components of the calf muscles. Squeeze test: cup calcaneus in palm of hand and squeeze (thenar eminence is against medial arch)—usually there is pain at medial arch if plantar fasciitis present. Arch stretch: neutral ankle position with passive dorsiflexion of all toes—pain at calcaneus sign of plantar fasciitis.

Differential diagnosis

1. Microfracture (stress) or avulsion of the calcaneus
2. Entrapment of the medial calcaneal branch of the posterior tibial nerve
3. Tarsal tunnel syndrome

Treatment. Taping (see Figure 33.7) arch support, low dye tape (see Figure 33.8), 1/4 inch heel lifts or heel cups without lift, correction of underlying foot biomechanics with shoe change and/or orthotics[1], and stretching the gastrocnemius and soleus. Also add ice massage, cross friction massage (massage is done by thumbs across, 90-degree angle to, longitudinal fibers of plantar fascia), and arch stretch (21). Treatment of any lower kinetic chain issues in the lower limb will also help. Night splints can be very helpful, especially in reducing morning pain (22). Iontophoresis with dexamethasone can be an additional palliative tool, leading to quick results (23). After pain is relieved, intrinsic strengthening is initiated. Surgical intervention for any type of calcaneal/hindfoot pain is a last resort. Surgical removal of calcaneal spurs has been less than satisfactory in the nonathletic population. It should be avoided in an injured athlete. Because the heel pain syndrome is self-limiting, patience may be the most important aspect of any treatment. Also, Achilles and gastrocnemius stretching are appropriate. Overuse protocols should be followed. Occasionally, steroid injections may be administered as well; however, resultant long-term relief is rare.

Extracorporeal shock wave therapy (ESWT) has also been studied in the treatment of plantar fasciitis; this may also be a useful tool in the treatment options for chronic plantar fasciitis (24–26). Some recent studies noted less successful results (27,28).

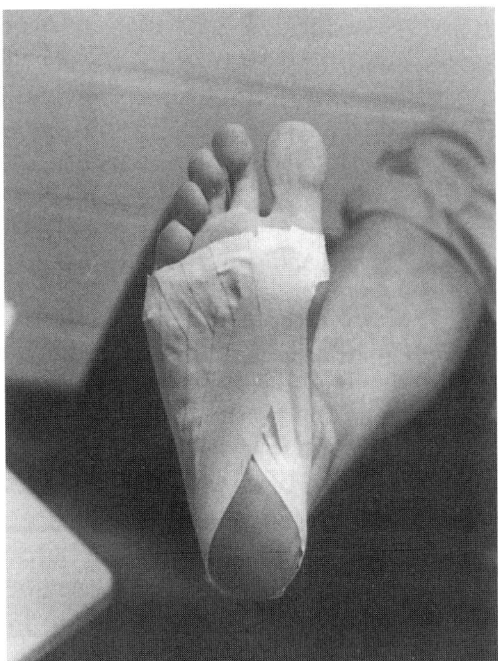

Figure 33.7 Taping for plantar fasciitis.

Calcaneal Stress Fracture

Epidemiology. Most commonly seen in beginning runners, runners who train on asphalt or concrete, or where there is a sudden increase in exercise time. The sports most likely to lead to this type of injury are running and jumping sports (poor landing mechanics increase the risk).

Signs and symptoms. Sudden onset of constant pain is seen with this injury. Percussion tenderness over the calcaneus; compression of the medial and lateral calcaneal tuberosities create extreme pain. The squeeze test (as in the preceding text) can also cause pain in distal calcaneal stress fractures.

[1] A word about orthotics—the authors suggest using soft, inexpensive orthotics, which will frequently alleviate the symptoms. The more expensive hard orthotics are often no more effective in the general athlete population. Although there is debate over which is the best method for measuring subtalar neutral, orthotics made from subtalar joint neutral position continue to provide high patient satisfaction and symptom relief (17). Also, the variation in the application of the research principles in orthotic fabrication can vary between treating professionals (18). Percy and Menz (19) suggest that orthotics do not seem to affect postural stability in athletes. Orthotics provide more than calcaneal and tibial skeletal control. Research continues to evaluate the effect of orthotics, as it is still debated: is it skeletal, proprioceptive, or muscle firing adaptation that occurs with wearing orthotics that decreases the symptoms (20)?

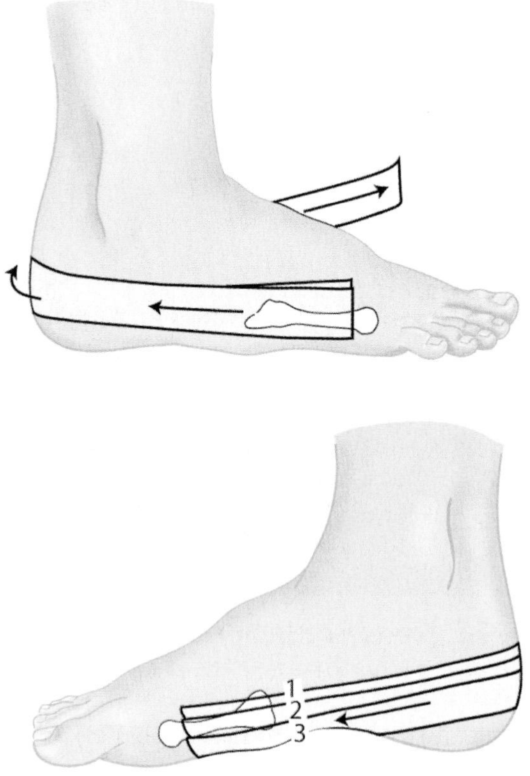

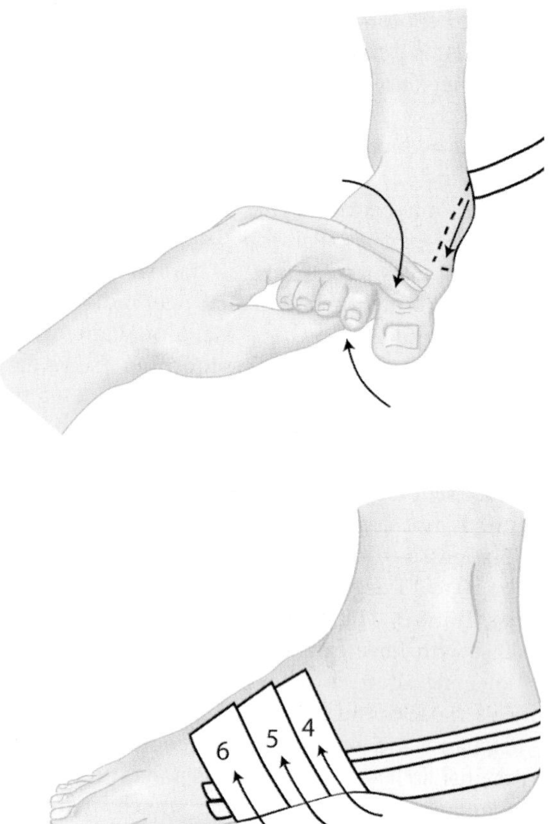

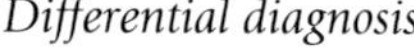

Figure 33.8 Low dye taping.

Differential diagnosis

1. Acute calcaneal fracture. Usually the result of trauma—falling on heel from heights
2. Plantar fasciitis. Pain not as constant, nor onset as sudden in this condition compared with a calcaneal stress fracture.
3. Calcaneal neuritis. Pain reproduced with pressure or compression over nerve branch; other tests are negative

Diagnostic aids. X-ray usually negative because of the lack of sensitivity of x-rays to pick up stress fractures earlier than 3 weeks, and an extremely thin calcaneal cortex. It takes up to 6 weeks before any sclerotic line or cortical change can be seen on x-ray (see Figure 33.9). Axial view is excellent for visualization of the calcaneus. Computed tomography (CT) scans can be helpful in characterizing complex calcaneal fractures. A triple phase nuclear medicine scan is helpful.

Treatment. Similar to any stress fracture. Ambulation should be encouraged if the patient is comfortable; if severe pain is present, consider non-weight bearing with crutches for ambulation. Alternate non–gravity-dependent sports such as swimming can be pursued to keep up cardiovascular fitness.

Return to competition. Consult overuse guidelines.

Os Trigonum Syndrome (Posterior Impingement-Type Syndrome)

Anatomy and epidemiology. Accessory ossicle at posterior talus. It is found in approximately 23% of the general population (29). The most common sports involved in symptomatic conditions are jumping and ballet (*en pointe*)—especially in young female dancers (30). Sports that cause distal load with forced full plantar flexion (i.e., soccer) can also be symptomatic. The os trigonum can be attached to the posterior tals (it is then called *Stieda's process*) (see Figure 33.10).

Signs and symptoms. Pain in back of ankle with extreme plantar flexion with axial load or distal load to foot. Examples are ballet (*en pointe*), soccer (kick ball with tip of foot), and runners (downhill run).

Differential diagnosis. This syndrome is a result of (a) acute os trigonum avulsion fracture, (b) irritation of a previous os trigonum fracture, or (c) congenital os trigonum nonunion with irritation. Imaging with lateral x-ray and making a comparison with opposite ankle can help differentiate Sheperd's fracture (avulsion fracture of the posterolateral process of talus). Also, ancillary lateral view of the ankle in maximum plantar flexion may help. Magnetic resonance

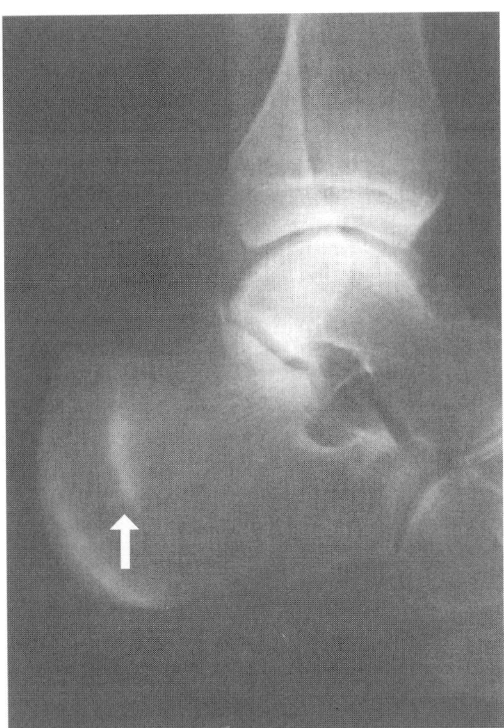

Figure 33.9 Calcaneal stress fracture evidenced by the sclerotic region (*arrow*).

imaging (MRI) is another tool that is useful in differential and treatment decisions.

Treatment. Evaluate for shoe wear that causes pressure to area. Taping may be done to limit forced terminal extension in sports that distally load into forced plantar flexion (kicking with tip of foot). Relative rest from aggravating activity, ice massage, intrinsic foot and ankle strengthening, and NSAIDs are recommended. A xylocaine injection into the posterior capsule can also be used as a diagnostic and treatment tool. Surgical excision of symptomatic os trigonum may be performed if there is no resolution; this is usually done in dancers if they are at least 16 years of age.

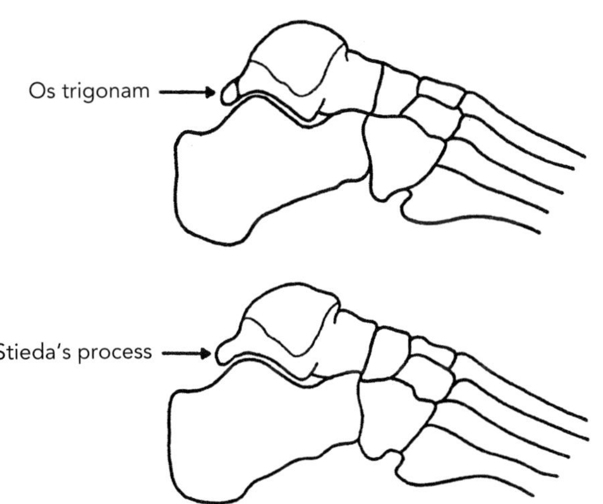

Figure 33.10 Os trigonum and Stieda's process (lateral view).

Calcaneo Apophysitis (Seiver's or Sever's Disease)

Epidemiology. Found most often in males between ages of 8 and 13. With increased participation in youth sports and early specialization in certain sports, this problem has become more common and is also increasingly seen in girls.

Biomechanics. Considered a traction injury eliciting stress from the Achilles tendon on a not-yet-fused posterior calcaneal apophysitis.

Symptoms. Pain usually occurs bilaterally with increased sensitivity to the back of the heel. Walking is usually painless but wearing shoes causes pain.

Diagnostic aids. X-ray is usually of little help, especially if the condition appears to be bilateral. At best, some cortical hypertrophy may be present.

Treatment. Symptomatic because the problem is self-limiting. Activities should be decreased to the point of comfort. Quarter inch heal lifts may take some pressure off the Achilles tendon attachment. Speed of symptom resolution can vary from 2 weeks to 3 months depending upon symptom stage when first treated and ability to "relatively rest" the athlete.

"Black-Dot" Heel

Epidemiology. Seen primarily in runners and athletes in walking casts where cotton padding has balled-up (31).

Biomechanics. Caused by pinching of skin at the bottom of heel between the heel counter and the sole of the shoe.

Signs and symptoms. Painless black or blue plaque on the posterior or posterolateral heel. Oval or circular lesions(s) are found lying just above thickened plantar skin. These lesions are not raised, but represent microhemorrhages of capillaries secondary to repetitive trauma.

Treatment. Self-limiting if insult is removed.

Prevention. Place felt inside shoe to smooth out heel counter/sole junction, change shoe, or replace cast.

Heel Bruise

Epidemiology. Repetitive, high impact.

Biomechanics. Calcaneal fat pad normally cushions the heel on impact. However, the quality of the fat pad can change with age and soften, offering less protection. This condition may predispose heel in the masters athlete, usually a runner, to bone bruising and subperiosteal bleeding. Runners with short overstrides or those who run downhill a great deal are predisposed to this condition.

Symptoms. Pain with compression of fat pad; not typically with squeezing of calcaneus.

Treatment. Firm heel counter or heel cup (worn in athletic and daily wear shoes). A donut pad may initially relieve the acute inflammatory pain. Correction may be made in training technique related to jump landing and heel strike during running.

Posterior Calcaneal Pain

Bursitis Subcutaneous (Retro-Achilles; "Pump Bump")

Epidemiology. Poor-fitting shoes. Also calcaneal changes related to Haglund's deformity (see subsequent text).

Signs and symptoms. Pain at superior calcaneal tuberosity. There may be redness, swelling, and significant pain localized to the area of the superficial bursa overlying the Achilles tendon (see Figure 33.11)—directly below position of the heel counter. You may be able to palpate the bursa if it is thickened or enlarged. Squeezing the area between the posterior part of the calcaneus and the Achilles tendon should elicit pain. Also check for decreased passive dorsiflexion.

Treatment. Change shoe or apply padding; ice massage, aspiration and steroid injection. Note that a "pump bump" may result from a chronically inflamed subcutaneous bursitis—small bony flakes or avulsions from the os calcis can form a hardened, thickened bony prominence in longtime running athletes. To treat this, increase padding, and look at heel counter for shape and fit; the athlete may need heel lifts or custom molded orthotics. Surgery is not indicated because of the close proximity of Achilles tendon.

Retrocalcaneal Bursitis

Epidemiology. Poor-fitting shoes—heel counter not snug or padding insufficient.

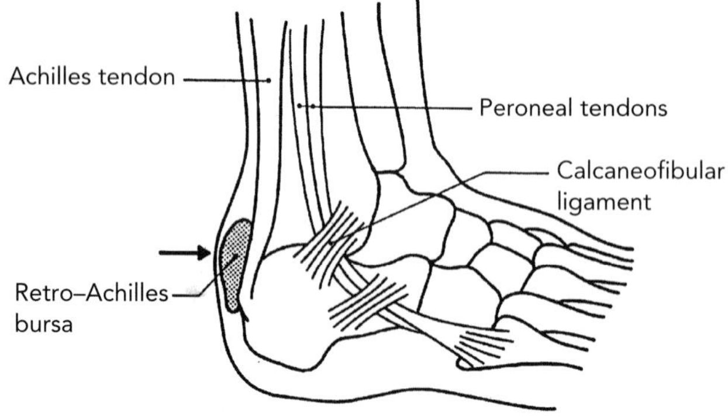

Figure 33.11 Retro-Achilles (subcutaneous) bursitis. Location of pain: The superior calcaneal tuberosity. Characteristics: tenderness located between the posterior part of the calcaneus, the Achilles tendon and skin. Look for swelling superficial to the Achilles tendon and a bony prominence (pump bump) directly beneath the position of the heel counter.

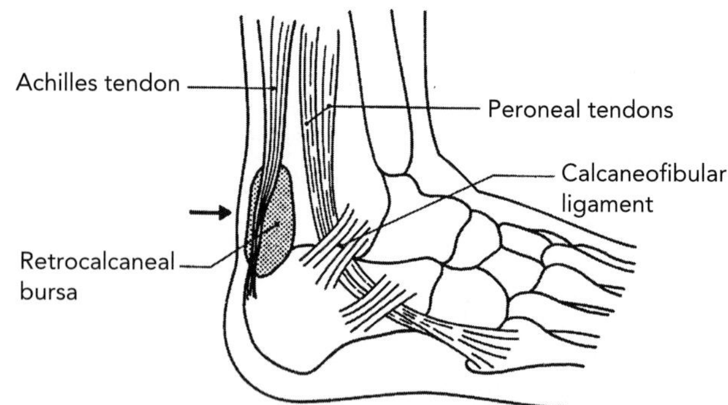

Figure 33.12 Retrocalcaneal bursitis. Location of pain: Either at the insertion of the Achilles tendon just distal to the tip of the tuberosity, or several centimeters proximal to that: between calcaneus and Achilles tendon. Characteristics: look for tenderness, swelling, and fullness in an area directly in front of the Achilles tendon and behind the calcaneus.

Signs and symptoms. Pain located in the posterior superior and usually lateral prominence of the calcaneus (see Figure 33.12), either at insertion of Achilles tendon just distal to the tip of the tuberosity or several centimeters proximal to that point. Pain is accentuated by activity and ultimately becomes so severe that the patients have difficulty walking. Frequently, athletes report that pain is worse at the beginning of activity and decreases as they warm up. Tenderness, swelling, and fullness occur in the area directly in front of the Achilles tendon and behind the calcaneus (done by applying pressure medially and laterally just anterior to the tendon and above its insertion into the calcaneus). Check for decreased passive dorsiflexion. Note that this is one of the few entities where marked inflammation can lead to complete degeneration of the bursae.

Treatment. Reduce pressure by lowering the edge of the heel counter, improving the fit of the heel, and padding the shoe. Try shoes without heel support or posterior strap (i.e., clogs). Adding a heel lift or cup could also help. Aspiration and steroid injection is considered in recalcitrant cases. Surgery is rarely needed. The athlete may have mechanics of foot ankle complex with stance phase of running and could benefit from orthotics to remove shear and asymmetrical loading to the Achilles tendon.

Haglund's Syndrome

Epidemiology. Protrusion of the posterior superior calcaneal angle with recurrent stress from low heel counter or sling-back shoes resulting in soft tissue prominence that is painful (32). It can look clinically like a "pump bump" (Figure 33.13).

Signs. Soft tissue swelling at insertion of Achilles tendon. Severe pain is noted with palpation of swelling; there may or may not be thickening of Achilles tendon.

Diagnostic aids. X-rays: true lateral with measurement of posterior calcaneal angle can help identify Haglund's

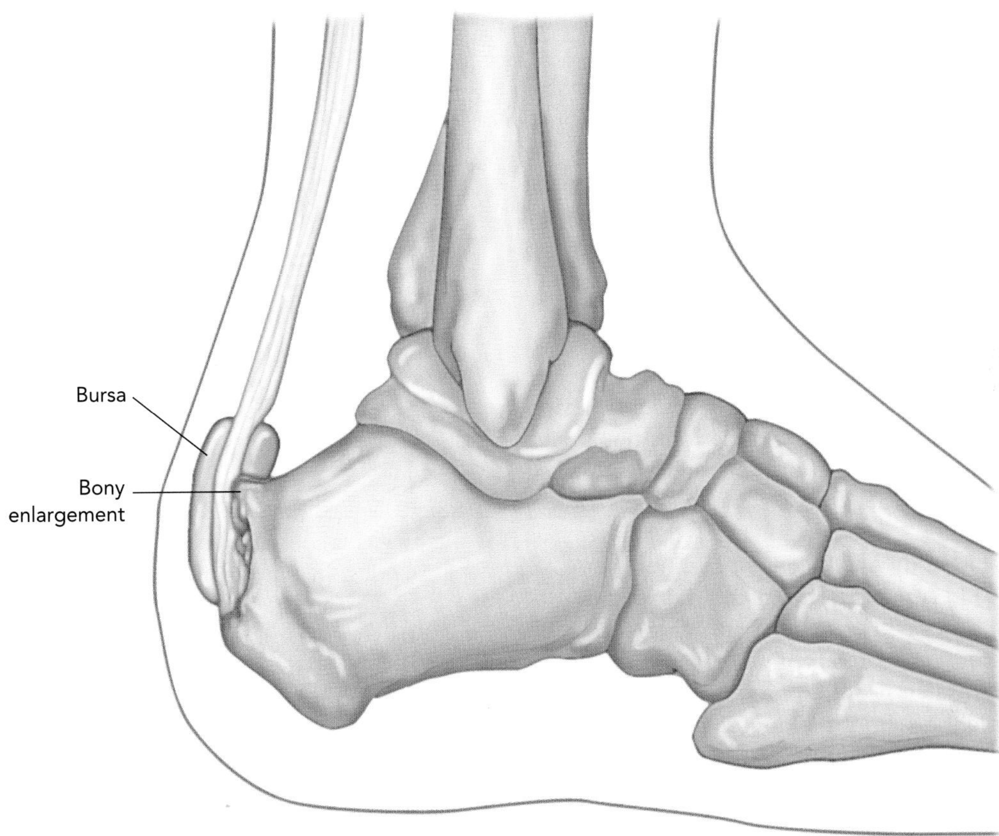

Figure 33.13 Haglund's deformity.

deformity. Loss of lucent retrocalcaneal recess is also noted.

Treatment. Increase padding, look at heel counter for shape and fit; possibly steroid injection into superficial tendo Achilles bursa will help. Surgery may be considered after failed conservative management.

Flexor Hallucis Longus Tendinitis

Epidemiology. Common in dancers owing to the positioning of the foot *en pointe*. This condition is known as the "Achilles tendon of the foot in a dancer" (33). The tendon passes through the tarsal tunnel, which acts as a pulley on it.

Signs and symptoms. Pain and tenderness behind the medial malleolus of the ankle, especially in dancers. Often pain will radiate beneath the medial arch and under the sustentaculum tali (34). The condition worsens with activity and is relieved by rest. Provocative testing involves active plantar flexion and passive dorsiflexion of ankle. There is pain on resisted plantar flexion of the great toe. Although often misdiagnosed as posterior tibial or Achilles tendinitis, pain is deeper than in the Achilles tendon (see Figure 33.14).

Differential diagnosis. Posterior tibialis tendinitis, Achilles tendinitis, tarsal tunnel syndrome.

Treatment. Ice, phonophoresis, ROM stretching. Taping techniques to limit MTP dorsiflexion may also help. This injury typically responds to conservative measures. NSAIDs can help. Please refer to Table 23.2 for treatment of generic overuse problems. Steroid injections into the tendon sheath should be avoided.

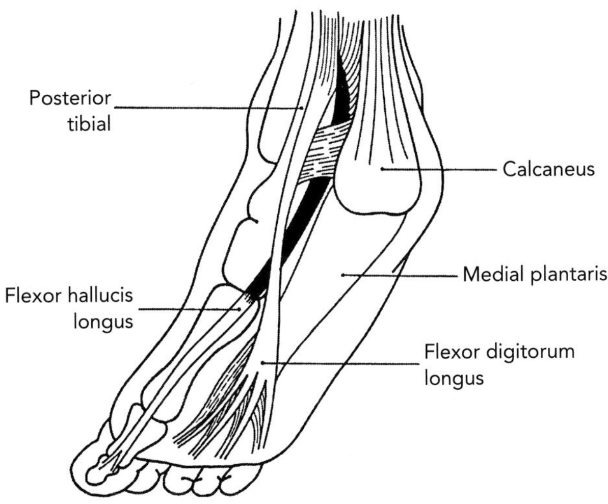

Figure 33.14 Flexor hallucis longus tendinitis. Location of pain: The medial side of the hindfoot. Characteristics: look for tenderness along the path of the flexor hallucis longus tendon (particularly tenderness that radiates beneath the medial arch and under the sustentaculum tali.)

MIDFOOT

Anatomy. The longitudinal arch is located across this portion of the foot. The roof of that arch is formed by the bones of the midfoot, and the floor by the plantar fascia and medial plantaris muscles. The joint motion between the bones of the midfoot is restricted by the shape of the bones, the taut ligaments between the bones, and the relatively constant contraction of intrinsic as well as extrinsic foot muscles.

Biomechanics. Although the motion between any two of these bones is small, the total motion of the midfoot can vary from a few degrees dorsiflexion to 15 degrees plantar flexion. The transitional area (border) between the midfoot and forefoot is located across the tarsometatarsal (TMT) joints. This joint is also called the *Lisfranc joint* and forms the transversus arch of the midfoot. Posterior tibial and peroneal tendons add support to this arch. The second TMT joint is recessed and therefore more stable, allowing a greater transfer and dissipation of force coming from the first metatarsal during running. A major factor in shaping the arch of the midfoot is the "truss" of plantar fascia that spans the midfoot. This truss acts as a mild shock absorber.

Epidemiology. Midfoot pain is common among athletes who wear lightweight shoes or foot coverings. This is especially true in gymnastics and competitive running. This footwear causes excessive pronation because the lack of support causes midtarsal joint synovitis and overuse tendinitis. One study noted that 29% of the foot injuries in offensive lineman were midfoot sprains (35).

Spring Ligament Sprain

Epidemiology. Found usually in a runner wearing light shoes and running for the first time on hard, frozen, uneven ground in the spring. The lesion is a sprain of the calcaneal navicular ligament. It is often referred to as a *medial midfoot sprain.*

Signs and symptoms. Creates deep midfoot aching and pain in the medial side. Other midfoot sprains involving lateral cuneiforms may be present. Weight-bearing x-rays will assist in seeing widening between tarsals and metatarsals present in these ligament tears; they are also helpful in identifying Lisfranc injury, with or without related fractures.

Treatment. Medial heel wedge of 1/8 to 1/4 inch; NSAIDs, ice massage, protocol for overuse, stretching of posterior calf muscle, strengthening of the intrinsic muscles of foot. Iontophoresis with xylocaine and hydrocortisone, among other treatments, has been helpful (36). Improve shoe fit. Prognostically, medially located midfoot pain is more severe than lateral midfoot pain. Medial midfoot sprains may require short-term immobilization more often and the patient needs a comparatively longer time to return to play (35).

Posterior Tibialis Tendinitis

Epidemiology. Athlete with concurrent plantar fasciitis that has altered gait mechanics, hyperpronator with poor heel counter stability or following a twisting injury to the foot. Training issues such as running on a crowned road can cause this condition.

Biomechanics. Posterior tibialis and gastrocnemius/soleus complex are strong inverters and beneficial in preventing pronation. Consider strain of these corresponding muscles when present. Sports that require eversion of hindfoot (i.e., ice hockey) place an athlete at risk.

Signs and symptoms. Pain at the insertion on the navicular bone and occasionally proximally along the tendon in the medial hindfoot. Pain is worse with activity and relieved by rest. Passive pronation and active supination of foot will aggravate the athlete's pain. Swelling may be seen in severe injury. Consider this condition if pain persists in the medial midfoot after resolution of other symptoms related to an eversion ankle sprain (see Figure 33.15).

Differential diagnosis. This is as noted in flexor hallucis longus (FHL) tendinitis.

Treatment. Medial heel wedge 1/8 to 1/4 inch; NSAIDs, ice massage, protocol for overuse, stretching of posterior calf muscle, strengthening of the intrinsic muscles of foot. Iontophoresis with xylocaine and hydrocortisone, among other treatments, has been helpful (36). Improve shoe fit. In severe tendinitis, recalcitrant to conservative treatment or surgical reconstruction may be necessary; generally, the flexor digitorum longus tendon is used in this repair.

Tarsal Tunnel Syndrome

Epidemiology. Recalcitrant plantar fasciitis with myofascial scarring; poor-fitting shoes; any alterations of foot

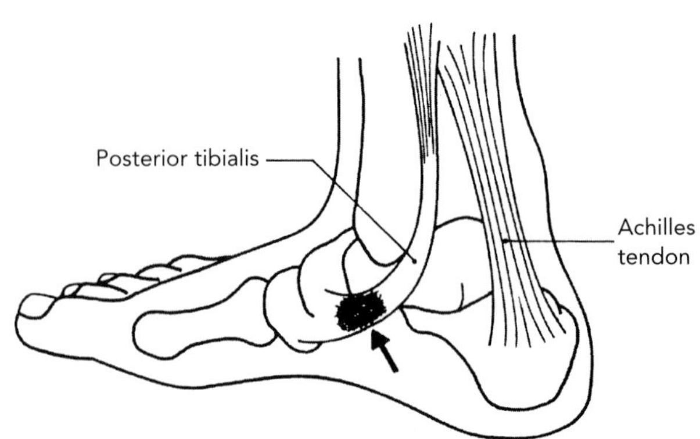

Figure 33.15 Posterior tibial tendinitis. Location of pain: The medial side of the hindfoot. Characteristics: look for tenderness along the path of the posterior tibial tendon (particularly at the insertion of the tendon on the navicular tuberosity).

biomechanics that increases stress on plantar fascia and flexor retinaculum; peripheral polyneuropathies of systemic origin (e.g., diabetes).

Anatomy. Tarsal tunnel contains tibialis posterior, flexor digitorum longus and FHL tendons, and the posterior tibial artery and nerve. Posterior tibial nerve branches include medial calcaneal, medial, and plantar nerves (proximal to distal).

Signs and symptoms. Pain may be present in midfoot, depending upon the branch of posterior tibial nerve involved. Pain is in the distal, inferior calcaneus region if the calcaneal branch is involved. Nocturnal symptoms are worse than those during daytime. Positive Tinel's over medial calcaneus is occasionally present. Paresthesias accompany pain in many cases. Numbness/paresthesias in sole of foot may be present.

Treatment. Improve shoe fit. Medial heel wedge is useful if rearfoot valgus is present. Electromyography (EMG) should be obtained if continuous numbness is present. Injection can be administered for pain relief if ice massage, transcutaneous electrical nerve stimulation (TENS), heel cup, or heel wedge is not helpful. Surgical lysis is rarely required.

Cuboid Syndrome

Epidemiology. Following lateral inversion ankle sprain, or lateral midfoot twisting injury while running on uneven terrain.

Signs and symptoms. Lateral foot pain over the cuboid, feeling of "weakness" or "instability" in the midfoot. Pain on palpation of plantar aspect of the cuboid is usually present. Decreased joint play in midfoot is often noted. Swelling may be present.

Diagnostic aids. X-rays are usually negative.

Treatment. Manipulation—(whip action) followed by low dye tape job is often effective. The athlete may also benefit from a pad under the medial portion of the cuboid with taping dorsolateral under the foot to depress the lateral portion of the cuboid (in more chronic cases where soft tissue components have accommodated cuboid).

ANATOMICAL VARIANTS (MIDFOOT)

The following are the more common anatomical variants of the foot (see Figure 33.16), either presenting primarily or caused by previous surgery or injury. All are predisposing factors to some of the foot pain problems mentioned in this section. They depend to a great extent on the ligamentous integrity of the subtalar and midtarsal joints.

Pronated Foot

Biomechanics. Concurrent heel valgus, descended or depressed arch and forefoot valgus may be noted.

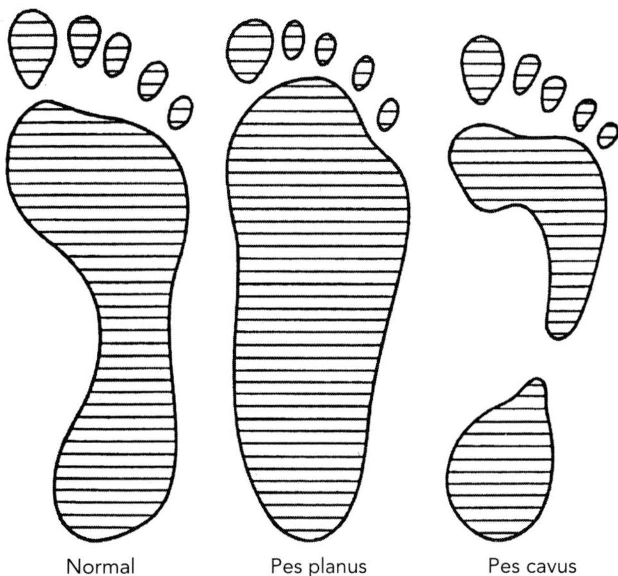

Figure 33.16 Anatomical variant footprints. A comparison of a normal footprint with one with pes planus, or flatfoot, and one with pes cavus, or high arch.

This clinical picture is a reflection of ligament laxity and sometimes termed a *flexible flat foot.* Although not necessarily pathological, this syndrome may be adaptive to accommodate a runner for spring and cushion to the heel in stance phase. The supple foot does not return to the rigid positioning for toe-off; flattening medially and eversion of the heel allows the toe-off. However, the adduction of the talus and abduction of the forefoot may lead to Achilles tendon problems. The hyperpronation seen may be compensating for genu varus, increased femoral rotation, or a tight gastroc-soleus complex (the most common coexisting problem).

Aspects of pronation and supination are evaluated extensively in the sports medicine arena as factors contributing to other symptoms in the lower extremity for runners. A conclusive relationship between increased foot pronation and exercise-related leg pain has not been well established across the athletic population (37–41). Treatment techniques for addressing symptomatic, excessive pronation include orthotics, medial longitudinal arch taping, and shoe changes (42).

Pes Planus (Flat Foot)

Epidemiology. Congenital, intrinsic muscle weakness, and neurological deficit.

Biomechanics. The height of the longitudinal arch is considerably reduced and the floor to navicular measurement in standing is reduced. Excessive pronation and outward rotation of the foot results in loss of shock absorption (see Figure 33.17). This can predispose to increased incidence of stress fractures (38). It may be noted that all infants up to 2 years of age

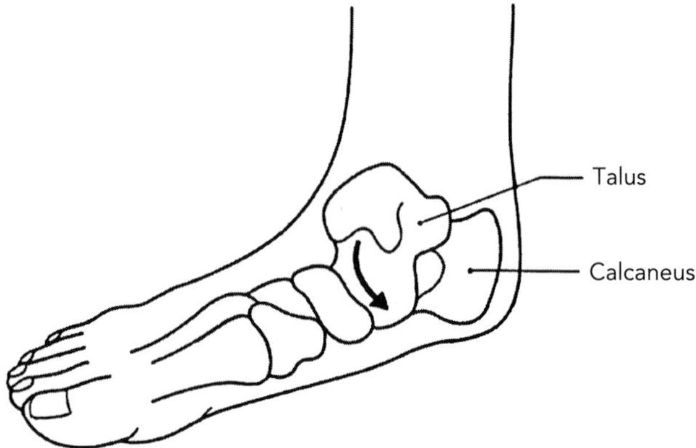

Figure 33.17 Pes planus—the talar head displaces medially and plantarward.

are flat-footed after they begin to stand. Talocalcaneal tarsal coalitions also may be considered in painful, stiff pes planus.

Diagnostic aids. X-rays occasionally demonstrate talocalcaneal tarsal coalitions, and posterior axial (Harris) view is notably helpful in the x-ray series. CT scan may be necessary to delineate the problem clearly (43).

Signs and symptoms. If present, there is diffuse pain in midfoot or sole. Flexible pes planus may not cause pain.

Treatment. If symptomatic, an arch support with medial heel wedge (rearfoot posting) is appropriate. Flexible flat feet may benefit from orthotic insert as well (44). Strengthening of the intrinsic muscles of the foot and extrinsic muscles of the lower leg and stretching of the gastroc-soleus complex are also important measures.

Pes Cavus

Epidemiology. Usually congenital; rarely neurological deficit can be the cause (HMSN).

Biomechanics. Higher than normal inflexible longitudinal arch (see Figure 33.18). This inflexible anatomical variation of the foot structure causes poor shock absorption, with an inability of the individual to tolerate much repetitive loading. During the gait cycle, as the heel strikes and weight transfers to the forefoot for toe-off, pronation may be inadequate, and the foot stays slightly supinated or arched and does not absorb shock well. Most of the weight will remain along the lateral border for impact. Inversion sprain is potential injury risk.

Signs and symptoms. If present, pain radiates from the proximal arch distally, as well as causing lateral knee and lateral lower leg problems. The patient is at high risk for fascial rupture, which creates great disability because healing of the plantar fascia is usually associated with scar tissue, which is much more painful and tighter that the original problem. Hammer toes, metatarsal (38), and sesamoid injuries may be more common in this foot structure. Flexible pes cavus may not cause pain in foot.

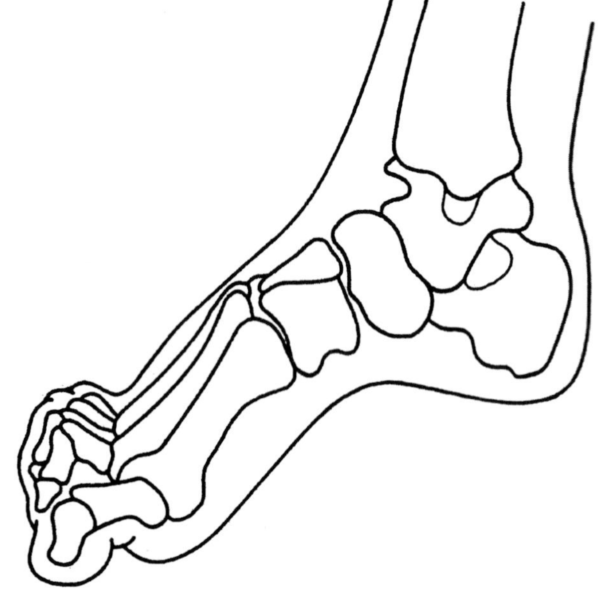

Figure 33.18 Pes cavus.

Treatment. If symptomatic, lightweight padding could be inserted to take pressure off the plantar fascial truss; provide arch support, and increase flexibility in Achilles tendon and arch. Increase strength in the flexor hallucis longus.

Morton's Foot

Anatomy. The second toe is longer than the first and is the result of a congenital anatomical foot with a short, highly mobile first ray (first multiple metatarsal [MT] and MTP and phalange).

Biomechanics. Hypermobility of the first metatarsal unit leads to overpronation with a shift of load dissipation from the first to the second metatarsal. The normal result is a painful callus under the second metatarsal head. Posterior displacement of sesamoids and thickening of the bone (x-ray) in second metatarsal shaft may also be seen. There is an increased incidence of pain and hallux rigidus in dancers with this condition (45).

Signs and symptoms. If present, there is pain along midfoot, callus under second MTP, and possible shear callus under first MTP base.

Treatment. If symptoms are present, foot insert with Morton's extension (extra padding proximal to second MT head) may be used, allowing first metatarsal to assume weight bearing in its normal sequence at toe-off phase of stance. Medial heel wedge and arch support may also be helpful.

DORSUM OF THE FOOT—MEDIAL TO LATERAL

Instep Bruise

Epidemiology. Trauma from a ball, shoe, or other equipment used in sport (hockey stick) that strikes the instep of the foot.

Signs and symptoms. Ecchymosis, maybe swelling, pain with palpation.

Treatment. Treat as soft tissue injury and bone contusion once fracture is ruled out using x-rays. Felt pad inside shoe and molded plastic shield instep guard for some sports (baseball/softball) are used.

Os Supranaviculare

Anatomy. The navicular bone of the midfoot is located at the apex of the arch of the foot. In an estimated 3.5%, an accessory ossification center of the navicular bone is located in the posterior superior aspect of the forefoot over the navicular bone.

Biomechanics. Athletic shoes without arch support and ill-fitting shoes will cause increased pronation and irritation of the accessory bone at the top of the shoe. Additionally, irritation of the bone can occur because shoelaces are too tight.

Signs and symptoms. Swelling and pain over the os prominence.

Treatment. Ice and steroid injection and rarely surgical removal.

Navicular Stress Fracture

Epidemiology. Rigid midfoot metatarsus adductus, decreased dorsiflexion, and/or decreased subtalar motion are risk factors. The condition occurs after repetitive longitudinal stress to the bone as it gets compressed between the talus and cuneiforms. Fracture occurs usually in the middle third, relatively avascular region. This is an uncommon fracture and is often overlooked.

Signs and symptoms. Insidious onset of vague pain at dorsomedial midfoot or medial arch; pain on palpation of navicular bone along the dorsal and sole; history of weight-bearing pain in a runner or jumper; decreased dorsiflexion due to pain.

Diagnostic aids. Coned down AP view of foot and can often be missed on standard x-ray views. Often CT scan, three phase, pinhole nuclear medicine scan, or MRI will be needed. Positioning is important because sagittal plane is typical location for stress fracture. Imaging does not correlate with clinical symptoms with long-term follow-up (46).

Treatment. Non–weight-bearing short leg cast 6 to 8 weeks. This may then be followed by 2 weeks in weight-bearing cast. If displaced, surgery may be considered.

Fracture of the Fifth Metatarsal

This condition is secondary to lateral inversion sprain of the ankle. If there is involvement of the proximal fifth metatarsal, one of three injuries can occur:

1. Strain of the insertion of the peroneus brevis muscle—many times caused by stepping on an uneven, unexpected surface. This is usually seen in running athletes (trail running, or, asphalt or cement surfaces).
2. Avulsion fracture of the base of the fifth metatarsal—this is an injury with bony involvement and has the same biomechanics as mentioned in the preceding text. Occasionally, os vesalianum, an accessory bone, can be located near base of fifth metatarsal and may be confused with a fracture fragment.
3. Jones fractures—a transverse fracture through the diaphysis of the fifth metatarsal (see Figure 33.19). This may have originated as a stress fracture commonly seen in sports such as basketball and volleyball that involve jumping (47). Jones fractures are notorious for their slow and often incomplete healing.

Treatment. According to injury:

1. Peroneus brevis strain—eversion strapping, ice, no cast necessary.
2. Avulsion fracture—immobilization and casting is necessary to prevent nonunion (a common occurrence).
3. Jones fracture—If only stress fracture is present, immobilization by casting for 4 weeks in a short leg cast, followed by reassessment. If the fracture is complete, the athlete can be placed in a non–weight-bearing cast for 4 to 6 weeks and reassessed; however, surgery is usually opted for decreasing the time taken to return to sports and for reliability of healing. Compression screw fixation is a typical selection, although the optimal surgical treatment is not yet established (48). If surgery is delayed, a bone graft may be needed. The risk is high for nonunion. In dancers, a spiral fracture of the fifth MT shaft can occur with inversion ankle injuries.

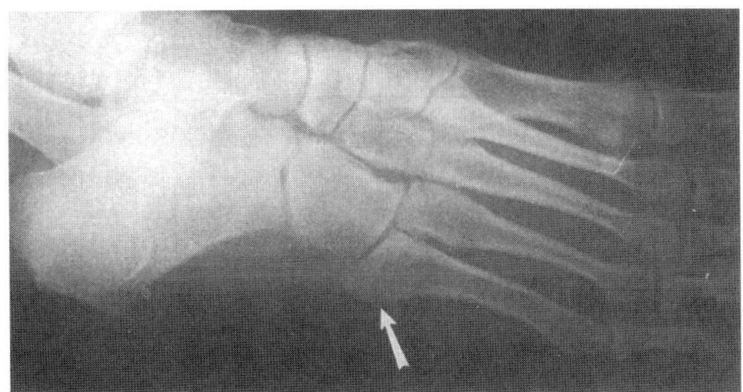

Figure 33.19 Jones fracture.

Dorsal Compression Neuropathy

Epidemiology. Most often seen in skiers and hunters. This condition is a neuropathy of the deep peroneal nerve as well as a synovitis of the extensor tendons. The area of the foot where this irritation typically occurs is at the nerve that lies beneath the extensor retinaculum of the ankle. This is also called *anterior tarsal tunnel syndrome*.

Biomechanics. Compression between bone and shoe/boot lead to the inflammatory or ischemic neuropathy and synovitis mentioned in the preceding text. This is different from the "numb toes" complaint voiced by treadmill or elliptical users where a brief period of paresthesia is felt in toes or foot during sustained workout. The latter is more likely due to repeated pressure on the ball of the foot, and moving the foot in shoe (safely) and ample width in toe box of shoe can help; with respect to elliptical, occasional backward motion can help by distributing pressure differently to foot.

Signs and symptoms. Numbness and tingling dorsal foot, occasionally into toes; may mimic compartment syndrome. Tinel's at anterior ankle is positive. Repeated active dorsiflexion/plantarflexion motion may also increase the symptoms.

Differential diagnosis. Compartment syndrome.

Treatment. Ice, elevation, increased padding at area, relacing shoe so that there is decreased pressure at localized point of dorsal foot and NSAIDs.

FOREFOOT, TOES

Anatomy

Practically all of the motion of the forefoot is located in the MTP joints. These joints adapt to uneven surfaces. Passive ROM of the first MTP joint is 30 degrees plantarflexion and up to 90 degrees dorsiflexion. With dorsiflexion, the MTP joints (because they are sliding joints) can become jammed and compressed. These joints can be actively or passively extended by external force past the normal dorsiflexion.

Metatarsal Area

Metatarsalgia

Epidemiology. This vague term used for describing pain in the metatarsal area has been clarified by Scranton (49) into three categories: (a) primary metatarsalgia—pain across the articulation secondary to imbalance in the weight distribution between the metatarsals and toes (calluses, hallux valgus, wearing high-heeled shoes); (b) secondary metatarsalgia—joint imbalance caused by issues other than MTP joint dysfunction (metatarsal stress fracture, sesamoiditis, excessive pronation, with forefoot valgus—toe extensors may increase effort for dorsiflexion of ankle leading to pain at lateral MTP joints); (c) forefoot pain caused by disorders of weight distribution unrelated to the MTP joint (Morton's foot, plantar fasciitis).

Treatment. Includes arch support for weight distribution and metatarsal pad behind the MTP, maybe a medial heel wedge.

Metatarsal Stress Fracture

Epidemiology. Most commonly occurs in the second metatarsal secondary to loading on push-off during running. It is more common in female athletes. This may be due to the systemic issues of the presence of female athlete triad in the athlete. This bone hypertrophies with long-term running and has been seen to be hypertrophied in swimmers who push off walls during turns. Fifty-five percent of stress fractures in the foot and ankle are in the first and second metatarsals (56).

Very often hypertrophy of the distal metatarsals, especially the metatarsal heads, is a result of bone remodeling (response to Wolff's law). In activities like dancing or long distance running, this radiographic change is common. The hypertrophy should be considered adaptive to the stresses involved. Amenorrheic dancers with persistent pain and tenderness in a metatarsal shaft should be considered as having a metatarsal stress fracture until proved otherwise (51). Predisposing factors to a second metatarsal fracture include amenorrhea/delayed menarche, theoretically the foot impact stress with Morton's foot, rigid cavus foot, and anterior ankle impingement.

Biomechanics. May be caused not only by overuse, but also by biomechanical adjustments for other foot injuries (blisters). Pes planus and pes cavus have also been suggested as factors. If biomechanical adjustments occur, the third to fifth metatarsals can be subject to stress fracture. Drez et al. (52) showed that the commonly held belief that a shorter than normal first metatarsal is not a contributing factor to metatarsal stress injury.

Signs and symptoms. Pain on palpation of plantar and dorsal surfaces of the specific metatarsal in question, in addition to less percentage with swelling localized to fracture site. There is pain with plantar- and dorsiflexion of involved metatarsal.

Diagnostic aids. X-ray may take up to 2 weeks to demonstrate periosteal change or cortical break; bone scan is diagnostic and usually positive 3 days postinjury (53).

Treatment. Follow-up protocol for overuse/stress fracture management (Table 23.2). See Figure 33.20 for MT pad placement.

Intermetatarsal Neuroma (Morton's)

Biomechanics. Metatarsals roll during hyperpronation, occasionally pinching a intermetatarsal nerve, usually the one between the second and third, or, the

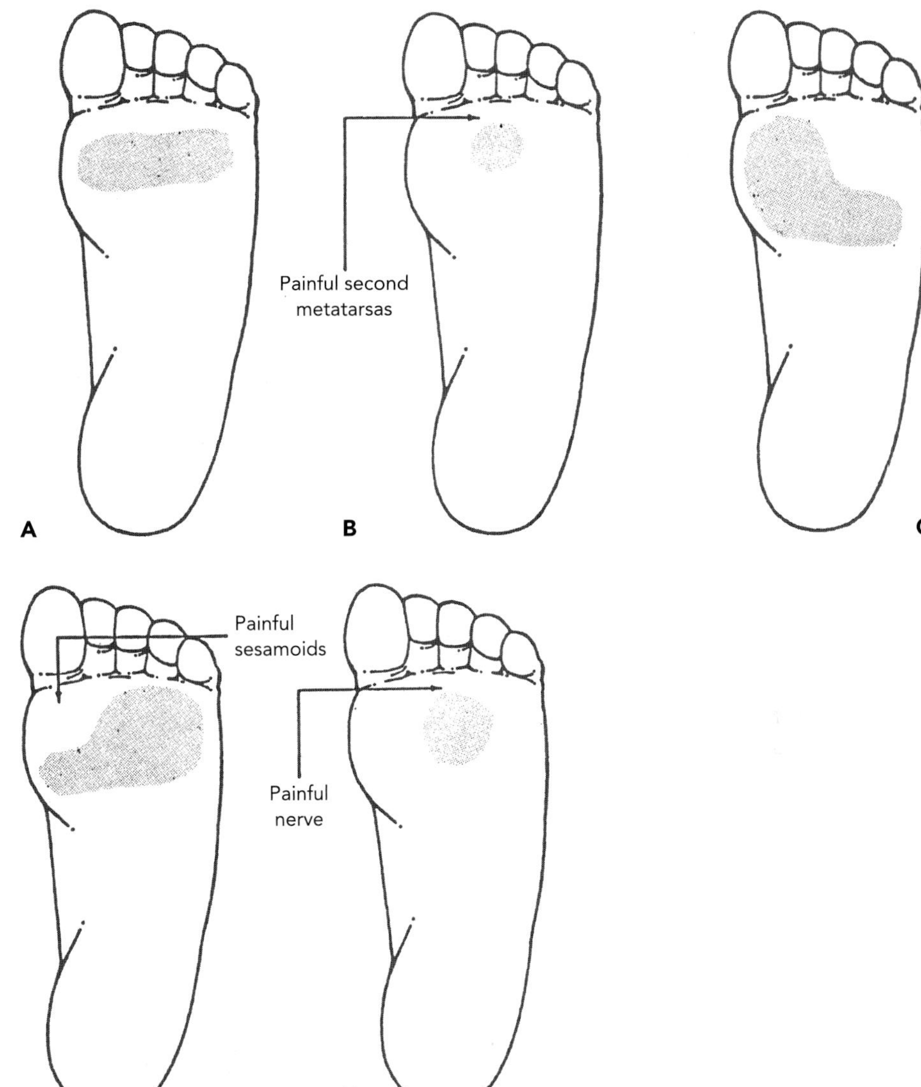

Figure 33.20 Metatarsal pad placement.

third and fourth toes (see Figure 33.21). In this area, the nerve is covered only by plantar skin. Morton's neuroma is truly not a neuroma but rather a thickening of the tissues (perineural fibrosis) surrounding the nerve, probably due to chronic trauma (54). This disorder is more common in women than in men (ratio 8:1).

Signs and symptoms. The patient complains of sharp, burning pain on impact with any uneven surface. The pain is well localized and sometimes radiates into the involved web space and inner side of adjacent toes. It is aggravated by wearing snug, thin-soled shoes. There is a sharp burning pain on impact. Reproduction of pain may be done by squeezing forefoot (metatarsal heads) together. A good clinical test is to inject a local anesthetic into the area to see if the pain dissipates.

Treatment. Procedures to decrease pronation, shoes with wider toe box, metatarsal bar to relieve and dissipate force. The patient may benefit from steroid injection. If patient fails to respond to conservative treatment, excision of the thickened nerve may provide relief. Usually the metatarsal head heals by "creeping substitution" with only minimal deformity (33). Occasionally, if the MTP joint becomes involved, surgical intervention may be necessary.

Interdigital Neuritis from Entrapment of Interdigital Nerves as they Pass Under Transverse Metatarsal Ligament

Epidemiology. Hyperextension of toes. It may be seen on long-term static machine use, that is, treadmill, where there is repetitive posture of extended toes, or in high heels.

Signs. Pain and tenderness with pressure between metatarsal heads and with hyperextension of toes.

Treatment. Avoiding position of toe hyperextension. Movement of toes is required with prolonged exercise.

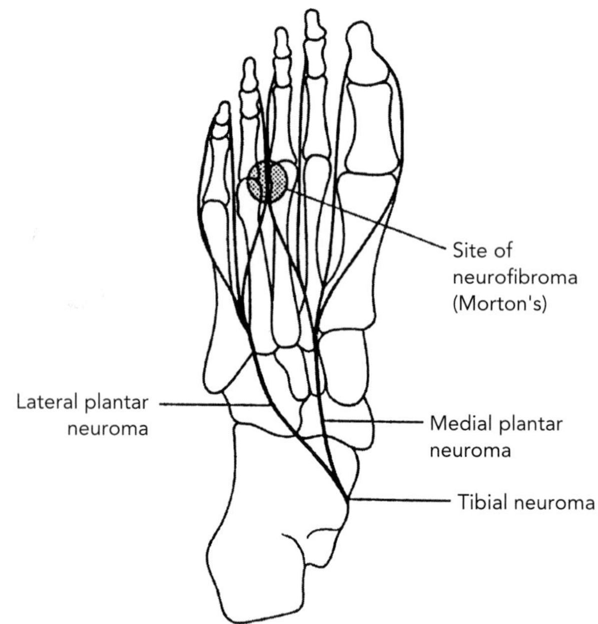

Figure 33.21 Morton's neuroma.

Osteochondrosis Metatarsal Head (Freiberg's Infarction)

Epidemiology. Vascular insult occurs to the primary growth center. This is usually in the second metatarsal head and occurs during the second decade of life. It has also been reported in adults (55).

Signs and symptoms. Localized tenderness; persistent pain with weight bearing.

Treatment. Metatarsal pad to relieve pressure (see Figure 33.20). Rocker sole or rigid foot plate in shoe may be used to provide rest to repetitive MTP joint flexion.

SESAMOID DISORDERS

Sesamoiditis

Epidemiology. Cleat placement in sports such as football, baseball, and soccer is under the sesamoids. Activity like aerobic dance, when a lot of time may be spent jumping on metatarsal heads.

Anatomy. The pair of sesamoids are in the tendon of the flexor hallucis longus.

Signs/symptoms. Pain with passive dorsiflexion at sesamoid bones; pain with palpation of sesamoids.

Treatment. Pad to unburden the first metatarsal head (see Figure 33.20).[2]

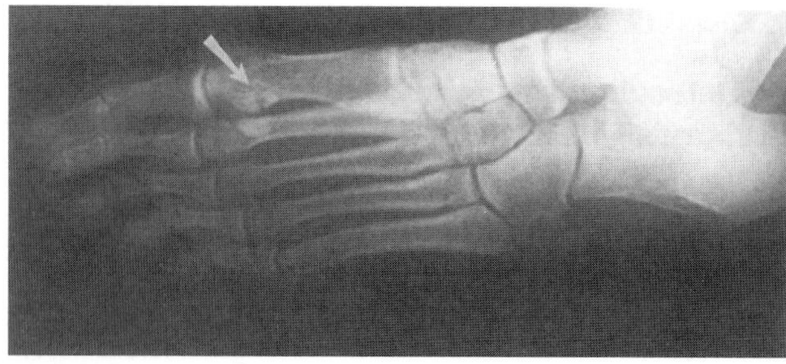

Figure 33.22 Sesamoid fracture.

Fracture of the Sesamoid

Epidemiology. Hyperextension of the first MTP joint can result in a fracture of the sesamoid (see Figure 33.22). This is seen in dancers. Medial is more common.

Signs and symptoms. Same as in preceding text.

Treatment. Treat like a turf toe. The patient may need short leg cast if pain is severe. Risk of nonunion can occur.[2]

Stress Fracture

Epidemiology. Seen in runners, basketball and tennis players, and dancers.

Diagnostic aids. X-ray is usually negative and bone scan is positive.

Treatment. Involves prolonged casting (6 weeks) (56).[2]

Bipartite/Tripartite Sesamoid

This is a normal variant that becomes clinically important only in differentiating between pathology and normality.

Differential diagnosis. For sesamoid fractures.

SKIN LESIONS OF THE FOREFOOT

Callus

Epidemiology. Reactive keratotic skin usually found in the feet of any weight-bearing sport such as running, football, or volleyball (Figure 33.21).

Differential diagnosis. Must differentiate from plantar warts and corns. Calluses lack "seeds" (thrombosed capillaries) that are seen in warts.

Treatment. Free distribution of weight-bearing forces by cushioning shoes on ball of foot or in heel. Frequent shaving of skin layers to prevent skin buildup is necessary to keep condition from getting worse. Skin lotion should be applied to soften skin. It may be

[2]Surgical intervention in sesamoid disorders: controversy surrounds the option of surgical intervention for sesamoid pain. This controversy is based on the unpredictable results and complications seen after sesamoidectomy. Although conservative treatment may take longer, this option is usually better. The one exception to the recommendations not to intervene surgically involves osteonecrosis of the sesamoids. Most often this occurs in the lateral sesamoid; its cause is unknown and its prognosis is often poor. This may be the one true indication for surgical intervention in sesamoid pain (33).

noted that a pinch callus on the great toe is associated with Morton's foot.

Blisters

Epidemiology. Blisters usually occur early in a season when the skin is soft or new equipment (shoes) is worn.

Biomechanics. Friction between shoe and skin because of sudden stopping creates a shearing force between the epidermis and dermis into which fluid accumulates and creates a blister.

Treatment. Felt padding (donut shape); if necessary, aspiration followed by the application of silver sulfadiazine (Silvadene), to control and prevent infection. If contamination of a blister does occur, it should be unroofed, thoroughly debrided, and aseptic soap (Betadine) applied.

Soft Corn

Epidemiology. Corns usually occur interdigital or under prominent MTP or other boney prominence.

Biomechanics. The compression of narrow toe box, repetitive weight-bearing force to the boney prominence or MTP, or toe deformity with subsequent toe overlap, and so on, contribute to reactive keratotic skin with a central firm core that causes pain.

Treatment. Corn pad between toes. Proper nail care is required to avoid sharp corner of end nail from pressing into adjacent toe. Ensure that proper fitting foot wear/toe box is used. Shaving keratotic skin layers and over-the-counter topical products for removal of keratotic skin will help. X-rays are needed to evaluate for boney issues contributing to corn recurrence if the above methods fail.

Warts

Etiology. Caused by the virus, verruca vulgaris. Usually this enters the skin through damaged areas.

Biomechanics. Because of pressure, warts tend to move inward as opposed to warts on non–weight-bearing surfaces like the hand, which grow outward.

Signs. "Seeds" (thrombosed capillaries).

Treatment. Shaving plus application of 40% salicylate plaster everyday; liquid nitrogen may be applied every 2 weeks.

TOES

Hallux Deformity

Limitus. Limited painful motion of the first MTP joint. This becomes a chronic problem when the athlete pushes off to run. Excessive pronation is also noted (57). Stretching and firm shoe soles or a metatarsal bar pad can help (see Figure 33.20).

Rigidus

Epidemiology. Hypermobility of the first metatarsocuneiform; more recently it is not considered as a primary cause (58).

Signs and symptoms. Limited and painful motion of first MTP joint. Functional rigidus refers to the limitation in motion increasing when foot is dorsiflexed and then MTP is tested. Completely fused first MTP joint becomes pain free.

Treatment. Firm-soled shoes. Over-the-counter OTC full-length orthotic with the first metatarsal area removed. Steroid injections should not be administered into the joint.

Valgus

Epidemiology. Hypermobility of the first metatarsocuneiform.

Signs and symptoms. Condition creating a bunion that is irritated by push off of the foot. It can create medial knee pain. It is attributed to tightness in toe box (narrow/pointed) or high heels. It has also been associated with stress fracture of the hallux (59).

Treatment. Taping great toe in position; orthotic bunion splint at night to decrease the progression of hallux valgus; shoes with wide toe box. The last resort is surgery.

Toe Fracture

Epidemiology. Kicking or "stubbing" toe; forced hyperextension.

Signs and symptoms. Pain, swelling, discoloration.

Treatment. Postoperative shoe, buddy taping (with padding between the toes taped). Surgery is recommended if interphalangeal joint or proximal phalanx of hallux is involved.

Turf Toe

Epidemiology. Most commonly seen in football offensive lineman, receivers, and defensive backs. It is usually more prevalent when unyielding playing surfaces like artificial turf are involved, with an incidence of 83% reported in professional football players (60).

Biomechanics. Sprain of the first MTP joint capsule due to flexible shoes causing the first MTP to undergo forced hyperextension. Decreased ankle dorsiflexion can also be a contributing factor (60).

Signs. Pain can be reproduced by passive extension of first MTP, specifically around the plantar joint capsule.

Differential diagnoses. Sesamoid injury.

Treatment. Firmer toebox in shoe; taping; immobilization using flat steel or orthoplast insert for forefoot; first metatarsal splint (see Figure 33.23) (restricting extension of first MTP).

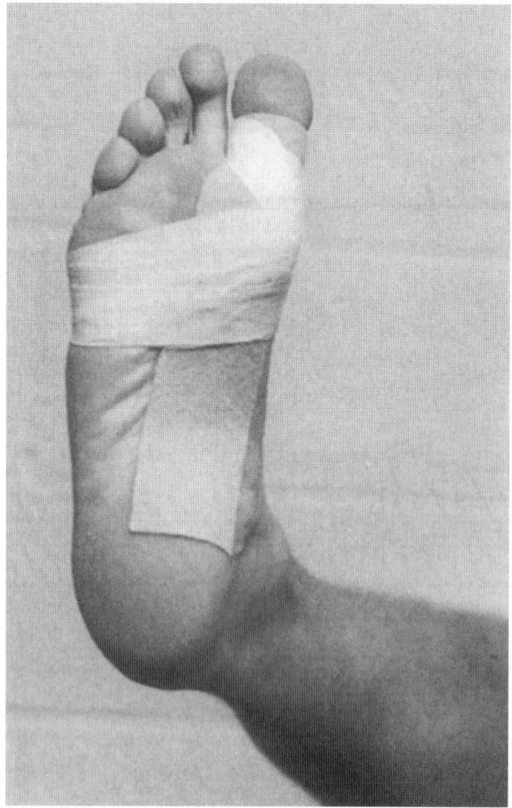

Figure 33.23 Turf toe.

Claw Toe

Anatomy. MTP joint extended, proximal interphalangeal (PIP) joint flexed (Figure 33.24).

Treatment. Strengthening of the intrinsic muscles of the foot with the use of towel pulls and marble pickup exercises.

Hammer Toe

Anatomy. Flexion of both PIP and distal interphalangeal (DIP) joints (Figure 33.25).

Biomechanics. Result of ill-fitting shoes.

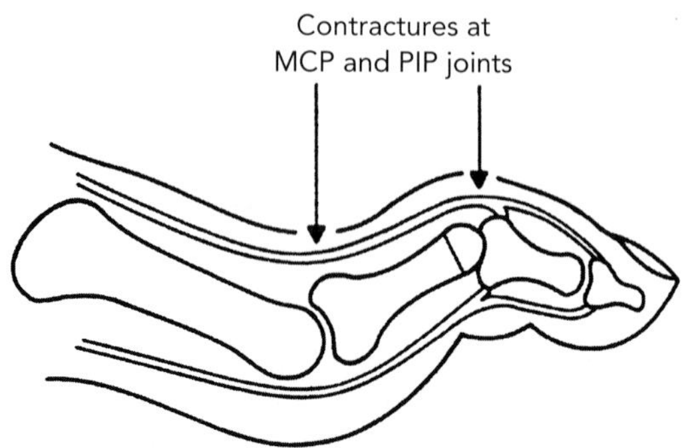

Figure 33.24 Claw toe deformity. MCP = metacarpalphalangeal; PIP = proximal interphalangeal.

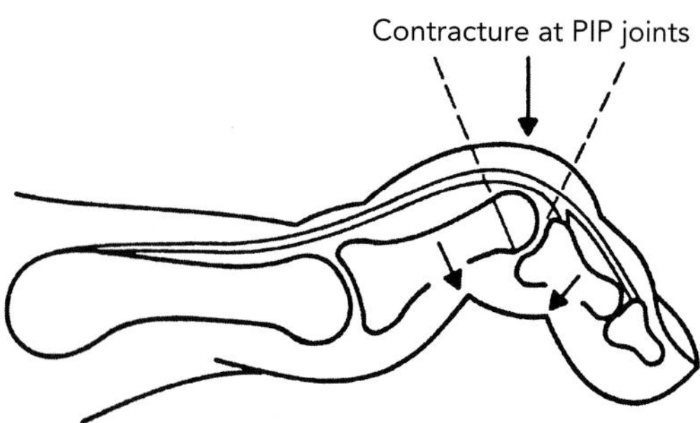

Figure 33.25 Hammer toe deformity. PIP = proximal interphalangeal.

Signs. Corns or calluses from on the dorsum of the PIP joints.

Treatment. Orthotic, deeper toe box, surgery.

Subungual Hematoma(Tennis Toe or Black Toe)

Epidemiology. Seen commonly in running and tennis and is caused by ill-fitting shoes.

Treatment. Hematoma can be relieved (if painful) by use of a sterile hot paper clip penetrating the nail distal to growth plate, or no. 11 scalpel blade.

Onchonychia (Ingrown Toenail)

Epidemiology. Ill-fitting or dirty shoes.

It may be noted that high school students often grow during a season. Shoe wear that was appropriately fitted at the start of the season may become too small later on.

Treatment. Hot soaks, lift edge of nail with cotton and pull back skin. If condition is chronic, a portion or an entire nail may need to be removed with in-office surgery.

Ganglion Cyst

Presents as a dorsal mass in the web space between the toes and increases in size during activity and decreases with rest. It is usually the result of evagination of the flexor tendon sheaths. Aspiration and steroid injection are indicated and surgery may be necessary.

REFERENCES

1. Matheson GO, Macintyre JG, Taunton JE, et al. Musculoskeletal injuries associated with physical activity in older adults. *Med Sci Sports Exerc* 1989;21(4):379–385.
2. Munro CF, Miller DI, Fuglevand AG. Ground reaction forces in running: a reexamination. *J Biomech* 1987;20:147–155.
3. Valian GA, Cavanagh PR. A study of landing from jump: implications for the design of a basketball shoe. In: Winter DA, ed. *Biomechanics IX*. Champaign, IL: Human Kinetics, 1983.
4. Nigg BM. The role of impact forces and foot pronation: a new paradigm. *Clin J Sport Med* 2001;11(1):2–9.
5. Waller JF. Hindfoot and midfoot problems of the runner. In: Mack RP, ed. *The foot and leg in running sports*. St. Louis, MO: AAOS, CV Mosby, 1982:64–72.

6. Nuber GW. Biomechanics of the foot and ankle during gait. *Clin Sports Med* 1988;7(1):1–13.
7. Garrick JF, Requa RK. The epidemiology of foot and ankle injuries in sports. *Clin Sports Med* 1988;7(1):29–36.
8. Nyland JA, Ullery LR, Caborn DN. Medial patellar taping changes the peak plantar force location and timing of female basketball players. *Gait Posture* 2002;15(2):146–152.
9. Mann RA, Moran GT, Daugherty SE. Comparative electromyography of the lower extremities in jogging, running, and sprinting. *Am J Sports Med* 1986;14:501.
10. Common sports related injuries and illnesses—pelvis and lower extremity. In: McKeag DB, Hough DO. *Primary Care Sports Medicine*. Dubuque, Brown & Benchmark: 1993:469.
11. Neptune RR, Zajac FE, Kautz SA. Muscle force redistributes segmental power for body progression during walking. *Gait Posture* 2004;19:194–205.
12. Graham CE. Painful heel syndrome. *J Musculoskel Med* 1986;3(10):42–47.
13. Rzonca EC, Baylis WJ. Common sports injuries to the foot and leg. *Clin Podiatr Med Surg* 1988;5:591–612.
14. Warren BL. Plantar fasciitis in runners: treatment and prevention. *Sports Med* 1990;10(5):338–345.
15. Riddle DL, Pulisic M, Pidcoe P, et al. Risk factors for plantar fasciitis: a matched case-control study. *J Bone Joint Surg Am* 2003;85A(5):872–877.
16. Leach R, Schepsis A. hindfoot pain in athletes: why, and what can be done? *J Musculoskel Med* 1985;2(10):16–25.
17. Morano J, Hodge W. Orthotic survey: preliminary results. *J Am Podiatr Med Assoc* 1993;83(3):139–148.
18. Guldemond NA, Leffers P, Schaper NC, et al. Comparison of foot orthoses made by podiatrists, pedorthists and orthotists regarding plantar pressure reduction in the The Netherlands. *BMC Musculoskelet Disord* 2005;6:61.
19. Percy ML, Menz HB. Effects of prefabricated foot orthoses and soft insoles on postural stability in professional soccer players. *J Am Podiatr Med Assoc* 2001;91(4):194–202.
20. Stacoff A, Reinschmidt C, Nigg BM, et al. Effects of foot orthoses on skeletal motion during running. *Clin Biomech (Bristol, Avon)* 2000;15(1): 54–64.
21. DiGiovanni BF, Nawoczenski DA, Lintal ME, et al. Tissue-specific plantar fascia-stretching exercise enhances outcomes in patients with chronic hell pain: a prospective, randomized study. *J Bone Joint Surg Am* 2003;85:1270–1277.
22. Wapner KL, Sharkey PF. The use of night splints for treatment of recalcitrant plantar fasciitis. *Foot Ankle* 1991;12(3):135–156.
23. Gudeman SD, Eisele SA, Heidt RS, et al. Treatment of plantar fasciitis by iontophoresis of 0.4% dexamethasone. A randomized, double-blind, placebo-controlled study. *Am J Sports Med* 1997;25(3):312–316.
24. Hyer CF, VanCourt R, Block A. Evaluation of ultrasound-guided extracorporeal shock wave therapy (ESWT) in the treatment of chronic plantar fasciitis. *Foot Ankle Surg* 2005;44(2):137–143.
25. Ogden JA, Cross GL, Williams SS. Bilateral chronic proximal plantar fasciopathy: treatment with electrohydraulic orthotripsy. *Foot Ankle Int* 2004;25:298–302.
26. Ogden J, Alvarez RG, Cross GL, et al. Plantar fasciopathy and orthotripsy: the effect of prior cortisone injection. *Foot Ankle Int* 2005;26:231–233.
27. Buchbinder R, Ptasznik R, Gordon J, et al. Ultrasound-guided extracorporeal shock wave therapy for plantar fasciitis: a randomized controlled trial. *JAMA* 2002;288:1364–1372.
28. Haake M, Buch M, Schoellner C, et al. Estracorporeal shock wave therapy for plantar fasciitis: randomized controlled multicentre trial. *Br Med J* 2003;327:75–79.
29. Cilli F, Akcaoglu M. The incidence of accessory bones of the foot and their clinical significance. *Acta Orthop Traumatol Turc* 2005;39(3):243–246.
30. Brown TD, Micheli LJ. Foot and ankle injuries in dance. *Am J Orthop* 2004;33(6):303–309.
31. Kuland DM. *The injured athlete*. Philadelphia: JB Lippincott Co, 1982:450.
32. Rossi F, La Cava F, Amato F, et al. The Haglund syndrome (H.s.): clinical and radiological features and sports medicine aspects. *J Sports Med* 1987;27:258–265.
33. Hamilton WG. Foot and ankle injuries in dancers. *Clin Sports Med* 1988;7(1):143–173.
34. Oloff LM, Schulhofer SD. Flexor hallucis longus dysfunction. *J Foot Ankle Surg* 1998;37(2):101–109.
35. Meyer SA, Callaghan JJ, Albright JP, et al. Midfoot sprains in collegiate football players. *Am J Sports Med* 1994;22(3):392–401.
36. Smith W, Winn F, Parette R. Comparative study using four modalities in shin-splint treatments. *J Orthop Sports Phys Ther* 1986;8:77–80.
37. Hreljac A, Marshall REN, Hume PA. Evaluation of lower extremity overuse injury potential in runners. *Med Sci Sports Exerc* 2000;32:1635–1641.
38. Kaufman KR, Brodine SK, Shafer RA, et al. The effect of foot structure and range of motion on musculoskeletal overuse injuries. *Am J Sports Med* 1999;27:585–593.
39. Reinking MF, Hayes AM. Intrinsic factors associated with exercise-related leg pain in collegiate cross-country runners. *Clin J Sport Med* 2006;16(1):10–14.
40. Wen DY, Puffer JC, Schmalzried TP. Injuries in runners: a prospective study of alignment. *Clin J Sports Med* 1998;8:187–194.
41. Willems TM, De Clercq D, Delbaere K, et al. A prospective study of gait related risk factors for exercise-related lower leg pain. *Gait Posture* 2006;23:91–98.
42. Vicenzino B, Franettovich M, McPoil T, et al. Initial effects of anti-pronation tape on the medial longitudinal arch during walking and running. *Br J Sports Med* 2005;39(12):939–943.
43. Herzenberg JE, Goldner L, Martinez S, et al. Computerized tomography of talocalcaneal tarsal coalition: a clinical and anatomic study. *Foot Ankle* 1986;6:273–288.
44. Esterman A, Pilotto L. Foot shape and its effect on functioning in Royal Australian Air Force recruits. Part 2: pilot, randomized, controlled trial of orthotics in recruits with flat feet. *Mil Med* 2005;170:629–633.
45. Ogilvie-Harris DJ, Carr MM, Fleming PJ. The foot in ballet dancers: the importance of second toe length. *Foot Ankle Int* 1995;16(3):144–147.
46. Burne SG, Mahoney CM, Forster BB, et al. Tarsal navicular stress injury: long-term outcome and clinicoradiological correlation using both computed tomography and magnetic resonance imaging. *Am J Sports Med* 2005;33(12):1875–1881.
47. Lehman R, Torg J, Pavlov H, et al. Fractures of the base of the fifth metatarsal distal to the tuberosity: a review. *Foot Ankle* 1987;7(4):242–252.
48. Porter DA, Duncan M, Meyer SJF. Fifth metatarsal Jones fracture fixation with a 4.5 mm cannulated stainless steel screw in the competitive and recreational athlete: a clinical and radiographic evaluation. *Am J Sports Med* 2005;33(5):726–733.
49. Scranton PE Jr. Metatarsalgia: diagnosis and treatment. *J Bone Joint Surg* 1980;62A:723.
50. McBryde AM Jr. Stress fractures. In: Baxter DE, ed. *The foot and ankle in sport*. St Louis: Mosby, 1995:81–93.
51. Warren MP, Brooks-Gunn J, Hamilton LH, et al. Scoliosis and fractures in young ballet dancers: relation to delayed menarche and secondary amenorrhea. *N Engl J Med* 1986;314:1348–1353.
52. Drez D, Young JC, Johnston RD, et al. Metatarsal stress fractures. *Am J Sports Med* 1980;8(2):123–125.
53. Santi M, Sartoris DG. Diagnostic imaging approach to stress fracture of the foot. *J Foot Surg* 1991;30:85–97.
54. Mann RA. Foot disorders symposium—introduction. *Postgrad Med* 1984;75(5):146–149.
55. Salvi AE, Metelli GP. A case of Freiberg's disease in an adult patient. *Chir Organi Mov* 2004;89(4):325–328.
56. McBryde AM, Anderson RB. Sesamoid foot problems in the athlete. *Clin Sports Med* 1988;7(1):51–60.
57. Lichiak JE. Hallux limitus in the athletes. *Clin Podiatr Med Surg* 1997;14:407–426.
58. Coughlin MJ, Shurnas PS. Hallux rigidus. *J Bone Joint Surg Am* 2004;86(Suppl 1):119–130.
59. Pitsis GC, Best JP, Sullivan MR. Unusual stress fractures of the proximal phalanx of the great toe: a report of two cases. *Br J Sports Med* 2004;38:31–33.
60. Rodeo SA, O'Brien S, Warren RF, et al. Turf-toe: an analysis of metatarsophalangeal joint sprains in professional football players. *Am J Sports Med* 1990;18(3):280–285.

4

Diagnostic Studies, Rehabilitation, and Associated Areas

Imaging in Sports Medicine

34

Jonathan A. Staser Kenneth A. Buckwalter

After history and physical examination, imaging may be the most important diagnostic tool in the assessment of patients with sports injuries. Imaging techniques for these patients include radiography, fluoroscopy, nuclear medicine scintigraphy, ultrasound (US), computed tomography (CT), and magnetic resonance imaging (MRI). In some patients, it may be necessary to use more than one technique. For example, the imaging workup of a shoulder injury might begin with plain radiographs, but requires an advanced imaging technique such as a MR arthrogram to confirm the diagnosis.

This chapter will review some of the indications and general approaches to imaging of sports-related injuries. A discussion of muscle tears will be followed by a more detailed review covering imaging of the knee, shoulder, elbow, and ankle, the most commonly injured joints encountered in practice.

RADIOGRAPHY

Radiography employs x-rays to create an image of the patient. Tissues, like bone, that absorb more of the x-ray beam are whiter on the image; tissues like fat absorb much less of the x-ray beam and are blacker on the image. Because radiography is projectional, a radiograph is a two-dimensional representation of a three-dimensional object. Overlap of structures can lead to confusion and, for this reason, a minimum of two orthogonal (perpendicular) projections are recommended for assessment of bony structures. For small joints in the extremities such as the hand and wrist, three views are recommended to reveal small fractures that may only be seen on a single view (1). The minor incremental cost and radiation exposure are justifiable in this context.

Radiography is unparalleled in its ability to demonstrate bony detail because it has the highest spatial resolution of any imaging technique. However, radiography has limited ability to visualize differences in soft tissue structures. Consequently, the strength of radiography lies in the detection of bony pathology such as fractures, not soft tissue injuries. Radiographs are also extremely useful in detecting soft tissue calcifications. For example, hydroxyapatite crystals seen in calcific bursitis are easy to identify on radiographs, but difficult to detect on MRI.

Although radiography traditionally has been performed using special x-ray film and film cassettes, advances in technology have facilitated the production of radiographs in digital format (2). The two main methods used are computed radiography (CR) and digital radiography (DR). CR uses special plates that are scanned by a laser after exposure to the x-ray beam, producing the radiographic image. DR captures the digital image directly. The ability to acquire, store, and transmit radiographic images allows for simultaneous multiple location display. The diagnostic quality of digital images is equivalent to conventional film-screen radiography and there are additional benefits such as reduced radiation exposure and efficiency that warrant installation of digital equipment in busy facilities.

It is important to recognize that radiography has limitations. In the case of suspected fracture, if initial radiographs are found to be normal, there are several options. The least expensive option is to obtain follow-up radiographs. Because bony remodeling is dependent on the patient's metabolic activity, radiographic changes will be visible sooner in children and adolescents (5–7 days) than adults (7–14 days); radiographic changes may be extremely difficult to detect in seniors, particularly those with osteoporosis.

For the high performance athlete, delayed radiographic imaging may be unacceptable because of the time constraints imposed by training or game play. In this situation, CT or MRI is performed next. If the working diagnosis is fracture, CT is recommended; if the working diagnosis is soft tissue injury, MRI is recommended. Because MRI is more sensitive in the detection of bone marrow edema and soft tissue damage, it is often obtained. MRI may not be able to distinguish a nondisplaced fracture from a large bone contusion. Additionally, small avulsion fractures often are occult on MRI. For these reasons, it is essential to remember that radiographs should always be obtained concurrently.

NUCLEAR MEDICINE

Bone scintigraphy is performed by injecting a radiopharmaceutical (typically Tc-methylene diphosphonate) intravenously followed by imaging in 1 to 2 hours. The radiopharmaceutical concentrates in metabolically active regions of the bone. A viable blood supply is necessary to deliver the agent to the target tissues. Because the radiopharmaceutical is radioactive, only a small quantity must localize in the bone for a positive result. Therefore, nuclear imaging is extremely sensitive in detecting bony remodeling. However, the radiopharmaceuticals used in skeletal imaging are nonspecific; a fracture could present a similar appearance as an infection or tumor.

Nuclear bone scans have other limitations. Although scintigraphy is extremely useful when a large region of the body needs to be surveyed for radiographically occult disease, detailed pictures of the anatomy are difficult to obtain. Because growing children have metabolically active growth plates, injuries to the growth plates may not be detectable on scintigraphy. Furthermore, imaging of the soft tissues such as ligaments, tendons, and cartilage is not possible with a bone scan, further limiting the usefulness of scintigraphy. In large part, scintigraphy has been supplanted by MRI, which is usually as sensitive as scintigraphy in assessing bone marrow disease, provides superior spatial resolution and facilitates visualization of soft tissue injuries.

Positron emission tomography (PET) is another nuclear imaging technique for skeletal and soft tissue imaging. Most of the current applications of PET are cardiac or oncologic, but the clinical experience continues to evolve. Newer PET devices are coupled with CT scanners: PET/CT. The addition of CT imaging to PET addresses the concerns that some physicians have regarding the limited spatial resolution of nuclear imaging. The short-lived radioisotopes for PET reduce the time between injection and imaging, increasing the usefulness of the technique. Although there is great potential for this imaging method, the role in sports imaging is unclear and the examinations are costly.

ULTRASOUND

US relies on the transmission and reception of high-frequency sound waves (4–15 mHz) to produce images of soft tissues. In most instances, the US transducer is placed on the skin overlying the symptomatic region. The depth of penetration of the beam is determined by the frequency of the transducer; lower frequencies penetrate deeper into the tissues. Spatial resolution is also determined by the frequency of the transducer; higher frequencies are associated with higher resolution. As a result, it is difficult to obtain detailed pictures of deep tissues, but superficial structures can be evaluated in great detail.

US images are limited to a small display field. Consequently, US images are difficult to orient and interpret. Some surgeons are reluctant to operate on the basis of US findings alone, which is another limitation of US. Furthermore, it is difficult to show a large anatomical region such as a thigh on a single image. US examinations typically are performed in real time by a physician or a technologist supervised by a physician. There is a steep learning curve for musculoskeletal imaging, further limiting the usefulness of US in sports injuries.

On the other hand, US imaging is ideal for interventional procedures, such as steroid injections of bursae, tendon sheaths, and joints. The real time capability of US makes it possible to do these procedures with ease. Additionally, US equipment is relatively inexpensive and the technology has continued to shrink so that portable US devices are now laptop computer–sized. Image quality for these smaller devices can be inferior to that produced by larger stand alone units, but the gap in quality between small and larger units continues to narrow. The role of US in diagnosis and intervention of musculoskeletal injuries is continuing to expand.

COMPUTED TOMOGRAPHY

CT is a widely available imaging technique. The strength of CT lies in its ability to image bony structures in high resolution. Additionally, CT imaging is tomographic, revealing the internal structure of patients by displaying two-dimensional cross-sections of the scanned anatomy. The cross-sectional display is helpful in eliminating the overlap of structures that limits radiography. Although CT is the workhorse of modern body imaging, discrimination of the soft tissues in the musculoskeletal system limits its application in extremity imaging. In general, intravenous contrast is not warranted unless there is a suspicion for mass or abscess.

Throughout most of its history, CT imaging was limited to the transverse plane. Because radiographs of joints are usually obtained in frontal and lateral projections, physicians are most comfortable assessing joints using sagittal or coronal planes; unfortunately, conventional CT is best suited for axial plane imaging. The development of multichannel computed tomography (MCCT) scanners

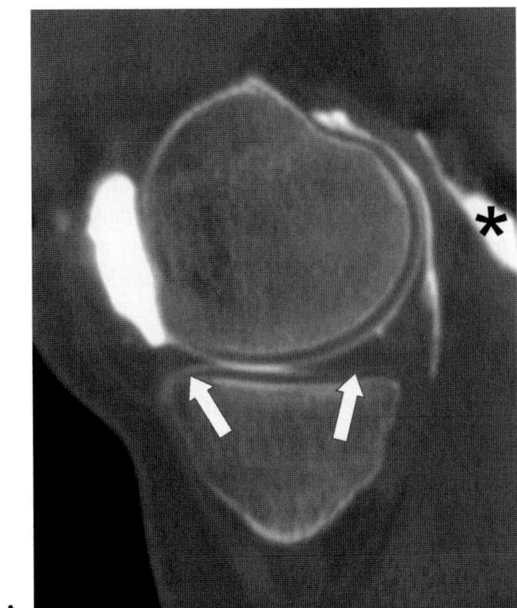

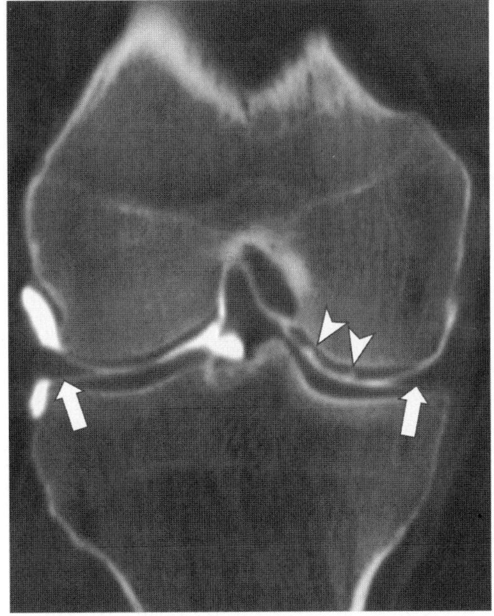

Figure 34.1 Computed tomographic arthrogram of the knee. **A:** Sagittal multiplanar reformation, anterior to the left of image, shows normal triangularly shaped horns of the medial meniscus (*arrows*). Contrast is seen leaking posteriorly from a ruptured Baker's (*asterisk*). **B:** Coronal multiplanar reformat, lateral to the left of image, shows the normal bodies of the medial and lateral menisci. Small partial thickness cartilage defects of the medial femoral condyle are outlined by contrast (*arrowheads*).

over the last decade has enabled submillimeter-thick imaging, which makes it possible to create sagittal and coronal multiplanar reformations of joints in detail similar to direct axial imaging (3).

Both CT and MCCT use x-rays to produce images of patients. Radiation dose is relatively low for most CT examinations, but it is not insignificant, especially when multiple follow-up examinations are performed. Radiation-sensitive tissues such as the gonads and thyroid are exposed when imaging the pelvis (hip joints) and the upper chest (shoulder and sternoclavicular joints), but most extremity imaging (elbow, wrist, knee, ankle, foot) can be performed without exposing radiation-sensitive tissues. In general, radiation exposure should be minimized in children and young adults, but should not be considered a contraindication. Pregnancy is a relative contraindication for a CT examination, particularly when direct exposure of the fetus would be incurred.

The availability of modern MCCT scanners has expanded the indications for CT imaging. In particular, imaging of patients with metal hardware is facilitated greatly by MCCT (4). Although metal artifacts may not be eliminated completely, most patients with orthopedic hardware can be imaged using MCCT. Types of hardware that do not interfere with bony visualization include intramedullary nails (rods), fixation plates, and small screws. Many patients with joint prostheses also can be imaged successfully. Additionally, patients with metal fragments such as shrapnel and gunshot debris are suitable candidates for CT examinations.

Another good application for MCCT is high resolution computed tomographic arthrography (CTA) (5). CTA can be performed in any joint using either single or double contrast technique. The indications for CTA include patients with the following conditions: metal in close proximity to a joint, MR incompatible implants, severe claustrophobia, failed MR examination (with or without an arthrogram), and morbid obesity. CTA provides excellent visualization of the articular surfaces and intra-articular structures such as the knee menisci (see Figure 34.1) and the glenoid labrum in the shoulder.

MAGNETIC RESONANCE IMAGING

MRI has revolutionized imaging of the musculoskeletal system. Similar to CT, MRI produces cross-sectional images of the relevant anatomy. Unlike CT, MRI uses no ionizing radiation. Instead, MRI uses radiowaves to produce images of the body. For most applications, the soft tissue contrast of MRI is much greater than that of CT, explaining the usefulness of this technique for musculoskeletal imaging. Additionally, depending on the radiofrequency pulse sequence, images can be made to emphasize different types of tissue contrast.

For conventional MRI, the hydrogen atom or proton is the most widely imaged nucleus. Tissue contrast is related to the T1 and T2 relaxation times of the target tissues as well as the concentration of protons in the tissue. Depending on the pulse sequence used, tissue signal intensities can

TABLE 34.1
RELATIVE TISSUE SIGNAL AND MR IMAGE WEIGHTING

Type of Image Weighting	Relative Tissue Signal Intensity from Dark to Bright
T1	cortical bone < ligaments < menisci < fluid < muscle < cartilage < fat
T2	cortical bone < ligaments < menisci < muscle < cartilage < fat < fluid
Proton density	cortical bone < ligaments < menisci < muscle < cartilage < fluid < fat

reflect T1, T2, or proton density weighting. Fluid is dark and fat is bright on T1- weighted images; fluid is brighter than fat on T2-weighted images; proton density weighted images are somewhere in between (see Table 34.1). In general, injuries are detected on MR images by alterations in anatomy, for example, a meniscal tear, or by the presence of edema, for example, a bone contusion. As a result, it is common practice to obtain sequences that show anatomical detail in conjunction with fluid-sensitive sequences in every imaging plane.

Chemical saturation (fat saturation) is a commonly used technique to reduce signal from fat. T2-weighted images produced with fat suppression increase the contrast between edema and bone marrow, making it easier to identify bone contusions in the intramedullary space. A similar effect can be achieved using the short inversion time inversion recovery (STIR) sequence (see Figure 34.2). Fat suppression applied to T1-weighted images increases image contrast on postgadolinium enhanced images.

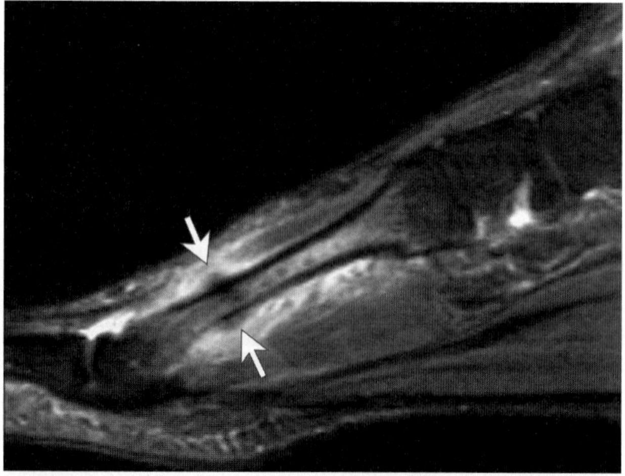

Figure 34.2 36-year-old woman with foot pain. Sagittal STIR image shows intense marrow edema of second metatarsal. Low signal intensity stress line and cloudy periosteal reaction (*arrows*) are evident. STIR = short inversion time inversion recovery.

Although MRI is very safe, the intense magnetic field used to produce images may not be safe for all patients. This magnetic field is tens of thousands of times stronger than the earth's magnetic field and the main MR magnet is always turned on. Therefore, exposure to the magnet may be harmful even if the patient is not being imaged at the time of exposure. Most orthopedic hardware is considered to be safe; however, metal implants in close proximity to the region of interest can obscure detail. Patients with pacemakers, specific kinds of heart valves, and certain venous filters may not be safe in close proximity to the magnet. Because some medical devices are MR safe, it is important to know as much as possible about the device before the examination including such details as device manufacturer and model number.

Intravenous contrast agents such as gadolinium can be helpful to document sites of active inflammation, for example, plantar fasciitis, and should be administered if a malignant soft tissue mass is suspected. For many examinations, contrast is not necessary. However, there are growing number of applications when intra-articular contrast is extremely useful. For a direct MRI arthrogram, the gadolinium agent is diluted and injected into the joint under fluoroscopy. If radiographic contrast media (iodine) is injected along with the gadolinium, CTA can be performed without another injection if the patient is unable to tolerate the MRI examination. It is also possible to perform an indirect MRI arthrogram by injecting the gadolinium contrast intravenously and performing delayed imaging within 20 to 60 minutes. This procedure eliminates the need for an arthrogram and is well tolerated by most patients. Indirect arthrography works well in joints like the knee that have a small to moderate sized effusion; however, indirect arthrography is not as useful in joints like the shoulder where distension of the joint is necessary for optimal visualization of labral tissue.

Presently, most imaging is performed at 1.5 Tesla (T) and there is a great deal of experience in this field strength. Clinical imaging is now possible at higher and lower field strengths. Imaging at 3.0 T is driven by neuroimaging and body applications; however, scanners currently are being delivered with musculoskeletal coils to facilitate musculoskeletal applications. Although there is potential for improved image quality at 3.0 T, care must be taken to address image artifacts such as chemical shift, which will offset the gains achieved by higher field strength imaging. Additionally, tissue heating limits the use of certain pulse sequences and image contrast can be different than that at 1.5 T. The clinical utility of 3.0 T imaging may take time to establish for routine bone and joint studies; except for specialized examinations, there is minimal incremental benefit at present.

Patient preferences for less confining magnets have led to the development of the open magnet scanner. A wide variety of field strengths are available from 0.2T to 1.0T. Advances in open imaging technology have improved image quality greatly; however, many systems may be operating without the benefit of a recent system upgrade. In general, higher field strengths are associated with higher image quality, and this is also true for open magnets (see Figure 34.3). When referring patients to any system, particularly an open system, it is worthwhile inquiring if the system has passed the American College of Radiology Accreditation standard; this is a standard required by some insurers and is a minimal quality guarantee (6).

MUSCLE AND TENDON TEARS

Muscle and tendon tears are extremely common sports injuries. Optimal treatment depends on accurate staging. The bone–tendon–muscle unit tears at its weakest point and this functional unit is analogous to a chain, which is only as strong as its weakest link. The weakest link varies with age; adolescents tend to avulse apophyses, adults tear the muscle, and mature adults often tear tendons. Knowledge of these injury patterns is helpful to guide the imaging assessment.

After the initial clinical evaluation, radiographs should be obtained. This is especially true for older children and adolescents presenting with an apophyseal injury, which may be diagnosed from the initial radiographs. Common sites of apophyseal injuries are the ischial tuberosity (hamstrings), the anterior inferior iliac spine (rectus femoris) and the anterior superior iliac spine (sartorius) (7,8). Further investigation of muscle and tendon injuries proceeds with US or MRI. US has a limited field of view and is best suited for focal abnormalities such as a distal Achilles tendon tear. Because many muscle tears may extend over tens of centimeters, MRI is suggested as the most effective imaging tool (9). MRI is a more comprehensive assessment than US and allows for the assessment of occult bone injuries such as stress fractures.

Muscle tears occur more often in muscles spanning two joints, muscles with a higher proportion of type II fibers, and with activities favoring eccentric muscle contraction (10). As a result, more muscle tears are seen in lower extremity muscles, such as the hamstring and quadriceps muscle groups in the thigh and the gastrocnemius muscle in the calf. Upper extremity tears are seen less often; most of them occur in the biceps muscle or tendon of the upper arm (see Figure 34.4). Other factors increasing the likelihood of tear include aging, prior injury, and steroid abuse.

At MR imaging, muscle tears are found at the myotendinous junction within the muscle body; this is the junction between muscle fascicles and the central tendon, not the anatomical junction between the muscle and tendon seen grossly at surgery. On cross-sectional views of muscle tears, the edema is seen around the central tendon of the muscle.

Muscle tears can be graded depending on the severity of the injury. A grade I or mild strain is characterized by low level diffuse muscle edema demonstrated on fat suppressed T2- weighted or STIR images. Perifascial edema is sometimes seen with a grade I strain. Conservative treatment is usually sufficient. A grade II or moderate strain

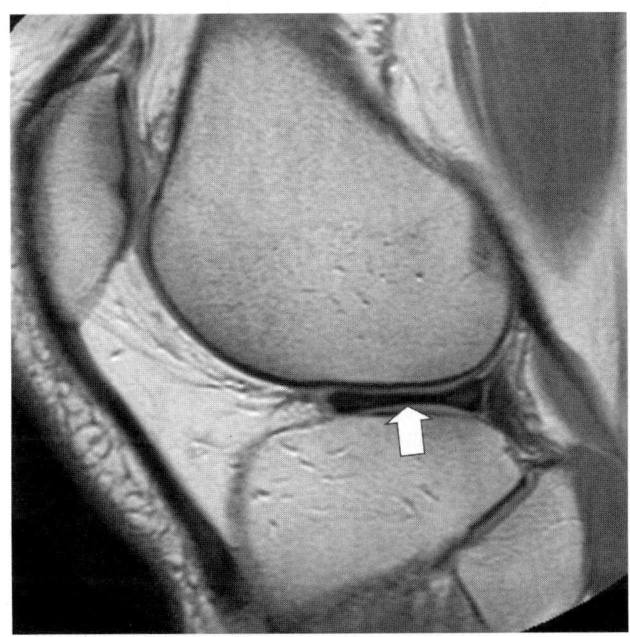

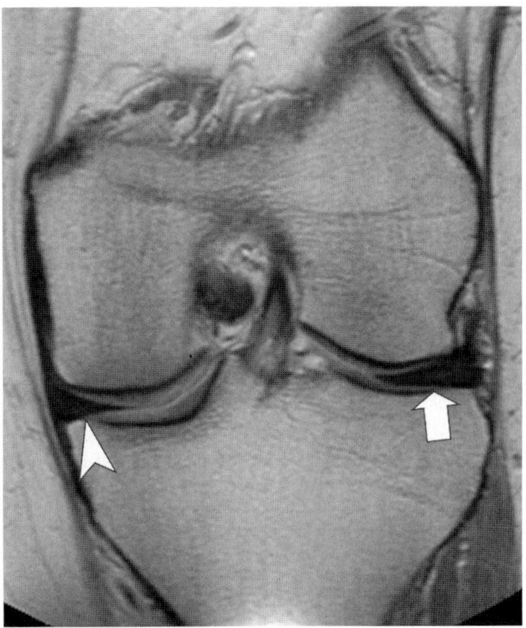

Figure 34.3 MRI of the knee, 1.0T extremity magnet. MRI = magnetic resonance imaging. **A:** Sagittal proton density image through the lateral meniscus (*arrow*) shows that it is possible to obtain excellent images on some open scanners. The "bowtie" shape of the meniscus was present on more than three consecutive images indicating a discoid meniscus. **B:** Coronal proton density image shows that the body of the lateral meniscus (*arrow*) is larger than the body of the medial meniscus (*arrowhead*). Both meniscal bodies are typically the same size on a mid coronal image like this.

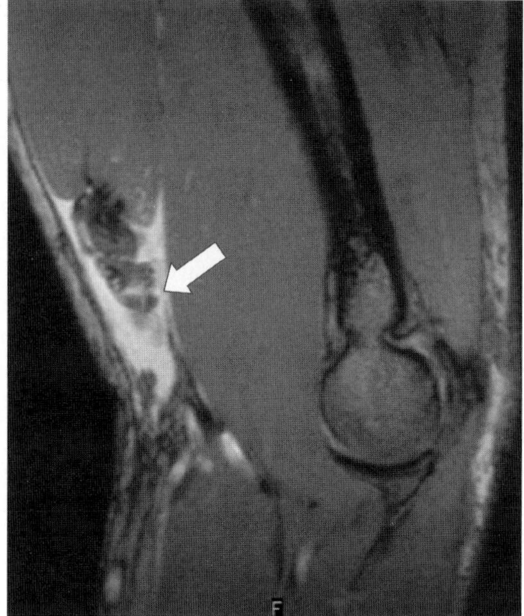

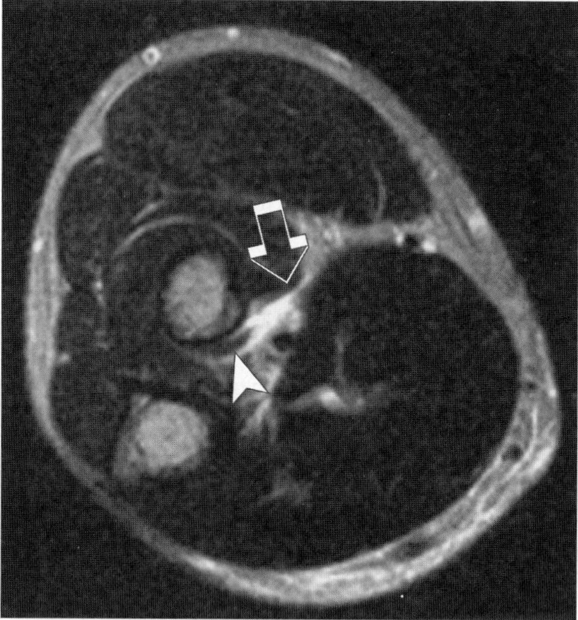

Figure 34.4 Distal biceps tear. **A:** Sagittal gradient echo image, anterior to image left, show retracted distal biceps muscle and tendon (*arrow*). Bright fluid and hemorrhages surround the distal muscle and tendon, tracking inferiorly to the insertion site. **B:** Axial T2-weighted image at the insertion site of the biceps tendon onto the radial tuberosity shows a tiny remnant of the distal tendon (*arrowhead*); distal fluid (*open arrow*) noted along the expected course of the tendon.

is characterized by a partial thickness tear associated with partial loss of strength. At MRI, a grade II strain presents as high signal at the myotendinous junction with perifascial edema. Most of these strains resolve in 10 to 12 days, but they are associated with an increased risk of future tear. Lastly, grade III strains are complete muscle tears with discontinuous muscle fibers; a hematoma may be visible in the gap (see Figure 34.5). Surgery may be indicated in the case of a grade III strain to prevent permanent retraction and muscle atrophy.

Older patients may present with tendon tears instead of a muscle injury. Other factors predisposing patients to tendon tears include metabolic diseases such as hyperparathyroidism and diabetes (see Figure 34.6). Lastly, patients on fluoroquinolone antibiotics can experience tendon disruption, particularly the Achilles tendon; comorbidities include obesity, renal disease and prior steroid injection (11).

A variety of conditions can mimic muscle tears. Delayed onset muscle soreness (DOMS) resembles a grade I muscle strain at MRI, but symptoms begin 1 to 2 days after exercise as opposed to the immediate symptoms of a grade I strain. Patients with poorly controlled type 1 diabetes can develop muscle infarcts that present clinically with calf or thigh pain, resembling a muscle strain. The edema pattern of infarcts is more diffuse than the peritendinous edema of a muscle strain, allowing differentiation. Patients with muscle abscess will present with muscle pain, but the clinical history and MR appearance should lead to the correct diagnosis. Rupture of a Baker's cyst can cause acute calf pain, resembling a muscle strain or deep venous thrombosis, but the edema of a ruptured cyst often extends to the intramuscular fascial planes, facilitating the correct diagnosis.

KNEE IMAGING

The knee is often injured in sport activities. Physical examination of the knee may be incomplete in the setting of an acute injury because of pain or guarding, increasing the importance of imaging. Radiographs are helpful to assess for fracture, effusion, and calcified loose bodies. In acute trauma, a cross-table lateral radiograph of the knee is preferred to a conventional lateral knee radiograph to look for the presence of a fat-fluid level which indicates an intra-articular fracture. Radiographs also are helpful to assess for small cortical fractures that may be difficult to detect on MRI. One example, the Segond fracture (see Figure 34.7), is a harmless looking chip fracture of the proximal lateral tibial plateau margin. This fracture represents an avulsion of the middle third lateral capsular ligament and has a high likelihood of an associated anterior cruciate ligament tear (ACL). Similar, but less common, the reverse Segond, is a medial tibial plateau fracture associated with a posterior cruciate ligament (PCL) tear and a medial meniscus tear.

If radiographs are normal or inconclusive and a serious injury remains a strong consideration, MRI or CT can be pursued as the next step. CT is helpful when assessing bony structures and CT is used most often to confirm or stage a fracture if surgical repair is planned. For most sport related trauma, MRI is the most commonly used imaging tool.

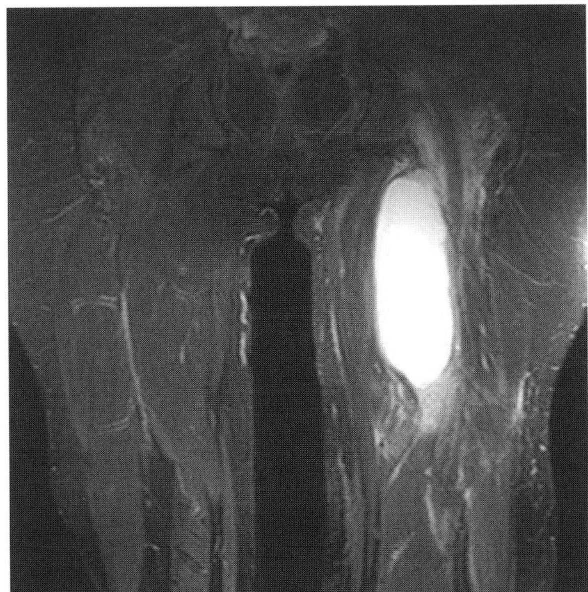

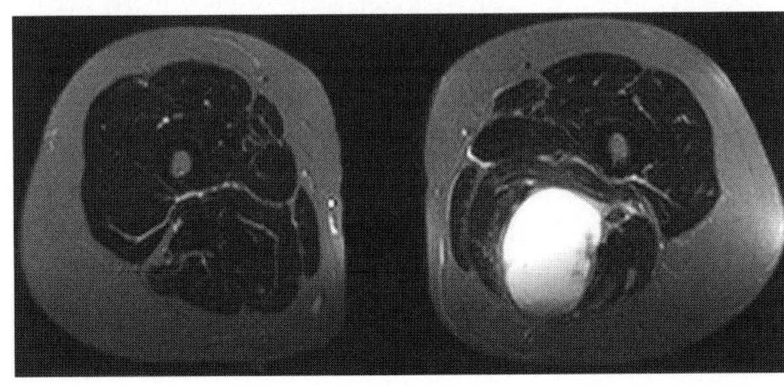

Figure 34.5 Grade III muscle strain. **A:** Coronal STIR image of the posterior thighs shows a large fluid-filled gap in the left hamstring bed. **B:** Axial inversion recovery image through the hamstring tear shows a small layering fluid–fluid level at the extreme posterior margin consistent with a hematoma. STIR = short inversion time inversion recovery.

Although MRI excels at soft tissue imaging, the bone marrow also can be assessed well with MRI. Bone marrow edema can be detected at MRI using fat suppressed T2-weighted or STIR images. Edema may indicate the presence of a contusion, stress fracture, infarct, or other pathological process. Following trauma, edema in the marrow space usually indicates a bone contusion which represents microscopic trabecular disruption and intraosseous hemorrhage. In general, avulsion injuries such as the Segond fracture are not associated with significant marrow edema; however, impaction injuries are associated with significant edema. Additionally, marrow signal changes, particularly those in the subchondral region, are nonspecific; some of these abnormalities represent stress-related changes or early degenerative cysts. A typical stress fracture seen in the distal femur is important to recognize as it was previously referred to as *spontaneous osteonecrosis of the knee* (SONK). This condition actually represents a subcortical insufficiency fracture of the femoral condyle (12). The typical patient is not a marathon runner, but a middle-aged adult, perhaps inspired by a new exercise program. Intense marrow edema is identified throughout most of the affected femoral condyle, associated with significant pain (see Figure 34.8). Many patients have associated chronic meniscus tears.

Meniscus tears are quite common and easily detected with MRI; sensitivity and specificities vary between 85% and 95% for the medial meniscus with similar, but slightly lower numbers for the lateral meniscus (13–16). The normal meniscus consists of fibrocartilage, which is dark on most MRI pulse sequences (see Figure 34.3). Each meniscus is C-shaped and is divided roughly into an anterior horn, a body, and a posterior horn. On sagittal and coronal images, the meniscus has a triangular shape. The point of the triangle is referred to as the *free edge* or *apex* and the base of the triangle is the peripheral margin. The remaining two surfaces articulate with the femoral condyle and the tibial plateau. The anterior and posterior horns are best seen on sagittal images; the meniscal body is best seen on coronal images. Tears are diagnosed by the presence of a line of increased signal extending to one or both of the articular surfaces (see Figure 34.9) (17). To decrease the number of false positives, the finding must be seen on a minimum of two images (18). An additional sign of tear is distortion of the meniscal shape with blunting or irregularity of the normal black triangle (see Figure 34.8B). Some meniscus signal changes are associated with parameniscal cysts and the presence of a cyst increases the likelihood of a tear.

There are varieties of types of meniscus tears including horizontal, vertical, and complex. Radial tears involve the free edge of the meniscus and may extend into the substance of the meniscus resulting in flap or parrot beak tears. Most significant is the bucket handle tear which is a vertical tear involving the entire meniscus (19). The free edge fragment, the "bucket handle", often displaces into the central notch of the knee, resulting in locking or other mechanical symptoms (see Figure 34.10). Less comprehensive tears may produce a free fragment which rotates or flips into another portion of the knee.

Occasionally, the meniscus is too large. This developmental abnormality usually occurs laterally and is termed a *discoid meniscus*; it can occur bilaterally. A discoid meniscus is more prone to tear than a normal meniscus, possibly related to the altered stresses induced by the abnormal meniscus shape. There are several subtypes, but on coronal images the mid-body of most discoid menisci extends beyond the medial or lateral compartment midline (see Figure 34.3). On sagittal images, the normal "bowtie" shape of the meniscus persists on three or more consecutive images.

Serious injuries of the knee may be associated with ligament tears. MRI is extremely reliable in the evaluation of ACL tears (20). There are numerous indirect signs of ACL injury (21). However, the most reliable sign of a complete ACL tear is nonvisualization of the ligament; a normal appearing ACL on MRI has near 100% accuracy in confirming that the ligament is intact (see Figure 34.11). Because valgus stress is associated with ACL injuries, it is common to see lateral compartment bone bruises in

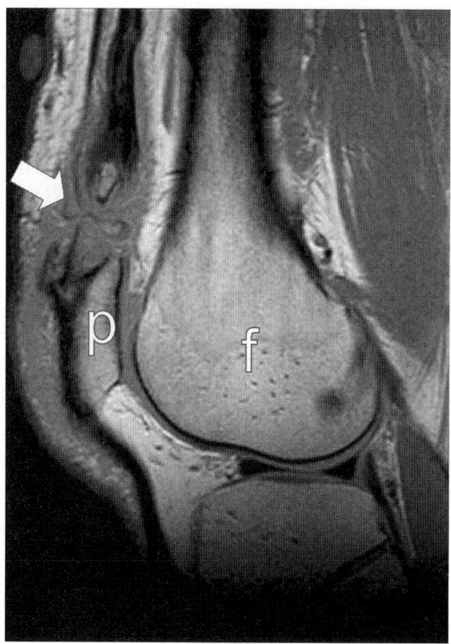

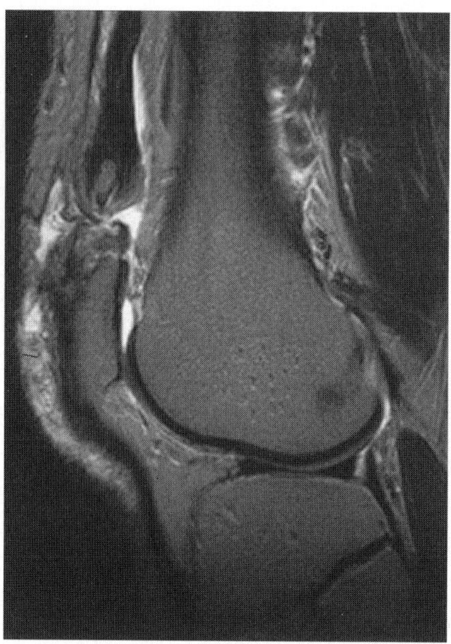

Figure 34.6 51-year-old man heard a pop and experienced severe knee pain during physical activity. Sagittal T1 (A) and T2 (B) weighted images of the knee; patella (p) and the distal femur (f) are visible. A fluid-filled gap representing a tear (*arrow*) of the distal quadriceps tendon is best seen on sagittal T2-weighted images (B). The patella is inferiorly subluxed because of the tear.

the setting of an ACL tear secondary to impaction of the lateral femoral condyle on the lateral tibial plateau. More severe valgus stress results in additional tears of the medial collateral ligament (MCL) and the medial meniscus, although there is some evidence to suggest that lateral meniscus tears are more common than medial meniscus tears in this setting (22). PCL tears are much less common than ACL tears and usually are associated with significant trauma; isolated PCL tears are uncommon (23,24).

Tears of the MCL and lateral collateral ligament (LCL) usually occur in association with other injuries (25,26). Injuries to the MCL are common, but injuries to the LCL are uncommon. These ligament tears or sprains can be graded according to severity. Grade I injuries are diagnosed by the presence of edema around the ligament, but ligament fibers are intact and conservative management is sufficient. With more stress, a grade II injury may occur, which is accompanied by the presence of a partial ligament tear (see Figure 34.12). The severity and location of injury guides management. A grade III injury is diagnosed when the ligament is completely disrupted.

Insertional tendinopathy or Jumper's knee (see Figure 34.13) usually is seen at the origin of the patellar tendon on the patella, but may also be seen at the quadriceps insertion on the patella. Injuries to these tendons may be seen in athletes involved in basketball, volleyball, and other jumping sports. On MRI, there is intermediate signal at the attachment site of these tendons on fluid-sensitive sequences. It is important to ignore similar signal changes at these sites on proton density and T1-weighted images because of a well-known MRI artifact, the magic angle artifact, which is responsible for producing these signal changes.

Disruption of the quadriceps or patellar tendon may be seen in the setting of extreme trauma, but is found more commonly in older individuals. In younger athletes, it is more common to encounter transient lateral patellar dislocation (27). The patella is pulled out of the trochlear groove as the femur rotates internally while the knee is in flexion. The patella usually spontaneously relocates. Patients present with a large knee effusion and extensive bone bruising of the anterior lateral femoral condyle (see Figure 34.14). The fibers of the medial patellar retinaculum may be torn and there can be significant cartilage damage to the surface of the patella as well as the femoral condyle.

Evaluation of the injured post operative knee is challenging. It is now common to see injured athletes who have undergone reconstructive surgery. Most of these patients can undergo an MR examination; however, metal hardware may obscure structures immediately adjacent to the hardware. MRI usually is effective in assessing the status of an ACL graft. MRI can evaluate the tibial and femoral tunnels for graft placement, disruption or laxity of the graft, notch impingement, and post operative ganglion formation.

MRI is less reliable in detecting meniscus tears in the setting of a prior meniscectomy (28). Often, the prior surgical history is unavailable at the time of imaging. If a limited meniscectomy has been performed (<25% of the meniscus has been resected), conventional diagnostic criteria can be applied for diagnosing a meniscus tear. If an extensive meniscectomy has been performed, it may be extremely difficult to confirm a persistent tear or a re-tear. MR arthrography has been proposed as a solution for this problem, but the results are disappointing (29). Although MR arthrography is not always helpful in the post operative meniscus patient, it is more effective than conventional MRI in documenting the presence of cartilage defects.

For those patients who cannot tolerate an MR examination, it is possible to perform a CTA. After the intra-articular injection of iodinated contrast media, a thin section CT examination is performed. Sagittal and coronal multiplanar

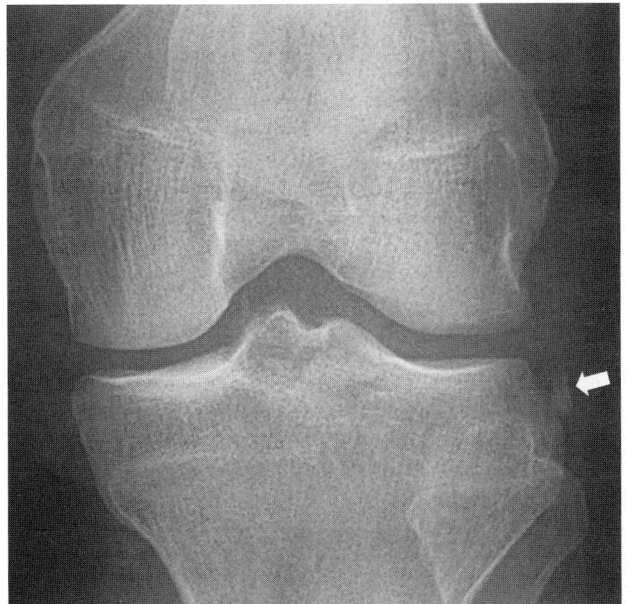

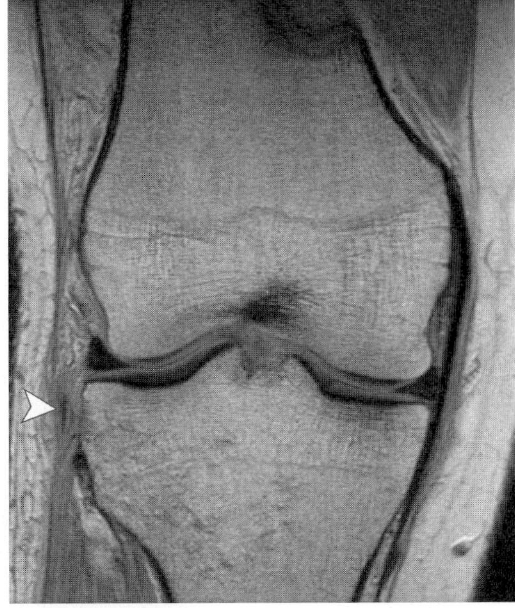

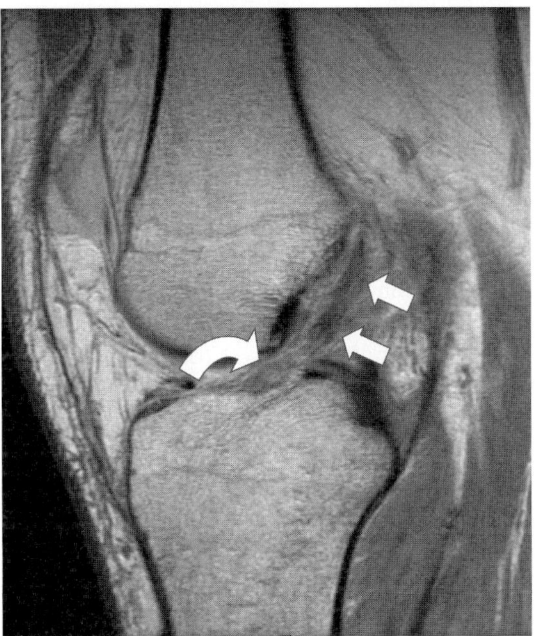

Figure 34.7 **A**: Segond fracture. Tiny chip fracture (*arrow*) represents avulsion of the mid third lateral capsular ligament. This seemingly insignificant fracture is often associated with an anterior cruciate ligament (ACL) tear. Magnetic resonance imaging (MRI) of this patient showed ACL disruption (not shown). **B**: Coronal proton density weighted image, different patient than in (**A**), shows a tiny flake of bone (*arrowhead*) representing the Segond fracture illustrating how difficult it can be to detect these fractures without corresponding radiographs. **C**: Same patient as in (**B**), sagittal proton density weighted image through the middle of the knee shows complete tear of the ACL (*arrows*) at the tibial attachment (*curved arrow*).

image reformations are created, which resemble sagittal and coronal MR images (see Figure 34.1). CTA performs as well as MRI in the detection of meniscus tears. Additionally, CTA is superior to MRI in detecting articular surface defects. Although the ACL fibers cannot be seen directly, the outline of the ACL can be assessed for redundancy or disruption and a complete ACL tear can be detected with CTA. Visualization of bone marrow and other soft tissue structures is limited. For some patients, a CTA is an acceptable means of evaluating the joint (5).

SHOULDER IMAGING

The shoulder joint is the most mobile joint in the body. This mobility comes at a cost: the joint is intrinsically unstable

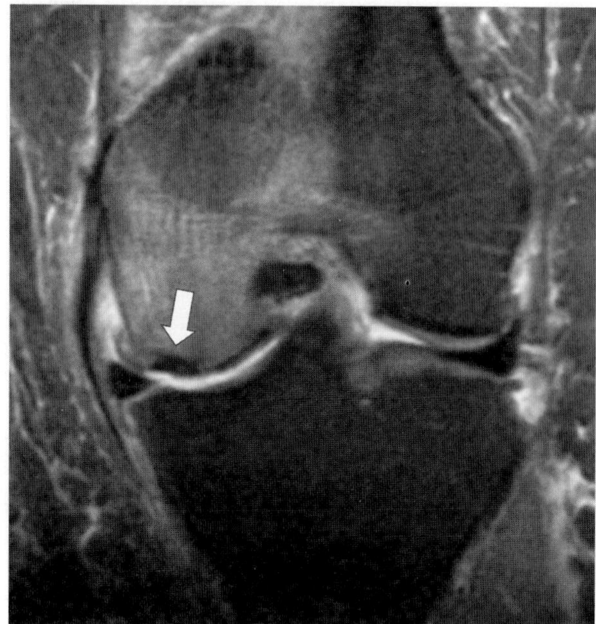

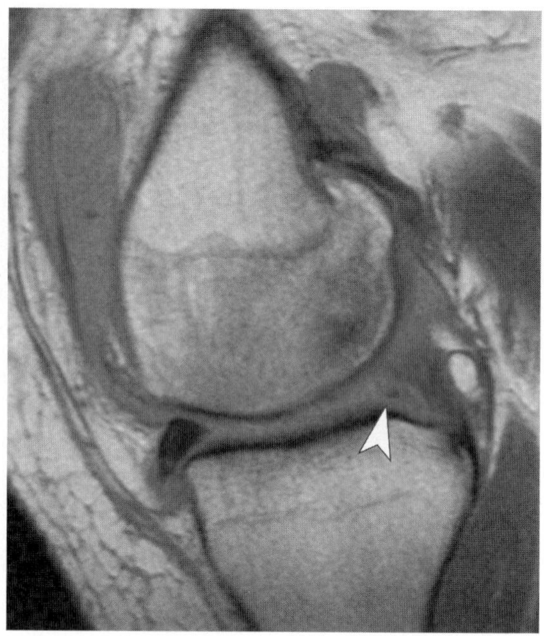

Figure 34.8 56-year-old woman with increasing knee pain. **A:** Coronal short inversion time inversion recovery (STIR) image of the knee shows intense marrow edema of the medial femoral condyle. Low signal line (*arrow*) in the subcortical region of the condyle represents insufficiency fracture, accounting for the intense marrow edema. **B:** Sagittal proton density weighted image demonstrates severe distortion of the posterior horn of the medial meniscus, representing a tear (*arrowhead*), which is often found in association with the insufficiency fracture.

because the glenoid fossa is relatively small compared to the size of the humeral head. Without the stabilization of the surrounding musculature, the humeral head could easily slip out of the glenoid fossa. Unfortunately, the mobility of the humeral head predisposes the glenoid and the labrum to damage, resulting in degeneration, tear, and, in some cases, fracture.

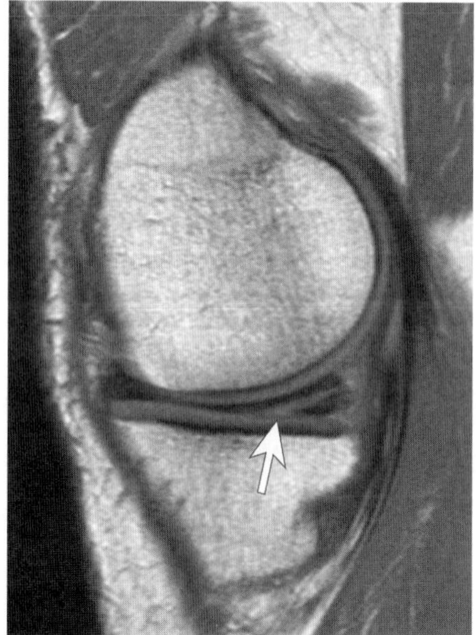

Figure 34.9 Sagittal proton density weighted image through the posterior horn of the medial meniscus shows a line of increased signal (*arrow*) extending to the inferior articular surface representing a tear.

Imaging of the shoulder begins with radiographs to assess for glenohumeral joint space narrowing, osteophytes, fracture, and calcific tendonitis. The importance of radiography must be emphasized as small tuberosity fractures and rotator cuff calcifications usually are not visible on MRI. Many radiographic projections of the shoulder are possible, but the following three views are recommended for a limited, yet comprehensive survey of the joint: true anteroposterior (AP) (Grashey), internal rotation AP, axillary view (see Figure 34.15). The Garth view can be obtained in lieu of the axillary view to assess the relationship of the humeral head to the glenoid when a dislocation is suspected; the Garth view may not be acceptable to some orthopedic surgeons when a fracture is present. If impingement symptoms are present, a supraspinatus outlet projection can be obtained in addition to the routine views to assess for acromioclavicular (AC) joint osteophytes.

MRI generally is considered the next step in the evaluation of the shoulder. If the patient presents with symptoms of rotator cuff disease, a non contrast shoulder MRI will suffice. If there is a concern about the status of the labrum or biceps anchor point, MR arthrography is recommended (30–32). If the patient has had prior reconstructive surgery, MRI generally will provide adequate visualization and MR arthrography is recommended to ensure distension of the joint spaces. Patients with large screws in the glenoid may be better served with a

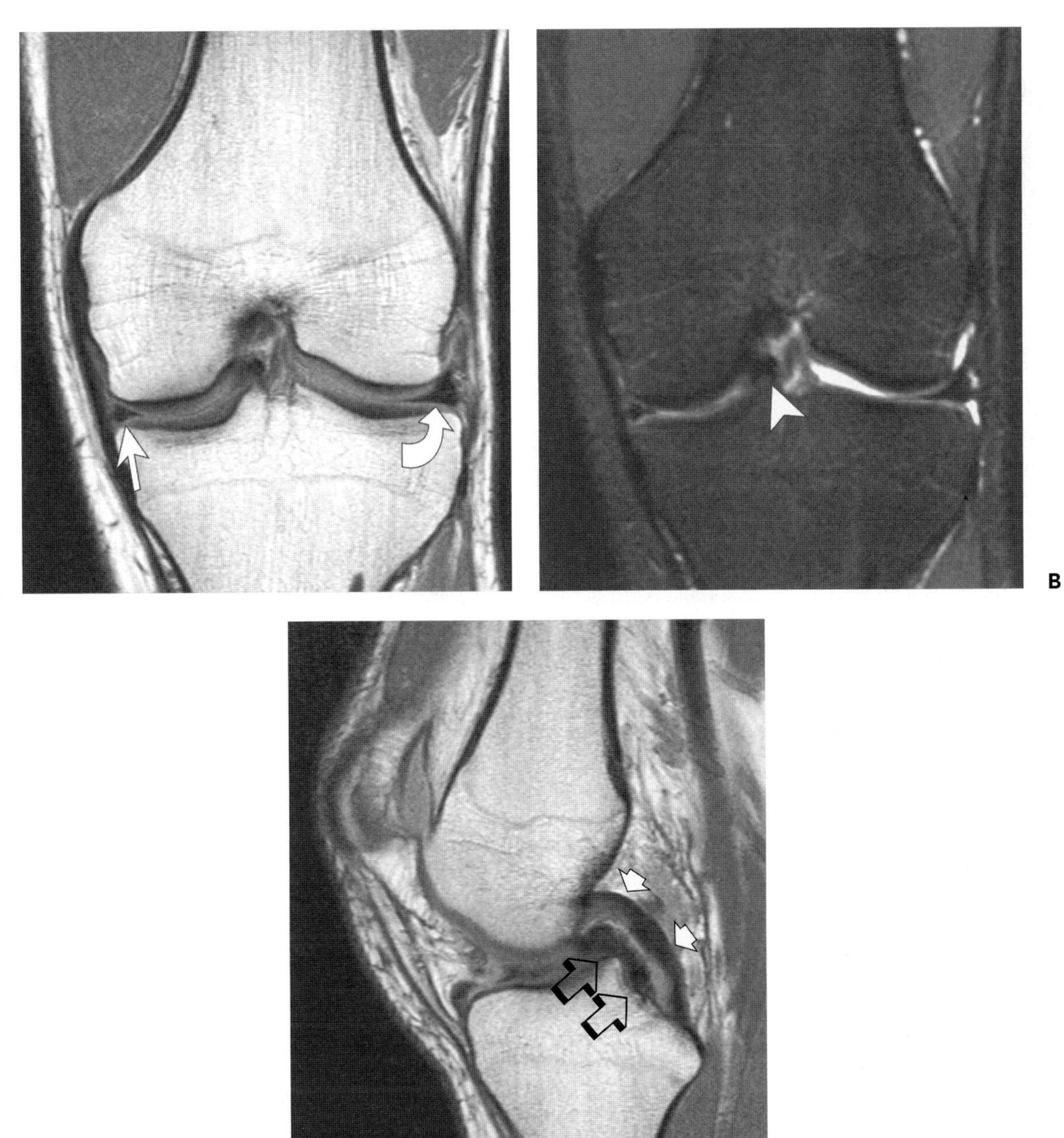

Figure 34.10 31-year-old man experienced a twisting injury during a basketball game 1 week before imaging. **A:** Coronal proton density weighted image of the knee shows that the body of the medial meniscus (*arrow*) is smaller than the body of the lateral meniscus (*curved arrow*). Normally, the bodies of both menisci are similarly sized. **B:** Coronal short inversion time inversion recovery (STIR) image, same location as A. shows the displaced bucket handle fragment (*arrowhead*) of the medial meniscus, explaining the small size of the body of the meniscus. **C:** Sagittal proton density weighted image shows the displaced bucket handle fragment (*open arrows*), immediately inferior to the posterior cruciate ligament (*wide arrows*). This is the "double posterior cruciate ligament (PCL) sign", a finding associated with bucket handle tears.

CTA. Exceptionally large patients, severely claustrophobic patients, and patients with MR incompatible hardware also are candidates for CTA (see Figure 34.16).

MRI of the shoulder consists of oblique coronal and oblique sagittal images to assess the rotator cuff tendon and muscles and axial images to evaluate the glenohumeral joint. The normal rotator cuff is mostly dark on all pulse sequences and is assessed primarily in the oblique coronal plane (see Figure 34.17). The superior surface of the rotator cuff tendon is referred to as the bursal surface and the inferior surface is the articular surface. The subacromial-subdeltoid bursa lies immediately superior to the bursal surface of the cuff and the glenohumeral joint lies inferior to the articular surface. The lateral 1 to 1.5 cm of the rotator

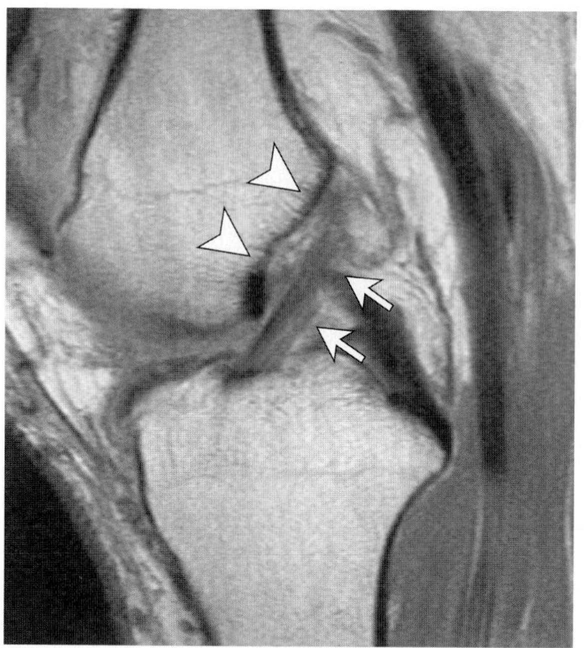

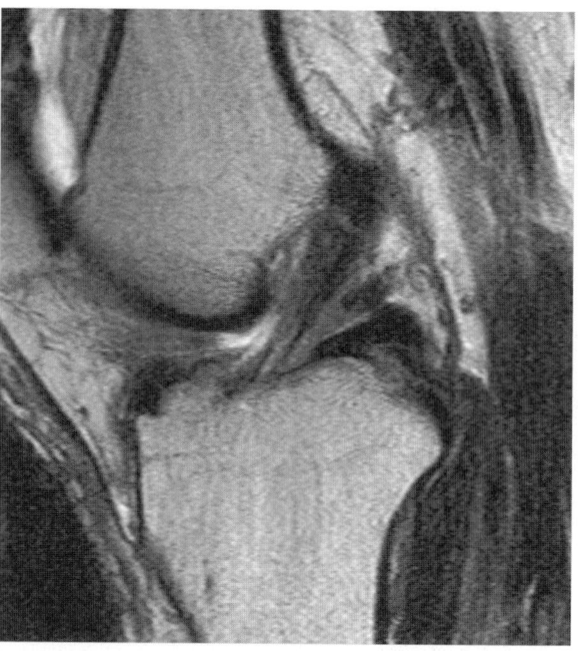

Figure 34.11 Sagittal proton density (**A**) and corresponding T2-weighted (**B**) images through a normal anterior cruciate ligament (compare with figure 34.7C). The normal anterior cruciate ligament (ACL) (*arrows*) is intermediate in signal on proton density weighted images and may appear striated. Signal intensity of the ligament decreases on T2- weighted images. The ligament is parallel or nearly parallel with the roof of the intercondylar notch (*arrowheads*) called *Blumensaat's line*.

cuff tendon is referred to as the *critical zone*. This region of the tendon is most vulnerable to damage because it is relatively avascular. Most tears occur in this region.

The diagnosis of a rotator cuff tear is made at MRI by identifying a fluid-filled gap in the tendon (see Figure 34.18A,B). If the tear extends from the articular surface to the bursal surface, it is termed a *full thickness tear*. Note that by this definition, a tiny perforation extending from articular to bursal surfaces qualifies as a full thickness tear. The extension of the tear in the anteroposterior dimension is referred to as the *width* of the tear. Therefore, a through and through tear involving the entirety of the

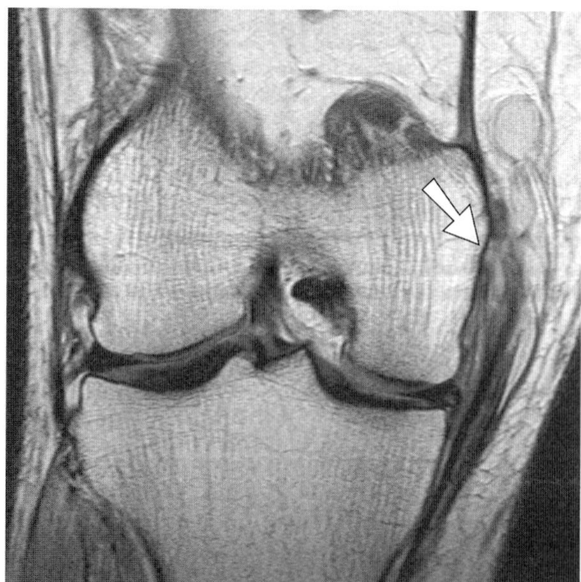

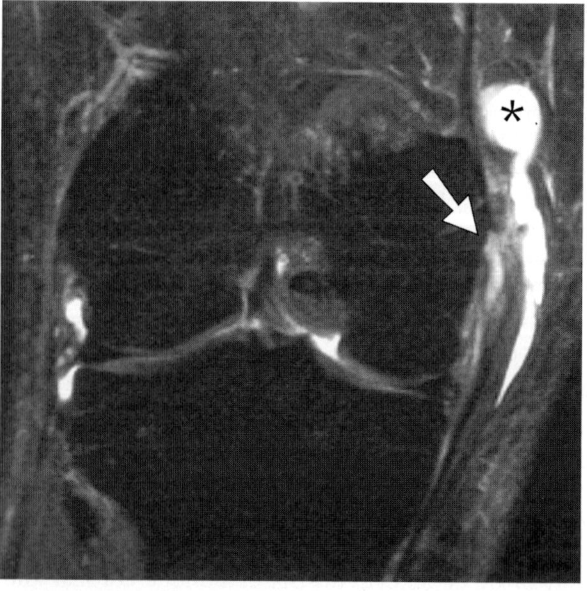

Figure 34.12 High grade proximal medial collateral sprain (*arrow*) is demonstrated on coronal proton density (**A**) and corresponding short inversion time inversion recovery (STIR) (**B**) images. Fluid leaking from the tear has formed an accessory bursa (*asterisk*).

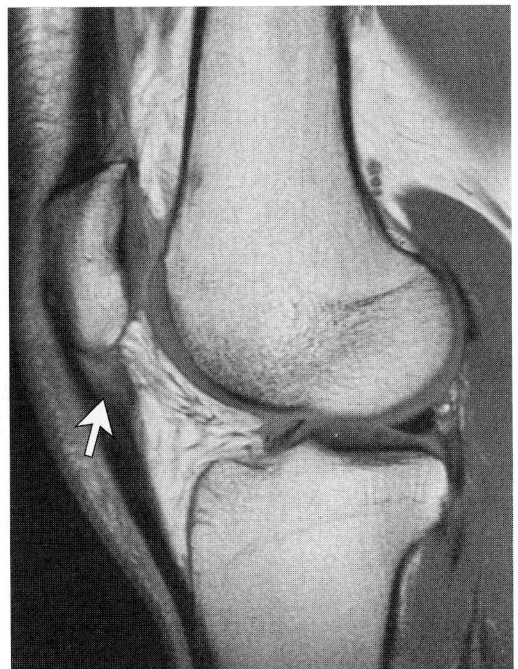

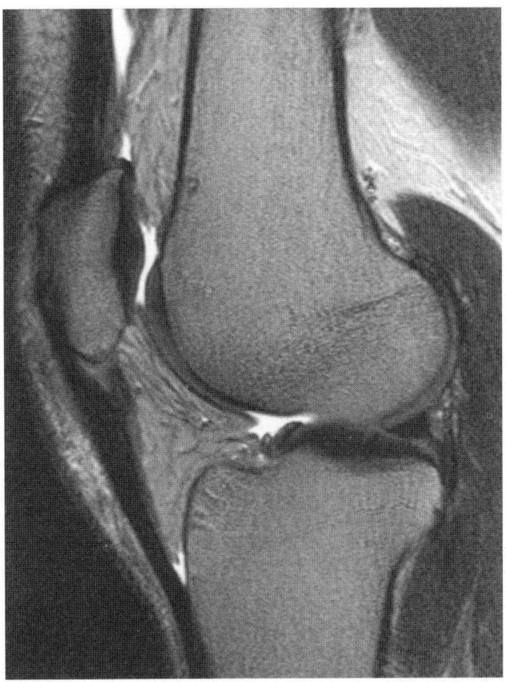

Figure 34.13 31-year-old man with anterior knee pain. Sagittal proton density (**A**) and T2-weighted (**B**) images of the knee through the level of the mid patellar tendon. Intermediate signal of the proximal patella on proton density image (*arrow*) persists on T2-weighted image (**B**). Focal tendinopathy is consistent with the diagnosis of Jumper's knee.

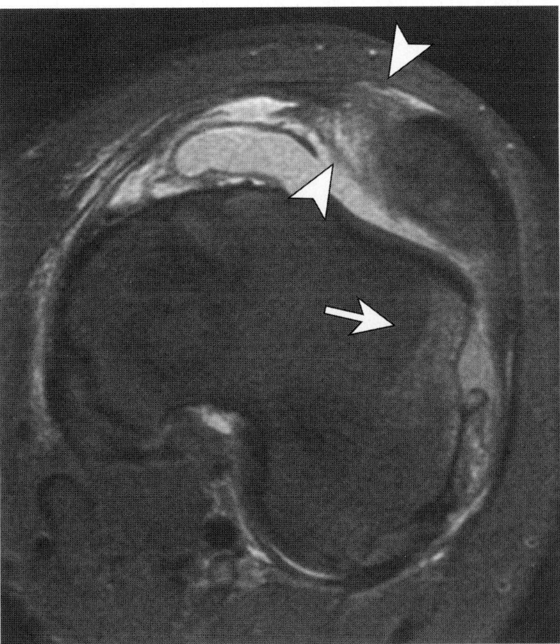

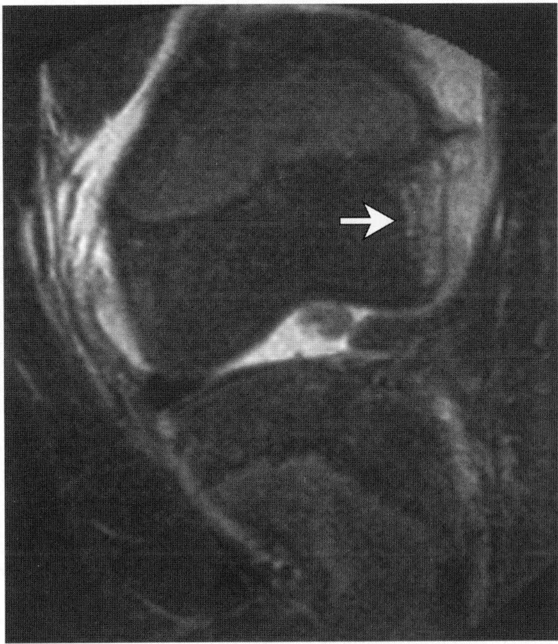

Figure 34.14 **A**: Axial inversion recovery weighted image shows anterior lateral femoral condyle bone bruise (*arrow*) and tear of the medial patellar retinaculum (*arrowheads*) secondary to transient lateral patellar dislocation. **B:** Coronal short inversion time inversion recovery (STIR) image through the anterior femoral condyles shows the distribution of the bone bruise (*arrow*) secondary to impaction of the medial patellar margin on the anterior margin of the lateral femoral condyle.

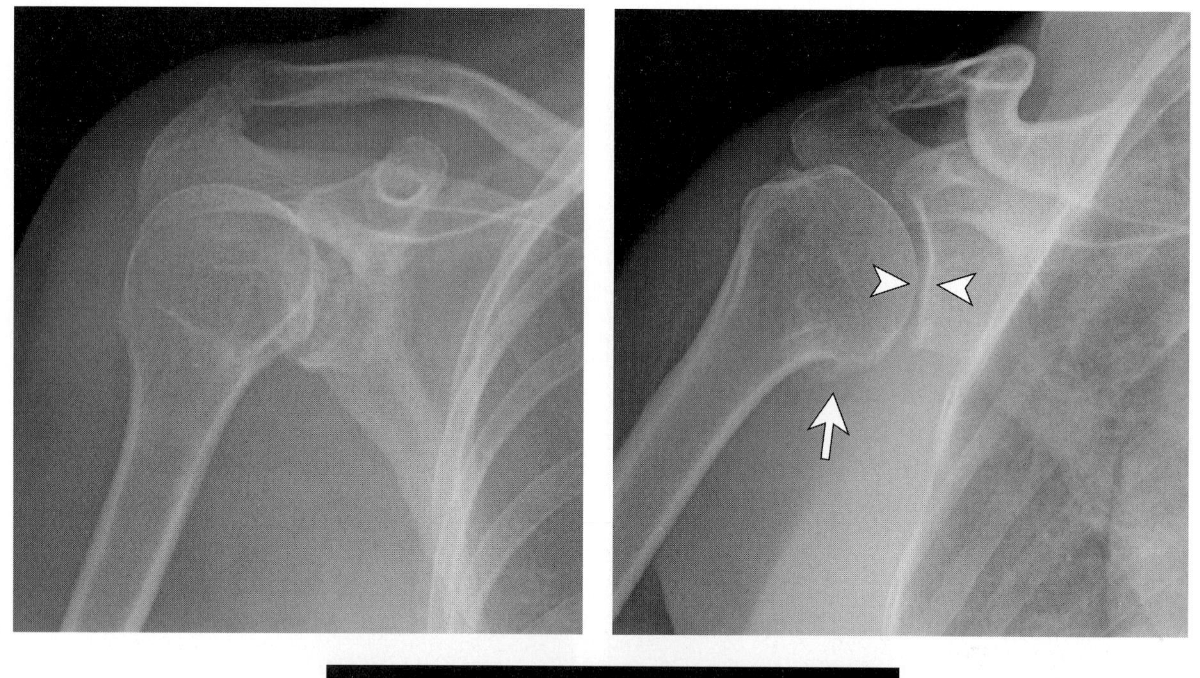

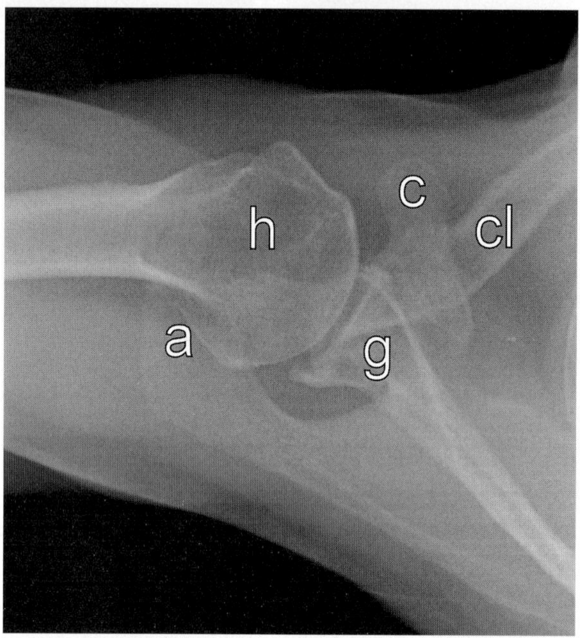

Figure 34.15 Routine 3 view shoulder series, 68-year-old woman with right shoulder pain. **A:** Anteroposterior (AP) view of the shoulder with the humerus in internal rotation is useful to evaluate the humeral head and to inspect the rotator cuff tendon for calcifications. **B:** Grashey or true AP view of the shoulder is obtained by simultaneously rotating the patient in a posterior oblique position and externally rotating the humerus. This view profiles the glenohumeral joint. Degenerative osteophytes of the humeral head (*arrow*) and glenohumeral joint narrowing (*arrowheads*) are well demonstrated. **C:** Axillary view of the shoulder, anterior at the top of the image. Humerus (h), glenoid (g), acromion (a), coracoid process of the scapula (c), and clavicle (cl) are annotated. The axillary view demonstrates the anterior posterior relationship of the humeral head to the glenoid and is helpful in assessing patients with suspected dislocations. The axillary view is obtained with the arm abducted and requires a cooperative patient.

supraspinatus tendon is referred to as a full thickness, full width supraspinatus tear. In general, dimensions of the tear are reported to assist with further management.

Oblique sagittal images are helpful in assessing the anteroposterior extent of tears, and also are helpful in identifying atrophy of the rotator cuff muscles (see Figure 34.18C); severe muscle atrophy is a relative contraindication for surgical repair. Extreme medial retraction of the cuff tendon following tear is a poor prognostic indicator if surgical repair is a consideration. If the cuff is

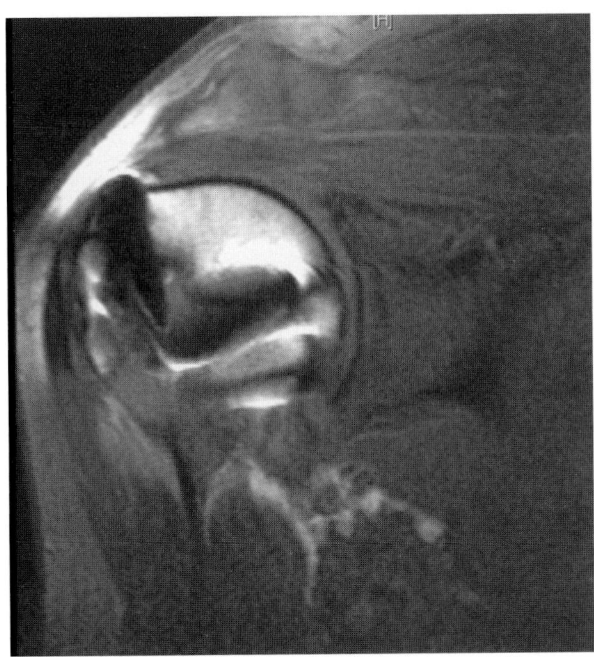

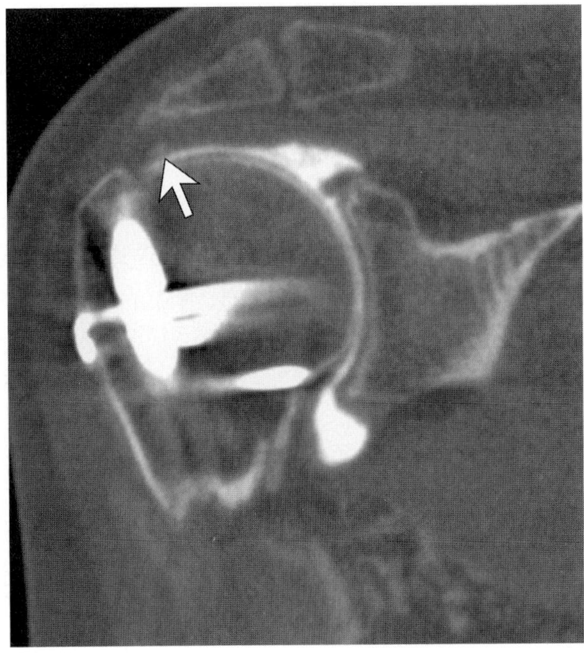

Figure 34.16 **A**: Patient with prior humeral fracture stabilized with long intramedullary nail presents with new shoulder pain. Coronal fat suppressed T1- weighted image obtained during magnetic resonance (MR) arthrogram fails to demonstrate the supraspinatus insertion onto the humeral head because of extensive metal artifact. Examination was nondiagnostic. **B:** Metal artifact on followup computed tomography (CT) arthrogram is less extensive, allowing visualization of a small undersurface tear (*arrow*) of the lateral supraspinatus tendon.

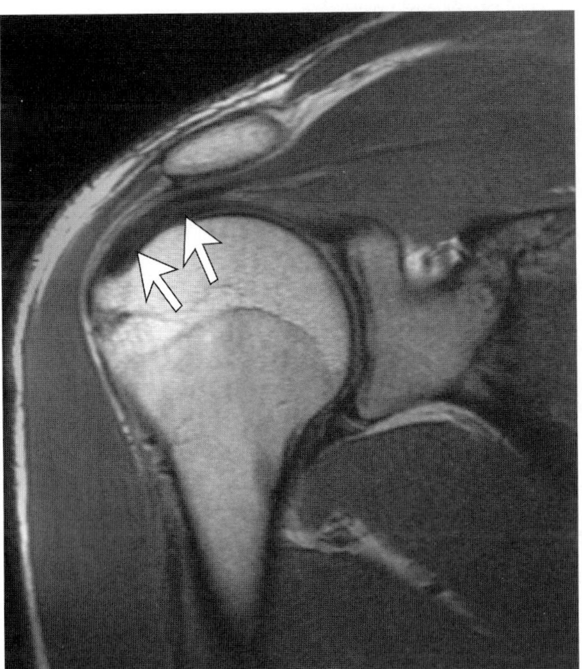

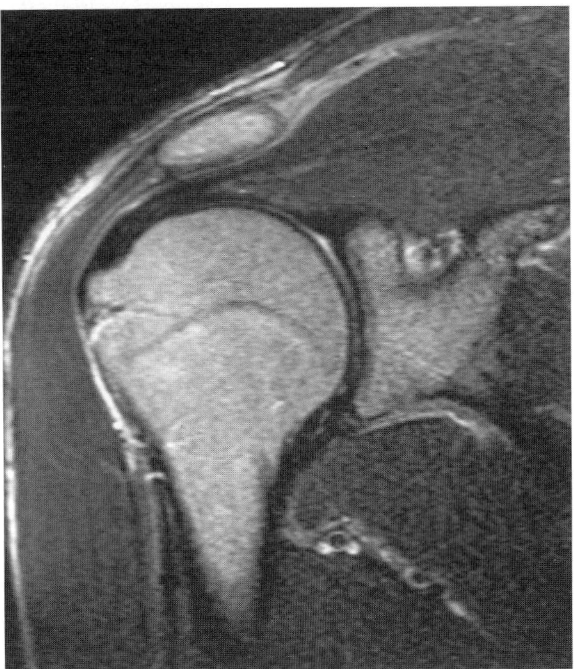

Figure 34.17 Oblique coronal proton density (**A**) and corresponding inversion recovery (**B**) weighted images through the mid supraspinatus tendon (*arrows*) show the low signal intensity appearance of the normal rotator cuff.

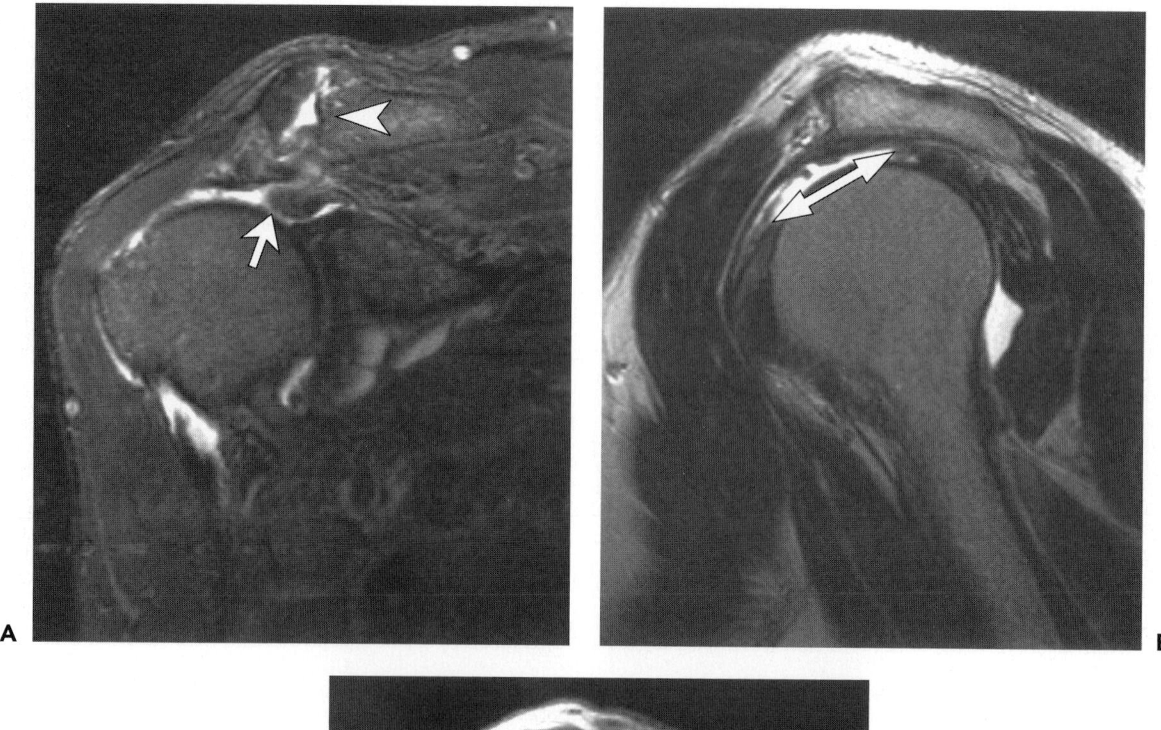

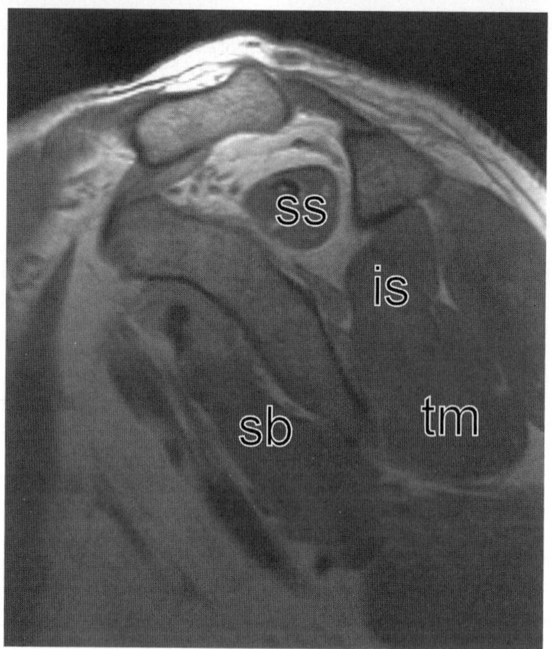

Figure 34.18 **A**: Oblique coronal inversion recovery weighted image demonstrates large full thickness tear of the supraspinatus tendon. The retracted tendon (*arrow*) is just lateral to the glenoid margin. Marked hypertrophic changes are present at the acromioclavicular (AC) joint (*arrowhead*). **B:** Oblique sagittal T2-weighted image shows that the tear of the supraspinatus tendon is full width; that is, the entire anterior to posterior extent of the tendon is torn (*double arrows*). **C**: Oblique sagittal proton density weighted image, medial to B. Moderate atrophy of the supraspinatus muscle (ss) is documented. Compare the thickness of the supraspinatus muscle with the remaining rotator cuff muscles; infraspinatus (is), subscapularis (sb), teres minor (tm).

retracted medial to the glenoid, surgical repair often is contraindicated. Oblique sagittal images are useful to document the shape of the acromion and to look for AC joint osteophytes, which may cause mechanical impingement.

Another problem affecting the AC joint is the os acromiale, a remnant of the acromial ossification center. Many patients with an os acromiale are asymptomatic; however, some patients develop a pseudoarthrosis, which can become symptomatic. A separate condition affecting the AC joint is lateral clavicle osteolysis. This can be seen with repetitive shoulder injuries and has been reported in weightlifters who are most symptomatic when performing bench press exercises. Radiographs may show progressive indistinctness of the lateral clavicle with progressive widening of the AC joint. MRI may show intense marrow edema, most notable on STIR or fat suppressed T2-weighted images (33). Symptoms can mimic rotator cuff pathology.

Partial thickness tears are diagnosed when fluid tracks from the bursal or the articular surface of the rotator cuff tendon into the substance of the tendon itself. Articular sided tears are more common than bursal sided tears. Small perforations of the cuff can track along the central tendon and extend medially as intramuscular cysts for several centimeters.

Tendinopathy of the rotator cuff is mucoid degeneration within the substance of the tendon and normally is found in the critical zone region. Tendinopathy is diagnosed at MRI if there is increased signal within the tendon on fluid-sensitive images. Because some low level signal can be seen normally within the tendon substance, focal thickening of the tendon can increase the likelihood that the signal changes represent true tendinopathy. Magic angle artifacts can cause spuriously high signals on T1-weighted and proton density images, so it is important to verify the pulse sequence type before establishing the diagnosis (34).

The glenoid labrum deepens the shallow fossa of the bony glenoid and represents focal thickening of the adjacent joint capsule. The labrum consists of fibrocartilage which is dark on all MR pulse sequences. Both gradient echo and fat suppressed proton density weighted sequences demonstrate the labrum well. The normal labrum is triangular in cross section and is seen best on oblique coronal and axial plane images.

Tears of the labrum can be difficult to diagnose because there are a wide variety of normal variants (35). Most of the normal variants occur in the anterior and superior quadrant of the labrum. One common variant in this location, the Buford complex, is a hypertrophied middle glenohumeral ligament accompanied by an absent labrum. The hypertrophic ligament is closely applied to the glenoid margin and provides a functionally equivalent substitute. Because the coracoid process is seen on axial images from the superior margin to the mid-glenoid, most abnormalities of the anterior labrum on the axial plane can be ignored if the coracoid is visible on the same image. The more inferior portion of the labrum should assume a triangular shape, if it is normal.

Rounding and blunting of the labrum at MRI may represent degenerative fraying. Unfortunately, internal rotation of the shoulder may result in deformity of the anterior labrum, simulating a tear. Despite all attempts to position patients optimally, some patients cannot be positioned in the confines of the scanner without some degree of internal rotation. Fluid signal seen within the labrum almost always represents a tear. Fluid may be present at the articular margin of the labrum as the labrum apposes the articular cartilage; this "undercutting" of the labrum is also a normal variant. However, fluid should never track completely through the base of the labrum (see Figure 34.19). Occasionally, a paralabral cyst will form and the presence of a cyst is associated with a high likelihood of a labral tear.

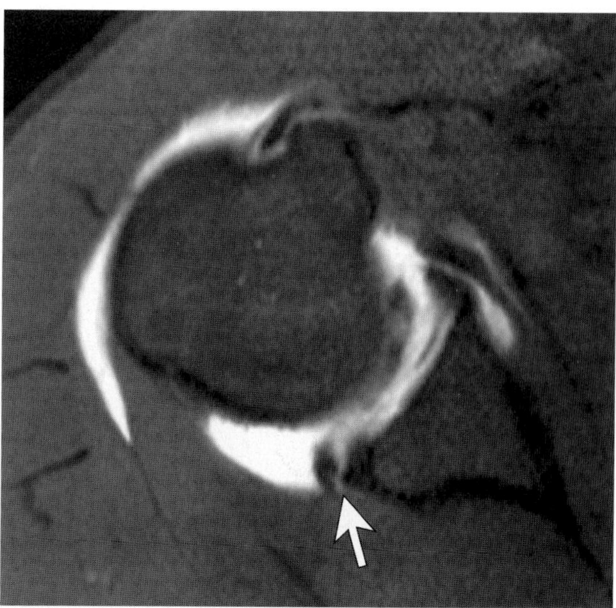

Figure 34.19 Axial fat suppressed T1-weighted image of the shoulder following intra-articular administration of dilute gadolinium solution (magnetic resonance (MR) arthrogram). Tear of the posterior labrum is diagnosed by identifying contrast tracking into the labrum (*arrow*).

Cysts located at the superior margin of the glenoid are particularly important if they extend into the suprascapular notch (see Figure 34.20). The scapular nerve passes through the notch, innervating the supraspinatus muscle, then continues along, sending a branch to the infraspinatus muscle. Masses in or adjacent to the notch can compress the nerve causing muscle atrophy. Depending on the compression level, either the infraspinatus muscle or both the supraspinatus and infraspinatus muscles will be affected. Initially, there will be denervation atrophy which presents as increased signal within the muscle. Later, fatty infiltration will occur followed by loss of muscle bulk. Patients with compression neuropathy can present with weakness that may simulate rotator cuff disease.

Shoulder dislocations are seen frequently, particularly in contact sports. Anterior dislocations are most common. Because posterior dislocations are relatively rare, a seizure disorder should be excluded if the patient has not experienced an unusual injury mechanism. Exceedingly rare, but exceptionally dramatic is *luxatio erecta*. Patients with this type of dislocation present with the arm overhead as if asking a question. This condition is important to recognize as these patients have serious associated injuries, often presenting with tuberosity fractures and large rotator cuff tears.

Following anterior dislocation, patients may develop an impaction fracture of the posterior superior humeral head, the Hill-Sachs lesion (see Figure 34.21). This has been described as a "hatchet" deformity and is best detected on

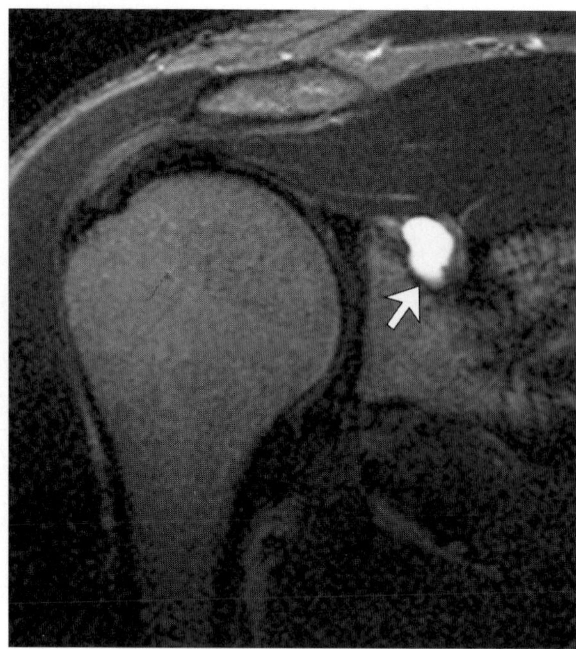

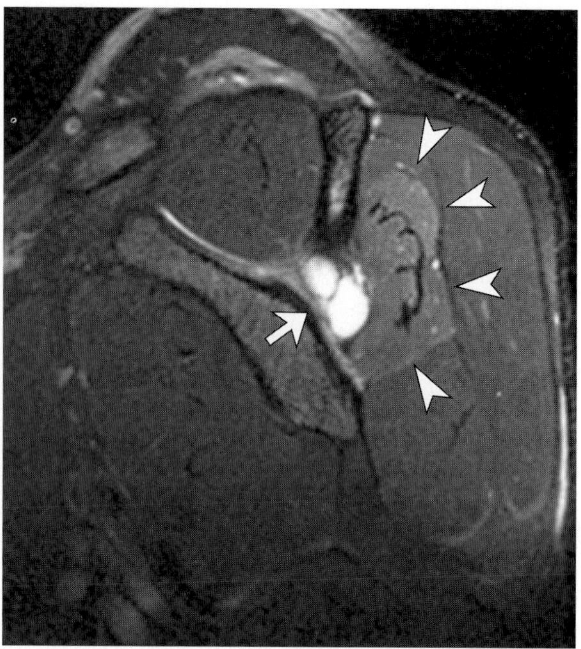

Figure 34.20 23-year-old man with shoulder weakness. **A:** Oblique coronal inversion recovery weighted image shows spinoglenoid notch ganglion (*arrow*) associated with superior labral tear (not shown). **B:** Oblique sagittal T2-weighted image illustrates that the ganglion (*arrow*) is inferior to the scapular spine. Compression of the scapular nerve at this location causes denervation edema of the infraspinatus muscle (*arrowheads*).

the internally rotated anteroposterior (AP) radiograph of the shoulder. Because the humeral head displaces anteriorly and inferiorly in an anterior dislocation, the head may damage the anterior inferior labrum and capsule. In a more extreme example, the inferior glenoid will fracture, called a *Bankart fracture.* A spectrum of associated abnormalities can be encountered including capsular stripping, tears of the inferior glenohumeral ligament, and cartilage defects that go by a variety of acronyms. These findings are best evaluated with an MR arthrogram which should include a series of images obtained with the shoulder in the abducted and externally rotated position, the ABER positioned view (36).

One interesting abnormality encountered in baseball pitchers is the Bennett lesion (thrower's exostosis). This is an extra-articular posterior capsular avulsive injury associated with labral tears and a posterior undersurface rotator cuff tear. The lesion should be suspected if there is unexplained posterior shoulder pain in a throwing athlete; a calcification paralleling the posterior interior rim of the glenoid is a helpful plain film finding and suggests trauma to the posterior band of the inferior glenohumeral ligament. It is important to recognize that not all of these lesions are symptomatic and correlation with the physical examination is necessary to establish the diagnosis. The imaging work-up proceeds with an MR arthrogram.

Another lesion seen in throwers is the superior labrum anterior and posterior tear (SLAP). In throwing athletes, the injury occurs during the acceleration phase of throwing. Patients complain of pain with overhead activity or throwing; some patients may complain of pain after a fall on the outstretched arm with the shoulder in abduction and forward flexion. In addition to throwers, SLAP tears can be seen in tennis players, volleyball players and weightlifters. There are multiple types of SLAP tears, depending on the site of tear as well as the extension into the biceps anchor point. Although these tears can be identified on routine MR imaging, MR arthrography is recommended if a SLAP tear is suspected (see Figure 34.22).

ELBOW IMAGING

The elbow is not injured as commonly as the shoulder or knee. However, with increasing numbers of people participating in racquet sports, injuries of this joint are becoming more prevalent. The imaging evaluation of an elbow injury begins with AP and lateral radiographs. These two views usually are adequate for demonstrating most elbow dislocations and fractures. The lateral view is particularly useful in identifying an elbow effusion, which is apparent when the normally hidden anterior and posterior fat pads become visible (see Figure 34.23). The presence of an effusion is associated with a high likelihood of fracture (37). In adults, the fracture usually involves the radial head, but in children the fracture most often occurs in the supracondylar region of the distal humerus.

The elbow joint consists of three separate articulations that share a common joint capsule. These articulations are the proximal radioulnar joint, the ulnohumeral joint,

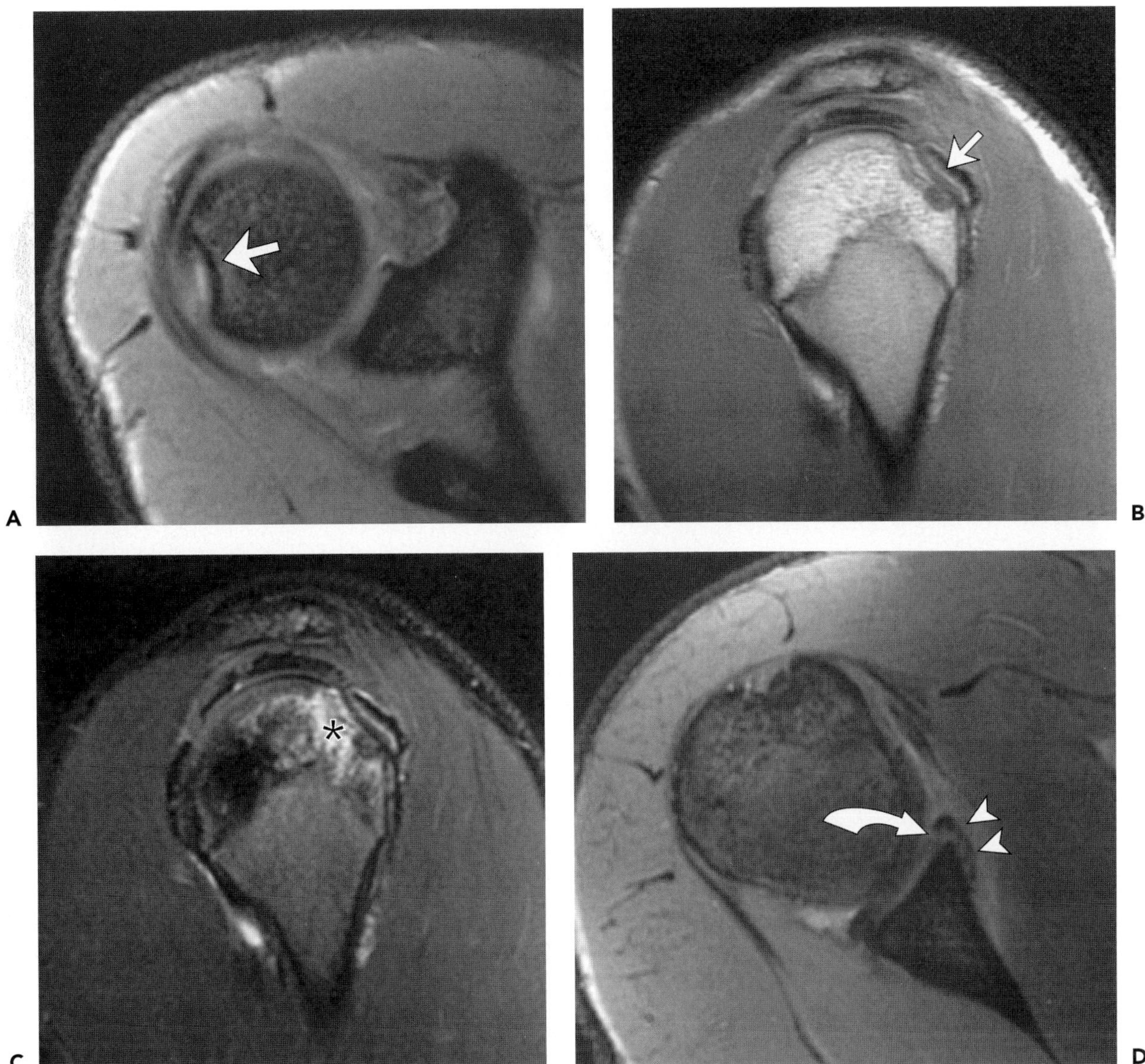

Figure 34.21 15-year-old adolescent with a history of recent anterior dislocation. **A:** Axial gradient echo image shows contour deformity (*arrow*) of the posterior superior humeral head representing the Hill-Sachs lesion. **B:** Oblique sagittal proton density weighted image shows extent of impaction fracture of the posterior humeral head (*arrow*). **C:** Oblique sagittal fat suppressed T2-weighted image shows bone marrow edema (*asterisk*) secondary to the impaction fracture. **D:** Axial gradient echo image through the inferior labrum shows fluid signal at the base of the anterior labrum (*curved arrow*) representing labral tear; there is associated capsular stripping (*arrowheads*) related to the dislocation and labral injury.

and the radiocapitellar joint. Elbow joints are the third most commonly dislocated joints in adults (after the glenohumeral joint and interphalangeal joints) and the elbow is the most commonly dislocated joint in children. The usual mechanism of injury is hyperextension secondary to a fall on an outstretched arm. If a proximal fracture of the ulna is encountered, it is important to recognize that some of these are associated with radial head dislocations (Monteggia fracture dislocation).

The elbow joint capsule is relatively thin anteriorly and posteriorly. The medial and lateral portions of the capsule are thickened and strengthened by the LCL and MCL. The LCL complex consists of the radial collateral ligament, the lateral ulnar collateral ligament, the annular ligament, and the accessory collateral ligament. The annular ligament surrounds the radial head and is the primary stabilizer of the proximal radioulnar joint. The radial collateral ligament arises from the lateral epicondyle and inserts into the annular ligament. The lateral ulnar collateral ligament also arises from the lateral epicondyle and inserts into the supinator crest of the ulna. The latter two ligaments are functionally the most important and provide lateral stabilization of the joint. MRI provides excellent anatomical detail of the ligaments of the elbow (38). The normal radial collateral and

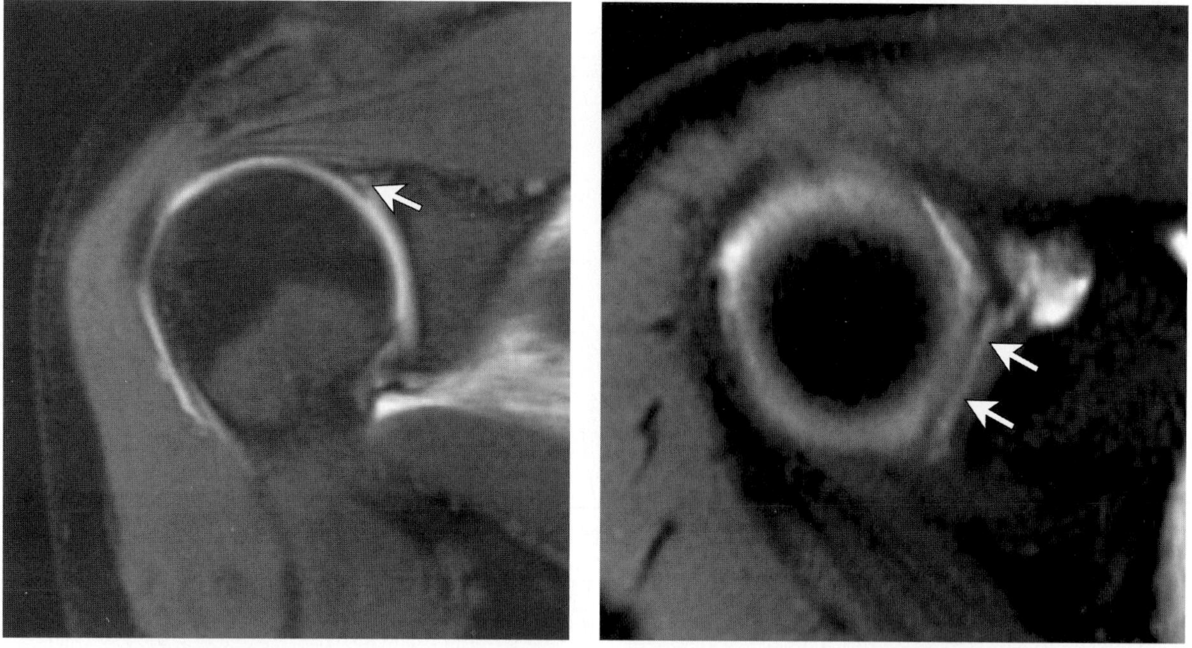

Figure 34.22 31-year-old woman with 12 years of shoulder pain and physical examination suggesting labral tear. Oblique coronal (**A**) and oblique sagittal (**B**) fat suppressed T1-weighted images show contrast tracking into the superior labrum (*arrows*) from the anterior to posterior aspects of the labrum representing a superior labrum anterior and posterior (SLAP) tear.

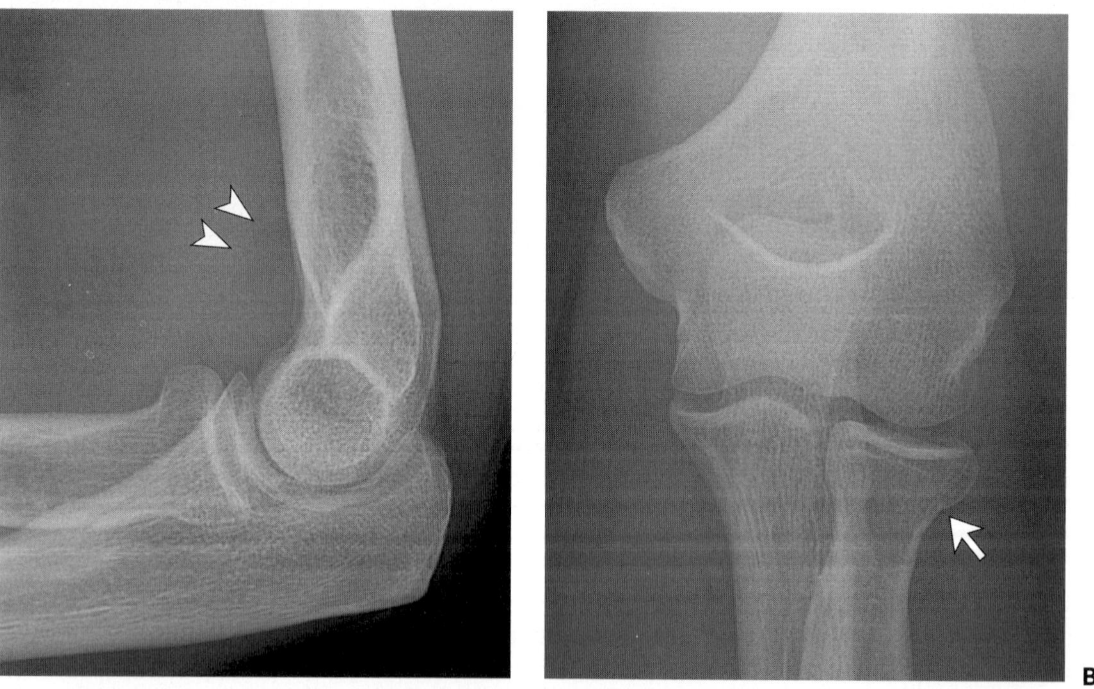

Figure 34.23 34-year-old man fell off a bicycle and sustained an elbow injury. **A:** Lateral radiograph of the elbow shows displaced anterior fat pad (*arrowheads*) indicating an effusion. **B:** Anteroposterior (AP) radiograph of the elbow shows nondisplaced fracture of the radial neck (*arrow*).

lateral ulnar collateral ligaments are best seen on coronal proton density or gradient echo images. Tears of the lateral ulnar collateral ligament usually occur proximally, and are apparent as a fluid gap on fluid-sensitive sequences.

The MCL complex consists of the anterior, posterior and transverse ligaments. Most important is the anterior ligament or anterior band which arises from the medial epicondyle and inserts onto the sublime tubercle of the ulna. This ligament provides the primary restraint to valgus stress and may be injured in athletes who participate in throwing sports. The anterior band is best visualized on coronal proton density images as a thin dark line. Tears of the anterior band are best seen on fluid-sensitive sequences (see Figure 34.24A,B).

The muscles of the elbow are commonly divided into anterior, posterior, medial, and lateral compartments. The anterior compartment muscles are the biceps and brachialis. The muscle attachments are best visualized on axial and sagittal proton density MR sequences. The biceps tendon runs superficial to the brachialis and inserts into the radial tuberosity; it is the most commonly injured tendon of the elbow (see Figure 34.4). The mechanism of injury is usually forceful overload during concentric contraction with the elbow near midflexion. The lacertus fibrosus is the aponeurosis of the biceps tendon, and it helps to keep the biceps tendon anchored to the radial tuberosity. Partial tears of the biceps tendon most commonly occur at the distal attachment, but minimal retraction of the tendon

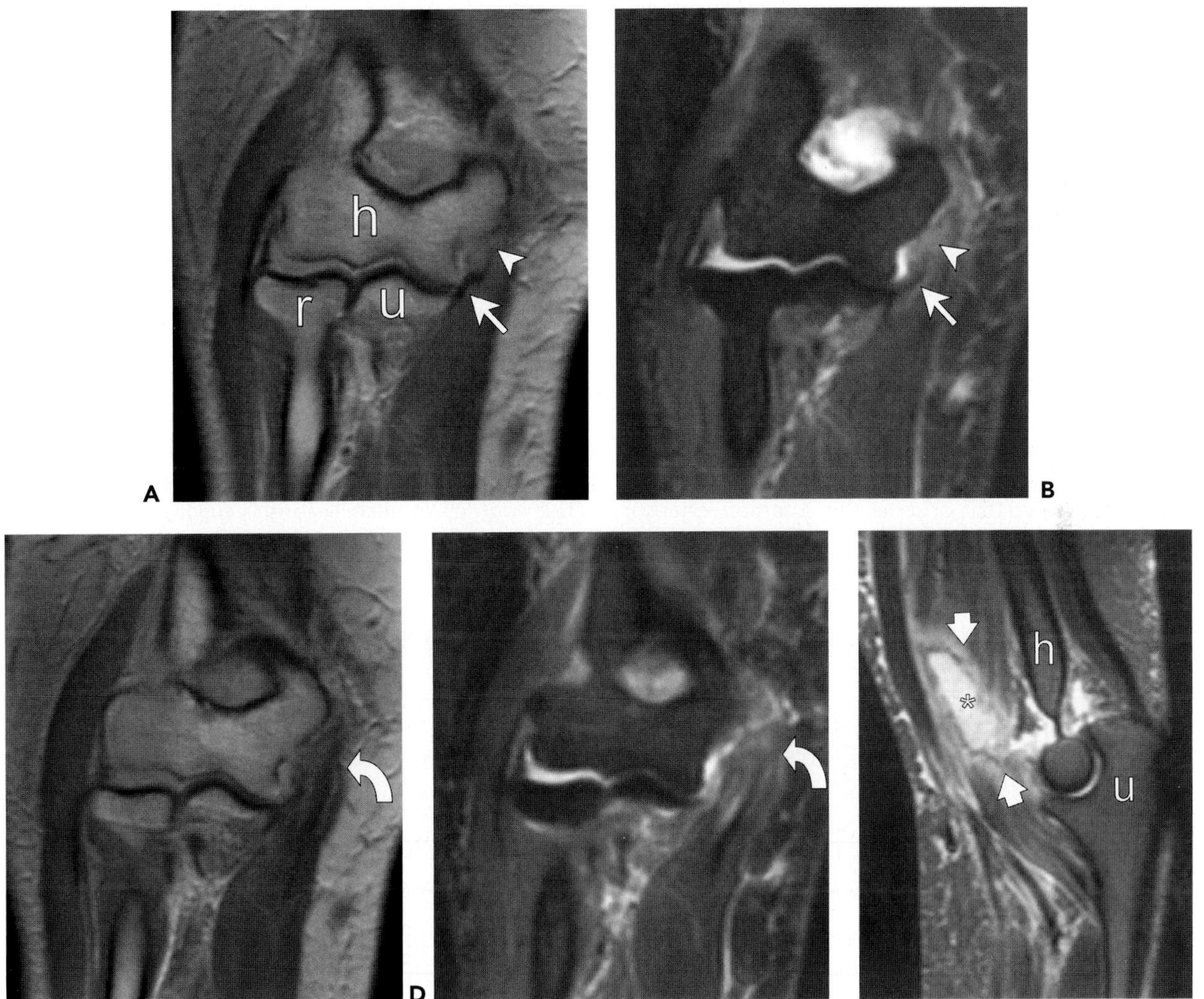

Figure 34.24 Patient injured elbow during a fall resulting in multiple soft tissue injuries to the joint capsule and surrounding structures. **A:** Coronal proton density weighted image of the elbow, radius (r), ulna (u), and humerus (h) marked for orientation. Tear (*arrowhead*) of the anterior band of the medial collateral ligament (*arrow*) is illustrated. **B:** Coronal short inversion time inversion recovery (STIR) image of elbow, same level as A. Edema surrounding tear (*arrowhead*) of the medial collateral ligament (*arrow*) is best seen on this fluid sensitive sequence. **C and D.** Coronal proton density (**C**) and STIR (**D**) images of the elbow, same orientation as figures (**A**) and (**B**) shows tear of the common flexor origin (*curved arrow*). **E:** Sagittal inversion recovery image shows a large tear (*thick arrows*) of the brachialis muscle. Hematoma (*asterisk*) in the gap indicates a high grade injury. Humerus (h) and ulna (u) marked for orientation.

may be noted at imaging because of the reinforcement by the lacertus fibrosus. Partial tears of the biceps tendon are best seen on sagittal and axial fluid-sensitive sequences that demonstrate abnormally increased fluid signal within the tendon. A complete tear is diagnosed by identifying a fluid gap and retraction of the two torn ends of the tendon (see Figure 34.4) (39,40).

The brachialis tendon inserts into the ulnar tuberosity, and is less commonly injured than the brachialis muscle, in part because the tendon is surrounded by muscle until its distal most insertion into the ulna. The brachialis tendon is injured by forceful supination or hyperextension (see Figure 34.24). Climber's elbow is a brachialis strain, and a coronal fluid–sensitive MR sequence will show abnormal fluid signal in the brachialis muscle.

The posterior compartment of the elbow contains the triceps and anconeus muscles. The triceps tendon inserts into the olecranon and is the least commonly ruptured tendon in the body (41,42). Tendinopathy also rarely affects the triceps. Injuries usually are the result of direct trauma. A partial tendon tear or tendinopathy are best evaluated on sagittal and axial fluid-sensitive sequences that will depict abnormally increased signal and enlargement of the triceps tendon. Like other tendons, a complete tear is diagnosed by identifying a fluid gap and retraction of the torn tendon ends. Hypertrophy of the triceps, an accessory triceps insertion, or an accessory muscle (epitrochlearis anconeus) can occur in the posterior compartment and have been reported in association with cubital tunnel syndrome (43,44).

The lateral compartment muscles of the elbow include the brachioradialis, supinator, and common extensors of the hand and wrist that arise as the common extensor tendon from the lateral epicondyle. These tendons are best seen on a coronal proton density MR sequence. An extremely common cause of lateral elbow pain is tennis elbow or lateral epicondylitis, which refers to degeneration and tear of the common extensor tendons (45,46). Typical patients with lateral epicondylitis are middle-aged and chronically overuse the common extensor tendons by playing racquet sports. The imaging diagnosis is straight forward, and coronal fluid–sensitive sequences often depict fluid signal within the common extensor tendons at their origin on the lateral epicondyle (see Figure 34.25).

The medial compartment muscles of the elbow include pronator teres, palmaris longus, and the common flexors of the hand and wrist that arise as the common flexor tendon from the medial epicondyle. As with the common extensor origin, the common flexor tendons are best seen on a coronal proton density MR sequence. Although not as common as lateral epicondylitis, medial epicondylitis afflicts those who repeatedly overload the common flexor tendons. Medial epicondylitis has also been termed *golfer's elbow* or *pitcher's elbow*, because these sports predispose athletes to degeneration or tear of the common flexor tendons (45). The clinical diagnosis is straightforward and the patients usually respond to conservative therapy. MR imaging is useful in patients who do not respond to rest and anti-inflammatory medications. Tendinopathy, partial thickness, and full-thickness tears are readily identified on fluid-sensitive sequences and any associated abnormalities such as a capsular ligament tear, can also be visualized.

Osteochondritis dissecans refers to an osteochondral fracture; in the elbow, this most commonly occurs in the anterior capitellum or the radial head (see Figure 34.26). The etiology of such lesions is unclear, but it has been hypothesized that repetitive trauma and ischemia are

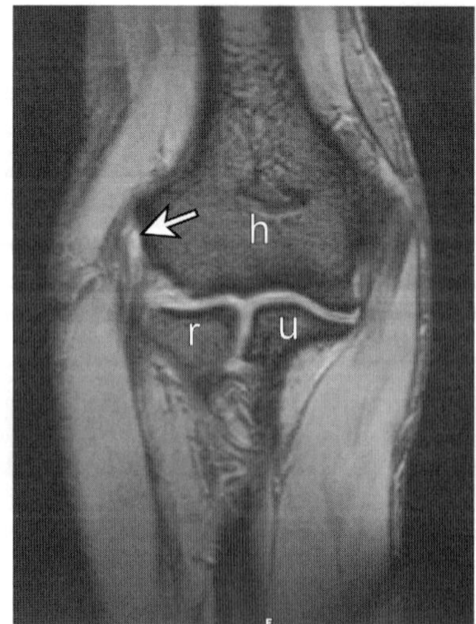

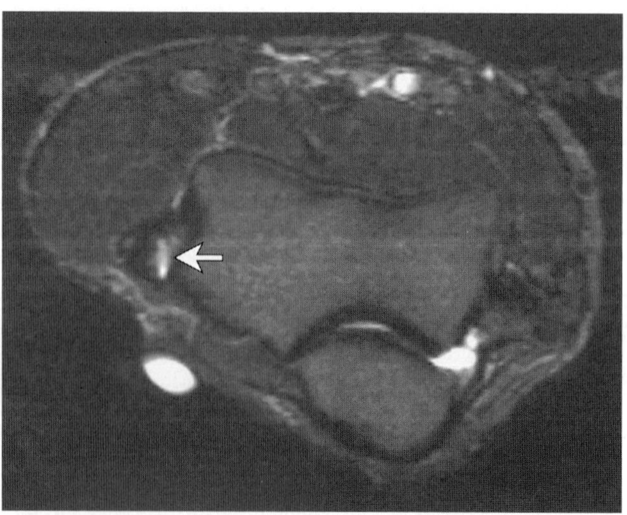

Figure 34.25 Patient complains of lateral epicondyle pain. Radiographs were normal (not shown). **A:** Coronal gradient echo image shows partial tear (*arrow*) of the common extensor origin; humerus (h), radius (r), and ulna (u) marked for orientation. **B:** Axial inversion recover image image shows fluid signal (*arrow*) at the common extensor origin, the site of tear. Posterior superficial skin marker (bright oval) placed by technologist correlates the finding with the site of maximum tenderness.

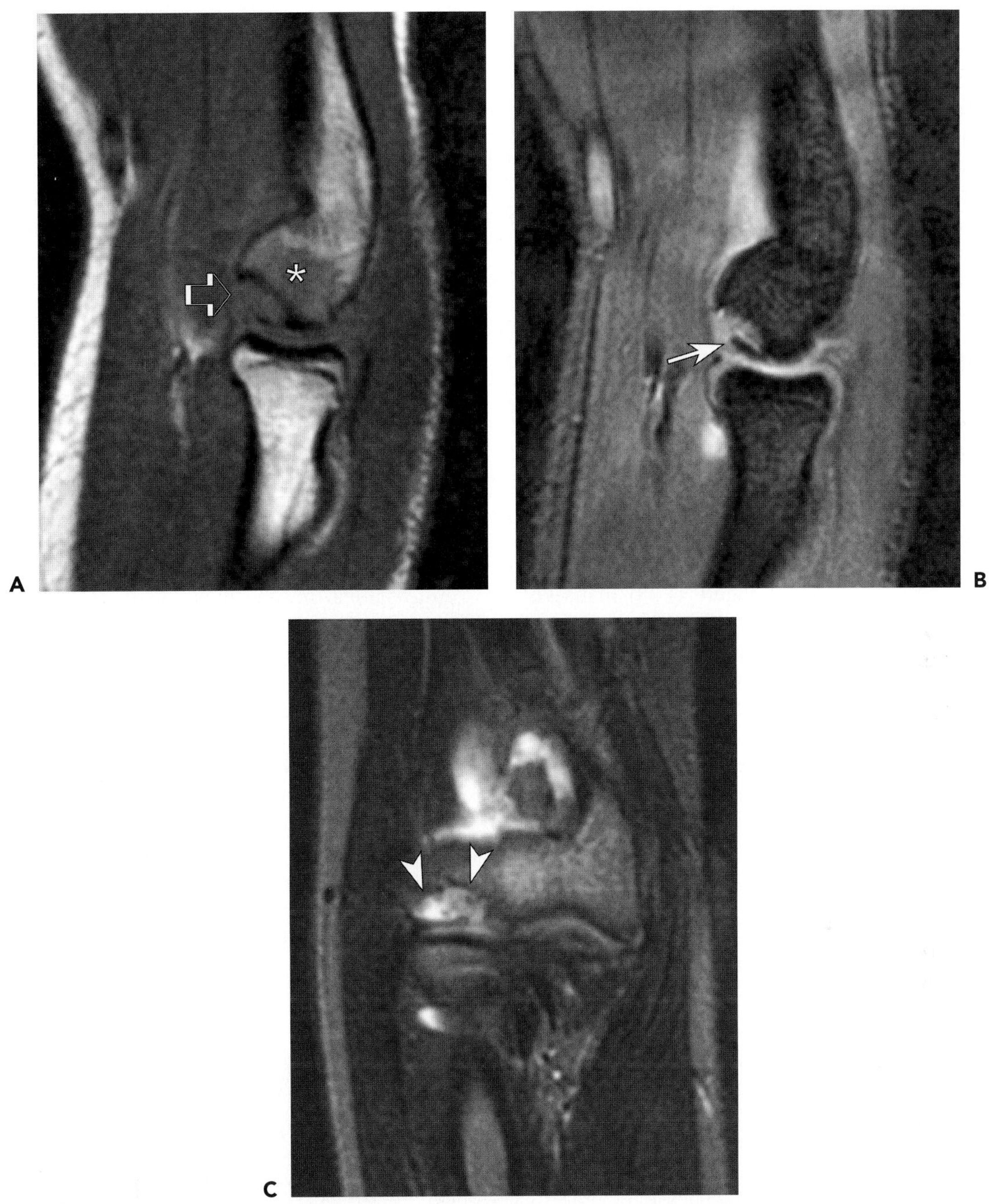

Figure 34.26 14-year-old adolescent girl with elbow pain. **A:** Sagittal T1-weighted image through the radiocapitellar joint shows edema of the capitellum. There is irregularity of the distal capitellum (*open arrow*). **B:** Sagittal gradient echo image, same level as in A. There is an osteochondral fragment of the capitellum (*arrow*) consistent with osteochondritis dissecans. **C:** Coronal inversion recovery weighted image through the anterior capitellum shows fluid and edema (*arrowheads*) at the base of the osteochondral lesion, highly suggestive of instability.

contributing factors. This type of injury is most often observed in baseball pitchers and gymnasts 12 to 16 years old. On plain radiography, a subchondral lucency may be seen in the capitellum or radial head.

MR imaging is useful to evaluate the stability of these lesions (47). Stable lesions usually demonstrate normal to minimally increased subchondral signal on sagittal or coronal fluid-sensitive sequences. The cartilage overlying the abnormal subchondral injury is intact and the risk of the subchondral injury progressing to become a loose intra-articular body is low. Unstable lesions are characterized by fluid at the base of the osteochondral defect with a concomitant increased risk for becoming intra-articular loose bodies. Loose bodies originating from the osteochondral lesion can migrate throughout the joint limiting motion, requiring surgical intervention.

Arthrography with CT or MRI is helpful to evaluate stability of an osteochondral lesion and to document the location of intra-articular loose bodies.

Similar to osteochondritis dissecans (OCD), Panner's disease is in the spectrum of osteochondral lesions of the elbow, but is distinguished by an earlier age of onset, occurring in children 5 to 10 years old who are involved in throwing sports (48). Panner's disease exclusively involves the anterior capitellum, possibly as a result of osteonecrosis or disordered endochondral ossification.

ANKLE IMAGING

Ankle injuries are common in all sports. Similar to the other joints discussed, imaging evaluation of ankle injuries begins with radiography. AP, lateral and the oblique mortise views are obtained to assess for fracture, dislocation and ankle mortise widening (see Figure 34.27). Fractures of the ankle are usually evident on plain films, but CT can be useful for fracture diagnosis and staging (see Figure 34.28). In cases of occult or stress fracture, MRI is useful to identify the marrow changes that accompany these sometimes subtle injuries. A stress fracture on MR is identified by a linear region of low signal on T1 sequences that is usually surrounded by high signal on fluid-sensitive sequences.

Ankle sprains account for approximately 75% of ankle injuries and should be suspected when there is widening of the ankle mortise. Sprains most often occur when there is a combination of plantar flexion and ankle inversion leading to ligament injury. Approximately 80% to 90% of ankle sprains involve the lateral stabilizing ligaments: the anterior talofibular, calcaneofibular, and posterior talofibular ligaments. Most commonly, the anterior talofibular ligament is torn (see Figure 34.29). With increasingly severe injuries, the remaining ligaments are torn sequentially so that the next to tear is the calcaneofibular ligament followed by the posterior talofibular ligament. Ankle sprains can be graded 1 to 3 both clinically and with imaging (49). Grade 1 sprains are clinically characterized by mild tenderness and swelling without functional loss or mechanical instability. In grade 1 sprains, fluid-sensitive MRI shows fluid surrounding one of the lateral stabilizer ligaments. Patients with grade 2 sprains have some loss of function and mild or moderate ankle instability. MRI demonstrates an incomplete tear of the ligaments. Grade 3 sprains are clinically characterized by loss of function and severe instability. At MRI, there will be complete ligament disruption. In most patients, imaging is not necessary for diagnosis and management.

Approximately 15% of ankle sprains result in mechanical or functional stability of the joint. There are several complications of ankle sprains, including anterolateral impingement syndrome, tears of the proneus brevis tendon, and sinus tarsi syndrome.

Anterolateral impingement syndrome typically occurs after a partial or complete tear of the anterior talofibular ligament, with secondary hemorrhage and synovial proliferation that involves the lateral gutter of the ankle (50). The lateral gutter is the space bounded by the anterior talofibular and tibiofibular ligaments anteriorly, by the fibula laterally, and by the tibia medially. MR imaging will reveal a mass (hypertrophic synovium or scar), which is usually intermediate signal intensity on T1 and fluid-sensitive sequences. MR arthrography can be helpful if this diagnosis is suspected (51). Patients with anterolateral impingement syndrome have anterolateral ankle pain and swelling, which is often difficult to distinguish from other conditions.

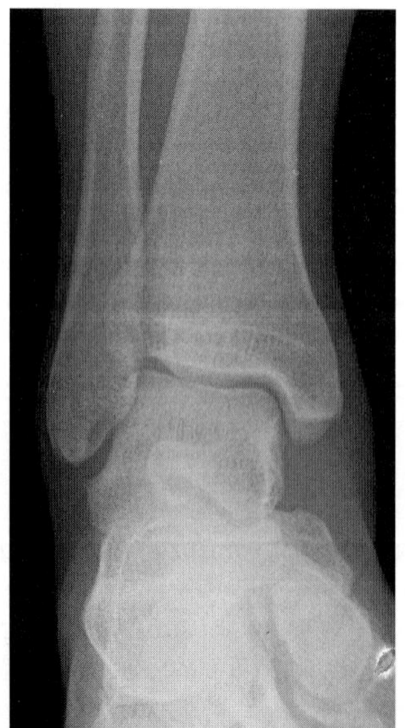

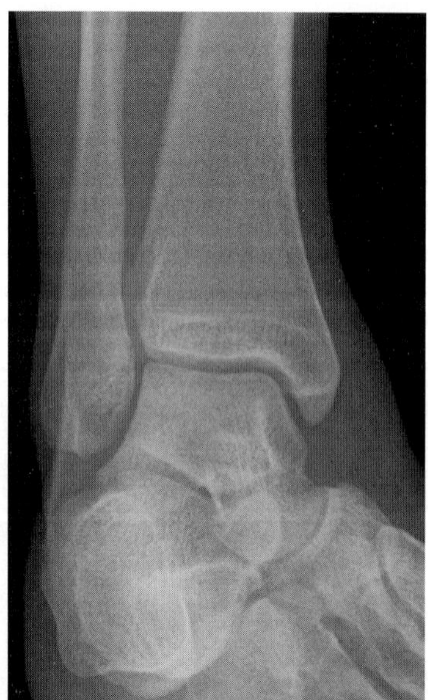

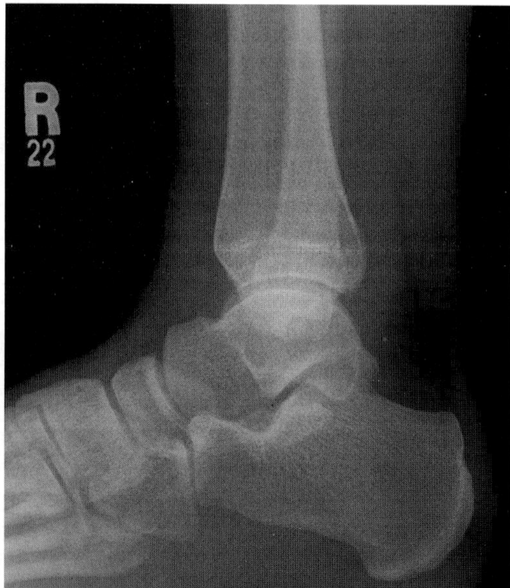

Figure 34.27 Routine 3 view ankle series, 20-year-old man with ankle pain. Normal anterposterior (AP) (A), mortise (B), and lateral (C) radiographs of the ankle.

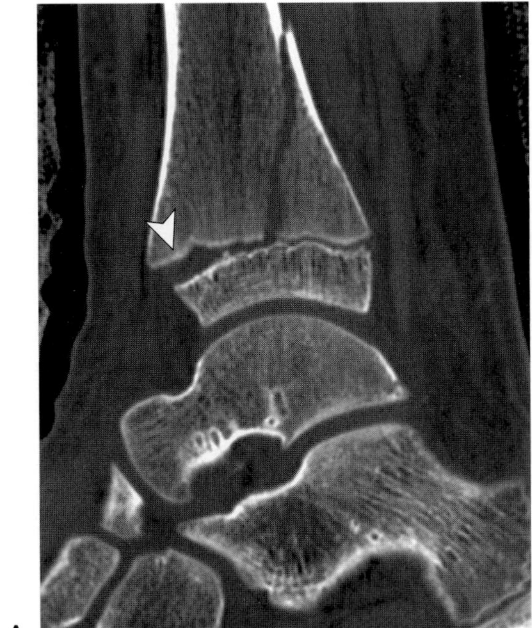

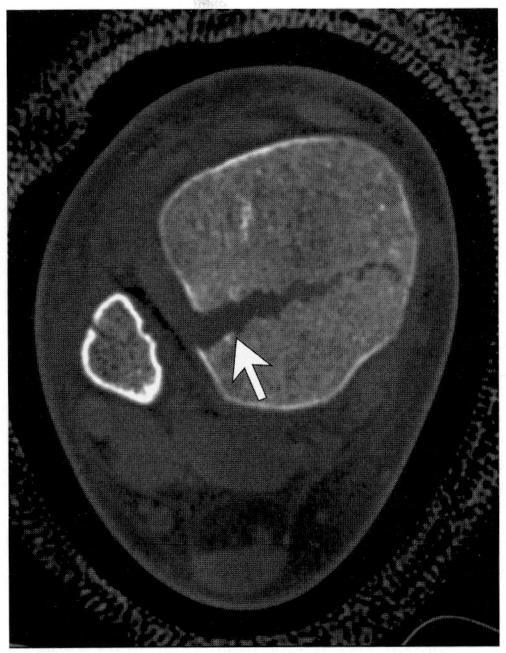

Figure 34.28 Salter II fracture of the distal tibia. Computed tomography (CT) allows for precise classification of fracture type and facilitates quantification of fracture fragment displacement. **A:** Sagittal reformation from the CT examination. The epiphysis is maximally distracted anteriorly (*arrowhead*). **B:** Axial CT image through the distal tibia shows that the metaphyseal segment is most distracted laterally (*arrow*).

The peroneus longus and brevis tendons are important lateral stabilizers of the ankle. A split tear of the peroneus brevis tendon is the term used to describe a longitudinal tear of the tendon (52). Split tears of the peroneus brevis tendon are commonly associated with sprains of the lateral ligaments of the ankle. The clinical diagnosis of a peroneal tendon tear is difficult to make because the symptoms may overlap with other ankle instability findings (see Figure 34.30). Partial tears occur more frequently than complete tears, and the diagnosis can be established with MRI.

The sinus tarsi is located between the posterior subtalar and talocalcaneonavicular joints and contains fat, neurovascular structures, and several ligaments. The ligaments

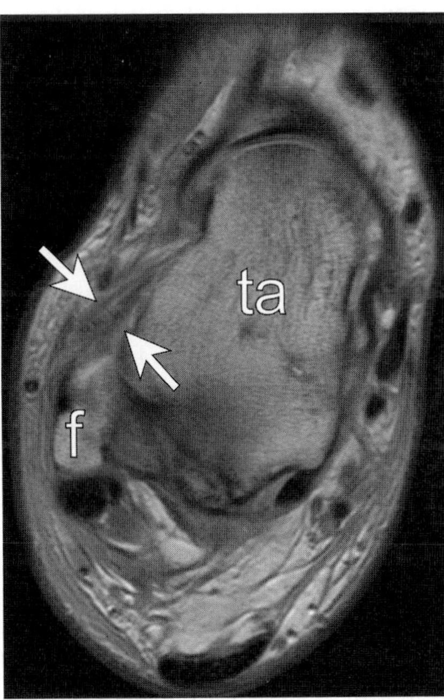

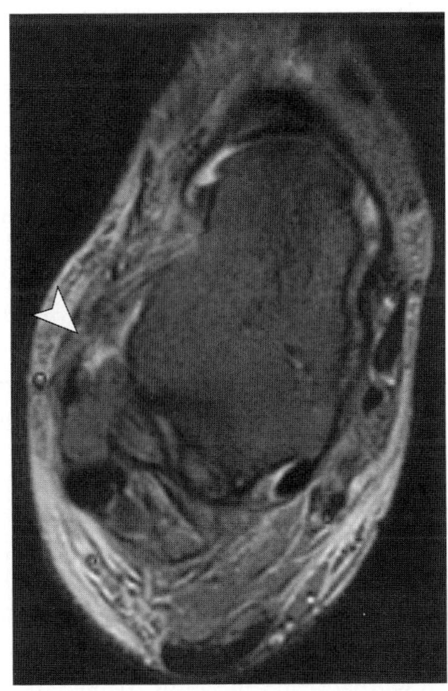

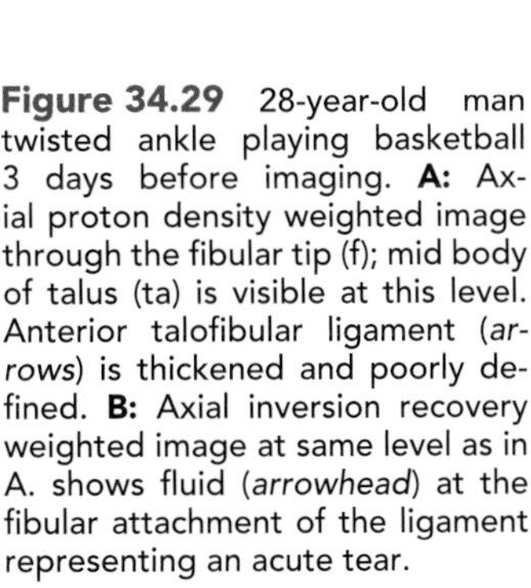

Figure 34.29 28-year-old man twisted ankle playing basketball 3 days before imaging. **A:** Axial proton density weighted image through the fibular tip (f); mid body of talus (ta) is visible at this level. Anterior talofibular ligament (*arrows*) is thickened and poorly defined. **B:** Axial inversion recovery weighted image at same level as in A. shows fluid (*arrowhead*) at the fibular attachment of the ligament representing an acute tear.

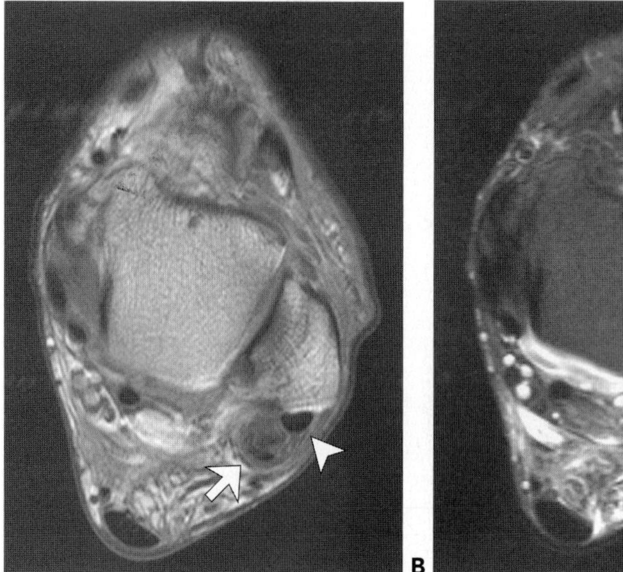

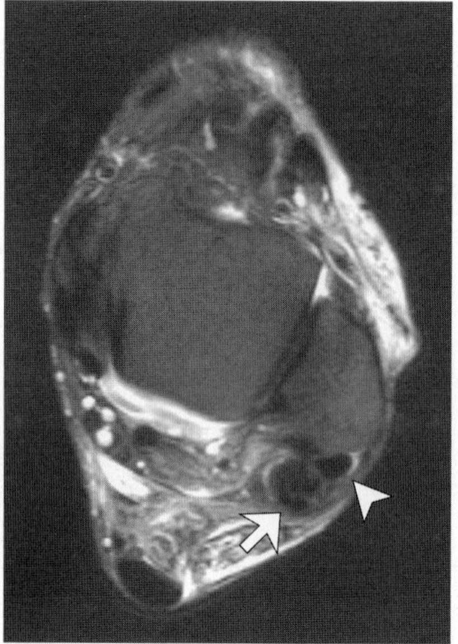

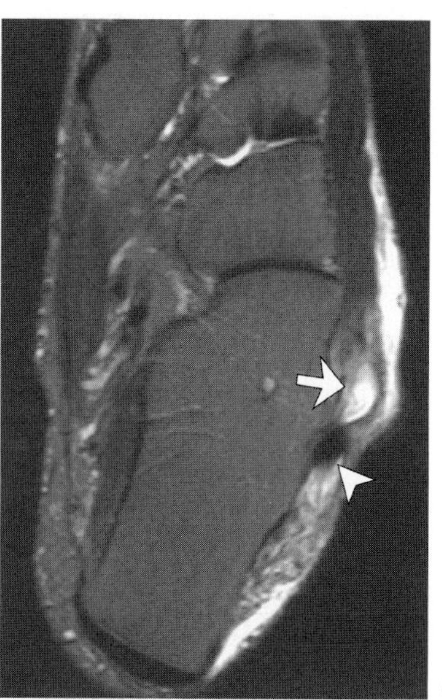

Figure 34.30 52-year-old man with prior ankle injury 1 week before imaging. Lateral pain with motion and weight bearing. **A:** Axial proton density weighted image at the level of the distal fibula shows abnormal thickening and heterogeneous signal of the peroneus brevis tendon (*arrow*). Compare with the adjacent normal sized peroneus longus tendon (*arrowhead*). **B:** Axial inversion recovery weighted image at same level as in A. shows that there is no fluid signal within the peroneus brevis tendon indicating that there is only severe tendinopathy in this portion of the tendon. Normal adjacent peroneus longus tendon is again demonstrated (*arrowhead*). **C:** Axial inversion recovery weighted image, several centimeters below that in B, shows the empty tendon sheath of the peroneus brevis tendon (*arrow*) indicating complete tendon tear. At this level in the foot, the normal peroneus longus tendon (*arrowhead*) can be seen posterior to the peroneus brevis.

of the sinus tarsi are important for maintaining hindfoot stability, whereas the nerve endings are important for proprioception. Injury to the structures contained within the sinus tarsi results in hindfoot instability and lateral foot pain (53,54). There is a high association between lateral ligament injury and sinus tarsi syndrome. A normal sinus tarsi contains abundant fat and will be bright on T1-weighted images. In patients with sinus tarsi syndrome, the normal fat is replaced with fibrous tissue, and the sinus tarsi signal becomes hypointense on T1 weighed images. Often, MRI can show evidence of prior injury to the lateral stabilizing ligaments of the ankle.

Tendon injuries are common in the ankle. Tendons are injured frequently because of their proximity to osseous structures in the ankle. Sports injuries of the ankle tendons include tendon tears, dislocation, and tenosynovitis. Tendon tears result from chronic repetitive microtrauma or acute major trauma. MRI is the most useful imaging modality for the evaluation of tendon injuries, although US performed by experienced individuals can be extremely helpful (53).

The Achilles tendon is the most frequently injured tendon of the ankle. It is the largest tendon in the body and it is formed from the soleus and gastrocnemius muscles. It is one of the few tendons in the body that does not have a tendon sheath. Instead, the Achilles tendon has a paratenon. Therefore, the Achilles tendon is not afflicted with tenosynovitis, but rather paratendinitis. On MRI, the normal Achilles tendon is low signal with a flat or concave anterior margin on axial T1 images. Sometimes, there is a vertically oriented thin line of high signal in the tendon, which represents the junction of the gastrocnemius and soleus muscles, and this should not be confused with a tendon tear. Most individuals have a small plantaris tendon anteromedial to the Achilles tendon. The fat plane between the Achilles and plantaris tendons is bright on T1 images, and this can be mistaken for a partial tear of the Achilles tendon.

Injuries of the Achilles tendon classically occur in "Weekend Warrior" athletes. These unconditioned individuals are more prone to partial and complete tears, and men are approximately five to six times more likely to suffer a traumatic Achilles tendon injury than women. Partial and complete tears occur most often within 2 to 6 cm of the insertion into the calcaneus, an area of relative avascularity (see Figure 34.31). MR findings of Achilles tears include partial or complete disruption of the fibers and intrasubstance high signal on T1 and fluid-sensitive sequences. With a complete tear, fluid and blood products can be identified within the tendon gap; MRI can be helpful in determining the gap between the ends of the torn tendon. US can also depict partial or complete tears of the Achilles tendon.

Osteochondral lesions can occur in the medial and lateral talar dome, often occurring after an inversion or eversion injury of the ankle (see Figure 34.32). These lesions occur when the tibia impacts the talus (55). Often

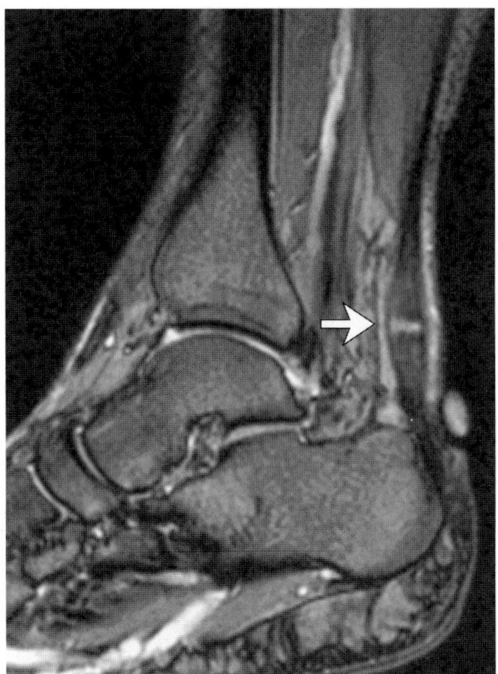

Figure 34.31 Sagittal gradient echo image of the ankle shows fusiform swelling of the distal Achilles tendon with a partial intrasubstance tear (*arrow*) in the mid portion of the swollen segment.

there is an associated ligamentous injury. Osteochondral lesions are well depicted by MRI, and involvement of the joint cartilage can be determined. MRI can determine whether an osteochondral lesion is stable or loose, although MR arthrography is recommended to assess stability of a known osteochondral lesion (56). MR characteristics of a loose (unstable) osteochondral lesion include high signal intensity surrounding the fragment on fluid-sensitive sequences, fissuring of the overlying cartilage, and migration of the osteochondral fragment that may be identified in the joint as a loose body. MRI is also helpful in depicting the associated injuries.

CONCLUSION

Imaging is an essential tool in the evaluation of sports injuries. Correct diagnosis can avoid delayed healing or permanent loss of joint function. A variety of imaging options are available, and it is important to understand when each modality is indicated. In general, radiographs are obtained initially to evaluate for fracture and joint dislocation. Radiographs are also useful for correlation with cross-sectional studies. CT is useful to assess and clarify the extent of a fracture, whereas MRI is best suited for evaluating the soft tissues of the joint as well as the bone marrow to assess for occult fracture.

Both MR and CT arthrography are adjunct techniques that can increase the visibility of intra-articular structures, helping to evaluate articular surfaces, osteochondral lesions, loose bodies, and capsular structures. Currently, the principal indication for arthrography is the assessment of the glenoid labrum of the shoulder, which is most comprehensively assessed with MR angiography (MRA). Indications for arthrography of other joints are less clear. Lastly, CTA should be considered a good tool for the assessment of the knee and shoulder joints, particularly for patients who cannot tolerate an MR examination because of claustrophobia, severe obesity, MR incompatible implanted devices or metal hardware in close proximity to the joint of interest.

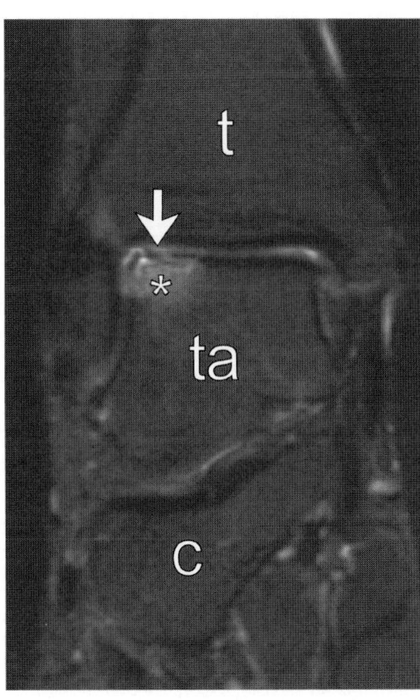

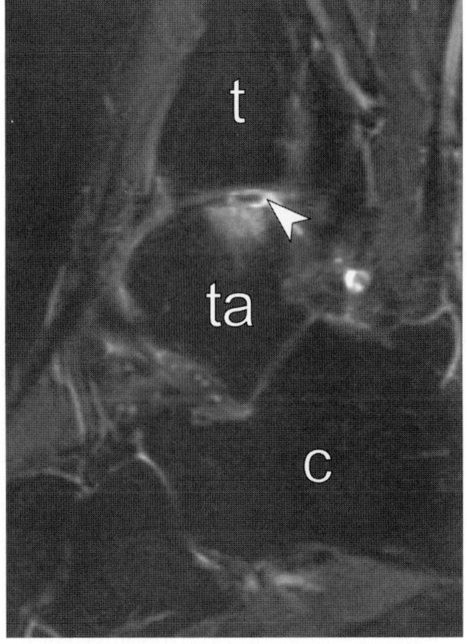

Figure 34.32 Osteochondral lesion of the talar dome. Talus (ta), tibia (t), and calcaneus (c) marked for orientation. **A:** Coronal inversion recovery image shows marked edema (*asterisk*) of the lateral talar dome. There is irregularity of the cortical margin (*arrow*). **B:** Sagittal short inversion time inversion recovery (STIR) image shows fluid beneath the margin of the osteochondral lesion (*arrowhead*) suggesting an unstable fragment. Appearance is consistent with osteochondritis dissecans.

APPENDIX 34.1
SUGGESTED SCREENING RADIOGRAPHIC PROJECTIONS

Region	Projections	Comments
Shoulder	AP internal rotation Grashey Axillary	Garth view in lieu of axillary, if patient cannot be positioned.
Elbow	AP Lateral	
Wrist	PA Oblique Lateral	
Hand	PA Oblique Fan Lateral (spread fingers)	For nontrauma (arthritis), substitute reverse oblique for fan lateral.
Hip	AP pelvis Lauenstein projection of affected hip	For suspected fracture, substitute surgical lateral for Lauenstein projection. For suspected osteonecrosis (AVN) or slipped capital epiphysis, substitute frog-leg view for Lauenstein projection.
Knee	Standing AP Lateral (tabletop[a])	For suspected fracture, cross-table lateral recommended and tabletop AP view. Semiflexed standing PA views can document cartilage loss more effectively than nonflexed views.
Ankle	AP Oblique Lateral	Base of fifth metatarsal should always be visible on lateral projection of ankle as fractures of the fifth metatarsal base may present with ankle symptoms.
Foot	PA Oblique Lateral	Lisfranc fractures are easily missed on radiographs; consider CT if this is a consideration.
Toe/finger	PA Oblique Lateral	Dedicated toe or finger projections are better for tiny chip fractures than foot or hand radiographs.
Cervical spine	AP Lateral	For trauma, add open mouth odontoid and swimmer's lateral view to see C7-T1 junction. Pillar or oblique views can be helpful. Consider CT instead of additional projections in severe trauma. Oblique projections are helpful when chronic nerve root symptoms are present.
Thoracic spine	AP Lateral	
Lumbar spine	AP Lateral Cone down lateral	Oblique views can be helpful for suspected spondylolysis, but radiation dose is high and CT may be more effective at near equivalent exposures.

PA = posterioanterior; AP = anterioposterior; CT = computed tomography; AVN = avascular necrosis.
[a]A tabletop projection is a view taken on the x-ray table rather than a wall-mounted film holder.

REFERENCES

1. De Smet AA, Doherty MP, Norris MA, et al. Are oblique views needed for trauma radiography of the distal extremity? *AJR Am J Roentgenol* 1991;172(6):1561.
2. Buckwalter KA, Braunstein EM. Digital skeletal radiography. *AJR Am J Roentgenol* 1992;158(5):1071–1080.
3. Buckwalter KA, Rydberg J, Kopecky KK, et al. Musculoskeletal imaging with multislice CT. *AJR Am J Roentgenol* 2001;176(4):979–986.
4. White LM, Buckwalter KA. Technical considerations: CT and MR imaging in the postoperative orthopedic patient. *Semin Musculoskelet Radiol* 2002;6(1):5–17.
5. Buckwalter KA. CT arthrography. *Clin Sports Med* 2006;25(4):899–915.
6. Weinreb JC. MR accreditation helps to assure quality service. *Diagn Imaging (San Franc)* 2000;22(7):39–43.
7. Rossi F, Dragoni S. Acute avulsion fractures of the pelvis in adolescent competitive athletes: prevalence, location and sports distribution of 203 cases collected. *Skeletal Radiol* 2001;30(3):127–131.
8. El-Khoury GY, Daniel WW, Kathol MH. Acute and chronic avulsive injuries. *Radiol Clin North Am* 1997;35(3):747–766.
9. Farber JM, Buckwalter KA. MR imaging in nonneoplastic muscle disorders of the lower extremity. *Radiol Clin North Am* 2002;40(5):1013–1031.
10. El-Khoury GY, Brandser EA, Kathol MH, et al. Imaging of muscle injuries. *Skeletal Radiol* 1996;25(1):3–11.
11. Khaliq Y, Zhanel GG. Fluoroquinolone-associated tendinopathy: a critical review of the literature. *Clin Infect Dis* 2003;36(11):1404–1410.
12. Kidwai AS, Hemphill SD, Griffiths HJ. Radiologic case study. Spontaneous osteonecrosis of the knee reclassified as insufficiency fracture. *Orthopedics* 2005;28(3):236, 333–336.
13. Crues JV, III, Mink J, Levy TL, et al. Meniscal tears of the knee: accuracy of MR imaging. *Radiology* 1987 Aug;164(2):445–8.
14. Polly DW, et al. The accuracy of magnetic resonance imaging compared with the findings of arthroscopy. *J Bone Joint Surg Am* 1988;70:192.
15. Cruz JV, et al. Meniscal tears of the knee: accuracy of MR imaging. *Radiology* 1987;164:445.

16. Mesgarzadeh M, et al. MR imaging of the knee: expanded classification and pitfalls to interpretation of meniscal tears. *Radiographics* 1993;13:489.
17. De Smet AA, Norris MA, Yandow DR, et al. MR diagnosis of meniscal tears: the importance of high signal in the meniscus that extends to the articular surface. *AJR Am J Roentgenol* 1993;161:101.
18. De Smet AA, Tuite MJ. Use of the "two-slice-touch" rule for the MRI diagnosis of meniscal tears. *AJR Am J Roentgenol* 2006;187(4):911–914.
19. Wright DH, De Smet AA, Norris M, et al. Buckle-handle tears of the medial and lateral meniscus: value of MR imaging in the detection of displaced fragments. *AJR Am J Roentgenol* 1995;165:621.
20. Moore SL. Imaging the anterior cruciate ligament. *Orthop Clin North Am* 2002;33(4):663–674.
21. Tung GA, Davis LM, Wiggins ME, et al. Tears of the anterior cruciate ligament: primary and secondary signs at MR imaging. *Radiology* 1993;188:661.
22. Shelbourne KD, Nitz PA. The O'Donoghue triad revisited. Combined knee injuries involving anterior cruciate and medial collateral ligament tears. *Am J Sports Med* 1991;19(5):474–477.
23. Sonin AH, Fitzgerald SW, Hoff FL, et al. Posterior cruciate ligament injury: MR imaging diagnosis and patterns of injury. *Radiology* 1995;190:455.
24. Sonin AH, et al. MR imaging of the posterior cruciate ligament: normal, abnormal, and associated injury patterns. *Radiographics* 1995;15:552.
25. Schweitzer MS, et al. Medial collateral ligament injuries: evaluation of multiple signs, prevalence, and location of associated bone bruises and assessment with MR imaging. *Radiology* 1995;194:825.
26. Seebacher J, et al. The structures of the posterolateral aspect of the knee. *J Bone Joint Surg Am* 1982;64:536.
27. Kirsch MD, Fitzgerald SW, Friedman H, et al. Transient lateral dislocation of the patella: diagnosis with MR imaging. *AJR Am J Roentgenol* 1993;161:109.
28. White LM, Kramer J, Recht MP. MR imaging evaluation of the postoperative knee: ligaments, menisci, and articular cartilage. *Skeletal Radiol* 2005;34(8):431–452.
29. White LM, Schweitzer ME, Weishaupt D, et al. Diagnosis of recurrent meniscal tears: prospective evaluation of conventional MR imaging, indirect MR arthrography, and direct MR arthrography. *Radiology* 2002;222(2):421–429.
30. Woertler K, Waldt S. MR imaging in sports-related glenohumeral instability. *Eur Radiol* 2006;16:2622–2636.
31. Beltran J, Rosenberg ZS, Chandnani VP, et al. Glenohumeral instability: evaluation with MR arthrography. *Radiol Clin North Am* 2002;40(2):217–234.
32. Palmer WE, Brown JH, Rosenthal DI, et al. Labral-ligamentous complex of the shoulder: evaluation with MR arthrography. *Radiology* 1994;190:645.
33. de la Puente R, Boutin RD, Theodorou DJ, et al. Post-traumatic and stress-induced osteolysis of the distal clavicle: MR imaging findings in 17 patients. *Skeletal Radiol* 2002;31(5):311.
34. Timins ME, Erickson SJ, Estowski LD, et al. Increased signal in the normal supraspinatus tendon on MR imaging: diagnostic pitfall caused by magic-angle effect. *AJR Am J Roentgenol* 1995;165:109.
35. De Maeseneer M, Van Roy F, Lenchik L, et al. CT and MR arthrography of the normal and pathologic anterosuperior labrum and labral-bicipital complex. *Radiographics* 2000;20:S67–S81.
36. Cvitanic O, Tirman PF, Feller JF, et al. Using abduction and external rotation of the shoulder to increase the sensitivity of MR arthrography in revealing tears of the anterior glenoid labrum. *AJR Am J Roentgenol* 1997;169(3):837–844.
37. Gaurav KG. The Fat Pad Sign. *Radiology* 2002;222(2):419–420.
38. Kaplan LJ, Potter HG. MR imaging of ligament injuries to the elbow. *Radiol Clin North Am* 2006;44(4):583–594.
39. Agins HJ, Chess JL, Hookstra DV, et al. Rupture of the distal insertion of the biceps tendon. *Clin Orthop* 1988;234:34.
40. Falchook JS, et al. Rupture of the distal biceps tendon: evaluation with MR imaging. *Radiology* 1994;190:659.
41. Sherman OH, Snyder SJ, Fox JM, et al. Triceps tendon avulsion in a professional body builder. *Am J Sports Med* 1984;12:485.
42. Tiger E, Mayer DP, Glazer R, et al. Complete avulsion of the triceps tendon: MRI diagnosis. *Comput Med Imaging Graph* 1993;17:51.
43. Aoki M, Kanaya K, Aiki H, et al. Cubital tunnel syndrome in adolescent baseball players: a report of six cases with 3- to 5-year follow-up. *Arthroscopy* 2005;21(6):758.
44. O'Hara JJ, Stone JH. Ulnar nerve compression at the elbow caused by a prominent medial head of the triceps and an anconeus epitrochlearis muscle. *J Hand Surg [Br]* 1996;21(1):133–135.
45. Kijowski R, Tuite M, Sanford M. Magnetic resonance imaging of the elbow. Part II: abnormalities of the ligaments, tendons, and nerves. *Skeletal Radiol* 2005;34(1):1–18.
46. Whiteside JA, Andrews JR. Tendinopathies of the elbow. *Sports Med Arthrosc Rev* 1995;3:195.
47. Kijowski R, De Smet AA. MRI findings of osteochondritis dissecans of the capitellum with surgical correlation. *AJR Am J Roentgenol* 2005;185(6):1453–1459.
48. Kobayashi K, Burton KJ, Rodner C, et al. Lateral compression injuries in the pediatric elbow: Panner's disease and osteochondritis dissecans of the capitellum. *J Am Acad Orthop Surg* 2004;12(4):246–254.
49. Schneck CD, Mesgarzadeh M, Bonakdarpour A. MR imaging of the most commonly injured ankle ligaments. Part II. Ligament injuries. *Radiology* 1992;184(2):507–512.
50. Robinson P, White LM. Soft-tissue and osseous impingement syndromes of the ankle: role of imaging in diagnosis and management. *Radiographics* 2002;22(6):1457–1469. discussion 1470–1471.
51. Robinson P, White LM, Salonen DC, et al. Anterolateral ankle impingement: mr arthrographic assessment of the anterolateral recess. *Radiology* 2001;221(1):186–190.
52. Bencardino JT, Rosenberg ZS, Serrano LF. MR imaging features of diseases of the peroneal tendons. *Magn Reson Imaging Clin N Am* 2001;9(3):493–505.
53. Nallamshetty L, Nazarian LN, Schweitzer ME, et al. Evaluation of posterior tibial pathology: comparison of sonography and MR imaging. *Skeletal Radiol* 2005;34(7):375–380.
54. Steinbach LS. Painful syndromes around the ankle and foot: magnetic resonance imaging evaluation. *Top Magn Reson Imaging* 1998;9(5):311–326.
55. Schachter AK, Chen AL, Reddy PD, et al. Osteochondral lesions of the talus. *J Am Acad Orthop Surg* 2005;13(3):152–158.
56. Cerezal L, Abascal F, Garcia-Valtuille R, et al. Ankle MR arthrography: how, why, when. *Radiol Clin North Am* 2005;43(4):693–707.

Rehabilitation

35

Michael D. Jackson

"Doc, when do you think I will be ready to play again?" This is one of the most common questions asked of physicians practicing sports medicine. The top priority of injured athletes typically is the length of time it will take before they can return to competition. Highly motivated athletes often have tunnel vision after an injury. In some cases they are willing to risk reinjury (and perhaps even more serious injury) in order to return to their sport as soon as possible. Once the correct diagnosis is made, the team physician's role is largely devoted to answering this basic question.

The primary intent of this chapter is to arm primary care physicians, who may be serving as team doctors for their community schools and/or caring for recreational athletes as part of their office practice, with the knowledge base necessary to answer questions regarding an athlete's ability to return to competition.

The time it takes to safely return to competition is critical. Factors that influence the length of the recovery phase and ultimate return to activity include the specific injury, level of competition, age and sex of the athlete, and the ability to carefully monitor the rehabilitation process. When the "return to competition" question is asked, it is tempting to reply with a specific date. Typically, the situation is not that clear-cut. Therefore, the appropriate response is to outline a progressive, functional, rehabilitation (PFR) protocol and informing the athlete that when specific and objective functional goals are met, they can expect to safely return to competition. It is also imperative that before the injured athlete leaves the training room or your office, it is clear to them that most of the responsibility for reaching these objectives is on their shoulders. An injured athlete who stops by the training room infrequently, forgets to take medications, or neglects to follow the rehabilitation protocol, must understand the consequences. The recovery time is prolonged each time there is a variation from the prescribed plan of action.

Without a good understanding of the importance of the team approach to athletic injuries, it may be difficult for everyone involved in the care of the athlete to exercise common sense and good judgment. Consequently, deciding when an athlete is ready to resume play becomes even more complex. An injured athlete may attempt to get one member of the sports medicine staff to allow him/her to return to competition before it is safe, so it is paramount that everyone involved understands the concept of PFR.

Before discussing when an injured athlete is ready to return to play, one should be familiar with the principles of sports medicine rehabilitation (see Table 35.1). After these principles are covered, several rehabilitation protocols for common athletic injuries are outlined. Because 80% to 90% of these injuries are due to disruption of soft tissue structures, the primary focus of this chapter will be on restoring the integrity of soft tissues and preventing reinjury.

PRINCIPLES OF REHABILITATION

Prevention of Injuries

It has been said that "an ounce of prevention is worth of pound of cure," and this is very appropriate with regard to athletic injuries. Injury prevention is extremely important to any team or individual. As team physicians, we attempt to minimize the overall impact that injuries may have during a season and one of the best ways to do so is to prevent them from occurring. Prevention is the fundamental axiom of sports medicine rehabilitation. All other guidelines stem from this primary concept. Table 35.2 gives the basic principles of injury prevention. A more thorough discussion is presented in Chapter 8.

Protection, Rest, Ice, Compression, Elevation

One of the most important concepts in managing acute athletic injuries is prompt intervention in order to mitigate the inflammatory response and resulting edema that follows soft-tissue trauma. The inflammatory response to

TABLE 35.1
PRINCIPLES OF REHABILITATION OF SOFT-TISSUE SPORTS INJURIES

Prevention of injuries
PRICE
Early Mobilization and Restoration of ROM
Modalities
Medications
Restoration of balanced muscle strength and endurance
Maintaining cardiovascular fitness
Proprioception, balance, and agility
Flexibility
Protective taping and bracing
Psychological support
Functional progressive rehabilitation

PRICE = protection, rest, ice, compression, and elevation; ROM = range of motion

soft-tissue damage is a cascade of chemical, metabolic, and vascular events that lead to an increase in capillary permeability (1–4). Initially, these events serve a necessary and useful purpose in promoting soft-tissue healing. However, excessive swelling within or around a joint leads to pain, decreased range of motion (ROM), joint laxity, and diminished proprioception (5,6). Prompt, aggressive action to minimize the inflammatory response may reduce recovery time and permit an earlier safe return to activity. The first few hours of treatment often determine how quickly an injury will heal. The basic early treatments therefore focus on protecting the injured area, reducing the swelling, and decreasing the inflammatory process. Protection, Rest, Ice, Compression, and Elevation (PRICE) make up the earliest methods of treatment in most cases.

TABLE 35.2
PRINCIPLES OF INJURY PREVENTION

Preparticipation evaluations
Complete rehabilitation of previous injuries
Balanced muscle strength and flexibility
Proper body mechanics
In-season and off-season conditioning
Aerobic and anaerobic fitness
Proper nutrition and hydration
Avoidance of overtraining and burnout
Appropriate warm-ups and cool-downs
Safe and appropriate equipment
Safe and appropriate field and court conditions
Protective Equipment, Taping and Bracing
Proper coaching techniques
Understanding the rules of various sports
Community education
Sports medicine network
Understanding the ethical dilemmas in sports medicine

Protection may involve several strategies. Temporary immobilization with a cast, splint, or brace is sometimes indicated; crutches to prevent or assist weight bearing on an injured lower extremity or a sling to support the upper extremity are both examples of protection. Preventing further injury to a joint or extremity is paramount. Placing an athlete with a Grade I or Grade II ankle sprain on crutches for 3 to 5 days after injury may seem a bit extreme. However, depending upon how much walking the athlete must do, the condition of the walking surfaces, and the reliability of the athlete, this protective step may be warranted. If there are any concerns regarding the potential for further injury, always err on the side of caution and protect the injured joint or extremity as much as possible.

Rest is probably the most difficult thing to convince an athlete to address, but it is very important in the early course of an acute injury. In some situations, relative rest is indicated as opposed to absolute rest. Some key points must be made about the type and amount of rest needed. First, repeated microtrauma to an already injured tissue can cause further injury and prolong healing. However, immobilization can lead to soft-tissue contracture, loss of ROM, muscle atrophy, and deconditioning. There is a fine line between too much rest and too much activity in any rehabilitation protocol. You can be assured that you are on the correct side of the line so long as progression through functional stages continues in the absence of increased pain, progressive joint instability, and/or swelling.

Ice is possibly the single most important part of any sports medicine staff's armamentarium. It is cheap, easy to use, readily available, and has few contraindications (7). Ice therapy causes vasoconstriction, decreasing edema and the metabolic demands of injured tissues. It decreases muscle spasticity and has a local analgesic effect. Ice helps limit the inflammatory response and thereby the extent of injury. The controversy over cold therapy versus heat therapy will be discussed later. The important thing to remember is that ice is the modality of choice for the initial treatment of acute soft-tissue injuries.

Compression is very useful in minimizing the extent of soft-tissue swelling (6,8). In fact, several authors believe that it is the single most effective deterrent (8,9). Again, the rationale is to control edema so as to reduce the recovery time. Figure 35.1(b–f) demonstrates how compression is used after an ankle injury. A foam pad is prewrapped to the lateral side of the ankle to prevent capillary leakage and enhance lymphatic drainage. A U-shaped foam pad (see Figure 35.1(b)) tailored to fit around the malleolus is probably most effective. Once the pad is applied, it is imperative to keep it in position. Ice packs can be placed on top of the pad but the pad itself should not be removed until the ecchymosis begins to turn yellowish. The change in

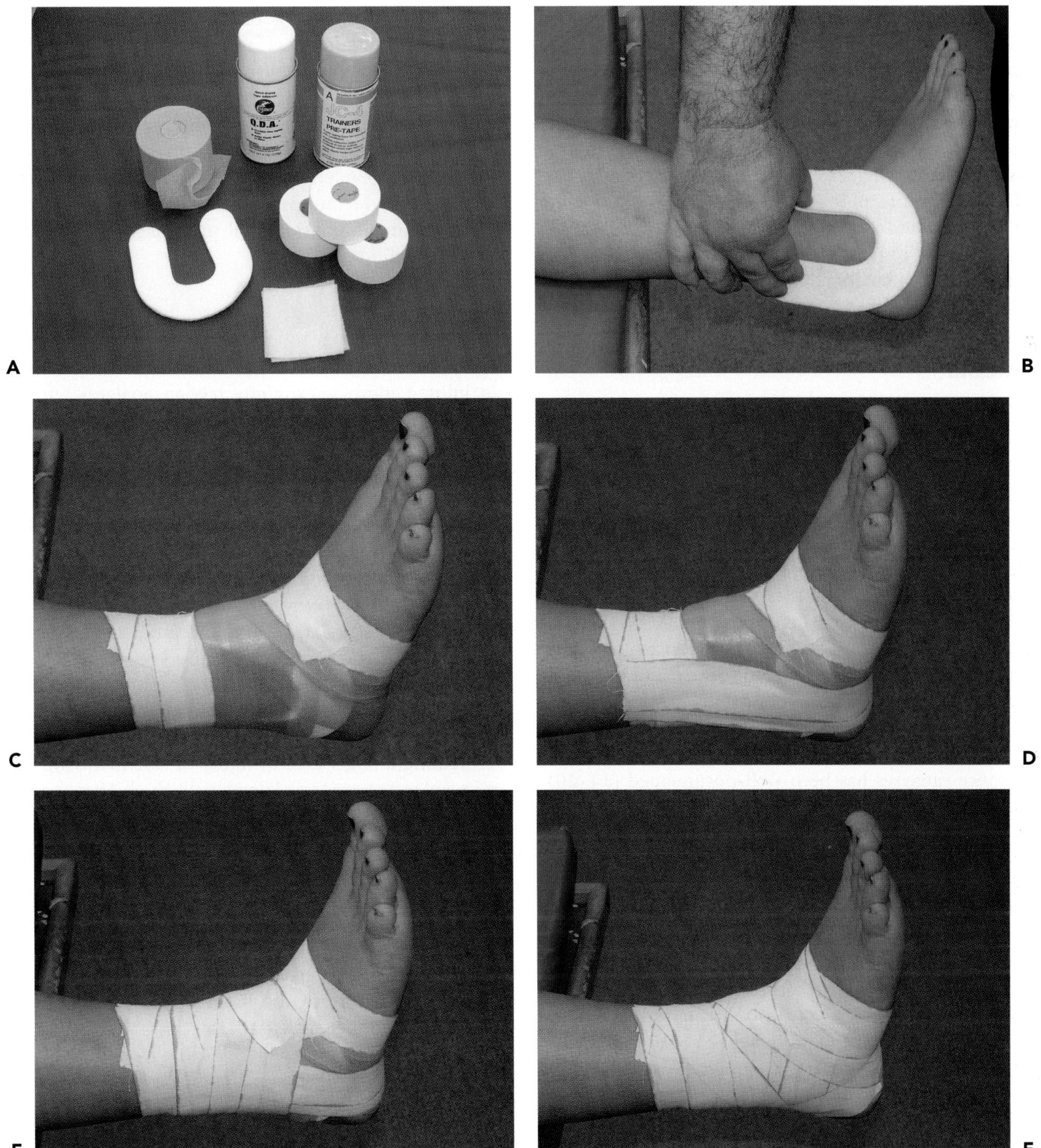

Figure 35.1 Ankle Taping. A: Materials needed: $1\frac{1}{2}$ inch adhesive tape, prewrap, tape adherent spray, pressure padding. B: Spray ankle with adherent, and then apply pressure pad(s). C: Apply prewrap beginning distally at the head of the metatarsals and continuing proximally to midcalf, then apply distal and proximal tape anchors. D: Apply *vertical* stirrups beginning slightly posterior to the malleoli. E and F: Completed ankle taping should be tight enough for support and protection and loose enough to allow for swelling.

skin coloration represents the breakdown of hemoglobin, and rebound swelling is unlikely at this stage.

This technique is much more effective in controlling edema than using standard elastic wrapping. Elastic wraps can be counterproductive. If wrapped too tightly and left on for prolonged periods, they can have a tourniquet effect. Once the appropriate compression wrap is placed, regular monitoring is essential to assure that edema is not increasing. A pneumatic compression device may also be very helpful for controlling edema.

Elevation plays an obvious role in minimizing swelling, but it is often forgotten. Rather than telling an athlete to go home and soak his/her newly sprained ankle in a bucket of ice water, explain that it would be more effective to wrap an ice pack around the ankle and elevate it. This is particularly true within the first 24 hours, when keeping the injured extremity elevated higher than the heart is essential.

The PRICE protocol is aimed at minimizing the swelling that accompanies acute trauma. Taken individually, each step may seem insignificant, but the summation of these interventions can be dramatic (4–11).

Early Mobilization and Restoration of Range of Motion

Early mobilization after soft-tissue injuries, fractures, and surgery is a topic that warrants considerable attention. Not everyone supports this concept. There is considerable controversy regarding the nonoperative management of ankle sprains (6,11–13). As noted earlier, temporary immobilization may be indicated, depending upon the athlete and the circumstances. However, long-term immobilization should be avoided whenever possible.

There are several reasons to begin gentle ROM exercises soon after an injury. Early motion enhances lymphatic drainage and clearing of the necrotic debris, and also helps maintain joint proprioception and muscle strength (11–13). Significant increases in the strength and thickness of ligamentous tissue as a result of early motion and endurance exercises has been well documented (14–20). Finally, and probably most important, early mobilization minimizes joint stiffness and inhibits the development of soft-tissue contractures due to excessive scar formation. Collagen proliferation is part of the inflammatory response. Appropriate stressing of this new tissue promotes optimal organization of collagen fibrils and limits randomized scar tissue from impeding joint motion (21). Recovery time can be prolonged for several days or even weeks if an injured joint develops stiffness and a significant loss of ROM. Immobilization may be needed initially for protection, but some movement can usually begin shortly after injury. Always work within the pain-free ROM. Joint stability should always be monitored because an unstable joint should not be subjected to excessive ROM exercises. As rehabilitation advances, flexibility exercises can be escalated. However, if there is prolonged postexercise pain, the ROM exercise regimen should be reduced to previous pain-free levels.

Therapeutic Modalities

Detailed discussions about the technical application of different modalities are often neglected in clinical settings. Many physicians have little knowledge of the principles behind the various modalities and their application, partly because this work generally falls under the domain of athletic trainers and therapists. Even so, a fundamental understanding of each modality is important. Every time one of the modalities is used, a specific, objective goal should be kept in mind, including the timing and sequence of their use. The intensity, duration, and frequency of application can be critical in expediting recovery.

Finally, many treatment regimes become popular without adequate evidence of their efficacy. Comprehensive review of the literature highlights how little we actually know about the physiological principles and efficacy of many modalities.

Cryotherapy

Cold therapy is one of the most common therapeutic interventions applied after acute athletic injury. Cooling an injured joint or extremity has an analgesic effect as well as retards secondary injury (4,22,23). Cryotherapy is also believed to reduce acute edema by decreasing blood flow (24,25), metabolic activity (22,24), and permeability of postcapillary venules (26).

There are several ways to apply cold therapy, including ice massage, ice water immersion in a whirlpool bath, an ice blanket or pack, or immersion in ice water slush. Coolant sprays in the form of ethychloride or fluromethane are used for topical anesthesia and in the techniques of spray and stretch.

Ice massage means local application of an ice cup in a circular motion for a period of 5 to 10 minutes. Ice water immersion, either in a whirlpool or ice water slush, is good for treating a larger area of injury or one involving bony or irregular surfaces (e.g., lateral malleolus). After analgesia occurs, the athlete can begin gentle ROM exercises while the injured part is immersed. This therapy should usually last up to 20 minutes and can be repeated every 1.5 to 2 hours. Ice packs are applied in a similar manner. Remember that the application of any form of cryotherapy for extended periods of time may cause temporary or even permanent injury to nervous tissue (27,28). The therapeutic effects of cold therapy are listed in Table 35.3 and the contraindications are given in Table 35.4.

A common recommendation is that ice should be used for the first 24 to 48 hours after acute soft-tissue injury, followed by heat. We caution against using any set period of time. So long as there is evidence that swelling is increasing, do not start heat therapy. Edema can easily continue after the first 48 hours in an injured joint that is not treated

TABLE 35.3
THERAPEUTIC EFFECTS OF COLD

Vasoconstriction
Decreased muscle spasm
Increased threshold of pain
Relative anesthesia

TABLE 35.4
CONTRAINDICATIONS TO COLD THERAPY

Raynaud's phenomenon
Raynaud's disease
Cold urticaria
Cryoglobulinemia
Paroxysmal hemoglobinuria
Cold presser response positive
Circulatory insufficiency
Anesthetic skin
Severe cardiopulmonary disease

appropriately. Heat in this situation would potentially worsen the edema. Use ice until you are convinced the swelling has stopped. This may take several days, depending upon the type and extent of injury. Ice application after activity may also be indicated after an athlete begins PFR. Too often, the use of ice is neglected after the athletes are allowed to return to activity. When this happens, a small amount of edema may recur and prolong the recovery time.

Heat Therapy

The application of heat can bring about analgesia and a decrease in muscle spasms. However, if applied too soon, heat may actually increase pain by increasing edema. Therefore, heat should *not* be considered for initial treatment of an acute injury. The desirable therapeutic effects of heat include reducing pain, relieving muscle spasm, increasing blood flow, decreasing joint stiffness, and increasing the elasticity of collagen fibers (7,29). The effective therapeutic temperature is 40°C to 45.5°C (104°F–113.9°F), which is a very narrow range, and it is essential to remember that there is a thin margin between the therapeutic range and the tissue damage range, which begins at 46°C (114.8°F). Therapeutic effects are determined by the duration of heating, total area treated, tissue temperature, and the rate of temperature rise in the tissues. The most effective duration is 3 to 30 minutes, depending upon the modality of application. Heat can be applied by convection (moist air cabinet, hydrotherapy), conduction (hot packs, paraffin), radiation (infrared), or conversion (diathermy, ultrasound). It can be applied in either superficial or deep form. The most common modalities for superficial heat are whirlpool baths and hydroculator packs. The most common modality for deep heat is ultrasound.

Superficial heat produces its highest temperature at the body surface but penetrates only a few millimeters into the tissue (7,29). Because the penetration of heat is minimal, superficial heat often is chosen for reflex muscle relaxation and its sedative effect. Immersing the trunk and all four extremities in a Hubbard tank will induce a mild fever in most people. Consequently, the maximum water temperature should not exceed 38°C (100.4°F). Immersion of a single extremity can be done safely up to 41°C (105.8°F). Remember that heating increases the metabolic demand of tissues. If ischemia is a problem (ischemic ulcer), keep the temperature at 35°C to 37°C (95°F–98.6°F). Heat application by hydrotherapy should be done in 20- to 30-minute periods because longer immersion may cause local tissue damage.

Hydroculator packs contain dried silica gel capable of absorbing and retaining water and heat. They are usually heated to a temperature of 65.5°C to 76.6°C (150°F–170°F) and then wrapped in several towels before being placed on the athlete. This helps control the transfer of heat by conduction. Treatment periods usually are 20 to 30 minutes long.

Another form of superficial heat is paraffin wax baths. The wax mixture usually consists of four to eight parts paraffin mixed with one part mineral oil. The mixture is heated and maintained at 50.5°C to 56.6°C (125°F–134°F) and can be applied by dipping or continuous immersion. Total treatment time usually is 20 to 30 minutes. This is a very effective method of treating injured joints of the hands and feet.

Radiant heat from infrared lamps has limited application in sports medicine; they are used mostly for dermatological conditions.

Deep heating modalities include short wave, microwave, and ultrasound. Ultrasound is the one most often used to apply deep heat for sports injuries.

Short wave diathermy is the therapeutic application of an electric current with a very high frequency that is converted to heat within the tissues. The two techniques of application are the condenser method and induction coil applicators. Treatment usually lasts 20 to 30 minutes and the highest temperature is obtained in the deep subcutaneous tissues of superficial muscles. It does not penetrate into deep joint structures.

A disadvantage of short wave diathermy is that it cannot be accurately dosed nor can the amount of energy transferred to the patient be monitored. The only safeguard against excessive heating is the athlete's perception of warmth and pain. In addition, the patient must be kept dry because perspiration, which contains electrolytes, can serve as an electrical conductor and cause burning of the skin (see Table 35.5).

Microwave diathermy is a deep heating modality using high frequency electromagnetic waves. As with short wave diathermy, there is no accurate way to monitor the dose. Because microwave applicators are small and cannot be used to treat very large areas, their effectiveness is limited at present.

Ultrasound is a form of acoustic energy produced by mechanical vibrations. Ultrasound waves are at frequencies that are inaudible to the human ear (above 2,000 cycles/second). To produce energy for therapeutic purposes, a machine requires a generator of high frequency current and an applicator sound head with a transducer that

TABLE 35.5
CONTRAINDICATIONS AND PRECAUTIONS IN THE USE OF SHORTWAVE OR MICROWAVE DIATHERMY

Use near cardiac pacemaker
Use over the eyes
Use over open wounds or moist dressings (risk of selective heating)
Use over areas of increased perspiration (risk of selective heating)
Use over epiphyseal growth plates in children
Use over an area of infection (risk of spread)
Use over subcutaneous fat deposits in obese persons (selective heating of subcutaneous fat)

receives electrical currents of sufficient frequency to cause it to vibrate and produce sound waves.

Ultrasound energy is transmitted to the tissues by this applicator. The waves do not pass easily through air, so an air-free medium must be interposed between the applicator and the skin. Mineral oil or a gel is the usual coupling medium. Ultrasound has the deepest penetration of any deep heating modalities. It is the only one that can directly increase deep tissue (muscle and bone interfaces) temperature to a therapeutic level (7,29–32), reportedly increasing temperatures at depths up to 5 cm (20,33–36). Deep heat can increase the elastic properties of collagen tissue, making it useful in the treatment of soft-tissue contracture, muscle spasm, and thrombolysis (37–47). When ultrasound is used with a gentle stretching and strengthening program, ROM is often returned to stiff and contracted joints. In addition to its role as a thermal agent, it has also been used therapeutically for healing wounds (17, 48,49), pain relief (50–52) and acceleration of fracture healing (1,53–58). Ultrasound can be more accurately dosed than short wave and microwave diathermy. The therapeutic range is 0.5 to 2 watts/cm^2 and usually is applied for a period of 4 to 8 minutes. It may cause a feeling of local warmth and tingling, but if pain occurs, too much energy is being used. Another advantage of ultrasound is that it can be used with whirlpool baths to deliver deep heat over irregular bony surfaces such as the lateral malleolus.

The therapeutic effects of heat are summarized in Table 35.6. Table 35.7 lists the contraindications to heat therapy.

Contrast Baths

Contrast therapy combines heat and cold modalities, typically alternating between immersion in warm and cold water. This technique, indicated in subacute and chronic conditions, is believed to produce a number of physiological effects, including increased tissue temperature and blood flow, blood flow changes in both the ipsilateral and contralateral extremities, hyperemia of the superficial blood vessels, decreased muscle spasm, reduced inflammation, and improved ROM.

TABLE 35.6
THERAPEUTIC EFFECTS OF HEAT

Increased blood flow
Increased visco elastic properties of collagen
Sedation
Analgesia
Muscle relaxation and decreased muscle spasm
Increased metabolic rate
Increases the suppurative process

Typically, the injured extremity is immersed for 10 minutes in hot water, 40.0°C to 43.3°C (104°F–110°F). The injured part is then placed in cold water between 10°C to 15.5°C (50°F–60°F) for 1 minute. The total treatment time of 30 minutes is an alternating process, with hot water immersion for 4 minutes followed by cold water immersion for 1 minute after the initial 10-minute period of heat. A second method calls for submerging the limb in an ice slush bath for 2 minutes and then in tepid water at 33.9°C to 37.7°C (93°F–98°F) for 30 seconds. The baths are alternated for 15 minutes, beginning and ending with cold immersion (53).

Electric Stimulation

Electrotherapy has become very popular in sports medicine (31,33,34,59,60). It is used to increase the strength of healing ligaments and tendons (60), prevent muscle atrophy (31), and control swelling and edema (33,59). In addition, electrotherapy is being used to introduce medications into subcutaneous tissues after they have been applied to the overlying skin (61), a process called *iontophoresis* (62). Even so, there is considerable debate about the effectiveness

TABLE 35.7
CONTRAINDICATIONS TO HEAT THERAPY

Impaired sensation or an anesthetic area
Noninflammatory edema
Ischemia in the area being treated
Malignancy in the area being treated
Metallic implants (except in ultrasound diathermy)
Application over the gonads
Exposure to a developing fetus
Skin disorders that are aggravated by heat
Altered level of consciousness
Hemorrhagic diathesis
Very young or very old patients

of electrotherapy, and its usefulness should *not* be oversold. Claims that electrical stimulation can actually reduce body fat, increase cardiorespiratory endurance, and build strength in muscle mass should be received with caution. A very good understanding of the applications and limitations of electrotherapy obviously is important.

Transcutaneous Electrical Nerve Stimulation

Perhaps the most widespread use of electrotherapy has been for pain control. Transcutaneous electrical nerve stimulation (TENS) is the application of controlled low voltage electrical pulses through skin electrodes. TENS is based on the "gate" theory of pain by Melzack and Wall (63). The endogenous opiate system of the central nervous system may also have a role in explaining how TENS therapy actually reduces pain (64). The effectiveness of TENS is controversial, including the correlation between the appropriate frequency, pulse, output intensity, and waveform of use. TENS can be applied for brief periods with very intense stimulation or for longer periods at lower intensity. In acute situations, TENS may be applied alone or with ice for 30-minute periods. This can be repeated every 2 to 3 hours. For chronic pain, TENS may be used on a more regular basis throughout the day. It should never be used to mask pain during competition. TENS has been used to control postoperative pain (34) and reduce postoperative muscular atrophy (60). Controlling pain after an injury and during the earlier phases of rehabilitation is essential for expediting recovery. Pain does play a protective role, so masking it in uncontrolled activities can lead to further and perhaps more serious injury.

High Voltage Pulsed Galvanic Stimulation

Another popular concept with reported effectiveness is high voltage pulsed galvanic stimulation (HVPGS). HVPGS is the use of high voltage (150—500 volts) pulsed direct current for the stimulation of local blood flow. The reported effects of HVPGS include reduction of pain, edema, and muscle spasm, as well as accelerated wound healing and prevention of muscle atrophy. It is supposed to have advantages over low voltage stimulators because it creates less caustic sensation due to the specific waveform and depth of penetration. However, there is very little research to support the claims. There have been many anecdotal reports of effectiveness. One study did show an increase in blood flow in healthy volunteers when HVPGS was used at the highest frequency and with negative polarity for 20 to 30 minutes (33).

Iontophoresis

Iontophoresis is a method by which ionized medication is driven through the skin by an electrical current. Corticosteriod preparations, local anesthetics, and salicylates are the most common medications used. It is indicated in the treatment of inflammatory soft-tissue injuries. The recommendation is that the current intensity should be no greater than 5 mA, and that the duration of treatment should not exceed 15 to 20 minutes. This form of therapy reportedly has several advantages over injections of anti-inflammatory medications, including more consistent drug delivery and a lower overall dose. Because the treatment is not invasive, it is supposed to be painless. Again, there is very little research to substantiate these claims. Some authors have found that the initial depth of penetration is less than 1 cm with this method (65). There is considerable disagreement about its efficacy and, if it proves to be useful, the question is whether the beneficial results are due to local responses or to systemic effects of the medications.

Phonophoresis

Phonophoresis is similar to iontophoresis. Whole molecules of medications are driven through the skin into the subcutaneous tissues by means of ultrasound. As with any other application of ultrasound, a coupling medium must be used in addition to the medicated cream preparations. As with iontophoresis, phonophoresis may be used to treat inflammatory soft-tissue injuries. The treatment period usually lasts approximately 10 minutes. Two authors have found that the depth of penetration with this modality is anywhere from 5 to 6 cm (41,65).

Many anecdotal reports exist touting phonophoresis as an effective method of treating a variety of soft-tissue injuries. However, there have been no controlled studies to substantiate these clinical observations. Phonophoresis may be a good treatment option for injuries to large musculo-tendon units (e.g., Achilles tendon) in which the risk of tendon damage secondary to local steroid injection must be weighed against the benefits. Corticosteroid, local anesthetics, aspirin and anti-inflammatory preparations can all be introduced into tissues by phonophoresis.

Light Therapy

Light therapy is a method by which energy is directed into the body tissue through visible or infrared (invisible) light. Light therapy is a recent addition to the group of therapeutic modalities. It utilizes light to trigger a series of chemical reactions within the body that ultimately help injured tissues return to optimal state and begin the healing process. Light therapy is indicated in the treatment of various conditions, including carpal tunnel syndrome, musculoskeletal injury, tendonitis, arthritis, and wound healing.

As a therapeutic modality, light therapy is a blanket term that includes low-level laser therapy (LLLT), super luminous diodes (SLDs), and light emitting diodes (LEDs). Each of these forms of therapy has different qualities and specifications and may vary regarding their application. The depth of penetration is believed to vary from superficial for LEDs up to 5 cm for LLLT. Treatment times and dosages also vary widely, depending on the injury being treated and the method of therapy being used. Benefits include it being noninvasive and generally painless (66).

Research surrounding light therapy is mixed, and its efficacy is under debate. Nevertheless, there are many light therapy devices currently being utilized to treat sport-related injuries, making it important to have some knowledge of this modality.

Massage, Tissue Mobilization, and Manipulation

Manual therapies such as soft-tissue mobilization and massage are used to reduce swelling and alleviate pain. Common forms of massage are stroking, compression, and percussion, all of which may produce sensations of pleasure, relaxation of muscle, and sedation. It also may be helpful in decreasing edema by increasing lymphatic drainage, stretching adhesions, and mobilizing accumulated fluids. Contraindications to massage include infection, deep vein thrombosis, skin disease, hemorrhagic diastases, and malignancy. Soft-tissue mobilization requires keen palpatory skills and a good understanding of manual techniques. It should only be done by individuals with knowledge of the fundamental concepts and experience in its use.

Manipulation is defined as the abrupt, passive movement of a joint beyond its physiological range but within its anatomical range. Most studies have focused on vertebral manipulation. A few studies have shown temporary relief of pain compared to other modalities, but there are no controlled studies to support many of the popular benefits ascribed to manipulation (67).

Traction

Traction is a technique in which a distracting force is applied to a particular part of the body to promote stretching of soft tissue and separation of joint surfaces. Traction may be intermittent or continuous and may be directed at any angle. Indications for traction include stretching muscles and ligaments, opening up vertebral foramina, and the distraction of vertebral bodies (68). Contraindications include spinal cord compression, extreme osteoporosis, atherosclerotic disease of the vertebral and/or carotid system, malignancy involving the vertebra, infectious diseases of the intervertebral disk or vertebral body, and rheumatoid arthritis with odontoid disease.

Clinically, the most effective application of traction is in the cervical spine to relieve pressure on cervical nerve roots. The patient sits on a chair with the neck at approximately 25 degrees of forward flexion. The weight of the head, approximately 10 lb, must be overcome before effective cervical traction occurs. Distraction of the cervical vertebra usually happens when the weight reaches 20 to 35 lb (68). If this treatment relieves the athlete's symptoms, a home program can be used several times a day.

The overall effectiveness of lumbosacral traction is controversial. It has been reported that traction forces that exceed 300 lb are necessary to achieve a significant degree of lumbar vertebral distraction (69). Therefore, lumbosacral traction has limited practical use in a clinical setting. Using 20 to 30 lb of pelvic traction while a person is lying in bed serves only to keep him/her still. Higher tolerable distraction forces can be achieved with intermittent traction. However, there is still considerable debate about whether significant distraction occurs.

Gravity inversion to achieve lumbar distraction has become popular, although there are serious potential complications such as hypertensive responses and increased intraocular pressure (70).

In summary, the use of therapeutic physical modalities is widespread in sports medicine. Specific objective goals (decrease swelling, increase ROM, or decrease pain) should guide every individual's therapy program.

The timing and sequence of heat and cold therapy are outlined in the protocols at the end of the chapter. It is worth noting that considerable research has been done on the general use and effects of heat and cold therapy, but very little of it has been done on the specific applications of particular modalities and their comparative effects. We are left with many anecdotal claims. The very nature of athletic competition makes sports medicine providers anxious to come up with an edge in treatment. Couple this general mind-set with today's advancing technology and enterprising marketing pressures, and it is easy to see the difficulty involved in making rational decisions about the use of these modalities. Resist being oversold.

Finally, there is the placebo effect. As long as commonsense prevails, we know we will see improvement in soft-tissue injuries regardless of which modality is used. Keep an open mind about trying different ways. Avoid cookbook routines; do not treat every sprained ankle alike. Also, if one combination is not working, do not be afraid to try a different approach.

Restoring Muscle Strength and Endurance

After an injury or surgery, restoring muscle strength and muscle endurance becomes a primary focus of rehabilitation. Strength can be defined as the maximum force exerted against an immovable object (isometric strength), the heaviest weight lifted against gravity (isotonic strength), or the maximum torque developed against an accommodating resistance at a constant velocity of joint motion (isokinetic strength). Muscle power is defined as the amount of force generated times the distance through which that force is generated per unit of time. Muscular endurance is the ability of a muscle to generate force repetitively.

The principles of strength training for conditioning or for rehabilitation are similar, except for the intensity of training. Some athletes are accustomed to spending time in weight training rooms for conditioning. However, strength training after an injury must be done in a controlled, supervised manner, with much less intensity. If the strengthening program is started too early or improperly done, the potential for reinjury is significant and the rehabilitation course may be prolonged.

In designing any strengthening program for rehabilitation, keep in mind the following five basic principles:

- The need to overload muscles in order to increase their strength
- The concept of progressive resistant exercises (PREs)

- Methods of strength training
- Specificity of training
- Achieving balanced strength while maintaining flexibility

The need to work muscles against resistance that is greater than normal in order to produce strength gains was popularized in the 1940s by DeLorme (28,29). Strength gains in human muscle fibers are primarily the result of hypertrophy of individual muscle fibers (73,74). With animal models, researchers have shown the actual number of muscle cells that increases as a result of training (74). Whether this will hold true for humans is yet to be shown.

DeLorme also popularized the concept of PREs, which is an extension of the overload principle. As strength increases, the initial resistance is no longer effective in providing a stimulus for overload. Therefore, resistance must be progressively increased. On the basis of this principle, a format was designed using three sets of 10 repetitions for weight training workouts. This format uses a repetitive maximum (RM), which is the maximum load a muscle or group of muscles can lift for a given number of times before fatigue. For instance, the 10-RM is the amount of weight an athlete can lift 10 times before fatigue. A common format for weight training used in training rooms across the country consists of 10 repetitions at three fourth of the 10-RM, and a final set of 10 repetitions at the 10-RM. The technique of PREs is a practical application of the overload principle and forms the basis of most weight training programs.

Methods of strength training are summarized in Table 35.8. There is considerable debate about the best method for increasing strength, and no single technique really can be considered superior to another (73,74). Isometrically trained muscles are stronger when measured isometrically. Similarly, isotonically trained muscles are stronger when measured isotonically. In deciding which strength training method to use, take into account the status of the athlete's injury, overall physical condition, and intended purpose of the strength training. Static or isometric strengthening is often useful when joint movements must be restricted or when movement still causes pain. Muller demonstrated that strength decreases by approximately 5%/day in the absence of contraction, but one isometric contraction a day at half the maximum strength is enough to prevent this loss (24). If isometric training is used to develop greater strength for a particular movement, these exercises must be done at several points throughout the ROM. In view of the availability of dynamic methods of strength training, this particular form of training may be extremely time consuming and compliance may be a problem. Also, there is a certain lack of carryover to specific motor skills (24). Despite these disadvantages, it is important to start isometric strength training as early as possible after an injury. This form of exercise can help prevent muscle atrophy in an injured extremity. As noted earlier, HVPGS may be useful by inducing isometric contraction of muscles, thereby preventing atrophy and maintaining strength.

TABLE 35.8
METHODS OF STRENGTH TRAINING

- Static
  - Isometric
- Dynamic
  - Constant resistance or isotonic (Universal Gym or free weights)
  - Variable resistance (DeLand Sports Medical Industries, David, Eagle, or Nautilus Equipment)
  - Accommodating resistance at fixed speeds or isokinetic (Cybex, Kin-Com, Lido, and Orthotron Machines)

Once swelling subsides and motion is almost pain-free, dynamic strengthening can begin. Isotonic strengthening is a dynamic exercise involving changes in muscle length as tension develops against a constant resistance. A concentric isotonic contraction is the type of muscular contraction that occurs when a muscle shortens as it develops tension (e.g., a barbell curl). An eccentric muscle contraction occurs when a muscle actually lengthens as it develops tension (e.g., lowering a weight to the floor with the arms). There are limitations to isotonic exercises. The amount of weight or resistance is fixed and is a function of the weakest part of the ROM of a particular lift. Simply stated, the muscles moving the weight are working at below maximum intensities throughout most of the ROM. Examples of this type of training include free weights and the Universal weight lifting system. Despite these limitations, free weights are the most affordable strength training equipment available to most athletes. Free weights have the advantage of allowing the user to isolate a specific muscle or muscles for strength training.

Methods of strength training using variable resistance are an attempt to increase the intensity of work for a group of muscles throughout the full ROM. Hydraulic or cam-shaped machines have been developed for this purpose (e.g., Nautilus, David Systems). Surgical tubing and elastic bands are simpler forms of this method. The resistance of the hydraulic or cam-shaped machines attempts to match the angle-specific strength of specific muscle groups. Advantages of this type of training include the ability to work muscles at a higher maximal rate, and to provide strengthening in both eccentric and concentric manner (remember that many athletic movements involve eccentric contractions). The principles of overload and PREs apply to the variable resistance methods of strength training as well as the constant resistance method.

Isokinetic strength training involves accommodating resistance (or "weight") at fixed speeds. The amount of resistance encountered accommodates to match the force applied. One advantage of this method is that an appropriate amount of resistance is encountered throughout the entire ROM. If there is pain, or a muscle becomes fatigued at any point in the ROM, the amount of resistance encountered decreases proportionally as the force applied decreases. That makes this mode of strength training very helpful early in the course of rehabilitation when safety is a concern. Examples of isokinetic equipment include Cybex, Kim-Com, and Lido.

Another advantage of isokinetic strengthening is that direct measurements of muscle power, torque, and endurance can be made. Serial measurements can be used to document the progress an athlete is making in rehabilitation. In addition, strength training can be done at speed settings ranging from 0 to 300 degrees/second. Many functional activities in athletics involve very fast joint ranges of motion (the elbow and shoulder may reach speeds of 5000–8000 degrees/second during the acceleration phase of pitching). Therefore, this method of strength training has the advantage of being able to develop strength at joint speeds that cannot be developed by other methods. In addition, once a particular amount of muscle strength is achieved, work can begin on muscle power and endurance. Muscle power is usually developed at slower speeds (180 degrees/second) and with fewer repetitions. Muscle endurance is developed at faster speeds (300 degrees/second) with multiple repetitions, often to the point of exhausting the muscle (24).

The following points summarize the advantages of isokinetic exercise. (a) It is the only way to load a contracting muscle to its maximum capacity through the full ROM. (b) More resistance than can be withstood is never given because the equipment accommodates resistance. (c) It allows accommodation of pain and fatigue throughout the ROM. (d) Exercise can occur at faster, more functional joint velocities. (e) There are decreased joint compressive forces at faster speeds, reducing the risk of articular cartilage injury. There is ongoing debate about the reproducibility, specificity, and accuracy of isokinetic testing, but this method comes closer to measuring muscle performance at functional speeds than any other method currently available. After an athlete undergoes a complete rehabilitation program, the injured extremity should be compared to the noninjured side and to the preinjury measurements if they are available.

Specificity of Training

This principle is based on the specific motor skill requirements for different sports. Athletes develop particular movement patterns that are characteristic of gross and fine motor skills needed to perform different athletic activities. Specificity of training should be utilized when incorporating strengthening programs into rehabilitation activities. This is based on the fact that all voluntary movements are a function not only of the strength of the muscles used in the movement but also on a finely regulated series of neuromuscular events. These include central and peripheral nervous system factors that cause the recruitment and coordination of firing of appropriate motor units. To illustrate this concept, note that strengthening activities for leg muscles, such as squats or deep knee bends, typically do not demonstrate the same increased ability to generate force when used in other movements such as jumping. Similarly, the strength and fine motor skills needed to swing a bat at a baseball are far different from the ones needed to swing a golf club.

The need for exercise protocols that re-educate muscles and joints in sports-specific patterns is illustrated by the concept of proprioceptive neuromuscular facilitation (PNF). PNF is a form of exercise in which the accommodating resistance is manually applied to various patterns of movement to strengthen and retrain the muscles that guide joint motion (25,75). PNF is based on stimulation of proprioceptors within the skin, muscle, and tendons to promote the re-education of muscles through rotational and diagonal patterns specific to the athlete's sport. This technique uses a contraction and relaxation phase that increases the flexibility of tight muscle groups. In addition to isometric contraction, relaxation and stretch sequence rotational and diagonal patterns are used with appropriate manual resistance to maintain facilitory sensory inputs and to recruit appropriate muscles throughout the sport specific pattern. Increasingly heavier gauges of surgical tubing or elastic band material can be used to raise the resistance level of specific functional patterns of movement (see Figure 35.2(a and b)).

Strengthening programs are frequently used after injury or surgery. However, injured athletes scheduled for surgery should be considered for preoperative strengthening programs to hasten recovery and mitigate the invariable loss of strength.

Sports-specific strength training can be extremely helpful in preventing injury. For example, football players should be encouraged to strengthen their neck muscles, quadriceps, and hamstrings in order to protect their necks and knees from serious injury. Swimmers, throwers, and tennis players should concentrate on achieving a balance of strength and flexibility in their shoulders.

Sequence of Exercises

In designing rehabilitation protocols, keep in mind not only the type and number of exercises to be done, but also their order. Take care to avoid exercising the same set of muscles without planned rest periods. Larger groups of muscles should be exercised first to avoid fatigue in smaller muscle groups. Exercising smaller groups first may limit the subsequent effectiveness of exercise intended to overload larger groups. The concept of circuit training illustrates sequencing. Circuit training is a series of strengthening exercises done in sequence to maximize strength gains and avoid muscle fatigue. As an injured athlete progresses through the rehabilitation program, the intensity and the number of repetitions per unit time can be increased.

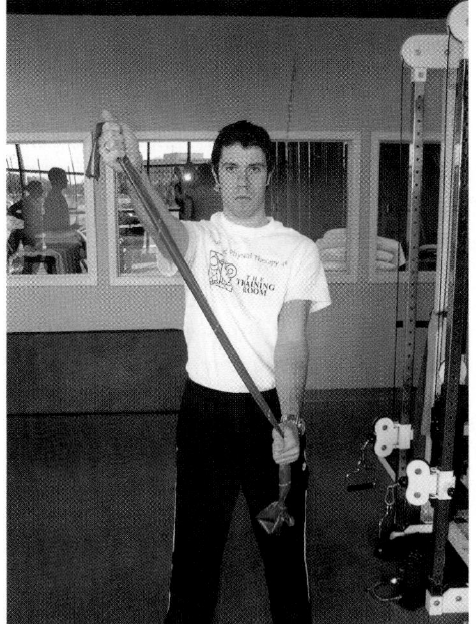
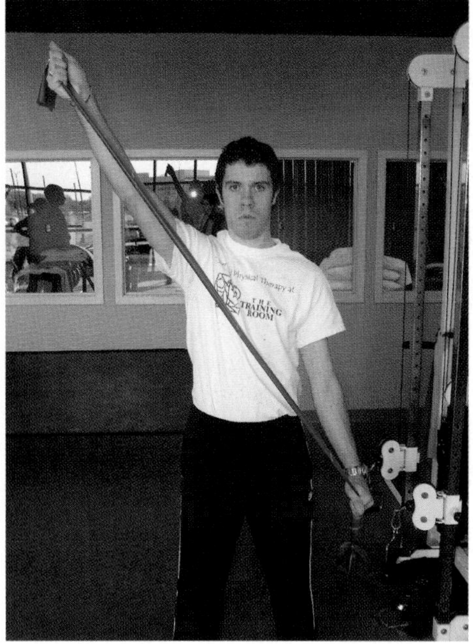

Figure 35.2 Demonstration of functional patterns of movement using varying gauges of elastic bands to increase resistance.

Achieving Balanced Strength and Maintaining Flexibility

It is easy for the athlete and the sports medicine staff to focus on strengthening a single set of muscles after an injury, but it is very important that balanced strength be regained, not only in the injured group of muscles, but also in the agonists and antagonists of the muscle group.

Regaining balanced strength is not enough. Regular stretching to increase and maintain full flexibility and ROM is paramount. Normal strength without complete joint motion can lead to reinjury or to new injuries. This is particularly true for injuries to the shoulders of throwing athletes and in spinal injury.

In summary, the postinjury program calls for improving muscle strength, endurance, and power, beginning with static or isometric strengthening at multiple joint angles. Dynamic resistive exercises should start when swelling has been controlled and 60% to 70% of pain-free ROM has been reestablished. During later stages of rehabilitation, there should be a progressive increase in the intensity of the workout. Specificity of strength training should be incorporated into the program, which should be individualized to the athlete's particular sports-specific movements. Isokinetic exercise is helpful initially to protect a joint from further damage secondary to pain or fatigue. In later stages, it can increase muscular power and endurance.

Progression through these stages in restoring normal muscle function should be monitored carefully. So long as the athlete is not experiencing increased pain, loss of (or excessive) ROM, or significant swelling, progression through the early, intermediate, and final stages of rehabilitation may safely continue. Remember that balanced strength and flexibility must be achieved before the final phases of rehabilitation can safely begin.

Maintaining Cardiovascular Fitness

After an injury, every effort should be made to maintain the preinjury aerobic fitness level. When an injury has been managed successfully, it is unfortunate if the return to competition must be delayed because the athlete has a diminished cardiopulmonary fitness level. The potential for reinjury or new injury secondary to deconditioning is considerable.

If an athlete has an upper extremity injury, fitness levels can be maintained by stationary cycling, jogging, or swimming. With lower extremity injuries, alternatives include one-legged bicycling, arm ergometry, or swimming. Remember that the benefits of aerobic conditioning are a function of training frequency, duration, and intensity. Regardless of the type of exercise, the target heart rate must be maintained for 30 to 45 minutes at least three times a week to prevent a significant loss of aerobic fitness.

Restoration of Balance and Agility

It stands to reason that an athlete who possesses good balance and agility will be less prone to injury. During the intermediate and later phases of rehabilitation, it is important to incorporate drills that increase balance and agility. Agility is a function of coordination, strength, power, endurance, reaction time, and speed of movement. Taken together, these variables determine how quickly

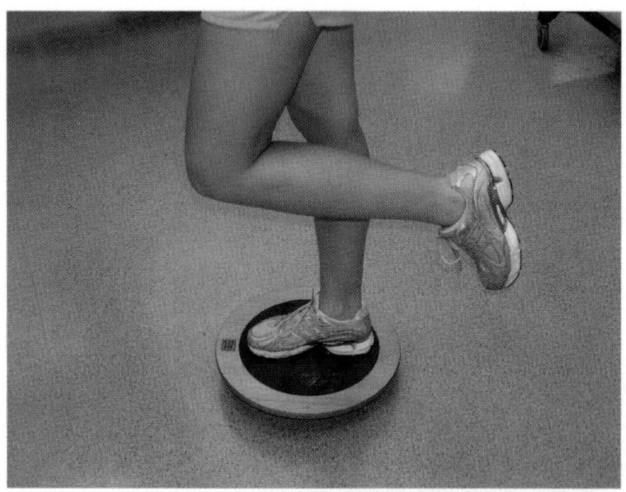

Figure 35.3 Use of a balance or tilt board to improve proprioception and reaction time.

the body is able to change direction. Balance is the maintenance of body position in relation to the forces of gravity. Balanced human movement is a finely regulated but complex mechanism involving the end-organ feedback to the central nervous system from muscle spindles, Golgi tendon organs, skin receptors, and proprioceptive receptors in the joints. The cerebellum is the primary integrating center that controls feedback from the peripheral receptors and cortex.

Immobilization, surgery, or an injury may compromise both balance and agility owing to interruption of this feedback mechanism (76). Balance and agility drills can be included in the functional progressive exercises discussed later (see section "Engram"). Balance activities include walking on a beam and hopping (one-legged, two-legged, and back and forth across a string, 6 to 10 in off the ground). Jumping rope is also a good activity for improving balance. Drills to improve the reaction time, the rate of acceleration, and maximum speed should also be included. Proprioception and reaction time can be improved in athletes who have recurring ankle sprains by using a balance or tilt board (see Figure 35.3).

Flexibility

There are no well-designed, controlled studies to support the principles that most sports staff uses as guides to promote increased flexibility for performance enhancement or to prevent and rehabilitate athletic injuries. Flexibility is a function of the structural properties of musculotendinous units and joint capsules, and also the neurophysiological principles of feedback and adjustment. Therefore, much of what we "know" about flexibility is intuitive and anecdotal. Theoretically, a lack of flexibility in tendons, muscles, and joint capsules predisposes athletes to injury. For example, tightness of the gastrocsoleus group can cause an athlete to excessively pronate the foot. Decreased flexibility in the hamstrings, quadriceps, tensor fascia lata, or gastrocsoleus group may interfere with reaction time in the knee joint and predispose it to injury. Therefore, maintenance of general flexibility is important both as a preventive measure and for injury rehabilitation. It is difficult to determine an optimal state of flexibility for any given athlete.

Flexibility exercises can be done individually or with a partner. Stretching should always involve warm-up and cool-down periods, and may be more effective after an activity is completed and the soft tissues are more distensible. Static stretching, which involves prolonged, gentle stretching at moderate tension, is believed to be safer and more effective than short term intermittent or ballistic stretching (77,78). In spite of the paucity of controlled data supporting the benefits of stretching and maintaining a state of flexibility, this concept warrants considerable attention, both for prevention and rehabilitation.

Taping and Bracing

Taping is one of the most useful tools of an athletic trainer. It can be considered both as an art and a science. It has been advocated for more than a century as a means of protecting ankle ligaments (68). Although many researchers dispute the benefits of ankle taping (79–81), recent studies have demonstrated its effectiveness in reducing new injuries (39,61,82–85) and excess motion (27,78,80,86–89). Taping has also been shown to restrict subtalar inversion (74,90,91), restrain anterolateral rotary subluxation of the talus in the presence of ligamentous laxity, and reduce strain on the anterior–inferior tibiofibular syndesmosis (68). Although tape loosens significantly after a short period of exercise (91), its restraining effect on extreme ankle motion is not lost during prolonged athletic activity (60,84,85,92–96).

The use of braces, particularly knee braces, also has received a considerable amount of attention and, like taping, their use is controversial (97). Currently available braces can be divided into three categories. The first category comprises braces used prophylactically to prevent knee injuries (McDavid, Don Joy, Iowa, and Anderson). Then there are knee braces that are used during rehabilitation after an injury or surgery (Bledsoe, Watco, OSI). Finally, there is a whole group of braces designed to protect unstable knees during athletic competition. These functional braces include the Don Joy Gold Point, one of the most commonly used.

As stronger and lighter weight materials are developed that provide functional stability without interfering with reaction time, speed of joint movement, and coordination, we find that athletes are more inclined to use them. Further clinical investigation needs to be done to substantiate their effectiveness. In spite of this lack of research data, bracing the knee after medial collateral, lateral collateral, and anterior cruciate ligament (ACL) injuries is strongly advised.

Psychological Support

The entire sports medicine staff must be aware of the potential psychological impact of surgery and/or injuries on an athlete (see Chapter 36). The athlete's level of confidence and self-esteem may suffer tremendously. It may be the first time that the athlete is in a situation in which he/she is not totally in control of factors affecting him/her. This may have a profound effect on the relationships he/she has with the family, coaches, and members of the sports medicine staff (42,98–100). This may be particularly true with young athletes of high caliber.

There are at least two important factors to keep in mind during rehabilitation. First, injured athletes need to feel that they are still a part of the team, so everything within reason should be done to allow them to attend practices and do their rehabilitation as part of the team. The athlete will want to attend team meetings and social functions. Second, every team physician should be aware of the athlete who is looking for a way out of competition. Frequent reoccurrence of injuries or new injuries should alert the physician to the possibility that a particular athlete may not want to continue. These situations must be handled very delicately as there may be many complicating factors that are involved (social and familial). Finally, during the later phases of rehabilitation, it is important for the athlete to have psychologically adjusted to the injury and feel ready to return to full competition before actually being allowed to do so. Any hesitation on the part of the athlete to return to competition should be recognized and addressed.

Functional Progressive Rehabilitation

We started this chapter with the basic question: "Doc, when do you think I'll be ready to play again?" We see that there is no easy answer. Reviewing the principles of rehabilitation should shed some light on the basic requirements of any rehabilitation protocol. Functional progressive rehabilitation is nothing more than the integration of these general principles we have been discussing into an organized, progressively more difficult sequence of exercises designed to meet the specific needs of an injured athlete's particular sport. These principles are outlined in Table 35.9.

After injury, the basic principles of early rehabilitation treatment should be followed. However, at some point, the injured extremity or joint must be put to a functional test. Functional tasks should begin during the intermediate phases of rehabilitation after comfortable weight bearing and/or pain-free ROM have been established.

Engrams

Engram programming is a process of retraining the neuromusculoskeletal system to invoke the desired, complex, and sports-specific motor movements in an "automatic" manner (100). Skilled movement patterns involve balance, feedback, and agility. Care must be taken to develop the desired motion slowly with supervised repetition to ensure that substitutional patterns and neuromuscular imbalances do not develop, thereby decreasing the risk of injury (101). It is indicative of inadequate rehabilitation if they do develop. In such a situation, look for subtle weakness of muscles, soft-tissue contractions causing restriction, joint motion, and/or other possible causes of pain with movement.

As functional progressive exercises are advanced, it is imperative to ensure that the specific motor skill in question remains "pure." Remember that it is important to establish proper form and motion before adding speed to the protocol. Each task begins at half speed, is advanced to three fourth speed, and then to full speed as intensity and frequency are also increased. A task is not considered complete until it can be done with sufficient repetitions at full speed without subsequent swelling, loss of ROM, pain, increased joint laxity, substitutional patterns, or hesitation on the part of the athlete. Progression along this continuum of increasingly more difficult tasks should continue only as the criteria are met. Do not permit the athlete to advance to a new and more difficult task until the previous task is successfully completed.

Developing functional progressive exercise protocols is not difficult so long as there is an understanding of the principles of rehabilitation, the extent of the injury and its subsequent constraints, and the demands of the athlete's particular sport. This type of exercise protocol allows the final phases of rehabilitation to be carefully monitored. If it appears that the athlete is being pushed too quickly, previous activity levels should be resumed and the intensity and frequency of the workout decreased. With this protocol, the athletes can psychologically adjust to the recovery phase and it makes them more aware of the timetable for returning to competition.

A number of articles have been published outlining rehabilitation programs for both upper and lower extremity injuries (35,40,54,57,66,80,102–110). In addition, several protocols are outlined here. Where appropriate, these include functional progressions that can be made a part of the overall rehabilitation. Do not try to follow a cookbook approach, because any protocol is, at best, only a guideline.

In the final stages of rehabilitation, observation of the athlete in practice situations is necessary to decide when to allow full participation under game conditions. The rule: "No practice by Thursday, no play on Saturday" is a good one. If the athlete is a football player, he/she is allowed to practice for a few days in a red jersey to remind his/her teammates not to hit him/her with full contact. After successfully completing this stage, he/she should participate in full contact team practices before being cleared to play in the next game.

Using this type of graduated program removes much of the burden of answering that ultimate question from the shoulders of the physician. The answer to the question regarding return to competition is usually readily apparent to the athlete, the sport medicine staff, and the physician.

TABLE 35.9

PHASES OF SPORTS MEDICINE REHABILITATION

- Early phase (1 to3 days)
  - PRICE
  - Early active ROM in an ice slush
  - Anti-inflammatories
  - Static (isometric) strengthening
  - Consider electrotherapy and pneumatic compression
  - Possible immobilization and non–weight-bearing status
- Intermediate phase (2 to 7 days)
  - Progressive weight bearing with protection
  - Continue ice until swelling stops
  - Consider contrast baths, electrotherapy and/or heat
  - Work toward full ROM
  - Continue anti-inflammatories
  - Begin dynamic strengthening when 60% to 70% of pain-free motion is present
  - Begin proprioceptive training
  - Begin exercises to maintain cardiopulmonary endurance
  - Once comfortable weight bearing has been achieved, begin functional progressions with protective taping and/or bracing
  - Engram programming begins
  - Continue ice after workouts
- Late phase (5 days to several weeks or even months)
  - Heat before workouts, ice afterwards
  - Establish full ROM. (heat may be very helpful to increase ROM)
  - Possibly discontinue anti-inflammatories
  - Advance muscle strengthening and include power and endurance training
  - Isokinetic training
  - Advance proprioceptive training, include balance and agility drills
  - Advance aerobic fitness activities
  - Advance engram programming
  - Advance functional progressions to competitive levels, testing strength, mobility, agility, speed, and balance
- Final phase (when an athlete is ready to return to competition)
  - Normal ROM
  - Symmetric, balanced muscle strength and endurance
  - Pain-free activity at functional levels
  - Successful completion of functional progressions
  - Appropriate Fitness Level
  - Has returned to a noncompetitive setting without difficulty (has practiced with the team)
  - Mentally and emotionally prepared to return to competition

PRICE = Protection, Rest, Ice, Compression, and Elevation; ROM = range of motion

Once an athlete does resume competition, it is imperative that rehabilitation continues for the duration of the competitive season. Soft tissues, particularly ligamentous structures, may take several months to heal completely (17,18). Strengthening, conditioning, agility drills, and protective bracing or taping will continue to be important.

REHABILITATION PROTOCOLS FOR SPECIFIC ATHLETIC INJURIES

The last section of this chapter contains several generic protocols outlining the rehabilitation of a few of the more common athletic injuries. Complete discussion of the rehabilitation for many of these injuries is beyond the scope of this chapter. Therefore, guidelines and general principles have been offered. More detailed references for specific injuries have been included. Each of these protocols is based on the fundamental phases of rehabilitation outlined in Table 35.9. Keep in mind that the key to a successful rehabilitation program is to start with a good base. Most successful therapists have developed "tricks of the trade" over time on the basis of their experiences with multiple injuries and physicians. Be mindful that the recovery time is determined on a case-by-case basis; included here are the normal ranges that can be expected.

Protocols for Rehabilitation

Knee Injuries

Athletes frequently injure their knees. It is a complex joint and many of the biochemical factors relating to its structure and function remain a mystery. Although clinical diagnosis of specific injuries may be difficult, the use of arthroscopy and magnetic resonance imaging (MRI) has greatly enhanced the precision of diagnosis. Treatment must be based an accurate diagnosis.

The treatment and rehabilitation of knee injuries has changed significantly in the past decade. Surgical philosophies about ligament tears and injuries to the meniscus have been re-evaluated, and there is a trend toward nonsurgical treatment. The role of the meniscus in knee joint stability and in maintaining proper biomechanics has received considerable attention (111). Noyes reported that patients with anterior cruciate-deficient knees, who also had a meniscectomy, demonstrated a two- to four-fold increase in swelling and pain with activity (112). Therefore, preserving the meniscus, or as much of it as possible, is very important.

In general, the evolution of knee injury rehabilitation has gone from prolonged immobilization to early, protected mobilization. The disadvantages of long-term immobilization have been well documented (17). A functionally progressive sequence is the cornerstone for the rehabilitation of knee injuries (see Table 35.10).

The approach to collateral ligament injuries also has changed dramatically. If the ACL is intact and the menisci are undamaged, then collateral ligament injuries often can be managed nonsurgically (37). Outlined in the subsequent text is a protocol for Grade I and II medial and lateral collateral ligament sprains.

Rehabilitation Guidelines Following Grade 1 and 2 Medial and Lateral Collateral Ligament Sprains

Day 1 through 5

1. PRICE
   - Knee immobilizer (especially at night)
   - Crutches with partial weight bearing
   - Ice 20 to 30 minutes every 3 to 4 hours
   - Compression dressing; loosen if ankle begins to swell
2. Protected ROM to pain tolerance (30 degrees of flexion to 90 degrees of flexion)
3. Isometric quadriceps exercises; three sets of 15—20 per day
4. Straight leg lifts; 3 sets of 20, three to five times per day
5. Analgesic or anti-inflammatory medications
6. Arm ergometry for cardiovascular conditioning
7. Modalities: electric muscle stimulation (EMS), pulsed ultrasound

Day 3 through 12

1. Progression from cryotherapy to contrast baths to heat therapy once swelling has stopped
2. Continue with crutches and immobilizer until swelling stops and complete pain-free ROM and weight bearing are established
3. Whirlpool bath with biking motion for ROM
4. Modalities: continuous ultrasound and EMS
5. Swimming with kickboard, doing gentle flutter kicks for 20 to 30 minutes
6. Continue isometrics
7. Continue medications as needed
8. Straight leg-raises with knee held straight
   - Work up to 10 RM three sets of ten per day
   - Incorporate hip flexion, extension and abduction/adduction exercises
9. Advance arm ergometry

Day 10 through 20

1. Heat before workout, ice afterwards
2. Wean off crutches; knee immobilizer may need to be worn at night
3. Continue whirlpool and/or swimming ROM exercises
4. If 90 degrees of comfortable knee flexion is present, begin stationary bicycling with toe clips (for hamstring work) 15 to 20 minutes/day
5. Running straight ahead in waist-deep water with good footing can begin for 15 to 20 minutes/day
6. Medications may be discontinued, depending upon pain and swelling
7. Begin hamstring curls; three sets of ten RM
8. Advanced quadriceps exercises or begin isokinetic work

Day 16 to Completion

1. Continue advancing strengthening program
2. Continue cardiovascular conditioning on the bicycle or running in the pool
3. Begin functional progressions
   - Walk/jog intervals (walk 1/4 mi, jog 1/8 mi, three sets/day for 1 to 3 days)
   - Jog/run intervals (jog 1/4 mi, run 1/8 mi, three sets/day from 1 to 3 days)
   - Hop/jump intervals (jump rope with both feet for three minutes; then left foot for 1 minute followed by the right foot for 1 minute. Three

TABLE 35.10
KNEE REHABILITATION

Walking
Running at half speed
Advance to full speed
Change of direction
Quick stops and starts
Protective bracing
Engram assembly and functional progressions
Practice in a controlled environment, simulating game conditions
Return to full activity

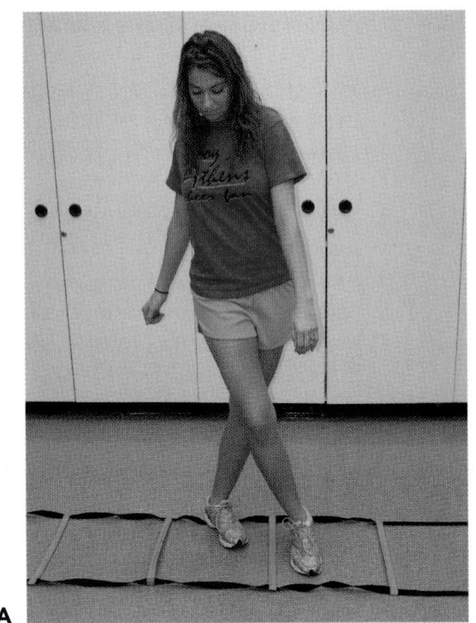
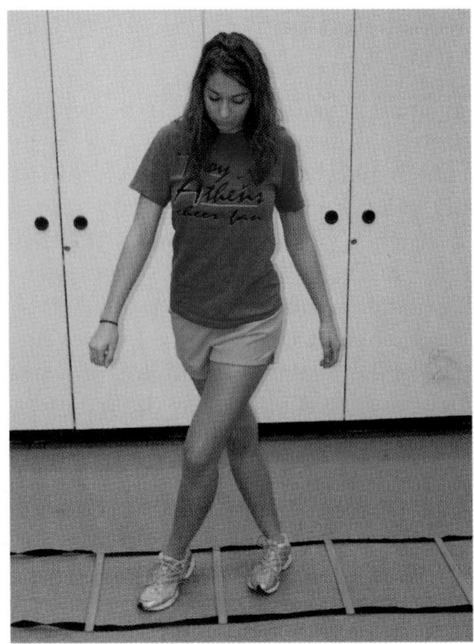

A B

Figure 35.4 Use of cutting or agility drills such as cross-overs or cariocas are useful in the rehabilitation of knee injuries.

sets, increasing the number of times, for 1 to 3 days)
- Sprint intervals (straight ahead sprints beginning at half speed advancing to full speed over 20 to 50 yd)
- Cutting/agility drills (large figure of 8s, advance to smaller figure of 8s, zigzag patterns, lateral shuffles, cariocas, tire drills, running pass routes, and dummy drills) (see Figure 35.4(a and b))
- Careful attention to slow, repetitions of sports-specific patterns is necessary to ensure proper engram assembly

4. Continue ice after workout
5. Isokinetic strength testing (the athlete can return to practice once 90%–100% strength is obtained)
6. Strengthening and agility must continue throughout the remainder of the season.

Rehabilitation Guidelines for Patello–Femoral Dysfunction

Patello–femoral dysfunction or knee extensor mechanism disorders are often incorrectly called *chondromalacia*. These disorders can be divided into the following three categories:

1. Malalignment of the spine, hip, and/or lower extremity, which results in altered knee biomechanics
2. Abnormalities of the patello–femoral joint articulation
3. An imbalance of strength and/or flexibility of the surrounding muscles, tendons, retinaculum, and ligaments (40)

This problem is often seen in runners and cyclists, it is also more common in males than females. A few of the more obvious predispositions include increased Q angle of the knee, excessive pronation of the foot, genu recurvatum, pelvic obliquity, scoliosis, femoral anteversion, iliotibial band tightness, "squinting" patellae, and relative weakness of the vastus medialis obliquis (VMO) muscle. There are many more subtle biochemical factors to be considered.

Nonsurgical treatment often is successful. The focus of treatment should not be on VMO strengthening alone. Increasing flexibility in tight antagonists (hamstrings) and the vastus lateralis is very important. Also, make sure there is no concomitant injury to these musculotendinous units, which may be causing reflex-inhibition. Manual patellar retraction is helpful in the early phases. Finally, slow repetitive practice of VMO contraction in sports-specific settings is important for proper engram coding. These functional steps should be undertaken once proper techniques have passed critical evaluation.

1. PRICE
   - Avoid compression around the knee; this may actually make the condition worse
   - Avoid deep knee bends, climbing stairs, squatting, and getting out of low chairs
   - If the condition is severe, the athlete may need to use crutches and be non–weight-bearing for several days
   - Avoid wearing high-heeled shoes
   - Rest is extremely important (Relative or absolute rest may be indicated.
   - Ice should be used frequently during the initial and intermediate phases of rehabilitation (consider TENS and deep friction massage)
2. Analgesic or anti-inflammatory medications (these are usually very helpful for this condition)

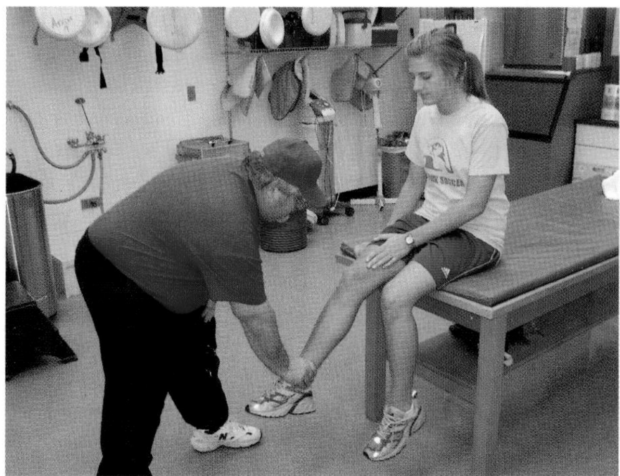

Figure 35.5 Slow, repetitive contractions of the vastus medialis obliquis.

3. Isometric quadriceps strengthening (with manual patellar retraction placing force on the lateral side of the patellar and pushing medially with each contraction)
4. Consider electrotherapy to the VMO
5. Increase flexibility of hamstrings, vastus lateralis, and iliotibial band
6. Short arc quadriceps to selectively strengthen the VMO muscle
   - Short arc quadriceps should be done in the last 15 to 20 degrees of extension
   - Begin with 1- to 2-lb weight boots or ankle weights and progress to 100 RM; three sets of 100 daily
   - Bent-knee leg-presses and partial squats may be done instead of short arc quads; this may cause less compressive force on the patellae
7. Slow, repetitive contractions of VMO to begin engram coding (see Figure 35.5)
8. Advanced, skilled coordinated movements using proprioceptive, neuromuscular techniques
9. Cardiovascular conditioning (arm ergometry, one-legged bicycling, or running in waist-deep water may be begun in the initial phases of rehabilitation)
10. Once functional progressions begin, a patellar knee sleeve may be helpful. A slow, progressive return to running may be begun when the athlete is pain-free, has good ROM, and good strength
    - Begin running in the pool
    - Advance by running on consistent indoor or outdoor surfaces
    - Avoid hill and speed work until the athlete's previous weekly mileage is obtained
11. Continue quadriceps strengthening and maintain hamstring flexibility after full activity has resumed

Rehabilitation Following Anterior Cruciate Ligament Injury

The treatment and subsequent rehabilitation of ACL injuries varies. These injuries may be treated nonoperatively or they may require surgery. Consideration must be on an individual basis. The athlete's level of competition or recreational pursuits, future demands, job requirements, and the ability to maintain compliance with a long-term rehabilitation program must be assessed and integrated into treatment decisions. If surgery is required, there are several different procedures, including a number of intra-articular and/or extra-articular repairs. The reader may wish to read some of the articles that have been written on this topic (16–19,40,55,57,104,106,108,112). Although there are many variables to any protocol for ACL rehabilitation, all of them contain certain key points. Also, regardless of the protocol, the total recovery time may be 4 to 12 months, depending upon the exact nature of the injury and the subsequent treatment. The therapist or trainer must understand the surgical procedure performed, so as to individualize the program for each athlete.

Early, protected mobilization is the current standard of care for many knee injuries. This also is true for ACL reconstructions, whereas a decade ago an athlete might have been immobilized in a cast for several weeks or months. Now, complete casting is often avoided and ROM exercises may begin in the recovery room, using continuous passive ROM (CPM) machines. Salter has shown that CPM reduces adhesions, decreases the incidence of postoperative hemathrosis, facilitates regeneration of articular cartilage, and increases joint nutrition (113). Paulo et al. have also studied early motion and documented the promotion of organized collagen healing as a result (114).

The basic premise behind ACL rehabilitation focuses on our evolving concept of ligamentous healing. The appropriate amount of stress is a matter of considerable debate. As a result, a reader can find several published "protocols" for ACL rehab that contain conflicting information. Paulos et al. divided their protocol into five phases (114). They recommended complete immobilization for the first 6 weeks of controlled motion. Steadman claims that the immobilization period should be 8 weeks and terminal knee extension should be avoided for at least 6 months (115). However, Steadman also has stated that earlier terminal knee extension may be done safely if the exercise involves a "closed kinetic chain." For example, an athlete with a repaired ACL may be encouraged to do half-squats to full standing exercises (and thereby achieving terminal extension of the knee) so long as the foot on the injured side is on the ground, creating a closed kinetic chain. Presumably due to the coactivation of the hamstrings, less torque is placed across the autograph than when the chain is "open" (i.e., when the knee is brought to full extension without the foot being on the ground).

The major source of controversy in ACL rehab is about the timing of terminal knee extension. It is hard to reconcile promoting patello–femoral joint motion and strength around the joint and protecting the newly repaired graft from undue stress. Jackson and Drez have shown that the anterior drawer forces placed upon the ACL increase dramatically after 40 degrees of knee flexion as the knee is brought to full extension in an "open" kinetic chain (18).

Also, animal studies have convinced many that the ACL in humans may take up to 24 months to reach full maturity and that ACL strength probably never returns completely without some augmentive repair (55).

So it is easy to see that designing a universally accepted ACL protocol is not easy. Regardless of which protocol the reader follows, bear in mind the general principles of rehabilitation outlined in Table 35.1. Also, remember that prolonged immobility should be avoided and healing tissues have stress limits and should not be overloaded.

Guidelines for Anterior Cruciate Ligament Rehabilitation Following Surgery

1. Explain the rehabilitation protocol and its timetable to the athlete before surgery. Depending upon the injury and the subsequent surgical repair, rehab may take 4 to 12 months.
2. Immobilization should be minimized. If there are no concomitant ligament or meniscus repairs, continuous passive ROM often can begin in the perioperative period.
3. Isometric strengthening can usually begin in the immediate postoperative phase. These should be done several times throughout the day. Electrical stimulation may be effective during the immobilization phase.
4. Immobilization should not exceed 6 to 8 weeks.
5. Immobilization with knee brace (instead of cast) permits controlled changes for eventual active ROM, wound inspection, and early patellar mobilization.
6. In the early phases of rehab, active knee extension is often controlled between 40 and 70 degrees of flexion to avoid excessive anterior drawer forces across the patella.
7. Terminal knee extension may be allowed early in the course of rehabilitation as long as it involves a "closed" kinetic chain.
8. In 2 to 4 months, most ROM should be established.
9. At 4 to 6 weeks, partial weight bearing, light strengthening, and endurance can begin.
10. PREs can begin at 6 to 8 weeks and should not be advanced too aggressively in the first 6 months.
11. Eccentric and concentric strength gains occur independently. Therefore, include exercises for both.
12. Isokinetic exercises may begin at 10 to 12 weeks as long as isotonic progressions have been pain-free without substituted patterns or recurrent effusions. Do not overload the healing tissues.
13. Monitoring the patello–femoral joint reaction forces during isokinetic exercise is difficult, therefore, care must be taken not to create patello–femoral pain or abnormal tracking that will prolong rehab.
14. An extension block may be needed with all forms of strengthening until the lateral phase of rehab.
15. Running straight ahead may usually begin at 4 to 6 months, depending upon progression thru the previous phases. Quadriceps strength should be 75% of total body weight (peak torques on isokinetic testing), or a minimum of 80% of the uninjured quadriceps, before running is allowed.
16. Progressive, functional tasks with cariocas, soft cutting, and backwards running can begin after successful completion of full speed straight ahead running. All running should be done in a protective brace.
17. Remember the final phases of all rehabilitation (see Table 35.9). These steps must be accomplished before full sports participation is allowed.

Rehabilitation Guidelines Following Grade 1 and 2 Lateral Ligament Sprains of the Ankle

This is the most common injury in sports medicine. Please refer to the discussions of Principles of Rehabilitation for further details.

Day 1 through 3

1. PRICE
   - Compression wrap with U-shaped pads (consider pneumatic compression with a Jobst pump [See Figure 35.1])
   - Spats brace or air splint
   - Possible use of crutches for temporary non—weight-bearing
   - Early ROM in an ice slush
   - Elevate as much as possible
2. Analgesic or anti-Inflammatory medications
3. Consider electrotherapy
4. Cardiovascular conditioning with arm ergometry, one-legged bicycling, or swimming

Day 3 through 7

1. Continue ice until swelling stops then consider contrast baths and heating modalities
2. Increase ROM both passively and actively (Thera-band or towel stretches)
3. Continue medications
4. Progressive weight bearing (continue to wear ankle brace)
5. Begin isometric strengthening of inverters, eveters, plantar, and dorsi flexors
6. Begin strengthening intrinsic foot muscles (pulling a weight on a towel toward the athlete with the toes, as in Figure 35.6; picking up marbles with the toes)
7. Achilles tendon stretching
8. Advanced cardiovascular conditioning
9. Proprioceptive exercises with a tilt board when pain-free ROM is present

Days 5 through 14

1. Use of heat before activities (whirlpool or ultrasound) and ice after activities
2. Consider discontinuing medications
3. Consider discontinuing air splint
4. Continue stretching and flexibility
5. Continue tilt board activities
6. Begin lower extremity functional progression and engram assembly (hopping, jumping rope, gentle cutting activities)

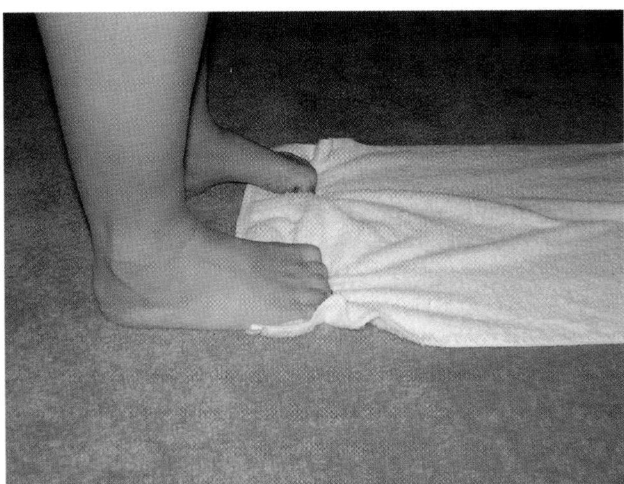

Figure 35.6 Strengthening of intrinsic foot musculature by pulling a weight on a towel with the toes.

7. Continue strengthening and flexibility exercises after return to competition
8. Protective taping before practice and competition

Rehabilitation Guidelines After Injuries to the Shoulder

The shoulder joint is unique. Because it is designed to allow maximum mobility, it has an inherent degree of structural instability. There is only one point where the shoulder girdle is attached to the axial skeleton: the sternoclavicular joint. Therefore, stability of the shoulder is maintained primarily by the surrounding muscles. This means that rehabilitation of an injured shoulder directly or indirectly involves increasing the strength and flexibility of the muscles surrounding the shoulder joint. Regardless of the injury, the important thing to remember is that a balance between strength and flexibility is necessary to prevent reinjury.

Throwing athletes, swimmers, gymnasts, tennis players, and wrestlers frequently injure the shoulder. Direct trauma to the shoulder causing glenohumeral dislocation or acromioclavicular separation is a common mechanism for injury. However, overuse injuries resulting from repetitive microtrauma are more common and often more difficult to treat.

Repetitive, efficient motion of the shoulder in carrying out sports-specific tasks is a finely orchestrated event involving more than glenohumeral biomechanics. This is particularly true when all five phases of throwing are considered: wind-up, cocking, acceleration, release deceleration, and follow-through (80). Throwing is a delicately balanced interplay of strength, flexibility, and neuromusculoskeletal engrams, which coordinate lower extremity, trunk, and arm motion while maintaining a very small center of glenohumeral joint rotation.

Injuries frequently occur when one small part of this finely orchestrated event breaks down. For instance, if a pitcher has a knee injury and loses quadricep strength, he may substitute a whipping motion of his arm in an attempt to make up the loss of one of his primary accelerators (his quadriceps) during the acceleration phase of throwing.

As with the knee, shoulder rehabilitation requires a working knowledge of fundamental biomechanical principles, which govern normal shoulder motion. Perry has addressed the biomechanics of the shoulder during sports-specific tasks (93).

Regardless of the type of shoulder injury, there are several key points to be kept in mind. If a setback occurs, it often can be traced to one or more of the following points:

- The rotator cuff muscles act primarily to maintain the center of rotation of the glenohumeral joint. An injury to one of the cuff muscles may allow repetitive, subtle subluxation.
- Acceleration of the throwing arm is primarily a function of trunk rotation, hip and knee extension, and conversion of stored energy in the glenohumeral capsule. The rotator cuff muscles are not accelerators.
- The posterior shoulder muscles, including the rotator cuff muscles, the biceps, brachialis, and brachioradialis, are the primary decelerators of the arm.
- Proper scapulothoracic motion is critical for fluid glenohumeral motion. Always evaluate scapulothoracic motion and look for substitutional patterns, decreased mobility, and myofascial pain syndromes of this joint as a cause of abnormal shoulder biomechanics.
- The deltoid and other large muscles surrounding the shoulder often create substantial subluxing shear forces across the glenohumeral joint in addition to their purposeful actions. This is a common cause of impingement syndromes.
- The supraspinatus and infraspinatus are the two key muscles that counter the shear force of the deltoid by maintaining joint compressions, and thereby the center of rotation.
- Along with the infraspinatus, the teres minor acts to offset the upward displacement caused by the initial deltoid action. Therefore, selective strengthening of these muscles may significantly increase a downward pulling force of the humerus and reduce impingement forces in the subacromial space.
- Injuries to the cervical spine, nerve roots, brachial plexus, and peripheral nerves of the upper extremity are often overlooked in shoulder injuries. Nerve entrapment or a chronic radiculopathy can cause weaknesses in any one of the key muscles of the shoulder and alter joint biomechanics and performance. Undiagnosed nerve injuries frequently cause delayed or unsuccessful rehabilitation. Electromyography (EMG) can be helpful in delineating these problems.
- Always ensure that proper form and motion are encoded in the engrams before working on increasing speed and delivery. This requires paying attention to strength, flexibility, and timely motion of the trunk and lower extremities.

- Conditioning should continue throughout the competitive season, including strengthening and flexibility.

The protocol for treating anterior dislocations of the glenohumeral joint and injuries to the rotator cuff is given next.

Rehabilitation Guidelines Following Anterior Dislocation of the Glenohumeral Joint

1. Immediately after an acute anterior dislocation of the shoulder, the joint should be reduced.
2. Place ice over the entire shoulder for 30 minutes every 2 to 3 hours while awake for the first 48 hours.
3. Analgesic or anti-inflammatory medications may be helpful and should be started immediately if there are no contraindications.
4. The arm should be placed in a sling in an internally rotated position with the elbow flexed at 90 degrees for comfort. It can be further immobilized by placing an ace wrap or swathe around the arm and trunk (see Figure 35.7).
5. The injured extremity should remain immobilized in a sling for a minimum of 3 weeks.
6. One week postinjury, while still in a sling, begin
   - isometric hand-grips or squeezing of a tennis ball
   - forearm ROM
   - isometric adduction and internal rotation
   - **external rotation and abduction are to be avoided**
   - begin aerobic conditioning with stationary bicycling
7. Three weeks postinjury, while out of the sling, begin
   - Codman's pendulum exercises
   - isometric internal rotation
   - finger-climbing
   - shoulder-shrugs and retraction
8. Four weeks postinjury, begin
   - evaluation of the shoulder muscle weakness and prescription for home strengthening exercises using surgical tubing (see Figure 35.8(a–c))

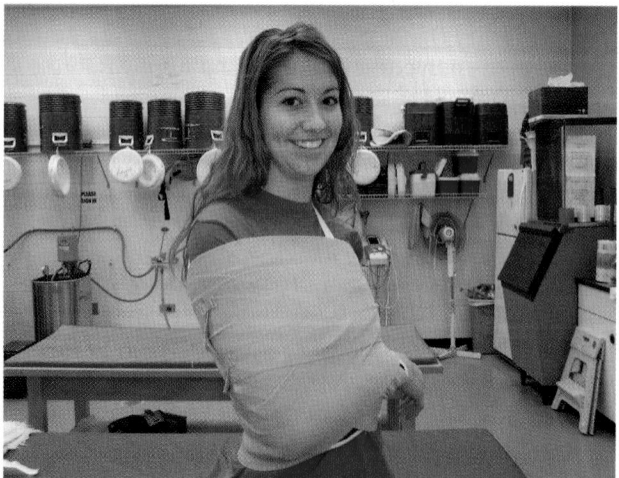

Figure 35.7 Immobilization of the acutely injured shoulder using an ace wrap.

9. Four to five weeks postinjury
   - external rotation exercises may be begun with light resistant surgical tubing
   - complete isokinetic program should be started to include strengthening of all muscles about the shoulder, particularly muscles of internal rotation and adduction
   - if an isokinetic machine is unavailable, simply advance the surgical tubing program by using heavier material, and increase the intensity and frequency of workouts
   - PNF should begin as long as there is pain-free ROM. This is the beginning of engram assembly
10. Nine to twelve weeks postinjury
    - isokinetic testing may be begun, comparing the uninjured shoulder to the injured shoulder
    - if 75% of strength is obtained, begin functional progressions, which could include progressive workouts on a swim bench, light throwing activities beginning with mirror throwing, then throwing a tennis ball at 10 ft, 20 ft, 30 ft, and so on, or in the case of hockey, an athlete might begin practicing wrist and slap shots at half speed. In addition, functional progressions may include medium and half speed workouts on an isokinetic machine. Make sure that substantial patterns do not occur and "contaminate" the encoded engram
    - advance functional progressions slowly until at least 90% strength is obtained in the injured shoulder compared to the uninjured side or preinjury data on the injured side. Advance throwing program to include light throwing at larger distances (100 ft or more), short tosses at half to three fourth the speed.
    - advance aerobic conditioning
    - return to competition once the final criteria of rehabilitation have been met
    - continue an active strengthening and stretching program after returning to competition

Rehabilitation Guidelines Following Rotator Cuff Injuries

The "pitcher's" or "swimmer's" shoulder often involves some type of injury to the rotator cuff. This could include a tear of the rotator cuff, tendonitis of one of the cuff tendons, a glenoid labrum tear, bursitis, or an impingement syndrome. Specific treatment depends on the exact nature and extent of the injury. Following the healing phase, rehabilitation should focus on balancing both strength and flexibility of the muscles around the shoulder girdle. An imbalance between these factors often leads to improper biomechanics and reinjury (42). A good understanding of the biomechanics of throwing is helpful in designing a rehabilitation protocol (80). Remember, the rotator cuff impingement syndrome may represent a spectrum of pathology ranging from rotator tears to bursitis and tendonitis.

Therefore, timetables for recovery may vary significantly, depending on the extent of the injury. Be sure your

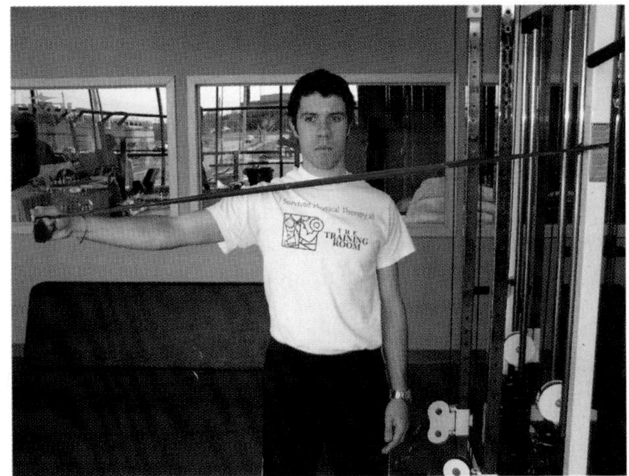
A

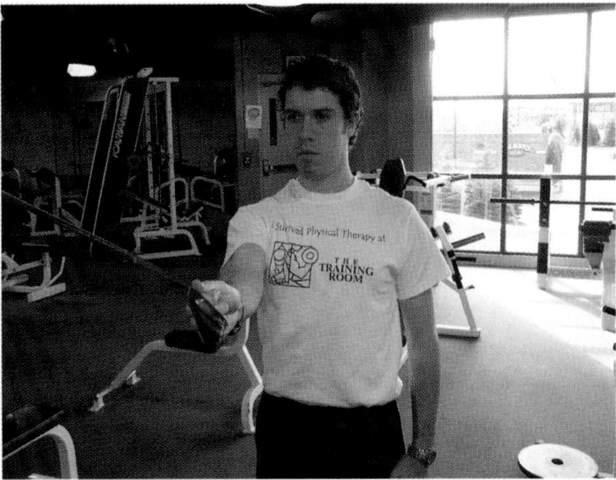
B

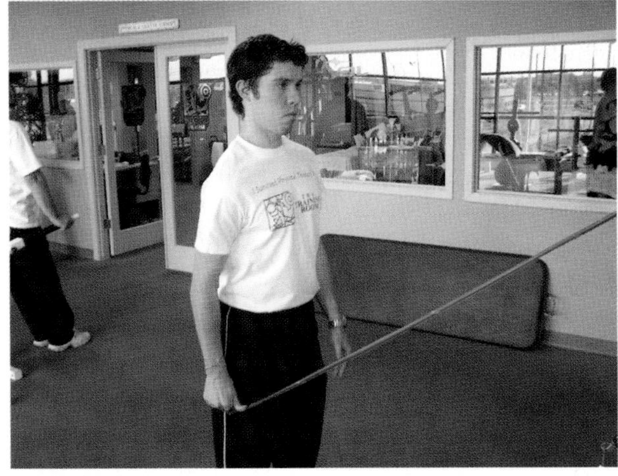
C

Figure 35.8 Shoulder strengthening exercises using surgical tubing attached to a post.

diagnosis is accurate and reassess it if recovery is prolonged or reinjury occurs.

The following list highlights some key points in the rehabilitation of rotator cuff injuries:

1. Sufficient rest should be ensured while tissue healing occurs.
2. Gentle ROM exercises must be carried out.
3. Analgesic or anti-inflammatory medications may be used to reduce swelling and to control pain.
4. Begin *isometric* strengthening within the first week, avoid excessive abduction, and external rotation.
5. Once pain-free ROM is established, begin PNF with emphasis on static stretching and diagonal movements of the shoulder.
6. Maximum flexibility in horizontal flexion, combined abduction, and external rotation should be established.
7. Dynamic strengthening should not begin until maximum flexibility and synchrony of motion is established. Dynamic strengthening can include physical tubing exercises, one to five pound weights or an isokinetic program. Frequent repetition with low weights or resistance is recommended initially. Particular attention should be directed toward the infraspinatus, teres minor, and subscapularis muscles (see Figures 35.9 and 35.10). These muscles act to create a downward pull on the humeral head, thereby increasing the suprahumeral space.
8. Improving muscle endurance, especially of the rotator cuff muscles, is critical. Therefore, high-speed isokinetic strengthening with low resistance should begin once the acute inflammatory stage is controlled.
9. Light throwing or swimming exercises can begin once a balance of strength and flexibility has been achieved.
10. Functional progression and initial engram encoding for throwing includes mirror throwing (slowly performing the act of throwing with a 1 lb weight in the hand while standing in front of a mirror). Advance to short distance throwing (starting by throwing with a tennis ball at 10 to 15 feet for no more than 10 minutes daily initially); long distance throwing can begin for 15 to 20 minutes at a time, and throwing distances should increase up to 120 feet.
11. Six to eight weeks postinjury, forearm pitching may be begun, allowing the athlete to begin throwing from the mound. Only the fast all should be thrown at first, and it should begin at half speed. Workouts

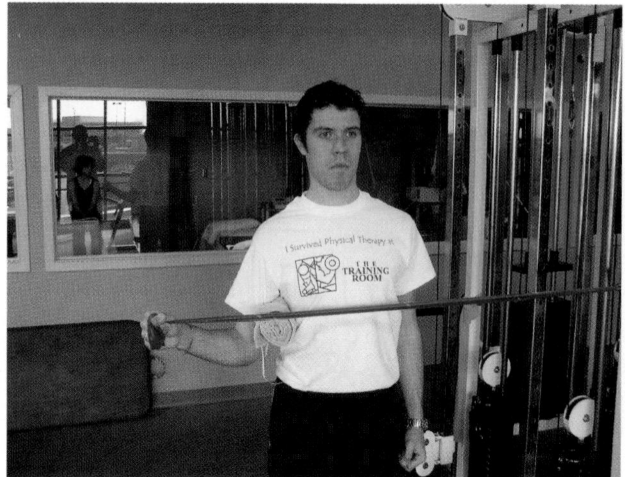

Figure 35.9 Strengthening of the infraspinatus and teres minor muscles using a resistance band. Placing a towel between the arm and chest wall will assist in maintaining proper technique.

should not last longer than 30 minutes initially. Functional progression should be done in stages, with maximum velocity and breaking balls gradually introduced toward the end of this phase.

12. Once the criteria for return to competition have been met, conditioning must continue with emphasis on maintaining flexibility and balanced strength of the rotator cuff muscles. Additionally, all throwing athletes should be on a regular off-season program to avoid injury or reinjury.
13. For swimmers, functional progressions are designed using the swim bench, beginning short distance swimming with a variety of strokes, progressing to use hand paddles for increased resistance, and finally increasing the duration and intensity of the workouts. As with the throwing athletes, swimmers must maintain a balance of strength and flexibility in the shoulder both during the season and off season. Excessive buildup of strength at the expense of flexibility may actually predispose swimmers and throwing athletes to rotator cuff injuries.

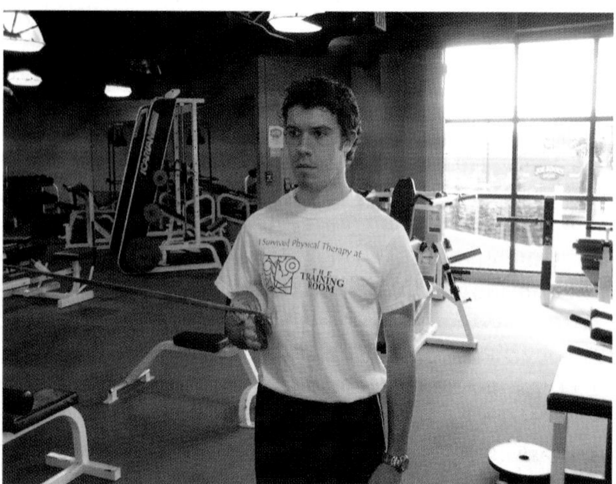

Figure 35.10 Strengthening of the subscapularis muscle using a resistance band.

Guidelines for Rehabilitation of Spine Injuries

Injuries to the spine are among the most difficult problems encountered by physicians. A central theme that has been emphasized here is that successful treatment is contingent upon accurate diagnosis.

Several articles have discussed traumatic injuries in the athletic settings, which result in vertebral fractures and dislocations (22,36,94,116–118). Torg's pioneering work has set out the biomechanical factors associated with traumatic cervical spine injuries and subsequent spinal cord damage (36,94,117,118). Because of these and other studies, the National Collegiate Athletic association (NCAA) and American High School Athletic Association adopted changes in rules in 1976, which outlawed spearing or using the head as a weapon during tackling. The result was that the incidence of quadriplegia from football injuries dropped from 28 in 1975 to five in 1984 (36,94,117,118). This data is based on approximately 1.75 million high school and college athletes participating in football on an annual basis.

Most spine injuries do not involve vertebral fractures or dislocation. Most of these injuries fall into a broad, nebulous diagnostic subset of soft-tissue injuries. Establishing a specific diagnosis on the basis of clear-cut pathological entities that cause pain and spinal dysfunction is a very difficult task. Table 35.11 outlines diagnostic categories of traumatic and overuse lumbar spine injuries encountered in sports.

Everyday static and dynamic functions of the spine are still somewhat mysterious, and some of the basic principles of spine biomechanics are not fully understood (22,36,94, 116–119). Therefore, injuries to the spine, particularly those in which repetitive motion is involved in sports-specific tasks, can be difficult to diagnose. A detailed discussion of spine anatomy biomechanics, differential diagnosis, diagnostic testing, and subsequent treatment is beyond the scope of this chapter, but there are many excellent sources in the literature (22,32,36,38,50,56,79, 92,94,116–125).

Because lumbar spine soft-tissue injuries are so common in athletes participating in football, wrestling, shooting sports, gymnastics, and dance, a brief discussion of the general approach to these injuries is in order. First, it is important to use a methodical diagnostic approach to establish a precise diagnosis so that the rationale for subsequent treatment plans is optimal. Table 35.11 lists the diagnostic categories that provide a framework for handling complaints of low back pain. It is important to obtain a history of the onset, timing, mechanism of injury, and response to previous treatment.

"Shot-gunning" workups for spine injuries can be very costly. Computed tomography (CT) Scans, MRI Scans, EMGs, Somatosensory evoked potentials (SSEPs),

TABLE 35.11
DIAGNOSTIC CATEGORIES OF TRAUMATIC AND OVERUSE LUMBAR SPINE INJURIES IN SPORTS

- Vertebral fractures and/or dislocations
  - With spinal cord injury
  - Without spinal cord injury
- Facet joint syndromes
- Spondylolysis and spondylolisthesis
- Malalignment syndromes
  - Pelvic and SI joint dysfunction due to an imbalance of muscle strength and flexibility
  - Scoliosis, hyperlordosis
  - Leg length discrepancies
  - Scheuermann's disease
- Disogenic: with and without nerve root irritation
  - Herniation
  - Annular tear
  - Internal disc disruption syndrome
- Segmental instabilities
  - With nerve root irritation
  - Without nerve root irritation
- Soft tissue
  - Acute and chronic myofascial pain syndrome
  - Interspinous ligament disruption with and without segmental instability
- Stenosis: central and lateral
  - Congenital vs. acquired
  - Dynamic vs. static lesion

SI joint = sacroiliac joint

myelograms, and diagnostic blocks may be needed to pinpoint the diagnosis, but it is important to approach the diagnostic workup methodically. Decide about the tests that are cost-effective and appropriate under the circumstances.

Most lumbar spine injuries in sports settings involve acute and chronic overloading of the facet joints, acute and chronic stress injuries to the pars interarticulars resulting in spondylolysis and spondylolisthesis, and malalignment problems. These injuries are the most common because athletes are often in a hyperlordotic position with an increased lumbosacral angle (LSA). This causes significantly increased axial and torsional loads to be placed upon the facets and other posterior elements (121,123).

Rehabilitation of lumbar spine injuries often requires retraining the athlete to obtain a more neutral spine, both in static and dynamic posturing, and correcting the imbalances of strength and flexibility in the soft tissue associated with lumbar spine and pelvic support. Much of what we know about these two principles is the result of research on low back injuries in industrial settings (32,38,50,56,79,92,121–126). They are worth emphasizing from the standpoint of both prevention and rehabilitation. In the case of our college and high school athletes, we have included an exercise protocol specifically to address these two principles, both during in-season and off-season training programs.

The concept of obtaining a more neutral spine addresses the issue of decreasing hyperlordosis and thereby mitigating the increased loads placed on the posterior elements of the spine. It also addresses many of the malalignment issues and the critical interplay between the lumbar spine and pelvis in both static and dynamic posturing. The muscles and soft tissues that interact to provide support for the spine and pelvis can dramatically alter the posture of both the spine and its base of support, the pelvis. The goal is not to eliminate all lumbosacral lordosis: "neutral" spine is a relative term that must be determined on an individual basis.

An athlete with a relatively tight hip flexors could have an increased LSA, subsequent hyperlordosis, and increased loading of their facet joints, resulting in low back pain. In such an example, a primary goal would be to correct this malalignment through proper strengthening of the antagonists (hip extensor muscles) and increase the flexibility of the hip flexors. This decreases both the LSA and the lordosis and achieves a more neutral spine. This approach is a bit oversimplified, but it illustrates the concept of "neutral" spine. Several other supporting structures also would need to be assessed and included in the treatment plan.

Using the example mentioned here, once a more neutral posture is determined for the individual in a static setting, the concept of maintaining a neutral spine would be carried over to their dynamic sports movements during functional progressions and engram assembly. This would be accomplished by carefully monitoring slow repetitions of the movement and reinforcing proper techniques as progressions advanced.

This is the principle of engram programming. For example, let us assume that the athlete is a pitcher. Once he/she obtains a more neutral spine, he/she is taught to pitch using these same principles. By lowering his/her center of gravity during delivery (which requires quadriceps strengthening), using the abdominal muscles, hip extensors, and muscles of the back, he/she is taught to concentrate on maintaining balance and proper posture throughout the five phases of pitching. This type of training continues after the athlete returns to full competition and also during the off-season to prevent recurrent back injury.

A finely orchestrated interplay among several key muscles and soft tissue supports helps achieve a more neutral spine. Outlined in the subsequent text, and illustrated in Figure 35.11, is the basic protocol that we use for our athletes to prevent and treat back injuries.

Remember that successful treatment depends on an accurate diagnosis. "Soft-tissue strain" is a broad and nebulous diagnostic category. Avoid using this protocol in a cookbook manner for all athletic back injuries.

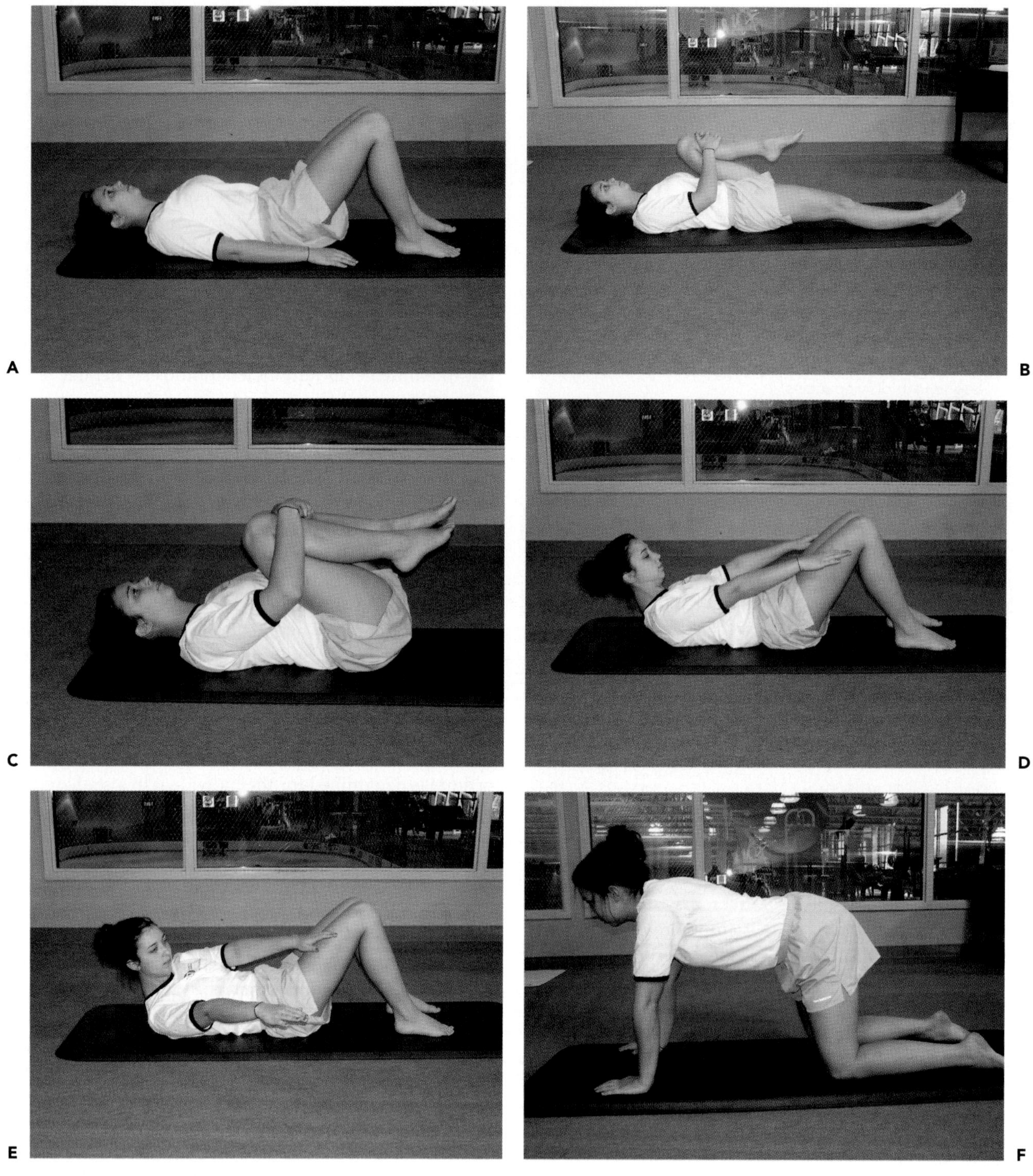

Figure 35.11 A: Pelvic tilt exercises for neutral spine training. B: Knee to chest exercises with one leg at a time. C: Knee to chest exercises with both knees flexed simultaneously. D: Partial sit-up position. E: Rotational sit-up position. F: Cat position of neutral spine training. G: Camel position. H: Trunk flexion in prone position. I and J: Trunk flexion in seated position. K: Prone extension position. L: Hamstring extension (Hurdler's position). M: Hamstring extension with knee extended. N: Quadricep stretching. To promote balance, this stretch can be performed without the use of a balance pole. Note the flat spine position. O: Hip flexor stretching position, note the flat spine position. P: Stretching of gastrocnemius muscles. Q: Stretching of the soleus muscle. R: Bridging exercise. S: Partial incline sit-ups with knees bent. T: Leg-raises that can be performed while hanging from elbows. U: Spine extensor strengthening exercise. V: Strengthening of the latissimus dorsi using weight machine; note the front pull-down position. W: Hip extensor strengthening using weight machine. X: Quadriceps strengthening using knee extension machine.

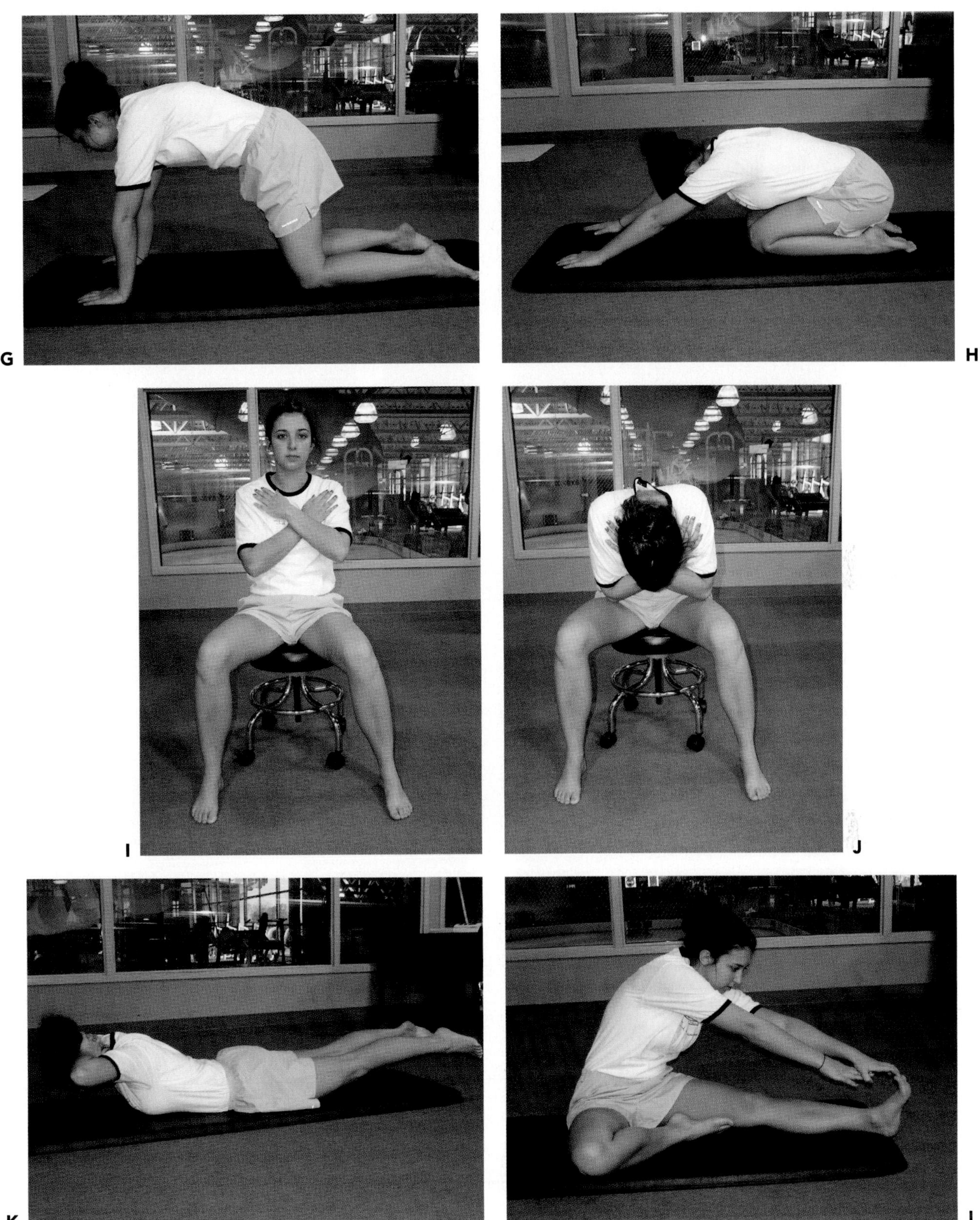

Figure 35.11 (*continued*)

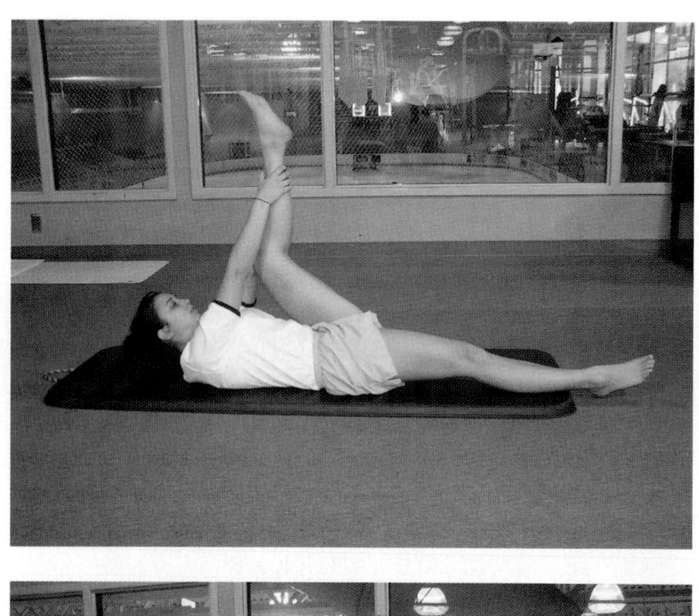
M

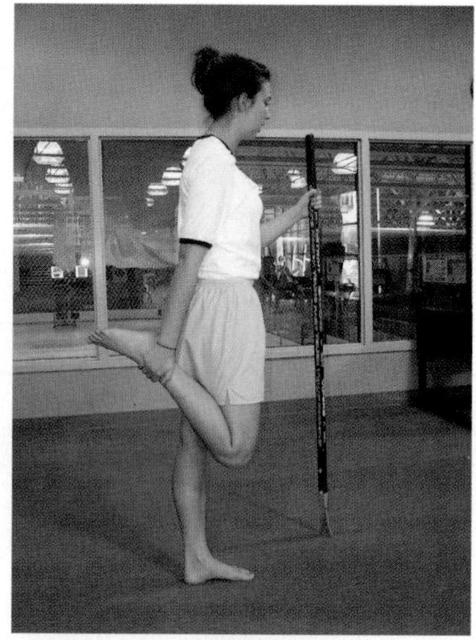
N

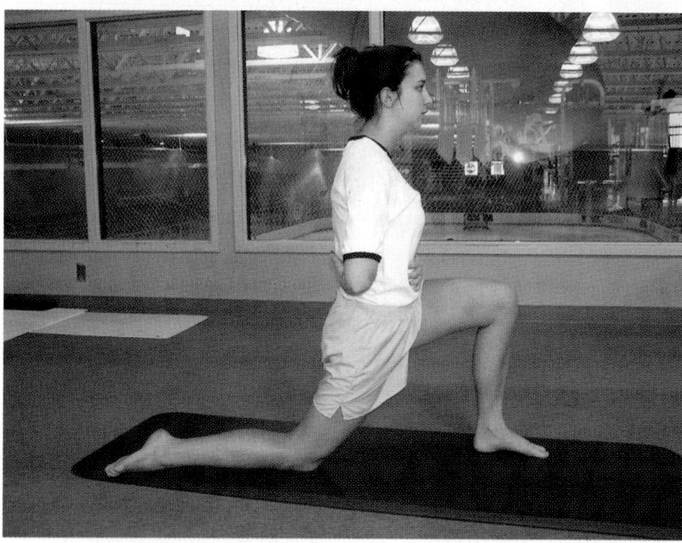
O

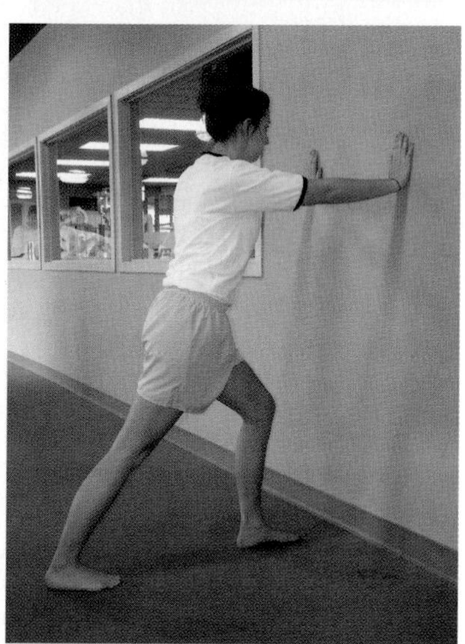
P

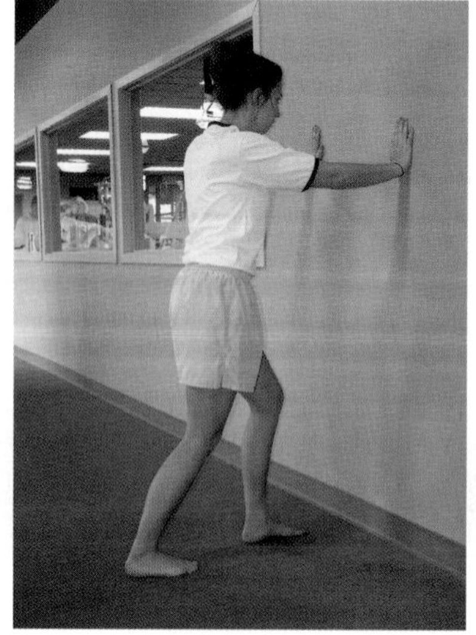
Q

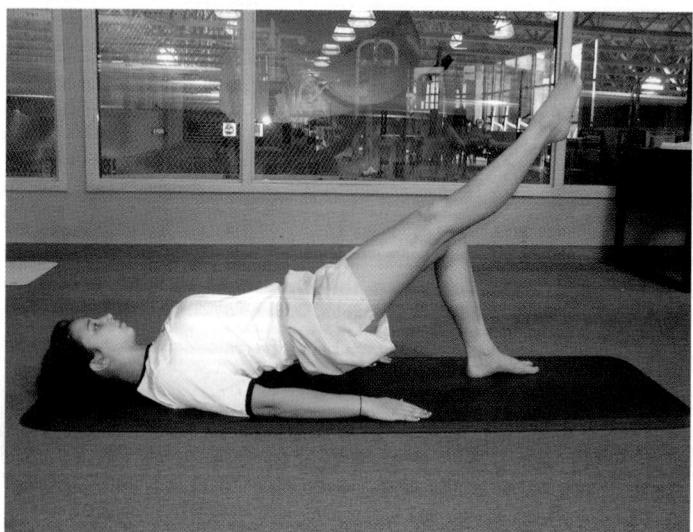
R

Figure 35.11 *(continued)*

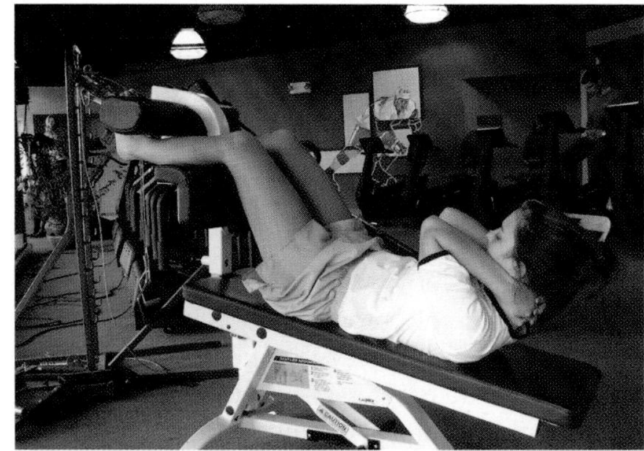

S

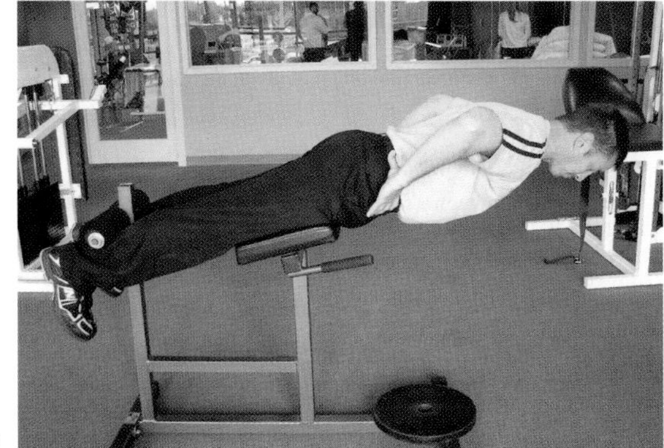

U

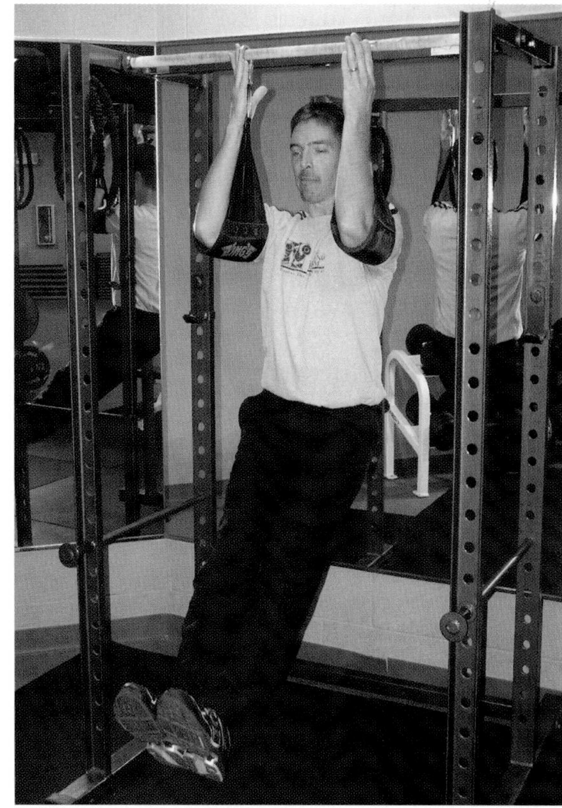

T

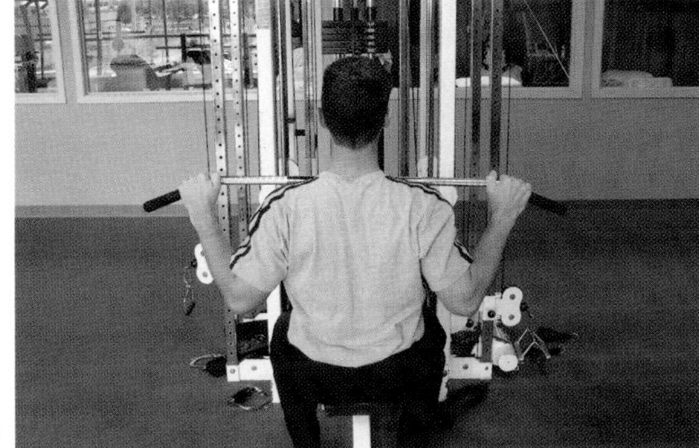

V

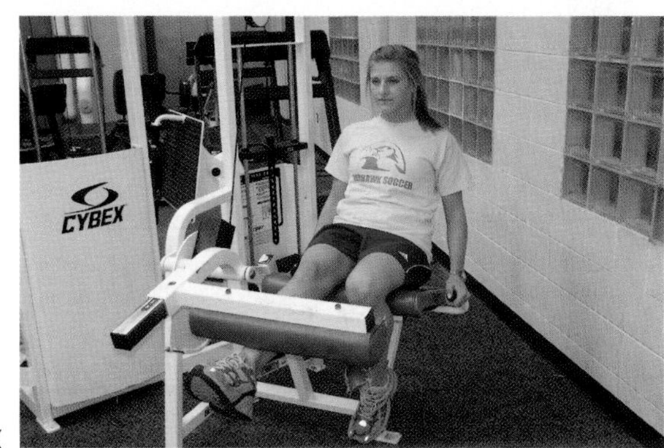

X

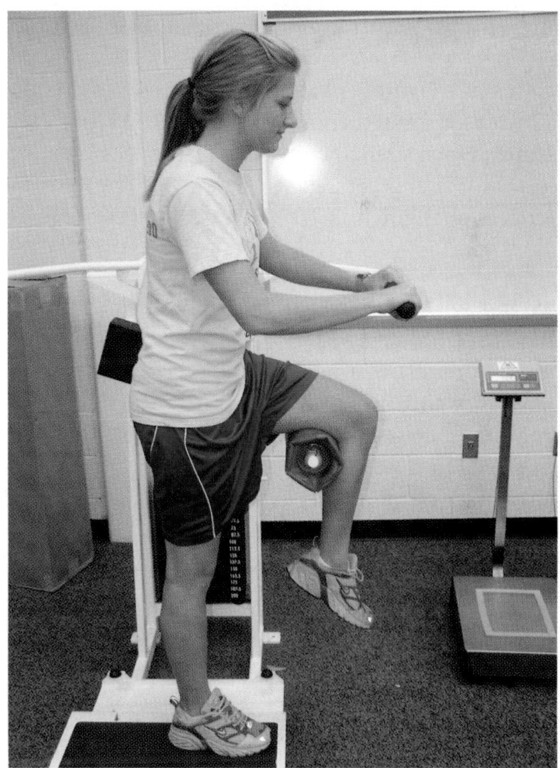

W

Figure 35.11 (*continued*)

Young, healthy appearing athletes can have significant underlying diseases. A methodical approach, with judicious use of diagnostic testing procedures, will lead to a precise diagnosis and help establish a rational approach to rehabilitation. Finally, all of the general principles of rehabilitation for controlling inflammation and pain, establishing relative rest but maintaining cardiovascular fitness, and so on, are a part of this protocol.

Guidelines for Rehabilitation of Lumbar Spine Injuries

Static Phase of Neutral Spine Training

1. Pelvic tilts (used as part of all the exercises shown in Figure 35.11, whenever possible) (see Figure 35.11(a))
2. Knee to chest (see Figure 35.11(b) and c)
3. Partial and rotational sit-ups (see Figure 35.11(d and e))
4. Cat and camel (see Figure 35.11(f and g))
5. Trunk flexion, prone and seated (see Figure 35.11(h, i, and j))
6. Prone extension (see Figure 35.11(k))
7. Hamstring stretching (see Figure 35.11(l, m))
8. Quadriceps stretching (see Figure 35.11(n))
9. Hip flexor stretching (see Figure 35.11(o))
10. Gastrocsoleus stretching (see Figure 35.11(p, q)
11. Bridging (see Figure 35.11(r))
12. Incline sit-ups, partial and rotational (see Figure 35.11(s))
13. Leg-raises (see Figure 35.11(t))
14. Spine extensor strengthening (see Figure 35.11(u))
15. Latissimus Dorsi strengthening (see Figure 35.11(v))
16. Hip extensor strengthening (see Figure 35.11(w))
17. Quadriceps strengthening (see Figure 35.11(x))

Dynamic Phase of Neutral Spine Training

1. Balance and agility training with neutral spine positioning (engram reinforcement)
2. Swimming (breaststroke and backstroke)
3. Stationary bicycling
4. Slow motion, sports-specific tasks once proper form has been achieved in slow motion
5. Advanced speed of sports-specific tasks once proper form has been achieved in slow motion
6. Full speed analysis of sports-specific tasks; videotape the activity if necessary

SUMMARY

We began this chapter with the question: "When will I be ready to play again?" We hope you are now ready to answer this question on a case-by-case basis. The key to successful rehabilitation is making a precise diagnosis. Once an accurate diagnosis is established, refer to a checklist of items (see Table 35.1) to review the principles of rehabilitation and to set up realistic guidelines for a given athlete.

Part of the job as a sports medicine physician is rehabilitation supervision, and it often becomes a difficult task. Even after a fine balance between relative rest and reconditioning is achieved, there may be outside pressures from the coaching staff, trainers, athletes, and parents to shorten the recovery period. A good working relationship among the sports staff is important, and a key ingredient in such a relationship is a consistent rehabilitation protocol that has measurable, progressive, and functional outcomes. With this framework, let everyone involved in the athlete's care observe the progresses or setbacks daily. A structured rehabilitation protocol removes the guesswork from the formula, enabling the athletes themselves to answer the question about rehabilitation.

REFERENCES

1. Einhorn TA. Enhancement of fracture healing. *J Bone Joint Surg Am* 1995;77:940–956.
2. Franklin B, Rubenfire M. Cardiac rehabilitation. *Clin J Sport Med* 1984;3:2.
3. Klatz RM, Goldman PM, Pinchunk BG, et al. The effects of gravity inversion procedures on systemic blood pressure, intraocular pressure, and central retinal arterial pressure. *J Am Osteopath Assoc* 1983;82:853–857.
4. Knight KL. *Cryotherapy in sports injury management*. Champaign, IL: Human Kinetics, 1995:3–12.
5. Bertolucci L. Introduction of anti-inflammatory drugs by iontophoresis: double-blind study. *J Orthop Sports Phys Ther* 1982;4:103–108.
6. McMaster W. Cryotherapy. *Phys Sportsmed* 1982;10(11):112–119.
7. Goodfellow J, Hyngerford DS, Zindel M. Patellofemoral joint mechanics and pathology: functional anatomy of the patellofemoral joint. *J Bone Joint Surg Br* 1976;58:287.
8. McKeag D, Brody H, Hough D. Medical ethics in sports. *Phys Sports* 1984;12(8):8, 145–150.
9. Hahn T. Corticosteriod-induced osteopenia. *Arch Intern Med* 1978;138: 882–885.
10. Guskiewicz KM, Riemann BL, Onate JA. Comparison of 3 methods of external support for management of acute lateral ankle sprains. *J Athl Train* 1999;34(1):5–10.
11. Knott M, Voss D. *Proprioceptive neuromuscular facilitation: patterns and techniques*. Harper & Row, 1985.
12. Brown S. Ankle edema and galvanic muscle stimulation. *Phys Sportsmed* 1980;8:79–86.
13. Kennedy JC, Baxter WR. The effects of local steroid injections on tendons. A biomechanical and microscopic correlative study. *Am J Sports Med* 1976;4:11–21.
14. Blinc A, Francis CW, Trudnowski JL, et al. Characterization of ultrasound-potentiated fibrolysis *in vitro*. *Blood* 1993;81:2636–2643.
15. Bunch RP, Bednarski K, Holland D, et al. Ankle joint support: a comparison of reusable lace-on braces with taping and wrapping. *Phys Sportsmed* 1985;13:59–62.
16. Cooper D, Fair J. Contrast baths and pressure treatment of ankle sprains. *Phys Sportsmed* 1977;5:51–55.
17. Jackson BA, Swane J, Starcher BC. Effect of ultrasound therapy on the repair of Achilles' tendon injuries in rats. *Med Sci Sports Exerc* 1991;23:171–176.
18. Jackson DW, Drez D Jr, eds. *The anterior cruciate deficient knee: new concepts in ligament repair*. St. Louis: CV Mosby, 1987.
19. Jokl P, Kaplan N, Stovell P, et al. Non-operative treatment of severe injuries to the medial and anterior cruciate ligaments of the knee. *J Bone Joint Surg* 1984;66A(5):741–744.
20. Lehmann JF, DeLateur BJ, Warren G, et al. Heating produced by ultrasound in bone and soft tissue. *Arch Phys Med Rehabil* 1993;17:247–251.
21. Ackerman G, Nolan C. Adrenocortical responsiveness after alternate-day corticosteroid therapy. *N Engl J Med* 1968;278(8), 405–409.
22. Knight K. The effects of hypothermia on inflammation and swelling. *Clin Sports Med* 1985;4(3):405–416.
23. Merrick MA. Secondary injury after musculoskeletal trauma; a review and update. *J Athl Train* 2002;37:209–217.
24. Ho SSW, Coel MN, Kagawa R, et al. The effects of ice on blood flow and bone metabolism in knees. *Am J Sports Med* 1994;22:537–540.
25. Knight KL, Londeree BR. Comparison of blood flow in the ankle of uninjured subjects during therapeutic applications of heat, cold, and exercise. *Med Sci Sports Exerc* 1908;12:76–80.
26. Rippe B, Grega GJ. Effects of isoprenaline and cooling on histamine-induced changes of capillary permeability in the rat hindquarter vascular bed. *Acta Physiol Scand* 1978;103:252–262.
27. Burks RT, Bean BG, Marcus R, et al. Analysis of athletic performance with prophylactic ankle devices. *Am J Sports Med* 1991;19:104–106.

28. Kennedy J, Alexander I, Hayes K. Nerve supply of the human knee and its functional importance. *Am J Sports Med* 1982;10:329–335.
29. Gracovetsky S, Farhan H. The optimum spine. *Spine* 1986;11(6):543–573.
30. Hayes BT, Merrick MA, Sandrey MA, et al. Three-Mhz ultrasound heats deeper into the tissues than originally theorized. *J Athl Train* 2004;39(3):230–234.
31. Higgins D, Kaminski TW. Contrast therapy does not cause fluctuations in human gastrocnemius intramuscular temperature. *J Athl Train* 1998;33(4):336–340.
32. Hong CZ, Shellock FG. Effects of a topically applied counterirritant (Eucalyptamint) on cutaneous blood flow and on skin and muscle temperature. *Am J Phys Med Rehabil* 1991;70:29–33.
33. Draper DO, Harris ST, Schulthies S, et al. Hot-pack and 1-Mhz ultrasound treatments have an additive effect on muscle temperature increase. *J Athl Train* 1998;33:21–42.
34. Duarte LR. The stimulation of bone growth by ultrasound. *Arch Orthop Trauma Surg* 1983;101:153–159.
35. Lehmann JF, DeLateur BJ, Silverman DR. Selective heating effects of ultrasound in human beings. *Arch Phys Med Rehabil* 1966;47:331–339.
36. Lehmann JF, DeLateur BJ, Stonebridge JB, et al. Therapeutic temperature distribution produced by ultrasound as modified by dosage and volume of tissue exposed. *Arch Phys Med Rehabil* 1967;48:662–666.
37. Draper DO, Sunderland S. Examination of the law of grotthus-draper: does ultrasound penetrate Subcutaneous fat in humans? *J Athl Train* 1993;28(3):246–250.
38. Francis SW, Onundarson PT, Carstensen EL, et al. Enhancement of fibrinolysis *in vitro*by ultrasound. *J Clin Invest* 1992;90:2063–2068.
39. Harpaz D, Chen X, Francis CW, et al. Ultrasound enhancement of thrombolysis and reperfusion *in vitro*. *J Am Coll Cardiol* 1993;21:1507–1511.
40. Higazi AA, Katz I, Mayer M, et al. The effect of ultrasonic irradiation and temperature on fibrinolytic activity *in vitro*. *Thromb Res* 1993;69:251–253.
41. Kornowski R, Metzler RS, Chernine A, et al. Does external ultrasound accelerate thrombolysis? Results from a rabbit model. *Circulation* 1994;89:339–344.
42. Kudo S. Thrombolysis with ultrasound effect. *Tokyo Jileikai Med J* 1989;104:1005–1012.
43. Lauer CG, Burge R, tang DB, et al. *Effect of ultrasound on tissue-type plasminogen activator-induced thrombolysis*. *Circulation* 2002;86:1257–1264.
44. Luo H, Steffen W, Crcek B, et al. Enhancement of thrombolysis by external ultrasound. *Am Heart J* 1993;125:1564–1569.
45. Nilsson AM, Odselius R, Roijer A, et al. Pro-and antifibrinolytic effects of ultrasound on streptokinase-induced thrombolysis. *Ultrasound Med Biol* 1995;21:833–840.
46. Noyes FR, Moar PA, Mathews DS, et al. The symptomatic anterior cruciate-deficient knee. *J Bone Joint Surg* 1983;65A:154.
47. Prentice WE. *Therapeutics modalities in sports medicine*, 2nd ed. St. Louis, MO: Time Mirror/Mosby, 1990:132.
48. Bly NN, McKenzie AL, West JM, et al. Low-dose ultrasound effects on wound healing: a controlled study with Yucatan pigs. *Arch Phys Med Rehabil* 1992;73:656–664.
49. Roche C, West J. A controlled trail investigating the effect of ultrasound on venous ulcers referred from general practitioners. *Physiotherapy* 1984;70:475–477.
50. Johns LD. Nonthermal effects of therapeutic ultrasound: the frequency resonance hypothesis. *J Athl Train* 2002;37(3):293–299.
51. Kitchen SS, Partridge CJ. A review of therapeutic ultrasound. *Clin Orthop* 1998;355(suppl):216–229.
52. Rubin D. Ultrasonic therapy: physiological basis and clinical application. *Calif Med* 1958;89:349–351.
53. Busse JW, Bhandari M, Kulkarni AV, et al. The effect of low-intensity pulsed ultrasound therapy on time to fracture healing: a meta-analysis. *Can Med Assoc J* 2002;166(4):437–441.
54. Draper DO, Prentice, WF. Therapeutic ultrasound. In: *Therapeutic modalities for allied health professionals*. New York: McGraw-Hill, 1998:263–309.
55. Draper DO, Sunderland S, Kirkendall DT, et al. A comparison of temperature rise in human calf muscles following application of underwater and topical gel ultrasound. *J Orthop Sports Phys Ther* 1993;17:247–251.
56. Heckman JD, Ryaby JP, McCabe J, et al. Acceleration of tibial fracture healing by non-invasive, low-intensity pulsed ultrasound. *J None Joint Surg Am* 1994;76:26–34.
57. Kahn J, ed. Ultrasound. In: *Principles and practice of electrotherapy*, 4th ed. New York: Churchill Livingstone, 2000:49–68.
58. Kristianstnsien TK, Ryaby JP, McCabe J, et al. Accelerated healing of distal radial fractures with the use of specific, low-intensity ultrasound: a multicenter, prospective, randomized, double blind, placebo-controlled study. *J Bone Joint Surg Am* 1997;79:961–973.
59. Binder A, Hodge G, Greenwood AM, et al. Is therapeutic ultrasound effective in treating soft tissue lesions? *Br Med J* 1986;290:512–514.
60. Laughman RK, Carr TA, Chao EY, et al. Three-dimensional kinematics of the taped ankle before and after exercise. *Am J Sports Med* 1980;8:425–431.
61. Abdenour TE, Saville WA, White RC, et al. The effect of ankle taping upon torque and range of motion. *Athl Train J Natl Athl Train Assoc* 1990;14:227–228.
62. Aronen J. Shoulder rehabilitation. *Clin J Sport Med* 1985;4(3):447–494.
63. Melzack R, Wall P. Pain mechanisms: a new theory. *Science* 1965;150:971.
64. Manfroy PP, Ashton-Miller JA, Wojtys EM. The effect of exercise, prewrap, and athletic tape on the maximal active and passive ankle resistance of ankle inversion. *Am J Sports Med* 1997;25:156–163.
65. Downey J, Darling R. *Physiological basis of rehabilitation medicine*. Philadelphia: WB Saunders, 1971.
66. Johnson D. *Phototherapy level 1: an introduction to light as a therapeutic modality*. Taylor, MI: SIR Video Concepts: D. Johnson, 2005–2006.
67. Glick J. The prevention and treatment of ankle injuries. *Am J Sports Med* 1976;4:4.
68. Gibney VP. Sprained ankle: a treatment that involves no loss of time, requires no crutches, and is not attended with an ultimate impairment of function. *N Y Med J* 1895;61:193–197.
69. Knight K. Guidelines for rehabilitation of sports injuries. *Athl Train* 1976;11(1):7.
70. Frank K. Clinical experience in 130 anterior cruciate ligament reconstructions. *Orthop Clin North Am* 1976;7:191–193.
71. Cabaud H, Chatty A, Gildengorin V, et al. Exercise effects on the strength of the rat anterior cruciate ligament. *Am J Sports Med* 1980;8:79–86.
72. Calabrese L, Rooney T. The use of nonsteroidal anti-inflammatory drugs in sports. *Phys Sportsmed* 1986;14(2):89–87.
73. Carson WG. Diagnosis of extensor mechanism disorders. *Clin Sports Med* 1985;4(2):231–245.
74. Greene TA, Wright CR. A comparative support evaluation of three ankle orthoses before, during, and after exercise. *J Orthop Sports Phys Ther* 1990;11:453–467.
75. Garrick JG, Requa RK. Role of external support in the prevention of ankle sprains. *Med Sci Sports* 1973;5:200–203.
76. Eldridge W. The importance of psychotherapy for athletic-related orthopedic injuries among adults. *Compr Psychiatry* 1983;24(3):271–277.
77. Akeson WH, Wo S, Amiel D, et al. Connective tissue response to immobility. *Clin Orthop* 1973;93:356–362.
78. Gehlsen GM, Pearson D, Bahamonde R. Ankle joint strength, total work, and ROM: comparison between prophylactic devices. *Athl Train J Natl Athl Train Assoc* 1991;26:62–63.
79. Hamill J, Knutzen KM, Bates Bt, et al. Evaluation of two ankle appliances using ground reaction force data. *J Orthop Sports Phys Ther* 1986;7:110–114.
80. Malina RM, Plagenz LB, Rarick GL. Effect of exercise upon the measurable supporting strength of cloth and tape ankle wraps. *Res Q Exerc Sport* 1963;34:158–165.
81. Rovere GD, Clark TJ, Yates CS, et al. Retrospective comparison of taping and ankle stabilizers in preventing ankle injuries. *Am J Sports Med* 1988;16:228–233.
82. DeLorme T. Restoration of muscle power by heavy resistance exercises. *J Bone Joint Surg* 1945;27:645.
83. Kirkaldy-Willis WH. *Managing low back pain*. New York: Churchill Livingstone, 1983.
84. Seitz CJ, Goldfuss AJ. The effect of taping and exercise on passive foot inversion and ankle plantar flexion. *Athl Train J Natl Athl Train Assoc* 1984;19:178–182.
85. Vaes P, Deboeck H, Handelberg F, et al. Comparative radiological study of the influence of ankle joint strapping and taping on ankle stability. *J Orthop Sports Phys Ther* 1985;7:110–114.
86. Fischer RD. The measured effect of taping, joint range of motion, and their interaction upon the production of isometric ankle torques. *Athl Train J Natl Athl Train Assoc* 1982;17:218–223.
87. Kozar B. Effects of ankle taping upon dynamic balance. *Athl Train* 1974;9:04.
88. Paris DL. The effect of the swede-o, new cross, and McDavid ankle braces and adhesive ankle taping on speed, balance, agility, and vertical jump. *J Athl Train* 1992;27:253–256.
89. Paris DL, Sullivan SJ. Isometric strength of rearfoot inversion and eversion in nonsupported, taped, and braced ankles assessed by a handheld dynamometer. *J Orthop Sports Phys Ther* 1992;15:229–235.
90. Morris HH, Musnicki W. The effect of taping on ankle mobility following moderate exercise. *J Sports Med* 1983;23:422–426.
91. Rarick GL, Bigley G, Karst R, et al. The measurable support of the ankle joint by conventional methods of taping. *J Bone Joint Surg Am* 1962;44A:1183–1191.
92. Alt W, Lohrer H, gollhofer A. Functional properties of adhesive ankle taping: neuromuscular and mechanical effects before and after exercise. *Foot Ankle Int* 1999;20:238–245.
93. Karlsson J. Andreasson, go. The effect of external ankle support in chronic lateral ankle stability. *Am J Sports Med* 1992;20:2570261.
94. Lohrer H, Alt W, Gollhofer A. Neuromuscular properties and functional aspects of taped ankles. *Am J Sports Med* 1999;27:69–75.
95. Pederson TS, Ricard MD, Merrill G, et al. The effects of spatting and ankle taping on inversion before and after exercise. *J Athl Train* 1997;32:29–33.
96. Wilkerson GB. Comparative biomechanical effects of the standard method of ankle taping and a taping method designed to enhance subtalar stability. *Am J Sports Med* 1991;19:588–595.
97. Kelley W. *Text book of rheumatology*, 2nd ed. WB Saunder, 1985.
98. Collins K, Storey M, Peterson K. Peroneal nerve palsy after cryotherapy. *Phys Sportsmed* 1986;14:105–108.

99. Griffin J, Karsellis T. *Physical agents for physical therapists*. Springfield, Ill: Charles C Thomas Publisher, 1978.
100. Huang H, Wolf SL, He J. Recent developments in biofeedback for neuromotor rehabilitation. *J Neuroeng Rehabil* 2006;3:11.
101. Myer GD, Ford KR, Hewett TE. Rationale and clinical techniques for anterior cruciate ligament injury prevention among female athletes. *J Athl Train* 2004;39:352–364.
102. Anderson B. *Stretching*. Bolinas, CA: Shelter Publications, 1980.
103. Clayton M, Miles J, Abdulla M. Experimental investigations of ligamentous healing. *Clin Orthop* 1968;61:146–153.
104. Delacerda FG. Effect of unwrap conditions on the supportive effectiveness of ankle strapping with tape. *J Sports Med Phys Fitness* 1978;18:77–81.
105. Dolan MD, Thornton RM, Fish DR, et al. Effects of cold water immersion on edema formation after blunt injury to the hand. *J Athl Train* 1997;32(3):233–237.
106. Duda N. Prevention and treatment of throwing-arm injuries. *Phy Sport Med* 1985;13(6):181–185.
107. Fumich RM, Ellison AE, Guerin GJ, et al. The measured effects of taping on combined foot and ankle motion before and after exercise. *Am J Sports Med* 1981;9:165–169.
108. Hadjiargyrou M, McLeod K, Ryaby JP, et al. Enhancement of fracture healing by low intensity ultrasound. *Clin Orthop* 1998;335(suppl):216–229.
109. Lehmann J. *Therapeutic heat and cold*, 3rd ed, Baltimore: Williams & Wilkins, 1982.
110. Mendel FC, Fish DR. New perspectives in edema control via electrical stimulation. *J Athl Train* 1993;28(1):63–74.
111. Hubbard TJ, Aronson SL, Denegar CR. Does cryotherapy hasten return to participation? A systematic review. *J Athl Train* 2004;39(1):88–94.
112. Jensen J, Conn R, Hazelrigg G, et al. The use of transcutaneous neurostimulation and isokinetic testing in arthroscopic knee surgery. *Am J Sports Med* 1985;13:27–32.
113. Kottke F, Pauley D, Ptak R. The rationale for prolonged stretching for correction of shortening of connective tissue. *Arch Phys Med Rehabil* 1966;47:345–352.
114. Paulos L, Noyes FR, Grood E, et al. Knee rehabilitation after anterior cruciate ligament reconstruction and repair. *Am J Sports Med* 1981;9:140–149.
115. Steadman JR. Rehabilitation of acute injuries in the anterior cruciate ligament. *Clin Orthop Rel Res* 1983;172:129–132.
116. LaRocca H, ed. Scientific approach to the assessment and management of activity-related spinal disorders—a monograph for physicians. *Spine* 1987;12:75.
117. Lehmann J, Warren C, Scham S. Therapeutic heat and cold. *Clin Orthop* 1974;99:207–245.
118. Lippitt AB. The facet joint and its role in spine pain. *Spine* 1984;9(7).
119. Denegar CR, Perrin DH. Effect of transcutaneous electrical nerve stimulation, cold, and a combination treatment on pain, decreased range of motion, and strength loss associated with delayed onset muscle soreness. *J Athl Train* 1992;27:200–206.
120. Bettencourt CM, Calstrom P, Brown SH, et al. Using work simulation to treat adults with back injuries. *Am J Occup Ther* 1986;40(1):12–18.
121. Brand RL, Black HM, Cox JS. The natural history of inadequately treated ankle sprains. *Am J Sports* 1977;5:248–249.
122. Calliet R. *Low back pain syndrome*, 3rd edi. Philadelphia: FA Davis Co, 1981.
123. Grant A. Massage with ice and treatment of painful conditions of the musculoskeletal system. *Arch Phys Med Rehabil* 1964;45:233–238.
124. Hopkins TJ, Ingersoll CD, Edwards J, et al. Cryotherapy and transcutaneous electric neuromuscular stimulation decrease arthrogenic muscle inhibition of the vastus medialis after knee joint effusion. *J Athl Train* 2001;37(1):25–31.
125. McKeag D. The primary care aspects of overuse syndromes in sports. *Prim Care* 1984;11(3):43–59.
126. Holden DL, Eggert AW, Butler JE. The non-operative treatment of Grade I and II medial collateral ligament injuries to the knee. *Am J Sports Med* 1983;11:340.

SUGGESTED READINGS

Mayer TG. Orthopedic conservation care: the functional restoration approach. *Spine: State Arts Rev* 1986;1(1).

Mayhew J, Riner W. Effects of ankle wrapping on motor performance. *Athl Train* 1974;9:27.

McArdle W, Kath F, Katch V. *Exercise physiology: energy nutrition, and human performance*. (Chapter 21) Lea & Febiger, 1981.

Messer J, Reitman D, Sack H, et al. Association of adrenocorticosteroid therapy and peptic ulcer disease. *N Engl J Med* 1983;309(1):41–47.

Moffett JA, Chase SM, Porteck BS, et al. A controlled prospective study to evaluate the effectiveness of a back school in the relief of chronic low back pain. *Spine* 1986;11(2):120–122.

Montgomery JB, Steadman JR. Rehabilitation of the injured knee. *Clin Sports Med* 1985;4(2):333–343.

Doyon J, Song AW, Karni A, et al. Experience-dependent changes in cerebellar contributions to motor sequence learning. *Proc Natl Acad Sci U S A* 2002;99(2):1017–1022.

Morrissey M, Brewster C, Shields C, et al. The effects of electrical stimulation on the quadriceps during post-operative knee immobilization. *Am J Sports Med* 1985;13(1):40–48.

Muller A. Influence of training and inactivity on muscle strength. *Arch Phys Med Rehabil* 1970;51:449–462.

Murphy R. The use and abuse of drugs in athletics. In: Scheider R, ed. *Sports injuries mechanisms, prevention and treatment*. Chapter 33. Williams & Wilkins, 1985.

Myburgh KH, Vaughan CL, Isaacs SK. The effects of ankle guards and taping on joint motion before, during, and after a squash match. *Am J sports Med* 1997;25:156–163.

Greipp J. Swimmer's shoulder: the influence of flexibility and weight training. *Sports Med* 1985;13(8):92–105.

Myrer JW, Draper DO, Durrant E. Contrast therapy and intramuscular temperature in the human leg. *J Athl Train* 1994;29:318–322.

Nachemson A. The influence of spinal movements on the lumbar intradiscal pressure and on the tensile stresses in the annulus fibrosis. *Acta Orthop Scand* 1963;33:183–207.

Nachemson A. Lumbar intradiscal pressure. *Acta Orthop Scand* 1960;(Supp 143):1–104.

Nachemson AL. The lumbar spine: an orthopedic challenged. *Spine* 1976;1:59.

Nideffer R. The injured athlete: psychological factors and treatment. *Orthop Clin North Am* 1983;14(2):373–385.

McIntyre DR, Smith MA, Denniston NL. The effectiveness of strapping techniques using prolonged dynamic exercise. *Athl Train J Natl Athl Train Assoc* 1983;18:52–55.

Noble J, Erat K. In defense of the meniscus. A prospective study of 200 meniscectomy patients. *J Bone Joint Surg Br* 1980;62-B(1):7–11.

Noyes F. Functional properties of knee ligaments and alterations induced by immobilization. A correlative biochemical and histological study in primates. *Clin Orthop* 1977;123:210–242.

Noyes F, Torvik PJ, Hyde WB, et al. Biomechanics of ligament failure II. An analysis of immobilization, exercise and reconditioning effects in primates. *J Bone Joint Surg Am* 1974;56A:1406–1418.

Holden D, Eggert A, Butler J. The non-operative treatment of grade I and II medial collateral ligament injuries to the knee. *Am J Sports Med* 1983;11(5):340–344.

Olsson SB, Johansson B, Nilsson AM, et al. Enhancement of thrombolysis by ultrasound. *Ultrasound Med Biol* 1994;20:375–382.

Owen BD. Posture, exercise can help prevent low back injuries. *Occup Health Safety* 1986;55(6):33–37.

Pappas A, Zawacki R, McCarthy C. Rehabilitation of the pitching shoulder. *Am J Sports Med* 1985;13(4):223–232.

Mattacola CG, Dwyer MK. Rehabilitation of the ankle after acute sprain or chronic instability. *J Athl Train* 2002;37:413–429.

Kottke F, Stillwell K, Lehmann J. *Krusen's handbook of physical medicine and rehabilitation*. 3rd ed. WB Saunders, 1982.

Cox J, Brand R. Evaluation and treatment of lateral ankle sprains. *Phys Sportsmed* 1977;5(6):51–55.

Perry J. Anatomy and biomechanics of the shoulder in throwing, swimming, gymnastics and tennis. *Clin Sports Med* 1983;2:247–270.

Potera C. Knee braces: questions raised about performances. *Phys Sportsmed* 1985;13(9).

Abeles M, Urman J, Rothfield N. Aseptic necrosis of bone in systemic lupus erythematosus. *Arch Intern Med* 1978;138(5):750–754.

Herring SA, et al. The effective use of rehabilitation modalities. In: *Functional rehabilitation of sports and musculoskeletal injuries* Aspen Publishers, 1998.

Prez D, Faust DC, Evans JP. Cryotherapy and nerve palsy. *Am J Sports Med* 1981;9:256–257.

Quillen W. An alternative management protocol for lateral ankle sprains. *Ortho Sports Phys Ther* 1981;2(4):187–190.

Quillen W. Phonophoresis: a review of the literature and technique. *Athl Train* 1980;15:109–110.

Rantanen J, Thorsson O, Wollmer P, et al. Effects of therapeutic ultrasound on the regeneration of skeletal myofibers after experimental muscle injury. *Am J Sports Med* 1999;27:54–59.

Rarick L. The measurable support of ankle joint by conventional methods of taping. *J Bone Joint Surg* 1962;44A:1183.

Brown FW, ed. *Symposium of the lumbar spine. American Academy of Orthopedic Surgeons*. St. Louis: Mosby, 1979.

Reher P, Elbeshir NL, Harvey W, et al. The stimulation of bone formation *in vitro* by therapeutic ultrasound. *Ultrasound Med Biol* 1997;23:1251–1258.

Reid D. Ankle injuries in sports. *Am J Sports Med* 1973;1:3.

Ricard MD, Sherwood SM, Schulthies SS, et al. Effects of tape and exercise on dynamic ankle inversion. *J Athl Train* 2000;35:31–37.

Markey K. Rehabilitation of the anterior cruciate deficient knee. *Clin Sports Med* 1985;4(3):513–526.

Rodnan GP, Schumacher HR, Zvaifler NS, eds. *Primer on the rheumatic diseases*. 8th ed. Arthritis Foundation, 1983.

Rogoff J. *Manipulation, traction and massages*. 2nd ed. Williams & Williams, 1980.

Rovere GD. Low back pain in athletes. *Phys Sportsmed* 1987;15(1):105–117.

Hecker B, Carron H, Schwartz D. Pulsed galvanic stimulation: effects of current frequency and polarity on blood flow in healthy subjects. *Arch Phys Med Rehabil* 1985;66(6):369–371.

Roy S, Irvin R. *Sports medicine prevention, evaluation, management and rehabilitation.* Chapter 8. Prentice-Hall, 1983.
Roy S, Irvin R. *Sports medicine prevention, evaluation, management and rehabilitation.* Prentice-Hall, 1983.
Giove T, Sayer J, Kent G, et al. Non-operative treatment of the torn anterior cruciate ligament. *J Bone Joint Surg* 1983;65A:184–192.
Ryan A. Ankle sprains, a roundtable. *Phys Sportsmed* 1986;14(2):101–118.
Salter RB, Hamilton SW, Wedge JH, et al. Clinical application of basic research on continuous passive motions for disorders of and injuries to synovial joints: a preliminary report. *J Ortho Res* 1984;1:325.
Sammarco J. Biomechanics of the ankle: surface velocity and instant center of rotation in the sagittal plane. *Am J Sports Med* 1977;5:6.
Deyo RA, ed. Occupational back pain. *Spine: State Art Rev* 1987;2(1).
Simon L, Mills J. Nonsteroidal anti-inflammatory drugs Part I. *N Engl J Med* 1980;302:1179–1185.
Simon L, Mills J. Nonsteroidal anti-inflammatory drugs Part II. *N Engl J Med* 1980;302:1327–1343.
Smith R. The dynamics in prevention of stress-induced burnout in athletics. *Prim Care* 1984;11(1):115–124.
Spencer CW, ed. Injuries to the spine. *Clin Sports Med* 1986;5:2.
Stanford B. The myth of electrical exercise. *Phys Sportsmed* 1983;11(12):144.
Stanish W, Rubinovich M, Kozey J, et al. The use of electricity of ligament and tendon repair. *Phys Sportsmed* 1985;13(8):109–116.
Sutter J. Rehabilitation of the knee following arthroscopic surgery. *Contemp Orthop* 1985;11(3):29–41.
Tipton C, Matthes R, Maynar J, et al. The influence of physical activity on ligaments and tendons. *Med Sci Sports* 1975;7(3):165–175.
Torg JS, ed. Head and neck injuries. *Clin Sports Med* 1987;6:1.
Torg JS, Quendenfeld TC, Burnstein A, et al. National football head and neck injury registry report on cervical quadriplegia: 1971–1975. *Am J Sports Med* 1977;7:127–132.
Torg JS, Quendenfeld TC, Theiler ER, et al. Collision with spring-loaded football tackling and blocking dummies. *JAMA* 1976;236:1270–1271.
Torg JS, Truex RC, Marshall J, et al. Spinal injury at the third and fourth cervical vertebrae from football. *J Bone Joint Surg* 1977;59A:1015–1019.
Travel J, Simons D. Myofascial pain and dysfunction. In: *The trigger pint manual.* Williams & Williams, 1983.
Unverferth LJ, Olix ML. The effect of local steroid injection on tendons. *J Sports Med* 1973;1:31–37.
Vaes P, DeBoeck H, Handleberg S, et al. Comparative radiologic study of the influence of ankle joint bandages on ankle stability. *Am J Sports Med* 1983;13:46–49.
DeLorme T, Watkins A. Techniques of progressive resistant exercise. *Arch Phys Med Rehabil* 1948;29:263.
White AH, ed. Failed back surgery syndrome. *Spine: State Art Rev* 1986;1(1).
Wilkerson G. External compression for controlling traumatic edema. *Phys Sportsmed* 1985;13(6):97–104.
Wilkerson GB. Biomechanical and neuromuscular effects of ankle taping and bracing. *J Athl Train* 2002;37:436–445.
Wilkerson G. Treatment of ankle sprains with external compressions and early mobilization. *Phys Sportsmed* 1985;13(6):83–90.
Matsen S, Krugmire R. The effect of externally applied pressure on post fracture swelling. *Clin Sports Med* 1985;4(3):513–526.
Wilson S, Cooke M. Double bandaging of sprained ankles. *Br Med J* 1998;317:1722–1723.
Zarins B, Andrews J, Carson W, eds. *Injuries to the throwing arm.* Philadelphia: WB Saunders Co, 1985.
Zarins B, Boyle J, Harris B. Knee rehabilitation following arthroscopic meniscectomy. *Clin Orthop Related Res* 1985;198:36–42.
Zimmerman M. Peripheral and central nervous mechanics of nociception, pain, and pain therapy: facts and hypotheses. In: Bonica J, ed. *Advances in pain research and therapy.* New York: Raven Press, 1979.

Sport Psychology

36

Christopher M. Carr

The field of sport and exercise psychology explores the relationship between psychological factors (e.g., cognition, affect) and optimal performance. Sport psychology is slowly becoming an integral aspect of the holistic care of the sports medicine patient. The sports medicine specialist should have some knowledge regarding the various facets of sport and performance psychology, as many of these skills are relevant to the care and management of an athletic population. For the purpose of this chapter, the areas of both "sport" and "performance" psychology will be discussed.

"Performance" Psychology is used in this chapter to represent the various environments under which mental skills enhancement can be useful. *"Sport" Psychology* represents the use of mental skills training within the sport and exercise domain. Many of the techniques utilized by elite athletes have had comparable successes with elite musicians, actors, and dancers. Therefore, the skills that are addressed in this chapter, although related in the sport environment, may be helpful for various forms of performance. The sports medicine professional can benefit his or her understanding of the diversity of performance issues and problems that may affect the patients by the material presented in this chapter.

Topics addressed in this chapter include a brief review of the history and current issues of sport psychology, a quick summary of "mental skills" training techniques, and a discussion of specific performance concerns related to the injured athlete. If a sports medicine professional is to establish a "holistic" philosophy of care, an understanding of underlying psychological processes along with a model of care, is necessary.

HISTORY AND CURRENT ISSUES

Sport psychology dates back to the turn of the twentieth century(Wiggins, 1984). The field of sport psychology is a relatively young discipline, yet it has a history unrealized by most. The historical path of sport psychology is patchy at best with roots in both applied and academic sport psychology, which are primarily housed in physical education/kinesiology. Rarely is "sport" psychology recognized as a specialty within psychology departments.

In the late 1800s and early 1900s, sport psychology had its beginning. It was Norman Triplett, who in 1897 conducted the first experiment in sport psychology by investigating the effect of cyclists on one another's performance. After finding that young children performed better on a rote motor task in the presence of other children, he concluded that cyclists would usually perform better in the presence of other cyclists. The results supported the hypothesis; when a cyclist performed with another cyclist on the track, they went faster than when they performed by themselves. Other studies taking place at about the same time include looking at motor behavior by exploring individual reaction times as well as how personality development was influenced by sport. However, none of these experiments and studies were directly applied to athletes or sporting realms (Wiggins, 1984).

Because the United States Olympic Committee (USOC) hired its first full-time sport psychologist in 1985, the applied realm of sport psychology has continued to grow tremendously (the USOC now has four full-time licensed psychologists representing its sport psychology services). Journals within the area of sport psychology were published and Division 47 (Exercise and Sport Psychology) in the American Psychological Association (APA) was established, for the first time in history recognizing the uniqueness offered to the field of psychology in sport. In addition, the first time that teams were accompanied by a sport psychologist was during the 1988 Olympic Games. Other advancements in the field included the establishment of the Association for the Advancement of Applied Sport Psychology (AAASP) in 1986 and the beginning of the Journal of Sport Psychology in 1979. In 1991, as a way to further advance this burgeoning field, the AAASP established criteria designating a "certified consultant" in the field of sport psychology to improve the clarity and understanding of a sport psychologist.

The applied realm of sport psychology has been growing rapidly in use and popularity during the 1990s. This use has not been limited to elite athletes such as those represented at the Olympic Games. Applied sport psychology is finding itself at the Olympic, professional, college, high school, and youth levels. Many well-known professional athletes in football, baseball, basketball, and golf have been sharing their beliefs in sport psychology as part of a performance, along with physical and technical skills, that makes a complete athlete. Some collegiate athletic departments now employ full-time psychologists for their student athletes. The amount of requests for sport psychology services at high school and elementary school levels and youth camps has grown tremendously in recent years.

Applied sport psychology covers all sports, not just those more visible, such as football, baseball, and basketball. Sport psychology is being utilized and sought after for race car drivers, as well as in mountain biking, rowing, soccer, and rifle and pistol shooting. Many physicians, attorneys, and corporate executives are requesting sport psychology principles be applied to the "performances" in their respective settings. The applied possibilities in performance psychology seem almost endless.

Although the field has come far in the last 10 years, especially in the area of applied sport psychology, it has not been without its controversies. Probably the largest debate in the field of sport psychology involves the question of what is a "sport psychologist" and who are able to identify themselves as such. Two primary groups identify themselves as sport psychologists, one from the academic side and the other from the applied side. The academicians and researchers in exercise and sport psychology and physical education are concerned with how an athlete can increase speed, motor control, and/or other physical capabilities to enhance performance. The sport psychologist in applied settings, on the other hand, has typically been concerned with the mental and emotional well-being of the athlete and utilizes psychological theory and concepts in the sport world.

In 1991, the AAASP identified requirements for being a "certified consultant" in the field of sport psychology as a step toward clarifying the training required to be a sport psychologist. Murphy (1995) summarizes the criteria as follows:

- A doctoral degree
- Knowledge of scientific and professional ethics and standards
- Three courses in sport psychology (graduate level preferred; advanced techniques)
- Courses in biomechanics or exercise physiology
- Courses in the historical, philosophical, social, or motor behavior bases of sport
- Course work in pathology and its assessment
- Training in counseling (e.g., coursework, supervised practice)
- Supervised experience with a qualified person in sport psychology
- Knowledge of skills and techniques in sport or exercise
- Courses in research design, statistics, and psychological assessment
- Knowledge of the biological bases of behavior
- Knowledge of the cognitive–affective bases of behavior
- Knowledge of the social bases of behavior
- Knowledge of individual behavior

MENTAL SKILLS IN SPORT

Many coaches and athletes attempt to put in a significant amount of physical practice to correct mistakes made during competition. Many times, however, the mistakes are due to mental breakdowns as opposed to physical or technical ones. In these cases the athlete needs to practice mental, not physical, skills. In the same way, physicians working in sports medicine facilities and/or with athletes sometimes forget or do not realize how mental skills can be used in their work.

Although coaches, athletes, and sports medicine physicians agree that more than 80% of the mistakes made in sport are mental, they still do not attempt to learn or teach mental skills that will assist athletes on the field or during rehabilitation. First, sports medicine physicians' lack of knowledge about mental skills prevents them from using them in their work with athletes. Although physicians may tell their athletes to "just relax" as they go through rehabilitation of an injury, they do not provide them with the knowledge of how to do so. Second, mental skills in sport are often viewed as part of an individual's personality and something that cannot be taught. Many physicians feel that injured athletes either have or do not have the mental toughness to progress through rehabilitation. Mental skills can be learned! Injured Olympic athletes report practicing mental training on a daily basis. Another reason why physicians working with athletes might neglect mental training is because of lack of time. However, these skills can not only be learned, but they do not require an excessive amount of time.

The following section briefly discusses some of the mental skills necessary for athletes to improve chances of optimal performance in their sports, whether on the field or in the training room. These skills are the basics and much more depth and detail, than this chapter allows, is needed to completely explain and understand the power of the mind in sport.

GOAL SETTING

Goal setting is one of the primary mental skills used by athletes. In fact, this skill is helpful and even necessary to develop other mental skills. Csikszentmihalyi (5) discusses goal-setting as one of the necessary components of achieving a "flow" experience. He describes "flow" as an experience in which a person achieves peak performance. Other terms used for this "flow" experience are "in the zone" and "playing unconscious."

It is not typically a problem to get athletes to identify goals. The difficulty comes in trying to help athletes set the right kind of goals—ones that provide direction, increase motivation, and guide them to achieving optimal performance. Athletes, and most people for that matter, do not need to be convinced that goals are important. They do, however, need instruction on setting *good* goals and a program that works to achieve them.

It is demonstrated in the empirical research that goal-setting can enhance recovery from injury. Research also demonstrates that certain types of goals are more effective in helping athletes achieve these goals. Several goal-setting principles have been identified that provide a strong base for building a solid goal-setting program (see Table 36.1).

1. *Set specific goals.* Research illustrates that setting **specific** goals produces higher levels of performance than planning no goals at all or setting goals that are too broad. Yet many times physicians tell athletes to "do their best" or "give everything you have" regarding their recovery. Although these goals are admirable, they are not specific and do not help athletes move toward optimal performance. Goal-setting needs to be **measurable** and stated in **behavioral** terms. Instead of an athlete setting his or her goal to "get better," sport medicine physicians can help these injured athletes set a more appropriate goal such as "increasing leg press weight by 25% over the next 2 weeks."
2. *Set realistic but challenging goals.* Goals should be challenging and difficult, yet attainable. Goals that are too easy do not present a challenge, and therefore, can lead to less than maximal effort. Goals that are too difficult may sometimes lead to failure, which results in frustration. This frustration leads to lower morale and motivation. In between these two extremes are challenging and realistic goals.

TABLE 36.1
GOAL-SETTING PRINCIPLES

1. Set specific goals
2. Set realistic but challenging goals
3. Set long- and short-term goals
4. Set performance goals
5. Write down goals
6. Develop goal-achievement strategies
7. Provide goal support
8. Evaluate goal achievement

3. *Set both long- and short-term goals.* Many times injured athletes discuss a long-term goal of returning to play after a serious injury. This goal is necessary and provides the final destination for the athletes. It is important, however, for physicians to help them focus on short-term goals as a way in which to attain long-term goals. For example, a physician can make certain that an injured athlete sets daily and weekly goals in the rehabilitation process. One way to employ this principle is to picture a staircase with the end or long-term goal at the top of the staircase, the present level of performance at the base of the stairs, and the short-term goals as the steps in between.
4. *Set performance goals.* It is important for sports medicine physicians to assist athletes in setting goals related to performance rather than outcomes (such as returning to play). Murphy (15) discusses "action goals" versus "result goals" being extremely important and often missed by physicians. With action-focused goals, athletes concentrate their energies on the "actions" of a task as opposed to the "outcome." Action goals give focus to the task on hand, are under the athlete's control, and produce confidence and concentration. Result-focused goals, however, are not productive and often lead to slower recovery. These types of goals give focus to irrelevant factors, things outside the control of the athlete, and tend to produce anxiety and tension. For example, if a collegiate tennis player is working back after a serious shoulder injury, physicians can help him or her by setting action goals, such as lifting a certain weight or obtaining a certain degree of flexibility that will lead to the outcome, full recovery.
5. *Write down goals.* Sport psychologists have recommended that goals be written down and placed where they can be easily seen on a daily basis. Athletes may choose to write them on index cards and place them in their locker, locker room, or bedroom. Many times physicians and athletes spend much time with goal-setting strategies only to see them end up discarded in some drawer. The manner in which goals are recorded is varied, but the important fact is that they remain visible and available to athletes on a daily basis. This type of goal-setting may be very effective in helping athletes identify recovery goals (e.g., degrees of flexion) early in their rehabilitation from athletic injury. For example, the physical therapist/athletic trainer could write down the athlete's rehabilitation goals for the week on a card and they could both review this card at the end of the week. If rehabilitation was successful in the short-term (weekly goals), such success should enhance an athlete's confidence and focus for recovery and eventual return to play.
6. *Develop goal achievement strategies.* This aspect of goal setting is often neglected, because goals are set without appropriate strategies to achieve them. An analogy to this faulty process is like taking a trip from San Diego to Buffalo without having a map. It will take one much longer to reach the final destination without a map. For example, physicians may encounter an athlete

with frequent flu-like symptoms. This athlete needs to employ appropriate strategies that will assist him or her in reducing the frequency of these symptoms, such as working on improving nutrition, sleep hygiene, stress management, and/or time management.

7. *Provide goal support.* Research in the sport psychology literature has demonstrated the vital importance that other significant people play in helping athletes achieve goals. In fact, it has been shown that exercise adherence is strongly affected by spousal support (6). Sports medicine physicians need to enlist the support and help of parents, faculty, friends, and others to help athletes focus on the actions required to achieve success (i.e., returning to play).
8. *Evaluate goal achievement.* Evaluating progress toward goals is one of the most important aspects of goal-setting, yet it is frequently overlooked. Injured athletes may spend considerable time in setting goals and devising programs, but it will be for naught if they do not regularly monitor their progress in achieving these goals. To draw an analogy from philosophy, just as an unexamined life in not worth living, unexamined goal-setting is not worth doing.

AROUSAL CONTROL

What is Arousal Control?

Have you ever watched the NCAA basketball finals and wondered how a player can make a free throw or last second shot with thousands of people screaming and millions of people watching on television? If you are like most, we wonder in amazement at how athletes are able to remain calm during such times of high pressure and anxiety. The fact is that these athletes **are** actually nervous. The skill they have developed is to utilize this anxiety as a way to perform their very best. Similarly, when athletes become injured, they typically experience much anxiety as well as physical pain and lose their place in the line-up, or are unable to perform something that has been a major part of their life for several years. Sports medicine physicians can help the athletes learn to utilize the anxiety surrounding their injury as a way to help them recover quicker.

The theories of arousal regulation are many. Some of the more common theories include (21) Inverted-U theory (7), Zone of Optimal Functioning (ZOF), the multidimensional theory of anxiety developed by Martins et al. (13), and catastrophe theory as proposed by Thom (1975) and mathematically applied by Hardy and Fazey (9).

AROUSAL REGULATION TECHNIQUES

Breathing

Perhaps the most simple and most important technique to regulating anxiety is breathing (10). It is common for athletes to take short, quick breaths when confronted with a stressful event or situation such as rehabilitating an injury. With such choppy breaths, the breathing system contracts and does not supply enough oxygen to the body, particularly the muscles. This action results in the muscles becoming tense and fatigued, both of which will prevent optimal performance in recovery. Taking slow, deep breaths allows athletes to supply their bodies with an adequate amount of oxygen that will assist them in better recovery.

Muscle Relaxation

One of the most potentially damaging aspects of anxiety for athletes is muscle tension (11). If an athlete's muscles are tense, he or she will not be able to perform the kinesthetic tasks required by their sport or rehabilitation process in a free-flowing and smooth manner. Therefore, for athletes to perform their best, they must learn to relax their muscles. If their muscles are not relaxed, the athlete's movements will be rigid, short, and tight.

How do athletes learn to relax their muscles? Edmund Jacobson's (1938) progressive relaxation technique laid the groundwork for most current relaxation procedures. His technique and other similar ones allow athletes to become aware of different muscle groups, how they hold tension in these areas, and also how to release this tension. Sports medicine physicians can be extremely helpful by teaching these athletes to perform this mental skill as a way of making their rehabilitation less painful and return to play more quickly.

ATTENTIONAL AND FOCUS SKILLS

Knowing *what* to focus on, and *when* to focus on it is essential for optimal athletic performance. Highly talented athletes often fail to achieve their best performance not because of lack of ability, but rather of an inability to focus on the "cues" that are necessary for optimal play. For example, a baseball pitcher may be able to throw an excellent 91 M.P.H. slider in his warm-up, but if he is unable to throw it in a game situation, he is not likely to have optimal performance.

Concentration skills can be enhanced through the use of mental skills, such as imagery, cognitive strategies, and attentional control strategies.

Imagery

What is the mystery in imagery that has helped elite athletes compete so well? There is no mystery at all. Imagery is a human capacity many people do not know about and/or have chosen not to use. It is a skill that very few athletes have developed to its full potential or realized its possible applications.

Imagery is a process by which sensory experiences are stored in memory and internally recalled and performed in the absence of external stimuli (Murphy, 1994). Imagery is more than visualization, more than just the sense of vision. To maximize its potential, imagery must be a multisensory event, involving as many of the senses as possible, including the sense of sound, touch, and movement.

Imagery has many uses for athletes, including regulating arousal level (3) and rehabilitation from injury (19). Imagery is useful for coping with pain and injury by speeding recovery as well as keeping athletic skills from deteriorating. It is difficult for athletes to go through an extended layoff, but instead of feeling sorry for themselves, they can imagine performing practice skills and thereby facilitate recovery.

Cognitive Strategies

Self-talk is one of several different cognitive strategies in sport. It occurs whenever an individual thinks, either internally or externally. Sport psychologists are concerned with the self-talk of athletes and how it influences their focus and concentration, arousal level, and performance. The preponderance of research supports the hypothesis that positive self-talk creates better or "no worse" performance.

Self-talk has a direct impact upon our emotional experience. If athletes are engaging in negative self-talk, their affective experience may be one of frustration, anger, or extreme anxiety. These emotional states will challenge breathing, increase muscle tension, and create a loss of concentration and focus, resulting in lower performance. However, if an athlete's self-talk is positive and relevant, the resulting emotional experience will be one of relaxation, calmness, and centeredness; as a result, the chances of good performance increase dramatically. Sports medicine physicians can assist athletes by teaching and discussing positive self-talk and the differences it can make to recovery.

Attentional Control Strategies

CONCENTRATION

Concentration is the ability to focus all of one's attention on the task at hand. For physicians and their athletes, concentration is being able to direct all attention to the recovery process. When athletes experience anxiety, however, maintaining attention on the task at hand becomes more difficult and concentration becomes narrow and internally directed toward worry, self-doubt, and other task-irrelevant thoughts (16).

Part of the definition of concentration involves paying attention to "relevant environmental cues". This ability to give one's full attention to only the relevant parts of a task is sometimes very difficult to do. Think about a football player recovering from a serious knee injury. What cues are relevant and what are irrelevant? Relevant cues include the rehabilitation process—keeping meetings with the physical therapist, good goal-setting, and following the physician's recommendations regarding treatment. Irrelevant cues, however, might include the thoughts of friends or the next opponent on the schedule. These cues have absolutely nothing to do with rehabilitation. The physical actions required to rehabilitate the knee do not change regardless of the next opponent.

Improving Concentration Skills

Physicians can be extremely beneficial in helping athletes maintain the concentration levels on the task at hand (i.e., rehabilitating an injury). First, sport physicians can remind the athletes that just as they are skilled to maintain focus in high-pressure situations (i.e., shooting free-throws to win a game), they can do this same thing in the recovery process.

Second, athletes can use cue words to help bring their full attention to the tasks in rehabilitation. For example, a tennis player recovering from an elbow injury might use the term *stay loose* as he or she lifts weights to strengthen the elbow or the word "breathe" to remind him or her that deep breathing will help relaxation during times of intense pain.

Research has demonstrated that routines can focus concentration and be extremely helpful in mental preparation (4,14,17). The mind can easily wander during rehabilitation. Injured athletes might worry about losing their position or the reactions of coaches and teammates. These are the times in which routines are ideal. For example, when an athlete is performing rehabilitation exercises, he or she might take a deep breath, imagine what he or she wants to do in the session, and then say one or two cues words to maintain this focus.

The importance of staying focused in the here and now cannot be overemphasized. Many times athletes get caught up in thinking about past injuries or what might happen to their position on the team after returning, causing them to lose focus on the relevant cues of the rehabilitation process at the present time.

In summary, to develop an effective mental skills plan, an athlete must incorporate the use of many specific and defined behavioral skills in a structured manner. This type of detailed skill development requires more than a "he just needs mental toughness" approach. Rather, it is a systematic plan of skills that are individualized to account for the athlete's age, skill level, sport-specific demands, and individual abilities.

PSYCHOLOGICAL FACTORS WITH ATHLETIC INJURY

An inevitable aspect of sports participation is the risk of athletic injury. Injuries ranging from lacerations to ligament sprains to fractured bones are an undeniable aspect of the sports world. Yet, to fully "treat" the injured athlete, what is done for his or her "psychological" (compared with "physical") recovery? For example, to inform a patient that he or she is to have an anterior cruciate ligament

(ACL) reconstruction that will require surgery followed by extensive rehabilitation before his/her return to play is one aspect of care. What if the injury occurs 2 weeks before a championship contest? What happens on the day before a national scouting combine where his/her individual talents will be assessed with the potential reward being millions of dollars? At this point, a significant emotional, mental, and behavioral dynamic will occur, which should be treated. A well-timed referral to a sport psychologist may enhance not only the emotional and mental recovery of the athlete, but also physical recovery.

The purpose of this brief section is to review some of the expected emotional, behavioral, and cognitive responses of the injured athletes. Heil (1993) presented a comprehensive text that addresses many of the psychological dynamics of the injured athlete. For purposes of this section, the following "stages" of response to athletic injury will be highlighted (Heil, 1993).

Point of Injury/Immediate Post-Injury

First, the most immediate emotional response at the point of injury is shock; the degree of shock may range from minor to significant, depending upon the severity of the injury. For example, an open fracture that is observed by the injured athlete may stimulate more of a shock response than a minor laceration. However, individual personality differences may impact the shock response. Second, there may be a pattern of emotional disorganization, where the individual may demonstrate atypical emotional responses to external or internal stimuli. For example, an injured athlete may become "giddy" on the sidelines during an examination. This response is an adaptive emotional response to a potentially traumatic event; it is a "normal" response to an abnormal event (injury trauma). Finally, the first denial response occurs, typically in an "I can't believe this happened" response. It is important to note that "denial" itself is an adaptive response that allows an individual to manage extreme emotional responses to situational stress.

As denial presents at the first stage of injury, it may resemble an attempt to recover. This may become an unrealistic expectation of recovery. For example, the athlete with a diagnosed ACL tear may tell an athletic trainer "I'll be ready to go next week"; in fact, the athlete may really believe this as truth during this stage. However, with little or no intervention, the reality of the injury will be confronted and the athlete will move to the second stage of response.

Treatment Decision and Implementation

This stage is filled with uncertainty for the athlete; lack of knowledge of medical treatments and potential rehabilitation may create excess anxiety. This "reactive" anxiety to the injury and treatment decision may become "anticipatory" anxiety as surgery dates get closer. These anxiety responses may be mild, moderate, or severe in regard to the disruption of daily functioning for the athlete. A psychological referral for even mild anxiety may facilitate more effective coping and response skills given the therapeutic relationship.

An additional factor to consider is the athlete's decision-making skills, as some athletes may not have a significant support system (e.g., parents) available at the time of making a decision about treatment. If surgery is required, and the athlete has no previous surgical experience, there will be an adaptive anxiety to manage the realities of anesthesia, pain, and physical restrictions. If the athlete is a collegiate student-athlete and far from home (e.g., cross country or foreign), there will be additional stressors due to the distance from their primary support network. It is often at this stage that a referral to a sport psychologist may best assist the athlete in their recovery. The athlete may be more open to support during this time of decision-making, and a psychologist can assist in not only the decision-making process, but for emotional support.

Early and Late Rehabilitative (Post-surgical)

Whether the intervention is surgical or non-surgical, there may be a series of emotional, behavioral, and cognitive responses, which follow the implementation of treatment. Primarily, there may be affective responses that appear "atypical" to the athlete's baseline behaviors. These emotional responses may be in the form of depression (acute), anger, confusion, and/or frustration. Again, individual differences will vary on the basis of the athlete's personality style, adaptive coping skills, and social (e.g., family) support network.

If there are delays in scheduled recovery times, or disruptions in the healing process (e.g., infection), anger or withdrawal may become the affective response. Although anger is a difficult emotion to manage, a nonbehavioral display of anger is an adaptive response. Because withdrawal is more "comfortable" for the health care provider, it may feel like an adaptation to injury; however, this withdrawal may exacerbate symptoms of depression, which may lead to further disruption in functioning.

Another factor to consider in the psychological rehabilitation of the injured athlete is social support networks. A team physician should be aware of the athlete's team "environment" during injury rehabilitation. If the environment is negative and punishing (athletes with some injuries are disregarded as "weak" or "faking"), the sports medicine personnel become more of a support network for the athlete. Make sure to educate coaches and hold them responsible for the behaviors of teammates attitudes/behaviors; however, it is primarily the coaching staff whose support is most needed (and often are most neglectful). The team physician and/or director of sports medicine should have a supportive process for informing, educating, communicating, and reinforcing an emotionally secure environment for the athlete to recover in.

Return to Play

This stage of injury rehabilitation often presents with the dynamics of fear and relief. These emotional responses may conflict with one another during what appears to be a desirable period for the athlete. . .returning to competition. Fear of reinjury and fear of being able to compete and perform are typical affective responses for the athlete. When discussed and identified as "normal" adaptations to the emotional demands of competition and recovery, many athletes move through this stage well. When the athlete ruminates or obsesses about his or her full recovery status, the feelings of fear may create inhibition in rehabilitation, or perhaps even questions about their abilities. If the athlete has been working with a psychologist, these emotional and cognitive beliefs will have been discussed and processed, so adaptive plans would be ongoing and implemented. If the athlete has had no opportunities to discuss emotional responses to the injury, these fears may create significant disruption to coping (e.g., compliance to rehabilitation decreases).

The use of mental imagery is often useful to facilitate the "relief" response and to visualize optimal performance in a healthy body. The use of imagery in injury healing, as well as return to play/action, can be an effective instrument in the psychological care of the injured athlete.

These "stages" of the injury process will display a variety of emotional (e.g., depression and anger), behavioral (e.g., rehabilitation non-compliance), and cognitive (e.g., negative beliefs about future performance) responses from any athlete. Although these responses may range from mild to severe, a psychological referral can be helpful in facilitating an adaptive processing of these psychological demands. The sports medicine professional who aspires to a "holistic" care of the athlete should have, or create, the appropriate referral network for the psychological health of the injured athlete. A psychologist can provide the supportive counseling/consultation to assist the athlete in his or her emotional and cognitive recovery from injury.

SPORT PSYCHOLOGY SERVICES WITHIN A SPORTS MEDICINE SETTING

A sports psychologist is an important component to any sports medicine team. His or her practice is devoted to the psychological care and consultation with the athletic population regardless of the level of competition (i.e., professional, elite amateur, collegiate, high school, and other youth athletes). Services are also provided for other elite-performance organizations, including the performing arts and the military.

Psychological services provided include individual and group counseling (private practice), which may be third-party reimbursable for diagnostic conditions (e.g., injured athletes with mood disorders). Often, the psychologist works in collaboration with primary care sports medicine physicians with medication management and counseling to provide the optimal level of care for some mood and anxiety disorders. Other individual consultations may include performance-enhancement counseling, which utilizes psychological skills to enhance athletic performance (e.g., imagery skills for golf). Although many of these consultations do not treat a specific Diagnostic and Statistical Manual of Mental Disorders, fourth edition (DSM - IV) diagnosis, the development of cognitive and behavioral skills to enhance composure, confidence, and focus are desirable by many elite-level performers.

A staff psychologist may also provide consultation with sports organizations, and address both personal and performance counseling issues. Additionally, educational and consultation work with coaching staffs, sports medicine staffs, and administrative staffs can enhance the development of optimal skills within the athletic environment. This "positive" psychology orientation also leads to lectures and workshops in the surrounding community, including work in educational systems, medical systems, and youth sport organizations. The role of a licensed psychologist with sport psychology training/experience is an invaluable adjunct to a comprehensive sports medicine staff. The need and demand for services continue to develop as athletes and other elite performers seek to gain the "mental edge" in their competitive venues.

SUMMARY

This chapter has briefly highlighted the area of sport psychology as it relates to performance psychology skills (mental training); these skills may be of interest to the practicing sports medicine professional. The issues related to the psychological rehabilitation of the injured athlete are of obvious importance to sports medicine staff; the overview of affective responses will assist in understanding the normal and adaptive responses of the injured athlete. Finally, a brief description of a psychologist's role within a sports medicine practice is presented.

The psychological issues that are present in the world of sport and elite performance are numerous, and not all are mentioned in this chapter. Issues of eating disorders, substance abuse, and psychological health with athletes should be explored by the sports medicine professional. This chapter may provide a brief introduction to the growing field of applied psychology within sports medicine.

REFERENCES

1. Botterill C. Goal setting for athletes with examples from hockey. In: Martin GL, Hrycaik D, eds. *Behavior modification and coaching: principles, procedures, and research*. Springfield: Charles C Thomas Publisher, 1983.
2. Carr C, Kays T. Survey of Ohio State Athletics; 1997.
3. Caudill D, Weinberg R, Jackson A. Psyching-up and track athletes. A preliminary investigation. *J Sport Psychol* 1983;5:231–235.
4. Cohn PJ, Rotella RJ, Lloyd JW. Effects of a cognitive behavioral intervention on the preshot routine and performance in golf. *Sport Psychol* 1990;4:33–47.
5. Csikszentmihalyi M. Flow. 1990.
6. Dishman RK, ed. *Exercise adherence: its impact on public health*. Champaign: Human Kinetics, 1988.

7. Hanin YL. A study of anxiety in sport. In: Straub WF, ed. *Sport psychology: an analysis of athlete behavior*. Ithaca: Mouvement, 1980.
8. Hardy CV, Richman JM, Rosenfeld LB. The role of social support in the life stress/injury relationship. *Sport Psychol* 1993;5:128–139.
9. Hardy, L, Fazey J. The inverted U-hypothesis: a catastrophe for sport psychology. *Paper presented at the annual meetings of the North American society for the psychology of sport and physical activity*. Vancouver, British Columbia, Canada, 1987.
10. Harris, DV. Relaxation and energizing techniques for regulation of arousal. In: Williams JM, ed. *Applied sport psychology: personal growth to peak performance*. Palo Alto: Mayfield, 1986.
11. Landers DM, Boutcher SH. Arousal-performance relationships. In: Williams JM, ed. *Applied sport psychology: personal growth to peak performance*. Palo Alto: Mayfield, 1986.
12. Locke EA, Latham GP. *A theory of goal setting and task performance*. Englewood Cliffs: Prentice Hall, 1990.
13. Martins R, Vealy RS, Burton D. *Competitive anxiety in sport*. Champaign: Human Kinetics, 1990.
14. Moore WE. Covert-overt service routines. The effects of a service routine training program on elite tennis players. Unpublished Doctoral Dissertation. University of Virginia, 1986.
15. Murphy S. *The achievement zone*. New York: GP Putnam's Sons, 1996.
16. Nideffer, RM. Concentration and attentional control training. In: Williams JM, ed. *Applied sport psychology: personal growth to peak performance*. Palo Alto: Mayfield, 1993.
17. Orlick T. *Psyching for sport: mental training for athletes*. Champaign: Leisure Press, 1986.
18. Van Raalte J, Brewer B. *Exploring sport and exercise psychology*. Washington: American Psychological Association, 1996.
19. Weinberg RS, Gould D. *Foundations of sport and exercise psychology*. Champaign: Human Kinetics, 1995.
20. Weinberg RS, Weigand D. Goal setting in sport and exercise: a reaction to locke. *J Sport Exerc Psychol* 15:88–95.
21. Yerkes RM, Dodson JD. The relation of strength and stimulus to rapidity of habit formation. *J Comp Neurol Psychol* 1908;18:459–482.

Drug Use

37

Richard T. Ferro

In the present society, use of ergogenic substances to enhance athletic performance is not just for those athletes involved in professional or Olympic sport. The 1994 deregulation of over-the-counter (OTC) "supplement" sales allowed pharmaceutical manufacturers and supplement companies to sell potentially harmful drugs without stringent U.S. Food and Drug Administration (FDA) safety and efficacy trials (1). As long as a company does not claim "to diagnose, prevent, mitigate, treat, or cure a specific disease" on the label of the supplement, the products are allowed to be sold OTC to individuals of all ages, including the adolescent population (1). In fact, anabolic agents including testosterone precursors, stimulants, and a plethora of products claiming to enhance size and strength, to decrease body fat, and to increase energy and sports performance are available by phone, over the Internet and OTC. Even prescription medications such as anabolic androgenic steroids (AAS), insulin, human growth hormone (hGH), and Epogen are easily obtainable without a prescription through numerous Internet companies that are willing to ship these products directly to your home.

Although the use of ergogenic substances is by no means a modern phenomenon, never before have they been so readily available and used by so many recreational athletes and young people. Supplements such as the testosterone precursors (dehydroepiandrosterone, androstenedione, and androstenediols), ephedrine derivatives, and countless combination "stacking" products of these potentially dangerous substances are placed in the hands of anyone willing to pay for them. The fact that many of these products are less expensive than they have been in the past compounds the problem. Despite dangerous side effects and numerous deaths linked with the use of these products, they are becoming more popular. Recently there has been a rash of highly publicized deaths of prominent athletes that were suspected to be due to the use of OTC ergogenic aids. Nonetheless, for some athletes, the potentially hazardous or fatal side effects of using ergogenic aids are a risk they are willing to take. In general, the line between illicit ergogenic aids and OTC supplements has been greatly distorted by all those hoping to profit from their sale, from the athletes who take a win-at-any-price attitude by using these substances to the drug manufacturers who want to make as much money as possible.

To help us better delineate and more easily understand this fine line, the International Olympic Committee (IOC) defined the use of ergogenic aids or "doping" in 1968. The IOC's action was in direct response to a number of deaths of prominent athletes using performance-enhancing substances, and the political outcry for control of such practices at that time. They defined the illegal use of ergogenic aids or "doping" as "the administration to, or the use by, a competing athlete of any substance foreign to the body or any physiological substance taken in abnormal quantity or by an abnormal route of entry into the body, with the sole intention of increasing in an artificial and unfair manner his performance in competition" (2). In light of this definition, it is quite obvious that most of the current day OTC supplements, including creatine monohydrate, fit the IOC's definition of a doping agent.

We live in an age where health care workers and physicians of all specialties need to be knowledgeable about supplements because of the potentially harmful or fatal side effects, as well as possible interactions with prescription medications. As a health care professional, whether a team physician, a primary care physician, an athletic trainer, a nurse, or a nutritionist, one must be qualified to discuss the possible benefits, as well as the potential short- and long-term sequelae of using such performance-enhancing drugs. No longer can we think of the supplements that our athletes, patients, and children take as benign or "natural" in any manner.

In this chapter we will specifically review categories of pharmacological agents that are being used to enhance athletic performance, and will discuss relevant examples in each class. Furthermore, we will explore the use of ergogenic aids in our society, their mechanisms of action, possible benefits, and associated risks. We will use the drug classification system established by the IOC and currently used by the World Anti-Doping Agency (WADA), as a framework in which to examine these ergogenic substances.

STIMULANTS

Ever since the ancient Olympic games, athletes have used a variety of substances, including stimulants, in their quest for enhancement of athletic performance. These practices ranged from the ingestion of mushrooms, which contained muscarine, to the consumption of bread laced with opium (3,4). By the 1800s, the extensive use of ergogenic substances such as caffeine, nitroglycerin, amphetamines, strychnine, and ephedrine were being reported, making it obvious that a win-at-any-price attitude had been established in athletics long before the modem "professionalization" of sports (3–5).

This category of prohibited substances encompasses a variety of central nervous system (CNS) stimulants including amphetamines, caffeine, clenbuterol, cocaine, and the sympathomimetics (ephedrine and pseudoephedrine). Stimulants have been used by athletes for centuries to reduce fatigue, enhance aggression and competitiveness, suppress appetite, decrease sensitivity to pain, and increase alertness, response time, and strength (6–8). Stimulants were some of the first drugs studied and used as ergogenic aids in the modem era of athletics as well (9). Many of these banned drugs are available without a prescription. Whether purposefully or inadvertently used, studies have revealed that in drug tests, half of the athletes' positive results for stimulants were due to OTC drugs (10). Despite the emphasis the media has placed on steroid use among athletes, studies have shown that the prevalence of amphetamine use by college athletes was about twice that of anabolic steroids (11,12).

Amphetamines

Amphetamines were originally developed in 1920. Their vasoconstrictive properties allowed them to be initially used for the treatment of nasal congestion (7). Their emergence as performance enhancers occurred during World War II when German soldiers used amphetamines to delay fatigue and enhance their alertness while on patrol duty (13).

Amphetamines are structurally similar to endogenous catecholamines such as epinephrine, and are believed to enhance the release of neurotransmitters, especially norepinephrine (8). Therefore, much of their ergogenic effects are believed to be due to stimulation of the sympathetic nervous system. Peak plasma concentration is achieved very rapidly after intravenous administration of amphetamines, whereas the maximum concentration after oral ingestion usually occurs within 2 hours (14). Although the question of whether amphetamines truly enhance athletic performance is debated in the literature, the available studies and anecdotal reports strongly suggest that amphetamines are truly efficacious for their purported uses, especially in sports where speed, power, and endurance are essential (9,13,15–18). Available research reveals that the ergogenic effects are partially obtained through (a) prolonging the time to exhaustion, (b) increasing tolerance to strenuous exercise, (c) blunting pain perception and symptoms of fatigue, and (d) increasing aggression, which may increase the potential for injury in contact sports (19).

Many possible adverse side effects of amphetamine use are related to their effects on the CNS. Neurological symptoms and behavioral effects include restlessness, insomnia, anxiety, tremor, confusion, agitation, irritability, paranoia, hallucinations, increased aggressiveness, and a potential for psychological addiction (9,17). Cardiovascular complications include a lower threshold for arrhythmias, provocation of angina, hypertension, headaches, tachycardia, and palpitations. Adverse gastrointestinal side effects include abdominal pain, decreased appetite, and vomiting. Thermoregulatory disturbances may be caused by a decrease in the ability to sense the body's limitation, and thereby may lead to the increased incidence of (or predisposition to) heat illness, including heatstroke (7,9,20). An abrupt cessation of amphetamines can result in chronic fatigue, lethargy, and depression (6,21). There have even been case reports where excessive doses have led to convulsions, coma, strokes, and death; while long-term exposure to amphetamines has resulted in dyskinesias, compulsive behavior, and paranoid delusional states (7–9,13,19,22).

It was not until the death of Danish cyclist Kurt Enemar Jensen at the 1960 Summer Olympic Games in Rome that a considerable international anti-doping movement was initiated (23). Many were stunned by the fact that Jensen and two of his fellow teammates became ill after ingesting amphetamine and Roniacol (a cough syrup) for performance enhancement. Jensen ultimately died and his two teammates were admitted to an Italian hospital in critical condition. In another incident, Tommy Simpson, a notable British cyclist, died during the thirteenth day of the Tour de France in 1967. At the time of his death, a vial of amphetamines was found in his possession (24). The following year, amphetamine abuse was believed to play a major role in the deaths of yet another cyclist, Yves Mottin, as well as a soccer player, Jean-Louis Quadri (24). These incidents helped generate considerable anti-doping sentiment and began a cascade of significant worldwide anti-doping legislation. From that point forward, a gradual evolution in collective thinking also began; drug use for performance enhancement was no longer considered just a matter of personal choice. Instead, it became an unethical act that clearly carried significant health risks. It also directly induced others to use ergogenic substances in order to compete equitably (25,26).

Caffeine

Caffeine is undoubtedly the most widely consumed stimulant in the world. This is in part due to its widespread social use, and availability to people of all ages. It is present in many different types of beverages, including coffee, cola drinks, hot chocolate, and tea (6,27). It may also be the most widely abused drug in sports, as it is routinely consumed by most sports competitors (28). Caffeine is a methylxanthine derivative related to theophylline and theobromine, which occurs naturally in many species of plants and is found in cocoa, coffee beans, and tea leaves. It is also found in many prescription and nonprescription medications such as analgesics, and weight-loss and cold preparations (27). Approximately 80% of the adult population in the United States drinks coffee or tea on a daily basis. Furthermore, coffee accounts for 90% of the caffeine consumed in the United States, where an average of approximately 210 mg of caffeine/person/day is consumed (29).

After ingestion, caffeine reaches peak blood levels in approximately 30 to 60 minutes (8). It acts as a potent CNS stimulant, increasing arousal or level of consciousness, reducing fatigue, and decreasing motor reaction time when concentrations of 85 to 200 mg are consumed (7). Most believe the ergogenic dose is between 250 and 350 mg (8). Therefore, the IOC and the National Collegiate Athletic Association (NCAA) initially placed limits on caffeine ingestion. At present, caffeine is treated as a controlled substance by the NCAA. Certain amounts are tolerated because of its presence in commonly ingested beverages, but excessive amounts constitute grounds for disqualification (30). Before the formation of WADA, the IOC's acceptable urine concentration was up to 12 μg/mL, whereas the NCAA's is currently up to 15 μg/mL. To reach these levels, most athletes would have to drink six to eight cups of coffee in one sitting (approximately 600–800 mg of caffeine), 2 to 3 hours before testing. Because the ergogenic effects are gained well below these accepted limits, some question these organizations' motives and raise ethical issues regarding the ergogenic use of caffeine (28). Furthermore, some argue that caffeine should be added to the banned substance list, which would thereby require athletes to abstain from caffeine ingestion 48 to 72 hours before competition. Interestingly however, caffeine is no longer prohibited at any concentration by WADA.

Over the years, there has been conflicting data in the literature concerning the *in vivo* reproducibility of caffeine's ergogenic effects. Although some have questioned the true ergogenic value of caffeine, athletes and coaches have believed in and used caffeine as an ergogenic aid for years. Only relatively recently has the true ergogenic value of caffeine, especially regarding short-term (<5 minutes) high-intensity (>100% maximal aerobic power [VO_2 max]) exercise (STHIX) been significantly borne out in published research. What the evidence has more clearly supported is the notion that caffeine is ergogenic during prolonged (>30 minutes), moderate intensity (~75%–80% $Vo_{2\ max}$) exercise. For example, in one study, the run time to exhaustion at 85% of $Vo_{2\ max}$ in elite runners increased by 44% following the ingestion of an acceptable, under-the-limit dose of caffeine (31).

Information concerning STHIX has often been dismissed, even when positive results were shown. The early *in vivo* studies on humans found little evidence for a performance-enhancing effect on STHIX. On the other hand, early animal *in vitro* and *in situ* studies revealed that caffeine could increase muscle force production through CNS stimulation, enhanced neuromuscular transmission, and/or enhanced muscle fiber contractility (32). More recently however, a number of well-controlled studies have indicated that caffeine can improve performance during STHIX and repeated bouts of STHIX. One such study examined the effects of caffeine ingested at 6 mg/kg on the performance of repeated bouts of cycling at 100% VO_2 max (33). This study showed that the cycle time to exhaustion was significantly improved with caffeine and that epinephrine and lactate (muscle and blood) levels were increased with use of caffeine. Interestingly, muscle glycogen stores did not vary between the placebo and caffeine groups. Therefore, the authors concluded that STHIX was not associated with glycogen sparing, and may in fact have been due to elevated epinephrine levels which increased muscle glycogenolysis at this intensity, thereby increasing anaerobic energy provision. Ultimately, although both adrenaline and lactate (muscle and blood) levels were elevated following caffeine ingestion and STHIX, the significance of these elevations is unclear. Caffeine also appears to influence electrolyte handling and substrate use, which may also further affect anaerobic performance (32).

There are three major theories that explain the ergogenic effects of caffeine. First, caffeine has a direct effect on the CNS, which alters our perception of effort and/or affects the propagation of neural signals somewhere between the brain and the neuromuscular junction (28). It thereby decreases fatigue and improves our level of consciousness. Second, caffeine is believed to increase muscle force production through direct CNS stimulation, enhanced neuromuscular transmission, and enhanced muscle fiber contractility. Caffeine causes this by increasing permeability of the sarcoplasmic reticulum to calcium, thereby increasing the amount of intracellular calcium available for muscular contraction (13). Third, caffeine has the ability to increase circulating levels of free fatty acids (FFA) because of an increase in lipolysis. Oxidation of fatty acids then provides the initial energy source, leaving glycogen available for later use (34). Caffeine thereby reduces an individual's dependence on muscle glycogen as a fuel source during prolonged exercise, and improves endurance (9). Ultimately, caffeine increases the production of plasma catecholamines, including epinephrine, which is undoubtedly linked to many of its purported effects. These effects include increased psychological arousal, increased cardiac output, enhanced muscle contractility, and an increased mobilization and utilization of FFA during exercise (30).

The possible adverse side effects of using caffeine include anxiety, irritability, restlessness, inability to focus, tremor, headaches, insomnia, diuresis leading to fluid imbalances, gastrointestinal disturbances, hypertension, cholesterol abnormalities, tachycardia, and hyperesthesia (8,9,13). Caffeine can be lethal at doses of 3 to 10 g, causing delirium, seizures, tachycardia, and/or ventricular dysrhythmias (7,28).

Although tolerance to the performance-enhancing effects of caffeine has not been extensively studied, it appears that the derived ergogenic benefits may be significantly hampered in habitual consumers of caffeine (35). It has been suggested that in order for athletes to obtain the maximal ergogenic effect of caffeine, they should abstain from caffeine use at least 4 days before their competition to avoid a tolerance phenomenon (34). Additionally, the ingestion of caffeine should take place 3 to 4 hours before an endurance exercise, during peak plasma concentrations of FFAs rather than 1 hour or less before an event. If ingested an hour or less before competition, only the peak plasma concentration of caffeine is reached (36,37). However, some speculate that using caffeine 1 hour before competition also provides an effective ergogenic mechanism, especially in shorter length races, because in these instances it not only increases levels of epinephrine, but also increases psychological stimulation (30).

Finally, studies have shown that doses of up to 9 mg caffeine/kg body weight will produce peak plasma concentrations, with urine concentrations generally below the 12 μg/mL IOC limit (38) The optimal dose for performance enhancement appears to be between 3 and 6 mg/kg (28). At this level, side effects appear to be minimized and urine concentrations will not approach illegal limits. Many studies have been performed on the appropriate ergogenic levels even before the American cycling team used caffeine suppositories for performance enhancement in the 1984 Olympics (39). Not surprisingly, given the research available at that time, none of the American cyclists tested positive for caffeine. In fact, only a few athletes with illegal caffeine levels have been detected in Olympic competitions. Those athletes included an Australian pentathlete in 1988, two German swimmers in 1992, and Italian cyclists in 1992 and 1994 (28).

Sympathomimetics

Sympathomimetic amines are CNS stimulants and include ephedrine, pseudoephedrine, norpseudoephedrine, and phenylpropanolamine (PPA). The prototypical sympathomimetics, ephedrine and PPA, were found in many OTC common cold remedies. PPA was also a common ingredient in diet pills, until it was taken off the market by the FDA because of an increased risk of hemorrhagic stroke in women (40). These drugs, also known as *amphetamine* look-alikes, were often combined with caffeine in the early 1970s. Unfortunately, use of these stimulants can have significant side effects, especially in larger doses. They include tachycardia, palpitations, arrhythmias, anginal pain, hypertension, intracranial hemorrhage, restlessness, anxiety, insomnia, headaches, anorexia, dizziness, confusion, delirium, respiratory difficulty, nausea, vomiting, urinary retention, hallucinations, psychosis, and possible addiction (13,41–43).

Ephedrine

Ephedrine is still used in the treatment of asthma, hay fever, sinusitis, allergic rhinitis, urticaria, and other allergic disorders. It is also used as a pressor agent in hypotensive states and is found in a variety of OTC supplements (13,43). Ephedrine continues to be used as an ergogenic aid, because it tends to have amphetamine-like effects. Accordingly, athletes who use ephedrine report a significant boost of energy that increases the quality of their workouts and enhances their performance (42). Athletes also report using ephedrine alkaloids, including ephedra and ma huang, not only for their stimulant-like effects, but also for their thermogenic, fat-burning properties (41). Ephedrine achieves this thermogenic effect by stimulating the thyroid gland to transform the weaker thyroxine (T4) hormone into the more potent triiodothyronine (T3). When combined with caffeine and aspirin (which is referred to as the *thermogenic stack*) the thermogenic effect is significantly enhanced. Recent studies have confirmed many of the purported ergogenic effects of ephedrine, including prolonged time to exhaustion and decreased perception of exertion (44). To the general public, the use of caffeine-ephedrine stacking appears to be a recent trend; however the use of amphetamine "look-alikes" or ephedrine alkaloids, combined with caffeine, were knowingly used as ergogenic aids earlier than the 1970s. One of the more notable Olympic cases involving sympathomimetic use occurred at the 1972 Games when Rick DeMont, an American swimmer, was disqualified for taking medication containing ephedrine, reportedly for asthma (45). It is interesting to see that the use of caffeine and ephedrine stacking has come full circle. These substances are now more widely used than ever before by the general population because of their prevalence in OTC supplements.

As is the case with many of the OTC supplements, there has been an increased incidence of adverse side effects and/or death from ephedrine alkaloid toxicity. This is often due to an accidental overdose prompted by exaggerated off-label claims, and a belief that "natural" medicinal agents are inherently safe. It is important for individuals to realize that just because a supplement is labeled "natural" or is from a herbal source, it is not necessarily safe. A recent example is the OTC herbal product kava kava that has been found to cause serious liver toxicity. The FDA is now advising consumers of the potential risk of severe liver injury associated with the use of kava-containing dietary supplements (46).

The use of ephedrine alkaloids has been linked to many episodes of ephedrine toxicity and ephedrine-related deaths, especially when taken in combination with caffeine (47). The FDA has received more than 80 reports of ephedra-linked deaths and at least 1,400 reports of adverse reactions since 1994 (48). One interesting study reviewed more than 140 documented cases submitted to the FDA (49). The authors found that 47% of these adverse events involved cardiovascular symptoms, with the most frequent being elevated blood pressure followed by palpitations, and/or tachycardia. Eighteen percent involved CNS side effects including stroke and seizure, 13 caused permanent disability, and at least 10 events resulted in death (49).

To reduce the number of adverse reactions due to nutritional supplements containing ephedrine, the FDA proposed appropriate marketing and labeling changes for these products in 1997 (50). Although their proposal did not ban OTC ephedrine-containing products, it was intended to make consumers more aware of safety concerns (50). Under the FDA's guidelines, ephedrine manufacturers had to: (a) refrain from making supplements that contained more than 8 mg of ephedrine alkaloids per serving, (b) avoid using labels that suggested the use of more than 8 mg of ephedrine alkaloids in a 6-hour period or the total daily intake of more than 24 mg, (c) instruct consumers not to use ephedrine for longer than 7 days, (d) refrain from combining other stimulant ingredients, including caffeine, with ephedrine alkaloids, and (e) warn consumers that taking more than the recommended dosage of this product may result in a heart attack, stroke, seizure, or death (50). Owing to significant lobbying by supplement manufacturers, the FDA has since withdrawn these guidelines. However, as with many OTC supplements with a paucity of long-term safety and efficacy trials, the "FDA remains concerned that adverse effects are associated with long-term consumption of such products and with consumption of such products in excess of labeled serving sizes" (51).

With the surge in use of OTC supplements containing ephedrine alkaloids, there were numerous reports of collegiate and professional athletes suffering severe side effects after using these products. These included the collapse of at least 10 Northwestern University football players, including Rashidi Wheeler, who died after a rigorous preseason workout during August 2001. Another death believed to be related to the use of ephedra includes that of former Florida State University freshman Devaughn Darling, who collapsed and died in February 2001 after a workout. Although autopsy results were inconclusive, they did reveal ephedrine in his system (48). On September 27, 2001, the National Football League (NFL) also banned the use of ephedrine-containing products, decades after the NCAA and IOC had done so. The decision was in direct response to the August 1, 2001, death of Minnesota Vikings' offensive lineman Korey Stringer, a professional football player who was believed to be using ephedrine during practice (52). Finally, following the national media frenzy that implicated ephedra in the death of a 23-year-old during a Baltimore Orioles training camp in February of 2003, along with the mounting evidence of more than 18,000 reports of adverse events and more than 100 deaths linked to the use of ephedra-containing products, the FDA banned its use on April 2, 2004.

ANABOLIC AGENTS

Anabolic Androgenic Steroids

Although there have been many discussions about the ethical and legal aspects of the use of AAS, a most poignant fact must not be forgotten—the use of AAS remains prevalent in the athletic community. Survey results among Americans indicate that AAS use is found in approximately 2% of students between the ages of 10 and 14, between 5% and 12% of high school males, and between 2% and 20% of college athletes (53–55). Estimates of AAS use in elite athletes (e.g., Olympians, professional football linemen) range from 44% to 99% (56). The 1993 Drug Abuse National Household Survey found that there are at least 1 million current or former AAS users in this country (others estimate >3 million), that males had higher levels of AAS use during their lifetime than females (0.9% and 0.1%, respectively), that the median age of first AAS use was 18 years, and, most alarmingly, that for the 12- to 17-year-old group the median age of initiation was 15 years (57). AAS use was highly correlated with self-reported aggressive behavior and crimes against property. Among the 12- to 34-year-old age group, steroid use was associated with the use of alcohol as well as illicit drugs (57). In another study, it was reported that 75% of all steroid users will have done so before their 17th birthday which means that most AAS use begins before high school ends (55).

It was reported to the NCAA that greater than 50% of college athletes who admitted to AAS usage began in high school (11). Buckley et al. conducted the first nationwide study of AAS use at the high school level in 1987 (55). AAS use was found in 6.6% of high school males. Of this group, approximately 40% reported doing five or more cycles, 38% had initiated use before age 16, 44% used more than one steroid at a time, and 38% used injectable AAS. No difference was found in rates between urban and rural areas. Interestingly, there was a significant difference by the size of enrollment, (i.e., the larger the high school, the higher the rate of reported AAS use). In a study of middle school students in Massachusetts (n = 965), 2.7% reported using steroids (58).

In 1985 Anderson and McKeag surveyed 2,039 NCAA athletes at 11 colleges and universities (11). The use of AAS was defined as use in the past 12 months. The greatest use was found among football players at 9%. Four percent of male track and field, and tennis and basketball players and 3% of male baseball players reported using AAS. The only women's sport in which AAS were used was women's swimming, in 1% of the athletes. In 1991 the survey was replicated (12). Again, 2,039 male and female athletes were surveyed from 11 colleges and universities (7 of the original 11 schools participated). AAS use had increased only slightly over the preceding 4 years. This time the incidence of reported AAS use was 10% among football players, 4% for male track and field athletes, and 2% each for baseball, basketball and tennis. The use of AAS had increased in women's sports. Now 1% of women who participated in track and field, basketball, and swimming admitted to AAS use. Among those athletes admitting to AAS use, 25% began using before college, 25% initiated use during the first year of college, and 50% began after the first year of college.

Why has the use of AAS become so prevalent among athletes? Yesalis' 1987 study identified several reasons why athletes use steroids: 47.1% do so to improve athletic performance, 26.7% use AAS to improve their appearance, and 10.7% reported they do so to treat athletic injuries (55). AAS help athletes achieve size and strength gains when they are used concurrently with a proper diet and training regimen (59). However, studies have shown long-term AAS use may have detrimental consequences (59,60).

AAS are synthetic hormones that are analogs of testosterone, which athletes use in supraphysiological doses to give them the effects of high levels of testosterone. Like testosterone, these hormones are synthesized from the parent compound cholesterol. Various modifications made to the cholesterol compound yield AAS with differing properties. AAS as a group of compounds have a common structure based on the steroid nucleus, which consists of three six-member carbon rings and one five-member carbon ring. The naturally occurring steroids include male and female sex hormones (androgens and estrogens), the adrenal cortex hormones (corticosteroids), progesterone, bile salts, and sterols (cholesterol).

Natural testosterone is not effective when taken orally because of rapid first-pass liver metabolism. Similarly, natural testosterone injections undergo a relatively rapid rate of breakdown in the liver. Therefore, in an attempt to develop a more purely anabolic steroid, AAS are molecularly altered to resist this metabolic breakdown. The efficacy of orally administered AAS is greatly improved by alkylation at the 17 position (C-17 alpha-alkalization). This change decreases the first-pass metabolism by the liver and increases the AAS potency, although it also significantly increases the level of hepatotoxicity. The efficacy of parenteral or injectable AAS is enhanced by esterification of the 17-hydroxyl group. This modification yields a more lipid-soluble compound with extended activity. Parenteral AAS are suspended in oil or water. Suspending AAS in oil for injection helps them remain in the body for weeks or months. For example, testosterone cypionate (Depo) is detectable for at least 6 to 12 months. Oil-based AAS can also be administered transdermally. Water-based AAS such as stanozolol (Winstrol) are detectable for 5 to 12 months.

In men, testosterone acts in two ways—anabolically by stimulating nitrogen retention and muscle growth and androgenically, by promoting the development of secondary sexual characteristics. Endogenous testosterone plays a role in determining male sex characteristics. *In utero*, testosterone brings facial hair and a deepening of the voice during puberty, regulates the release of follicle stimulating-hormone (FSH) and luteinizing hormone (LH), increases protein synthesis, increases aggression, and increases sex drive. Testosterone is produced primarily by the Leydig cells of the testes and to some extent by the adrenals (usually <10% in males). Most of the daily testosterone production comes from the peripheral metabolism of prehormones (61,62). Serum testosterone levels are regulated by a negative feedback loop in response to low testosterone levels. In this loop, the hypothalamus releases gonadotrophin-releasing hormone that stimulates the pituitary to release gonadotrophins, which then act upon testosterone-producing sites (the testes and adrenals in males, and the ovaries and adrenals in females). FSH then downregulates the number of LH receptors.

The effects that compel athletes to take AAS stem from their anabolic nature. Anabolic refers to promoting the process of assimilation of nutritive matter and its conversion into living substance as well as promoting tissue growth by increasing the metabolic processes involved in protein synthesis. The anabolic effects that are sought by athletes include increased protein synthesis, decreased cortisol and adrenocorticotropic hormone (ACTH) release that is related to the inhibition of catabolic effects on skeletal muscle, promotion of a positive nitrogen balance that increases muscle mass, increased strength or force of muscle contraction (which may be a permanent increase if weight training is paired with a high protein diet [2.2 gm/kg/day]), inhibition of protein catabolism that may hasten recovery from injury; and stimulation of erythropoiesis that increases endurance due to the increase in red blood cell (RBC) mass. AAS use may also allow faster recovery time from repetitive, high-intensity workouts, enhance performance by increasing aggressiveness, and produce euphoria, thereby decreasing the sense of fatigue during training (59,60,63). Therefore, AAS can contribute to increases in lean body weight, strength, and endurance, if coupled with a proper diet and high-intensity exercise (64–67). Furthermore, the strength building effects of AAS are greater in athletes who have trained before AAS use than in those who have not trained (65). Two additional mechanisms theorized to result in the anabolic effects of AAS include increased messenger RNA and intracellular calcium concentration through the cAMP pathway, and increased acetylcholine release at the neuromuscular junction in the brain, thereby increasing monoamine levels which in turn increases aggression and energy (61,68).

For athletes, the less desirable effects of AAS stem from their androgenic properties. Androgenic refers to masculinization (i.e., stimulation of the development of male sex hormones and male secondary sexual characteristics). Androgenic effects include increased body and facial hair, deepening of the voice, increased sex drive, increased aggressiveness, male pattern baldness, and acne. Ultimately, AAS bind to androgen receptors, stimulate production of RNA, and are anticatabolic because they improve the utilization of protein and inhibit the catabolic effect of glucocorticoids (59).

Athletes use AAS according to different regimens. One regimen is stacking or simultaneously using an average of five different AAS, in both oral and injectable forms, in 6- to 12- week cycles. Stacking is done because AAS users believe it will activate and saturate multiple steroid receptor sites, decrease the amount of each AAS necessary, decrease associated side effects, and provide synergistic benefits. Cycling is done to avoid developing a tolerance to AAS, avoid detection, decrease the incidence of harmful side effects associated with long-term AAS use, and allow the body to return to normal function between cycles. This last rationale for cycling is logical, given that endogenous testosterone levels, sperm production, and the entire hypothalamic-pituitary-gonadal axis are affected by AAS use; therefore, off-cycling allows these processes to return to normal. A type of drug regimen that involves stacking increasingly larger dosages of AAS, is commonly referred to as *stacking the pyramid*. There are numerous AAS regimens out there and they are becoming increasingly more complex.

AAS users employ dosages that may range from 40 to 100 times what is medically prescribed (63). The daily dose and route of AAS usage will depend on the cycle and stacking method used. AAS in dosages ranging from 50 to more than 200 mg/day are not unusual. The oral AAS preparations with shorter half-lives are typically taken up to three times daily. Parenteral injections vary anywhere from daily to weekly. AAS are taken along with other kinds of drugs that will prevent or counteract their androgenic effects, as well as extend their anabolic effects. Human chorionic gonadotrophin (hCG) is taken to counteract testicular atrophy; diuretics are taken to block water retention, create the "ripped" look and to circumvent detection; tamoxifen and other anti-estrogens are taken to block gynecomastia due to aromatization of the androgens; and antiacne medications are taken to resolve the acne that may develop in some AAS users (63). There have been reports that endocrinologists and steroid users have experimented with the use of prednisone to retard the anabolic gains that are lost after coming off AAS (69). While this is counterintuitive because cortisol is catabolic, the catabolic link may have more to do with endogenous ACTH. Not all of the combinations of AAS and other drugs are safe. In fact, some can be deadly. The riskiest use of AAS involves athletes who take multiple substances at one time while engaging in other self-destructive behaviors (63).

To avoid detection, athletes adjust their regimens according to the current knowledge of drug testing and discontinue use in a "safe" time period, make steroid alterations, and/or utilize masking techniques. Experienced users are knowledgeable about detection methods and event testing and can generally beat the system. Annual use patterns vary with the sport and the likelihood of being tested. Bodybuilders typically cycle on and off several times per year for several years, in a very systematic manner around competition dates. The typical 12-week cycle will include a pyramid with at least three to four different AAS. The athlete will then continue on other drugs which stop the rebound physiological bottoming out, prolong the anabolic and positive nitrogen balance, maintaining muscle and strength increases gained during the cycle.

Gains produced with AAS use are not made without significant risks. In one study, male mice were exposed for 6 months to four different types of AAS in levels that correspond to those that humans take (70). In addition to a control group that was not given any AAS, mice were given doses of AAS at 20 or 5 times the normal level for mice. One year after the end of the AAS exposure, 52% of the 20-time group had died, compared with only 35% of the 5-time group, and 12% of the control group.

AAS use leads to many cardiovascular side effects, including hypertension, in susceptible individuals (71). AAS use may lead to concentric left ventricular hypertrophy with decreasing ventricular compliance without affecting cardiac function (72,73). AAS use has also led to an increased incidence of myocardial infarction and arterial thrombosis by stimulating thrombus formation and accelerating atherosclerosis. This appears to be caused by suppressing prostacyclin production in arterial smooth muscle cells (74,75). AAS also appear to negatively effect lipid profiles. AAS increase low-density lipoprotein (LDL) levels and decrease high-density lipoprotein (HDL) levels, although these effects are reversible after discontinuation.

Sachtleben et al. (67) reported on the effects of AAS use on serum lipoprotein and apolipoprotein levels (67). They demonstrated a relationship between elevated levels and (a) an increased incidence of coronary artery disease and (b) an increased risk of myocardial infarction. They also showed that cardiovascular risk was intensely altered by AAS use through negative changes in the cholesterol to HDL-C ratio (from 4.8 mg/dL user-off to 6.8 mg/dL user-on). Not only did they detect significant alterations in serum lipid values, they also observed that the alterations were maintained for at least 8 weeks even after AAS use was stopped. They concluded that AAS users seem to be at risk for the development of early atherosclerosis (67).

Not all studies have shown significant effects on lipid levels. Cohen et al. (76) studied 18 competitive bodybuilders (10 AAS users, 8 nonuser controls) and found that serum lipoprotein-A levels actually decreased and total cholesterol and triglyceride levels remained the same in AAS users (76). This was despite the higher dietary intake of cholesterol in the steroid group and the high doses taken of potent AAS such as Anadrol, Deca-Durabolin, Winstrol, Dianabol, Sostenon 250, Primobolan, and Anavar. In fact, because lipoprotein-A levels greater than 30 mg/dL translate into a twofold greater chance of coronary artery disease, AAS users were found to have an advantage: only 30% of AAS users exhibited levels greater than 30 mg/dL as compared with 88% of the "clean" subjects.

Other studies have shown more detrimental sequelae to AAS use (59,70,72,73,77,78). Because there are testosterone receptors in most tissues of the human body, AAS exert effects on nearly every system. In the liver, AAS (especially oral agents) cause elevated liver enzymes such as serum glutamic-oxaloacetic transaminase (SGOT), serum glutamate pyruvate transaminase (SGPT), bilirubin (cholestatic jaundice), and alkaline phosphatase; increased risk of liver tumors such as benign hepatocellular adenoma, peliosis hepatitis (which is seen in patients taking AAS for chronic medical conditions and does not usually present in athletes), and hepatocellular carcinoma of which there are several reported cases among athletes, especially those taking AAS for long periods (56,79). Other reported side effects were an increase in libido, irritability, headaches, nausea, muscle spasm resulting in chest pain, nervousness, increased hunger, kidney tumors, hyperinsulinemia, and diabetes secondary to impaired glucose tolerance (80).

Other potential side effects of AAS use include an increased incidence in tendon rupture and ligament sprains. The most frequently reported AAS-related musculotendinous injuries are in the quadriceps femoris and the triceps brachii (56). There are two theories to explain these injuries. AAS use may lead to a decrease in connective tissue strength causing tendinoligamentous failure. However, most believe that what is actually responsible for the connective tissue failure is the sudden relative increase in muscle strength and size obtained by AAS use (81).

AAS have a pronounced effect on the immune system, as well. Studies have shown humeral immunity may be impaired; immunoglobulin G (IgG), IgM, and IgA levels may be decreased and killer T-cell function may be altered (82). There does not appear to be any clinical correlation with these changes and the significance is unknown. There have been anecdotal reports of leukemia, lymphoma, and melanoma in young athletes using AAS (83). There has been one reported case of AIDS due to the sharing of needles (84).

Males who use AAS experience many side effects. AAS use leads to decreases in FSH, LH, natural testosterone, and spermatogenesis; testicular atrophy (which usually reverses within 2–16 months of discontinuation), scrotal pain, difficulty urinating (prostatic hypertrophy), and adenocarcinoma of the prostate (64,85,86). This last effect poses a serious potential risk in males because the prostate is a very specific target tissue for androgens and prostate cancer is androgen sensitive. However, recent studies do not confirm evidence that AAS use alters the risk of prostate cancer (87).

The effects of prolonged AAS use on female physiology are most poignantly detailed in an article that delves into the former German Democratic Republic's experimentation with AAS (60). In girls and women, the higher performance levels gained after using AAS and increasing muscle strength do not return to their pre-AAS levels after the steroids are withdrawn (60). In fact, women experience side effects similar to those experienced by men including decreased FSH, LH, and natural estrogen levels; breast tissue atrophy; muscle tightness; body weight increases; muscle cramps; irregular menstruation including amenorrhea; acne; alteration of libido, and fertility; edema; diarrhea; constipation; functional and structural liver damage; hepatocellular tumors which tend to be larger and more malignant than spontaneous adenomas; peliosis hepatitis; and water retention in muscle (60,65). Irreversible changes include deepening of the voice through laryngeal hypertrophy, arrest of body growth in adolescents, clitoromegaly, squaring of the jaw, hirsutism, and male pattern baldness.

High school studies on the prevalence of AAS use are particularly worrisome, due to the effects exerted by these drugs on the developing adolescent. Premature epiphyseal closure is a permanent side effect (64). AAS affect the pituitary gland and testes, greatly reducing endogenous testosterone and suppressing spermatogenesis in males. Though discontinuation of AAS by mature males results in an eventual return to normal hormonal activity, this has not been established for immature males or females (88).

Some believe the most significant "acute" effects of AAS are psychological. A 1988 Pope and Katz retrospective study revealed that 22% of AAS users interviewed displayed manic or depressive symptomatology while taking the drugs, another 12% had transiently become psychotic, 3% to 9% became manic or hypomanic, and 7% suffered from major depression. The depression usually occurred 6 weeks after withdrawal from AAS during which some athletes felt that they were shrinking, getting weaker, and could not workout as intensely as they could while on AAS. Overall, 12% to 15% became addicted to AAS (77). Some studies suggest that among AAS users up to 40% will suffer from affective disorders and up to 40% will become addicted (89). AAS use increases aggression and hostility and has resulted in homicides and suicides (59,90–92). Others believe that many AAS users have significant personality disorders and psychiatric problems and that psychoactive drugs may put them over the edge (92).

Despite the considerable evidence that shows the adverse effects of AAS use, Street et al. (1996) concluded that the risk of permanent serious health complication is low with the use of injectable steroids at "moderate" dosages of 200 to 300 mg/week for 6 to 12 weeks/year (56). However, they do warn that the use of oral 17-alkylated AAS are associated with the greatest health risks. Most athletes currently supplement with a variety of stacking techniques to decrease side effects, and will often use more water-based, short-acting AAS along with insulin and hGH.

Beta Agonists

This family of drugs derives its name from its ability to stimulate Beta adrenoceptors found on the surface of muscle cells, which naturally act as triggers for the metabolic effects of adrenaline. Since the 1970s, $Beta_2$ agonists have been used worldwide in the treatment of asthma because they cause the smooth muscle found in the airways to relax, resulting in bronchodilation. They are usually administered in relatively small doses directly into the lungs through an inhaler. In this manner, only a small amount of the drug is actually absorbed systemically causing little effect on other tissues. However, by the mid 1980s it was discovered that when higher doses of Beta$_2$ agonists were given by mouth, the drugs caused a rapid and marked increase in the growth of skeletal muscle and a reduction in body fat (93). These effects have been seen in a variety of animals including fish, mice, rats, rabbits, poultry, sheep, cattle, and most importantly humans (94,95). It appears that every major pharmaceutical company has developed its own patented β_2 agonist drug.

Clenbuterol

Beta adrenergic agents, including clenbuterol, are commonly used to treat the approximate 10% to 15% of athletes that are believed to have exercise-induced bronchospasm and asthma. However, clenbuterol is thought to be the most commonly abused of these substances because of its more potent ergogenic effects. It was not long after more stringent drug testing was utilized to deter the use of AAS that clenbuterol became a more popular ergogenic aid. By the 1990s, clenbuterol use was rampant among elite athletes. In 1996, U.S. hammer thrower Jud Logan and shot-putter Bonnie Dasse, were disqualified for clenbuterol use at the Barcelona Summer Olympics. It has been estimated that up to one third of elite athletes have used it as an ergogenic aid, and there are many more anecdotal reports that the true prevalence of clenbuterol abuse in sport is much greater than this (96).

Clenbuterol is a β_2 agonist that is prescribed in Mexico and Europe as a bronchodilator (97). In the United States it has not been approved by the FDA for human or even animal use (96). Compared with the β_2 agonists that are marketed in the United States, clenbuterol has a longer half-life and greater potency (98). Although there have been no published studies on the effects of clenbuterol on humans, the purported benefits of clenbuterol use are drawn from animal studies and animal husbandry in other countries, where it is used as a repartitioning and potent anabolic agent (96–98). Repartitioning agents manipulate growth and body composition, enhancing deposition of body protein, and decreasing fat (98). Clenbuterol's ergogenic effects are purported to be: (a) an increase in lean muscle mass through the direct promotion of lipolysis and the retardation of adipose tissue deposition and (b) an increase in the rate of muscle protein deposition (96,97). In rats, clenbuterol causes rapid hypertrophy of skeletal and cardiac muscle but not hyperplasia (96,98). Muscle growth is postulated to be related to the ratio of protein synthesis to protein degradation (96). Clenbuterol suppresses both synthesis and degradation, but seems to have a greater effect on degradation with the net result being increased synthesis (96). Clenbuterol also increases heat production in the mitochondria of muscle and possibly brown fat, thereby increasing energy expenditure (98). From studies on rats, it has been determined that the growth-promoting effect lasts for a limited time and appears to level off with prolonged treatment (96). It has been speculated that this may be the result of downregulation of receptor numbers and receptor responsiveness (27,96).

Athletes who use clenbuterol prefer capsules or tablets rather than the inhalant form, which is also available. Athletes usually take twice the dosage recommended for the treatment of bronchospasm (recommended dose 0.04–0.06 mg). Dosage follows a 3-week on/off cycle (96). During the on-cycle, clenbuterol is taken for 2 days and discontinued for 2 days to avoid any diminishing effects caused by downregulation of receptor numbers and receptor responsiveness (96). Despite such precautions, there is a rapid attenuation of clenbuterol's effectiveness after a few weeks of use (27). Because niacin improves muscle blood flow, it is often taken concurrently with clenbuterol to hasten distribution (96). When AAS are discontinued before a competition, clenbuterol is used to slow down the loss of muscle mass and to promote lipolysis of subcutaneous fat (known as *stripping*), thereby improving muscle definition (96).

Side effects that have been reported with clenbuterol use include muscle tremor, palpitations, muscle cramps, transient tachycardia, anxiety, headaches, peripheral vasodilation, anorexia, insomnia, and adrenergic tremor (20). Another side effect, myocardial hypertrophy, has been reported in animal studies and when it occurs in humans who abuse clenbuterol could lead to outlet obstruction and ultimately sudden death (96). Other potentially life-threatening side effects are hyperthermia, myocardial infarction, stroke, and dysrhythmia (27).

Incidents of clenbuterol food poisoning have been reported resulting from the consumption of animals treated with clenbuterol (99). Clenbuterol is unique as a β_2 agonist because it is not rapidly broken down in the body and is prone to form high concentrations in both adipose tissue and liver (100). In one incident in Italy, meat samples contained clenbuterol at 4.5 mg/kg. People who ate 10 to 20 g of meat ingested therapeutic dosages of clenbuterol whereas the amount of meat found in a normal meal, approximately 100 gram, resulted in the ingestion of five times the therapeutic dosage levels (99). In another incident in Spain, 35 people were reported to have been hospitalized following an outbreak of clenbuterol poisoning caused by contaminated calf liver (100). Effects caused by eating this contaminated food included those mentioned in the preceding text, as well as gastrointestinal disturbances, vertigo, myalgia-arthralgia, cephalalgia, weakness, and confusion. The average duration of symptoms was 48 hours (99).

Cimaterol

Cimaterol is in the β_2 agonist family of phenylethanolamines along with other popular fat loss drugs, including ephedrine and clenbuterol. Although Cimaterol, 2-amino-5-1-hydroxy-2-1-methylethyl-aminoethyl or anthranilonitrile, has been researched for its anabolic and anticatabolic properties in both animals and humans since at least the 1980s, it is relatively unknown among athletes, even at the professional and elite levels. It is touted as the most effective fat stripping or repartitioning agent currently not being used extensively in the sports world. In fact, cimaterol may be a more powerful β agonist than clenbuterol (101). Only those on the cutting edge of sports doping have been experimenting with cimaterol. Because it is not extensively used, the most common short- and long-term (and potentially lethal) side effects experienced by humans are not yet known. Many speculate that the side effects should be similar to those experienced with the use of clenbuterol. Some fear that because cimaterol's $Beta_2$ agonist properties are much more powerful than clenbuterols, its adverse side effect profile might be much worse as well. It may turn out to be a much more dangerous drug for athletes to use, and possibly lead to many more fatalities than clenbuterol.

Because β_2-agonists were discovered to have anabolic properties while also stimulating basal metabolism, human studies have focused on the use of cimaterol as both an anticatabolic agent and anabolic agent. Cimaterol has been used in human studies to prevent muscle loss in cancer patients (tumor-induced catabolism) and to prevent muscle catabolism in burn victims (94,101). In one study, researchers found that in as little as a 20-day period of time, those receiving cimaterol experienced an average of 10% muscle weight gain (102). Research has shown that at a subcutaneous dose of 0.15 mg/kg, cimaterol inhibits muscle catabolism in burn victims, enhances protein accretion (the net uptake of amino acids into muscle cells) by up to 260% greater than control and enhances muscle protein synthesis even in states of severe stress.

At present, the suggested human dosing extracted from animal experimentation is 20 to 50 mg/day, which is estimated to cost less than a dollar, and like clenbuterol, makes it a very inexpensive and effective anabolic agent (103). Fortunately, there are existing methods for detecting the use of cimaterol in humans (104,105). Despite the fact that most of the data on β_2-agonists result from studies on animals and that all of the short- and long-term health consequences are unknown, many athletes use these drugs for fat loss and muscle growth. In short, cimaterol is currently viewed as an ideal β_2-agonist by some athletes because it stimulates fat loss, helps retain muscle, promotes protein synthesis at the muscle cell level, is inexpensive and appears to be safe enough that it is being researched in cancer patients and burn victims.

PEPTIDE HORMONES, MIMETICS, AND ANALOGS

As a class, these drugs are banned because of the chemical interactions and effects they have on the production of endogenous forms of testosterone and similar compounds.

Insulin

Insulin is a peptide hormone produced in the pancreas by the cells of the islets of Langerhans. This protein hormone is best known for its ability to regulate the amount of glucose in the blood. The IOC banned insulin in 1998 because of its abuse as an ergogenic aid. However, this ban does not apply to diabetic athletes who obviously depend upon insulin for regulation of their blood glucose levels. Insulin has many important physiological functions, in addition to this ability to promote glucose utilization. It also increases amino acid transport and stimulates ribosomal protein production, thereby increasing protein synthesis in muscle (106). Athletes looking for an ergogenic edge use insulin, a hormone integral in the body's process of energy utilization, for its anabolic characteristics and for its ability to reverse the catabolic effects in the postexercise state. It does this by increasing the formation of protein, triglyceride, and very low-density lipoprotein by the liver (106).

Bodybuilders are believed to have pioneered the use of insulin as an ergogenic aid decades ago. However, because of more stringent drug testing and the relatively low androgenic side effect profile for women, it has had a resurgence on the world doping scene. Recent trends suggest that a greater proportion of elite athletes are beginning to use insulin to enhance their performance not only because of its efficacy, but because certain forms of exogenous insulin are difficult to detect using present testing methods (107). Certain exogenous forms have half-lives of as little as 4 minutes, and even if they are detected, can be difficult to distinguish from endogenous insulin (108).

Insulin can help athletes in several ways. It can be used alone or as a stacking agent where it works alongside other anabolic agents such as testosterone or hGH to synergistically enhance strength and muscle size gains. In one study, it was purported that insulin used as a sole agent results in rapid muscle weight gain (10 lb), without concurrent fat gain, over a period of as little as 1 month (109). In this article, the author recommends not only using several units of insulin at least two times per day, but also recommends limiting carbohydrate intake to 100 mg/day and increasing protein intake to 600 mg/day, which fortunately is not a typical use pattern by most athletes. Interestingly, the author warns that, "This program can be very dangerous if done incorrectly. . .if you try this theoretical approach to insulin use, you understand that you may seriously harm yourself or die, thereby forfeiting your rights to hold anyone responsible but yourself!" (109)

Most athletes will use insulin as one component of a larger program of ergogenic drug use, although women may use it as a single agent. To prevent the adverse side effects of hypoglycemia, most athletes will take insulin and glucose simultaneously. One advanced technique used by endurance athletes (such as middle-distance runners and track athletes) to bolster performance is to follow a method called a *hyperinsulinaemic clamp*. During this technique, athletes infuse glucose and insulin simultaneously over several hours, which enables them to glycogen load their muscles before and between events. Experiments by Sonksen and others suggest that hyperinsulinaemic clamps can increase the rate of glucose metabolism up to 12-fold and greatly enhance muscle glycogen stores, thereby providing a great ergogenic advantage (107).

There are many potential side effects to using exogenous insulin, especially in individuals who do not suffer from a lack of endogenous insulin supply or from insulin insensitivity. The risks of insulin use are similar to those encountered by insulin-dependent diabetics. These risks include hypoglycemia, effects from low blood-glucose concentration (confusion, unusual behavior, neurological deficits, convulsions, coma, and death), effects from epinephrine release (vasoconstriction, tachycardia, profuse sweating, fear, and tension), lipodystrophy, lipoatrophy, insulin allergy, insulin resistance, immunological response, and the production of autoantibodies against insulin (106). Furthermore, insulin use combined with rigorous exercise can also result in unexpected hypoglycemic attacks, which may continue despite the cessation of insulin use (106).

Insulin is almost impossible to detect using standard drug tests. Worse, the hormone could easily kill if wrongly administered. It has been shown that insulin sensitivity increases both during and after exercise (109, 110). Therefore with exercise, less insulin is necessary to process a given load of carbohydrate (109,110). In one study that looked at the influence of physical activity on the level of insulin in sedentary and physically trained older men, it was found that insulin levels were higher in the sedentary subjects, than in the physically trained subjects after the administration of an effort test (111). While exercising, the liver decreases glucose production, the pancreas becomes more efficient, more glucose than fat cells are used by an increased number of muscle cells and there is an overall weight decrease (110). Because of the increased insulin sensitivity after exercise, insulin-dependant diabetics and athletes using insulin supplementation for ergogenic purposes must be careful not to experience severe hypoglycemia, also known as *postexercise late-onset hypoglycemia* or *PEL*.

Human Growth Hormone and Recombinant Growth Hormone

hGH consists of a single chain polypeptide of 191 amino acids stabilized by two disulfide bonds (7,112). The molecular mass is 22,000 daltons. The half-life of hGH in plasma ranges from 17 to 45 minutes and it is metabolized in the liver (113). hGH is synthesized by anterior pituitary somatotropes and is secreted in a pulsatile manner by the adenohypophysis found in the pituitary gland (27,112,114). Growth hormone-releasing hormone (GHRH) and somatotropin release-inhibiting hormone, which are produced by the hypothalamus, regulate the release of hGH (63). hGH release is also affected by a variety of factors including exercise, diet, drugs, nutrition, stress, sleep, cardiorespiratory fitness, and feedback mechanisms (7,27,63,114). The mean production of hGH is 500 to 875 μg/day (112). The secretion of hGH increases in response to exercise, hypoglycemia, and most of all, sleep, with the largest amount secreted approximately 60 to 90 minutes after its onset (27,63). Endogenous L-arginine, L-lysine, and omithine also stimulate the production of hGH (63). It is interesting to note that short bouts of intense exercise such as a 400-yd dash, tend to increase hGH secretion dramatically, although levels peak and subside gradually (112,114,115). In general, the amount of hGH that is released because of exercise is directly related to the intensity of the exercise (63). Glucose loading and obesity blunt the release of hGH during exercise (7). Suppression of hGH is further caused by increased blood levels of hGH, increased blood levels of insulin-like growth factor (IGF-1), hyperglycemia, and hypothermia (63).

The consumption of recombinant growth hormone (rGH) has become easier to achieve mainly because biotechnological advances have increased availability and safe supplies of the drug (112,115). Athletes take one of two available forms of rGH, which are structurally related to hGH. rGH also consists of a single amino acid chain, although one form has 192 amino acids instead of 191 (115). The range of medically prescribed dosages of rGH varies between 0.06 mg/kg to 0.1 mg/kg three times weekly depending on whether the 191 or 192 amino acid rGH is used (7,27). There have been reports that athletes use up to 20 times the medically prescribed dosages, sometimes using from four units three times per week to as much as 10 units/day for many weeks (114,115). rGH is taken by intramuscular injection in 6 to 12 cycles and is coadministered with AAS (63). Athletes also attempt to stimulate endogenous hGH secretion by taking clonidine, levodopa, and vasopressin, which may do so by acting directly on the pituitary gland, or by acting indirectly through the stimulation of GHRH (113,116). Arginine, omithine, L-lysine, and tryptophan are also used to attempt to stimulate endogenous hGH release.

The desired anabolic properties of rGH are identical to those that result from the effects of endogenous hGH on the human body. hGH primarily serves to foster growth through the stimulation of the secretion of somatomedins by the liver and other organs, which in turn regulate the activities of other hormones (27,114). Along with the somatomedin IGF-1, hGH facilitates muscle, bone and cartilage growth; increases protein deposition; facilitates all aspects of cellular amino acid uptake; facilitates cell protein synthesis and simultaneously reduces protein catabolism; inhibits glucose uptake in muscle; and decreases protein metabolism by lipolysis (27,63). Administration of rGH results in increased FFAs, increased hepatic lipid stores, and decreased peripheral fat stores with the ultimate result being decreased body fat and increased lean body mass (27). All of this is achieved without the risk of detection because there are currently no IOC-approved urine or blood tests for the detection of doping with rGH (27,115,117).

Some of the ergogenic benefits of rGH use, although popularly touted, are, in practice, limited in scope. While it has been shown that rGH use increases the size and strength of muscles in hGH-deficient individuals, its impact on nondeficient users is less dramatic (118). In fact, research has shown that increases in muscle size do occur in nondeficient individuals, but increases in *strength* do not (113) The reason for this has been postulated to involve ribonucleic acid (RNA). Muscle growth induced by rGH depends on increases in the rate and translation of existing RNA, whereas muscle growth resulting from exercise depends on the synthesis of new RNA (7). Therefore, rGH use results in increases in muscle size but not strength (113). Other limited effects of rGH administration include minimal gains in lean body mass in athletes who do not have a large fat mass. Interestingly, in athletes who have a large fat mass, rGH use does lead to increases in lean body mass.

Given such large doses, the resulting side effects are not surprising. In adolescents, the administration of rGH causes gigantism due to overstimulation of the open physes (63). In adults, side effects include acromegaly that results in the overgrowth of a variety of organs, bones, facial features, fingers, toes, and coarsening of the skin; diabetes; coronary heart disease; cardiomyopathy; congestive heart failure; hypertension; thyroid disease; peripheral neuropathy; decreased libido; impotence; menstrual disorders; osteoporosis; abnormal growth of melanocytic nevi; decreases in HDL-cholesterol and apolipoprotein A-1; and a shortened life span (7,27,63,114). Some of the side effects of rGH use may be irreversible. Other consequences of rGH use can be deadly (27,63). For example, acromegaly can lead to cardiac failure which is one of the major causes of death in individuals with this syndrome (63). Although the availability of synthetic rGH has ostensibly precluded the possibility of contracting Creutzfeldt-Jakob disease, it should be noted that cadaver-originated hGH may still be available on the black market. Therefore, the possibility of contracting this disease from hGH, which is sold as rGH, is still a very real danger (7). Other risks in obtaining rGH involve quality and purity of the drug as well as legitimacy. The DEA estimates that 30% to 50% of rGH products are phony (119).

Human Chorionic Gonadotrophin

hCG is a hormone that is used for its multifaceted properties involving its complicated relationship with both exogenous and endogenous testosterone (120). Male athletes use hCG to promote endogenous testosterone production. Its use is considered equivalent to exogenous testosterone administration by the IOC (60,121). The same cellular response that enables LH to stimulate endogenous testosterone production also enables hCG to do so (120). hCG is also used to prevent testicular atrophy and shutdown during prolonged periods of exogenous AAS use. Furthermore, the simultaneous administration of hCG and AAS leads to the normalization of the testosterone to epitestosterone (T/E) ratio that is used to detect the presence of exogenous AAS. Without this coadministration of hCG and AAS, the T/E ratio would be greater than the internationally agreed upon ratio of 6:1, and AAS would be detected. For females who take hCG to promote ovarian steroidogenesis, hCG is not as effective as in males and will probably have little if any effect on their athletic performance (120,122,123). Also in females, the presence of high levels of hCG does not necessarily indicate that exogenous hCG has been taken because this hormone can be found in the urine during normal or abnormal pregnancy.

Endogenous and Recombinant Human Erythropoietin and Blood Doping

Endogenous and recombinant human erythropoietin (EPO and rHuEPO, respectively) has similar structures: one polypeptide chain of 166 amino acids with two disulfide bonds and four polysaccharide chains. Another erythropoieses-stimulating protein, darbepoetin alfa (Aranesp, manufactured by Amgen) is similar in structure to EPO and rHuEPO, but has two additional N-linked oligosaccharide chains, an increased molecular weight, and a greater negative charge (124–126). EPO is the human hematopoietic hormone that regulates RBC production in bone marrow (127–129). RBCs carry oxygen to skeletal muscle and aid in the maintenance of acid–base status (130). When renal oxygenation is decreased, oxygen-sensor cells in the kidney stimulate EPO release (127,128). The plasma half-life of rHuEPO is 20 hours when administered subcutaneously by injection and its effects have been known to last for 2 weeks (128). Owing to the added carbohydrate side chains, darbepoetin alfa has a terminal half-life approximately three times longer than rHuEPO, which allows less frequent dosing (124–126,131). Because blood doping, as defined by the IOC, is the administration of blood, RBCs, and related blood products to an athlete, the use of rHuEPO and darbepoetin would obviously fall into this prohibited category. Therefore, the terms *rHuEPO administration* and *blood doping* are used interchangeably throughout this section (121).

The athletic community, especially in sports where endurance is the key to winning, has been using rHuEPO for years for its obvious effects on the circulatory/oxygen energy system (30). An estimated 3% to 7% of elite endurance sport athletes utilize rHuEPO (132). Darbepoetin alfa use surfaced in the 2002 Salt Lake City Winter Olympics. More RBCs lead to increased total hemoglobin, hemoglobin concentration, hematocrit, and RBC mass (30,127,132,133). These changes lead to an increased oxygen carrying capacity of the blood (each gram of hemoglobin carries approximately 1.34 mL of oxygen), which consequently increases oxygen delivery to working muscles, enhances VO_2 max, and thereby enhances endurance performance (30,127,128,130,132). rHuEPO's ability to increase RBC mass over several hours is extraordinary when it is noted that even a 5% increase in RBC mass usually takes months of adaptation to endurance training (130).

Improved submaximal performance also occurs after rHuEPO intake and stems from the reduced physiological strain, which is characterized by lower heart rate, lower venous and arterial lactate, higher venous and arterial pH values, and lower ratings of perceived exertion following rHuEPO doping (30,130). In one study of the effects of rHuEPO, 15 recreationally trained men received 20 to 40 IU of rHuEPO/kg injected three times a week for 6 to 7 weeks. rHuEPO use led to a linear increase in hemoglobin levels (0.28 g/wk), which were 11% greater after 6 weeks of administration, an increase in VO_2 max and a 17% increase in treadmill run time to exhaustion (134). Administration of rHuEPO may also improve performance in distance races. It has been shown that an increase in RBC by blood doping decreases 10-km run times by approximately 69 seconds, 3-mi run times by approximately 24 seconds, and 1,500-m run times on a track by approximately 5 seconds (135–137). Ergogenic responses to rHuEPO administration vary from person to person and depend on physiological factors such as training state, level of fitness, and genetics (130).

Administration of rHuEPO has definite ergogenic benefits for athletes exercising in heat (130). Because rHuEPO enables greater oxygen carrying capacity of the blood, a given submaximal exercise can be performed with decreased muscle blood flow (130). In the heat, this would decrease the competition between circulatory oxygen delivery and circulatory heat dissipation, allowing the latter to be more effective (130). In one study involving heat acclimated men, 300 mL of RBC were administered 2 to 4 days before and after these men walked in the heat while (a) normally hydrated and (b) dehydrated by 5% of their body weight on another day. The increased RBC resulted in lowered heart rates, sweating thresholds, and core temperatures; an increased sweating sensitivity; and an overall thermoregulatory advantage in either condition (138). It was concluded that blood doping results in a thermoregulatory advantage, which is greatest for heat acclimated individuals and slight for unacclimated people (130).

Although the use of rHuEPO and darbepoetin alfa seems to have positive effects, such as enhanced heat dissipation, it also has many adverse effects. Major side effects could stem from the use of improper dosages of rHuEPO or darbepoetin alfa. The amount of rHuEPO or darbepoetin alfa that is normally prescribed, for example to cure renal anemia, would only add up to several milligrams for 1 year of treatment (127). Because athletes typically use ergogenic aids in dosages that are several times those which are usually prescribed, the probability exists that there may be individuals who are using dangerously high levels of rHuEPO or darbepoetin alfa. In one case report, an individual had been using 2000 U of rHuEPO every 2 days for 3 months (133). Such levels could stimulate large increases in RBC mass, especially because RBC increase is dose dependent, with a concomitant result of dangerously high hematocrit levels (139). Because hematocrit increases above 30% force blood viscosity to rise exponentially, there would also be a dramatic rise in blood viscosity (140). The subsequent increase in viscosity would lead to an increase in vascular resistance, which would make the heart contract more forcefully to circulate blood. Moreover, because viscosity tends to increase with dehydration, there would be a potential for increased risk of coronary and cerebral occlusions, thrombosis, bradycardia, and pulmonary emboli resulting in death (18,133,141). Additional side effects of rHuEPO and darbepoetin alfa administration include hyperkalemia, hypertension directly related to dosage, flu-like symptoms, and an inhibition in the endogenous production of EPO (128,130).

OVER-THE-COUNTER SUPPLEMENTS

Dehydroepiandrosterone

Dehydroepiandrosterone (DHEA) is an androgen steroid produced primarily in the adrenal glands from acetate and is the major adrenal steroid of young adults. In 1996 the FDA banned the sale of DHEA for any indication because of insufficient evidence of its safety and value. Since that time it has become a popular OTC nutritional supplement (142). DHEA in its free, sulfated, and lipoidal forms is the most abundant steroid secreted by the adult human adrenal (128). Although a small amount of DHEA is converted to the more potent androgens testosterone and dihydrotestosterone, as well as androstenedione in peripheral tissues, the true role and physiological functions of DHEA have yet to be fully uncovered. In fact, while DHEA is most often referred to as an *adrenal androgen* because it can be converted in the periphery to testosterone, DHEA itself does not interact with androgen receptors, but with separate DHEA-specific receptors (143). Studies show that at the lowest doses, DHEA has effects on neurological and immunological tissues, suggesting that these two types of sites may be physiological targets. DHEA also affects cardiological and metabolic functions as well as tumor growth, but such actions require higher doses and may reflect "pharmacologic" activities (128,143,144). It is proposed that DHEA's pattern of activity represents a new class of steroid hormones, the "regnantoids." (143)

Research investigating the ergogenicity of DHEA is somewhat limited at present. There is a considerable amount of anecdotal support from athletes in a variety of sports that proclaim its athletic enhancing qualities. It has been hypothesized that supplementation with DHEA will aid, maintain, or increase testosterone levels, reduce body fat accumulation, reduce the risk of atherosclerosis as one ages, and possibly protect against certain cancers (144–146). One study has actually helped confirm some of the purported beneficial effects, where untrained healthy men (mean age 24 years old) were supplemented with 1,600 mg of DHEA per day for 28 days (147). Although testosterone levels were not significantly affected, both DHEA and androstenedione levels were increased. There was also a 31% reduction in percent body fat and a decrease in serum cholesterol levels. Additionally, a double-blind, placebo-controlled study done in 1993 using etiocholanedione, a metabolite of DHEA, found that doses of 32 mg/kg/day also produced significant weight loss in subjects (148). Furthermore, animal studies fully support this ergogenic effect.

The underlying physiological mechanism of weight loss with DHEA use is not known. One researcher believes the underlying cause of weight loss with DHEA supplementation to be an increase in mitochondrial respiration (149). However, most of the animal studies were done using high doses of DHEA over a period of weeks to months. Although DHEA has clear antiobesity actions in obese animals, subsequent studies on humans have failed to show changes in either body fat or weight (150,151).

An interesting fact about DHEA use is that even at high doses (50 times the suggested OTC supplement dose), there have not been any reported dose-limiting side effects (152). Long-term effects are yet to be determined, but overall, users of DHEA report few adverse effects, most of which are secondary to androgen excess. Notable irreversible side effects include virilization or voice deepening, hair loss, clitoromegaly, and hirsutism in women and gynecomastia in men (63). Potential adverse consequences of DHEA use include tumorigenesis, specifically hepatic tumors, hepatomegaly, elevation in liver enzymes, increased cardiac risk factors in women (altered glucose tolerance and elevated lipid levels), elevated PSA levels in men, acne, as well as other androgenic side effects (153–156). Furthermore, some researchers believe that unopposed prolonged estrogen and testosterone secretion may increase the risk of uterine and prostate cancers (157).

Whether DHEA is a member of a prior unreported and distinct class of steroid hormones that exerts unique physiological actions is still debated. Research reveals that there is some truth to its potential ergogenic effects, especially at higher doses (143). It is very apparent that the research regarding the ergogenic effects of DHEA in athletes is lacking at present. While OTC nutritional supplement manufacturers purport effects with doses of DHEA between 50 (the physiological dose in young adults) to 200 mg/day, as with many other OTC supplements, neither the ergogenicity nor safety of long-term use of DHEA in humans has been irrefutably demonstrated.

Creatine Monohydrate

Creatine monohydrate is not only one of the most popular ergogenic aids, it is also one of the most researched performance enhancing supplements. It is commonly used by high school, college, professional, and Olympic athletes. Creatine was first introduced in the United States as a potential OTC ergogenic aid in 1992. Since then its use has grown significantly. In fact, the NCAA study of Substance Use and Abuse Habits of College Student-Athletes found that at least 13.3% of college athletes surveyed reported using creatine (158).

Creatine is an organic compound made by the liver, kidneys, and pancreas from three amino acids—glycine, methionine, and arginine. In addition to being synthesized by the body, creatine is also obtained through consumption of meat and fish products. Approximately 1 g of creatine per day is made in the body and another gram per day is consumed in the diet (159). Creatine is then transported from these synthesis sites to the skeletal muscles. Creatine exists in two forms in muscle—as free creatine and as creatine phosphate, which makes up two thirds of the total creatine in the body.

Creatine appears to play a major role in energy production during quick bursts of activity. In fact, during explosive sprinting exercise, the energy supplied to rephosphorylate adenosine diphosphate (ADP) to adenosine triphosphate (ATP) is largely determined by the amount of phosphocreatine (PC) stored in the muscle (160,161). When muscles contract, ATP is used as the fuel for movement. ATP provides energy by releasing one of its phosphate molecules and is thereby transformed into ADP. Because muscle has only enough ATP stored to perform high-intensity muscle contractions for approximately 10 seconds, more ATP must subsequently be synthesized for the muscle to continue contracting. Essentially, PC will give up its phosphate molecule to ADP to create additional ATP. Therefore, the ability to regenerate ATP, to some degree, depends on the supply of PC in the muscles (158). PC is a major source of muscular energy during STHIX bouts lasting from approximately 2 to 30 seconds (162). As PC stores become depleted during these explosive exercises, performance is likely to rapidly deteriorate because of the inability to resynthesize ATP at the required rate (163). Consequently, studies suggest that increasing muscle creatine content through supplementation may increase the availability of PC, and allow for an actual accelerated rate of ATP resynthesis in myocardial and skeletal muscle during and/or after STHIX. Additionally, creatine supplementation is thought to act by buffering the intracellular hydrogen ions that are associated with lactate production and muscle fatigue (164–168). These effects should significantly influence the amount of energy generated during brief periods or repeated bouts of STHIX, thereby increasing the force of muscular contraction and prolonging anaerobic exercise, and theoretically improving repetitive sprint performance capacity.

Creatine is purported to increase strength, produce greater and faster lean-tissue muscle gains, increase energy, improve sprint performance, delay fatigue, and aid in fat loss. Research indicates that to maximize creatine stores, a "loading phase" of supplementation with 20 to 25 g of creatine monohydrate per day for 2 to 7 days is necessary.

Creatine loading increases total creatine content by 15% to 30% and intramuscular PC stores by 10% to 40% (169). After this "loading phase," a "maintenance phase" of 3 to 5 g/day is all that is needed to maintain these levels. Any extra supplement ingested will only be excreted by the kidneys.

A number of studies corroborate creatine's performance-enhancing benefits. Research has shown improvement in strength, power, sprint performance, and work performed during multiple sets of maximal effort muscle contractions. For example, one study reported an increased amount of work performed during five sets of bench press and jump squats after "loading phase" of creatine (25 g/day for 7 days) (170). Other studies have shown significant improvements in single-effort sprint performance in sprints lasting 6 to 30 seconds (171,172). Another study reported that sprint performance during a series of 300- and 1,000-m runs was significantly improved with a 30 g/day for 6 days loading phase (163). A study testing off-season college football players found significant increases in repetitive sprint performance (in the first 5 of 12 by 6-second sprints with 30 seconds rest between sprints) and isotonic lifting volume from maximal effort repetition tests on the bench press, squat, and power clean (173). Reported ergogenic effects include increased one-repetition maximum and/or peak power, improved vertical jump and repetitive-jump performance, increased work during repetitive sets of maximal-effort muscle contractions, enhanced sprint performance in sprints lasting 6 to 30 seconds, improved repetitive-sprint performance, and improved high-intensity exercise performance in events lasting 90 to 600 seconds. Studies in support of these hypotheses indicate that creatine loading may improve high-intensity exercise performance in a variety of athletic activities such as rowing, running, cycling, swimming, and resistance exercise (163,168,170,171,174–182).

Not all studies investigating the ergogenic value of creatine supplementation have reported enhanced exercise performance. Several field studies reported a lack of significant ergogenic effect after creatine supplementation (182–192). Overall, creatine supplementation appears to be less ergogenic when initial loading regimens are less than 20 g/day for 5 days, when low dose (2–3 g/day) regimens without a loading period are used, and when there is less than a 5-week period of time in between crossover experiments to allow complete washout of exogenous creatine. In addition, studies tend to show that creatine does not enhance endurance exercise or effect performance in sprints lasting 6 to 60 seconds when prolonged recovery periods of 5 to 25 minutes are given between sprint trials (30).

The only side effect of creatine monohydrate supplementation in clinical investigations has been weight gain (162,169). However, clinical investigations have reported modest elevations in serum creatinine, blood urea nitrogen (BUN), creatine kinase (CK), lactate dehydrogenase (LDH), and aspartate amino transferase (AST) (193,194). The significance of these elevations is unknown, but they appear to normalize with cessation of creatine monohydrate supplementation. Additionally, there is concern over whether creatine supplementation may cause long-term suppression of endogenous creatine synthesis, liver damage, increased renal stress, increased thermal stress, dehydration, and muscle strains and pulls. Repeated anecdotal reports by numerous athletes, trainers, and physicians, seem to support the idea that supplementation with creatine monohydrate does cause significant side effects, most specifically muscle pulls (particularly in the hamstrings and biceps), dehydration, and severe muscle cramping. (Personal communication from Chief Iron Bear (World's Strongest Man Competitor), Special Olympics Symposium, July 1, 1999, Raleigh, NC.)

Although there is a significant amount of research regarding its ergogenic qualities, the literature that effectively evaluates the adverse health effects and medical safety of short- and long-term creatine supplementation is relatively sparse. Further unbiased clinical research needs to be completed. Until then, creatine monohydrate's widespread use will undoubtedly continue to flourish in the athletic arena, especially because it appears to be an effective ergogenic aid that is currently allowed by most athletic governing bodies.

CONCLUSIONS

Now that drug testing includes the use of blood, antidoping programs will undoubtedly be much more effective as revealed by the positive test results at the 2002 Winter Olympic Games and in cycling competitions throughout Europe in the same year to the Tour de France winner in 2006. We applaud the formation of an independent drug testing council for the Olympics, WADA, so the world's best athletes can truly become positive role models for our children, and follow the Olympic creed of "Stronger, Higher, Faster"...without drugs! Unfortunately, there remains a constant in our society that if there are laws and regulations governing drug use in sports, there will be people willing to break them in order to win, especially when millions of dollars are at stake.

The newest frontier in doping in sports lies in genetic engineering and cloning, whereby super athletes are created through manipulation of their genetic code (195). Anticipating the tremendous impact this might have on fair sports competition, the WADA has added gene therapy as one of its prohibited methods in the second draft of its World Anti-Doping Code (196). WADA states that "gene or cell doping is defined as the non-therapeutic use of genes, genetic elements and/or cells that have the capacity to enhance athletic performance." (191) In spite of these preventive measures, there are those who postulate that a new breed of genetically engineered super athletes will be competing in professional and Olympic sport by the year 2008 (197).

A change in our society must occur where we once again adopt moral and ethical standards which are not based on monetary reward, and we once again value sporting achievements obtained through hard work and training, without the use of drugs or genetic manipulation. Until such a time, or until drug testing technologies are developed which make it possible to detect lifetime drug use, sporting activities at all levels will go hand and hand with ergogenic drug use.

REFERENCES

1. U. S. Food and Drug Administration. *Dietary supplement health and education act of 1994*, Public Law 103–417, 103rd Congress, Approved October 25, 1994.
2. Barnes L. Olympic drug testing: improvements without progress. *Phys Sports Med* 1980;8:21–24.
3. Catlin DH, Hatton CK. Use and abuse of anabolic and other drugs for athletic enhancement. *Adv Intern Med* 1991;36:399–424.
4. Puffer JC. The use of drugs in swimming. *Clin Sports Med* 1986;5:77–89.
5. Ferro RT, McKeag DB. Drug testing in sports. In: Garrett WE, Kirkendall DT, Squire DL, eds. *Principles and practice of primary care sports medicine*, Philadelphia: Lippincott Williams & Wilkins, 2001:151–190.
6. MacAuley D. Drugs in sport. *Br J Med* 1996;313:211–215.
7. Knapp WD, Wang TW, Bach BR. Ergogenic drugs in sports. *Clin Sports Med* 1997;16:375–392.
8. Ghaphery NA. Performance-enhancing drugs. *Orthop Clin North Am* 1995;26:433–442.
9. Wagner JC. Enhancement of athletic performance with drugs: an overview. *Sports Med* 1991;12:250–265.
10. Mottram DR. Banned drugs in sport does the International Olympic Committee (IOC) list need updating? *Sports Med* 1999;27:1–10.
11. Anderson WA, McKeag DB. *The substance use and abuse habits of college student-athletes*. (Report No. 2). Mission: The National Collegiate Athletic Association, 1985.
12. Anderson WA, Albrecht RR, McKeag DB, et al. A national survey of alcohol and drug use by college athletes. *Phys Sports Med* 1991;19:91–104.
13. Wadler GI, Hainine B. *Drugs and the athlete*. Philadelphia: FA Davis Co, 1989:75.
14. Eskridge KD, Guthrie SK. Clinical issues associated with urine testing of substances of abuse. *Pharmacotherapy* 1997;17:497–510.
15. Chandler JV, Blair SN. The effect of amphetamines on selected physiological components related to athletic success. *Med Sci Sports Exerc* 1980;12:65–69.
16. Karpovich PV. Effect of amphetamine sulfate on athletic performance. *JAMA* 1959;170:558–561.
17. Smith GM, Beecher HK. Amphetamine sulfate and athletic performance. *JAMA* 1959;170:542–557.
18. Wadler GI. Drug use update. *Med Clin North Am* 1994;78:439–455.
19. Smith DA, Perry PJ. The efficacy of ergogenic agents in athletic competition. Part II: other performance-enhancing agents. *Ann Pharmacother* 1992;26:653–659.
20. Melibn MG, Walsh WM, Shelton GL. *The team physician's handbook*. Philadelphia: Henley & Belfus, 1997:219.
21. Weiner N. Norepinephrine, epinephrine, and the sympathomimetic-amines. In: Gilman AG, Goodman LA and Gilman A, eds. *Goodman and Gillman's the pharmacological basis of therapeutics*. New York: Macmillan, 1985.
22. Langston JW, Langston EB. Neurological consequences of drug abuse. In: Asbury AK, McKhann GM, McDonald WI, eds. *Diseases of the nervous system: clinical neurobiology*, Philadelphia: WB Saunders, 1986:1333.
23. Beckett AH, Cowan DA. Misuse of drugs in sport. *Br J Sports Med* 1979;12:185–194.
24. Landry GL, Kokotallo PK. Drug screening in the athletic setting. *Curr Probl Pediatr* 1994;24:344–359.
25. Fuentes RJ, Davis A, Sample B, et al. Sentinel effect of drug testing for anabolic steroid abuse. *J Law Med Ethics* 1994;22:224–230.
26. Beckett AH, Tucker GT, Moffat AC. Routine detection and identification in urine of stimulants and other drugs, some of which may be used to modify performance in sport. *J Pharm Pharmacol* 1967;19:273–294.
27. Thein LA, Thein JM, Landry GL. Ergogenic aids. *Phys Ther* 1995;75:426–439.
28. Spriet LL. Caffeine and performance. *Int J Sport Nutr* 1995;5:584–599.
29. Williams JH. Caffeine, neuromuscular function and high-intensity exercise performance. *J Sports Med Phys Fitness* 1991;31:481–489.
30. Williams MH. Ergogenic aids: a means to citius, altius, fortius, and Olympic gold? *Res Q Exerc Sport* 1996;67:1–8.
31. Graham T, Spriet L. Performance and metabolic responses to a high caffeine dose during prolonged exercise. *J Appl Physiol* 1991;71:2292–2298.
32. Doherty M. Caffeine: effects on short-term, high-intensity exercise. *J Perform Enhanc Drugs* 1996;1:135–143.
33. Jackman M, Wending P, Friars D, et al. Metabolic catecholamine, and endurance responses to caffeine during intense exercise. *J Appl Physiol* 1996;81(4):1658–1663.
34. Nehlig A, Debry G. Caffeine and sports activity: a review. *Int J Sports Med* 1994;15:215–222.
35. Fisher SM, McMurray RG, Berry M, et al. Influence of caffeine on exercise performance in habitual caffeine users. *Int J Sports Med* 1986;7:276–280.
36. Flinn S, Gregory J, McNaughton LR, et al. Caffeine ingestion prior to incremental cycling to exhaustion in recreational cyclists. *Int J Sports Med* 1990;11:188–193.
37. Weir J, Noakes DT, Myburgh K, et al. A high carbohydrate diet negates the metabolic effects of caffeine during exercise. *Med Sci Sports Exerc* 1987;19:10–105.
38. Van Soeren MH, Sathasivam P, Spriet LL, et al. Caffeine metabolism and epinephrine responses during exercise in users and non-users. *J Appl Physiol* 1993;75:805–812.
39. Cadarette BS, Levine L, Berube CL, et al. Effects of varied doses of caffeine on endurance performance to fatigue. *Biochem Exerc* 1983;13:871–877.
40. Keman WN, Viscoii CM, Brass LM, et al. Phenylpropanolamine and the risk of hemorrhagic stroke. *N Engl J Med* 2000;343:1826–1832.
41. Duchaine D. *Underground body opus militant weight loss and recomposition*. Carson: Xipe Press, 1996.
42. Grundig P, Badrnann M. *World anabolic review*. Houston: MB Muscle Books, 1995.
43. Ephedrine (001149). *Mosby's genRx: the complete reference for generic and brand drugs*, 11th ed. St. Louis: Mosby, 2001.
44. McGuire MJ, Spivak JL. Erythrocytosis and polycythemia. In: Spivak JL Eichner ER, eds. *The fundamentals of clinical hematology*, 3rd ed. Baltimore: The Johns Hopkins University Press, 1993:117–128.
45. Bell DG, Jacobs I, Zamecnik J. Effects of caffeine, ephedrine and that combination on time to exhaustion during high-intensity exercise. *Eur J Appl Physiol* 1998;77:427–433.
46. Sidney KH, Lefcoe WM. The effects of ephedrine on the physiological and psychological responses to submaximal and maximal exercises in man. *Med Sci Sports* 1977;9:95.
47. U. S. Food and Drug Administration Center for Food Safety and Applied Nutrition Consumer Advisory. *Kava-containing dietary supplements may be associated with severe liver injury*. March 25, 2002. http://www.cfsan.fda.gov/≃dms/addskava.html.
48. Gurley BJ, Garber SF, White LM, et al. Ephedrine pharmacokinetics after the ingestion of nutritional supplements containing Ephedra sinica (ma huang). *Ther Drug Monit* 1998;20(4):439–445.
49. O'Keefe M. Supplement is linked to player death. *New York Daily News* Aug 12, 2001.
50. Haller CA, Benowitz NL. Adverse cardiovascular and central nervous system events associated with dietary supplements containing ephedra alkaloids. *N Engl J Med* 2000;343:1833–1838.
51. U. S. Food and Drug Administration. Dietary supplements containing ephedrine alkaloids; proposed rule June 4, 1997. *Fed Regist* 1997;62(107):30677–30724.
52. U. S. Food and Drug Administration. Dietary supplements containing ephedrine alkaloids; withdrawal in part federal register. 2000;65(64): 17474–17477.
53. Hobson K. *Danger at the gym: popular workout-boosting pills and drinks with ephedra get tagged with new health warnings*. U. S. News & World Report, http://www.usnews.com/usnews/nycu/health/articles/020121/21ephecta.htm, January 21, 2002.
54. Duda M. Drug testing challenges: college and pro athletes. *Phys Sports Med* 1983;11:647.
55. Yesalis C. Incidence of anabolic steroid use: a discussion of methodological issues. In: Yesalis C, ed. *Anabolic steroids in sport and exercise*. Champaign: Human Kinetics Publishers, 1993:49–69.
56. Buckley W, Yesalis C, Fried K, et al. Estimated prevalence of anabolic steroid use among male high school seniors. *JAMA* 1988;260:3441–3445.
57. Street C, Antonio J, Cudlipp D. Androgen use by athletes: a reevaluation of the health risks. *Can J Appl Physiol* 1996;21:421–440.
58. Yesalis CE, Kennedy NJ, Kopstein AN, et al. Anabolic-androgenic steroid use in the United States. *JAMA* 1993;270:1217–1221.
59. Faigenbaum AD, Zalchkowsky LD, Gardener DE, et al. Anabolic steroid use by male and female middle school students. American Academy of Pediatrics Committee on Sports Medicine and Fitness. Adolescents and anabolic steroids: a subject review. *Pediatrics* 1997;99:904–908.
60. Franke WW, Berendonk B. Hormonal doping and androgenization of athletes: a secret program of the German Democratic Republic Government. *Clin Chem* 1997;43:1262–1279.
61. Griffin JE, Wislon JD. Disorders of the testes. In: Fauci AS, Brauoveld E, Issebacher KJ, eds. *Harrison's principles of internal medicine*. New York: McGraw-Hill, 1998:2087–2097.
62. Wu FCW. Endocrine aspects of anabolic steroids. *Clin Chem* 1997;43: 1289–2192.
63. Stusnd JE, Diorio DJ. Anabolic agents. *Clin Sports Med* 1998;17:261282.
64. American College of Sports Medicine. Position stand: the use of anabolic-androgenic steroids in sports. *Sports Med Bull* 1984;19:13–18.
65. Honour JW. Steroid abuse in female athletes. *Curr Opin Obstet Gynecol* 1997;9:181–186.
66. Bhasin S, Storer TW, Berman N, et al. The effects of supraphysiological doses of testosterone on muscle size and strength in normal men. *N Engl J Med* 1996;335:1–7.
67. Sachtleben TR, Berg KE, Cheatham JP, et al. Serum lipoprotein patterns in long-term anabolic steroid users. *Res Q Exerc Sport* 1997;68:110–115.

68. Haupt HA. Anabolic steroids and growth hormone. *Am J Sports Med* 1993;21:468–474.
69. *Muscle Media 2000*. Notes from the underground. 1996; 108–114.
70. Bronson FH, Matheme CM. Exposure to anabolic androgenic steroids shortens life span of male mice. *Med Sci Sports Exerc* 1997;29:615–619.
71. Freed DLJ, Banks AJ, Longson D, et al. Anabolic steroids in athletics: crossover double-blind trial on weightlifters. *Br Med J* 1975;2:471–473.
72. Dickerman RD, McConathy WJ, Schaller F, et al. Echocardiography in fraternal twin bodybuilders with one abusing steroids. *Cardiology* 1997;88:50–51.
73. Dickerman RD, Schaller F, Zachariah NY, et al. Left ventricular size and function in elite bodybuilders using anabolic steroids. *Clin J Sports Med* 1997;7:90–93.
74. Ferenchidc GS, Adelman S. Myocardial infarction associated with anabolic steroid use in a previously healthy 37-year-old weightlifter. *Am Heart J* 1992;124(2):507–508.
75. Ferenchick G, Schwartz D, Ball M, et al. Androgenic-anabolic steroid abuse and platelet aggregation: a pilot study in weightlifters. *Am J Med Sci* 1992;303:78–92.
76. Cohen LI, Hartford CG, Rogers GG. Upoproteln(a) and cholesterol in body builders using anabolic androgenic steroids. *Med Sci Sports Exerc* 1996;28:176–179.
77. Pope HG, Katz DL. Psychiatric and medical effects of anabolic-androgenic steroid use. *Arch Gen Psychiatry* 1994;51:375–382.
78. Patti S, Ungurean A, Vecsei L. Basilar artery occlusion associated with anabolic-steroid abuse in a 17-year-old bodybuilder. *Eur Neurol* 1997;27:190–191.
79. Overly WL, Dankoff JA, Wang BK, et al. Androgens and hepatocellular carcinoma in an athlete. *Ann Intern Med* 1984;100:58.
80. Haffner SM. Sex hormone-binding protein, hyperinsulinemia, insulin resistance and noninsulin-dependent diabetes. *Horm Res* 1996;45:233–237.
81. Laseter JT, Russell JA. Anabolic steroid-induced tendon pathology: a review of the literature. *Med Sci Sports Exerc* 1991;23:1–3.
82. Calabrese LH, Kleiner SM, Barana BP, et al. The effects of anabolic steroids and strength training on the human immune response. *Med Sci Sports Exerc* 1989;21:386–392.
83. Haupt HA, Rovere GD. Anabolic steroids: a review of the literature. *Am J Sports Med* 1984;12:469–484.
84. Sklarek H, Mantovani RP, Erens E, et al. AIDS in a bodybuilder using anabolic steroids. *N Engl J Med* 1984;311:1701.
85. Aiache AE. Surgical treatment of gynecomastia in the body builder. *Plast Reconstr Surg* 1989;83:61–66.
86. Roberts JT, Essenhigh DM. Adenocarcinoma of prostate in a 40 year old body-builder. *Lancet* 1986;8509:742.
87. Jin B, Turner L, Walters WAW, et al. Androgen or estrogen effects on human prostate. *J Clin Endocrinol Metab* 1996;81:4290–4295.
88. Korkia P. Anabolic steroid use in adolescents. *Sports Exerc Inj* 1996;2:36–140.
89. Brower KJ, et al. Anabolic-androgenic steroid dependence. *J Clin Psychiatry* 1989;50:31–33.
90. Schwerin MJ, Corcoran KJ. Beliefs about steroids: user vs. non-user comparisons. *Drug Alcohol Depend* 1996;40:221–225.
91. Brower KJ, Blow FC, Ellopulos GA, et al. Anabolic androgenic steroids and suicide. *Am J Psychiatry* 1989;146:1075.
92. Corrigan B. Anabolic steroids and the mind. *Med J Aust* 1996;165:222–226.
93. Emery PW, Rothwel NJ, Stock MJ, et al. Chronic effects of beta 2 adrenergic agonists on body composition and protein synthesis in the rat. *Biosci Rep* 1984;4(1):83–91.
94. Stallion A, Foley-Nelson T, Chance WT. Anticatabolic effect of the beta-2-agonist cimaterol *in vivo* in tumor-bearing animals. *J Surg Res* 1995;59(3):387–392.
95. Kitaura T, Tsunekawa N, Kraemer W. Inhibited longitudinal growth of bones in young male rats by clenbuterol. *Med Sci Sports Exerc* 2002;34:67–273.
96. Prather ID, Brown DE, North P, et al. Clenbuterol: a substitute for anabolic steroids? *Med Sci Sports Exerc* 1995;27:1118–1121.
97. Spann C, Winter ME. Effect on clenbuterol on athletic performance. *Ann Pharmacother* 1995;29:75–77./
98. DiPasquale MG. Stimulants and adaptogens: Part 1. *Drugs Sports* 1992;1: 8–10.
99. Brambilia G. Food poisoning following consumption of clenbuterol-treated veal in Italy. *JAMA* 1997;278:635.
100. Meyer HH, Rinke LM. The pharmacokinetics and residues of clenbuterol in veal calves. *J Anim Sci* 1991;69(11):4538–4544.
101. Nelson JL, Chalk CL, Warden GD. Anabolic impact of cimaterol in conjunction with enteral nutrition following burn trauma. *J Trauma-Inj Infect Crit Care* 1995;38(2):237–241.
102. Byrem TM, Beermann DH, Robinson TF. The beta-agonist cimaterol directly enhances chronic protein accretion in skeletal muscle. *J Anim Sci* 1998;76(4):988–998.
103. Kalman D. Cimaterol Is it the best fat burner? *Muscular Dev* 2002; 100–103.
104. Bazylaic G, Nagels U. Integrated acquisition of analytical and biopharmaceutical screening data for beta-adrenergic-drugs employing diversified macrocycle supported potentiometric detection in HPLC systems. *Curr Med Chem* 2002;9(16):1547–1566.
105. Van Vyncht G, Preece S, Gaspar P, et al. Gas and liquid chromatography coupled to tandem mass spectrometry for the multiresidue analysis of beta-agonists in biological matrices. *J Chromatogr A* 1996;750(1–2):43–49.
106. Willey JW. Insulin as an anabolic aid? A danger for strength athletes. *Phys Sportsmed* 1997;25(10):103–104.
107. Sonksen PH. Insulin, growth hormone and sport. *J Endocrinol* 2001;170: 13–25.
108. Starr O. The ultimate "no fat gain" insulin program. *Muscle Month* 2000;1.
109. Zinker BA. Nutrition and exercise in individuals with diabetes. *Clin Sports Med* 1999;18(3):585–606.
110. Bielak KM, Merket RM. Exercise. *Clin Fam Pract* 2000;2(2):407–421.
111. Tissandier O, Peres G, Fiet J, et al. Testosterone, dehydroepiandrosterone, insulin-like growth factor 1, and insulin in sedentary and physically trained aged men. *Eur J Appl Physiol* 2001;85(12):177–184.
112. Saugy M, Cardis C, Schweizer C, et al. Detection of human growth hormone doping in urine: out of competition tests are necessary. *J Chromatogr B Biomed Appl* 1996;687:201211.
113. Macintyre JG. Growth hormone and athletes. *Sports Med* 1987;4:129–142.
114. Cowart VS. Human growth hormone: the latest ergogenic aid? *Phys Sports Med* 1988;16:175–185.
115. Kicman AT, Mali JP, Teale JD, et al. Serum IGF-1 and IGF binding proteins 2 and 3 as potential markers of doping with human GH. *Clin Endocrinol* 1997;47:43–50.
116. Cutter L. The regulation of growth hormone secretion. *Endocrinol Metab Clin North Am* 1996;25:541–571.
117. Di Luigi L, Guidetti L. IGF-1, IGFBP-2, and -3: do they have a role in detecting rhGH abuse in trained men? *Med Sci Sports Exerc* 2002;34(8):1270–1278.
118. Yarasheski KE. Growth hormone effects on metabolism, body composition, muscle mass, and strength. *Exerc Sport Sci Rev* 1994;22:285–312.
119. Schrof JM. *Pumped up*. US News and World Report, June 1, 1992.
120. Laidler P, Cowan DA, Hider RC, et al. New decision limits and quality-control material for detecting human chorionic gonadotrophin misuse in sports. *Clin Chem* 1994;40:1306–1311.
121. United States Olympic Committee. *National anti-doping program policies and procedures*. Colorado Springs: USOC Drug Control Administration.
122. Delbeke FT, Van Eenoo P, De Backer P. Detection of human chorionic gonadotrophin misuse in sports. *Int J Sports Med* 1998;19:287–290.
123. De Boer D, De Jong EG, Van Rossum JM, et al. Doping control of testosterone and human chorionic gonadotrophin: a case study. *Int J Sports Med* 1991;12:46–51.
124. Thompson CA. Once-weekly erythropoiesis-stimulating protein enters market. *Am J Health Syst Pharm* 2001;58(22):2120–2121.
125. Nissenson AR. Novel erythropoiesis stimulating protein for managing the anemia of chronic kidney disease. *Am J Kidney Dis* 2001;38(6):1390–1397.
126. Egrie JC, Browne JK. Development and characterization of novel erythropoiesis stimulating protein (NESP). *Nephrol Dial Transplant* 2001;16(Suppl. 3):3–13.
127. Choi D, Kim M, Park J. Erythropoietin: physico - and biochemical analysis. *J Chromatogr B Biomed Appl* 1996;687:189–199.
128. Strider PR. Other ergogenic agents. *Clin Sports Med* 1998;17:283–297.
129. Harris BA, Epstein PE Jr. Out of thin air the evolving enigma of erythropoietin and neocytolysis. *Ann Intern Med* 2001;134(8):710–712.
130. American College of Sports Medicine. The use blood doping as an ergogenic aid (position statement). *Med Sci Sports Exerc* 1996;28:1–8.
131. *Am J Nurs*. New Drugs. 2002;102(1):24.
132. Wilber RL. Detection of DNA-recombinant human epoetin-alfa as a pharmacological ergogenic aid. *Sports Med* 2002;32(2):125–142.
133. Lage JM, Panizo C, Masdeu J, et al. Cyclist's doping associated with cerebral sinus thrombosis. *Neurology* 2002;58(4):665.
134. Ekblom BG, Berglund B. Effect of erythropoietin administration on maximal aerobic power. *Scand J Med Sci Sports* 1991;1:88–93.
135. Brien AJ, Simon TL. The effect of red blood cell reinfusion on 10-km race time. *JAMA* 1987;257:2761–2765.
136. Brien AJ, Harris RJ, Simon TL. The effects of an autologous Infusion of 400 mL red blood cells on selected hematological parameters and 1,500 m race time in highly trained runners. *Bahrain Med Bull* 1989;11:6–16.
137. Goforth HW, Campbell NL, Hogdon JA, et al. Hematologic parameters of trained distance runners following induced erythrocythemia. *Med Sci Sports Exerc* 1982;14:174.
138. Sawka MN, Gonzalez RR, Young AJ, et al. Polycythemia and hydration: effects on thermoregulation and blood volume during exercise heat stress. *Am J Physiol* 1988;225:R456–R463.
139. Eschbach JW, Egrie JC, Downing MR, et al. Correction of the anemia of end-stage renal disease with recombinant human erythropoietin. *N Engl J Med* 1987;316:73–78.
140. McGuire MJ, Spivak JL. Erythrocytosls and polycythemia. In: Spivak JL, Eicher ER, eds. *The fundamentals of clinical hematology*, 3rd ed. Baltimore: The Johns Hopkins University Press, 1993:117–128.
141. Pimay F. Doping in sports. *Rev Med Liege* 2001;56(4):265–268.
142. Abramowicz M. The medical letter: dehydroepiandrosterone (DHEA). 1996;38:91–92.
143. Svec F, Porter JR. The actions of exogenous dehydroepiandrosterone in experimental animals and humans (44285). *Proc Soc Exp Biol Med* 1998;218:174–191.

144. Kreider RB. Dietary supplements and the promotion of muscle growth with resistance exercise. *Sports Med* 1999;27:97–110.
145. Gordon GB, Shantz LM, Talalay P. Modulation of growth, differentiation, and carcinogenesis by dehydroepiandrosterone. *Adv Enzyme Regul* 1987;26:355–382.
146. Heinonen PK, Kolvula T, Pystynen P. Decreased serum level of dehydroepiandrosterone sulfate in postmenopausal women with ovarian cancer. *Gynecol Obstet Invest* 1987;23:271–273.
147. Nestier JE, Barlascini CO, Clore JN, et al. Dehydroepiandrosterone reduces serum low density lipoprotein levels and body fat but does not alter insulin sensitivity in normal men. *J Clin Endocrinol Metab* 1988;66:57–61.
148. Zumoff B, Strain GW, Heymsfleld SB, et al. A randomized double-blind crossover study of the antiobesity effects of etiocholanedione. *Obes Res* 1993;2:13–18.
149. Cleary MP. The antiobesity effect of dehydroepiandrosterone in rats. *Proc Soc Exp Biol Med* 1991;196:8–16.
150. Usiskin KS, Butterworth S, Clore JN, et al. Lack of effect of dehydroepiandrosterone in obese men. *Int J Obes Relat Metab Disord* 1990;14:457–463.
151. Welle S, Jozefowicz R, Statt M. Failure of dehydroepiandrosterone to influence energy and protein metabolism in humans. *J Clin Endocrinol Metab* 1990;71:1259–1264.
152. Dyner TS, Lang W, Geaga J, et al. An open-label dose-escalation trial of oral dehydroepiandrosterone tolerance and pharmacokinetics in patients with HIV disease. *J Acquir Immune Defic Syndr Hum Retrovirol* 1993;6:459–465.
153. Barrett-Connor E, Goodman-Gruen D. Dehydroepiandrosterone sulfate does not predict cardiovascular death in postmenopausal women: the Rancho Bemardo Study. *Circulation* 1995;91:1757–1760.
154. Rao MS, Subbarao V, Yeldandi AV, et al. Inhibition of spontaneous testicular leydig cell tumor development in F-344 rats by dehydroepiandrosterone. *Cancer Lett* 1992;65:123–126.
155. Rao MS, Subbarao V, Kumar S, et al. Phenotypic properties of liver tumors induced by dehydroepiandrosterone In F-344 rats. *Jpn J Cancer Res* 1992;83:1179–1183.
156. Larkin M. DHEA: will science confirm the headlines? *J Lancet* 1998;352:206.
157. Armsey TD, Green GA. Nutrition supplements: science vs hype. *Phys Sportsmed* 1997;25:77–92.
158. Fontenot B. The creatine craze: such ergogenic promise—but at what price? *Nutrition Forum* 1998;15:11–12.
159. Bolotte CP. Creatine supplementation in athletes: benefits and potential risks. *J La State Med Soc* 1998;50:325–327.
160. Chanutin A. The fate of creatine when administered to man. *J Biol Chem* 1926;67:29–41.
161. Hultman E, Bergstrom J, Spriet LL. Energy metabolism and fatigue. In: Taylor A, Gollnick P, Green H, eds. *Biochemistry of exercise VII*, Vol. 27. Champaign: Human Kinetics Publishers, 1990:73–92.
162. Williams MH, Branch JD. Creatine supplementation and exercise performance: an update. *J Am Coll Nutr* 1998;17:216–234.
163. Harris RC, Vim M, Greenhaff PL, et al. The effect of oral creatine supplementation on running performance during maximal short term exercise in man. *J Physiol* 1993;467:74P.
164. Constantin-Teodosiu D, Greenhaff PL, Gardiner SM, et al. Attenuation by creatine of myocardial metabolic stress in Brattleboro rats caused by chronic Inhibition of nitric oxide synthase. *Br J Pharmacol* 1995;116:328892.
165. Gordon A, Hultman E, Kauser L, et al. Creatine supplementation in chronic heart failure increases skeletal muscle creatine phosphate and muscle performance. *Cardiovasc Res* 1995;30:413–418.
166. Greenhaff PL, Bodin K, Harris RC, et al. The influence of oral creatine supplementation on muscle phosphocreatine resynthesis following intense contraction in man. *J Physiol* 1993;467:75P.
167. Greenhaff PL, Bodin K, Soderlund K, et al. Effect of oral creatine supplementation on skeletal muscle phosphocreatine resynthesis. *Am J Physiol* 1994;266:E725–E730.
168. Lemon P, Boska M, Brodie D, et al. Effect of oral creatine supplementation on energetics during repeated maximal muscle contraction. *Med Sci Sports Exerc* 1995;27:S204.
169. Kreider R. Creatine supplementation: analysis of ergogenic value, medical safety, and concerns. *J Exerc Physiol Online* 1998;1:1–11.
170. Volek J, Kraemer W, Bush J, et al. Creatine supplementation enhances muscular performance during high-intensity resistance exercise. *J Am Diet Assoc* 1997;97:765–770.
171. Balsom PD, Soderlund K, Sjodin B, et al. Skeletal muscle metabolism during short duration high-intensity exercise: influence of creatine supplementation. *Acta Physiol Scand* 1995;1154:303–310.
172. Casey A, et al. Creatine ingestion favorably affects performance and muscle metabolism during maximal exercise in humans. *Am J Physiol* 1996;271:E31–E37.
173. Kreider R, Ferreira M, Wilson M, et al. Effects of creatine supplementation on body composition, strength and sprint performance. *Med Sci Sports Exerc* 1998;30:73–82.
174. Balsom PD, Ekblom B, Soderlund K, et al. Creatine supplementation and dynamic high-intensity intermittent exercise. *Scand J Med Sci Sports* 1993;3:143–149.
175. Birch R, Noble D, Greenhaff PL. The influence of dietary creatine supplementation on performance during repeated bouts of maximal isokinetic cycling in man. *Eur J Appl Physiol* 1994;69:268–270.
176. Davison B, Cutler M, Moody A, et al. Effects of oral creatine loading on single and repeated maximal short sprints. *Aust J Sci Med Sport* 1995;27:56–61.
177. Earnest CP, Snell PG, Rodriguez R, et al. The effect of creatine monohydrate ingestion on anaerobic power indices, muscular strength and body composition. *Acta Physiol Scand* 1995;153:207–209.
178. Greenhaff PL, Casey A, Short AH, et al. Influence of oral creatine supplementation of muscle torque during repeated bouts of maximal voluntary exercise in man. *Clin Sci* 1993;84:565–571.
179. Grindstaff PD, Kreider RB, Bishop R, et al. Effects of creatine supplementation on repetitive sprint performance and body composition in competitive swimmers. *Int J Sport Nutr* 1997;7:330–348.
180. Jacobs I, Bleue S, Goodman J. Creatine ingestion increases maximal accumulated oxygen deficit and anaerobic exercise capacity. *Med Sci Sports Exerc* 1995;27:S204.
181. Rossiter HB, Cannell ER, Jakeman PM. The effect of oral creatine supplementation on the 1000-m performance of competitive rowers. *J Sports Sci* 1996;14:175–179.
182. Stout JR, Eckerson J, Noonan D, et al. The effects of a supplement designed to augment creatine uptake on exercise performance and fat-free mass in football players. *Med Sci Sports Exerc* 1997;29:S251.
183. Goldberg PG, Bechtel PJ. Effects of low dose creatine supplementation on strength, speed and power events by male athletes. *Med Sci Sports Exerc* 1997;29:S251.
184. Stroud MA, Holliman D, Bell D, et al. Effect of oral creatine supplementation on respiratory gas exchange and blood lactate accumulation during steady-state incremental treadmill exercise and recovery in man. *Clin Sci* 1994;87:707–710.
185. Mujika I, Chatard JC, Lacoste L, et al. Creatine supplementation does not improve sprint performance in competitive swimmers. *Med Sci Sports Exerc* 1996;28:1435–1441.
186. Redondo D, Dowling EA, Graham BL, et al. The effect of oral creatine monohydrate supplementation on running velocity. *Int J Sport Nutr* 1996;6:213–221.
187. Balsom PD, Harridge SDR, Sbderlund K, et al. Creatine supplementation per se does not enhance endurance exercise performance. *Acta Physiol Scand* 1993;149:521–523.
188. Bamett C, Hinds M, Jenkins DG. Effects of oral creatine supplementation on multiple splint cycle performance. *Aust J Sci Med Sport* 1996;28:35–39.
189. Burke LM, Pyne DB, Telford RD. Effect of oral creatine supplementation on single-effort sprint performance in elite swimmers. *Int J Sport Nutr* 1998;6:222–233.
190. Cooke WU, Grandjean PW, Barnes WS. Effect of oral astatine supplementation on power output and fatigue during bicycle ergometry. *J Appl Physiol* 1995;78:670–673.
191. Febbraio MA, Flanagan TR, Snow RJ, et al. Effect of creatine supplementation on intramuscular TCr, metabolism and performance during intermittent, supramaximal exercise in humans. *Acta Physiol Scand* 1995;155:387–395.
192. Odland LM, MacDougall JD, Tarnopolsky M, et al. The effect of oral creatine supplementation on muscle phosphocreatine and power output during a short-term maximal cycling task. *Med Sci Sports Exerc* 1994;26:S23.
193. Almada A, Mitchell T, Earnest C. Impact of chronic creatine supplementation on serum enzyme concentrations. *FASEB J* 1996;10:A791.
194. Earnest C, Aknada A, Mitchel T. Influence of chronic creatine supplementation on hepatorenal function. *FASEB J* 1996;10:A790.
195. Dyer G, Firn D. *Gene doping threatens to transform sport in the final part of our series, Geoff Dyer and David Firn examine the dangers to sport from medical advances*, Section: Drugs in Sport, 2nd ed. London: Financial Times, May 31, 2002:5.
196. World Anti Doping Agency. *Prohibited classes of substances and prohibited methods 2003*. Available at http://www.wada-ama.org, Draft dated September 27, 2002:5.
197. Adam D. Gene therapy may be up to speed for cheats at 2008 Olympics. *Nature* 2001;414(6864):569–570.

5
Sports Medicine and Your Community

Building a Sports Medicine Practice and Network

38

Christopher Madden

Establishing a good sports medicine network is pivotal to the success of a sports physician. The term *network* may be defined as an interconnected or interrelated chain, group, or system (1). An effective sports medicine network functions at both local and national levels. A network offers many advantages: facilitates delivery of quality comprehensive care to athletes in a timely manner; unites sports medicine professionals in the community to work as a "sports medicine team"; serves as the basis for a local referral network; facilitates relationships at physician, school, community, and national levels; fosters continuing education through colleague interaction, structured continuing medical education (CME), and sometimes through writing and public outreach activities. Personal network requirements will be closely related to personal goals and to the individual characteristics of each sports practice.

When establishing a network, maintain an awareness that the meaning of sports medicine may vary greatly among individuals and organizations. To individual sports physicians it usually encompasses the duties of a team physician, and it almost always includes office-based and other community activities directly related to sports. The primary care sports physician frequently interacts with athletes as a primary care provider in addition to serving as a team physician (2). Additionally, many primary care sports physicians apply concepts of health promotion and disease prevention to increase fitness in the general patient population (3). Primary care physicians (PCPs) may frequently encounter public and professional opinion that sports medicine is made up primarily of orthopedics and physical therapy, but through their actions in the community, the valuable and unique contributions of the primary care sports physician become obvious.

SELECTION OF THE "IDEAL SETTING"

The first question a sports physician should entertain is "What type of sports practice do I want?" Many variables factor in the decision of how and where to practice medicine, but defining your "ideal practice" is a good place to start (see Table 38.1).

Sports settings vary, but options usually include working in a private practice as a primary care and sports medicine physician (primary care or orthopedic office), working as a sports medicine physician only (mainly musculoskeletal) in a private office (usually orthopedic or sports medicine center), working in an academic setting with sports medicine opportunities (family medicine residency or sports medicine fellowship), or working at a collegiate student health center with team physician responsibilities. Selecting an "ideal practice" will help guide physicians in determining the type of network they need to build or enter.

When changing jobs, or when leaving residency or fellowship, start looking for the "ideal job" early. Sports medicine colleagues, journal advertisements, local resources (hospitals, practice groups, physician networks, independent physician organizations, managed care organizations), state and regional resources (state

TABLE 38.1

THINGS TO THINK ABOUT WHEN CHOOSING AN "IDEAL PRACTICE"

How much sports medicine do I want to practice?
How much primary care do I want to practice?
Is my practice philosophy compatible with the group's philosophy?
Which sports teams do I want to work with, and at which level(s) (recreational, high school, college, professional)?
Do I want to teach?
Do I want an academic affiliation?
Is the area I am considering receptive to primary care sports medicine?
Is there a "sports medicine team" in the area?
What is the quality of the sports medicine team? What are its expectations?
Are there untapped sports opportunities in the area?
Is a good sports medicine referral network available?
Where do I want to live?
What will make my family happy?
What are my commitments outside of the office?
What is my salary?
What is the ideal setting to achieve my goals?

TABLE 38.2

PRACTICE SETTINGS AMONG PRIMARY CARE SPORTS MEDICINE PHYSICIANS

	%
Solo	11
Private group practice	33
Multispecialty group	14
University-based	23
Residency-based	10
Others	9

Source: Hoffman D. *Primary care sports medicine—the realities (conference proceeding)*. San Diego: American Medical Society for Sports Medicine, 2000.

medical society, physician recruiters), and national resources (American Academy of Family Physicians [AAFP], American Medical Society for Sports Medicine [AMSSM], American College of Sports Medicine [ACSM]) may be good sources for job opportunities. The World Wide Web is a useful communication link for physicians looking for job opportunities. Three useful web sites that list career opportunities are: www.aafp.org, www.amssm.org, and www.acsm.org. Actively seek out and make job opportunities for yourself. Send a query letter and/or curriculum vitae to offices or institutions in areas of special interest, and follow up written communications with a phone call. Visit groups and communities with attractive sports medicine opportunities. A phone call to the local head athletic trainer often helps identify important sports medicine figures and organizations in the area. Phone conversations with sports medicine (primary care and orthopedic) physicians, physical therapists, and athletic trainers may help assess local attitudes, sports medicine politics and structure, and openness to a new sports physician's skills.

Published sports medicine demographic studies are limited. A recent survey of primary care sports medicine (PCSM) physicians indicates that most (71%) PCSM physicians are family practice doctors, and that internists, pediatricians, physical medicine and rehabilitation physicians, and emergency medicine physicians also practice PCSM. Among those surveyed, practice settings are diverse (see Table 38.2). Fifty six percent report practicing their primary specialty more than sports medicine, 23% report practicing more sports medicine than their primary specialty, 15% practice mostly sports medicine, and 3% practice mostly primary care (4).

An earlier questionnaire devised to ascertain sports medicine practice content indicates that 45% of responding family physicians serve as team physicians in one or more sports at varying levels (see Table 38.3) (5). A 1987 Physician and Sportsmedicine survey revealed that 46% of team physicians were family doctors and general practitioners, 17% were orthopedists, and other specialties (pediatrics, internal medicine, osteopathy, general surgery, obstetrics/gynecology) made up a smaller percent (6).

The AMSSM recently published surveys to its web site that address current practice demographic, salary, credentialing, and membership trends of AMSSM members in sports medicine (7–9). The surveys and additional sports medicine business practice resources may be accessed by members of AMSSM at www.amssm.org under Sports Medicine Practice Tools, a resource developed by AMSSM's Economics Committee. Table 38.4 highlights pertinent survey points.

A survey addressing potential gender differences in sports medicine illustrates no significant differences with regard to practice types, location, and time spent in sports

TABLE 38.3

FAMILY PRACTICE TEAM PHYSICIANS BY LEVEL OF COMPETITION

Competition	Number
Elementary school	31
Middle school	40
High school	93
College or university	11
Community league	8

Source: Mellion MB. The sports medicine content of family practice. *J Fam Pract* 1985;21(6):473–478.

TABLE 38.4

AMERICAN MEDICAL SOCIETY FOR SPORTS MEDICINE PRACTICE, SALARY, AND MEMBERSHIP—PARTIAL SURVEY RESULTS

Number of patients seen per half day in office: 46%, 10–15; 29%, 5–10; 15%, 15–20
Number of consultations seen per half day in office: 77%, 0–5; 18%, 5–10
Gender of survey participants (Practice and Salary Survey): 83% male, 17% female
Board certification in sport medicine (Practice and Salary Survey): 96% yes, 4% no
Primary board certification (Practice and Salary Survey): 79% family medicine, 8% pediatrics, 8% internal medicine, 1% emergency medicine, 0.5% physical medicine and rehabilitation
Completed sports medicine fellowship: 75% yes, 25% no
Weekly hours spent performing inpatient care: 88%, 0–5; 4%, 5–10
Weekly hours spent performing training room duties: 63%, 0–5; 20%, 5–10
Weekly hours spent teaching: 50%, 0–5; 20%, 5–10
Weekly hours spent doing research: 88%, 0–5; 6%, 5–10
Hold academic rank: 66% yes, 34% no
Most common academic rank: assistant professor 20%, associate professor 12%
Clinical practice setting: 58% sports medicine clinic, 25% orthopedic surgery clinic, 42% family medicine clinic, 18% student health, 4% pediatric clinic[a]
Salary range (Practice and Salary Survey): 70,000 > 300,000 dollars
Most frequent salaries (reported in hundred thousand): 8%, 110–120; 9%, 120–130; 13%, 130–140; 9%, 140–150; 13%, 150–160; 6%, 160–170; 4%,170–180; 6%, 190–200; 7%, 200–210
Credentialing with insurance company: 12% orthopedics, 65% family medicine, 71% sports medicine, 3% physical medicine, 6% podiatrics, 6% internal medicine, 2% emergency medicine, 3% others
Do area insurance companies allow dual credentialing (e.g., primary specialty and sports medicine): 28% yes, 13% no, 47% do not know[a]
Is there a need for dual credentialing in your area and why: 20% need for reimbursement problems, 6% need for advertisement/marketing, 10% no need, 47% do not know
Teams covered (membership survey): 39% recreational, 74% high school, 17.5% community college, 15% NCAA Division III, 11% NCAA Division II, 45% NCAA Division I, 29% Professional, 8. 5% NAIA
Reimbursed by team or athletic organization (Membership Survey): 54% not reimbursed, 25% stipend or part of salary, 1.4% hourly rate for training room, 3% hourly rate for game coverage, 11% benefits (team gear, etc.), 2.2% employer pays for right to deliver medical care to team, 2.2% employed solely by team or athletic organization[a]

[a]Percentages total >100% because some survey participants appropriately selected more than one option when applicable to specific setting.
Source: American Medical Society for Sports Medicine. *AMSSM practice and salary survey.* http://www.amssm.org/AMSSMEconomySurvey.pdf, 2006; American Medical Society for Sports Medicine. *Membership survey.* http://www.amssm.org/AMSSMMembershipSurvey2004.pdf, 2006; American Medical Society for Sports Medicine. *Economics committee pilot survey: insurance company credentialing and website recognition.* http://www.amssm.org/EconomicsCommitteePilotSurvey.pdf, 2006.

medicine with the exception of training room and event coverage, where males were more likely to cover all types of sporting events and were more likely to cover all levels of training rooms except Division I (10).

A mail survey of 250 sports medicine centers across the United States indicates that a "typical" sports medicine facility is corporate owned, but that ownership, ownership background, and management varies (Table 38.5) (11). The same survey indicates that most patients at the sports medicine centers are recreational athletes, but that many other types of athletes attend the center (Table 38.6) (11).

A slightly different client distribution was reported in a prior survey, where most patients were high school athletes (12). Most sports medicine centers employ physical therapists, some employ athletic trainers. Treatment of acute injures, injury prevention, and especially rehabilitation are the primary goals of the centers (11–13). The surveys (10–12) focused on a limited number of "sports medicine centers" in the United States and likely do not reflect the increasingly prevalent sports medicine practices of PCPs, especially in smaller settings and primary care–based offices.

ESTABLISHING A LOCAL SPORTS MEDICINE NETWORK

Identifying the Sports Medicine Team

One of the first steps to establishing a successful sports medicine practice, independent of practice demographics, involves identifying the local "sports medicine team." The team may exist on two levels locally: community and

TABLE 38.5
CHARACTERISTICS OF SPORTS MEDICINE FACILITY OWNERSHIP, ADMINISTRATION, AND MANAGEMENT

	%
Ownership	
Corporate	40
Partnership	29
University	21
Hospital	8
	8
Professional Background of Owner	
PT only	22
MD only	20
PT and MD	9
Other, including combinations of PT, MD. and other health professionals	49
Director of Day-to-Day Operations	
PT	45
PT/ATC	17
Orthopedist	13
Exercise physiologist	8
Others	17

PT = physical therapist; MD = medical doctor; ATC = certified athletic trainer.
Source: American Medical Society for Sports Medicine. *Membership survey*. http://www.amssm.org/AMSSMMembershipSurvey2004.pdf, 2006.

scholastic (usually high school or college) (see Figures 38.1 and 38.2).

Providing quality medical care for athletes is often challenging, and it frequently involves multiple individuals representing various professional disciplines (14). The primary care sports medicine physician may play a pivotal role, and often serves as a "gatekeeper" for his or her personal patients in the community model. On a community level, the primary care sports medicine physician may use his or her unique position and comprehensive understanding of medicine and sports medicine to help direct care for athletes. So, the term *team physician* may refer to the "activity of a sports physician in providing medical surveillance and care to a team of athletes, or to activities in coordinating a team of medical and paramedical professionals in the care of one or more athletes (14)."

The depth and breadth of the sports medicine team varies with each community, and some smaller communities may not even have a team physician, let alone a larger network of sports physicians and other sports professionals. The sports medicine physician should attempt to identify all "players" in the sports medicine arena, and the local school is a good place to start. Developing a successful relationship with the athletic trainer(s), coach(es), athletic director(s), and other pertinent school administrators sets the groundwork for becoming a team physician at the scholastic level and contributes to the development of a local sports medicine network. On a broader scale, the new team physician should actively and simultaneously develop relationships with local orthopedists, physicians and other consultants with interests in sports, and with other nonphysician sports and health professionals. If a network already exists on one or both levels, the new physician is faced with figuring out the best way to enter the network, and then how to function within and, if needed, to improve an already existing sports medicine system.

TABLE 38.6
CLIENT PROFILE OF 250 RANDOMLY SELECTED SPORTS MEDICINE CENTERS IN THE UNITED STATES

	Percentage of Patients
Amateur athletes	13
Recreational athletes	30
High school athletes	20
Public	19
Professional athletes	1
College athletes	10
Industrial injuries	7

Source: American Medical Society for Sports Medicine. *Membership survey*. http://www.amssm.org/AMSSMMembershipSurvey2004.pdf, 2006.

Marketing Strategies for a Sports Practice

A recent survey of 200 randomly selected sports medicine centers throughout the United States (from a directory of sports centers published in the Physician and Sportsmedicine, 1992) indicates that communication with physicians and referral sources may be one of the most effective marketing strategies. Lunches, meetings, phone calls, thank-you notes, and other general communications are all effective forms of networking. Other successful strategies mentioned in the survey include advertising in newspapers and other sources, high school contracts, word of mouth, and providing good service (13).

Announce your arrival. Arrange to have your picture taken, and if you are joining a group, it may be a good idea to have a picture taken of you with the group for the local newspaper. An immediate publicly recognized association with a good group can be a powerful starter for a new practice. Follow up the advertisement with a reminder advertisement 3 to 6 months after starting your practice. Join or establish a web page that allows you to describe your unique interests and skills. Researching through phone calls and personal meetings with other sports physicians before you arrive will facilitate an understanding of the sports medicine structure and politics in the area. Word your introductory announcement or

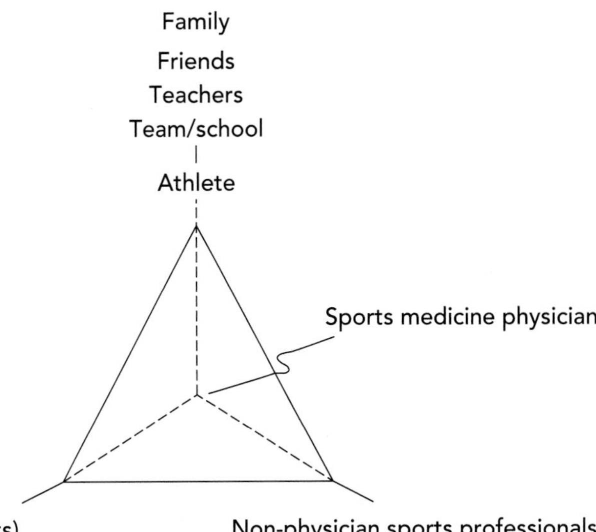

Physicians (specialists)

Orthopaedists
Primary care sports medicine physicians
Neurologists
Neurosurgeons
Physical medicine and rehabilitation physicians
Sports psychiatrists
Osteopaths
Other sports specialists

Non-physician sports professionals

Athletic trainers
Physical therapists
Sports psychologists
Sports dentists
Podiatrists and/or pedorthotists
Nutritionists
Exercise physiologists
kinesiologists
Other health educators

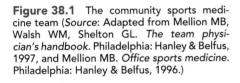

Figure 38.1 The community sports medicine team (*Source*: Adapted from Mellion MB, Walsh WM, Shelton GL. *The team physician's handbook*. Philadelphia: Hanley & Belfus, 1997, and Mellion MB. *Office sports medicine*. Philadelphia: Hanley & Belfus, 1996.)

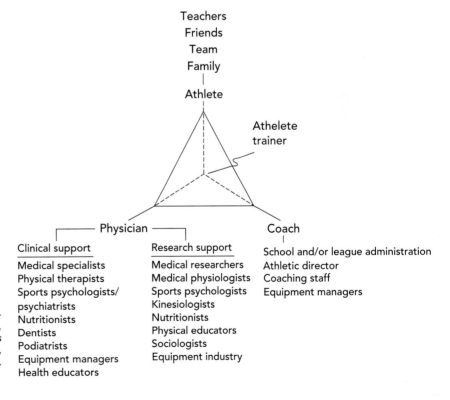

Figure 38.2 The scholastic sports medicine team (*Source*: Adapted from Mellion MB, Walsh WM, Shelton GL. *The team physician's handbook*. Philadelphia: Hanley & Belfus, 1997, and Mellion MB. *Office sports medicine*. Philadelphia: Hanley & Belfus, 1996.)

article appropriately, and do not overtoot your own horn. Attempt to facilitate cohesiveness among your sports colleagues, and to minimize competition, although it is likely that both elements will be present in most settings.

Meet your colleagues as soon as you arrive (see Figure 38.1). Find a network of orthopedists that you trust, and remember that not all orthopedists share equal training in sports medicine (15). Make the orthopedists aware of your skills and interests, and explain to them what benefits you may be able to provide to them and to the community (15). Seeing "overflow" patients in a busy orthopedic office may benefit the office by preventing patients from seeking another orthopedist, may keep patients happy by offering timely care, and will contribute to a strong relationship between primary care and orthopedic offices. Use insight from partners, physical therapists, athletic trainers, and word of mouth to develop quality referral groups. Schedule lunch time or early morning meetings and drop by offices (if appropriate) during "down time," which can be an issue the first few months of starting a new practice. Use any spare time to make additional phone calls to those who may not be able to meet with you in the near future. Tour physical therapy offices and meet with the therapists. Visit local schools and training rooms and meet the athletic trainers, coaches, and other administrators. Visit other fitness facilities, including local health clubs, and meet local nutritionists, exercise physiologists, and other sports professionals.

Be visible in the community and make yourself available to anyone asking for help with sports coverage. Offer to help with preseason, preparticipation physical examinations. Attend local sporting events, and if not already assigned a team, attempt to arrange assisted coverage so the other sports physicians become aware of your skills. Speak at every appropriate public opportunity, and pass out cards to everyone you meet (15). A few presentations addressing pertinent topics (e.g., head injuries before or during football preseason) may easily be arranged as CME talks at the local hospital, and they are a good way to meet a large number of physicians in your community, as well as to introduce them to your interests and skills.

Advertise in newspapers. Before you arrive, develop business cards that list your skills. Develop or modify letterhead pertinent to your sports practice, and come up with your own logo. For example, if you are joining a family medicine office with the existing letterhead, you may want to use the old letterhead (e.g., "Mountain View Family Practice") for family practice communications, but you may want to modify the letterhead to include your sports designation and the family practice name (e.g., Logo + "Sports Medicine at Mountain View Family Practice") for sports communications. Develop physical therapy referrals, prescription pads, handouts, and notepads that carry your logo and name.

Building an Office Practice

"Negotiating the labyrinth of managed care is increasingly part of the PCSM physician's job description, especially if he or she is a team physician" (2). Work closely with your new office staff to get approved on as many insurance plans as possible. The insurance companies frequently have panels that meet on a regular interval (e.g., quarterly), so start early (6–9 months). Your new partners' approval on various plans is often your ticket for successful and timely approval. If you are starting in a new office or as a solo provider, getting approved may be more difficult. Start even earlier (9–12 months). Apply for a state license at least a year in advance. Identify any organizations, especially independent physician associations (IPAs), that have established bargaining power with insurance companies and local physician networks. Each managed care plan is unique, and each has its own provider panel, reimbursement schedule, rules, and referral panel (16). Become familiar with your insurance plans (diagnostic services covered and who may order them, referral systems, etc.), communicate effectively (be able to discuss referrals to various designations), and designate a referral specialist within your office (2). Be aware that capitated contracts may financially hurt a sports medicine physician because of the increased need for diagnostic imaging and physical therapy services. Attempt to maintain a dual designation as a PCP and as a sports medicine specialist, especially in health maintenance organization (HMO)-driven environments. Know your CPT and ICD-9 codes well, including consultation codes (e.g., 99241–99245) and be able to use modifiers effectively (e.g., a modifier-25 links a procedure code with a visit code and increases the likelihood of both codes being paid). Track reimbursements from all insurance companies, and flag problem patterns so that they may be effectively addressed. Additional resources are available for further education in sports medicine business practice, billing and coding, and other economics at amssm.org (Sports Medicine Business Practice Tools), and with further reading (17–19). Some physicians may want to develop a sports medicine program within a larger insurance plan (2).

Work as a sports consultant and as a PCP if possible. Attempt to get paid for both designations with HMOs. HMOs may not reimburse consultations from sports medicine physicians credentialed to be in family practice only (with insurance company) because the rules of some plans do not allow patients to receive care in different primary care offices. Consultations are usually successfully reimbursed with non-HMO payers because patients are less restricted when seeking care (18). Success in this arena will vary among insurance companies because they each have unique rules and behaviors. A PCSM physician is often in an opportune position to work as a consultant within an office, and sometimes within a community. Many PCPs are uncomfortable managing common musculoskeletal and other sports problems, and having an "in-house" referral system may keep both patients and physicians happy (4,20, 21). Referrals may be generated within an office where the sports physician is already approved on all insurance plans.

Consultations must meet certain criteria. Another physician must formally request (verbally or in writing) an opinion or advice regarding evaluation and/or management of a specific problem, and this request must be documented in the patient record. The consultant must then document his or her opinion and any services that were ordered or performed in the patient record, and he or she should write a brief report to the physician requesting the consultation. For subsequent visits for the same problem, consultation codes should not be used (22). Note that PCPs may charge consultations without a specialty designation if a visit meets criteria for a consultation (18).

Charging for consultations may be approached in one of two ways: simply charge the insurance company for a consultation, and wait to see if the reimbursement arrives, or attempt to gain dual credentials as a sports medicine physician and as a PCP/family doctor with HMOs ahead of time to ensure reimbursement for subspecialty services. The problem with the latter approach is that you may flag yourself by saying, "I am a PCP, but I also want to be paid as a specialist." Common sense predicts what most insurance companies may do. By simply charging for a consultation with a patient within your group, the insurance company may not flag you, and you may be successfully reimbursed without the hassle of political negotiations. Most consultation reimbursement problems will arise in HMO-driven settings. With HMOs, accepting "lateral referrals" (between PCPs) within a primary care group may be easier than accepting them from somewhere outside the primary office. In non-HMO environments, consultations are frequently reimbursed with less hassle and without the need for dual credentialing. Remember, according to the consultation rules, specialty designation is not a consultation requirement ?this becomes an issue with HMOs and some other types of managed care contracts that have their own sets of rules. Choose your battles, and if problems arise, spend time debating your skills and the reimbursements requested on an as-needed basis. If you are entering an HMO-saturated setting, you may need to enter into negotiations in advance, before starting your practice. Set up your office to run as an efficient sports medicine practice and, if applicable, primary care medicine practice. Some sports physicians expand their practices by offering occupational medicine services (23). Open routes for patients to know about your practice: advertise, consider setting up appointments using the Internet, schedule "get-to-know" visits in the mornings, over lunches, or at the end of your days, give the back line number to sports colleagues, and run a message machine after hours so that all new patient calls may be tracked and returned. Make your own rehabilitation handouts and hand them out frequently—communicating with pictures and in writing facilitates better patient understanding and frequently results in better outcomes, and at the same time facilitates mass advertising. Rehabilitation teaching takes time, and time may be charged for—factor this into your CPT evaluation and management codes. Specific physical therapy codes (e.g., 97110) may be used when appropriate. Other frequently used printed documents may include preprinted prescription pads, scribble pads, physical therapy referral forms, and various protocols and progressions pertinent to sports medicine. Assemble an "injection tray" that may be carried from room to room for joint injections and arthrocentesis. Work with a local medical supply company to arrange an orthotic and brace cabinet for frequently used items (Table 38.7). Insurance companies will not often reimburse physicians for durable medical equipment (DME), and physicians frequently cannot charge patients for the items without breaching insurance contracts. Stocking DME items from a local supply company that rents a space in a physician's office can effectively remove the physician from the billing and profit arena. Develop a disclosure statement that makes the patient aware of DME options (pay medical supply company now vs. work through insurance company on your own later), and that demonstrates lack of physician's vested interests. Sports medicine physicians should own a current Healthcare Common Procedural Coding System (HCPCS) manual to assist in finding appropriate DME and prosthetic codes (24).

TABLE 38.7
CONTENTS OF A BRACE AND ORTHOTIC CABINET

Slings
Alumifoam
Stax splints
Orthoplast and heater
Wrist splints
Thumb spica splints
Tennis elbow pneumatic counterforce braces
Patellofemoral braces
Hinged knee braces
Ankle braces
Cast boots
Surgical shoes
Orthotic and other foot accessories (e.g., metatarsal pads, etc.)

Use community resources to enhance your office practice. Establish effective lines of communication with other provider groups within your referral network. Carefully select consultants on the basis of known competence and skill, attitude toward sports and athletes, and commitment to maximal functional return in minimal time (14). Make a directory of nonphysician health professionals pertinent to sports medicine in the area (e.g., nutritionists, exercise physiologists, neuropsychologists, etc.) Become familiar with retail stores that carry sports equipment, and know where to send patients for specific items (e.g., over-the-counter orthotics, shoes, etc.). Find out if there is a good orthotist or pedorthotist in the area, and observe the type of work he or she does. Familiarize yourself with sporting or recreational clubs or groups, and with local health clubs and membership options. Awareness of local fitness resources will facilitate exercise and health promotion counseling.

Building a Community Sports Practice

Choose one ore more schools, leagues, or teams to work with. Coverage opportunities will vary, and some school programs may not have an established relationship with a team physician and may have a minimally developed sports program, whereas others may have comprehensive sports medicine programs involving certified athletic trainers, established facilities, and a well-established relationship with a team or multiple team physicians. Colleges frequently have established programs, but the quality of programs at the high school level is more inconsistent. Do not assume that you will be able to work with the best school programs, and be willing to work with underprivileged schools and typically "noncovered" less popular events (e.g., track, swimming, cross country, etc.) (8,15).

Figure out whether you need to develop a new program or plug into an existing program. Persons responsible for obtaining the services of a team physician frequently include athletic directors, athletic trainers, and business managers or other officers from a team (25). Working with a certified athletic trainer is usually instrumental in setting up a new sports medicine program at a school. The relationship of the team physician to the institution (school, league, or team) should be established formally in writing. Job description, monetary arrangements, a statement of expectations, and any fiscal arrangements should be addressed (18). Documentation of athlete encounters is important, especially if other PCPs or consultants are involved in the athlete's care. Simple sideline or training room encounter forms are helpful. Resources are available that will help team physicians set up, evaluate, and if needed, modify scholastic sports medicine programs (25–28). To access coverage in some situations, a new team physician may have to cover a sport alongside an existing head team physician, or he or she may have to offer "fill-in" services. If no scholastic programs or existing sports medicine teams show interest in your skills, consider getting involved with recreational leagues, sporting clubs (e.g., running, cycling, triathlon, etc.), and health clubs. Volunteering for event coverage (e.g., races, special Olympics, camps, etc.) is another rewarding way to become involved in the local sports medicine community. You may have to start small, but if you show motivation and dedication, and if you provide and maintain a high standard of care, your attributes will likely be recognized, and your sports medicine responsibilities in the community will increase (15).

"The team physician addresses the physical, emotional, and spiritual needs of the athlete in the context of the sport and the needs of the team (25)." Be acutely aware of team physician duties when establishing a sports medicine network at a school and community level. Availability on the sidelines, in the training room, in the office, and on nights and weekends, established personally or through a well-organized coverage system, is one of the highest priorities of a team or sports physician (25). Team physicians medically supervise athletes in a variety of settings and situations. Supervision starts with the preparticipation physical examination (PPPE) and evaluation, and it extends to medical management of injuries and illnesses on and off the field, rehabilitation, and return-to-play decisions. Team physicians serve as administrators, liaisons (athlete–coach, athlete–parents, athlete–athlete's PCP, athlete–consultants, athlete or event–media), and educators at varying levels (14,25). Six major professional associations concerned about clinical sports medicine issues collaborated to develop "The Team Physician Consensus Statement," a concise and well-written document that should serve as a reference for all team physicians (29).

Become involved in "nonevent" activities in the community. Volunteering for community PPPEs is a good place to start. Participating with PPPEs often allows you to meet other sports medicine physicians, athletic trainers, coaches, athletes, and sometimes parents and other administrators. Establish or volunteer at a training room for a local school or team. The training room facilitates injury and illness prevention, ensures proper follow-up of injuries, and strengthens the relationship between physicians and athletes. Other community involvement may include free injury clinics at your office (e.g., Monday morning before clinic starts) or at a local health club, outreach activities at local sporting clubs, and continuing education workshops or lectures with physical therapists, athletic trainers, and other sports and health professionals at private offices, schools, local hospitals, and health and wellness clubs.

Be aware of legal issues involved with a sports medicine practice and network. "Good Samaritan" laws apply to most volunteer physicians acting at an athletic event, practice, or game at the high school level, but the laws may vary from one jurisdiction to another. "Good Samaritan" laws only protect physicians who do not act in a willful manner, who do not show gross negligence, and who serve without compensation. Put everything possible in writing—athlete encounters, and school, league, and team contracts that specify expectations, job description and responsibilities, and compensation agreements. Always notify your malpractice insurance carrier of the involvement of your team physician and other "non-office" sports medicine personnel. Legal counsel may be helpful when developing contracts and forms, especially those used outside the office setting.

ESTABLISHING A NATIONAL SPORTS MEDICINE NETWORK

Involvement with national sports medicine organizations, fellowship training and continuing education, and, for some sports physicians, formal collaboration on a national level and academic writing, offers valuable support for a local sports medicine network and practice and may provide great personal satisfaction.

National Sports Medicine Organizations

Organizations that will most likely be pertinent to a sports practice include the American College of Sports Medicine (ACSM), the American Medical Society for Sports Medicine (AMSSM), the American Orthopaedic Society for Sports Medicine (AOSSM), the American Osteopathic Academy of Sports Medicine (AOASM), and the National Association of Athletic Trainers (NATA).

The ACSM, founded in 1954, is an association of people and professions sharing the commitment to explore the use of medicine and exercise to make life healthier for all Americans. The ACSM is committed to the diagnosis, treatment, and prevention of sports-related injuries and to the promotion of physical activity. The ACSM's mission is to "promote and integrate scientific research, education, and practical applications of sports medicine and exercise science to maintain and enhance physical performance, fitness, health, and quality of life." The ACSM has a useful internet web site (www.acsm.org) that contains a certification and career center, ACSM health activity updates (history, news, comments), meetings and continuing education, member services center (ACSM regional chapters, fellowships and committees, interest groups), partnerships and sponsorships, research grants and scholarships, and publications (ACSM publications, positions stands, advertising). The ACSM's national yearly conference is well-attended and serves a broad audience ranging from basic science researchers to sports physicians and other sports and health professionals.

The AMSSM, formed in 1991, is an association of PCSM physicians (also includes some emergency medicine, physical medicine and rehabilition (PM&R), and OB/GYN physicians) "interacting to improve individual expertise in sports medicine, and to raise the standard of care in sports medicine practice in general" (mission). Goals of the AMSSM are listed in Table 38.8. The AMSSM has a web site (www.amssm.org) that provides information about the organization, publications and position statements, fellowships in sports medicine, membership, conferences, sports medicine business practice tools, board of directors and committees, and sports medicine positions. The site defines a sports medicine physician, contains various sports medicine forums (fellowship, team physician, etc.), establishes links to various helpful sports medicine resources, and hosts a database of AMSSM physicians that may be searched by location ("Find a Sports Medicine Doc"). Additionally, the AMSSM hosts an active internet forum titled "AMSSM Web" (www.amssm.net) that fosters discussion among sports medicine professionals and can be an excellent interactive educational resource. The AMSSM's yearly conference is popular among sports medicine physicians, PCPs, sports medicine fellows, and other health professionals for its continuing education and networking opportunities.

TABLE 38.8
GOALS OF THE AMERICAN MEDICAL SOCIETY FOR SPORTS MEDICINE

Goals of the American Medical Society for Sports Medicine, Inc. are as follows:

- To develop and maintain a national society of primary care sports medicine physicians who share a common philosophy, body of knowledge, and expertise related to sports medicine and its practice
- To provide multidisciplinary educational opportunities for primary care sports medicine physicians using meetings, video and printed materials, and similar educational tools
- To encourage and support research in the area of sports medicine
- To work with the American Medical Society for Sports Medicine Foundation
- To encourage and support the development and regular review of the knowledge base in sports medicine
- To develop and lead in formulating position statements, guidelines, and educational materials about sports medicine topics for both professional and public use
- To provide a venue for ideas and information sharing among colleagues about the practical aspects of sports medicine practice and care delivery
- To represent primary care sports medicine physicians in all issues and arenas affecting sports medicine, sports medicine physicians, and their ability to offer high-quality care to the public
- To promote the health and safety of athletes and physically active individuals through education of all involved in their care

Source: With permission from the American Society for Sports Medicine.

The AOASM, established in 1977, is an association of osteopathic physicians "dedicated to the art and science of sports medicine and emphasizing osteopathic principles in the practice of comprehensive health care" (mission statement). The AOASM addresses goals of the osteopathic sports medicine physician's practice on its web site (www.aoasm.org). The site addresses board certification, fellowships and residencies, membership, publications, position statements, the annual conference, and has a "find a sports medicine Doc" engine.

The AOSSM, established in 1972 primarily as a forum for education and research, is a national organization of orthopedic surgeons specializing in sports medicine that works closely with various primary care specialties, athletic trainers, and physical therapists to improve the identification, prevention, treatment, and rehabilitation of sports injuries. The AOSSM has a web site (www.aossm.org) that provides a calendar of events, lists orthopedic sports medicine fellowships, contains grant applications for research, has a "find a doctor" section, and addresses membership. The site contains information about its publications, hosts an "ask the doctor" forum, and holds a "media room" where pertinent press releases and documents are listed.

The NATA, founded in 1950, is an association of athletic trainers "dedicated to enhance the quality of health care for athletes and those engaged in physical activity, and to advance the profession of athletic training through education and research in the prevention, evaluation, management, and rehabilitation of injuries" (mission statement). NATA's web site (www.nata.org) contains various athletic trainer resources, employment opportunities, a list of accredited athletic training programs, membership information, position statements and press releases, information about publications, and a schedule of meeting and conventions.

Conferences and Continuing Education

Sports medicine physicians must stay current with evolving principles that affect sports medicine standards of care. This is especially important in an era where clinical decision making should rely on evidenced-based medicine whenever possible. Each physician should develop a process of study and review that best suits his or her situation and goals. Frequent self-appraisal will allow for adjustment of the process when needed. Most sports physicians enlist in a variety of resources including conferences, workshops, forums, committee work, and journal and text reviews. Recommended journals for regular review are listed in Table 38.9.

Many sports medicine conferences and workshops are offered nationwide. In addition to providing top quality continuing education, they offer an opportune ground for networking and for building collegiality and friendship. The AMSSM annual meeting and the ACSM annual meeting are probably the two most important conferences for sports physicians to attend. Conference dates, goals, content, and registration information may be reviewed on each organization's respective web site, or material may be obtained by calling the organizations individually.

TABLE 38.9
RECOMMENDED SPORTS MEDICINE JOURNALS (AND RESPECTIVE ORGANIZATIONS)

Journal
Clinical Journal of Sports Medicine (AMSSM)[a]
American Journal of Sports Medicine (AOSSM)[a]
Medicine and Science in Sports and Exercise (ACSM)[a]
British Journal of Sports Medicine[a]
Clinics in Sports Medicine[a]
Sports Medicine
International Journal of Sports Medicine
Journal of Bone and Joint Surgery
Journal of Orthopaedic & Sports Physical Therapy

[a]Recommended for regular review.

SUMMARY

Establishing a sports medicine network on local and national levels is important for developing a successful sports medicine practice that offers a high standard of care. Each personal network will vary depending on specific interests of the sports physician and on the needs of the sports community. Strong sports medicine networks offer advantages for everyone participating in sports and sports medicine. Great care and planning should be applied to the development of a strong network, and constant reappraisal of the network will allow for appropriate changes to meet evolving needs.

REFERENCES

1. *Merriam webster's collegiate dictionary*, 10th ed. Springfield: Merriam-Webster, Incorporated, 1993.
2. Henehan M, Jones R. Primary care sports medicine in the managed care environment: coping in today's culture. *Phys Sportsmed* 1997;25(6):96–106.
3. Vereschagin KS. Expanding sports medicine's role in primary care. *Phys Sportsmed* 1993;21(5):121–124.
4. Hoffman D. *Primary care sports medicine—the realities (conference proceeding)*. San Diego: American Medical Society for Sports Medicine, 2000.
5. Mellion MB. The sports medicine content of family practice. *J Fam Pract* 1985;21(6):473–478.
6. Samples P. The team physician: no official job description. *Phys Sportsmed* 1988;16(1):169–175.
7. American Medical Society for Sports Medicine. *AMSSM practice and salary survey*. http://www.amssm.org/AMSSMEconomySurvey.pdf, 2006.
8. American Medical Society for Sports Medicine. *Membership survey*. http://www.amssm.org/AMSSMMembershipSurvey2004.pdf, 2006.
9. American Medical Society for Sports Medicine. *Economics committee pilot survey: insurance company credentialing and website recognition*. http://www.amssm.org/EconomicsCommitteePilotSurvey.pdf, 2006.
10. McShane PA. Gender influences on career opportunities, practice choices, and job satisfaction in a cohort of physician with certification in sports medicine. *Clin J Sport Med* 2001;11(2):96–102.
11. Cerny FJ, Patton DC, Ehieldon TJ, et al. An organizational model of sports medicine facilities in the united states. *J Orthop Sports Phys Ther* 1992;15(2):80–86.
12. Esterson PS. Sports medicine centers in the United States: the personnel, patients and services. *J Orthop Sports Phys Ther* 1980;1:222–228.
13. Olsen D. A descriptive survey of management and operations at selected sports medicine centers in the United States. *J Orthop Sports Phys Ther* 1996;24(4):315–322.
14. Howe W. The team physician. *Prim Care* 1991;18(4):763–775.
15. Dec K, Fagan K, Fields K. *Lessons learned in establishing a sports medicine practice (conference proceeding)*. San Diego: American Medical Society for Sports Medicine, 2000.
16. .Miller R, Luft H. Managed care plans: characteristics, growth, and premium performance. *Annu Rev Public Health* 1994;15:437–439.
17. Madden C, Macintyre J, Joy E. Sports medicine practice economics, part 1: coding basics. *Phys Sportsmed* 2005;33(5):21–32.
18. Madden C, Macintyre J, Joy E. Sports medicine practice economics, part 2: consultations, modifiers, and other codes. *Phys Sportsmed* 2005;33(6):32–45.
19. Madden C, Macintyre J, Joy E. Sports medicine practice economics, part 3: billing, collecting, appeals, and related tasks. *Phys Sportsmed* 2005;33(7):32–45.
20. Connolly J, DeHaven K, Mooney V. Primary care management of musculoskeletal disorders. *J Musculoskeletal Med* 1998;15(8):28–38.
21. Buckler DGW. General practitioners' training for, interest in, and knowledge of sports medicine organizations. *Br J Sports Med* 1999;33(5):360–363.
22. American Medical Association. *Current procedural terminology CPT 2006*, Standard ed. Chicago: AMA Press, 2006.
23. White J. Sports medicine in the workplace: adapting—and expanding—your practice. *Phys Sportsmed* 1996;24(11):91–95, 101–103.

24. Medical Management Institute. *HCPCS level II professional coding manual,* 13th ed. Alpharetta: Medical Management Institute, 2006.
25. Mellion M, Walsh W, Madden C, et al. The team physician. In: Mellion M, Walsh W, Madden C, et al., eds. *The team physician's handbook,* 3rd ed. Philadelphia: Hanley and Belfus, 2002:1–11.
26. Rice S. The high school athlete: setting up a high school sports medicine program. In: Mellion M, Walsh W, Madden C, et al., eds. *The team physician's handbook,* 3rd ed. Philadelphia: Hanley and Belfus, 2002:67–76.
27. Niedfeldt M, Young C, Leshan L. Establishing a high-school-based training room clinic. *Wis Med J* 1996;95(6):356–360.
28. Dyment P, ed. *Health care for young athletes (see: self-appraisal checklist for health supervision in scholastic athletic programs),* 2nd ed. Elk Grove Village: American Academy of Pediatrics, Committee on Sports Medicine, 1991.
29. Project-based alliance for the advancement of clinical sports medicine, comprised of the American Academy of Family Physicians, the American Academy of Orthopaedic Surgeons, the American College of Sports Medicine, the American Medical Society for Sports Medicine, the American Orthopaedic Society for Sports Medicine, and the American Osteopathic Academy of Sports Medicine. Team Physician Consensus Statement; 2000;32(4):877–878.

39

Patient and Community Education on Physical Fitness

Eric D. Zemper

The emphasis of this final chapter is on patient and community education. It is important for the primary care physician to be involved in educating people about the need for physical fitness activities, to raise patient and public awareness, and to motivate people to act on this information.

IMPORTANCE OF BEING INVOLVED IN PATIENT AND COMMUNITY EDUCATION

During the first half of the twentieth century, the morbidity and mortality rates of Americans shifted away from acute infectious diseases to predominantly chronic illnesses related to lifestyle. Of the approximately 2.4 million deaths in the United States in 2003, 28% were due to cardiovascular disease, 23% were due to cancer, and 6% were due to cerebrovascular disease. There is good evidence that personal lifestyle (what and how much we eat and drink, amount and type of exercise we engage in, whether we smoke, and how we deal with daily stress) is strongly related to these three leading causes of death.

Some still hope that the way to reduce the magnitude of chronic disease lies in improved medical technology, but an increasingly prevalent view is that technology can play only a limited role. Although there have been several spectacular technological successes (e.g., organ transplants), these achievements generally affect a relatively small number of people. Despite these advances and the increase in our knowledge about chronic diseases, there has been little change in the last 40 to 50 years in the rates of these major diseases (1). Many physicians now believe that advances in medical technology will have little impact on the overall health of Americans, and that control of the current major health problems depends directly on modification of individual behavior and lifestyle habits (2). For the physician, this will involve more than telling patients with high blood pressure to cut back on salt or writing a prescription for a calcium channel blocker. The patients will need to know how to read nutrition labels and, specifically, how to monitor their sodium intake. It will involve more than telling patients with high cholesterol to cut out fats from their diets or writing a prescription for a statin. They will need to know the difference between saturated and unsaturated fats and specifically how to monitor them in their diets. In addition, in a country where half the population is overweight and one fourth of the population is obese, it will involve a lot more than just telling obese patients to cut down their calorie intake and get more exercise.

Therefore, primary care physicians who want to have a long-term impact on the health of their patients must become involved in educating them and helping them change their behavior. In fact, the U.S. Preventive Services Task Force and the American Heart Association recently have recommended that all primary care providers counsel all their patients about healthy diets and regular physical activity (3,4). You may wonder why primary care physicians have not been more involved in prevention efforts against the major lifestyle-related diseases. The answer is complex, but some reasons are clear. Few medical schools include the necessary training for young physicians to assume these roles. Historically, emphasis has been on treating sick patients, and the rewards in terms of money, prestige, and a sense of accomplishment act as powerful reinforcements for physicians to maintain their focus almost exclusively on these aspects of medical practice. Despite the shift from acute to chronic diseases and the obvious logic inherent in prevention, it will be quite difficult to change the situation very rapidly because the reward system in medicine is so heavily geared toward waiting until people are ill to treat them. For now, the impetus for change will have to come from individual physicians who decide to put their emphasis on preventing diseases.

Most physicians do not realize that their every word and action can be regarded as a form of health education, not only by patients and their families but also by the whole community. It is not a question of whether primary care physicians are providing health education for their community, but whether they are doing it well or poorly. Primary care physicians should speak out about the benefits of physical activity and other aspects of a healthy lifestyle. They should be a major community resource for health education, and they should be involved in coordinating access to other community health resources and organizations.

The call for changing destructive lifestyle habits comes from many sources, but primary care physicians have one of the best opportunities to help people initiate positive change or prevent the formation of negative habits because of the respect that their role has in our culture and their potential to influence the health practices of families. New attitudes and skills will be required of physicians who choose this path. They will need the ability to confront without being judgmental. They must recognize that old, unhealthy habits are hard to change and there are numerous social inducements and pressures to maintain or start these habits and discourage the adoption of healthier ones. Dealing with discouragement by both the patient and physician will be a necessary part of the effort. However, it has been demonstrated repeatedly that patients *can* change habits and lifestyles with the help of their physicians and the support of their families.

A study of access to health care (5) indicated that 90% of the American population has a usual source of health care and that 80% had seen a physician within the previous 12 months. Another study (6) indicated that 54% of all patient encounters involved primary care physicians (family practice, general practice, pediatrics, or internal medicine). The average encounter is sufficiently long to allow at least some minimal counseling on fitness and activity, even if such counseling is not directly related to the reason the patient is seeing the physician. Even so, physicians did this in less than 10% of these encounters. Several studies have shown that patients expect their physicians to be concerned about their health habits and to actively encourage appropriate lifestyle changes, including recommending fitness activities (7,8). Given the number of people that have contact with (9) and can be influenced by primary care physicians (10), the potential impact on the total health picture in our society can be enormous.

Much work remains to be done to define the impact of habitual physical activity and exercise on various chronic diseases, but a clear and consistent picture is emerging with regard to several major diseases (11–18). The relation of physical activity to coronary heart disease (CHD) has received the most attention so far. Many studies have shown that physical inactivity and lack of exercise are associated with increased risk of CHD, whereas habitually active individuals have reduced risk of CHD and sudden cardiac death (11,19–29). These associations hold good even when other risk factors such as age, smoking, hypertension, family history, and obesity are taken into account. In a variety of ways, it was shown that "Selection" (i.e., sick or unfit persons are less active) was not an explanation for these findings. There is a transient rise in the risk of a cardiac event during vigorous exercise, but this risk is outweighed by an overall reduction of risk during nonexercise periods (30). A number of recent studies indicate that habitual activity is associated with decreased risk of stroke (31–34). Paffenbarger et al. (35) report that mortality rates from all causes are reduced by one fourth to one third in individuals who expend 2,000 or more kcal during exercise per week as compared with those who are less active. A major conclusion of this study is that regular exercise does increase life expectancy.

Other chronic diseases for which exercise appears to have an ameliorating effect include hypertension, diabetes, and osteoporosis. Several studies indicate that habitual activity is associated with decreased risk of hypertension (36,37), and these studies also suggest that exercise may improve hypertension control. Other studies have shown that exercise helps type 2 diabetic patients by reducing blood glucose levels, increasing sensitivity of insulin receptors, and increasing the effectiveness of insulin (38–44). Although few controlled studies have been completed on whether exercise will prevent or postpone the development of type 2 diabetes, such a possibility is strongly implied by the metabolic and hormonal effects produced by regular exercise. There is a lack of research data on the effects of exercise in insulin-dependent diabetic patients, but physical activity is generally recommended as an important part of an overall treatment program. There is evidence that exercise and physical activity are inversely related to the development of specific types of cancers (45–51). The same is true for osteoporosis (52–56). These studies do indicate that the protective effect of exercise holds true only for weight-bearing activities; non–weight-bearing activities such as swimming apparently do not reduce bone loss.

Regular exercise also appears to effect mental health (57–60). Taylor et al. (61) reviewed a number of studies and concluded that physical activity and exercise are associated with improved self-concept and confidence, alleviation of symptoms of mild-to-moderate depression, reduction of anxiety, and alteration of some aspects of the stress response and coronary prone (type A) behavior.

Regular aerobic exercise has been increasingly recognized as an important factor in the prevention and control of obesity (62–67). Aerobic exercise is a vital element, in conjunction with dietary measures, in the weight loss programs that are most likely to achieve long-term success. It is becoming more apparent that exercise or diet alone is not likely to produce long-term weight loss, as is an appropriate combination of the two together.

Research on the effects of exercise on the various conditions has now reached sufficient quantity that extensive review articles and meta-analyses summarizing the findings (see [68–74]), including the importance of exercise and diet in treating metabolic syndrome, are beginning to appear (75). In a review of the effect of physical fitness (as opposed to just physical activity) on total mortality, Erikssen states that a sedentary lifestyle may be as detrimental to health as smoking (76).

There is still room for debate on some of the specifics related to the impact of habitual activity and exercise on various chronic diseases, but evidence from reviews such as those cited above and from longer term studies such as Paffenbarger et al. (35) indicates it is a reasonable assumption that physical activity and exercise have a positive effect on health, longevity, and prevention of chronic illnesses. At the very least, an appropriate exercise program will not shorten life and will likely improve its quality through positive effects on psychological and physical factors. Moreover, current research indicates that it is not necessary to have been exercising all your life to reap the benefits. Many positive effects can be gained from beginning a moderate program at any age. However, it is only logical that more benefits will be gained and fewer negative effects of being sedentary will accrue if good exercise habits are developed early in life (and yet physical education requirements continue to be reduced or eliminated in school curricula, where life-long exercise habits should be established).

The intensity of exercise does not have to be great to gain benefits (77). It is now recommended that adults should accumulate 30 minutes or more of moderate-intensity physical activity on most, preferably all, days of the week (16). This does not have to be one continuous 30-minute exercise bout, but can be an accumulation of shorter bouts. Earlier recommendations involved doing more intense exercise at 60% or more of aerobic capacity. This figure was based on earlier short-term studies on young men, but it came to be regarded as a minimal standard for everyone. Now it is apparent that exercise at less than 60% of aerobic capacity also produces beneficial effects, although it may take longer (77). This is an important point when a physician is trying to achieve a permanent change in a patient to a more active lifestyle, because exercises at a lower intensity are more acceptable and any associated medical risk will be much less. It also is important to note that the overall impact of adopting an exercise program will be much greater for sedentary individuals who successfully adopt a lower intensity program than for reasonably active individuals who adopt a more intensive exercise program (77).

Given the evidence that regular physical activity is an important part of a healthy lifestyle and will reduce the occurrence or severity of some chronic illnesses (see Table 39.1), it should be apparent that primary care physicians need to be aware of the basic approaches to educating individual patients and the general community about the desirability of being physically active.

RAISING PATIENT AND PUBLIC AWARENESS

The primary care physician can work at two levels to raise public awareness about the need for a healthy, active lifestyle: at the level of the individual patients when they are seen by the physician, and at the level of the community at large. While the emphasis here is on the value of being physically active, the same principles apply to promoting other aspects of a healthy lifestyle, such as proper nutrition, smoking cessation, and other factors that reduce the risk of cardiovascular disease, cancer, and cerebrovascular disease. All these elements should be covered in a prevention-oriented medical practice.

The primary care physician should initiate a systematic program of health risk assessment for all patients (79). This involves completing a thorough patient history that includes questions about diet, genetic background, prior physical condition, and attitudes toward health and fitness. Several health risk assessment packages, such as the Health Hazard Appraisal (80), are available commercially in the medical literature or on the Internet. A thorough health risk appraisal will produce a wealth of data that must not be just filed away. The risk assessment should be used as an educational tool as well as a data-gathering tool. The results of the health risk assessment are the first step in educating the patient and guiding him/her to a realization of the options available. The guidance and support of the physician will be crucial in the early stages of lifestyle adjustment.

The beginning stages of the patient education process generally take place on a one-to-one basis, but the patient's family should be involved as soon as possible when major changes are being contemplated. Spousal support has a major influence on adherence to exercise programs (81). The need for family support is most evident in smoking cessation or alcoholism intervention, but it is no less important in adopting a physically active lifestyle. In fact, it is likely that one or more other family members should be making similar changes. Once change is underway, many of the continuing elements of patient education can be handled by the office staff, but the physician should continue to monitor the progress. The patient education process and encouragement of necessary

TABLE 39.1
REFERENCE LITERATURE FOR EFFECTS OF EXERCISE ON VARIOUS DISEASES AND CONDITIONS

Diseases/Conditions	Source	References
Obesity	Blair, Jacobs, and Powell (1985)	(62)
	Leermakers et al. (2000)	(63)
	McInnis (2000)	(64)
	Ross et al. (2000)	(65)
	Schmitz et al. (2000)	(66)
	Sothern (2001)	(67)
BP/hypertension	Blair, et al. (1984)	(36)
	Roman, et al. (1981)	(37)
Stroke	Abbott et al. (1994)	(31)
	Agnarsson et al. (1999)	(32)
	Hu et al. (2000)	(33)
	Sacco et al. (1998)	(34)
CHD risk	Berlin and Colditz (1990)	(19)
	Blair, Kampert et al. (1996)	(11)
	CDC (1993)	(20)
	Garcia-Palmeri, et al. (1982)	(21)
	Kelley, Kelley and Tran (2004)	(69)
	Lakka et al. (1994)	(22)
	Lewis and Hoeger (2005)	(68)
	Manson et al. (1999)	(23)
	Morris, et al. (1980)	(24)
	Mozaffarian et al. (2004)	(78)
	Paffenbarger and Hale (1975)	(25)
	Paffenbarger, Wing, and Hyde (1978)	(26)
	Powell et al. (1987)	(27)
	Salonen, Puska, and Tuomilehto (1982)	(28)
	Siscovick, et al. (1982)	(29)
Blood glucose levels (diabetes)	Burchfiel et al. (1995)	(38)
	Creviston and Quinn (2001)	(39)
	Helmrich et al. (1991)	(40)
	Horton (1986)	(41)
	Laakso (2005)	(72)
	Lynch et al. (1996)	(42)
	Richter and Schneider (1981)	(43)
	Ryan (2000)	(44)
	Ryan (2003)	(70)
	Schulze and Hu (2005)	(71)
Osteoporosis	Aloia (1981)	(52)
	Chalmers and Ho (1980)	(53)
	Dalen and Olsson (1974)	(54)
	Krolner et al. (1983)	(55)
	Snow-Harter and Marcus (1991)	(56)
Mental health status	Brown and Wang (1992)	(57)
	Camacho, Roberts, and Lazarus (1991)	(58)
	Farmer et al. (1988)	(59)
	Stephens (1988)	(60)
	Taylor, Sallis, and Needle (1985)	(61)
Cancer	Coogan et al. (1997)	(45)
	Gotay (2005)	(74)
	Hardman (2001)	(46)
	Rockhill et al. (1999)	(47)
	Stein and Colditz (2004)	(73)
	Sternfeld (1992)	(48)
	Thune et al. (1997)	(49)
	Verloop et al. (2000)	(50)
	White et al. (1996)	(51)

CHD = coronary heart disease.

behavioral changes involve more information than can be presented here. Such information is available from a number of sources, including articles by Shapiro (82), Tapp et al. (83), and a program from the Centers for Disease Control and Prevention, called *PACE* (Physical Activity Counseling and Evaluation) (84). Preliminary results from studies of the PACE program indicate that it is practical and effective in the primary care setting (85). Part II of this book also contains information on prescribing appropriate exercises for patients.

Given the current perception of the importance of physician's involvement in counseling patients in nutrition and exercise, it is an unfortunate fact that most physicians have little or no training in these areas. While some physicians may feel comfortable getting into detailed discussions regarding the type, frequency, duration, and intensity of exercises for an individual patient, most are not, and fewer are ready to tackle the equally important areas of nutrition, such as how to read nutrition labeling, and details of planning, shopping for, and preparing appropriate meals. These areas are too important for the physician to take the easy way out by just handing the patient a brochure, which usually has little impact because of the lack of sufficiently detailed information. In addition to the necessity of the physician taking the time to learn more about exercise and nutrition counseling (the most appropriate approach for a prevention-oriented practice), adjunct approaches include having a nurse on the staff who is knowledgeable in these areas and can take on much of the responsibility of detailed counseling activities. The advantage in this approach is that nurses usually are better trained in behavior modification and motivation. Another alternative is to arrange an appointment for the patient with a fitness trainer or nutritionist. However, from the patient's perspective, this is not always an ideal alternative since it usually involves having to take more time off from work for another appointment. The likelihood of a successful intervention is considerably increased if the initial counseling and intervention activities are undertaken by the physician and staff in the physician's office.

The primary care physician also should be involved in making the entire community aware of the impact of lifestyle on health and longevity. The physician can work individually or act as a catalyst in promoting action. It might mean speaking to the local civic, social, or church groups, providing brochures, and using slides, movies, or videotapes. If used appropriately, the mass media can be quite effective in informing and motivating the community to act on health maintenance (86). The physician's role is to ensure that what is presented is accurate and will not be misinterpreted by those it is supposed to inform and motivate.

Other approaches include participating in local health fairs or contests, either as a separate activity through a local hospital or in conjunction with yearly county or state fairs. Videotapes and slides can be used in displays, and brochures can be provided. Various attention-getting activities, such as measuring blood pressures, or demonstrating health and cancer self-screens, or how to take a heart rate in monitoring exercise levels, can be used to raise awareness.

The physician should become involved with local school programs. Health education and physical education in the schools are important factors in long-term improvement of health in the general population (87). Unfortunately, the recent trend in local schools is to cut back on these programs. The physician should take a leading role in seeing that school health and physical education programs are improved and strengthened. Physical education should not consist of just playing games, but should have a specified teaching curriculum with emphasis on the importance of lifetime physical activity and fitness habits and basic instruction in individual sports that provide necessary aerobic fitness, which then can be pursued and enjoyed beyond the school years. The availability of adult fitness and activity courses through the local school district or other community education organizations also should be encouraged.

MOTIVATING PEOPLE TO ACT ON INFORMATION

Possession of knowledge is a necessary factor, but it is not always sufficient to induce action on matters of personal health. There are several current theories to explain individual health behavior, such as the Health Belief Model (88). According to this model, a person will take action to avoid disease if they have the following beliefs: (a) they are personally susceptible to the disease; (b) having the disease will have at least a moderately severe impact on some component of their life; and (c) taking a particular action will be beneficial by reducing their personal susceptibility to the disease or to its severity. A corollary to the third condition is that the action taken does not require overcoming one or more psychological barriers like cost, inconvenience, pain, or embarrassment.

On the basis of this theory, the physician who is trying to encourage a patient to adopt an active lifestyle must address all three conditions. The second condition is relatively easy; few would deny that having cardiovascular disease would have a major impact on their life. The first condition is a little more difficult. People tend to deny that they are susceptible to cardiovascular disease or any other lifestyle-related disease. It may be true that a particular individual is less susceptible, but no one can be positive that they are immune. The physician should point out the incidence of the disease using national statistics and, if possible, local statistics. A health risk assessment can be used to great effect. The third condition is the most difficult. The physician must convince the patient that a physically active lifestyle and regular exercise will reduce the risk of cardiovascular and other diseases and contribute to a longer, healthier life. Using research results may help with some individuals, although it seems that those who would benefit the most are often the most resistant. Interventions may be more successful if they focus on helping patients feel good about themselves rather than focusing entirely on the health benefits of exercise (81). Related to this is the important notion of self-efficacy. Patients should always be encouraged to feel that they really are capable of making the necessary changes in exercise or nutrition patterns, no matter what their current situation is or how difficult it may seem.

The physician should help the patient decide the type and amount of exercise, being careful to minimize the previously mentioned psychological barriers (89). The most popular fitness activities are done alone or in groups, without special classes or facilities. Of the approximately 20% of the adult population that is active at a minimal level to maintain cardiovascular fitness, only a small percentage is in organized formal exercise programs (90). However, some patients may need the support offered in a group setting. The physician's knowledge of the patient and of the results of the health risk assessment regarding the patient's attitudes toward health and fitness may help in making these decisions.

The ultimate responsibility for managing a patient's behavior is in the hands of the patient, but this does not preclude a role for the physician (and the office staff) in evaluating the progress and success of a behavior change. After a change is instituted, both patient and physician will be involved with monitoring, recording, and reinforcing the efforts over a period. Three levels of outcome can be measured in the efforts to change behavior to prevent disease (91). The first level comprises changes in the target behavior. For example, how many days during the past week did the patient go for a brisk walk or take part in other aerobic exercise, and how many total minutes were spent on these activities? The second level comprises short-term and medium-term physiological changes, such as lowered resting heart rate, improved work capacity, or lowered blood pressure. Finally, there are long-term changes in morbidity and mortality, such as prevention or delay of onset of cardiovascular disease as a result of regular exercise and its physiological adaptations. The first level of outcomes, changes in target behavior, usually is monitored and recorded by the patient (an activity or exercise log) and reviewed with the physician periodically. Short-term, physiological changes normally will be monitored in the physician's office. Time and history will record the third level changes in morbidity and mortality. The physician-recorded outcome measures of short-term and medium-term physiological changes provide the patient with important reinforcement and feedback on the success (or failure) of his/her efforts. Failures exposed by the first or second level evaluations should not be used as an accusatory tool against a noncomplying patient. Rather, it should signal a need for the physician to review the goals, strategies, support, and rewards for the lifestyle change being attempted. Shelton and Rosen (92) have outlined a number of techniques and considerations in using patient self-monitoring.

An important tool that should be developed and maintained in the office of a primary care physician is a community resource file. This file, on 3 × 5 cards or in a notebook or in computer memory, should contain listings of resources available within the community that can be mobilized to help patients make lifestyle changes, whether it be maintaining a regular exercise program, changing nutrition and eating patterns, or practicing regular self-screens for various forms of cancer. The resource file should list the resources, their location within the community, their cost (and whether they are cheaper in volume), and how to gain access. In addition to the sources of information, the file should contain educational materials, information on groups like Weight Watchers or Alcoholics Anonymous, screening labs, and exercise groups, to name a few examples. A review of this community resource file may reveal gaps and, if any of the missing resources are important enough, the physician may want to work for their establishment. A search of the Internet can turn up many additional resources for patient education, which can be viewed by patients on a computer in the physician's office, or the web addresses can be listed on handouts so that patients can access the recommended web sites at home. One source for extensive patient information on exercise and nutrition is www.americanheart.org.

There will be times when the physician has done all that normally would be necessary to induce a patient to adopt a healthier lifestyle, including reviewing a health risk assessment with the patient, educating the patient about susceptibility to cardiovascular or other diseases, developing an acceptable fitness program, and encouraging family support, and yet the patient does not take that final step and actually implement the change. It may take an additional cue or catalyst to prompt these patients to make the effort. This can be as simple as an occasional telephone call from the physician or office staff to see how the plan is going. Another effective catalyst or "trigger" is using examples of famous people or local people who have successfully adopted a physically active lifestyle. These examples can show that the barriers to regular exercise are not insurmountable. An example of the impact of a trigger on adoption of a healthy habit is the increase in requests for instruction in breast self-examination after the publicity surrounding the breast cancers of Betty Ford and Happy Rockefeller, the wives of the President and Vice President, some years ago.

IMPORTANCE OF THE PHYSICIAN, STAFF, AND OFFICE ENVIRONMENT IN PROMOTING HEALTHY LIFESTYLES

In some instances it may not be the absence of an appropriate cue that causes a patient to fail to make lifestyle improvements, but rather the presence of negative cues from the physician, office staff, or even the office environment. This happens not because of a planned, systematic learning effort, but rather through unplanned, unknowing instructions given to patients by the daily health behaviors of the physician and office staff members. Patients pick up the behavioral lessons being taught by an overweight physician or the receptionist who smokes.

Whether they intend to be or not, the physician and other health care professionals are role models for their patients and other members of the community, who know them as "doctor" or "nurse." A conscientious commitment to good health practices by the physician and staff members is necessary. The staff must show concern for their own health if patients are to see them as credible sources of preventive health information. A physician or other health professional who has health habits that run counter to the recommendations given to patients should attempt to correct them and be ready to answer patient questions, sometimes unspoken, about those habits.

The environment in the medical office is an extension of the health practices modeled by the physician and staff. A prohibition against smoking in the waiting room or reception area is a must. Posters and signs encouraging healthful practices extend the educational strategies and reinforce the role modeling. Apparently insignificant aspects of the office environment contribute or detract from the preventive health messages. For example, the choice of magazines for the public areas of the office can have an impact. *Reader's Digest* is a good choice because its editorial board stopped carrying cigarette advertisements in the 1950s when smoking was correlated with major health problems. Magazines that contain many advertisements for tobacco and alcohol products would be a poor choice. Subtle aspects of the office environment such as these may not be obvious to the patient, but they can be mentioned in brochures given to patients to help highlight the commitment to the maintenance of a healthy lifestyle. However, the physician remains the key individual in promoting appropriate health habits and he/she must be cognizant of that role when dealing with patients. Although medicine can be a stressful profession, a physician should neither maintain poor health habits nor use self-destructive behaviors for coping with stress (93,94).

We have briefly touched upon a very extensive topic that is very important in the primary care setting. The primary care physician must be able to care for the acute medical needs of physically active patients, and this has been the focus of the clinical chapters that comprise most of this book. However, the physician must also meet the long-term needs of all patients by encouraging the adoption of a healthier and more active lifestyle. The primary care physician must not only be concerned with his/her own patients, but also take an active part in encouraging and providing proper sports medicine care for all members of the community. In essence, because of his/her special knowledge and expertise, the primary care physician has an obligation to get involved with the community.

REFERENCES

1. Thomas L. On the science and technology of medicine. In: Knowles JH, ed. *Doing better and feeling worse*. New York: W. W. Norton & Company, 1977.
2. Knowles JH. The responsibility of the individual. In: Knowles JH, ed. *Doing better and feeling worse*. New York: W. W. Norton & Company, 1977.
3. Grundy SM, Balady GJ, Criqui MH, et al. Guide to primary prevention of cardiovascular disease: a statement for health care professionals from the task force on risk reduction. *Circulation* 1997;95:2329–2331.
4. U.S. Preventive Services Task Force. *Guide to clinical preventive services*, 2nd ed. Baltimore: Lippincott-Raven, 1996.
5. Robert Wood Johnson Foundation. Updated report on access to health care for the American people. Princeton, 1983.
6. Robert Wood Johnson Foundation. America's health care system: A comprehensive portrait. Princeton, 1978.
7. David AK, Boldt JF. A study of preventive health attitudes and behaviors in a family practice setting. *J Fam Pract* 1980;11:77.
8. Hyatt JD. Perception of the family physician by patients and family physicians. *J Fam Pract* 1980;10:295.
9. U.S. Department of Health and Human Services. *Physician visits: volume and interval since last visit, United States, 1980*. Hyattsville: National Center for Health Statistics, DHHS Publication PHS 83–1572, 1983.
10. Lewis BS, Lynch WD. The effect of physician advice on exercise behavior. *Prev Med* 1993;22:110–121.
11. Blair SN, Kampert JB, Kohl HW, et al. Influences of cardiorespiratory fitness and other precursors on cardiovascular disease and all-cause mortality in men and women. *JAMA* 1996;276:205–210.
12. Blair SN, Horton E, Leon AS, et al. Physical activity, nutrition, and chronic disease. *Med Sci Sports Exerc* 1996;28(3):335–349.
13. Blair SN, Kohl HW, Paffenbarger RS, et al. Physical fitness and all-cause mortality: a prospective study of healthy men and women. *JAMA* 1989; 262:2395–2401.
14. Booth FW, Gordon SE, Carlson CJ, et al. Waging war on modern chronic diseases: primary prevention through exercise biology. *J Appl Physiol* 2000; 88:774–787.
15. Lee IM, Paffenbarger RS. Associations of light, moderate, and vigorous intensity physical activity with longevity: the Harvard Alumni Health Study. *Am J Epidemiol* 2000;151:293–299.
16. Pate RR, Pratt M, Blair SN, et al. Physical activity and public health: a recommendation from the centers for disease control and prevention and the American College of sports medicine. *JAMA* 1995;273(5):402–407.
17. Powell KE, Blair SN. The public health burdens of sedentary living habits: theoretical but realistic estimates. *Med Sci Sports Exerc* 1994;26(7):851–856.
18. Siscovick DS, LaPorte RE, Newman JM. The disease-specific benefits and risks of physical activity and exercise. *Public Health Rep* 1985;100(2):180.
19. Berlin JA, Colditz GA. A meta-analysis of physical activity in the prevention of coronary heart disease. *Am J Epidemiol* 1990;132:612–628.
20. Centers for Disease Control. Physical activity and the prevention of coronary heart disease. *MMWR Morb Mortal Wkly Rep* 1993;42:669–672.
21. Garcia-Palmeri MR, et al. Increased physical activity: a protective factor against heart attacks in Puerto Rico. *Am J Cardiol* 1982;50:749.
22. Lakka TA, Venalainen JM, Rauramaa R, et al. Relation of leisure-time physical activity and cardiorespiratory fitness to the risk of acute myocardial infarction. *N Engl J Med* 1994;330:1549–1554.
23. Manson JE, Hu FB, Rich-Edwards JW, et al. A prospective study of walking as compared with vigorous exercise in the prevention of coronary heart disease in women. *N Engl J Med* 1999;341:650–658.
24. Morris JN, et al. Vigorous exercise in leisure-time: protection against coronary heart disease. *Lancet* 1980;2(8206):1207–1210.
25. Paffenbarger RS, Hale WE. Work activity and coronary heart mortality. *N Engl J Med* 1975;292:545.
26. Paffenbarger RS, Wing AL, Hyde RT. Physical activity as an index of heart attack risk in college alumni. *Am J Epidemiol* 1978;108:161.
27. Powell KE, Thompson PD, Caspersen CJ, et al. Physical activity and the incidence of coronary heart disease. *Annu Rev Public Health* 1987;8:253–287.
28. Salonen JT, Puska P, Tuomilehto J. Physical activity and risk of myocardial infarction, cerebral stroke and death: a longitudinal study in Eastern Finland. *Am J Epidemiol* 1982;115:526.
29. Siscovick DS, et al. Physical activity and primary cardiac arrest. *JAMA* 1982;243:3113.
30. Siscovick DS, et al. The incidence of primary cardiac arrest during vigorous exercise. *N Engl J Med* 1984;311:874.
31. Abbott RD, Rodriguez BL, Burchfiel CM, et al. Physical activity in older middle-aged men and reduced risk of stroke: the Honolulu Heart Program. *Am J Epidemiol* 1994;139:881–893.
32. Agnarsson U, Thorgeirsson G, Sigvaldason H, et al. Effects of leisure-time physical activity and ventilatory function on risk for stroke in men: the Reykjavik study. *Ann Intern Med* 1999;130:987–990.
33. Hu FB, Stampfer MJ, Colditz GA, et al. Physical activity and risk for stroke in women. *JAMA* 2000;283:2961–2967.
34. Sacco RL, Gan R, Boden-Albala B, et al. Leisure-time physical activity and ischemic stroke risk: the Northern Manhattan Stroke Study. *Stroke* 1998;29(2):380–387.
35. Paffenbarger RS, et al. Physical activity, all-cause mortality, and longevity of college alumni. *N Engl J Med* 1986;314:605.

36. Blair SN, et al. Physical activity and incidence of hypertension in healthy normotensive men and women. *JAMA* 1984;252:487.
37. Roman O, et al. Physical training program in arterial hypertension: a long-term prospective follow-up. *Cardiology* 1981;67:230.
38. Burchfiel CW, Scharp DS, Curb JD, et al. Physical activity and incidence of diabetes: the Honolulu Heart Program. *Am J Epidemiol* 1995;141:360–368.
39. Creviston T, Quinn L. Exercise and physical activity in the treatment of type 2 diabetes. *Nurs Clin North Am* 2001;36(2):243–271.
40. Helmrich SP, Ragland DRLeung W, et al. Physical activity and reduced occurrence of noninsulin-dependent diabetes mellitus. *N Engl J Med* 1991; 325:147–152.
41. Horton ES. Exercise and physical training: effects on insulin sensitivity and glucose metabolism. *Diabetes Metab Rev* 1986;2:1–17.
42. Lynch J, Helmrich SP, Lakka TA, et al. Moderately intense physical activities and high levels of cardiorespiratory fitness reduce the risk of non-insulin-dependent diabetes mellitus in middle-aged men. *Arch Intern Med* 1996;156:1307–1314.
43. Richter EA, Schneider SH. Diabetes and exercise. *Am J Med* 1981;70:201.
44. Ryan AS. Insulin resistance with aging: effects of diet and exercise. *Sports Med* 2000;30(5):327–346.
45. Coogan PF, Newcomb PA, Clapp RW, et al. Physical activity in usual occupation and risk of breast cancer. *Cancer Causes Control* 1997;8(4):626–631.
46. Hardman AE. Physical activity and cancer risk. *Proc Nutr Soc* 2001;60(1): 107–113.
47. Rockhill B, Willett WC, Hunter DJ, et al. A prospective study of recreational physical activity and breast cancer risk. *Arch Intern Med* 1999;159: 2290–2296.
48. Sternfeld B. Cancer and the protective effect of physical activity: the epidemiologic evidence. *Med Sci Sports Exerc* 1992;24:1195–1209.
49. Thune I, Brenn T, Lund E, et al. Physical activity and the risk of breast cancer. *N Engl J Med* 1997;336:1269–1275.
50. Verloop J, Rookus RA, van der Kooy K, et al. Physical activity and breast cancer risk in women aged 20–54 years. *J Natl Cancer Inst* 2000;92:128–135.
51. White E, Jacobs EJ, Daling JR. Physical activity in relation to colon cancer in middle-aged men and women. *Am J Epidemiol* 1996;144:42–50.
52. Aloia JF. Exercised skeletal health. *J Am Geriatr Soc* 1981;29:104.
53. Chalmers J, Ho KC. Geographical variations in senile osteoporosis: the association of physical activity. *J Bone Joint Surg* 1980;52:667.
54. Dalen N, Olsson KE. Bone mineral content and physical activity. *Acta Orthop Scand* 1974;45:170.
55. Krolner B, et al. Physical exercise as a prophylaxis against involuntary bone loss. *Clin Sci* 1983;64:541.
56. Snow-Harter C, Marcus R. Exercise, bone mineral density, and osteoporosis. *Exerc Sport Sci Rev* 1991;19:351–388.
57. Brown DR, Wang Y. The relationships among exercise training, aerobic capacity, and psychological well-being in the general population. *Med Exerc Nutr Health* 1992;1:125–142.
58. Camacho TC, Roberts RE, Lazarus NB, et al. Physical activity and depression: evidence from the alameda county study. *Am J Epidemiol* 1991;134:220–231.
59. Farmer ME, Locke BZ, Moscicki EK, et al. Physical activity and depressive symptoms: the NHANES I Epidemiologic Follow-up Study. *Am J Epidemiol* 1988;128:1340–1351.
60. Stephens T. Physical activity and mental health in the United States and Canada: evidence from four population surveys. *Prev Med* 1988;17:35–47.
61. Taylor CB, Sallis JF, Needle R. The relation of physical activity and exercise to mental health. *Public Health Rep* 1985;100(2):195.
62. Blair SN, Jacobs DR, Powell KE. Relationships between exercise or physical activity and other health behaviors. *Public Health Rep* 1985;100(2):172–180.
63. Leermakers EA, Dunn AL, Blair SN. Exercise and management of obesity. *Med Clin North Am* 2000;84(2):419–440.
64. McInnis KJ. Exercise and obesity. *Coronary Art Dis* 2000;11(2):111–116.
65. Ross R, Freeman JA, Jannsen I. Exercise alone is an effective strategy for reducing obesity and relate comorbidities. *Exerc Sport Sci Rev* 2000;28(4): 165–170.
66. Schmitz KH, Jacobs DR, Leon AS, et al. Physical activity and body weight: associations over ten years in the CARDIA study. Coronary artery risk development in young adults. *Int J Obes* 2000;24(11):1475–1487.
67. Sothern MS. Exercise as a modality in the treatment of childhood obesity. *Pediatr Clin North Am* 2001;48(4):995–1015.
68. Lewis V, Hoeger K. Prevention of coronary heart disease: a nonhormonal approach. *Semin Reprod Med* 2005;23(2):157–166.
69. Kelley GA, Kelley KS, Tran ZV. Aerobic exercise and lipids in women: a meta-analysis of randomized controlled trials. *J Womens Health* 2004; 13(10):1148–1164.
70. Ryan DH. Diet and exercise in the prevention of diabetes. *Int J Clin Pract* 2003;134(suppl):28–35.
71. Schulze MB, Hu FB. Primary prevention of diabetes: what can be done and how much can be prevented? *Annu Rev Public Health* 2005;26:445–467.
72. Laakso M. Prevention of type 2 diabetes. *Curr Mol Med* 2005;5(3):365–374.
73. Stein CJ, Colditz GA. Modifiable risk factors for cancer. *Br J Cancer* 2004; 90(2):299–303.
74. Gotay CC. Behavior and cancer prevention. *J Clin Oncol* 2005;23(2):301–310.
75. Wagh A, Stone NJ. Treatment of metabolic syndrome. *Expert Rev Cardiovasc Ther* 2004;2(2):213–228.
76. Erickssen G. Physical fitness and changes in mortality: the survival of the fittest. *Sports Med* 2001;31(8):571–576.
77. Haskell WL, Montoye HJ, Orenstein D. Physical activity and exercise to achieve health-related physical fitness components. *Public Health Rep* 1985;100(2):202.
78. Mozaffarian D, Fried LP, Burke GL, et al. Lifestyles of older adults: Can we influence cardiovascular risk in older adults? *Am J Geriatr Cardiol* 2004; 13(3):153–160.
79. Rodnick J. Health screening: What should you do? *Fam Pract Recertif* 1980;2:45.
80. Robbins LC. A system for indications for preventive medicine: health hazard appraisal. In: Kane RL, ed. *The behavioral sciences and preventive medicine*. Washington: U.S. Government Printing Office, DHEW Publication No. NIH 76–878, 1974.
81. Dishman RK, Sallis JF, Orenstein DR. The determinants of physical activity and exercise. *Public Health Rep* 1985;100(2):158.
82. Shapiro J. Development of family self-control skills. *J Fam Pract* 1981; 12(1):67.
83. Tapp JT, et al. The application of behavior modification to behavior management: guidelines for the family physician. *J Fam Pract* 1978;6(2):293.
84. Centers for Disease Control. *Project PACE: physician's manual: physician-based assessment and counseling for exercise*. Atlanta: Centers for Disease Control, 1992.
85. Long BJ, Calfas KJ, Sallis JF. et al. Evaluation of patient physical activity after counseling by primary care providers. *Med Sci Sports Exerc* 1994; 26(5)(Suppl):S4.
86. Marshall CL. *Toward an educated health consumer: mass communication and quality in medical care*. Washington: U.S. Government Printing Office, DHEW Publication No. (NIH) 77–81, 1977.
87. Kolbe LJ, Gilbert GG. Involving the schools in the national strategy to improve the health of Americans. *Proceedings of prospects for a healthier America: achieving the Nation's health promotion objectives*. Washington: U.S. Department of Health and Human Services/Public Health Service, 1984.
88. Rosenstock IM. The health belief model and preventive health behavior. In: Becker MH, ed. *The health belief model and personal health behavior*. Thorofare: Charles B. Slack, 1976.
89. Martin JE, Dubbert PM. Behavioral management strategies for improving health and fitness. *J Cardiopulm Rehabil* 1984;4:200.
90. Iverson DC, et al. The promotion of physical activity in the United States population: the status of programs in medical, worksite, community, and school settings. *Public Health Rep* 1985;100(2):212.
91. Pomerleau O, Bass F, Crown V. Role of behavior modification in preventive medicine. *N Engl J Med* 1975;292:1277.
92. Shelton JL, Rosen GM. Self-monitoring by patients. In: Rosen GM Geyman JP Layton RH, eds. *Behavioral science in family practice*. New York: Appleton-Century-Crofts, 1980.
93. Freeman AM, Sach RL, Berger PA. *Psychiatry for the primary care physician*. Baltimore: JB Lippincott, 1979.
94. Shangold MM. The health care of physicians: 'Do as I say and not as I do.'. *J Med Educ* 1979;54:668.

Index

Note: Page numbers followed by *f* indicate figures; those followed by *t* indicate tables; those followed by *n* indicate notes.

E

F

Q

R